BRITISH
NATIONAL
FORMULARY

September 1996

BRITISH NATIONAL FORMULARY

Number 32
(September 1996)

British Medical Association
and
Royal Pharmaceutical Society of Great Britain

Copies may be obtained through any bookseller or, in case of difficulty, direct from the publishers:

British Medical Association
Tavistock Square
London WC1H 9JP, England

The Pharmaceutical Press
PO Box 151
Wallingford
Oxon OX10 8QU, England

Comments and constructive criticism will be welcome, and should be sent to:
Executive Editor, British National Formulary,
c/o Royal Pharmaceutical Society of Great Britain,
1 Lambeth High Street, London SE1 7JN.

ISBN: 0 85369 362 5. ISSN: 0260–535X

The text for this edition was generated from an in-house database (designed by Quartet Software Ltd). Typeset from disk by Create Publishing Services Ltd, Bath, Avon BA2 3DZ, printed and bound by The Bath Press, Bath

Joint Formulary Committee
1996–97

Chairman
Charles F. George, BSc, MD, FRCP, FFPM

Deputy Chairman
Nicholas L. Wood, BPharm, FRPharmS

Committee Members

Alison Blenkinsopp, PhD,
    BPharm, MRPharmS
Peter Clappison, MB, ChB
Ann Lewis, LLB, FRPharmS,
    MCPP, MHSM, Barrister
Frank P. Marsh, MA, MB, BChir,
    FRCP

George M. Mitchell, OBE, KStJ, MB,
    ChB, FRPharmS
Jane Richards, MB BS, MRCS,
    LRCP, FRCGP,
    D(Obst)RCOG, DCH
James Smith, BPharm, PhD,
    MRPharmS, MCPP, MIInfSc
Patrick C. Waller, MD, FRCP

Joint Secretaries
Stella R. Lowry, MB, ChB, BSc

Ainley Wade, BPharm, MPhil, FRPharmS

Executive Editor

Dinesh K. Mehta, BPharm, MSc, MRPharmS (from May 1996)

Anne B. Prasad, MBE, FRPharmS (until May 1996)

Senior Assistant Editor

Sheenagh M. Townsend-Smith, BSc, DipLib

Assistant Editors

John Martin, BPharm, PhD, MRPharmS

Anjana Patel, BPharm, MSc, PhD, MRPharmS

Staff Editors

Ann M. Hargreaves, MRPharmS

Bryony Jordan, BSc, MRPharms, DipPharmPract

Sunayana A. Shah, BPharm, MRPharmS

Mark J. Timmis, BPharm, MRPharmS

Executive Secretary

Susan M. Thomas, BSc(Econ), MA

Contents

Arrangement of Information

Guidance on prescribing
This part includes information on prescription writing, controlled drugs and dependence, prescribing for children and the elderly, and prescribing in palliative care. Advice is given on the reporting of adverse reactions.

Emergency treatment of poisoning
The main intention of this chapter is to provide information on the management of acute poisoning when first seen in the home, although aspects of hospital-based treatment are mentioned.

Classified notes on drugs and preparations
The main text consists of classified notes on drugs and preparations. These notes are divided into 15 chapters, each of which is related to a particular system of the human body or to an aspect of medical care. Each chapter is then divided into sections which begin with appropriate *notes for prescribers*. These notes are intended to provide information to doctors, pharmacists, nurses, and other health professionals to facilitate the selection of suitable treatment. The notes are followed by details of relevant drugs and preparations.

DRUGS appear under pharmacopoeial or other non-proprietary titles. When there is an *appropriate current monograph* (Medicines Act 1968, Section 65) preference is given to a name at the head of that monograph; otherwise a British Approved Name (BAN), if available, is used. If the International Non-proprietary Name (INN) differs from the British Approved Name it follows the title in brackets.

PREPARATIONS usually follow immediately after the drug which is their main ingredient. They are printed in text-sized type but those considered by the Committee to be less suitable for prescribing are described in smaller type. Small type is also used for the entries describing foods for special diets, stoma and urinary appliances, and wound management products. Preparations are included under a non-proprietary title if:
    (a) they are marketed under such a title,
    (b) they are not otherwise prescribable under the NHS, or
    (c) they may be prepared extemporaneously.
  If proprietary preparations are of a distinctive colour this is stated, but flavour is not usually mentioned.
  In the case of compound preparations the indications, cautions, contra-indications, side-effects, and interactions of all constituents should be taken into account in prescribing.

PREPARATIONS NOT AVAILABLE FOR NHS PRESCRIPTION. The symbol NHS has been placed against those preparations included in the BNF that are not prescribable under the NHS. Those prescribable only for specific disorders have a foot-note specifying the condition(s) for which the preparation remains available. Prescribers are reminded that some preparations which are not *prescribable* by brand name under the NHS may nevertheless be *dispensed* using the brand name in question providing that the prescription has been written in the form of an appropriate non-proprietary name.

PRESCRIPTION-ONLY MEDICINES. The symbol PoM has been placed against those preparations that are available only on medical or dental prescription. For more detailed information see *Medicines, Ethics and Practice*, No. 16, London, Pharmaceutical Press, 1996 (and subsequent editions as available). The symbol CD indicates that the preparation is subject to the prescription requirements of the Misuse of Drugs Act. For regulations governing prescriptions for such preparations see pages 7–9.

PRICES have been calculated from the basic cost used in pricing NHS prescriptions dispensed in March 1996 or later, see p. 1 for further details.

Appendixes and indexes
The appendixes include information on interactions, liver disease, renal impairment, pregnancy, breast-feeding, intravenous additives, borderline substances, appliances, and cautionary and advisory labels for dispensed medicines. They are designed for use in association with the main body of the text.
  The Dental Practitioners' List and the Nurse Prescribers' List are also included in this section. The indexes consist of the Index of Manufacturers and the Main Index.

Preface

The BNF is a joint publication of the British Medical Association and the Royal Pharmaceutical Society of Great Britain. It is published under the authority of a Joint Formulary Committee which comprises representatives of the two professional bodies and of the Department of Health. It is available both as a pocket book version and as an identical electronic version.

An improved 'browser' version of the electronic BNF has now been developed and thanks are due to Quartet Software Ltd for their continued work on the design of the software, to T. Benson, C. Gordon, I. Herbert, D. Markwell and I. Purves for their advice on the project, and to M. Davis, C. Dewse, P. M. Mason and A. Tarr for additional checks on the data.

The Joint Formulary Committee also acknowledges the help of individuals and organisations that provided information or advised on specific matters. The principal contributors for this edition were S. P. Allison, D. G. Arkell, C. G. Barnes, S. Bazire, L. Beeley, R. H. Behrens, R. J. Buckley, I. Burgess, A. J. Camm, C. M. Castleden, D. A. Chamberlain, B. T. Colvin, W. A. M. Cutting, C. Diamond, R. Dinwiddie, S. Dover, A. J. Duxbury, G. H. Elder, A. M. Geddes, A. H. Ghodse, E. C. Gordon-Smith, I. A. Greer, J. Guillebaud, C. H. Hawkes, D. F. Hawkins, R. M. Jones, J. Kirwan, P. Kopelman, M. J. S. Langman, T. H. Lee, P. N. Leigh, W. A. Littler, G. M. Mead, J. M. Neuberger, A. J. Nunn, D. J. Oliver, L. P. Ormerod, L. E. Ramsay, F. Reynolds, P. A. Routledge, R. S. Sawers, M. C. Sheppard, S. D. Shorvon, T. Southwood, I. Stockley, A. Tattersfield, R. N. Thin, G. R. Thompson, D. G. Waller, D. A. Warrell, P. Watkins, G. B. Wyatt. The Committee wishes to record its particular thanks to members of the British Association of Dermatologists Therapy Guidelines and Audit Working Party, M. W. Greaves (Chairman), S. M. Breathnach, W. J. Cunliffe, D. J. Gawkrodger, C. E. H. Grattan, M. L. Price, H. C. Williams, M. Benham (Secretariat), for invaluable discussions and advice. The Committee also wishes to express its thanks to J. E. F. Reynolds and staff, for valuable access to the *Martindale* data bank and files. The Committee also wishes to express its thanks to correspondents in the pharmaceutical industry who provided information and made numerous comments on points of detail, to colleagues who have advised members of the Committee and the editorial staff on specific matters, and to T. M. Roberts and J. Ruddle for clerical assistance. Finally, the Committee would like to thank those doctors, pharmacists, nurses, and others who sent comments and suggestions.

The BNF is intended for rapid reference and cannot always contain all the information necessary for prescribing and dispensing. It should be supplemented as necessary from specialised publications and by reference to the manufacturers' data sheets. Within the space available the monographs in the BNF reflect the information in the manufacturers' data sheets, which are prepared in accordance with the Medicines (Data Sheet) Regulations 1972; they are available for most proprietary medicines. Less detail is given in some areas such as those dealing with obstetrics, malignant disease, and anaesthesia, as it is expected that those undertaking treatment will have specialised knowledge and will consult specialist literature. Supplementary information may be available from local drug information services.

Anne B. Prasad MBE FRPharmS

On the retirement of Mrs Anne B Prasad MBE FRPharmS, the Joint Formulary Committee wishes to record its deep appreciation of her outstanding tenure as the Executive Editor of the British National Formulary. The improvement in the quality and coverage during the eleven years of her editorship has firmly established the BNF's role as an indispensable resource for the practising prescriber and pharmacist.

Mrs Prasad also initiated the electronic BNF project and saw through the first phase of its development. She implemented a robust strategy for future electronic development thus ensuring that the BNF will continue to play a key role as the professions begin to embrace information technology.

The editorial team joins the Committee in paying tribute to an exceptional editor. It is a rare privilege to work with somebody of such uncompromising standards.

Changes

The BNF is revised twice yearly and numerous changes are made between issues. All copies of BNF No. 31 (March 1996) should therefore be withdrawn and replaced by BNF No. 32 (September 1996).
   Significant changes have been made in the following sections for BNF No. 32:

Paraquat poisoning [charcoal now recommended as first-line adsorbent], Emergency Treatment of Poisoning

Treatment of snake bites [text], Emergency Treatment of Poisoning

Beta-blockers [sotalol licensed for arrhythmias only], section 2.4

Fibrinolytic drugs [repeat administration of streptokinase and anistreplase], section 2.10

Allergic emergencies [self-administration of adrenaline], section 3.4.3

Centrally acting appetite suppressants [text], section 4.5.2

Leprosy [text], section 5.1.10

Glucocorticoids [reorganisation of text], section 6.3.2

Menorrhagia [significant changes], section 6.4.1.2

Preparations for acne [significant changes and reorganisation], section 13.6

Dose Changes

Preparations affected by changes in dose statements introduced into BNF No. 32:

Alprostadil, p. 350

Alteplase [regimen], p. 111

Antidepressants [text, duration of treatment], p. 171

Chlorothiazide, p. 61

Didronel PMO® [duration], p. 321

Ephedrine [reversal of hypotension in anaesthesia], p. 103

Fosfestrol, p. 367

Granisetron, p. 187

Lansoprazole [maintenance], p. 40

Ondansetron [postoperative], p. 188

Primidone [child], p. 207

Propofol, p. 521

Rowatinex®, p. 348

Sevredol®, p. 195

Sotalol [arrhythmias], p. 80

Thioridazine [child], p. 166

Vigabatrin [West's syndrome], p. 210

Classification Changes

1.6.2 *Picolax*® now in section 1.6.5

1.6.4 *Citramag*® now in section 1.6.5

1.6.5 Bowel cleansing solutions [new section]

6.3.2 Glucocorticoid therapy [title change]

6.3.3 and 6.3.4 no longer exist [text in section 6.3.2]

Electronic BNF

An improved version of the **electronic BNF**, with an extensive **browser facility** is available in parallel with this edition of the BNF. The browser has been developed to present the data as a direct and immediate reflection of the BNF database which permits rapid searching of its familiar layout.
   The eBNF can be searched *by drug* or *by preparation* or *by key word*, and can browse *the classification* and *the index*. *Interactions* hot-links and full *index-to-book* hot-links are provided. Hot links have now also been introduced in the text.
   The eBNF can also be linked into other Windows software. It also now includes the facility to add user-defined annotations and bookmarks..
   An annual subscription to the stand-alone eBNF includes two issues of the database together with eBNF Browser software. Prices start at £50 per annum for a single user with reductions for network users.

Hardware requirements are:
Microsoft Windows 3.1 or higher and at least a 386 processor with 4 megabytes of RAM (8 megabytes recommended) and takes up 12 megabytes of hard disk space (extra space may be needed during installation). It can be networked and will operate on any Windows supported network.

Work is now also well advanced on the development of a more elaborate version of the database to allow it to operate as part of an *intelligent decision-support* and *prescribing tool.*

New Preparations
Preparations included in appropriate sections of BNF No. 32

Acular, p. 441
Adizem-XL Plus, p. 96
Alphaparin, p. 106
Ametop, p. 537
Aquasept, p. 491
BDP Spacehaler, p. 134
Bettamousse, p. 463
Calcichew D3 Forte, p. 402
Campral EC, p. 221
CellCept, p. 363
Climesse, p. 306
Curatoderm, p. 469
Elleste-Duet, p. 307
Elleste-Solo, p. 308
Entocort CR, p. 45
EpiPen, p. 144
Estraderm MX, p. 308
Fareston, p. 370
Fleet Micro-enema, p. 52
Fleet Phospho-Soda, p. 53
Flomax MR, p. 345
Gonal F, p. 316
Humalog, p. 288
Improvera, p. 308
Konakion MM Paediatric, p. 403
Livostin eye-drops, p. 434

Livostin nasal spray, p. 447
Lithofalk, p. 56
Locoid Crelo, p. 462
Methadose, p. 224
Movicol, p. 51
MXL, p. 196
Nimbex, p. 531
NovoSeven, p. 112
Ophthalin, p. 442
Paradote, p. 192
Physiotens, p. 84
Progynova TS, p. 309
Quellada M, p. 487
Rilutek, p. 220
Salbutamol Spacehaler, p. 122
Salofalk suppositories and enema, p. 44
Skelid, p. 323
Sporanox liquid, p. 265
Taxotere, p. 362
Timoptol-LA, p. 438
Tomudex, p. 358
Tramake, p. 200
Vectavir, p. 485

Discontinued Preparations
Preparations discontinued during the compilation of BNF No. 32

Algipan spray
Aureocort cream
Bolvidon
Brocadopa
Capitol
Cedocard IV
Ceporex paediatric drops
Combantrin
Conova 30
Decortisyl
Epifoam
Fefol-Vit
Ferrocap-F 350
Gastron
Genisol

Haelan-C
Hydrocortistab cream and ointment
Ilosone suspension
Mithracin
Monuril Paediatric
Neocon 1/35
Neo-Medrone
Nipride
Ortho-Gynol
Psoradrate
Rapolyte
Savlon bath oil
Staycept
Tetrabid-Organon
Tribiotic

Drug Information Services

Information on any aspect of drug therapy can be obtained, free of charge, from Regional and District Drug Information Services. Details regarding the *local* services provided within your Region can be obtained by telephoning the following numbers.

England

Birmingham		0121-311 1974	Direct Line
	or	0121-378 2211	Extn 2296/2297
Bristol		(0117) 928 2867	Direct Line
Ipswich		(01473) 704430	Direct Line
	or	(01473) 704431	Direct Line
Leeds		(0113) 243 0715	Direct Line
Leicester		(0116) 255 5779	Direct Line
Liverpool		0151-794 8112/3/5/7	Direct Line
London			
Guy's Hospital		0171-955 5000	Extn 3594/5892
	or	0171-378 0023	Direct Line
Northwick Park Hospital		0181-869 3973	Direct Line
Royal London Hospital		0171-377 7487	Direct Line
	or	0171-377 7489	Direct Line
Manchester		0161-225 2063	Direct Line
	or	0161-276 6270	Direct Line
Newcastle		0191-232 1525	Direct Line
Southampton		(01703) 796908	Direct Line
	or	(01703) 796909	Direct Line

Wales

Cardiff	(01222) 742979	Direct Line

Scotland

Aberdeen		(01224) 681818	Extn 52316
Dundee		(01382) 60111	Extn 2351
Edinburgh		0131-536 2843	Direct Line
Glasgow		0141-552 4726	Direct Line
Inverness		(01463) 234151	Extn 288
	or	(01463) 220157	Direct Line

Northern Ireland

Belfast	(01232) 248095	Direct Line
Londonderry	(01504) 45171	Extn 3262

Southern Ireland

Dublin		Dublin 473 0589	Direct Line
	or	Dublin 453 7941	Extn 2348

National Teratology Information Services
0191-232 1525

Poisons Information Services

Belfast	(01232) 240503
Birmingham	0121-507 5588/9
Cardiff	(01222) 709901
Dublin	Dublin 837 9964 *or* Dublin 837 9966
Edinburgh	0131-536 2300
Leeds	(0113) 243 0715 *or* (0113) 292 3547
London	0171-635 9191 *or* 0171-955 5095
Newcastle	0191-232 5131

Note. Some of these centres also advise on laboratory analytical services which may be of help in the diagnosis and management of a small number of cases

Patient Packs

On January 1 1994, EC Directive 92/27/EEC came into force, outlining requirements for the labelling of medicines and for the format and content of user leaflets to be supplied with each medicine.

In the UK, packs which conform to the Directive are termed **patient packs**. They consist of a ready-to-dispense pack containing a patient information leaflet approved by the Medicines Control Agency (MCA).

All new medicines are required to comply with the Directive and when the licences of established medicines come up for renewal, they too will be required to comply with the Directive.

This transition to patient packs began in December 1995 and will be phased in gradually. It is anticipated that all medicines in the UK will comply by January 1999.

Most patient packs will contain enough medicine for *one month*, but special packs will be available for medicines that are regularly used in *shorter or longer* courses. If a patient still needs a *precise quantity* not allowed for in a pack, then the specific quantity can be indicated (otherwise arrangements are being made for the pharmacist to supply the nearest sized pack). Special arrangements will be made for *controlled drugs*.

Many medicines are already available in a manufacturer's original pack (often complete with a patient information leaflet). Amounts listed in the BNF correspond to these packs.

During the revision of each edition of the BNF careful note is taken of the information that appears on the patient information leaflets. Where it is considered appropriate to alert a prescriber to some specific limitation appearing on the patient information leaflet (for example, in relation to pregnancy) this advice now appears in the BNF.

The patient information leaflet also includes details of all inactive ingredients in the medicine. A list of common E numbers and the inactive ingredients to which they correspond is now therefore included in the BNF (see *inside back cover*).

Guidance on Prescribing

Prices in the BNF

Basic **net prices** have been introduced into the BNF in order to provide better indications of relative cost. Where there is a choice of suitable preparations for a particular disease or condition the relative cost may be used in making a selection. It should be emphasised, however, that cost-effective prescribing must take into account other factors (such as dose frequency and duration of treatment) that affect the total cost. The use of more expensive drugs is justified if it will result in better treatment of the patient or a reduction of the length of an illness or the time spent in hospital.

Prices have generally been calculated from the net cost used in pricing NHS prescriptions dispensed in March 1996, but where available later prices have been included; unless an original pack is available these prices are based on the largest pack size of the preparation in use in community pharmacies. The price for an extemporaneously prepared preparation has been omitted where the net cost of the ingredients used to make it would give a misleadingly low impression of the final price.

The unit of 20 is still sometimes used as a basis for comparison, but where suitable original packs or patient packs are available these are priced instead.

Gross prices vary as follows:

1. Costs to the NHS are greater than the net prices quoted and include professional fees and overhead allowances;

2. Private prescription charges are calculated on a separate basis;

3. Over-the-counter sales are at retail price, as opposed to basic net price, and include VAT.

BNF prices are NOT, therefore, suitable for quoting to patients seeking private prescriptions or contemplating over-the-counter purchases.

A fuller explanation of costs to the NHS may be obtained from the Drug Tariff.
It should be noted that separate Drug Tariffs are operative in England and Wales, Scotland, and Northern Ireland. Prices in the different tariffs may vary.

PACT and SPA

PACT (Prescribing Analyses and Cost) and SPA (Scottish Prescribing Analysis) automatically provide general practitioners with information about their prescribing. The information is sent on a quarterly basis direct from the Prescription Pricing Authority (and may be obtained for individual months on request). It is now available as a 'standard report' which replaces the previous *level 1* and *level 2 reports*. The previous *level 3 report* is replaced by a 'catalogue' which provides the data in a more helpful manner and is available on request for periods of one or more months.

General Guidance

Medicines should be prescribed only when they are necessary, and in all cases the benefit of administering the medicine should be considered in relation to the risk involved. This is particularly important during pregnancy where the risk to both mother and fetus must be considered (for further details see Prescribing in Pregnancy, Appendix 4).

ABBREVIATION OF TITLES. In general, titles of drugs and preparations should be written *in full*. Unofficial abbreviations should not be used as they may be misinterpreted; obsolete titles, such as Mist. Expect. should not be used.

NON-PROPRIETARY TITLES. Where non-proprietary ('generic') titles are given, they should be used in prescribing. This will enable any suitable product to be dispensed, thereby saving delay to the patient and sometimes expense to the health service. The only exception is where bioavailability problems are so important that the patient should always receive the same brand; in such cases, the brand name or the manufacturer should be stated. Non-proprietary titles should **not** be invented for the purposes of prescribing generically since this can lead to confusion, particularly in the case of compound and modified-release preparations.

Titles used as headings for monographs may be used freely in Great Britain and Northern Ireland but in other countries may be subject to restriction.

Many of the non-proprietary titles used in this book are titles of monographs in the European Pharmacopoeia, British Pharmacopoeia or British Pharmaceutical Codex 1973. In such cases the preparations must comply with the standard (if any) in the appropriate publication, as required by the Medicines Act (section 65).

PROPRIETARY TITLES. Names followed by the symbol ® are or have been used as proprietary names in the United Kingdom. These names may in general be applied only to products supplied by the owners of the trade marks.

DOSES. The doses stated in the BNF are intended for general guidance and represent, unless otherwise stated, the usual range of doses that are generally regarded as being suitable for adults. In general the *doses, indications, cautions, contra-indications and side-effects* in the BNF reflect those in the manufacturers' data sheets which, in turn, reflect those in the corresponding Product Licences. On the few occasions that an unlicensed drug is included in the BNF, this is now indicated in brackets after the entry. Where a use (or route) is recommended outside the licensed indication of an available product this too is indicated. It has been noted (*Drug and Therapeutics Bulletin*, 1992, *30*, 97–99) that prescribing of licensed medicines outside the recommendations of the Product Licence alters (and probably increases) the doctor's professional responsibility.

ORAL SYRINGES. An **oral syringe** is supplied when oral liquid medicines are prescribed in doses other than multiples of 5 mL. The oral syringe is marked in 0.5-mL divisions from 1' to 5 mL to measure doses of less than 5 mL. It is provided with an adaptor and an instruction leaflet. The *5-mL spoon* is used for doses of 5 mL (or multiples thereof).

STRENGTHS AND QUANTITIES. The strength or quantity to be contained in capsules, lozenges, tablets, etc. should be stated by the prescriber.

If a pharmacist receives an incomplete prescription for a systemically administered preparation other than a prescription for a controlled drug and considers it would not be appropriate for the patient to return to the doctor, the following procedures will apply:

(a) an attempt must always be made to contact the prescriber to ascertain the intention;

(b) if the attempt is successful the pharmacist must, where practicable, subsequently arrange for details of quantity, strength where applicable, and dosage to be inserted by the prescriber on the incomplete form;

(c) where, although the prescriber has been contacted, it has not proved possible to obtain the written intention regarding an incomplete prescription, the pharmacist may endorse the form 'p.c.' (prescriber contacted) and add details of the quantity and strength where applicable of the preparation supplied, and of the dose indicated. The endorsement should be initialled and dated by the pharmacist;

(d) where the prescriber cannot be contacted and the pharmacist has sufficient information to make a professional judgment the preparation may be dispensed. If the quantity is missing the pharmacist may supply sufficient to complete up to 5 days' treatment; except that where a combination pack (i.e. a proprietary pack containing more than one medicinal product) or oral contraceptive is prescribed by name only, the smallest pack shall be dispensed. In all cases the prescription must be endorsed 'p.n.c.' (prescriber not contacted) the quantity, the dose, and the strength (where applicable) of the preparation supplied must be indicated, and the endorsement must be initialled and dated;

(e) if the pharmacist has any doubt about exercising discretion, an incomplete prescription must be referred back to the prescriber.

ADDITIVES. Oral liquid preparations in the BNF that do not contain *fructose, glucose* or *sucrose* are labelled 'sugar-free'. Preparations containing hydrogenated glucose syrup, mannitol, or sorbitol are also marked 'sugar-free' since there is evidence that they are not cariogenic.

Where information on the presence of *aspartame, gluten, tartrazine, arachis (peanut) oil* or *sesame oil* is available, this is indicated in the BNF against the relevant preparation; the manufacturer should be contacted in the absence of information on additives in the BNF and in the product literature, if it is essential to check details.

Information is provided on *preservatives* in eye-drops and on *selected additives* in skin preparations (see section 13.1). Pressurised metered aerosols containing *chlorofluorocarbons* (CFCs) have also been identified throughout the BNF (see also pp. 118 and 123)

EXTEMPORANEOUS PREPARATION. The BP direction that a preparation must be *freshly prepared* indicates that it must be made not more than 24 hours before it is issued for use. The direction that a preparation should be *recently prepared* indicates that deterioration is likely if the preparation is stored for longer than about 4 weeks at 15° to 25°.

DRUGS AND DRIVING. Prescribers should advise patients if treatment is likely to affect their ability to drive motor vehicles. This applies particularly to drugs with sedative effects and patients should be warned that these effects are increased by alcohol. See also Appendix 9.

NOTICE CONCERNING PATENTS. In the BNF certain drugs have been included notwithstanding the existence of actual or potential patent rights. In so far as such substances are protected by Letters Patent, their inclusion in this Formulary neither conveys, nor implies, licence to manufacture.

HEALTH AND SAFETY. When handling chemical or biological materials particular attention should be given to the possibility of allergy, fire, explosion, radiation, or poisoning. Some substances, including corticosteroids, antibiotics, phenothiazines, and many cytotoxics, are irritant or very potent and should be handled with caution. Contact with the skin and inhalation of dust should be avoided.

SAFETY IN THE HOME. Patients must be warned to keep all medicines out of the reach of children. All solid dose and all oral and external liquid preparations must be dispensed in a reclosable *child-resistant container* unless:

(i) the medicine is in an original pack or patient pack such as to make this inadvisable;

(ii) the patient will have difficulty in opening a child-resistant container;

(iii) a specific request is made that the product shall not be dispensed in a child-resistant container;

(iv) no suitable child-resistant container exists for a particular liquid preparation.

All patients should be advised to dispose of *unwanted medicines* by returning them to a supplier for destruction.

NAME OF MEDICINE. The name of the medicine should appear on the label unless the prescriber indicates otherwise.

1. Subject to the conditions of paragraphs 4 and 6 below, the name of the prescribed medicine is stated on the label unless the prescriber deletes the letters 'NP' which appear on NHS prescription forms.

2. The strength is also stated on the label in the case of tablets, capsules, and similar preparations that are available in different strengths.

3. If it is the wish of the prescriber that a description such as 'The Sedative Tablets' should appear on the label, the prescriber should write the desired description on the prescription form.

4. The arrangement will extend to approved names, proprietary names or titles given in the BP, BPC, BNF, or DPF. The arrangement does not apply when a prescription is written so that several ingredients are given.

5. The name written on the label is that used by the prescriber on the prescription.

6. If more than one item is prescribed on one form and the prescriber does not delete the letters 'NP', each dispensed medicine is named on the label, subject to the conditions given above in paragraph 4. If the prescriber wants only selected items on such a prescription to be so labelled this should be indicated by deleting the letters 'NP' on the form and writing 'NP' alongside the medicines to be labelled.

7. When a prescription is written other than on an NHS prescription form the name of the prescribed preparation will be stated on the label of the dispensed medicine unless the prescriber indicates otherwise.

8. The Council of the Royal Pharmaceutical Society advises that the labels of dispensed medicines should indicate the total quantity of the product dispensed in the container to which the label refers. This requirement applies equally to solid, liquid, internal, and external preparations. If a product is dispensed in more than one container, the reference should be to the amount in each container.

Scope of the BNF

The BNF is intended for the guidance of medical practitioners, pharmacists, dentists, nurses, and others who have the necessary training and experience to interpret the information it provides. It is intended as a reference for the pocket, and should be supplemented by a study of more detailed publications when required.

Security and validity of prescriptions

The Councils of the British Medical Association and the Royal Pharmaceutical Society have issued a joint statement on the security and validity of prescriptions.

In particular, prescription forms should:

(i) not be left unattended at reception desks;

(ii) not left in a car where they may be visible; and

(iii) when not in use, be kept in a locked drawer within the surgery and at home.

Where there is any doubt about the authenticity of a prescription, the pharmacist should contact the prescriber. If this is done by telephone, the number should be obtained from the directory rather than relying on the prescription form information, which may be false.

Prescription Writing

Prescriptions[1] should be written legibly in ink or otherwise so as to be indelible[2], should be dated, should state the full name and address of the patient, and should be signed in ink by the prescriber[3]. The age of the patient should preferably be stated, and is a legal requirement in the case of prescription-only medicines for children under 12 years of age.

In general practice the following should be noted:

(a) The unnecessary use of decimal points should be avoided, e.g. 3 mg, not 3.0 mg.

Quantities of 1 gram or more should be written as 1 g etc.

Quantities less than 1 gram should be written in milligrams, e.g. 500 mg, not 0.5 g.

Quantities less than 1 mg should be written in micrograms, e.g. 100 micrograms, not 0.1 mg.

When decimals are unavoidable a zero should be written in front of the decimal point where there is no other figure, e.g. 0.5 mL, not .5 mL.

Use of the decimal point is acceptable to express a range, e.g. 0.5 to 1 g.

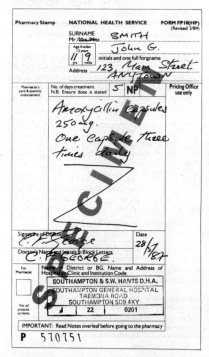

(b) 'Micrograms' and 'nanograms' should **not** be abbreviated. Similarly 'units' should **not** be abbreviated.

(c) The term 'millilitre' (ml or mL)[4] is used in medicine and pharmacy, and cubic centimetre, c.c., or cm[3] should not be used.

(d) Dose and dose frequency should be stated; in the case of preparations to be taken 'as required' a **minimum dose interval** should be specified.

When doses other than multiples of 5 mL are prescribed for *oral liquid preparations* the dose-volume will be provided by means of an **oral syringe**, see p. 2 (except for preparations intended to be measured with a pipette).

Suitable quantities:

Elixirs, Linctuses, and Paediatric Mixtures (5-mL dose), 50, 100, or 150 mL

Adult Mixtures (10-mL dose), 200 or 300 mL

Ear Drops, Eye-drops, and Nasal Drops, 10 mL (or the manufacturer's pack)

Eye Lotions, Gargles, and Mouth-washes, 200 mL

(e) For suitable quantities of dermatological preparations, see section 13.1.

(f) The names of drugs and preparations should be written clearly and **not** abbreviated, using approved titles **only** (see also advice in box on p. 5 to **avoid** creating generic titles for modified-release preparations).

(g) The symbol 'NP' on NHS forms should be deleted if it is required that the name of the preparation should not appear on the label. For full details see p. 3.

(h) The quantity to be supplied may be stated by indicating the number of days of treatment required in the box provided on NHS forms. In most cases the exact amount will be supplied. This does not apply to items directed to be used as required—if the dose and frequency are not given the quantity to be supplied needs to be stated.

When several items are ordered on one form the box can be marked with the number of days of treatment providing the quantity is added for any item for which the amount cannot be calculated.

(i) Although directions should preferably be in **English without abbreviation**, it is recognised that some Latin abbreviations are used (for details see Inside Back Cover).

(j) A prescription for a preparation that has been withdrawn or needs to be specially imported for a named patient should be handwritten. The name of the preparation should be endorsed with the prescriber's signature and the letters 'WD' (withdrawn or specially-imported drug); there may be considerable delay in obtaining a withdrawn medicine.

---

1. The above recommendations are acceptable for **prescription-only medicines** (PoM). For items marked **CD** see also Controlled Drugs and Drug Dependence p. 7.

2. It is permissible to issue carbon copies of NHS prescriptions as long as they are signed in ink.

3. Computer-generated facsimile signatures do not meet the legal requirement.

4. The use of capital 'L' in mL is a printing convention throughout the BNF; both mL and ml are recognised abbreviations for SI units.

Computer-issued Prescriptions

For computer-issued prescriptions the following recommendations of the Joint Computing Group of the General Medical Services Committee and the Royal College of General Practitioners should also be noted:

1. The computer must print out the date[1], the patient's surname, one forename, other initials, and address, and may also print out the patient's title. The age of children under 12 years must be printed in the box available; a facility may exist to print out the age of older children and adults as well.

2. The doctor's name[2] must be printed at the bottom of the prescription form; this will be the name of the doctor responsible for the prescription (who will normally sign it). The doctor's surgery address, reference number, and Health Authority (HA)[3] are also necessary. In addition, the surgery telephone number should be printed.

3. When prescriptions are to be signed by trainees, assistants, locums, or deputising doctors, the name of the doctor printed at the bottom of the form must still be that of the responsible principal. To avoid difficulties for the pharmacist checking the prescription, the name of the signing doctor may be printed in the signature box, to be signed over on prescribing.

4. Names of medicines must come from a dictionary held in the computer memory, to provide a check on the spelling and ensure that the name is written in full. The computer can be programmed to recognise both the non-proprietary and the proprietary name of a particular drug and to print out the preferred choice, but must not print out both names. For medicines not in the dictionary, separate checking mechanisms are required—the user must be warned that no check was possible and the entire prescription must be entered in the lexicon.

5. The dictionary may contain information on the usual doses, formulations, and (where relevant) pack sizes to produce standard predetermined prescriptions for common preparations, and to provide a check on the validity of an individual prescription on entry.

6. The prescription must be printed in English without abbreviation; information may be entered or stored in abbreviated form. The dose must be in numbers, the frequency in words, and the quantity in numbers in brackets, thus: 40 mg four times daily (112).

It must also be possible to prescribe by indicating the length of treatment required, see (h) above.

7. The BNF recommendations should be followed as in (a), (b), (c), (d), and (e) above.

8. Checks may be incorporated to ensure that all the information required for dispensing a particular drug has been filled in. Instructions such as 'as directed' should be avoided. For the instruction 'when required' the maximum daily dose should normally be specified.

9. Numbers and codes used in the system for organising and retrieving data must never appear on the form.

10. Supplementary warnings or advice should be written in full, should not interfere with the clarity of the prescription itself, and should be in line with any warnings or advice in the BNF; numerical codes should not be used.

11. A mechanism (such as printing a series of non-specific characters) may be incorporated to cancel out unused space, or wording such as 'no more items on this prescription' may be added after the last item. Otherwise the doctor should delete the space manually.

12. To avoid forgery the computer may print on the form the number of items to be dispensed (somewhere separate from the box for the pharmacist). The number of items per form need be limited only by the ability of the printer to produce clear and well-demarcated instructions with sufficient space for each item and a spacer line before each fresh item.

13. Handwritten alterations should only be made in exceptional circumstances—it is preferable to print out a new prescription. Any alterations that are made must be written in the doctor's own handwriting and countersigned.

14. Prescriptions for controlled drugs cannot be produced by a printer[4]. If there is a record of such a prescription in the computer, it must not be printed. Instead the computer may print out a blank form with the doctor's name[1] and other details printed at the bottom.

15. The strip of paper on the side of the FP10[5](Comp) may be used for various purposes but care should be taken to avoid including confidential information. It may be advisable for the patient's name to appear at the top, but this should be preceded by 'confidential'.

16. In rural dispensing practices prescription requests (or details of medicines dispensed) will normally be entered in one surgery. The prescriptions (or dispensed medicines) may then need to be delivered to another surgery or location; if possible the computer should hold up to 10 alternatives.

Generic names of **compound preparations** which appear in the BNF are those approved by the British Pharmacopoeia Commission; whenever possible they reflect the names of the active ingredients.

Prescribers should avoid creating their own compound names for the purposes of generic prescribing; such names do not have an approved definition and can be misinterpreted.

Special care should be taken to avoid errors when prescribing compound preparations; in particular the hyphen in the prefix 'co-' should be retained.

Special care should also be taken to avoid creating generic names for **modified-release** preparations where the use of these names could lead to confusion between formulations with different lengths of action.

---

1. The exemption for own handwriting regulations for phenobarbitone does not apply to the date; a computer-generated date need not be deleted but the date must also be added by the prescriber.
2. Except in Scotland where it does not appear.
3. Health Board in Scotland.
4. Except in the case of phenobarbitone (but see also footnote 1) or where the prescriber has been exempted from handwriting requirements, for details see Controlled Drugs and Drug Dependence p. 7.
5. GP10 in Scotland.

Emergency Supply of PoM at Patient's Request[1]

The Medicines (Products Other Than Veterinary Drugs) (Prescription Only) Order 1983, as amended, allows exemptions from the Prescription Only requirements for emergency supply to be made by a person lawfully conducting a retail pharmacy business provided:

(a) that the pharmacist has interviewed the person requesting the prescription-only medicine and is satisfied:

(i) that there is immediate need for the prescription-only medicine and that it is impracticable in the circumstances to obtain a prescription without undue delay;

(ii) that treatment with the prescription-only medicine has on a previous occasion been prescribed by a doctor[2] for the person requesting it;

(iii) as to the dose which it would be appropriate for the person to take;

(b) that no greater quantity shall be supplied than will provide five days' treatment except when the prescription-only medicine is:

(i) an ointment, cream, or preparation for the relief of asthma in an aerosol dispenser when the smallest pack can be supplied;

(ii) an oral contraceptive when a full cycle may be supplied;

(iii) an antibiotic in liquid form for oral administration when the smallest quantity that will provide a full course of treatment can be supplied;

(c) that an entry shall be made in the prescription book stating:

(i) the date of supply;

(ii) the name, quantity and, where appropriate, the pharmaceutical form and strength;

(iii) the name and address of the patient;

(iv) the nature of the emergency;

(d) that the container or package must be labelled to show:

(i) the date of supply;

(ii) the name, quantity and, where appropriate, the pharmaceutical form and strength;

(iii) the name of the patient;

(iv) the name and address of the pharmacy;

(v) the words 'Emergency supply'.

(e) that the prescription-only medicine is not a substance specifically excluded from the emergency supply provision, and does not contain a Controlled Drug specified in schedules 1, 2, or 3 to the Misuse of Drugs Regulations 1985 except for phenobarbitone or phenobarbitone sodium for the treatment of epilepsy: for details see *Medicines, Ethics and Practice*, No. 16, London, Pharmaceutical Press, 1996 (and subsequent editions as available).

ROYAL PHARMACEUTICAL SOCIETY'S GUIDELINES

(1) The pharmacist should consider the medical consequences of *not* supplying.

(2) If the patient is not known to the pharmacist, the patient's identity should be established by way of appropriate documentation.

(3) It may occasionally be desirable to contact the prescriber, e.g. when the medicine requested has a potential for misuse or the prescriber is not known to the pharmacist.

(4) Care should be taken to ask whether the patient's doctor has stopped the treatment, or whether the patient is taking any other medication.

(5) Except for conditions which occur infrequently (e.g. hay fever, asthma attack or migraine), a supply should not be made if the item requested was last prescribed more than 6 months ago.

(6) Consideration should be given to supplying less than 5 days' quantity if this is justified.

(7) Where a prescription is to be provided later, a record of emergency supply as required by law must still be made. It is good practice to add to the record the date that the prescription is received on. Payment for the medicine supplied is not a legal requirement, but may help to minimise the abuse of the emergency supply exemption. If an NHS prescription is to be provided, a refundable charge may be made.

---

1. For emergency supply at the request of a doctor see *Medicines, Ethics and Practice*, No. 16, London, Pharmaceutical Press, 1996 (and subsequent editions as available).
2. The doctor must be a UK-registered doctor.

> **Plasma concentrations** in the BNF are expressed in mass units per litre (e.g. mg/litre). The approximate equivalent in terms of amount of substance units (e.g. micromol/litre) is given in brackets.

Approximate Conversions and Units

lb	kg	stones	kg	ml	fl. oz
1	0.45	1	6.35	50	1.8
2	0.91	2	12.70	100	3.5
3	1.36	3	19.05	150	5.3
4	1.81	4	25.40	200	7.0
5	2.27	5	31.75	500	17.6
6	2.72	6	38.10	1000	35.2
7	3.18	7	44.45		
8	3.63	8	50.80		
9	4.08	9	57.15		
10	4.54	10	63.50		
11	4.99	11	69.85		
12	5.44	12	76.20		
13	5.90	13	82.55		
14	6.35	14	88.90		
		15	92.95		

Mass

1 kilogram (kg)	= 1000 grams (g)
1 gram (g)	= 1000 milligrams (mg)
1 milligram (mg)	= 1000 micrograms
1 microgram	= 1000 nanograms
1 nanogram	= 1000 picograms

Volume

1 litre	= 1000 millilitres (mL)
1 millilitre	= 1000 microlitres
1 pint	≈ 568 mL

Other units

1 kilocalorie (kcal)	= 4186.8 joules (J)
1000 kilocalories (kcal)	= 4.1868 megajoules (MJ)
1 megajoule (MJ)	= 238.8 kilocalories (kcal)
1 millimetre of mercury (mmHg)	= 133.3 pascals (Pa)
1 kilopascal (kPa)	= 7.5 mmHg (pressure)

Controlled Drugs and Drug Dependence

PRESCRIPTIONS. Preparations which are subject to the prescription requirements of the Misuse of Drugs Regulations 1985, i.e. preparations specified in schedules 2 and 3, are distinguished throughout the BNF by the symbol **CD** (Controlled Drugs). The principal legal requirements relating to medical prescriptions are listed below.

Prescriptions ordering Controlled Drugs subject to prescription requirements must be *signed* and *dated*[1] by the prescriber and specify the prescriber's *address*. The prescription must always state *in the prescriber's own handwriting*[2] in ink or otherwise so as to be indelible:

1. The name and address of the patient;
2. In the case of a preparation, the form[3] and where appropriate the strength[4] of the preparation;
3. The total quantity of the preparation, or the number of dose units, *in both words and figures;*[5]
4. The dose.[6]

A prescription may order a Controlled Drug to be dispensed by instalments; the amount of the instalments and the intervals to be observed must be specified.[7] Prescriptions ordering 'repeats' on the same form are **not** permitted.

It is an offence for a doctor to issue an incomplete prescription and a pharmacist is **not** allowed to dispense a Controlled Drug unless all the information required by law is given on the prescription. Failure to comply with the regulations concerning the writing of prescriptions will result in inconvenience to patients and delay in supplying the necessary medicine.

DEPENDENCE AND MISUSE. The most serious drugs of addiction are **cocaine**, **diamorphine** (heroin), **morphine**, and the **synthetic opioids**. For arrangements for prescribing of diamorphine, dipipanone or cocaine for addicts, see p. 9.

Despite marked reduction in the prescribing of **amphetamines** there is concern that abuse of illicitly produced amphetamine and related compounds is widespread.

Owing to problems of widespread abuse additional controlled drug requirements have been placed on **temazepam** (but it remains exempt from the additional prescribing requirements).

The principal **barbiturates** are now Controlled Drugs, but phenobarbitone and phenobarbitone sodium or a preparation containing either of these are exempt from the handwriting requirement but must fulfil all other controlled drug prescription requirements (**important: the own handwriting exemption does not** apply to the date; a computer-generated date need not be deleted but the date must also be added by the prescriber). Moreover, for the treatment of epilepsy phenobarbitone and phenobarbitone sodium are available under the emergency supply regulations (p. 6).

Cannabis (Indian hemp) has no approved medicinal use and cannot be prescribed by doctors (except under licence from the Home Secretary). Its use is illegal but has become widespread in certain sections of society. Cannabis is a mild hallucinogen seldom accompanied by a desire to increase the dose; withdrawal symptoms are unusual. **Lysergide** (lysergic acid diethylamide, LSD) is a much more

---

1. A prescription is valid for 13 weeks from the date stated thereon.
2. Does not apply to prescriptions for temazepam. Otherwise applies unless the prescriber has been specifically exempted from this requirement or unless the prescription contains no controlled drug other than phenobarbitone or phenobarbitone sodium or a preparation containing either of these; the exemption does **not** apply to the date—a computer-generated date need not be deleted but the date must also be added by the prescriber.
3. The dosage form (e.g. tablets) must be included on a Controlled Drugs prescription irrespective of whether it is implicit in the proprietary name (e.g. *MST Continus*) or of whether only one form is available.
4. When more than one strength of a preparation exists the strength required must be specified.
5. Does not apply to prescriptions for temazepam.
6. The instruction 'one as directed' constitutes a dose but 'as directed' does not.
7. A special form, FP10(HP)(ad), in Scotland HBP(A), is available to doctors in NHS drug treatment centres for prescribing cocaine, dextromoramide, diamorphine, dipipanone, methadone, morphine, or pethidine by instalments for addicts (see also Terms of Service, paragraph 43). In Scotland general practitioners can prescribe by instalments on form GP10. In England and Wales forms FP10 and FP10(HP) are not suitable for this purpose but form FP10(MDA) is available. **Important:** in all cases a special licence is necessary to prescribe cocaine, diamorphine, or dipipanone for addicts except for treatment of organic disease or injury, for details see p. 9.

Sample NHS prescription form (FP10(HP)) made out to Jane M Jones, 23 Wide Road, Elsewhere; Diamorphine hydrochloride 30mg ampoules, supply 6 (six) ampoules, 60mg daily by subcutaneous infusion over 24 hours; signed by Dr C. F. George, dated 25/2/94; Southampton & S.W. Hants D.H.A., Southampton General Hospital, Tremona Road, Southampton SO9 4XY.

B 060501

potent hallucinogen; its use can lead to severe psychotic states in which life may be at risk.

PRESCRIBING DRUGS LIKELY TO CAUSE DEPENDENCE OR MISUSE. The prescriber has three main responsibilities:

1. To avoid creating dependence by introducing drugs to patients without sufficient reason. In this context, the proper use of the morphine-like drugs is well understood. The dangers of other controlled drugs are less clear because recognition of dependence is not easy and its effects, and those of withdrawal, are less obvious. Perhaps the most notable result of uninhibited prescribing is that a very large number of patients in the country take tablets which do them neither much good nor much harm, but are committed to them indefinitely because they cannot readily be stopped.

2. To see that the patient does not gradually increase the dose of a drug, given for good medical reasons, to the point where dependence becomes more likely. This tendency is seen especially with hypnotics and anxiolytics (for CSM advice see section 4.1). The prescriber should keep a close eye on the amount prescribed to prevent patients from accumulating stocks that would enable them to arrange their own dosage or even that of their families and friends. A minimal amount should be prescribed in the first instance, or when seeing a new patient for the first time.

3. To avoid being used as an unwitting source of supply for addicts. Methods include visiting more than one doctor, fabricating stories, and forging prescriptions. A doctor should therefore be wary of prescribing for strangers and may be able to get information about suspected opioid addicts from the Home Office (for details see p. 9).

Patients under temporary care should be given only small supplies of drugs unless they present an unequivocal letter from their own doctors. Doctors should also remember that their own patients may be doing a collecting round with other doctors, especially in hospitals. It is sensible to decrease dosages steadily or to issue weekly or even daily prescriptions for small amounts if it is apparent that dependence is occurring.

The stealing and misuse of prescription forms could be minimised by the following precautions:

(a) do not leave unattended if called away from the consulting room or at reception desks; do not leave in a car where they may be visible; when not in use, keep in a locked drawer within the surgery and at home;
(b) draw a diagonal line across the blank part of the form under the prescription;
(c) write the quantity in words and figures when prescribing drugs prone to abuse; this is obligatory for controlled drugs (see Prescriptions, above);
(d) alterations are best avoided but if any are made they should be clear and unambiguous; add initials against altered items;
(e) if prescriptions are left for collection they should be left in a safe place in a sealed envelope.

TRAVELLING ABROAD. Prescribed drugs listed in schedules 4 and 5 to the Misuse of Drugs Regulations 1985 are not subject to import or export licensing but doctors are advised that patients intending to carry Schedule 2 and 3 drugs abroad may require an export licence. This is dependent upon the amount of drug to be exported and further details may be obtained from the Home Office by telephoning 0171-273 3806. Applications for licences should be sent to the Home Office, Drugs Branch, Queen Anne's Gate, London SW1H 9AT.

There is no standard application form but applications must be supported by a letter from a doctor giving details of:

the patient's name and current address;
the quantities of drugs to be carried;
the strength and form in which the drugs will be dispensed;
the dates of travel to and from the United Kingdom.

Ten days should be allowed for processing the application.

Individual doctors who wish to take Controlled Drugs abroad while accompanying patients, may similarly be issued with licences. Licences are not normally issued to doctors who wish to take Controlled Drugs abroad solely in case a family emergency should arise.

These import/export licences for named individuals do not have any legal status outside the UK and are only issued to comply with the Misuse of Drugs Act and facilitate passage through UK Customs control. For clearance in the country to be visited it would be necessary to approach that country's embassy or High Commission in the UK.

Misuse of Drugs Act

The Misuse of Drugs Act, 1971 prohibits certain activities in relation to 'Controlled Drugs', in particular their manufacture, supply, and possession. The penalties applicable to offences involving the different drugs are graded broadly according to the *harmfulness attributable to a drug when it is misused* and for this purpose the drugs are defined in the following three classes:

Class A includes: alfentanil, cocaine, dextromoramide, diamorphine (heroin), dipipanone, lysergide (LSD), methadone, morphine, opium, pethidine, phencyclidine, and class B substances when prepared for injection
Class B includes: oral amphetamines, barbiturates, cannabis, cannabis resin, codeine, ethylmorphine, glutethimide, pentazocine, phenmetrazine, and pholcodine
Class C includes: certain drugs related to the amphetamines such as benzphetamine and chlorphentermine, buprenorphine, diethylpropion, mazindol, meprobamate, pemoline, pipradrol, most benzodiazepines, androgenic and anabolic steroids, clenbuterol, chorionic gonadotrophin (HCG), non-human chorionic gonadotrophin, somatotropin, somatrem, and somatropin

The Misuse of Drugs Regulations 1985 define the classes of person who are authorised to supply and possess controlled drugs while acting in their professional capacities and lay down the conditions under which these activities may be carried out. In the regulations drugs are divided into five schedules each specifying the requirements governing such activities as import, export, production, supply, possession, prescribing, and record keeping which apply to them.

Schedule 1 includes drugs such as cannabis and lysergide which are not used medicinally. Possession and supply are prohibited except in accordance with Home Office authority.

Schedule 2 includes drugs such as diamorphine (heroin), morphine, pethidine, quinalbarbitone, glutethimide, amphetamine, and cocaine and are subject to the full controlled drug requirements relating to prescriptions, safe custody (except for quinalbarbitone), the need to keep registers, etc. (unless exempted in schedule 5).

Schedule 3 includes the barbiturates (except quinalbarbitone, now schedule 2), buprenorphine, diethylpropion, mazindol, meprobamate, pentazocine, phentermine, and temazepam. They are subject to the special prescription requirements (except for phenobarbitone and temazepam, see p. 7) but not to the safe custody requirements (except for buprenorphine, diethylpropion, and temazepam) nor to the need to keep registers (although there are requirements for the retention of invoices for 2 years).

Schedule 4 includes in Part II 33 benzodiazepines (temazepam is now in schedule 3) and pemoline which are subject to minimal control. Part I includes androgenic and anabolic steroids, clenbuterol, chorionic gonadotrophin (HCG), non-human chorionic gonadotrophin, somatotropin, somatrem, and somatropin. Controlled drug prescription requirements do not apply and Schedule 4 Controlled Drugs are not subject to safe custody requirements.

Schedule 5 includes those preparations which, because of their strength, are exempt from virtually all Controlled Drug requirements other than retention of invoices for two years.

Notification of Addicts

The Misuse of Drugs (Notification of and Supply to Addicts) Regulations 1973 require that any doctor who attends a person who the doctor considers or has reasonable grounds to suspect, is addicted to any of the 14 notifiable drugs (see below) shall, within seven days of the attendance, furnish in writing particulars of that person to:

Chief Medical Officer,
Home Office, Drugs Branch,
Queen Anne's Gate,
London SW1H 9AT.

The drugs to which the Regulations apply are:

Cocaine	Methadone
Dextromoramide	Morphine
Diamorphine	Opium
Dipipanone	Oxycodone
Hydrocodone	Pethidine
Hydromorphone	Phenazocine
Levorphanol	Piritramide

Note. Dipipanone is only legally available as Diconal® Tablets. These have been much misused by opioid addicts in recent years; only medical practitioners with a special licence may now prescribe them for addicts to treat addiction. Doctors and others should be suspicious of young people who ask for them, especially as temporary residents.

Particulars[1] to be notified to the Chief Medical Officer are:
Name and address
Sex
Date of birth
National Health Service number (if known)
Date of attendance
Name of drugs of addiction
Whether patient injects any drug (whether or not notifiable)

Notification must be confirmed annually in writing if the patient is still being treated by the practitioner. Notified information is incorporated in an Index of Addicts which is maintained in the Home Office and information from this is available on a confidential basis to doctors; in fact, it is good medical practice to check all new cases of addiction or suspected addiction with the Index before prescribing or supplying controlled drugs since this is a safeguard against addicts obtaining supplies simultaneously from two or more doctors. Enquiries can be made either in writing to the Chief Medical Officer or, preferably, by telephoning 0171-273 2213. To keep notified information confidential, such enquiries are normally answered by means of a return telephone call. The reply will come from lay staff who are not qualified to give guidance on the clinical handling of cases; a recorded telephone service is available for out-of-office hours.

The preceding paragraph applies only to medical practitioners in England, Scotland, and Wales. In Northern Ireland notification should be sent to:

Chief Medical Officer,
Department of Health and Social Services,
Dundonald House,
Belfast BT4 3SB.
Enquiries should also be made to that Department, telephone (01232) 520000 extension 24323.

Prescribing of diamorphine (heroin), dipipanone, and cocaine for addicts

The Misuse of Drugs (Notification of and Supply to Addicts) Regulations 1973 also provide that only medical practitioners who hold a special licence issued by the Home Secretary may prescribe diamorphine, dipipanone (Diconal®), or cocaine for addicts; other practitioners must refer any addict who requires these drugs to a treatment centre. Whenever possible the addict will be introduced by a member of staff from the treatment centre to a pharmacist whose agreement has been obtained and whose pharmacy is conveniently sited for the patient. Prescriptions for weekly supplies will be sent to the pharmacy by post and will be dispensed on a daily basis as indicated by the doctor. If any alterations of the arrangements are requested by the addict, the portion of the prescription affected must be represcribed and not merely altered. *General practitioners and other doctors may still prescribe diamorphine, dipipanone, and cocaine for patients (including addicts) for relief of pain due to organic disease or injury without a special licence.*

For prescription-writing guidelines, see p. 7.

---

1. Only the particulars of which the doctor has knowledge need be notified immediately; the remainder may be notified at a later date. Private doctors, police surgeons and prison medical officers may continue to notify the Home Office using form HS2A/1(Rev), available from their Health Authority (HA) or their Health Board in Scotland.

All other doctors, including general practitioners, hospital doctors and those practising in treatment centres, should use notification forms which can be obtained from their Regional Health Authority Drugs Misuse Database administrator.

Adverse Reactions to Drugs

Any drug may produce unwanted or unexpected adverse reactions. Detection and recording of these is of vital importance. Doctors are urged to help by reporting adverse reactions to:

CSM
Freepost
London SW8 5BR
(0171-627 3291)

Yellow prepaid lettercards for reporting are available from the above address or by dialling 100 and asking for 'CSM Freefone'; also, forms are bound in this book (inside back cover).

A 24-hour Freefone service is now available to all parts of the United Kingdom, for doctors seeking advice and information on adverse reactions; it may be obtained by dialling 100 and asking for 'CSM Freefone'. Outside office hours a telephone-answering machine will take messages.

The following regional centres also collect data:

CSM Mersey	CSM Wales
Freepost	Freepost
Liverpool L3 3AB	Cardiff CF4 1ZZ
(0151-236 4620 Extn 2126)	(01222 744181 Direct Line)
CSM Northern	CSM West Midlands
Freepost 1085	Freepost SW2991
Newcastle upon Tyne	Birmingham B18 7BR
NE1 1BR	[No telephone number]
(0191-232 1525 Direct Line)	

Suspected adverse reactions to *any* therapeutic agent should be reported, including drugs (those taken for *self medication* as well as those *prescribed*), blood products, vaccines, X-ray contrast media, dental or surgical materials, intra-uterine devices, and contact lens fluids.

ADROIT

Adverse Drug Reactions On-line Information Tracking (ADROIT) has now been introduced to facilitate the monitoring of adverse drug reactions.

NEWER DRUGS. These are indicated by the sign ▼. Doctors are asked to report *all* suspected reactions (i.e. any adverse or any unexpected event, however minor, which could conceivably be attributed to the drug). Reports should be made despite uncertainty about a causal relationship, irrespective of whether the reaction is well recognized, and even if other drugs have been given concurrently.

ESTABLISHED DRUGS. Doctors are asked to report *all* serious suspected reactions, including those that are fatal, life-threatening, disabling, incapacitating, or which result in or prolong hospitalisation; they should be reported even if the effect is well recognised.

Examples include anaphylaxis, blood disorders, endocrine disturbances, effects on fertility, haemorrhage from any site, renal impairment, jaundice, ophthalmic disorders, severe CNS effects, severe skin reactions, reactions in pregnant women, and any drug interactions. Reports of serious adverse reactions are required to enable risk/benefit ratios to be compared with other drugs of a similar class. For established drugs doctors are asked not to report well-known, relatively minor side-effects, such as dry mouth with tricyclic antidepressants, constipation with opioids, or nausea with digoxin.

Special problems

Delayed drug effects. Some reactions (e.g. cancers, chloroquine retinopathy, and retroperitoneal fibrosis) may become manifest months or years after exposure. Any suspicion of such an association should be reported.

The elderly. Doctors are asked to be particularly alert to adverse reactions in the elderly.

Congenital abnormalities. When an infant is born with a congenital abnormality or there is a malformed aborted fetus doctors are asked to consider whether this might be an adverse reaction to a drug and to report all drugs (including self-medication) taken during pregnancy.

Vaccines. Doctors are asked to report all suspected reactions to both new and established vaccines. The balance between risks and benefits needs to be kept under continuous review.

Prevention of adverse reactions

Adverse reactions may be prevented as follows:

1. Never use any drug unless there is a good indication. If the patient is pregnant do not use a drug unless the need for it is imperative.
2. It is very important to recognise allergy and idiosyncrasy as causes of adverse drug reactions. Ask if the patient had previous reactions.
3. Ask if the patient is already taking other drugs *including self-medication*; remember that interactions may occur.
4. Age and hepatic or renal disease may alter the metabolism or excretion of drugs, so that much smaller doses may need to be prescribed. Pharmacogenetic factors may also be responsible for variations in the rate of metabolism, notably of isoniazid and the tricyclic antidepressants.
5. Prescribe as few drugs as possible and give very clear instructions to the elderly or any patient likely to misunderstand complicated instructions.
6. When possible use a familiar drug. With a new drug be particularly alert for adverse reactions or unexpected events.
7. If serious adverse reactions are liable to occur warn the patient.

Defective Medicines

During the manufacture or distribution of a medicine an error or accident may occur whereby the finished product does not conform to its specification. While such a defect may impair the therapeutic effect of the product and could adversely affect the health of a patient, it should **not** be confused with an Adverse Drug Reaction where the product conforms to its specification.

The Defective Medicines Report Centre operates a 24-hour service to assist with the investigation of problems arising from licensed medicinal products thought to be defective, and to co-ordinate any necessary protective action. Reports on suspect defective medicinal products should include the brand or the non-proprietary name, the name of the manufacturer or supplier, the strength and dosage form of the product, the product licence number, the batch number or numbers of the product, the nature of the defect, and an account of any action already taken in consequence. The Centre can be contacted at:

The Defective Medicines Report Centre
Medicines Control Agency
Room 1801, Market Towers
1 Nine Elms Lane
London SW8 5NQ
0171-273 0574 (weekdays 9.00 am–5.00 pm)
or 0171-210 5368 or 5371 (any other time)

Prescribing for Children

All children, and particularly neonates, differ from adults in their response to drugs. Special care is needed in the neonatal period (first 30 days of life) and doses should always be calculated according to weight. At this age, the risk of toxicity is increased by inefficient renal filtration, relative enzyme deficiencies, differing target organ sensitivity, and inadequate detoxifying systems causing delayed excretion. In childhood dosage should be adjusted for weight until 50 kg or puberty is reached.

Whenever possible painful intramuscular injections should be **avoided** in children.

PRESCRIPTION WRITING. Prescriptions should be written according to the guidelines in Prescription Writing (p. 4). Inclusion of age is a legal requirement in the case of prescription-only medicines for children under 12 years of age, but it is preferable to state the age for **all** prescriptions for children.

It is particularly important to state the strengths of capsules or tablets. Although liquid preparations are particularly suitable for children, many contain sucrose which encourages dental decay. When taken over a long period, sugar-free tablets and liquid medicines should be used when possible.

When a prescription for a liquid oral preparation is written and the dose ordered is smaller than 5 mL, the preparation will no longer be diluted. Instead an **oral syringe** will be supplied, for full details, see p. 2. Parents should be advised not to add any medicines to the contents of the infant's feeding bottle, since the drug may interact with the milk or other liquid in it; moreover the ingested dosage may be reduced, if the child does not drink all the contents.

Parents must be warned to keep **all** medicines out of the reach of children, see Safety in the Home, p. 3.

Rare paediatric conditions

Information on substances such as *biotin* and *sodium benzoate* used in rare metabolic conditions can be obtained from:

Drug Information Centre, Alder Hey Children's Hospital, Liverpool L12 2AP (Tel. 0151-252 5381);
Pharmacy, Hospital for Sick Children, Great Ormond St, London, WC1N 3JH (Tel. 0171-405 9200)

Dosage in Children

Children's doses in the BNF are stated in the individual drug entries as far as possible, except where paediatric use is not recommended or there are special hazards.

Doses are generally based on body-weight (in kilograms) or the following age ranges:

first month (neonate)
up to 1 year (infant)
1–5 years
6–12 years

Where a single dose is quoted for a given range, it applies to the middle of the age range and some extrapolation may be necessary to obtain doses for ages at the lower and upper limits of the stated range.

DOSE CALCULATION. Children's doses may be calculated from adult doses by using age, body-weight, or body-surface area, or by a combination of these factors. The most reliable methods are those based on body-surface area.

Body-weight may be used to calculate doses expressed in mg/kg. Young children may require a higher dose per kilogram than adults because of their higher metabolic rates. Other problems need to be considered. For example, calculation by body-weight in the obese child would result in much higher doses being administered than necessary; in such cases, dose should be calculated from an ideal weight, related to height and age.

Body-surface area (BSA) estimates are more accurate for calculation of paediatric doses than body-weight since many physical phenomena are more closely related to body-surface area. The average body-surface area of a 70-kilogram human is about $1.8\,m^2$. Thus, to calculate the dose for a child the following formula may be used:

Approximate dose for patient =

$$\frac{\text{surface area of patient } (m^2) \times \text{adult dose}}{1.8}$$

The **percentage method** below may be used to calculate paediatric doses of commonly prescribed drugs that have a wide margin between the therapeutic and the toxic dose

Age	Ideal body-weight kg	lb	Height cm	in	Body-surface m^2	Percentage of adult dose
Newborn*	3.4	7.5	50	20	0.23	12.5
1 month*	4.2	9	55	22	0.26	14.5
3 months*	5.6	12	59	23	0.32	18
6 months	7.7	17	67	26	0.40	22
1 year	10	22	76	30	0.47	25
3 years	14	31	94	37	0.62	33
5 years	18	40	108	42	0.73	40
7 years	23	51	120	47	0.88	50
12 years	37	81	148	58	1.25	75
Adult						
Male	68	150	173	68	1.80	100
Female	56	123	163	64	1.60	100

* The figures relate to full term and not preterm infants who may need reduced dosage according to their clinical condition.

More precise body-surface values may be calculated from height and weight by means of a nomogram (e.g. J. Insley, *A Paediatric Vade-Mecum*, 12th Edition, London, Edward Arnold, 1990).

DOSE FREQUENCY. Doses for antibiotics are usually stated as every 6 hours. Some flexibility should be allowed in antibiotics to avoid waking them during the night. For example, the night-time dose may be given at the parent's bedtime.

Where new or potentially toxic drugs are used, the manufacturers' recommended doses should be carefully followed.

Prescribing in Palliative Care

In recent years there has been increased interest in providing better treatment and support for patients with terminal illness. The aim is to keep them as comfortable, alert, and free of pain as possible. It may also be necessary to direct attention to emotional, financial, social, or family problems. The patient's minister or the hospital chaplain may give invaluable help.

DOMICILIARY CARE. If they wish, whenever possible, patients should end their days in their own homes. Although families may at first be afraid of caring for the patient at home, they will usually do so if extra support from district nursing services, social services and voluntary agencies is provided. Families may be reassured if an assurance is given that the patient will be admitted to a hospital or hospice if they cannot cope.

HOSPITAL OR HOSPICE CARE. The most important lesson to be drawn from the experience of hospices is that both doctors and nurses must give time to listen to the patient. This gives great support and comfort to a patient who may otherwise suffer intolerable loneliness. Often problems come to light that can easily be dealt with—adjusting a blind in the late afternoon, an irritating noise to be avoided, drinks to be placed in easier reach, someone to read the newspaper, or the TV to be replaced by radio. The staff should not exclude the family from contributing to the patient's care; if prevented they may be resentful or subsequently suffer a feeling of guilt.

DRUG TREATMENT. The number of drugs should be as few as possible, for even the taking of medicine may be an effort. Oral medication is usually satisfactory unless there is severe nausea and vomiting, dysphagia, weakness, or coma, in which case parenteral medication may be necessary.

PAIN

Analgesics are always more effective in preventing the development of pain than in the relief of established pain.

The **non-opioid** analgesics **aspirin** or **paracetamol** given regularly will often make the use of opioids unnecessary. Aspirin (or other NSAIDs if preferred) may also control the pain of *bone secondaries*; naproxen, flurbiprofen, and indomethacin (see section 10.1.1) are valuable and if necessary can be given rectally. **Corticosteroids, radiotherapy** or radioactive isotopes of **strontium** (Metastron® available from Amersham) are also often useful for pain due to bone metastases.

Morphine is the most useful of the **opioid analgesics**. In addition to relief of pain, it confers a state of euphoria and mental detachment.

ORAL ROUTE. Morphine is given *by mouth* as an oral solution regularly every 4 hours, the initial dose depending largely on the patient's previous treatment. A dose of 5–10 mg is enough to replace a weaker analgesic (such as paracetamol or co-proxamol), but 10–20 mg or more is required to replace a strong one (comparable to morphine itself). If the first dose of morphine is no more effective than the previous analgesic it should be increased by 50%, the aim being to choose the lowest dose which prevents pain. Although a dose of 5–20 mg is usually adequate there should be no hesitation in increasing it to 30–60 mg or occasionally to 90–150 mg or higher if necessary. If pain occurs between doses the next dose due is increased; in the interim an additional dose is given.

Modified-release tablets of morphine (MST Continus® tablets or Oramorph® SR tablets) are an alternative to the oral solution; they have the advantage that they need only be taken every 12 hours. The starting dose of MST Continus® tablets or Oramorph® SR tablets is usually 10–20 mg every 12 hours if no other analgesic (or only paracetamol) has previously been taken, but to replace a weaker opioid analgesic (such as co-proxamol) the starting dose is usually 20–30 mg every 12 hours. Increments should be made to the dose, not to the frequency of administration, which should remain at every 12 hours.

The effective dose of MST Continus® tablets or Oramorph®SR tablets can alternatively be found by giving the oral solution of morphine every 4 hours in increasing doses until the pain has been controlled, and then transferring the patient to the same total 24-hour dose of morphine given as the modified-release tablet (divided into two portions for 12-hourly administration). The first dose of the modified-release tablet is given 4 hours after the last dose of the oral solution[1].

Modified-release capsules of morphine sulphate (MXL®) are available which need to be taken only once every 24 hours. This may aid compliance, but the patient's 24-hour morphine requirements should be found before starting this preparation; morphine, as oral solution or tablets, should be prescribed for breakthrough pain.

PARENTERAL ROUTE. If the patient becomes unable to swallow, the equivalent intramuscular dose of morphine is half the oral solution dose; in the case of the modified-release tablets it is half the total 24-hour dose (which is then divided into 6 portions to be given every 4 hours). **Diamorphine** is preferred for injection because being more soluble it can be given in a smaller volume. The equivalent intramuscular (or subcutaneous) dose of diamorphine is only about a quarter to a third of the oral dose of morphine; *subcutaneous infusion via syringe driver* can be useful (for details, see p. 14).

RECTAL ROUTE. Morphine is also available for *rectal administration* as suppositories; alternatively **oxycodone** suppositories can be obtained on special order.

---

1. Studies have indicated that administration of the last dose of the *oral solution* with the first dose of the *modified-release tablets* is not necessary.

TRANSDERMAL ROUTE. Transdermal preparations of fentanyl are now available, see section 4.7.2. Careful conversion from oral morphine to transdermal fentanyl is necessary; a 25 micrograms/hr patch is equivalent to a total dose of morphine up to 135 mg/24 hours

GASTRO-INTESTINAL PAIN. The pain of *bowel colic* may be reduced by loperamide 2–4 mg 4 times daily. Hyoscine hydrobromide may also be helpful, given sublingually at a dose of 300 micrograms 3 times daily as Kwells® (Roche Consumer Health) tablets. For the dose by *subcutaneous infusion* using a syringe driver, see p. 14.

Gastric distension pain due to pressure on the stomach may be helped by a preparation incorporating an antacid with an antiflatulent (see section 1.1.1) and by domperidone 10 mg 3 times daily before meals.

MUSCLE SPASM. The pain of muscle spasm can be helped by a muscle relaxant such as diazepam 5–10 mg daily or baclofen 5–10 mg 3 times daily.

NERVE PAIN. Pain due to *nerve compression* may be reduced by a corticosteroid such as dexamethasone 8 mg daily, which reduces oedema around the tumour, thus reducing compression.

Dysaesthetic or stabbing pain resulting from *nerve irritation* may be reduced by amitriptyline 25–75 mg at night, or by carbamazepine 200 mg 3 times daily.

Nerve blocks may be considered when pain is localised to a specific area. **Transcutaneous electrical nerve stimulation (TENS)** may also provide useful relief of pain.

MISCELLANEOUS CONDITIONS

Non-licensed indications or routes
Several recommendations in this section involve non-licensed indications or routes.

RAISED INTRACRANIAL PRESSURE. Headache due to *raised intracranial pressure* often responds to a high dose of a corticosteroid, such as dexamethasone 16 mg daily for 4 to 5 days, subsequently reduced to 4–6 mg daily if possible.

INTRACTABLE COUGH. *Intractable cough* may be relieved by moist inhalations or may require regular administration of an oral morphine hydrochloride (or sulphate) solution in an initial dose of 5 mg every 4 hours. Methadone linctus should be avoided as it has a long duration of action and tends to accumulate.

DYSPNOEA. *Dyspnoea* may be relieved by regular oral morphine hydrochloride (or sulphate) solution in carefully titrated doses, starting at 5 mg every 4 hours. Diazepam 5–10 mg daily may be helpful; a corticosteroid, such as dexamethasone 4–8 mg daily, may also be helpful if there is *bronchospasm* or *partial obstruction*.

EXCESSIVE RESPIRATORY SECRETION. *Excessive respiratory secretion* (death rattle) may be reduced by subcutaneous injection of hyoscine hydrobromide

400–600 micrograms every 4 to 8 hours; care must however be taken to avoid the discomfort of dry mouth. For the dose by *subcutaneous infusion* using a syringe driver, see next page.

RESTLESSNESS AND CONFUSION. *Restlessness and confusion* may require treatment with haloperidol 1–3 mg by mouth every 8 hours. Chlorpromazine 25–50 mg by mouth every 8 hours is an alternative, but causes more sedation. Methotrimeprazine is also used occasionally for restlessness. For the dose by *subcutaneous infusion* using a syringe driver, see next page

HICCUP. *Hiccup due to gastric distension* may be helped by a preparation incorporating an antacid with an antiflatulent (see section 1.1.1). If this fails, metoclopramide 10 mg every 6 to 8 hours by mouth or by intramuscular injection can be added; if this also fails, chlorpromazine 10–25 mg every 6 to 8 hours can be tried.

ANOREXIA. *Anorexia* may be helped by prednisolone 15–30 mg daily or dexamethasone 2–4 mg daily.

CONSTIPATION. *Constipation* is a very common cause of distress and is almost invariable after administration of an opioid. It should be prevented if possible by the regular administration of laxatives; a faecal softener with a peristaltic stimulant (e.g. co-danthramer), or lactulose solution with a senna preparation should be used (see sections 1.6.2 and 1.6.3).

FUNGATING GROWTH. *Fungating growth* may be treated by cleansing with a mixture of 1 part of 4% povidone-iodine skin cleanser solution and 4 parts of liquid paraffin. Oral administration of metronidazole (see section 5.1.11) may eradicate the anaerobic bacteria responsible for the odour of fungating tumours; topical application (see section 13.10.1.2) is also used.

CAPILLARY BLEEDING. *Capillary bleeding* may be reduced by applying gauze soaked in adrenaline solution (1 in 1000).

DRY MOUTH. *Dry mouth* may be associated with candidiasis which can be treated by nystatin oral suspension or pastilles, amphotericin lozenges, or miconazole oral gel after food (see section 12.3.2); alternatively, fluconazole can be given by mouth (see section 5.2). Morphine sulphate and antimuscarinic drugs (such as hyoscine) may cause dry mouth.

PRURITUS. *Pruritus*, even when associated with *obstructive jaundice*, often responds to simple measures such as emollients. In the case of obstructive jaundice, further measures include administration of cholestyramine or an anabolic steroid, such as stanozolol 5–10 mg daily; antihistamines can be helpful (see section 3.4.1).

CONVULSIONS. Patients with *cerebral tumours* or *uraemia* may be susceptible to convulsions. Prophylactic treatment with phenytoin or carbamazepine (see section 4.8.1) should be considered. When oral medication is no longer possible, diazepam as suppositories 10–20 mg every 4 to 8 hours, or phenobarbitone by injection 50–200 mg twice daily is continued as prophylaxis. For the use of midazolam by *subcutaneous infusion* using a syringe driver, see next page.

DYSPHAGIA. A corticosteroid such as dexamethasone 8 mg daily may help, temporarily, if there is an obstruction due to *tumour*. See also under Dry Mouth.

NAUSEA AND VOMITING. *Nausea and vomiting* are very common in patients with advanced cancer. The cause should be diagnosed before treatment with anti-emetics (see section 4.6) is started. Octreotide (see section 8.3.4.3), which stimulates water and electrolyte absorption and inhibits water secretion in the small bowel, can be used by subcutaneous infusion, in a dose of 300–600 micrograms/24 hours to reduce intestinal secretions and vomiting.

Nausea and vomiting may also occur in the initial stages of morphine therapy but can be prevented by giving an anti-emetic such as haloperidol or prochlorperazine. An anti-emetic is usually only necessary for the first 4 or 5 days therefore fixed-combination opioid preparations containing an anti-emetic are not recommended since they lead to unnecessary anti-emetic therapy (often with undesirable drowsiness). For the administration of anti-emetics by *subcutaneous infusion* using a syringe driver, see below.

INSOMNIA. Patients with advanced cancer may not sleep because of discomfort, cramps, night sweats, joint stiffness, or fear. There should be appropriate treatment of these problems before hypnotics are used. Benzodiazepines, such as temazepam, may be useful (see section 4.1.1).

HYPERCALCAEMIA. See section 9.5.1.2.

SYRINGE DRIVERS

Although drugs can usually be administered *by mouth* to control the symptoms of advanced cancer, the parenteral route may sometimes be necessary. If the parenteral route is necessary, repeated administration of *intramuscular injections* can be difficult in a cachectic patient. This has led to the use of a portable syringe driver to give a *continuous subcutaneous infusion*, which can provide good control of symptoms with little discomfort or inconvenience to the patient.

Indications for the **parenteral route** are:

the patient is unable to take medicines by mouth owing to *nausea and vomiting, dysphagia, severe weakness,* or *coma;*

there is *malignant bowel obstruction* in patients for whom further surgery is inappropriate (avoiding the need for an intravenous infusion or for insertion of a nasogastric tube);

occasionally when the patient *does not wish* to take regular medication by mouth.

NAUSEA AND VOMITING. **Haloperidol** is given in a *subcutaneous infusion* dose of 2.5–10 mg/24 hours.

Methotrimeprazine causes sedation in about 50% of patients; it is given in a *subcutaneous infusion dose* of 25–200 mg/24 hours.

Cyclizine is particularly liable to precipitate if mixed with diamorphine or other drugs (see under

Mixing and Compatibility, below); it is given in a *subcutaneous infusion dose* of 150 mg/24 hours.

Metoclopramide may cause skin reactions; it is given in a *subcutaneous infusion dose* of 30–60 mg/24 hours.

BOWEL COLIC OR EXCESSIVE RESPIRATORY SECRETIONS. **Hyoscine hydrobromide** effectively reduces respiratory secretions and is sedative (but occasionally causes paradoxical agitation); it is given in a *subcutaneous infusion dose* of 0.6–2.4 mg/24 hours.

Hyoscine butylbromide is effective in bowel colic, is less sedative than hyoscine hydrobromide, but is not always adequate for the control of respiratory secretions; it is given in a *subcutaneous infusion dose* of 20–60 mg/24 hours (**important:** this dose of *hyoscine butylbromide* must not be confused with the much lower dose of *hyoscine hydrobromide*, above).

RESTLESSNESS AND CONFUSION. **Haloperidol** has little sedative effect; it is given in a *subcutaneous infusion dose* of 5–30 mg/24 hours.

Methotrimeprazine has a sedative effect; it is given in a *subcutaneous infusion dose* of 50–200 mg/24 hours.

Midazolam is a sedative and an antiepileptic, and is therefore suitable for a very restless patient; it is given in a *subcutaneous infusion dose* of 20–100 mg/24 hours.

CONVULSIONS. If a patient has previously been receiving an antiepileptic *or* has a primary or secondary cerebral tumour *or* is at risk of convulsion (e.g. owing to uraemia) antiepileptic medication should not be stopped. **Midazolam** is the benzodiazepine antiepileptic of choice for *continuous subcutaneous infusion*, and is given in a dose of 20–40 mg/24 hours.

PAIN CONTROL. **Diamorphine** is the preferred opioid since its high solubility permits a large dose to be given in a small volume (see under Mixing and Compatibility, below). The table on the next page gives the approximate doses of *morphine by mouth* (as oral solution or standard tablets or as modified-release tablets) equivalent to *diamorphine by injection* (intramuscularly or by subcutaneous infusion).

MIXING AND COMPATIBILITY. The general principle that injections should be given into separate sites (and should not be mixed) does not apply to the use of syringe drivers in palliative care. Provided that there is evidence of compatibility, selected injections can be mixed in syringe drivers. Not all types of medication can be used in a subcutaneous infusion. In particular, **chlorpromazine, prochlorperazine** and **diazepam** are **contra-indicated** as they cause skin reactions at the injection site; to a lesser extent **cyclizine** and **methotrimeprazine** may also sometimes cause local irritation.

In theory injections dissolved in **water for injections** are more likely to be associated with pain (possibly owing to their hypotonicity). The use of **physiological saline** (sodium chloride 0.9%) however increases the likelihood of precipitation when more than one drug is used; moreover subcutaneous infusion rates are so slow (0.1–0.3 mL/hour) that pain is not usually a problem when water is used as a diluent.

Diamorphine can be given by subcutaneous infusion in a strength of up to 250 mg/mL; up to a strength of 40 mg/mL either *water for injections* or *physiological saline* (sodium chloride 0.9%) is a suitable diluent—above that strength only *water for injections* is used (to avoid precipitation).

The following can be mixed with *diamorphine:*

Cyclizine[1]
Dexamethasone[2]
Haloperidol[3]
Hyoscine butylbromide
Hyoscine hydrobromide
Methotrimeprazine
Metoclopramide[4]
Midazolam

Subcutaneous infusion solution should be monitored regularly both to check for precipitation (and discoloration) and to ensure that the infusion is running at the correct rate.

PROBLEMS ENCOUNTERED WITH SYRINGE DRIVERS. The following are problems that may be encountered with syringe drivers and the action that should be taken:

if the subcutaneous infusion runs *too quickly* check the rate setting and the calculation;

if the subcutaneous infusion runs *too slowly* check the start button, the battery, the syringe driver, the cannula, and make sure that the injection site is not inflamed;

if there is an *injection site reaction* make sure that the site does not need to be changed—firmness or swelling at the site of injection is not in itself an indication for change, but pain or obvious inflammation is.

Syringe driver rate settings. Staff using syringe drivers should be **adequately trained** and different rate settings should be **clearly identified** and **differentiated**; incorrect use of syringe drivers is a common cause of drug errors.

1. Cyclizine may precipitate at concentrations above 10 mg/mL *or* in the presence of physiological saline *or* as the concentration of diamorphine relative to cyclizine increases; mixtures of diamorphine and cyclizine are also liable to precipitate after 24 hours.
2. Special care is needed to avoid precipitation of dexamethasone when preparing.
3. Mixtures of haloperidol and diamorphine are liable to precipitate after 24 hours if haloperidol concentration is above 2 mg/mL.
4. Under some conditions metoclopramide may become discoloured; such solutions should be discarded.

Equivalent doses of morphine sulphate by mouth (as oral solution or standard tablets *or* as modified-release tablets) *or* of diamorphine hydrochloride by intramuscular injection *or by* subcutaneous infusion

These equivalences are approximate only and may need to be adjusted according to response

ORAL MORPHINE		PARENTERAL DIAMORPHINE	
Morphine sulphate oral solution or standard tablets	Morphine sulphate modified-release tablets	Diamorphine hydrochloride by intramuscular injection	Diamorphine hydrochloride by subcutaneous infusion
every 4 hours	**every 12 hours**	**every 4 hours**	**every 24 hours**
5 mg	20 mg	2.5 mg	15 mg
10 mg	30 mg	5 mg	20 mg
15 mg	50 mg	5 mg	30 mg
20 mg	60 mg	7.5 mg	45 mg
30 mg	90 mg	10 mg	60 mg
40 mg	120 mg	15 mg	90 mg
60 mg	180 mg	20 mg	120 mg
80 mg	240 mg	30 mg	180 mg
100 mg	300 mg	40 mg	240 mg
130 mg	400 mg	50 mg	300 mg
160 mg	500 mg	60 mg	360 mg
200 mg	600 mg	70 mg	400 mg

If breakthrough pain occurs give a subcutaneous (preferable) or intramuscular injection of diamorphine equivalent to one-sixth of the total 24-hour subcutaneous infusion dose. It is kinder to give an intermittent bolus injection *subcutaneously*—absorption is smoother so that the risk of adverse effects at peak absorption is avoided (an even better method is to use a subcutaneous butterfly needle).

To minimise the risk of infection no individual subcutaneous infusion solution should be used for longer than 24 hours.

Prescribing for the Elderly

Old people, especially the very old, require special care and consideration from prescribers.

POLYPHARMACY. Elderly patients are apt to receive multiple drugs for their multiple diseases. This greatly increases the risk of drug interactions as well as other adverse reactions. Moreover, symptoms such as headache, sleeplessness, and light-headedness which may be associated with social stress, as in widowhood, loneliness, and family dispersal can lead to further prescribing, especially of psychotropics. The use of drugs in such cases can at best be a poor substitute for effective social measures and at worst pose a serious threat from adverse reactions.

FORM OF MEDICINE. Elderly patients may have difficulty swallowing tablets; if left in the mouth, ulceration may develop. They should always be encouraged to take their tablets or capsules with enough fluid, and in some cases it may be advisable to prescribe liquid if available.

MANIFESTATIONS OF AGEING. In very old subjects, manifestations of normal ageing may be mistaken for disease and lead to inappropriate prescribing. For example, drugs such as prochlorperazine are commonly misprescribed for giddiness due to age-related loss of postural stability. Not only is such treatment ineffective but the patient may experience serious side-effects such as drug-induced parkinsonism, postural hypotension, and mental confusion.

SELF-MEDICATION. Self-medication with over-the-counter products or with drugs prescribed for a previous illness (or even for another person) may be an added complication. Discussion with relatives and a home visit may be needed to establish exactly what is being taken.

SUSCEPTIBILITY. The ageing nervous system shows increased *susceptibility* to many commonly used drugs, such as opioid analgesics, benzodiazepines, and antiparkinsonian drugs, all of which must be used with caution.

PHARMACOKINETICS

While drug distribution and metabolism may be significantly altered, the most important effect of age is reduction in renal clearance, frequently aggravated by the effects of prostatism, nephrosclerosis, or chronic urinary tract infection. Many aged patients thus possess only *limited reserves of renal function, excrete drugs slowly*, and are *highly susceptible to nephrotoxic drugs*. Acute illness may lead to rapid reduction in renal clearance, especially if accompanied by dehydration. Hence, a patient stabilised on a drug with a narrow margin between the therapeutic and the toxic dose (e.g. digoxin) may rapidly develop adverse effects in the after-math of a myocardial infarction or a respiratory tract infection.

The net result of pharmacokinetic changes is that tissue concentrations are commonly increased by over 50%, and aged and debilitated patients may show even larger changes.

ADVERSE REACTIONS

Adverse reactions often present in the elderly in a vague and non-specific fashion. *Mental confusion* is often the presenting symptom (caused by almost any of the commonly used drugs). Other common manifestations are *constipation* (with antimuscarinics and many tranquillisers) and postural *hypotension* and *falls* (with diuretics and many psychotropics).

HYPNOTICS. Many hypnotics with long half-lives have serious hangover effects of drowsiness, unsteady gait, and even slurred speech and confusion. Those with short half-lives should be used but they too can present problems (see section 4.1.1). Short courses of hypnotics are occasionally useful for helping a patient through an acute illness or some other crisis but every effort must be made to avoid dependence.

DIURETICS. Diuretics are overprescribed in old age and should **not** be used on a long-term basis to treat simple gravitational oedema which will usually respond to increased movement, raising the legs, and support stockings. A few days of diuretic treatment may speed the clearing of the oedema but it should rarely need continued drug therapy.

NSAIDs. Bleeding associated with *aspirin* and *other NSAIDs* is more common in the elderly, and the outcome tends to be more serious. NSAIDs are also a special hazard in patients with cardiac disease or renal impairment which may again place the elderly at particular risk.

OTHER DRUGS. Other drugs which commonly cause adverse reactions are *antiparkinsonian drugs, antihypertensives, psychotropics*, and *digoxin*; the usual maintenance dose of digoxin in very old patients is 125 micrograms daily (62.5 micrograms is often inadequate, and toxicity is common in those given 250 micrograms).

Drug-induced blood disorders are much more common in the elderly. Therefore drugs with a tendency to cause bone marrow depression (e.g. co-trimoxazole, mianserin) should be avoided unless there is no acceptable alternative.

The elderly generally require a lower maintenance dose of *warfarin* than younger adults; once again, the outcome of bleeding tends to be more serious.

GUIDELINES

First always question whether a drug is indicated at all.

LIMIT RANGE. It is a sensible policy to prescribe from a limited range of drugs and to be thoroughly familiar with their effects in the elderly.

REDUCE DOSE. Dosage should generally be substantially lower than for younger patients and it is common to start with about 50% of the adult dose. Some drugs (e.g. chlorpropamide) should be avoided altogether.

REVIEW REGULARLY. Review repeat prescriptions regularly. It may be possible to stop the drug (e.g. digoxin can often be withdrawn) or it may be necessary to reduce the dose to match diminishing renal function.

SIMPLIFY. Simplify regimens. Elderly patients cannot normally cope with more than three different drugs and, ideally, these should not be given more than twice daily. In particular, regimens which call for a confusing array of dosage intervals should be avoided.

EXPLAIN CLEARLY. Write full instructions on every prescription (*including* repeat prescriptions) so that containers can be properly labelled with full directions. Avoid imprecisions like 'as directed'. Child-resistant containers may be unsuitable.

REPEATS AND DISPOSAL. Instruct patients what to do when drugs run out, and also how to dispose of any that are no longer necessary. Try to prescribe matching quantities.

If these guidelines are followed most elderly people will cope adequately with their own medicines. If not then it is essential to enrol the help of a third party, usually a relative or a friend.

Emergency Treatment of Poisoning

TOXBASE is an on-line database which provides information about routine diagnosis, treatment and management of patients exposed to drugs, household products, and industrial and agricultural chemicals. It is available via a Viewdata system to authorised users including Accident and Emergency Departments (contact 0131-536 2303 for further information). **Important:** for more specialised information telephone the Poisons Information Centres.

TICTAC is a computer-aided tablet and capsule identification system. It is available to authorised users including Regional Drug Information Centres (see p. xiii) and Poisons Information Centres.

POISONS INFORMATION CENTRES (consult day and night)

Belfast		01232 240503
Birmingham		0121-507 5588
	or	0121-507 5589
Cardiff		01222 709901
Dublin		Dublin 837 9964
	or	Dublin 837 9966
Edinburgh		0131-536 2300
Leeds		0113 243 0715
	or	0113 292 3547
London		0171-635 9191
	or	0171-955 5095
Newcastle		0191-232 5131

Note. Some of these centres also advise on laboratory analytical services which may be of help in the diagnosis and management of a small number of cases

These notes are only guidelines and it is strongly recommended that **poisons information centres** (see above) be consulted in cases where there is doubt about the degree of risk or about appropriate management.

HOSPITAL ADMISSION. All patients who show features of poisoning should generally be admitted to hospital. Patients who have taken poisons with delayed actions should also be admitted, even if they appear well; delayed-action poisons include aspirin, iron, paracetamol, tricyclic antidepressants, co-phenotrope (diphenoxylate with atropine, *Lomotil*®), and paraquat; this also applies to modified-release capsules or tablets. A note should be sent of what is known and what treatment has been given.

It is often impossible to establish with certainty the identity of the poison and the size of the dose. Fortunately this is not usually important because only a few poisons (such as opioids, paracetamol, and iron) have specific antidotes and few patients require active removal of the poison. Most patients must be treated symptomatically. Nevertheless, knowledge of the type of poisoning does help in anticipating the course of events. Patients' reports may be of little help, as they may be confused or may only be able to say that they have taken an undefined amount, possibly of mixed drugs. Parents may think a child has taken something which could be poisonous and may exaggerate or underplay the risks out of anxiety or guilt. Sometimes symptoms are due to an illness such as appendicitis. Accidents can arise from a number of domestic and industrial products (the contents of which are not generally known).

General care

The **poisons information centres** (see above) will provide advice on all aspects of poisoning day and night

RESPIRATION

Respiration is often impaired in unconscious patients. An obstructed airway requires immediate attention. Pull the tongue forward, remove dentures and oral secretions, hold the jaw forward, insert an oropharyngeal airway if one is available, and turn the patient semiprone. The risk of inhaling vomit is minimised with the patient positioned semiprone and head down.

Most poisons that impair consciousness also depress respiration. Assisted ventilation by mouth-to-mouth or Ambu bag inflation may be needed. Oxygen is not a substitute for adequate ventilation, though it should be given in the highest concentration possible in poisoning with carbon monoxide and irritant gases.

Respiratory stimulants do not help and are **potentially dangerous**.

BLOOD PRESSURE

Hypotension is common in severe poisoning with central nervous system depressants. A systolic blood pressure of less than 70 mmHg may lead to irreversible brain damage or renal tubular necrosis. The patient should be carried head downwards on a stretcher and nursed in this position in the ambulance. Oxygen should be given to correct hypoxia and an intravenous infusion should be set up if at all practicable. Vasopressor drugs should **not** be used.

Fluid depletion without hypotension is common after prolonged coma and after aspirin poisoning due to vomiting, sweating, and hyperpnoea.

HEART

Cardiac conduction defects and arrhythmias may occur in acute poisoning, notably with tricyclic antidepressants. Arrhythmias often respond to correction of underlying hypoxia or acidosis. Ventricular arrhythmias that have been confirmed by emergency ECG and which are causing serious hypotension may require treatment with lignocaine (see p. 72). Supraventricular arrhythmias are seldom life-threatening and drug treatment is best withheld until the patient reaches hospital.

BODY TEMPERATURE

Hypothermia may develop in patients of any age who have been deeply unconscious for some hours particularly following overdose with barbiturates or phenothiazines. It may be missed unless temperature is measured rectally using a low-reading rectal thermometer. It is best treated by wrapping the patient in blankets to conserve body heat. Hot-water bottles are of little value and may cause burns.

CONVULSIONS

Single short-lived convulsions do not require treatment. Diazepam, up to 10 mg by slow intravenous injection, preferably in emulsion form, should be given if convulsions are protracted or recur frequently; it should not be given intramuscularly.

Removal and elimination

REMOVAL FROM THE STOMACH

The dangers of attempting to empty the stomach have to be balanced against the toxicity of the ingested poison, as assessed by the quantity ingested, the inherent toxicity of the poison, and the time since ingestion. Gastric emptying is clearly unnecessary if the risk of toxicity is small or if the patient presents too late.

Emptying the stomach by **gastric lavage** is of doubtful value if attempted more than 1–2 hours after ingestion. However, a worthwhile recovery of salicylates may be achieved up to 4 hours after ingestion. The chief danger of gastric aspiration and lavage is inhalation of stomach contents, and it

should **not** be attempted in drowsy or comatose patients unless there is a good enough cough reflex or the airway can be protected by a cuffed endotracheal tube. Stomach tubes should **not** be passed after corrosive poisoning.

Petroleum products are more dangerous in the lungs than in the stomach and therefore removal from the stomach is **not** advised because of the risk of inhalation.

On balance gastric lavage is seldom practicable or desirable before the patient reaches hospital.

Emesis induced by **ipecacuanha** (Paediatric Ipecacuanha Emetic Mixture BP) has been used in adults and children, but is of very limited value. There is no evidence that it prevents clinically significant absorption (even if used within 1–2 hours) and its adverse effects may often complicate diagnosis particularly in iron poisoning. It should only be considered if the patient is fully conscious, if the poison ingested is neither corrosive nor a petroleum distillate, if it is not adsorbed by activated charcoal, or if gastric lavage is inadvisable or refused (for advice call a poisons information centre).

Salt solutions, copper sulphate, apomorphine, and mustard are dangerous and should **not** be used.

IPECACUANHA

Indications: induction of emesis in selected patients, see notes above

Cautions: avoid in poisoning with corrosive or petroleum products owing to risk of aspiration (see notes above); also avoid if risk of aspiration, in shock, or if risk of convulsions; cardiovascular disease

Side-effects: excessive vomiting and mucosal damage; cardiac effects if absorbed

Dose: see under preparation below

Ipecacuanha Emetic Mixture, Paediatric (BP)

Paediatric Ipecacuanha Emetic

Note. Paediatric Ipecacuanha Emetic Mixture is equivalent in strength to Ipecac Syrup USP

Mixture, ipecacuanha liquid extract 0.7 mL, hydrochloric acid 0.025 mL, glycerol 1 mL, syrup 10 mL

Dose: ADULT 30 mL; CHILD 6–18 months 10 mL, older children 15 mL; the dose is followed by a tumblerful of water and repeated after 20 minutes if necessary

PREVENTION OF ABSORPTION

Given by mouth, **activated charcoal** can bind many poisons in the stomach, thereby *reducing their absorption*. The **sooner** it is given the **more effective** it is, but it may still be effective up to 2 hours after ingestion—longer in the case of modified-release preparations or of drugs with antimusarinic (anticholinergic) properties. It is relatively safe and is particularly useful for the prevention of absorption of poisons which are toxic in small amounts, e.g. antidepressants.

For the use of charcoal in active elimination techniques, see below.

Carbomix® (Penn)

Powder, activated charcoal, net price 25-g pack = £8.50, 50-g pack = £11.90

Dose: reduction of absorption, 50 g; CHILD, 25 g (50 g in severe poisoning)

Active elimination, see below

Medicoal® (Torbet)

Granules, effervescent, activated charcoal 5 g/sachet. Net price 5-sachet pack = £4.14, 30-sachet pack = £20.83

Dose: reduction of absorption, initially 1–2 sachets repeated every 15–20 minutes until dose of charcoal given is 5–10 times that of poison ingested (if amount known) *or* (if amount not known) until max. 10 sachets have been given; each sachet suspended in approx. 100 mL water (volume of suspension may need to be reduced for children)

ACTIVE ELIMINATION TECHNIQUES

Repeated doses of **activated charcoal** by mouth *enhance the elimination* of some drugs after they have been absorbed; repeated doses are given after overdosage with:

Aspirin	Phenobarbitone
Carbamazepine	Quinine
Dapsone	Theophylline

The usual adult dose of activated charcoal is 50 g initially then 50 g every 4 hours.

Other techniques intended to enhance the elimination of poisons after absorption are only practicable in hospital and are only suitable for a small number of severely poisoned patients. Moreover, they only apply to a limited number of poisons. Examples include:

Haemodialysis for salicylates, phenobarbitone, methyl alcohol (methanol), ethylene glycol, and lithium

Haemoperfusion for medium- and short-acting barbiturates, chloral hydrate, meprobamate, and theophylline.

Forced alkaline diuresis is no longer recommended.

Specific drugs

ALCOHOL

Acute intoxication with alcohol (ethanol) is common in adults but also occurs in children. The features include ataxia, dysarthria, nystagmus, and drowsiness, which may progress to coma, with hypotension and acidosis. Aspiration of vomit is a special hazard and hypoglycaemia may occur in children and some adults. Patients are managed supportively with particular attention to maintaining a clear airway and measures to reduce the risk of aspiration of gastric contents. The blood glucose is measured and glucose given if indicated.

ANALGESICS (NON-OPIOID)

ASPIRIN. Absorption of aspirin and other salicylates may be delayed, especially if enteric-coated tablets have been taken; blood concentrations taken within the first 6 hours may therefore be misleadingly low.

The chief features of poisoning are hyperventilation, tinnitus, deafness, vasodilatation, and sweating. Coma is uncommon but indicates very severe poisoning. The associated acid-base disturbances are complex.

Gastric emptying can achieve a worthwhile recovery of salicylates up to 4 hours after ingestion. Treatment must be in hospital where plasma salicylate, pH, and electrolytes can be measured. Fluid losses are replaced and sodium bicarbonate (1.26%) given to enhance urinary salicylate excretion when the plasma-salicylate concentration is greater than

500 mg/litre (3.6 mmol/litre) in adults *or* 350 mg/litre (2.5 mmol/litre) in children.

Haemodialysis is the treatment of choice for severe poisoning and should be seriously considered when the plasma salicylate concentration is greater than 700 mg/litre (5.1 mmol/litre).

NSAIDs. Mefenamic acid is an important member of this group encountered in overdosage. Convulsions are the most important feature of toxicity and are treated with diazepam.

Ibuprofen may cause nausea, vomiting, and tinnitus, but more serious toxicity is very uncommon. Gastric emptying is indicated if more than 100 mg/kg has been ingested within the preceding 2 hours, followed by symptomatic measures.

PARACETAMOL. As little as 10–15 g (20–30 tablets) of paracetamol may cause severe hepatocellular necrosis and, less frequently, renal tubular necrosis. Nausea and vomiting, the only early features of poisoning, usually settle within 24 hours. Persistence beyond this time, often associated with the onset of right subcostal pain and tenderness, usually indicates development of hepatic necrosis. Liver damage is maximal 3–4 days after ingestion and may lead to encephalopathy, haemorrhage, hypoglycaemia, cerebral oedema, and death.

Therefore, despite a lack of significant early symptoms, patients who have taken an overdose of paracetamol should be transferred to hospital urgently.

Gastric emptying is carried out if the overdose was taken within 2 hours of admission.

Antidotes such as **acetylcysteine** and **methionine** protect the liver if given within 10–12 hours of ingestion; acetylcysteine is effective up to and possibly beyond 24 hours but expert advice is **essential**.

Patients at risk of liver damage and therefore requiring treatment can be identified from a single measurement of the plasma-paracetamol concentration, related to the time from ingestion, provided this time interval is not less than 4 hours; earlier samples may be misleading. The concentration is plotted on a paracetamol treatment graph of a reference line ('normal treatment line') joining plots of 200 mg/litre (1.32 mmol/litre) at 4 hours and 6.25 mg/litre (0.04 mmol/litre) at 24 hours (see below). Those whose plasma-paracetamol concentrations are above the *normal treatment line* are treated with acetylcysteine by intravenous infusion (or, provided the overdose has been taken within **10–12 hours**, with methionine by mouth). Patients on enzyme-inducing drugs (e.g. carbamazepine, phenobarbitone, phenytoin, rifampicin, and alcohol) or who are malnourished (e.g. in anorexia, in alcoholism, or those who are HIV-positive) may develop toxicity at **lower** plasma-paracetamol con-

Patients whose plasma-paracetamol concentrations are above the **normal treatment line** should be treated with acetylcysteine by intravenous infusion (or, provided the overdose has been taken **within 10–12 hours**, with methionine by mouth). Patients on enzyme-inducing drugs (e.g. carbamazepine, phenobarbitone, phenytoin, rifampicin, and alcohol) or who are malnourished (e.g. in anorexia, in alcoholism, or those who are HIV-positive) should be treated if their plasma-paracetamol concentrations are above the **high-risk treatment line**.

centrations and should be treated if concentrations are above the *high-risk treatment line* (which joins plots that are at 50% of the plasma-paracetamol concentrations of the normal treatment line).

In remote areas methionine (2.5 g) should be given by mouth since it is seldom practicable to give acetylcysteine outside hospital. Once the patient reaches hospital the need to continue treatment with the antidote will be assessed from the plasma-paracetamol concentration (related to the time from ingestion).

See also Co-proxamol, under Analgesics (opioid).

ACETYLCYSTEINE

Indications: paracetamol overdosage (see notes above)

Cautions: asthma

Side-effects: rashes, anaphylaxis

Dose: by intravenous infusion, in glucose intravenous infusion 5%, initially 150 mg/kg in 200 mL over 15 minutes, followed by 50 mg/kg in 500 mL over 4 hours, then 100 mg/kg in 1000 mL over 16 hours

PoM **Parvolex®** (Evans)

Injection, acetylcysteine 200 mg/mL. Net price course of 12 amps of 10 mL = £31.75

METHIONINE

Indications: paracetamol overdosage, see notes above

Dose: by mouth, 2.5 g initially, followed by 3 further doses of 2.5 g every 4 hours

Methionine (Non-proprietary)
Tablets, DL-methionine 250 mg. Net price course of 40 tabs = £11.94
Available from Norton

ANALGESICS (OPIOID)

Opioids (narcotic analgesics) cause varying degrees of coma, respiratory depression, and pinpoint pupils. The specific antidote **naloxone** is indicated if there is coma or bradypnoea. Since naloxone is short-acting repeated injections are necessary according to the respiratory rate and depth of coma. Alternatively, it may be given by continuous intravenous infusion, the rate of administration being adjusted according to response.

CO-PROXAMOL. Combinations of dextropropoxyphene and paracetamol (co-proxamol) are frequently taken in overdosage. The initial features are those of acute opioid overdosage with coma, respiratory depression, and pinpoint pupils. Patients may die of acute cardiovascular collapse before reaching hospital (particularly if alcohol has also been consumed) unless adequately resuscitated or given **naloxone** as antidote to the dextropropoxyphene. Paracetamol hepatotoxicity may develop later and should be anticipated and treated as indicated above.

NALOXONE HYDROCHLORIDE

Indications: overdosage with opioids; for postoperative respiratory depression, see section 15.1.7
Cautions: physical dependence on opioids; cardiac irritability; naloxone is short-acting, see notes above
Dose: by *intravenous injection*, 0.8–2 mg repeated at intervals of 2–3 minutes to a max. of 10 mg if respiratory function does not improve (then question diagnosis); CHILD 10 micrograms/kg; subsequent dose of 100 micrograms/kg if no response
By *subcutaneous or intramuscular injection*, as intravenous injection but only if intravenous route not feasible (onset of action slower)
By *continuous intravenous infusion*, 2 mg diluted in 500 mL intravenous infusion solution at a rate adjusted according to the response

PoM **Naloxone** (Non-proprietary)
Injection, naloxone hydrochloride 400 micrograms/mL. Net price 1-mL amp = 73p
Available from Antigen, David Bull
PoM **Min-I-Jet® Naloxone** (IMS)
Injection, naloxone hydrochloride 400 micrograms/mL. Net price 1-mL disposable syringe = £5.23; 2-mL disposable syringe = £9.74
PoM **Narcan®** (Du Pont)
Injection, naloxone hydrochloride 400 micrograms/mL, net price 1-mL amp = £4.79
Neonatal preparations —see section 15.1.7

ANTIDEPRESSANTS

Tricyclic and related antidepressants cause dry mouth, coma of varying degree, hypotension, hypothermia, hyperreflexia, extensor plantar responses, convulsions, respiratory failure, cardiac conduction defects, and arrhythmias. Dilated pupils and urinary retention also occur. Metabolic acidosis may complicate severe poisoning; delirium with confusion, agitation, and visual and auditory hallucinations, is common during recovery.

Symptomatic treatment and activated charcoal by mouth may reasonably be given in the home before transfer but hospital admission is strongly advised, and supportive measures to ensure a patent airway and adequate ventilation during transfer are mandatory. Intravenous diazepam may be required for control of convulsions (preferably in emulsion form). Although arrhythmias are worrying, some will respond to correction of hypoxia and acidosis; the use of anti-arrhythmic drugs is best avoided. Diazepam given by mouth is usually adequate to sedate delirious patients but large doses may be required.

ANTIMALARIALS

Overdosage with chloroquine and hydroxychloroquine is extremely hazardous and difficult to treat. Urgent advice from a poisons information centre is essential. Life-threatening features include arrhythmias (which can have a very rapid onset) and convulsions (which can be intractable). Quinine overdosage is also a severe hazard and calls for urgent advice from a poisons information centre.

BETA-BLOCKERS

Therapeutic overdosages with beta-blockers may cause lightheadedness, dizziness, and possibly syncope due to impaired circulation secondary to bradycardia and hypotension; heart failure may be precipitated or exacerbated. These complications are most likely in patients with pre-existing conduction system disorders or impaired myocardial function. Bradycardia is the most common arrhythmia caused by beta-blockers, but sotalol occasionally induces ventricular tachyarrhythmias (sometimes of the torsades de pointes type). The effects of massive overdosage may vary from one beta-blocker to another; propranolol overdosage in particular may cause coma and convulsions.

Acute massive overdosage must be managed in hospital and expert advice should be obtained. Maintenance of a clear airway and adequate ventilation is mandatory. An intravenous injection of atropine is required to treat bradycardia and hypotension (3 mg for an adult, 40 micrograms/kg for a child). Cardiogenic shock unresponsive to atropine is probably best treated with an intravenous injection of glucagon 50–150 micrograms/kg [unlicensed indication and dose] in glucose 5% (with precautions to protect the airway in case of vomiting). A further dose of glucagon (or an intravenous infusion) may be required if the response is not maintained. If glucagon is not available, intravenous isoprenaline or intravenous prenalterol [not on UK market] are alternatives to glucagon.

HYPNOTICS AND ANXIOLYTICS

BARBITURATES. These cause drowsiness, coma, respiratory depression, hypotension, and hypothermia. The duration and depth of cerebral depression vary greatly with the drug, the dose, and the tolerance of the patient. The severity of poisoning is often greater with a large dose of barbiturate hypnotics than with the longer-acting phenobarbitone. The majority of patients survive with supportive measures alone. Charcoal haemoperfusion is the treatment of choice for the small minority of patients with very severe barbiturate poisoning who fail to improve, or who deteriorate despite good supportive care.

BENZODIAZEPINES. Benzodiazepines taken alone cause drowsiness, ataxia, dysarthria, and occasionally minor and short-lived depression of consciousness. They potentiate the effects of other central nervous system depressants taken concomitantly. Flumazenil, a benzodiazepine antagonist, may be used in the *differential diagnosis* of unclear cases of multiple drug overdose but expert advice is **essential** since adverse effects may occur (e.g. convulsions in patients dependent on benzodiazepines).

IRON SALTS

Iron poisoning is commonest in childhood and is usually accidental. The symptoms are nausea, vomiting, abdominal pain, diarrhoea, haematemesis, and rectal bleeding. Hypotension, coma, and hepatocellular necrosis occur later. Mortality is reduced with intensive and specific therapy with **desferrioxamine**, which chelates iron. The stomach should be emptied at once by gastric lavage. The serum-iron concentration is measured as an emergency and intravenous desferrioxamine given to chelate absorbed iron in excess of the expected iron binding capacity. In **severe toxicity** intravenous desferrioxamine should be given *immediately* without waiting for the result of the serum-iron measurement (contact a poisons information centre for advice).

DESFERRIOXAMINE MESYLATE

Indications: removal of iron from the body in poisoning; for use in chronic iron overload, see section 9.1.3

Cautions: avoid prochlorperazine

Side-effects: anaphylactic reactions, and hypotension when given too rapidly by intravenous injection

Dose: *By continuous intravenous infusion*, up to 15 mg/kg/hour; max. 80 mg/kg in 24 hours

PoM **Desferal®** (Ciba)
Injection, powder for reconstitution, desferrioxamine mesylate. Net price 500-mg vial = £3.70

LITHIUM

Most cases of lithium intoxication occur as a complication of long-term therapy and are caused by reduced excretion of the drug due to a variety of factors including dehydration, deterioration of renal function, infections, and co-administration of diuretics or NSAIDs (or other drugs that interact). Acute deliberate overdoses may also occur with delayed onset of symptoms (12 hours or more) due to slow entry of lithium into the tissues and continuing absorption from modified-release formulations.

The early clinical features are non-specific and may include apathy and restlessness which could be confused with mental changes due to the patient's depressive illness. Vomiting, diarrhoea, ataxia, weakness, dysarthria, muscle twitching, and tremor may follow. Severe poisoning is associated with convulsions, coma, renal failure, electrolyte imbalance, dehydration, and hypotension.

Therapeutic lithium concentrations are within the range of 0.4–1.0 mmol/litre; concentrations in excess of 2.0 mmol/litre are usually associated with serious toxicity and such cases may need treatment with haemodialysis (if there is renal failure). In acute overdosage much higher serum concentrations may be present without features of toxicity and measures to increase urine production are usually all that are necessary. Otherwise treatment is supportive with special regard to electrolyte balance, renal function, and control of convulsions.

PHENOTHIAZINES AND RELATED DRUGS

Phenothiazines cause less depression of consciousness and respiration than other sedatives. Hypotension, hypothermia, sinus tachycardia, and arrhythmias (particularly with thioridazine) may complicate poisoning. Dystonic reactions can occur with therapeutic doses, (particularly with prochlorperazine and trifluoperazine) and convulsions may occur in severe cases. Arrhythmias may respond to correction of hypoxia and acidosis but drugs may also be needed. Dystonic reactions are rapidly abolished by injection of drugs such as benztropine or procyclidine (see section 4.9.2).

STIMULANTS

AMPHETAMINES. These cause wakefulness, excessive activity, paranoia, hallucinations, and hypertension followed by exhaustion, convulsions, hyperthermia, and coma. The early stages can be controlled by chlorpromazine and, if necessary, beta-blockers. Later, tepid sponging, anticonvulsants, and artificial respiration may be needed. Amphetamine excretion can be increased by forced acid diuresis but this is seldom necessary.

COCAINE. Cocaine can be smoked, sniffed, or injected. It stimulates the central nervous system causing agitation, dilated pupils, tachycardia, hypertension, hallucinations, hypertonia, and hyperreflexia. Convulsions, coma and metabolic acidosis may develop in the worst cases. Sedation, with intravenous diazepam, may be all that is necessary (and will also control convulsions); intravenous propranolol may be indicated for severe arrhythmias (labetalol may be preferred if there is associated hypertension).

THEOPHYLLINE

Theophylline and related drugs are often prescribed as modified-release formulations and toxicity may therefore be delayed. They cause vomiting (which may be severe and intractable), agitation, restlessness, dilated pupils, and sinus tachycardia. More serious effects are haematemesis, convulsions, and supraventricular and ventricular arrhythmias. **Profound hypokalaemia** may develop rapidly.

The stomach should be emptied if the patient presents within 2 hours. Elimination of theophylline may be enhanced by repeated doses of activated charcoal by mouth (see also under Active Elimination Techniques). Hypokalaemia is corrected by intravenous infusion of potassium chloride and may be so severe as to require 60 mmol/hour (high doses under ECG monitoring). Convulsions should be controlled by intravenous administration of diazepam (emulsion preferred). Sedation with diazepam may be necessary in agitated patients.

Providing the patient is **not** an asthmatic, extreme tachycardia, hypokalaemia, and hyperglycaemia may be reversed by intravenous administration of propranolol (see section 2.4).

Other poisons

> Consult poisons information services day and
> night—p. 18.

CYANIDES

Cyanide antidotes include dicobalt edetate, given alone, and sodium nitrite, followed by sodium thiosulphate. These antidotes are held for emergency use in hospitals as well as in centres where cyanide poisoning is a risk such as factories and laboratories.

DICOBALT EDETATE

Indications: acute poisoning with cyanides

Cautions: owing to toxicity to be used only when patient tending to lose, or has lost, consciousness; not to be used as a precautionary measure

Side-effects: hypotension, tachycardia, and vomiting

Dose: by intravenous injection, 300 mg (20 mL) over 1 minute (5 minutes if condition less serious) followed immediately by 50 mL of glucose intravenous infusion 50%; if response inadequate a second dose of both may be given; if no response after further 5 minutes a third dose of both may be given

PoM **Kelocyanor®** (Cambridge)

Injection, dicobalt edetate 15 mg/mL. Net price 20-mL (300-mg) amp = £6.88

SODIUM NITRITE

Indications: poisoning with cyanides (used in conjunction with sodium thiosulphate)

Side-effects: flushing and headache due to vasodilatation

PoM **Sodium Nitrite Injection**

Injection, sodium nitrite 3% (30 mg/mL) in water for injections

Dose: 10 mL by intravenous injection over 3 minutes, followed by 25 mL of sodium thiosulphate injection 50%, by intravenous injection over 10 minutes

'Special-order' [unlicensed] product: contact Martindale or regional hospital manufacturing unit

SODIUM THIOSULPHATE

Indications: poisoning with cyanides (used in conjunction with sodium nitrite)

PoM **Sodium Thiosulphate Injection**

Injection, sodium thiosulphate 50% (500 mg/mL) in water for injections

Dose: see above under Sodium Nitrite Injection

'Special-order' [unlicensed] product: contact Martindale or regional hospital manufacturing unit

HEAVY METALS

Heavy metal antidotes include dimercaprol, penicillamine, and sodium calciumedetate.

DIMERCAPROL
(BAL)

Indications: poisoning by antimony, arsenic, bismuth, gold, mercury, possibly thallium; adjunct (with sodium calciumedetate) in lead poisoning

Cautions: hypertension, renal impairment (discontinue or use with extreme caution if impairment develops during treatment), elderly, pregnancy and breast-feeding

Contra-indications: not indicated for iron, cadmium, or selenium poisoning; severe hepatic impairment (unless due to arsenic poisoning)

Side-effects: hypertension, tachycardia, malaise, nausea, vomiting, salivation, lachrymation, sweating, burning sensation (mouth, throat, and eyes), feeling of constriction of throat and chest, headache, muscle spasm, abdominal pain, tingling of extremities; pyrexia in children; local pain and abscess at injection site

Dose: by intramuscular injection, 2.5–3 mg/kg every 4 hours for 2 days, 2–4 times on the third day, then 1–2 times daily for 10 days or until recovery

PoM **Dimercaprol** (Knoll)

Injection, dimercaprol 50 mg/mL. Net price 2-mL amp = £15.00

Note. Contains arachis oil as solvent

PENICILLAMINE

Indications: poisoning by certain toxic metal ions, particularly by copper and lead

Cautions; Contra-indications; Side-effects: see section 10.1.3

Dose: 1–2 g daily in divided doses before food until urinary lead is stabilised at less than 500 micrograms/day; CHILD 20 mg/kg daily

Preparations
See section 10.1.3

SODIUM CALCIUMEDETATE

Indications: poisoning by heavy metals, especially lead

Cautions: renal impairment

Side-effects: nausea, cramp; in overdosage renal damage

Dose: *by intravenous infusion*, adults and children, up to 40 mg/kg twice daily in sodium chloride intravenous infusion 0.9% or glucose intravenous infusion 5% for up to 5 days, repeated if necessary after 48 hours

PoM **Ledclair®** (Sinclair)

Injection, sodium calciumedetate 200 mg/mL. Net price 5-mL amp = £4.38

NOXIOUS GASES

CARBON MONOXIDE. Carbon monoxide poisoning is now usually due to inhalation of smoke, car exhaust, or fumes caused by blocked flues or incomplete combustion of fuel gases in confined spaces. Its toxic effects are entirely due to hypoxia.

Immediate treatment is essential. The person should be removed into the fresh air, the airway cleared, and **oxygen** 100% administered as soon as available. Artificial respiration should be given as necessary and continued until adequate spontaneous breathing starts, or stopped only after persistent and efficient treatment of cardiac arrest has failed. Admission to hospital is desirable because complications may arise after a delay of hours or days. Cerebral oedema should be anticipated in severe poisoning and is treated with an intravenous infusion of mannitol (see section 2.2.5). Referral for hyperbaric oxygen treatment should be discussed with the poisons information services if the victim is or has been unconscious, or has a blood carboxyhaemoglobin concentration of more than 20%, or is pregnant.

SULPHUR DIOXIDE, CHLORINE, PHOSGENE, AMMONIA. The immediate effect of all except phosgene is coughing and choking. Pulmonary oedema, with severe breathlessness and cyanosis may develop suddenly up to 36 hours after exposure. Death may occur. Patients are kept under observation and those who develop pulmonary oedema are given corticosteroids and oxygen. Assisted ventilation may be necessary in the most serious cases.

PESTICIDES

PARAQUAT. Concentrated liquid paraquat preparations (e.g. Gramoxone®), available to farmers and horticulturists, contain 10–20% paraquat and are extremely toxic. Granular preparations, for garden use, contain only 2.5% paraquat and have caused few deaths.

Paraquat has local and systemic effects. Splashes in the eyes irritate and ulcerate the cornea and conjunctiva. Copious washing of the eye and instillation of antibacterial eye-drops, should aid healing but it may be a long process. Skin irritation, blistering, and ulceration can occur from prolonged contact both with the concentrated and dilute forms. Inhalation of spray, mist, or dust containing paraquat may cause nose bleeding and sore throat but not systemic toxicity.

Ingestion of concentrated paraquat solutions is followed by nausea, vomiting, and diarrhoea. Painful ulceration of the tongue, lips, and fauces may appear after 36 to 48 hours together with renal failure. Some days later there may be dyspnoea with pulmonary fibrosis due to proliferative alveolitis and bronchiolitis.

Treatment should be started immediately. The single most useful measure is oral administration of repeat-dose **activated charcoal**; the first dose of 100 g is given with a laxative, followed by 50 g every 4 hours until the charcoal is seen in the stool. Gastric lavage is of doubtful value. **Fuller's earth** and **bentonite** given by mouth have also been used as adsorbents. A suspension of Fuller's earth 30% was used in three doses of 200–500 mL given at two-hour intervals; magnesium sulphate or mannitol were given with Fuller's earth to promote diarrhoea and empty the gut. Intravenous fluids and analgesics are given as necessary. Oxygen therapy should be avoided if possible since this may exacerbate damage to the lungs. Measures to enhance elimination of absorbed paraquat are probably valueless but should be discussed with the poisons information services who will also give guidance on predicting the likely outcome from plasma concentrations. Paraquat absorption can be confirmed by a simple qualitative urine test.

ORGANOPHOSPHORUS INSECTICIDES. Organophosphorus insecticides are usually supplied as powders or dissolved in organic solvents. All are absorbed through the bronchi and intact skin as well as through the gut and inhibit cholinesterase activity thereby prolonging and intensifying the effects of acetylcholine. Toxicity between different compounds varies considerably, and onset may be delayed after skin exposure.

Anxiety, restlessness, dizziness, headache, miosis, nausea, hypersalivation, vomiting, abdominal colic, diarrhoea, bradycardia, and sweating are common. Muscle weakness and fasciculation may develop and progress to generalised flaccid paralysis including the ocular and respiratory muscles. Convulsions, coma, pulmonary oedema with copious bronchial secretions, hypoxia, and arrhythmias occur in severe cases. Hyperglycaemia and glycosuria without ketonuria may also be present.

Further absorption should be prevented by emptying the stomach, removing the patient to fresh air, or removing soiled clothing and washing contaminated skin. In severe poisoning it is vital to ensure a clear airway, frequent removal of bronchial secretions, and adequate ventilation and oxygenation. **Atropine** will reverse the muscarinic effects of acetylcholine and is given in a dose of 2 mg as atropine sulphate injection (intramuscularly or intravenously according to the severity of poisoning) every

20 to 30 minutes until the skin becomes flushed and dry, the pupils dilate, and tachycardia develops.

Pralidoxime mesylate (P2S), a cholinesterase reactivator, is indicated, as an adjunct to atropine, in moderate or severe poisoning but is only effective if given within 24 hours. It may be obtained from designated centres, the names of which are held by the poisons information centres (see p. 18). A dose of 30 mg/kg (diluted with 10–15 mL water for injections) by slow intravenous injection should produce improvement in muscle power within 30 minutes but repeated doses or, in severe cases, an intravenous infusion of up to 500 mg/hour may be required.

PRALIDOXIME MESYLATE

Indications: adjunct to atropine in the treatment of organophosphorus poisoning

Cautions: renal impairment, myasthenia gravis

Contra-indications: poisoning due to carbamates and to organophosphorus compounds without anticholinesterase activity

Side-effects: drowsiness, dizziness, disturbances of vision, nausea, tachycardia, headache, hyperventilation, and muscular weakness

Dose: by slow intravenous injection (diluted to 10–15 mL with water for injections and given over 5–10 minutes), 30 mg/kg initially followed by 1–2 further doses if necessary; usual max. 12 g in 24 hours

CHILD 20–60 mg/kg as required depending on severity of poisoning and response

Note. Pralidoxime mesylate doses in BNF may differ from those in data sheet

PoM Pralidoxime Mesylate

Injection, pralidoxime mesylate 200 mg/mL

Available as 5-mL amps (from designated centres)

SNAKE BITES AND INSECT STINGS

SNAKE BITE. Acute envenoming from snake bite is rare in the UK and the only indigenous venomous snake is the adder (*Vipera berus*). The bite may cause local and systemic effects. Local effects include pain, swelling, bruising, and tender enlargement of regional lymph nodes. Systemic effects include early transient hypotension with syncope, angioedema, abdominal colic, diarrhoea, and vomiting, with later persistent or recurrent hypotension, ECG abnormalities, spontaneous systemic bleed-

ing, coagulopathy, adult respiratory distress syndrome, and acute renal failure. There is a small risk of fatal envenoming especially in children and the elderly.

Indications for antivenom treatment include systemic envenoming, especially hypotension (see above), vomiting, haemostatic abnormalities, polymorphonuclear leucocytosis and local envenoming if, after bites on the hand or foot, swelling extends beyond the wrist or ankle within 4 hours of the bite. The contents of one vial (10 mL) of **European viper venom antiserum** (available from Farillon) is given *by intravenous injection* over 10–15 minutes or *by intravenous infusion* over 30 minutes after diluting in sodium chloride intravenous infusion 0.9% (use 5 mL diluent/kg body-weight). The **same dose** should be used for **adults** and **children**. The dose can be repeated in 1–2 hours if symptoms of **systemic envenoming** persist. Adrenaline injection must be immediately to hand for treatment of anaphylactic antivenom reactions (for full details see section 3.4.3).

Antivenom is available for certain foreign snakes, spiders and scorpions. For information on identification, management, and supply, telephone:

Oxford	(01865) 220968
or	(01865) 221332
or	(01865) 741166
Liverpool	0151-708 9393
Liverpool (Fazakerley Hospital Pharmacy)	
(supply only)	0151-525 5980
London	0171-635 9191

INSECT STINGS. Stings from ants, wasps, hornets, and bees, cause local pain and swelling but seldom cause severe direct toxicity unless many stings are inflicted at the same time. If the sting is in the mouth or on the tongue marked swelling may cause respiratory distress. The stings from these insects are usually treated by cleaning the area, applying a cooling lotion (such as a calamine preparation), and giving an antihistamine by mouth. Bee stings should be removed by scraping them off with a finger nail or knife before cleaning the area. Anaphylactic reactions require treatment with intramuscular **adrenaline**. Inhalation of adrenaline (Medihaler-epi®, see section 3.4.3) may be sufficient only for mild bronchospasm, and self-administered intramuscular adrenaline (e.g. EpiPen®) is the best first-aid treatment for patients with severe hypersensitivity. For full details of the management of anaphylaxis, see section 3.4.3.

Classified Notes on Drugs and Preparations

Doping Classes and Methods of the International Olympic Committee Medical Commission 1996

The following are examples of classes and methods prohibited in sport

Classes	**Stimulants** eg. amphetamine, caffeine (above 12mg/L), cocaine, ephedrine. **Narcotics** eg. dextropropoxyphene, diamorphine (heroin), morphine, methadone, pethidine. **Anabolic Agents** eg. methandienone, nandrolone, stanozolol, testosterone, clenbuterol. **Diuretics** eg. acetazolamide, frusemide, hydrochlorothiazide, triamterene. **Peptide & Glycoprotein Hormones & Analogues** eg. growth hormone, corticotrophin, chorionic gonadotrophin, erythropoietin.
Methods	**Blood Doping** **Pharmacological, Chemical & Physical Manipulation** eg. substances or methods which alter the integrity and validity of the urine.
Classes subject to certain restrictions	A) **Alcohol** ⎫ restricted in certain sports, refer to regulations B) **Marijuana** ⎭ of international sports federations. C) **Local Anaesthetics** route of administration restricted to local or intra-articular injection*. D) **Corticosteroids** route of administration restricted to topical, inhalation*, local or intra-articular injection*. E) **Beta Blockers** restricted in certain sports, refer to regulations of international sports federations.

*written notification of administration should be given to relevant medical authority eg. governing body medical officer.

Treatment Guidelines
Examples of permitted and prohibited substances
(based upon the International Olympic Committee Doping Classes 1996)

	ALLOWED	BANNED
ASTHMA	salbutamol inhaler*, terbutaline inhaler*, salmeterol inhaler*.	products containing sympathomimetics (eg. ephedrine, fenoterol, isoprenaline).
COUGH	all antibiotics, steam and menthol inhalations, cough mixtures containing antihistamines, pholcodine, guaiphenesin, dextromethorphan.	products containing sympathomimetics (eg. ephedrine, phenylpropanolamine).
DIARRHOEA	diphenoxylate, loperamide, products containing electrolytes (eg. Dioralyte, Rehidrat).	products containing opioids (eg. morphine).
HAYFEVER	antihistamines, nasal sprays containing a corticosteroid* or xylometazoline, eye drops containing sodium cromoglycate.	products containing ephedrine, pseudoephedrine.
PAIN	aspirin, codeine, dihydrocodeine, ibuprofen, paracetamol, all non-steroidal anti-inflammatories.	products containing opioids (eg. dextropropoxyphene) or caffeine.
VOMITING	domperidone, metoclopramide.	

WARNING. The substances listed are only examples of substances currently permitted or prohibited by the IOC. Not all sports adopt the IOC Medical Code. If in doubt check with your governing body or with the Sports Council's Doping Control Unit—Drug Information Hotline 0171-383 2244

Supplies of this card are available from:
   Doping Control Unit, Sports Council, Walkden House, 3–10 Melton Street, London NW1 2EB
A similar card detailing classes of drugs and doping methods prohibited by the Football Association (1996–97 season) is also available

1: Drugs acting on the
GASTRO-INTESTINAL SYSTEM

The drugs and preparations in this chapter are described under the following sections:

1.1 Antacids
1.2 Antispasmodics and other drugs altering gut motility
1.3 Ulcer-healing drugs
1.4 Antidiarrhoeal drugs
1.5 Treatment of chronic diarrhoeas
1.6 Laxatives
1.7 Preparations for haemorrhoids
1.8 Stoma care
1.9 Drugs affecting intestinal secretions

1.1 Antacids

1.1.1 Aluminium- and magnesium-containing
1.1.2 Sodium bicarbonate
1.1.3 Calcium- and bismuth-containing

Antacids are still useful for treating gastro-intestinal disease; they can often relieve symptoms in both *ulcer* and *non-ulcer dyspepsia*, and in *reflux oesophagitis*. They are best given when symptoms occur or are expected, usually between meals and at bedtime, four or more times daily; additional doses may be required up to once an hour. Conventional doses e.g. 10 mL three or four times daily of liquid magnesium–aluminium antacids promote ulcer healing, but less well than antisecretory agents (section 1.3); proof of a relationship between healing and neutralising capacity is lacking. Liquid preparations are more effective than solids.

INTERACTIONS. Antacids should preferably not be taken at the same time as other drugs as they may impair their absorption. Antacids may also damage enteric coatings designed to prevent dissolution in the stomach. See also **Appendix 1** (antacids and adsorbents).

1.1.1 Aluminium- and magnesium-containing antacids

Aluminium- and **magnesium-containing** antacids, such as magnesium carbonate, hydroxide and trisilicate, and aluminium glycinate and hydroxide, being relatively insoluble in water, are long-acting if retained in the stomach. They are suitable for most antacid purposes. Magnesium-containing antacids tend to be laxative whereas aluminium-containing antacids may be constipating. Aluminium accumulation does not appear to be a risk if renal function is normal (see also Appendix 3).

Compound preparations have no clear advantages over simpler preparations: neutralising capacity may be the same.

Complexes such as **hydrotalcite** confer no special advantage.

Low Na⁺
The words low Na⁺ added after some preparations indicate a sodium content of less than 1 mmol per tablet or 10-mL dose.

ALUMINIUM HYDROXIDE
Indications: dyspepsia; for use in hyperphosphataemia, see section 9.5.2.2
Cautions: see notes above; **interactions:** Appendix 1 (antacids and adsorbents)
Contra-indications: hypophosphataemia

Aluminium-only preparations
Aluminium Hydroxide (Non-proprietary)
Tablets, dried aluminium hydroxide 500 mg. Net price 20 = 28p
Dose: 1–2 tablets chewed 4 times daily and at bedtime or as required
Mixture (gel), about 4% w/w Al_2O_3 in water, with a peppermint flavour. Net price 200 mL = 41p
Dose: antacid, 5–10 mL 4 times daily between meals and at bedtime or as required; CHILD 6–12 years, up to 5 mL 3 times daily
Note. The brand name NHS Aludrox® (Pfizer Consumer) is used for aluminium hydroxide mixture; net price 200 mL = £1.17. NHS Aludrox® tablets also contain magnesium.
Alu-Cap® (3M)
Capsules, green/red, dried aluminium hydroxide 475 mg (low Na⁺). Net price 120-cap pack = £4.22
Dose: antacid, 1 capsule 4 times daily and at bedtime; CHILD not recommended for antacid therapy

Co-magaldrox
Co-magaldrox is a mixture of aluminium hydroxide and magnesium hydroxide; the proportions are expressed in the form *x/y* where *x* and *y* are the strengths in milligrams per unit dose of magnesium hydroxide and aluminium hydroxide respectively
Maalox® (Rhône-Poulenc Rorer)
Suspension, sugar-free, co-magaldrox 195/220 (magnesium hydroxide 195 mg, dried aluminium hydroxide 220 mg/5 mL (low Na⁺)). Net price 500 mL = £1.97
Dose: 10–20 mL 20 minutes–1 hour after meals and at bedtime or when required; CHILD under 14 years not recommended
Maalox TC® (Rhône-Poulenc Rorer)
Tablets, co-magaldrox 300/600 (magnesium hydroxide 300 mg, dried aluminium hydroxide 600 mg (low Na⁺)). Net price 100 = £3.86
Suspension, sugar-free, co-magaldrox 300/600 (magnesium hydroxide 300 mg, dried aluminium hydroxide 600 mg/5 mL (low Na⁺)). Net price 500 mL = £3.86
Dose: antacid, 1–2 tablets chewed or 5–10 mL suspension 4 times daily 20 minutes–1 hour after meals and at bedtime; duodenal ulcer, 3 tablets or 15 mL suspension 4 times daily (treatment) *or* twice daily (prevention of recurrence)

Mucogel® (Pharmax)

Suspension, sugar-free, co-magaldrox 195/220 (magnesium hydroxide 195 mg, dried aluminium hydroxide 220 mg/5 mL (low Na⁺)). Net price 500 mL = £1.91

Dose: 10–20 mL 3 times daily, 20 minutes–1 hour after meals, and at bedtime or when required; CHILD under 12 years not recommended

> For **preparations** containing aluminium and magnesium on sale to the public and not prescribable on the NHS, see p. 31

MAGNESIUM CARBONATE

Indications: dyspepsia

Cautions: renal impairment; see also notes above; **interactions:** Appendix 1 (antacids and adsorbents)

Contra-indications: hypophosphataemia

Side-effects: diarrhoea; belching due to liberated carbon dioxide

Aromatic Magnesium Carbonate Mixture, BP

(Aromatic Magnesium Carbonate Oral Suspension)

Oral suspension, light magnesium carbonate 3%, sodium bicarbonate 5%, in a suitable vehicle containing aromatic cardamom tincture. Extemporaneous preparations should be recently prepared according to the following formula: light magnesium carbonate 300 mg, sodium bicarbonate 500 mg, aromatic cardamom tincture 0.3 mL, double-strength chloroform water 5 mL, water to 10 mL. Contains about 6 mmol Na⁺/10 mL. Net price 200 mL = 59p

Dose: 10 mL 3 times daily in water

Preparations on sale to the public
For **preparations** also containing aluminium, see above.

MAGNESIUM TRISILICATE

Indications: dyspepsia

Cautions; Contra-indications: see under Magnesium Carbonate

Side-effects: diarrhoea

Magnesium Trisilicate Tablets, Compound, BP

Tablets, magnesium trisilicate 250 mg, dried aluminium hydroxide 120 mg

Dose: 1–2 tablets chewed when required

Magnesium Trisilicate Mixture, BP

(Magnesium Trisilicate Oral Suspension)

Oral suspension, 5% each of magnesium trisilicate, light magnesium carbonate, and sodium bicarbonate in a suitable vehicle with a peppermint flavour. Extemporaneous preparations should be recently prepared according to the following formula: magnesium trisilicate 500 mg, light magnesium carbonate 500 mg, sodium bicarbonate 500 mg, concentrated peppermint emulsion 0.25 mL, double-strength chloroform water 5 mL, water to 10 mL. Contains about 6 mmol Na⁺/10 mL

Dose: 10 mL 3 times daily in water

Magnesium Trisilicate Oral Powder, Compound, BP

Oral powder, magnesium trisilicate 250 mg, chalk 250 mg, heavy magnesium carbonate 250 mg, sodium bicarbonate 250 mg/g. Contains about 3 mmol Na⁺/g. Label: 13

Dose: 1–5 g in liquid when required

Preparations on sale to the public
For **preparations** also containing aluminium, see above .

ALUMINIUM-MAGNESIUM COMPLEXES

HYDROTALCITE

Aluminium magnesium carbonate hydroxide hydrate

Indications: dyspepsia

Cautions: see notes above; **interactions:** Appendix 1 (antacids and adsorbents)

Hydrotalcite (Roussel)

Tablets, hydrotalcite 500 mg (low Na⁺). Net price 56-tab pack = 81p

Dose: 2 tablets chewed between meals and at bedtime; CHILD under 6 years not recommended, 6–12 years 1 tablet

Suspension, hydrotalcite 500 mg/5 mL (low Na⁺). Net price 500-mL pack = £1.96

Dose: 10 mL between meals and at bedtime; CHILD under 6 years not recommended, 6–12 years 5 mL

Note. The brand name NHS Altacite® was formerly used for hydrotalcite suspension and tablets; for Altacite Plus® preparations, see pp. 30 and 31.

OTHER COMPOUND PREPARATIONS FOR DYSPEPSIA AND REFLUX OESOPHAGITIS

Activated dimethicone (simethicone), given alone or added to an antacid as an antifoaming agent to relieve flatulence, is of uncertain value. Alginates added as protectants against *reflux oesophagitis* may be useful, but surface anaesthetics (e.g. oxethazine) added to improve symptom relief are of doubtful efficacy. The amount of additional ingredient or antacid in individual preparations varies widely, as does their sodium content, so that preparations may not be freely interchangeable.

Preparations containing activated dimethicone with an antacid may be useful for the relief of *hiccup in palliative care.*

See also section 1.3 for drugs used in the treatment of peptic ulcer.

Algicon® (Rhône-Poulenc Rorer)

Tablets, aluminium hydroxide-magnesium carbonate co-gel 360 mg, magnesium alginate 500 mg, heavy magnesium carbonate 320 mg, potassium bicarbonate 100 mg, sucrose 1.5 g (low Na⁺). Net price 60-tab pack = £2.40

Caution: diabetes mellitus (high sugar content)

Dose: 1–2 tablets 4 times daily (chewed after meals and at bedtime); CHILD under 12 years not recommended

Suspension, yellow, aluminium hydroxide-magnesium carbonate co-gel 140 mg, magnesium alginate 250 mg, magnesium carbonate 175 mg, potassium bicarbonate 50 mg/5 mL (low Na⁺). Net price 500 mL (lemon and mint-flavoured) = £2.79

Dose: 10–20 mL 4 times daily (after meals and at bedtime); CHILD under 12 years not recommended

Altacite Plus® (Roussel)
Suspension, sugar-free, co-simalcite 125/500 (activated dimethicone 125 mg, hydrotalcite 500 mg)/5 mL (low Na⁺). Net price 500 mL = £1.85

Dose: 10 mL between meals and at bedtime when required; CHILD 8–12 years 5 mL

NHS *Tablets*, see p. 31

Asilone® (Seton)
Suspension, sugar-free, dried aluminium hydroxide 420 mg, activated dimethicone 135 mg, light magnesium oxide 70 mg/5 mL (low Na⁺). Net price 500 mL = £1.95

Dose: 5–10 mL after meals and at bedtime or when required up to 4 times daily; CHILD under 12 years not recommended

NHS *Tablets*, see p. 31
NHS *Liquid*, see p. 31

Diovol® (Pharmax)
Suspension, sugar-free, aluminium hydroxide 200 mg, dimethicone 25 mg, magnesium hydroxide 200 mg/5 mL (low Na⁺). Net price 300 mL = £1.13

Dose: 5–10 mL 3 times daily between meals and at bedtime or when required

Gastrocote® (Seton)
Tablets, alginic acid 200 mg, dried aluminium hydroxide 80 mg, magnesium trisilicate 40 mg, sodium bicarbonate 70 mg. Contains about 1 mmol Na⁺/tablet. Net price 100-tab pack = £3.67

Dose: 1–2 tablets chewed 4 times daily (after meals and at bedtime); CHILD under 6 years not recommended

Caution: diabetes mellitus (high sugar content)

Liquid, sugar-free, peach-coloured, dried aluminium hydroxide 80 mg, magnesium trisilicate 40 mg, sodium alginate 220 mg, sodium bicarbonate 70 mg/5 mL. Contains 1.8 mmol Na⁺/5 mL. Net price 500 mL = £2.79

Dose: 5–15 mL 4 times daily (after meals and at bedtime)

Gaviscon® (R&C)
Tablets, sugar-free, alginic acid 500 mg, dried aluminium hydroxide 100 mg, magnesium trisilicate 25 mg, sodium bicarbonate 170 mg. Contains 2 mmol Na⁺/tablet. Net price 60-tab pack (peppermint or lemon flavour) = £2.25

Dose: 1–2 tablets chewed after meals and at bedtime, followed by water; CHILD 2–6 years 1 tablet (on doctor's advice only) and 6–12 years 1 tablet

Liquid, sugar-free, sodium alginate 250 mg, sodium bicarbonate 133.5 mg, calcium carbonate 80 mg/5 mL. Contains about 3 mmol Na⁺/5 mL. Net price 500 mL (aniseed- or peppermint-flavour) = £2.70

Dose: 10–20 mL after meals and at bedtime; CHILD 2–6 years (on doctor's advice only) and 6–12 years 5–10 mL

NHS *Gaviscon 250® and Gaviscon 500® Tablets*, see p. 31

Infant Gaviscon® (R&C)
Oral powder, sugar-free, sodium alginate 225 mg, magnesium alginate 87.5 mg, dried aluminium hydroxide 112.5 mg with colloidal silica and mannitol/dose (half dual-sachet). Contains 0.92 mmol Na⁺/dose. Net price 15 dual-sachets (30 doses) = £2.46

Dose: INFANT under 4.5 kg 1 dose (half dual-sachet) mixed with feeds (or water in breast-fed infants) when required; over 4.5 kg 2 doses (1 dual-sachet); CHILD 2 doses (1 dual-sachet) in water after each meal

Note. Not to be used in premature infants, or where excessive water loss likely (e.g. fever, diarrhoea, vomiting, high room temperature), or if intestinal obstruction

IMPORTANT. Each half of the dual-sachet is identified as 'one dose'. To avoid errors prescribe as 'dual-sachet' with directions in terms of 'dose'

Maalox Plus® (Rhône-Poulenc Rorer)
Suspension, sugar-free, dried aluminium hydroxide 220 mg, activated dimethicone 25 mg, magnesium hydroxide 195 mg/5 mL (low Na⁺). Net price 500 mL = £1.97

Dose: 5–10 mL 4 times daily (after meals and at bedtime or when required); CHILD under 5 years 5 mL 3 times daily, over 5 years appropriate proportion of adult dose

NHS *Tablets*, see p. 31

PoM **Mucaine®** (Wyeth)
Suspension, sugar-free, aluminium hydroxide mixture 4.75 mL, magnesium hydroxide 100 mg, oxethazaine 10 mg/5 mL. Net price 200-mL pack = 76p

Dose: 5–10 mL (without fluid) 3–4 times daily (15 minutes before meals and at bedtime or when required); CHILD not recommended

Note. Products containing oxethazaine can be sold to the public provided packs do not contain more than 400 mg (max. single dose 10 mg, max. daily dose 30 mg)

Topal® (Novex)
Tablets, alginic acid 200 mg, dried aluminium hydroxide 30 mg, light magnesium carbonate 40 mg with lactose 220 mg, sucrose 880 mg, sodium bicarbonate 40 mg (low Na⁺). Net price 42-tab pack = £1.67

Dose: 1–3 tablets chewed 4 times daily (after meals and at bedtime); CHILD half adult dose

> For **preparations** containing aluminium and magnesium on sale to the public and not prescribable on the NHS, see p. 31

DIMETHICONE ALONE

Infacol® (Pharmax)
Liquid, sugar-free, activated dimethicone 40 mg/mL (low Na⁺). Net price 50 mL = £1.67. Counselling, use of dropper

Dose: gripes, colic or wind pains, INFANT 0.5–1 mL before feeds

1.1.2   Sodium bicarbonate

Sodium bicarbonate, being soluble in water, is rapid-acting, but absorbed bicarbonate can cause alkalosis in excessive doses. Like other carbonate-containing antacids it liberates carbon dioxide which causes belching. Sodium bicarbonate and antacid preparations with a high sodium content, such as magnesium trisilicate mixture, should be avoided in patients on salt-restricted diets (in heart failure and in hepatic and renal impairment).

SODIUM BICARBONATE

Indications: rapid relief of dyspepsia; urinary tract, section 7.4.3; acidosis, sections 9.2.1.3 and 9.2.2

Cautions: hepatic and renal impairment, cardiac disease, pregnancy; patients on sodium-restricted diet; elderly; avoid prolonged use; **interactions:** Appendix 1 (antacids and adsorbents)

Side-effects: belching, alkalosis on prolonged use

Dose: see under preparations, below

Sodium Bicarbonate, BP, contains about 12 mmol Na⁺/g.
Label: 13
Dose: 1–5 g in water when required

Sodium Bicarbonate Tablets, Compound, BP,
(Soda Mint Tablets), sodium bicarbonate 300 mg. Contains about 4 mmol Na⁺/tab
Dose: 2–6 tablets sucked when required

Indigestion **preparations** on sale to the public (not prescribable on the NHS) include:

Actal® (alexitol = aluminium), **Actonorm Gel**® (aluminium, magnesium, dimethicone, peppermint oil), **Actonorm Powder**® (see section 1.2), **Altacite**® (hydrotalcite = aluminium, magnesium), **Altacite Plus Tablets**® (co-simalcite = aluminium, magnesium, dimethicone; suspension is prescribable), **Aludrox Liquid**® (aluminium), **Aludrox Tablets**® (aluminium, magnesium), **Aluhyde**® (see section 1.2), **Andrews Antacid**® (calcium, magnesium), **APP**® (see section 1.2), **Asilone Liquid**® (aluminium, dimethicone, magnesium; suspension is prescribable), **Asilone Tablets**® (aluminium, dimethicone)

Barum Antacid® (calcium), **Bellocarb**® (see section 1.2), **Birley**® (aluminium, magnesium), **Bismag**® (magnesium, sodium bicarbonate), **Bisma-Rex**® (bismuth, calcium, magnesium, peppermint oil), **Bisodol Extra Tablets**® (calcium, magnesium, sodium bicarbonate, dimethicone), **Bisodol Heartburn Tablets**® (alginic acid, magaldrate, sodium bicarbonate), **Bisodol Powder**® (magnesium, sodium bicarbonate), **Bisodol Tablets**® and **Bisodol Extra Strong Mint Tablets**® (calcium, magnesium, sodium bicarbonate), **Boots Double Action Indigestion**® (aluminium, magnesium, dimethicone), **Boots Headache and Indigestion Relief**® (sodium bicarbonate, sodium carbonate, paracetamol), **Boots Indigestion Tablets**® (calcium, magnesium, sodium bicarbonate)

Carbellon® (magnesium, charcoal, peppermint oil)

De Witt's Antacid Powder® (calcium, magnesium, sodium bicarbonate, light kaolin, peppermint oil), **De Witt's Antacid Tablets**® (calcium, magnesium, peppermint oil), **Dijex**® (aluminium, magnesium), **Dynese**® (magaldrate = aluminium, magnesium)

Entrotabs® (aluminium, attapulgite, pectin)

Gaviscon 250® and **500**® **Tablets** (alginic acid, aluminium, magnesium, sodium bicarbonate; **Gaviscon**® **Tablets** are prescribable), **Gelusil**® (aluminium, magnesium)

Maalox Plus Tablets® (aluminium, magnesium, dimethicone; suspension is prescribable), **Maclean**® (aluminium, calcium, magnesium), **Magnatol**® (alexitol, magnesium, potassium bicarbonate, xanthan gum), **Milk of Magnesia Tablets**® (magnesium; liquid is prescribable), **Moorland**® (aluminium, bismuth, calcium, magnesium, light kaolin)

Novasil Plus® (aluminium, magnesium, dimethicone), **Nulacin**® (calcium, magnesium, peppermint oil; *contains gluten*)

Opas® (calcium, magnesium, sodium bicarbonate)

Pepto-Bismol® (bismuth), **Premiums**® (aluminium, calcium, magnesium, peppermint oil)

Rap-eze® (calcium), **Remegel**® (calcium), **Rennie**® (calcium, magnesium), **Rennie Gold**® (calcium), **Roter**® (bismuth, magnesium, sodium bicarbonate, frangula)

Setlers Extra® (calcium, magnesium), **Setlers Liquid**® (aluminium, magnesium), **Setlers Tablets**® (calcium, magnesium), **Setlers Tums**® (calcium), **Simeco**® (aluminium, magnesium, dimethicone), **Sovol**® (aluminium, magnesium, dimethicone)

Unigest® (aluminium, dimethicone)

Windcheaters® (dimethicone)

1.1.3 Calcium- and bismuth-containing antacids

Bismuth-containing antacids (unless chelates) are best avoided because absorbed bismuth can be neurotoxic, causing encephalopathy; they tend to be constipating. Calcium-containing antacids can induce rebound acid secretion: with modest doses the clinical significance is doubtful, but prolonged high doses also cause hypercalcaemia and alkalosis, and can precipitate the milk alkali syndrome. **Interactions:** Appendix 1 (antacids and adsorbents). For **preparations** on sale to the public (not prescribable on the NHS), see opposite

1.2 Antispasmodics and other drugs altering gut motility

The smooth muscle relaxant properties of antimuscarinic and other antispasmodic drugs may be useful as adjunctive treatment in *non-ulcer dyspepsia*, in the *irritable bowel syndrome*, and in *diverticular disease*. The gastric antisecretory effects of conventional antimuscarinic drugs are of little practical significance since dosage is limited by atropine-like side-effects. Moreover, they have been superseded by more powerful and specific antisecretory drugs, including the histamine H₂-receptor antagonists and the selective antimuscarinic pirenzepine.

The dopamine-receptor antagonists metoclopramide and domperidone, and the acetylcholine-release promoter cisapride all tend to stimulate transit in the gut.

ANTIMUSCARINICS

The antimuscarinics (less correctly termed 'anticholinergics') can be divided into atropine and its related alkaloids (including the belladonna alkaloids), and synthetic antimuscarinics. The synthetic antimuscarinics can, in turn, be divided into **tertiary amine** (dicyclomine hydrochloride) and **quaternary ammonium compounds** (poldine methylsulphate and propantheline bromide). Dicyclomine hydrochloride has a much less marked antimuscarinic action than atropine and may also have some direct action on smooth muscle.

Quaternary ammonium compounds are less lipid soluble than atropine and so may be less likely to cross the blood–brain barrier; they are also less well absorbed. Although central atropine-like side-effects, such as confusion, are thereby reduced, peripheral atropine-like side-effects remain common with dry mouth, difficult visual accommodation, hesitant micturition, and constipation at doses which act as gut neuromuscular relaxants or inhibitors of acid secretion. The elderly are particularly susceptible; glaucoma and urinary retention may occur.

Antimuscarinics tend to relax the oesophageal sphincter and should be avoided in patients with symptomatic reflux; all antispasmodics should be avoided in paralytic ileus. Despite these side-effects antimuscarinics are nevertheless useful in some *dyspeptics*, in the *irritable bowel syndrome*, and in *diverticular disease*. Nonselective antimuscarinics

---

(e.g. belladonna alkaloids) are outmoded as ulcer treatments, any clinical virtues being outweighed by atropinic side-effects.

The quaternary ammonium compound, **hyoscine butylbromide** is advocated as a gastro-intestinal antispasmodic, but it is poorly absorbed; the injection is useful in endoscopy and radiology.

ATROPINE SULPHATE and BELLADONNA ALKALOIDS

Indications: see notes above; atropine sulphate, see also section 15.1.3

Cautions: elderly; urinary retention, prostatic enlargement, tachycardia, cardiac insufficiency, paralytic ileus, ulcerative colitis, and pyloric stenosis; may aggravate gastro-oesophageal reflux; pregnancy and breast-feeding; **interactions:** Appendix 1 (antimuscarinics)

Contra-indications: closed-angle glaucoma

Side-effects: dry mouth with difficulty in swallowing and thirst, dilatation of the pupils with loss of accommodation and sensitivity to light, increased intra-ocular pressure, flushing, dry skin, bradycardia followed by tachycardia, palpitations and arrhythmias, difficulty with micturition, and constipation; rarely fever, confusional states and rashes

Indigestion **preparations** on sale to the public (not prescribable on the NHS) containing belladonna and related alkaloids include:

Actonorm Powder® (atropine, aluminium, calcium, magnesium, sodium bicarbonate, peppermint oil), **Aluhyde**® (belladonna, aluminium, magnesium), **APP**® (homatropine, aluminium, bismuth, calcium, magnesium) **Bellocarb**® (belladonna, magnesium) **Enterosan**® (belladonna, morphine, kaolin) **Opazimes**® (belladonna, morphine, aluminium, kaolin)

DICYCLOMINE HYDROCHLORIDE
(Dicycloverine Hydrochloride)

Indications: adjunct in gastro-intestinal disorders characterised by smooth muscle spasm

Cautions; Contra-indications; Side-effects: see under Atropine Sulphate; contra-indicated in infants under 6 months

Dose: 10–20 mg 3 times daily; CHILD 6–24 months 5–10 mg up to 3–4 times daily, 15 minutes before feeds, 2–12 years 10 mg 3 times daily

PoM [1] **Merbentyl**® (Merrell)

Tablets, dicyclomine hydrochloride 10 mg. Net price 20 = 57p

Syrup, dicyclomine hydrochloride 10 mg/5 mL. Net price 100 mL = 86p

1. Dicyclomine hydrochloride can be sold to the public provided that the maximum single dose is 10 mg and the maximum daily dose is 60 mg

PoM Merbentyl 20® (Merrell)

Tablets, dicyclomine hydrochloride 20 mg. Net price 84-tab pack = £4.77

Compound preparations
Kolanticon® (Merrell)

Gel, sugar-free, dicyclomine hydrochloride 2.5 mg, dried aluminium hydroxide 200 mg, light magnesium oxide 100 mg, activated dimethicone (simethicone USP) 20 mg/5 mL. Net price 200 mL = £1.52; 500 mL = £1.85

Dose: 10–20 mL every 4 hours when required

HYOSCINE BUTYLBROMIDE

Indications: adjunct in gastro-intestinal disorders characterised by smooth muscle spasm (but see notes above); dysmenorrhoea (but see p. 190)

Cautions; Contra-indications; Side-effects: see under Atropine Sulphate and notes above; avoid in porphyria (see section 9.8.2)

Dose: by mouth, 20 mg 4 times daily; CHILD 6–12 years, 10 mg 3 times daily

By intramuscular or intravenous injection (acute spasm), 20 mg, repeated after 30 minutes if necessary

PoM [1] **Buscopan**® (Boehringer Ingelheim)

Tablets, coated, hyoscine butylbromide 10 mg. Net price 56-tab pack = £2.59 (not recommended, see notes above)

1. Can be sold to the public provided single dose does not exceed 20 mg, daily dose does not exceed 80 mg, and pack does not contain a total of more than 240 mg. Net price 24 × 10 mg-tab pack = £1.90

Injection, hyoscine butylbromide 20 mg/mL. Net price 1-mL amp = 20p

POLDINE METHYLSULPHATE
(Poldine Metilsulfate)

Indications: adjunct in gastro-intestinal disorders characterised by smooth muscle spasm

Cautions; Contra-indications; Side-effects: see under Atropine Sulphate and notes above

Dose: 2–4 mg 4 times daily

PoM Nacton® (Pharmark)

Tablets, scored, poldine methylsulphate 2 mg. Net price 112-tab pack = £12.29

Tablets forte, orange, scored, poldine methylsulphate 4 mg. Net price 112-tab pack = £21.66

PROPANTHELINE BROMIDE

Indications: adjunct in gastro-intestinal disorders characterised by smooth muscle spasm; for use in urinary frequency, see section 7.4.2

Cautions; Contra-indications; Side-effects: see under Atropine Sulphate and notes above

Dose: 15 mg 3 times daily at least 1 hour before meals and 30 mg at night, max. 120 mg daily; CHILD not recommended

PoM Pro-Banthine® (Baker Norton)

Tablets, pink, s/c, propantheline bromide 15 mg. Net price 100-tab pack = £4.56. Label: 23

OTHER ANTISPASMODICS

Alverine, **mebeverine**, and **peppermint oil** are believed to be direct relaxants of intestinal smooth muscle and may relieve pain in the *irritable bowel syndrome* and *diverticular disease*. They have no serious adverse effects but, like all antispasmodics, should be avoided in paralytic ileus. Peppermint oil occasionally causes heartburn.

ALVERINE CITRATE

Indications: adjunct in gastro-intestinal disorders characterised by smooth muscle spasm; dysmenorrhoea

Contra-indications: intestinal obstruction, colonic atony, faecal impaction, combination with sterculia also contra-indicated if difficulty in swallowing; pregnancy and breast-feeding

Side-effects: nausea, headache, pruritus, rash and dizziness reported

Dose: see under preparations

Spasmonal® (Norgine)

Capsules, blue/grey, alverine citrate 60 mg. Net price 20 = £2.18

Dose: 1–2 capsules 1–3 times daily; CHILD not recommended

Note. A proprietary brand of alverine citrate 60 mg (Relaxyl®) is on sale to the public for irritable bowel syndrome

Compound preparations
Alvercol® (Norgine)

Granules, beige, coated, sterculia 62%, alverine citrate 0.5%. Net price 500 g = £12.19. Label: 25, 27, counselling, see below

Dose: irritable bowel syndrome, 1–2 heaped 5-mL spoonfuls swallowed without chewing with water once or twice daily after meals; CHILD 6–12 years, half adult dose

COUNSELLING. Preparations that swell in contact with liquid should always be carefully swallowed with water and should not be taken immediately before going to bed

MEBEVERINE HYDROCHLORIDE

Indications: adjunct in gastro-intestinal disorders characterised by smooth muscle spasm

Cautions: paralytic ileus; pregnancy and breast-feeding; avoid in porphyria (see section 9.8.2.)

PoM Colofac® (Solvay)

Tablets, s/c, mebeverine hydrochloride 135 mg. Net price 20 = £1.67

Dose: ADULT and CHILD over 10 years, 1 tablet 3 times daily preferably 20 minutes before meals

Note. Tablets containing mebeverine hydrochloride 135 mg also available from APS, Berk (Fomac®), Cox, Evans, Generics, Hillcross, Lagap, Norton

Liquid, yellow, sugar-free, mebeverine hydrochloride 50 mg (as embonate)/5 mL. Net price 300 mL = £3.50

Dose: ADULT and CHILD over 10 years, 15 mL 3 times daily preferably 20 minutes before meals

Compound preparations
PoM Fybogel® Mebeverine (R&C)

Granules, buff, effervescent, ispaghula husk 3.5 g, mebeverine hydrochloride 135 mg/sachet. Contains 7 mmol K⁺/sachet (caution in renal impairment). Net price 60 sachets = £15.00. Label: 13, 22, counselling, see below

Dose: irritable bowel syndrome, ADULT, 1 sachet in water morning and night 30 minutes before food; an additional sachet may also be taken before the midday meal if necessary; CHILD not recommended

COUNSELLING. Preparations that swell in contact with liquid should always be carefully swallowed with water and should not be taken immediately before going to bed

PEPPERMINT OIL

Indications: relief of abdominal colic and distension, particularly in irritable bowel syndrome

Cautions: rarely sensitivity to menthol

Side-effects: heartburn, rarely, allergic reactions (including rash, headache, bradycardia, muscle tremor, ataxia)

LOCAL IRRITATION. Capsules should not be broken or chewed because this would release peppermint oil causing irritation of mouth or oesophagus

Colpermin® (Pharmacia)

Capsules, m/r, e/c, light blue/dark blue, blue band, peppermint oil 0.2 mL. Net price 100-cap pack = £10.96. Label: 5, 22, 25

Dose: 1–2 capsules, swallowed whole with water, 3 times daily 30–60 minutes before meals for up to 2–3 months if necessary; CHILD under 15 years not recommended

Mintec® (Monmouth)

Capsules, e/c, green/ivory, peppermint oil 0.2 mL. Net price 100-cap pack = £12.80. Label: 5, 22, 25

Dose: 1–2 capsules swallowed whole with water, 3 times daily before meals for up to 2–3 months if necessary; CHILD not recommended

Note. Mintec® is on sale to the public for irritable bowel syndrome

MOTILITY STIMULANTS

Metoclopramide and **domperidone** are dopamine antagonists which stimulate gastric emptying and small intestinal transit, and enhance the strength of oesophageal sphincter contraction. Metoclopramide is used in some patients with *non-ulcer dyspepsia*, for speeding the transit of barium during intestinal follow-through examination, and as accessory treatment for *oesophageal reflux*; domperidone is also used in *non-ulcer dyspepsia*. Both metoclopramide and domperidone are useful in non-specific and in cytotoxic-induced nausea and vomiting. Metoclopramide and occasionally domperidone may induce an acute dystonic reaction, particularly in young women and children—for further details of this and other side-effects, see section 4.6.

Cisapride is a motility stimulant believed to promote release of acetylcholine in the gut wall; it does not have dopamine-antagonist properties. It is of use in treating *oesophageal reflux* and *gastric stasis*

and in the short-term management of *non-ulcer dyspepsia*. Concomitant administration with drugs which inhibit the metabolism of cisapride can increase plasma concentration of cisapride leading to disturbances of cardiac rhythm (see under cisapride below for recommendations).

CISAPRIDE

Indications: see under dose

Cautions: halve dose initially in hepatic and renal impairment; elderly; cardiac disorders; **interactions:** Appendix 1 (cisapride); **important:** see also Arrhythmias, below

ARRHYTHMIAS. Concomitant administration of cisapride with drugs that inhibit its metabolism can raise plasma-cisapride concentrations, which may result in QT prolongation and serious ventricular arrhythmias (including torsades de pointes); reports have been received (from abroad) with co-administration involving clarithromycin, erythromycin, fluconazole, itraconazole, ketoconazole, and miconazole.

Recommendations are: *not to exceed* recommended dose of cisapride, *to use with caution* in conditions leading to QT prolongation such as uncorrected electrolyte disturbances (particularly hypokalaemia and hypomagnesaemia), *to use with caution* in congenital QT prolongation, *to use with caution* in patients taking medication known to prolong QT interval; and *to avoid* concomitant administration of cisapride with oral or parenteral formulations of clarithromycin, erythromycin, fluconazole, itraconazole, ketoconazole, or miconazole.

Contra-indications: where gastro-intestinal stimulation dangerous; pregnancy and breast-feeding

Side-effects: abdominal cramps and diarrhoea, occasional headaches and lightheadedness; convulsions, extrapyramidal effects and increased urinary frequency; liver function abnormalities (and possibly cholestasis) also reported; **important:** ventricular arrhythmias (including torsades de pointes) have been reported, for recommendations see Arrhythmias above

Dose: ADULT and CHILD over 12 years

Symptoms and mucosal lesions associated with gastro-oesophageal reflux, 10 mg 3–4 times daily *or* 20 mg twice daily (12-week course recommended); maintenance treatment, 20 mg at bedtime *or* 10 mg twice daily (20 mg twice daily if initial lesions were very severe) (halve 20-mg dose and double frequency of administration if severe abdominal cramps)

Symptoms of impaired gastric motility secondary to disturbed and delayed gastric emptying associated with diabetes, systemic sclerosis and autonomic neuropathy, 10 mg 3–4 times daily initially for 6 weeks (but longer treatment may be necessary)

Symptoms of dyspepsia (peptic ulcer or other lesions excluded), 10 mg 3 times daily (usual course 4 weeks)

COUNSELLING. Advise patient to take 15–30 minutes before meals and at bedtime (for night symptoms)

PoM Prepulsid® (Janssen)

Tablets, scored, cisapride (as monohydrate) 10 mg, net price 120-tab pack = £37.60. Counselling, administration, see above (also available as Alimix®)

Suspension, cisapride (as monohydrate) 5 mg / 5 mL. Net price 500 mL = £15.60. Counselling, administration, see above

DOMPERIDONE

Indications: functional dyspepsia; nausea and vomiting, see section 4.6

CHILDREN. Use in children is restricted to nausea and vomiting following cytotoxics or radiotherapy

Cautions; Side-effects; Dose: see section 4.6

Preparations

See section 4.6

METOCLOPRAMIDE HYDROCHLORIDE

Indications: see notes above; nausea and vomiting, see section 4.6

PATIENTS UNDER 20 YEARS. Use restricted to severe intractable vomiting of known cause, vomiting of radiotherapy and cytotoxics, aid to gastro-intestinal intubation, pre-medication

Cautions; Side-effects; Dose: see section 4.6

Preparations

See section 4.6

1.3   Ulcer-healing drugs

1.3.1   H$_2$-receptor antagonists
1.3.2   Selective antimuscarinics
1.3.3   Chelates and complexes
1.3.4   Prostaglandin analogues
1.3.5   Proton pump inhibitors
1.3.6   Other ulcer-healing drugs

Peptic ulceration commonly involves the stomach, duodenum, and lower oesophagus; after gastric surgery it involves the gastro-enterostomy stoma.

Healing can be promoted by general measures, stopping smoking and taking antacids and by antisecretory drug treatment. Relapse is common when treatment ceases, but long-term healing of duodenal and gastric ulcers can be obtained by eradicating associated infection with *Helicobacter pylori*.

HELICOBACTER PYLORI INFECTION

The ideal treatment is not yet clear (see examples in the table below). Triple therapy regimens provide higher eradication rates than dual therapy (but compliance may be a problem) and one-week regimens may be preferred. Eradication of infection commonly results in long-term ulcer remission. Antibiotic-induced colitis is a possible (but uncommon) risk and *H. pylori* reinfection can occur.

EXAMPLES OF HELICOBACTER PYLORI-ERADICATION REGIMENS

Triple therapy (one-week regimens)

Amoxycillin 500 mg 3 times daily
plus
Metronidazole 400 mg 3 times daily
plus
Omeprazole 20 mg twice daily *or* 40 mg once daily
for 7 days
Total net price = £19.18
> Note. Consider as a first choice; substitute clarithro-mycin 250 mg 3 times daily where metronidazole has been used before

Clarithromycin 250 mg twice daily
plus
Metronidazole 400 mg (*or* tinidazole 500 mg) twice daily
plus
Omeprazole 20 mg twice daily *or* 40 mg once daily
for 7 days
Total net price = £29.55 (metronidazole-containing regimen), £37.01 (tinidazole-containing regimen)
> Note. Consider as a first choice

Amoxycillin 1 g twice daily
plus
Clarithromycin 500 mg twice daily
plus
Omeprazole 20 mg twice daily *or* 40 mg once daily
for 7 days
Total net price = £41.76

Lansoprazole 30 mg twice daily
*plus **two** of the following:*
Amoxycillin 1 g twice daily
Clarithromycin 250 mg twice daily
Metronidazole 400 mg twice daily
for 7 days
Total net price = £30.97 (regimen containing amoxycillin and clarithromycin), £20.32 (regimen containing amoxycillin and metronidazole), £30.01 (regimen containing clarithromycin and metronid-azole)
> Note. These regimens are also licensed for eradication of *H. pylori* associated with gastritis

Triple therapy (two-week regimens)

Tetracycline 500 mg 4 times daily
plus
Metronidazole 400 mg 3 times daily
plus
Tripotassium dicitratobismuthate 120 mg 4 times daily
for 14 days
Total net price = £18.17
> Note. May be poorly tolerated; amoxycillin 500 mg 4 times daily has been substituted for tetracycline

Amoxycillin 750 mg 3 times daily
plus
Metronidazole 500 mg 3 times daily
plus
Ranitidine 300 mg at night (or 150 mg twice daily)
for 14 days
Total net price = £20.06
> Note. This dosage regimen has been licensed with a 500-mg dose of metronidazole, which would involve divid-ing the tablets to achieve the specified dose

Ranitidine bismuth citrate 400 mg twice daily
plus either
Amoxycillin 500 mg 4 times daily
or
Clarithromycin 250 mg 4 times daily (*or* 500 mg 3 times daily)
for 14 days
Total net price = £29.11 (amoxycillin-containing regimen), £70.96–£93.47 (clarithromycin-contain-ing regimens)

Dual therapy (two-week regimens)

Clarithromycin 500 mg 3 times daily
plus
Omeprazole 20 mg twice daily *or* 40 mg once daily
for 14 days
Total net price = £102.92
> Note. Lower eradication rates than with triple therapy regimens

Amoxycillin 750 mg (*or* 1 g) twice daily
plus
Omeprazole 20 mg twice daily *or* 40 mg once daily
for 14 days
Total net price = £38.94
> Note. This regimen is also licensed for gastric ulcer dis-ease; lower eradication rates than with triple therapy regimens

A total of 4–8 weeks of antisecretory treatment (with a H_2-receptor antagonist or omeprazole) may be con-sidered for ulcer healing

1.3.1 H_2-receptor antagonists

All H_2-receptor antagonists heal *gastric and duo-denal ulcers* by reducing gastric acid output as a result of H_2-receptor blockade; like cimetidine and ranitidine, the newer ones (famotidine and nizati-dine) can also be expected to relieve *peptic oeso-phagitis*. High doses of H_2-receptor antagonists have been used in the *Zollinger–Ellison syndrome*, but omeprazole may now be preferred.

Maintenance treatment with half doses prevents *ulcer relapse*, but does not modify the natural course of the disease when treatment has ceased and *H. pylori* eradication should be considered instead. Maintenance treatment is best suited to those with frequent severe recurrences and to the elderly who suffer ulcer complications.

Treatment of *undiagnosed dyspepsia* may be acceptable in younger patients but is undesirable in older people because the diagnosis of gastric cancer may be delayed.

Therapy can promote healing of *NSAID-associated ulcers* but there is no proof that the ulcer complications are prevented.

Treatment has not been shown to be beneficial in *haematemesis* and *melaena*, but prophylactic use reduces the frequency of bleeding from gastroduodenal erosions in *hepatic coma*, and possibly in other conditions requiring *intensive care*. Treatment also reduces the frequency of *acid aspiration* in obstetric patients at delivery (Mendelson's syndrome).

SIDE-EFFECTS. H_2-receptor antagonists are well tolerated and side-effects are uncommon with few significant differences between available drugs. Dizziness, somnolence or fatigue, and rash have occasionally been reported with all of them, and there are rare reports of headache, liver dysfunction, and blood disorders. Other rare reports include bradycardia or AV block, confusion, interstitial nephritis (cimetidine), and urticaria and angioedema. Cimetidine is also associated with occasional gynaecomastia and rare reports of impotence and myalgia. Causal relationships of other reports, such as pancreatitis, are unclear.

INTERACTIONS. Cimetidine retards oxidative hepatic drug metabolism by binding to microsomal cytochrome P450. It should be avoided in patients stabilised on warfarin, phenytoin, and theophylline (or aminophylline), but other interactions (see **Appendix 1**) may be of less clinical relevance. Famotidine, nizatidine, and ranitidine do not share the drug metabolism inhibitory properties of cimetidine.

CIMETIDINE

Indications: benign gastric and duodenal ulceration, stomal ulcer, reflux oesophagitis, Zollinger-Ellison syndrome, other conditions where gastric acid reduction is beneficial (see notes above and section 1.9.4)

Cautions: see notes above; renal and hepatic impairment (reduce doses, see Appendixes 2 and 3); pregnancy and breast-feeding; preferably avoid intravenous injection (infusion is preferable) particularly in high dosage (may rarely cause arrhythmias) and in cardiovascular impairment; **interactions:** Appendix 1 (histamine H_2-antagonists) and notes above

Side-effects: altered bowel habit, dizziness, rash, tiredness; reversible confusional states, reversible liver damage, headache; rarely, blood disorders (including thrombocytopenia, agranulocytosis, and aplastic anaemia), muscle or joint pain, hypersensitivity, bradycardia and AV block; interstitial nephritis and acute pancreatitis reported; gynaecomastia is also an occasional problem with cimetidine (but usually only in high dosage), and reversible impotence has also been reported (see also notes above)

Dose: by mouth, 400 mg twice daily (with breakfast and at night) *or* 800 mg at night (benign gastric and duodenal ulceration) for at least 4 weeks (6 weeks in gastric ulceration, 8 weeks in NSAID-associated ulceration); when necessary the dose may be increased to 400 mg 4 times daily or rarely (e.g. as in stress ulceration) to a max. of 2.4 g daily in divided doses; INFANT under 1 year, 20 mg/kg daily in divided doses has been used; CHILD over 1 year, 25–30 mg/kg daily in divided doses

Maintenance, 400 mg at night *or* 400 mg morning and night

Reflux oesophagitis, 400 mg 4 times daily for 4–8 weeks

Zollinger-Ellison syndrome (but see notes above), 400 mg 4 times daily or occasionally more

Gastric acid reduction (prophylaxis of acid aspiration; do not use syrup), obstetrics 400 mg at start of labour, then up to 400 mg every 4 hours if required (max. of 2.4 g daily); surgical procedures 400 mg 90–120 minutes before induction of general anaesthesia

Short-bowel syndrome, 400 mg twice daily (with breakfast and at bedtime) adjusted according to response

To reduce degradation of pancreatic enzyme supplements, 0.8–1.6 g daily in 4 divided doses according to response 1–1½ hours before meals

By intramuscular injection, 200 mg every 4–6 hours; max. 2.4 g daily

By slow intravenous injection, 200 mg given over at least 2 minutes; may be repeated every 4–6 hours; if a larger dose is needed or there is cardiovascular impairment, the dose should be diluted and given over at least 10 minutes (infusion is preferable); max. 2.4 g daily

By intravenous infusion, 400 mg in 100 mL of sodium chloride 0.9% intravenous infusion infused over ½–1 hour (may be repeated every 4–6 hours) *or* by continuous infusion at an average rate of 50–100 mg/hour over 24 hours, max. 2.4 g daily; INFANT under 1 year, *by intramuscular injection or slow intravenous injection or infusion*, 20 mg/kg daily in divided doses has been used; CHILD over 1 year, 25–30 mg/kg daily in divided doses

PoM [1] **Cimetidine** (Non-proprietary)

Tablets, cimetidine 200 mg, net generic prescription price 120-tab pack = £6.76; 400 mg, 60-tab pack = £6.94; 800 mg, 30-tab pack = £7.31

Available from APS, Ashbourne (Peptimax®), Berk (Ultec®), BHR (Phimetin®), Bioglan, Cox, CP, Eastern (Zita®), Galen (Galenamet®), Lagap, Norton, Opus (Acitak®)

1. Cimetidine can be sold to the public for adults and children over 16 years (provided packs do not contain more than 2 weeks' supply) for the short-term symptomatic relief of heartburn, dyspepsia, and hyperacidity (max. single dose 200 mg, max. daily dose 800 mg); for the prophylactic management of nocturnal heartburn (single night-time dose 100 mg); a proprietary brand (Tagamet 100® containing cimetidine 100 mg) is on sale to the public

PoM **Dyspamet®** (SK&F)

Chewtab® (chewable tablets), sugar-free, cimetidine 200 mg. Net price 120-tab pack = £18.40. Counselling, chew thoroughly

Note. Each chewable tablet contains aspartame 3 mg (see section 9.4.1)

Suspension, sugar-free, cimetidine 200 mg/5 mL. Contains sorbitol 2.79 g/5 mL. Net price 600 mL = £24.08

PoM **Tagamet®** (SK&F)

Tablets, all green, f/c, cimetidine 200 mg, net price 120-tab pack = £19.58; 400 mg, 60-tab pack = £22.62; 800 mg, 30-tab pack = £22.62

Effervescent tablets, sugar-free, cimetidine 400 mg. Contains 17.6 mmol Na+/tablet. Net price 60-tab pack = £20.56. Label: 13

Note. Each effervescent tablet contains aspartame 70 mg (see section 9.4.1)

Syrup, orange, cimetidine 200 mg/5 mL. Net price 600 mL = £28.49

Injection, cimetidine 100 mg/mL. Net price 2-mL amp = 32p

Intravenous infusion, cimetidine 4 mg/mL in sodium chloride intravenous infusion 0.9%. Net price 100-mL infusion bag = £2.05

Cimetidine with alginate

PoM **Algitec®** (SK&F)

Chewtab® (chewable tablets), off-white, cimetidine 200 mg, alginic acid 500 mg. Contains 2.05 mmol Na+/tablet. Net price 120-tab pack = £22.50. Counselling, chew thoroughly

Note. Each chewable tablet contains aspartame 5 mg (see section 9.4.1)

[1]*Suspension*, cimetidine 100 mg, sodium alginate 250 mg/5 mL. Contains 1.43 mmol Na+/5 mL. Net price 600 mL = £15.41

Dose: gastro-oesophageal reflux disease, 1 tablet chewed or 10 mL suspension 4 times daily (after meals and at bedtime), increased if necessary to 2 tablets or 20 mL suspension 4 times daily; to be taken for 4–8 weeks

[1]A proprietary brand (Tagamet® Dual Action containing cimetidine 100 mg, sodium alginate 250 mg/5 mL) can be sold for adults and children over 16 years (provided packs do not contain more than 2 weeks supply) for the short-term symptomatic relief of heartburn (max. single dose 10 mL, max. daily dose 40 mL)

FAMOTIDINE

Indications: see under Dose

Cautions: see under Cimetidine; does not inhibit hepatic microsomal drug metabolism

Side-effects: see under Cimetidine and notes above

Dose: benign gastric and duodenal ulceration, treatment, 40 mg at night for 4–8 weeks; maintenance (duodenal), 20 mg at night; CHILD not recommended

Reflux oesophagitis, 20–40 mg twice daily for 6–12 weeks; maintenance, 20 mg twice daily

Zollinger–Ellison syndrome (but see notes above), 20 mg every 6 hours (higher dose in those who have previously been receiving another H2-antagonist); doses up to 800 mg daily in divided doses have been used

PoM [1] **Pepcid®** (Morson)

Tablets, famotidine 20 mg (beige), net price 28-tab pack = £14.00; 40 mg (brown), 28-tab pack = £26.60

1. Famotidine can be sold to the public for adults and children over 16 years (provided packs do not contain more than 2 weeks' supply) for the short-term symptomatic relief of heartburn, dyspepsia, and hyperacidity (max. single dose 10 mg, max. daily dose 20 mg); a proprietary brand (Pepcid AC® containing famotidine 10 mg) is on sale to the public

NIZATIDINE

Indications: see under Dose

Cautions: see under Cimetidine; does not inhibit hepatic microsomal drug metabolism

Side-effects: see under Cimetidine and notes above; sweating also reported; rare reports of gynaecomastia

Dose: by mouth, benign gastric and duodenal ulceration, treatment, 300 mg at night *or* 150 mg twice daily for 4–8 weeks (up to 8 weeks in NSAID-associated ulceration); maintenance, 150 mg at night for up to 1 year; CHILD not recommended

Reflux oesophagitis, 150–300 mg twice daily for up to 12 weeks

By intravenous infusion, for short-term use in peptic ulcer hospital inpatients as alternative to oral route, *by intermittent intravenous infusion* over 15 minutes, 100 mg 3 times daily, *or by continuous intravenous infusion*, 10 mg/hour; max. 480 mg daily; CHILD not recommended

PoM **Axid®** (Lilly)

Capsules, nizatidine 150 mg (pale yellow/dark yellow), net price 30-cap pack = £11.34; 300 mg (pale yellow/brown), 30-cap pack = £21.74

Note. Capsules containing nizatidine 150 mg and 300 mg also available from Ashbourne (Zinga®)

Injection, nizatidine 25 mg/mL. For dilution and use as an intravenous infusion. Net price 4-mL amp = £1.20

RANITIDINE

Indications: benign gastric and duodenal ulceration, stomal ulcer, reflux oesophagitis, Zollinger–Ellison syndrome, other conditions where reduction of gastric acidity is beneficial (see notes above and section 1.9.4)

Cautions: see under Cimetidine; does not significantly inhibit hepatic microsomal drug metabolism; avoid in porphyria (section 9.8.2)

Side-effects: see under Cimetidine and notes above; rare reports of breast swelling and tenderness in men; erythema multiforme reported

Dose: by mouth, 150 mg twice daily (morning and night) *or* 300 mg at night (benign gastric and duodenal ulceration) for 4 to 8 weeks, up to 6 weeks in chronic episodic dyspepsia, and up to 8 weeks in NSAID-associated ulceration; in duodenal ulcer 300 mg can be given twice daily for 4 weeks to achieve a higher healing rate; CHILD (peptic ulcer) 2–4 mg/kg twice daily, max. 300 mg daily

Maintenance, 150 mg at night

Duodenal ulcer associated with *H. pylori*, 300 mg at night *or* 150 mg twice daily may be given with amoxycillin 750 mg 3 times daily and metronidazole 500 mg 3 times daily for 2 weeks; ranitidine treatment should be continued for a further 2 weeks

Note. This dosage regimen has been licensed with a 500-mg dose of metronidazole, which would involve dividing the tablets to achieve the specified dose

Prophylaxis of NSAID-induced duodenal ulcer, 150 mg twice daily

Reflux oesophagitis, 150 mg twice daily *or* 300 mg at night for up to 8 weeks, or if necessary 12 weeks (moderate to severe, 150 mg 4 times daily for up to 12 weeks); long-term treatment of healed oesophagitis, 150 mg twice daily

Zollinger–Ellison syndrome (but see notes above), 150 mg 3 times daily; doses up to 6 g daily in divided doses have been used

Gastric acid reduction (prophylaxis of acid aspiration) in obstetrics, *by mouth*, 150 mg at onset of labour, then every 6 hours; surgical procedures, *by intramuscular or slow intravenous injection*, 50 mg 45–60 minutes before induction of anaesthesia (intravenous injection diluted to 20 mL and given over at least 2 minutes), or *by mouth*, 150 mg 2 hours before induction of anaesthesia, and also, when possible on the preceding evening

By intramuscular injection, 50 mg every 6–8 hours

By slow intravenous injection, 50 mg diluted to 20 mL and given over at least 2 minutes; may be repeated every 6–8 hours

By intravenous infusion, 25 mg/hour for 2 hours; may be repeated every 6–8 hours

Prophylaxis of stress ulceration, initial slow intravenous injection of 50 mg (as above) then *continuous infusion*, 125–250 micrograms/kg per hour (may be followed by 150 mg twice daily *by mouth* when oral feeding commences)

PoM [1] **Zantac®** (Glaxo)

Tablets, f/c, ranitidine (as hydrochloride) 150 mg, net price 60-tab pack = £27.89; 300 mg, 30-tab pack = £27.43

Effervescent tablets, pale yellow, ranitidine (as hydrochloride) 150 mg (contains 14.3 mmol Na+/tablet), net price 60-tab pack = £27.88; 300 mg (contains 20.8 mmol Na+/tablet), 30-tab pack = £27.42. Label: 13

Note. The effervescent tablets contain aspartame (see section 9.4.1)

Syrup, sugar-free, ranitidine (as hydrochloride) 75 mg/5 mL. Net price 300 mL = £22.32

Injection, ranitidine 25 mg (as hydrochloride)/mL. Net price 2-mL amp = 64p

1. Ranitidine can be sold to the public for adults and children over 16 years (provided packs do not contain more than 2 weeks' supply) for the short-term symptomatic relief of heartburn, dyspepsia, and hyperacidity (max. single dose 75 mg, max. daily dose 300 mg); a proprietary brand (Zantac® 75 containing ranitidine (as hydrochloride) 75 mg) is on sale to the public

RANITIDINE BISMUTH CITRATE

(Ranitidine Bismutrex)

Indications: see under Dose

Cautions: see under Cimetidine; does not significantly inhibit hepatic microsomal drug metabolism; **interactions:** Appendix 1 (histamine H_2-antagonists)

Contra-indications: severe renal impairment; porphyria (section 9.8.2)

Side-effects: see under Ranitidine and notes above; rare reports of breast tenderness and swelling in men; see also under Tripotassium Dicitratobismuthate

Dose: 400 mg twice daily for 8 weeks in benign gastric ulceration or 4–8 weeks in duodenal ulceration; CHILD not recommended

Duodenal ulceration associated with H. pylori, 400 mg twice daily with *either* amoxycillin 500 mg 4 times daily for 2 weeks or with clarithromycin 250 mg 4 times daily (*or* 500 mg 3 times daily) for 2 weeks; ranitidine bismuth citrate treatment should be continued for a further 2 weeks; long-term (maintenance) treatment not recommended (max. total of 16 weeks treatment in any 1 year); CHILD not recommended

COUNSELLING. May darken tongue and blacken faeces

▼ **PoM** **Pylorid®** (Glaxo)

Tablets, blue, f/c, ranitidine bismuth citrate 400 mg. Net price 28-tab pack = £26.00; 56-tab pack = £52.00. Counselling (discoloration tongue and faeces)

1.3.2   Selective antimuscarinics

Pirenzepine is a selective antimuscarinic drug which inhibits gastric acid and pepsin secretion with fewer peripheral side-effects than the drugs in section 1.2. As it does not cross the blood-brain barrier it is unlikely to have central effects. It is as effective as H_2-receptor antagonists in healing *gastric and duodenal ulcers* and may also be useful in maintenance treatment. It has also been used in conjunction with H_2-receptor antagonists in resistant cases.

PIRENZEPINE

Indications: benign gastric and duodenal ulceration

Cautions: renal impairment

Contra-indications: prostatic enlargement, pyloric stenosis, paralytic ileus, closed-angle glaucoma; pregnancy

Side-effects: occasionally dry mouth and visual disturbances; agranulocytosis and thrombocytopenia have been reported

Dose: 50 mg twice daily, increased if necessary to a max. of 150 mg daily in 3 divided doses, for 4–6 weeks, or in resistant cases for up to 3 months; CHILD not recommended

PoM **Gastrozepin®** (Knoll)
Tablets, scored, pirenzepine hydrochloride, equivalent to anhydrous pirenzepine hydrochloride, 50 mg. Net price 60 = £27.50. Label: 22

1.3.3 Chelates and complexes

Tripotassium dicitratobismuthate is a bismuth chelate effective in healing *gastric and duodenal ulcers*. It may act by a direct toxic effect on gastric *Helicobacter pylori*, or by stimulating mucosal prostaglandin or bicarbonate secretion. The healing tends to be longer lasting than with H_2-receptor antagonists but relapse still occurs and regimens have now been developed involving co-administration of antibiotics (see p. 35). The bismuth content is low but absorption has been reported; encephalopathy (described with older high-dose bismuth preparations) has not been reported. Tablets are as effective as the liquid and more palatable.

Sucralfate is another effective treatment for *gastric and duodenal ulcers* and may act by protecting the mucosa from acid-pepsin attack. It is a complex of aluminium hydroxide and sulphated sucrose but has minimal antacid properties.

TRIPOTASSIUM DICITRATOBISMUTHATE

(Bismuth Chelate)
Indications: benign gastric and duodenal ulceration
Cautions: see notes above; **interactions:** Appendix 1 (tripotassium dicitratobismuthate)
Contra-indications: renal impairment, pregnancy
Side-effects: may darken tongue and blacken faeces; nausea and vomiting reported

De-Nol® (Yamanouchi)
Liquid, red, tripotassium dicitratobismuthate 120 mg/5 mL. Net price 560 mL = £20.51. Counselling, see below
Dose: 10 mL twice daily *or* 5 mL 4 times daily; taken for 28 days, followed by further 28 days if necessary; maintenance not indicated but course may be repeated after interval of 1 month; CHILD, not recommended
COUNSELLING. Each dose to be diluted with 15 mL of water; twice daily dosage to be taken 30 minutes before breakfast and main evening meal; four times daily dosage to be taken as follows: one dose 30 minutes before breakfast, midday meal and main evening meal, and one dose 2 hours after main evening meal; milk should not be drunk by itself during treatment but small quantities may be taken in tea or coffee or on cereal; antacids should not be taken half an hour before or after a dose; may darken tongue and blacken faeces
De-Noltab® (Yamanouchi)
Tablets, f/c, tripotassium dicitratobismuthate 120 mg. Net price 112-tab pack = £29.37. Counselling, see below
Dose: 2 tablets twice daily *or* 1 tablet 4 times daily; taken for 28 days followed by further 28 days if necessary; maintenance not indicated but course may be repeated after interval of 1 month; CHILD, not recommended
COUNSELLING. Each dose to be swallowed with half a tumblerful of water then as above under De-Nol®

SUCRALFATE

Indications: see under dose
Cautions: renal impairment (avoid if severe, see Appendix 3); pregnancy and breast-feeding; **interactions:** Appendix 1 (sucralfate)
Side-effects: constipation; diarrhoea, nausea, indigestion, gastric discomfort, dry mouth, rash, pruritus, back pain, dizziness, headache, vertigo and drowsiness
Dose: 2 g twice daily (on rising and at bedtime) *or* 1 g 4 times daily 1 hour before meals and at bedtime, taken for 4–6 weeks or in resistant cases 12 weeks; max. 8 g daily; CHILD not recommended
Prophylaxis of stress ulceration (suspension), 1 g 6 times daily (max. 8 g daily)
COUNSELLING. Tablets may be dispersed in 10–15 mL of water; antacids should not be taken half an hour before or after a dose

PoM **Antepsin®** (Wyeth)
Tablets, scored, sucralfate 1 g. Net price 112 = £9.80. Label: 5, counselling, see dose above
Suspension, sucralfate, 1 g/5 mL. Net price 560 mL = £9.80. Label: 5, counselling, antacids

1.3.4 Prostaglandin analogues

Misoprostol, a synthetic prostaglandin analogue has antisecretory and protective properties, promoting *gastric and duodenal ulcer* healing. It can prevent NSAID-associated ulcers, its use being most appropriate for the frail or very elderly from whom NSAIDs cannot be withdrawn.

MISOPROSTOL

Indications: see notes above and under Dose
Cautions: conditions where hypotension might precipitate severe complications (e.g. cerebrovascular disease, cardiovascular disease)
Contra-indications: pregnancy or planning pregnancy (increases uterine tone)—**important:** women of childbearing age, see also below, and breast-feeding
WOMEN OF CHILDBEARING AGE. Manufacturer advises that misoprostol should not be used in women of childbearing age unless the patient requires non-steroidal anti-inflammatory (NSAID) therapy and is at high risk of complications from NSAID-induced ulceration. In such patients it is advised that misoprostol should only be used if the patient takes *effective contraceptive measures* and has been advised of the *risks of taking misoprostol if pregnant*.
Side-effects: diarrhoea (may occasionally be severe and require withdrawal, reduced by giving single doses not exceeding 200 micrograms and by avoiding magnesium-containing antacids); also reported: abdominal pain, dyspepsia, flatulence, nausea and vomiting, abnormal vaginal bleeding (including intermenstrual bleeding, menorrhagia, and postmenopausal bleeding), rashes, dizziness

Dose: benign gastric and duodenal ulceration and NSAID-associated ulceration, 800 micrograms daily (in 2–4 divided doses) with breakfast (or main meals) and at bedtime; treatment should be continued for at least 4 weeks and may be continued for up to 8 weeks if required

Prophylaxis of NSAID-induced gastric and duodenal ulcer, 200 micrograms 2–4 times daily taken with the NSAID

CHILD not recommended

PoM **Cytotec®** (Searle)

Tablets, scored, misoprostol 200 micrograms. Net price 56-tab pack = £10.40; 112-tab pack = £20.80. Label: 21

With diclofenac or naproxen
See section 10.1.1

1.3.5   Proton pump inhibitors

The proton pump inhibitors **omeprazole** and **lansoprazole** inhibit gastric acid by blocking the hydrogen-potassium adenosine triphosphatase enzyme system (the 'proton pump') of the gastric parietal cell. They are the treatment of choice for *stricturing and erosive oesophagitis,* lesser degrees usually responding to life-style change, H_2-receptor antagonists, antacids, or motility stimulants. Omeprazole and lansoprazole are used in combination with antibiotics for the eradication of *H. pylori* (see p. 35); omeprazole and lansoprazole are effective short-term treatments for *gastric and duodenal ulcer.* Omeprazole is effective in the treatment of the *Zollinger-Ellison syndrome* (including cases resistant to other treatment).

OMEPRAZOLE

Indications: see under Dose

Cautions: exclude gastric malignancy; severe liver disease (see Appendix 2); avoid in pregnancy and breast-feeding; **interactions:** Appendix 1 (proton pump inhibitors)

Side-effects: rashes, urticaria, pruritus, bullous eruption, erythema multiforme, angioedema, alopecia and photosensitivity reported; diarrhoea, headache (both may be severe); also nausea, constipation, flatulence, abdominal pain, dizziness, faintness, vertigo, somnolence, malaise, insomnia and paraesthesia; muscle and joint pain, blurred vision, peripheral oedema, increased sweating, gynaecomastia and rarely impotence, loss of taste, stomatitis, gastro-intestinal candidiasis, leucopenia, thrombocytopenia, fever, bronchospasm, interstitial nephritis, liver enzyme changes and liver dysfunction also reported (and encephalopathy in pre-existing severe liver disease); reversible mental confusion, agitation, depression and hallucinations have been noted in the severely ill

Dose: benign gastric and duodenal ulcers (including those complicating NSAID therapy), 20 mg daily for 4 weeks in duodenal ulceration or 8 weeks in gastric ulceration; in severe or recurrent cases increase to 40 mg daily; maintenance for recurrent duodenal ulcer, 20 mg daily; prevention of relapse in duodenal ulcer, 10 mg daily increasing to 20 mg daily if symptoms return

Duodenal ulcer associated with *H. pylori,* see eradication regimens on p. 35 (amoxicillin with omeprazole regimen also licensed for benign gastric ulcer disease)

Zollinger–Ellison syndrome, initially 60 mg once daily; usual range 20–120 mg daily (above 80 mg in 2 divided doses)

Gastric acid reduction during general anaesthesia (prophylaxis of acid aspiration), 40 mg on the preceding evening then 40 mg 1–4 hours before surgery

Reflux oesophagitis, 20 mg daily for 4 weeks, followed by a further 4–8 weeks if not fully healed; 40 mg daily has been given for 8 weeks in reflux oesophagitis refractory to other treatment; may be continued at 20 mg daily

Acid reflux disease (long-term management), 10 mg daily increasing to 20 mg daily if symptoms return

CHILD not recommended

PoM **Losec®** (Astra)

Capsules, enclosing e/c granules, omeprazole 10 mg (pink), net price 28-cap pack = £19.95 (also 7-cap pack, hosp. only); 20 mg (pink/brown), 28-cap pack = £35.45 (also 7-cap pack, hosp. only); 40 mg (brown), 14-cap pack = £35.45 (also 7-cap pack, hosp. only). Label: 25

Note. Should be dispensed in original container (which contains a desiccant)

LANSOPRAZOLE

Indications: see under Dose

Cautions; Side-effects: see under Omeprazole

Dose: benign gastric ulcer, 30 mg daily in the morning for 8 weeks

Duodenal ulcer, 30 mg daily in the morning for 4 weeks; maintenance 15 mg daily

Duodenal ulcer or gastritis associated with *H. pylori,* see eradication regimens on p. 35.

Reflux oesophagitis, 30 mg daily in the morning for 4 weeks, followed by a further 4 weeks if not fully healed; maintenance 15–30 mg daily

CHILD not recommended

▼ PoM **Zoton®** (Lederle)

Capsules, enclosing e/c granules, lansoprazole 15 mg (yellow), net price 28-cap pack = £18.95, 56-cap pack = £37.90; 30 mg (lilac/purple), 14-cap pack = £16.68, 28-cap pack = £33.36, 56-cap pack = £66.72 (also 7-cap pack, hosp. only). Label: 5, 23, 25

1.3.6   Other ulcer-healing drugs

Carbenoxolone is a synthetic derivative of glycyrrhizinic acid (a constituent of liquorice).

The only oral preparation of carbenoxolone remaining on the UK market is in the form of a combination with antacids for *oesophageal ulceration and inflammation*.

However, side-effects (commonly sodium and water retention and occasionally hypokalaemia) may cause or exacerbate hypertension, oedema, cardiac failure, and muscle weakness. For these reasons other drugs are preferred; if used regular monitoring of weight, blood pressure, and electrolytes is advisable during treatment. Carbenoxolone may act by protecting the mucosal barrier from acid–pepsin attack and increasing mucosal mucin production.

Deglycyrrhizinised liquorice is free from the above side-effects but is of doubtful efficacy.

LIQUORICE, DEGLYCYRRHIZINISED
Indications; Cautions; Contra-indications; Side-effects: see under Caved-S (below)

Caved-S® (Pharmacia)
Tablets, brown, deglycyrrhizinised liquorice 380 mg, dried aluminium hydroxide 100 mg, bismuth subnitrate 100 mg, magnesium carbonate 200 mg, sodium bicarbonate 100 mg. Net price 180-tab pack = £10.97. Label: 24
Dose: benign gastric and duodenal ulceration, treatment, 2 tablets chewed 3 times daily (for duodenal ulceration increased if necessary to 6 times daily); maintenance, 1 tablet chewed 3 times daily (gastric ulceration), 2 tablets chewed 3 times daily (duodenal ulceration); CHILD no longer recommended
Note. Caved-S® tablets are contra-indicated in renal impairment and in pregnancy since they contain bismuth subnitrate; long-term use should be avoided, see also section 1.1.3; side-effects include mild diarrhoea; **interactions:** see Appendix 1 (antacids and adsorbents)

CARBENOXOLONE SODIUM
Indications: benign gastric ulceration in young and middle-aged adults (see also under preparation)
Cautions: cardiac disease, hypertension, hepatic and renal disease (see contra-indications); elderly (see under preparation); not recommended in children. See also notes above; **interactions:** Appendix 1 (carbenoxolone)
Contra-indications: hypokalaemia, cardiac failure and in those receiving cardiac glycosides (unless electrolyte levels monitored weekly and measures taken to avoid hypokalaemia); hepatic and renal impairment (see Appendixes 2 and 3); pregnancy
Side-effects: sodium and water retention (provoking hypertension and cardiac failure), hypokalaemia (leading to impaired neuromuscular function and muscle damage and to renal damage if prolonged)

Compound preparation
PoM **Pyrogastrone®** (Sanofi Winthrop)
Tablets, chewable, carbenoxolone sodium 20 mg, alginic acid 600 mg, dried aluminium hydroxide 240 mg, magnesium trisilicate 60 mg, sodium bicarbonate 210 mg (Na+ 3 mmol/tablet). Net price 100-tab pack = £24.85. Label: 21, 24
Liquid, carbenoxolone sodium 10 mg, dried aluminium hydroxide 150 mg (Na+ 0.85 mmol, K+ 1.5 mmol)/5 mL when reconstituted with water. Net price 500 mL = £12.39. Label: 21
Dose: for oesophageal inflammation and ulceration, 1 tablet, chewed, 3 times daily after meals, and 2 at night, for 6–12 weeks or 10 mL liquid 3 times daily after meals and 20 mL at night, for 6–12 weeks; not recommended for children or for adults over 75 years

1.4   Antidiarrhoeal drugs

1.4.1   Adsorbents and bulk-forming drugs

1.4.2   Antimotility drugs

The **first line** of treatment in acute diarrhoea, as in gastro-enteritis, is prevention or treatment of fluid and electrolyte depletion. This is particularly important in infants and in frail and elderly patients. For details of **oral rehydration preparations**, see section 9.2.1.2. Severe dehydration requires immediate admission to hospital and urgent replacement of fluid and electrolytes.

Antispasmodics (section 1.2) are occasionally of value in treating abdominal cramp associated with diarrhoea but they should **not** be used for primary treatment. Antispasmodics and antiemetics should be **avoided** in young children with gastro-enteritis as they are rarely effective and have troublesome side-effects.

Antibiotics and sulphonamides are generally unnecessary in simple gastro-enteritis, even when a bacterial cause is suspected, because the complaint will usually resolve quickly without such treatment, and infective diarrhoeas in the UK are often caused by viral infections. Systemic bacterial infection does, however, need appropriate systemic treatment. **Erythromycin** (see section 5.1.5) or **ciprofloxacin** (see section 5.1.12) can be used for treating Campylobacter enteritis. For drugs for shigellosis and salmonellosis, see section 5.1, table 1. The general use of sulphonamides in treating diarrhoea of travellers is inadvisable because of the risks of rash and agranulocytosis. Poorly absorbed drugs such as dihydrostreptomycin, neomycin, and sulphaguanidine should be **avoided** altogether in gastro-intestinal infection. They prolong rather than shorten the time taken to control diarrhoea by causing masked bacterial diarrhoea, carrier states, or antibiotic-associated colitis (pseudomembranous colitis). Clioquinol should also be **avoided** as it is neurotoxic; both it and lactobacillus preparations are valueless.

Cholestyramine and **aluminium hydroxide mixture** (section 1.1.1), bind unabsorbed bile salts and provide symptomatic relief of diarrhoea following ileal disease or resection, in bacterial colonisation of the small bowel, and in post-vagotomy diarrhoea.

1.4.1   Adsorbents and bulk-forming drugs

Adsorbents such as kaolin are **not** recommended for *acute diarrhoeas*. Bulk-forming drugs, such as ispaghula, methylcellulose, and sterculia (see section 1.6.1) are useful in controlling faecal consistency in ileostomy and colostomy, and in controlling diarrhoea associated with diverticular disease.

KAOLIN, LIGHT

Indications: diarrhoea but see notes above

Cautions: **interactions:** Appendix 1 (antacids and adsorbents)

Kaolin Mixture, BP

(Kaolin Oral Suspension)

Oral suspension, light kaolin or light kaolin (natural) 20%, and 5% each of light magnesium carbonate and sodium bicarbonate in a suitable vehicle with a peppermint flavour.

Dose: 10–20 mL every 4 hours

Note. Kaolin-containing preparations on sale to the public include Kaopectate® and KLN®

1.4.2   Antimotility drugs

In *acute diarrhoeas* antimotility drugs have a very limited role as adjuncts to fluid and electrolyte replacement (see section 9.2.1.2); they are **not** recommended for acute diarrhoeas in young children.

For comments on their role in *chronic diarrhoeas* see section 1.5.

CODEINE PHOSPHATE

Indications: see notes above

Cautions; Contra-indications; Side-effects: see section 4.7.2; not for use in conditions where inhibition of peristalsis should be avoided, where abdominal distension develops, or in acute diarrhoeal conditions such as acute ulcerative colitis or antibiotic-associated colitis; not recommended for children; tolerance and dependence may occur with prolonged use; **interactions:** Appendix 1 (opioid analgesics)

Dose: see under Preparations

PoM **Codeine Phosphate** (Non-proprietary)

Tablets, codeine phosphate 15 mg, net generic prescription price 20 = 35p; 30 mg, 20 = 38p; 60 mg, 20 = 97p. Label: 2

Dose: 30 mg 3–4 times daily (range 15–60 mg); CHILD not recommended

Note. Travellers needing to take codeine phosphate tablets abroad may require a doctor's letter explaining why they are necessary.

PoM **Diarrest®** (Galen)

Liquid, yellow, codeine phosphate 5 mg, dicyclomine hydrochloride 2.5 mg, potassium chloride 40 mg, sodium chloride 50 mg, sodium citrate 50 mg/5 mL. For diarrhoea, vomiting, and cramp. Net price 200 mL = £3.34

Dose: 20 mL 4 times daily with water; CHILD 4–5 years 5 mL, 6–9 years 10 mL, 10–13 years 15 mL but see cautions and notes above

NHS **Kaodene®** (Knoll)

Suspension, codeine phosphate 5 mg, light kaolin 1.5 g/5 mL. Net price 250 mL = £1.06

Dose: 20 mL 3–4 times daily; CHILD under 5 years not recommended, over 5 years 10 mL but see cautions and notes above

CO-PHENOTROPE

A mixture of diphenoxylate hydrochloride and atropine sulphate in the mass proportions 100 parts to 1 part respectively

Indications: adjunct to rehydration in acute diarrhoea (but see notes above); chronic mild ulcerative colitis

Cautions; Contra-indications; Side-effects: see notes above and under Codeine Phosphate; young children are particularly susceptible to OVERDOSAGE and symptoms may be delayed so that observation is needed for at least 48 hours after ingestion; in addition the presence of subclinical doses of atropine may give rise to the side-effects of atropine in susceptible individuals or in overdosage; **interactions:** Appendix 1 (opioid analgesics)

PoM **Lomotil®** (Searle)

Tablets, co-phenotrope 2.5/0.025 (diphenoxylate hydrochloride 2.5 mg, atropine sulphate 25 micrograms). Net price 20 = £1.57

Dose: initially 4 tablets, followed by 2 tablets every 6 hours until diarrhoea controlled; CHILD under 4 years not recommended, 4–8 years 1 tablet 3 times daily, 9–12 years 1 tablet 4 times daily, 13–16 years 2 tablets 3 times daily, but see also notes above

Liquid, red, sugar-free, co-phenotrope 2.5/0.025 (diphenoxylate hydrochloride 2.5 mg, atropine sulphate 25 micrograms)/5 mL. Net price 100 mL = £3.73

Dose: initially 20 mL, followed by 10 mL every 6 hours until diarrhoea controlled; CHILD under 4 years not recommended, 4–8 years 5 mL 3 times daily, 9–12 years 5 mL 4 times daily, 13–16 years 10 mL 3 times daily, but see also notes above

Note. Co-phenotrope 2.5/0.025 tablets are also available from Mepra-pharm (Diarphen®) and Norgine (Tropergen®)

LOPERAMIDE HYDROCHLORIDE

Indications: adjunct to rehydration in acute diarrhoea in adults and children over 4 years (but see notes above); chronic diarrhoea in adults only

Cautions; Contra-indications: see notes above and under Codeine Phosphate (except dependence)

Side-effects: abdominal cramps and skin reactions, including urticaria reported; paralytic ileus and abdominal bloating also reported

Dose: acute diarrhoea, 4 mg initially followed by 2 mg after each loose stool for up to 5 days; usual dose 6–8 mg daily; max. 16 mg daily; CHILD under 4 years not recommended, 4–8 years 1 mg 3–4 times daily for up to *3 days only*, 9–12 years 2 mg 4 times daily for up to 5 days

Chronic diarrhoea in adults, initially, 4–8 mg daily in divided doses, subsequently adjusted according to response and given in 2 divided doses for maintenance; max. 16 mg daily

PoM ¹ **Loperamide** (Non-proprietary)

Capsules, loperamide hydrochloride 2 mg. Net generic prescription price 30 = £1.62

Available from Berk (Diocaps®), Cox, Generics, Hillcross, Norgine (LoperaGen®), Norton, Tillomed (Normaloe®), Unichem

---

PoM [1] **Imodium®** (Janssen)

Capsules, green/grey, loperamide hydrochloride 2 mg. Net price 30 = £2.17

Syrup, red, sugar-free, loperamide hydrochloride 1 mg/5 mL. Net price 100 mL = £1.90

1. Loperamide can be sold to the public, for adults and children over 12 years, provided it is licensed and labelled for the treatment of acute diarrhoea; proprietary brands (NHS Arret® capsules, Diasorb® capsules and NHS Diocalm Ultra® capsules) are on sale to the public

MORPHINE

Indications: see notes above

Cautions; Contra-indications; Side-effects: see notes above and under Codeine Phosphate, sedation and the risk of dependence are greater

Kaolin and Morphine Mixture, BP

(Kaolin and Morphine Oral Suspension)

Oral suspension, light kaolin or light kaolin (natural) 20%, sodium bicarbonate 5%, and chloroform and morphine tincture 4% in a suitable vehicle. Contains 550 to 800 micrograms of anhydrous morphine/10 mL.

Dose: 10 mL every 4 hours in water

1.5   Treatment of chronic diarrhoeas

Once tumours are ruled out individual complaints need specific treatment including dietary manipulation as well as drug treatment and the maintenance of a liberal fluid intake.

IRRITABLE BOWEL SYNDROME

Irritable bowel syndrome can present with pain, constipation, or diarrhoea, all of which may benefit from a high-fibre diet with bran or other agents which increase stool bulk (section 1.6.1) if necessary. In some patients there may be important psychological aggravating factors which respond to reassurance. Antimotility drugs such as **loperamide** (see section 1.4.2) may relieve diarrhoea and antispasmodic drugs (see section 1.2) may relieve pain. Opioids with a central action such as codeine are better avoided because of the risk of dependence.

MALABSORPTION SYNDROMES

Individual conditions need specific management and also general nutritional consideration. Thus coeliac disease (gluten enteropathy) usually needs a gluten-free diet (Appendix 7) and pancreatic insufficiency needs pancreatin supplements (section 1.9.4).

ULCERATIVE COLITIS

For *acute attacks* of ulcerative colitis topical **corticosteroid** treatment such as prednisolone enemas or suppositories for localised rectal disease will induce remission; foam preparations are especially useful where patients have difficulty retaining liquid enemas. More extensive disease requires oral corticosteroid treatment and severe extensive or fulminant disease needs hospital admission and intravenous corticosteroid administration.

Sulphasalazine, a chemical combination of sulphapyridine and 5-aminosalicylic acid ('5-ASA') is useful in mild symptomatic disease requiring oral treatment; it is also available as suppositories for rectal disease. Activity resides in the 5-aminosalicylic acid moiety; sulphapyridine acts only as a carrier to the colonic site of action (but it still causes side-effects). Newer alternatives include **mesalazine** (5-aminosalicylic acid itself) and **olsalazine** (2 molecules of 5-aminosalicylic acid bonded together, separating in the lower bowel). Sulphonamide-related side-effects of sulphasalazine are avoided, but 5-aminosalicylate alone can still cause a range of adverse effects including blood disorders and lupoid phenomenon seen with sulphasalazine. Olsalazine may also be particularly prone to cause watery diarrhoea.

Corticosteroids are unsuitable for *maintenance treatment* because of side-effects. Sulphasalazine, mesalazine, and olsalazine all have value in preventing relapse and choice is related in part to their different side-effects. In resistant cases **azathioprine** (see section 8.2.1), 2 mg/kg daily, given under close supervision may be helpful [unlicensed indication].

Laxatives are required to facilitate bowel movement when proctitis is present but a high-fibre diet and bulk-forming drugs such as **methylcellulose** are more useful in adjusting faecal consistency (section 1.6.1).

Antimotility drugs such as codeine and loperamide should not be used in severe colitis as they can precipitate paralytic ileus and megacolon. They have limited value in mild disease, but treatment of the inflammation is more logical. For similar reasons antispasmodics should **not** be used in ulcerative colitis.

CROHN'S DISEASE

Treatment of Crohn's disease (particularly of colonic disease) is similar to that for ulcerative colitis. In small bowel disease the **aminosalicylates** may have marginal value. **Oral corticosteroids** (e.g. prednisolone) suppress inflammation, and **metronidazole** may be beneficial possibly through antibacterial activity. Other antibacterials should be given if specifically indicated and for managing bacterial overgrowth in the small bowel.

In both colitis and Crohn's disease general nutritional care and appropriate supplements are essential.

ANTIBIOTIC-ASSOCIATED COLITIS

Antibiotic-associated colitis (pseudomembranous colitis) is caused by colonisation of the colon with *Clostridium difficile* which may follow antibiotic therapy. It is usually of acute onset, but may run a chronic course; it is a particular hazard of clindamycin but few antibiotics are free of this side-effect. Oral **vancomycin** (see section 5.1.7) or **metronidazole** (see section 5.1.11) are used as specific treatment; vancomycin may be preferred for very sick patients.

DIVERTICULAR DISEASE

Diverticular disease is treated with a high-fibre diet, **bran supplements**, and **bulk-forming drugs**. **Antispasmodics** may provide symptomatic relief when colic is a problem (section 1.2). **Antibiotics** are used only when the diverticula in the intestinal wall become infected (specialist referral). **Antimotility** drugs which slow intestinal motility, e.g. codeine, diphenoxylate, and loperamide could possibly exacerbate the symptoms of diverticular disease and are **contra-indicated**.

AMINOSALICYLATES

CSM recommendation (blood disorders)
The CSM has recommended that patients receiving mesalazine, olsalazine or sulphasalazine should be advised to report any unexplained bleeding, bruising, purpura, sore throat, fever or malaise that occurs during treatment. A blood count should be performed and the drug stopped immediately if there is suspicion of a blood dyscrasia.

MESALAZINE

Indications: induction and maintenance of remission in ulcerative colitis
Cautions: pregnancy and breast-feeding
BLOOD DISORDERS. See CSM recommendation above
Contra-indications: salicylate hypersensitivity; renal impairment (nephrotoxic)
Side-effects: nausea, diarrhoea, and abdominal pain; headache; exacerbation of symptoms of colitis; rarely reversible pancreatitis, hepatitis, and interstitial nephritis; leucopenia, neutropenia, thrombocytopenia and aplastic anaemia reported; myocarditis, lupus phenomenon, fibrosing alveolitis also reported
Dose: see under preparations, below

PoM Asacol® (SK&F)
Tablets, red, e/c, mesalazine 400 mg. Net price 120-tab pack = £39.62. Label: 5, 25, counselling, blood disorder symptoms (see CSM recommendation above)
Dose: acute attack, 6 tablets daily in divided doses; maintenance 3–6 tablets daily in divided doses; CHILD not recommended
Note. Preparations that lower stool pH (e.g. lactulose) may prevent release of mesalazine
Foam enema, mesalazine 1 g/metered application. Net price 14 g (14 applications) with disposable applicators and plastic bags = £39.60. Counselling, blood disorder symptoms (see CSM recommendation above)
Dose: acute attack affecting the rectosigmoid region, 1 metered application (mesalazine 1 g) into the rectum daily for 4–6 weeks; CHILD not recommended
Acute attack affecting the descending colon, 2 metered applications (mesalazine 2 g) into the rectum daily for 4–6 weeks; CHILD not recommended

Suppositories, mesalazine 250 mg, net price 20-suppos pack = £6.50; 500 mg, 10 = £6.50. Counselling, blood disorder symptoms (see CSM recommendation above)
Dose: 3–6 suppositories of 250 mg (max. 3 suppositories of 500 mg) daily in divided doses, with last dose at bedtime; CHILD not recommended

PoM Pentasa® (Yamanouchi)
Slow Release tablets, m/r, both scored, mesalazine 250 mg, net price 200-tab pack = £32.28; 500 mg (grey), 100-tab pack = £32.28. Counselling, administration, see dose, blood disorder symptoms (see CSM recommendation above)
Dose: acute attack, up to 4 g daily in 2–3 divided doses; maintenance, 1.5 g daily in 2–3 divided doses; tablets may be dispersed in water, but should not be chewed; CHILD not recommended
Retention enema, mesalazine 1 g in 100-mL pack. Net price 7 enemas = £19.45. Counselling, blood disorder symptoms (see CSM recommendation above)
Dose: 1 enema at bedtime; CHILD not recommended
Suppositories, mesalazine 1 g. Net price 28-suppos pack = £44.68. Counselling, blood disorder symptoms (see CSM recommendation above)
Dose: ulcerative proctitis, acute attack, 1 suppository daily for 2–4 weeks; maintenance, 1 suppository daily; CHILD under 15 years not recommended

PoM Salofalk® (Thames)
Tablets, e/c, yellow, mesalazine 250 mg. Net price 100-tab pack = £17.50. Label: 5, 25, counselling, blood disorder symptoms (see CSM recommendation above)
Dose: acute attack, 6 tablets daily in 3 divided doses; maintenance 3–6 tablets daily in divided doses; CHILD not recommended
Suppositories, mesalazine 500 mg. Net price 30-suppos pack = £19.43. Counselling, blood disorder symptoms (see CSM recommendations above)
Dose: acute attack, 1–2 suppositories 2–3 times daily adjusted according to response; CHILD not recommended
Enema, mesalazine 2 g in 59-mL pack. Net price 7 enemas = £38.50. Counselling, blood disorder symptoms (see CSM recommendations above)
Dose: acute attack *or* maintenance, 1 enema daily at bedtime; CHILD not recommended

OLSALAZINE SODIUM

Indications: induction and maintenance of remission in ulcerative colitis
Cautions: pregnancy and breast-feeding
BLOOD DISORDERS. See CSM recommendation above
Contra-indications: salicylate hypersensitivity; renal impairment
Side-effects: watery diarrhoea, abdominal cramps, headache, nausea, dyspepsia, arthralgia, and rash; rarely reversible pancreatitis
Dose: acute attack, 1 g daily in divided doses after meals increased if necessary over 1 week to max. 3 g daily (max. single dose 1 g)
Maintenance, 500 mg twice daily after meals

PoM **Dipentum®** (Pharmacia)

Capsules, brown, olsalazine sodium 250 mg. Net price 100-cap pack = £25.63. Label: 21, counselling, blood disorder symptoms (see CSM recommendation above)

Tablets, yellow, scored, olsalazine sodium 500 mg. Net price 60-tab pack = £30.76. Label: 21, counselling, blood disorder symptoms (see CSM recommendation above)

SULPHASALAZINE

(Sulfasalazine)

Indications: induction and maintenance of remission in ulcerative colitis; active Crohn's disease; rheumatoid arthritis, see section 10.1.3

Cautions: history of allergy; hepatic and renal disease; G6PD deficiency; slow acetylator status; risk of haematological and hepatic toxicity (differential white cell, red cell and platelet counts initially and at monthly intervals for first 3 months, liver function tests at monthly intervals for first 3 months; upper gastro-intestinal side-effects common over 4 g daily; pregnancy and breast-feeding (see Appendixes 4 and 5); porphyria (see section 9.8.2)

BLOOD DISORDERS. See CSM recommendation above

Contra-indications: salicylate and sulphonamide hypersensitivity; CHILD under 2 years of age

Side-effects: nausea, vomiting, epigastric discomfort, headache, rashes; *occasionally:* fever, minor haematological abnormalities such as Heinz-body anaemia, reversible neutropenia, folate deficiency; reversible oligospermia; *rarely:* pancreatitis, hepatitis, exacerbation of colitis, thrombocytopenia, agranulocytosis, aplastic anaemia, Stevens–Johnson syndrome, neurotoxicity, photosensitisation, lupus erythematosus-like syndrome, and fibrosing alveolitis; proteinuria, crystalluria, haematuria, and nephrotic syndrome; urine may be coloured orange; some soft contact lenses may be stained

Dose: by mouth, acute attack 1–2 g 4 times daily (but see **cautions**) until remission occurs (if necessary corticosteroids may also be given), reducing to a maintenance dose of 500 mg 4 times daily; CHILD over 2 years, acute attack 40–60 mg/kg daily, maintenance dose 20–30 mg/kg daily

By rectum, in suppositories, alone or in conjunction with oral treatment 0.5–1 g morning and night after a bowel movement. As an enema, 3 g at night, retained for at least 1 hour

PoM **Sulphasalazine** (Non-proprietary)

Tablets, sulphasalazine 500 mg. Net generic prescription price 100 = £6.54. Label: 14, counselling, blood disorder symptoms (see CSM recommendation above), contact lenses may be stained

Available from APS, Berk, Cox, Lagap

PoM **Salazopyrin®** (Pharmacia)

Tablets, yellow, scored, sulphasalazine 500 mg. Net price 20 = £1.45. Label: 14, counselling, blood disorder symptoms (see CSM recommendation above), contact lenses may be stained

EN-Tabs® (= tablets e/c), yellow, f/c, sulphasalazine 500 mg. Net price 100-tab pack = £10.81. Label: 5, 14, 25, counselling, blood disorder symptoms (see CSM recommendation above), contact lenses may be stained

Suspension, yellow, sulphasalazine 250 mg/5 mL. Net price 500 mL = £16.44. Label: 14, counselling, blood disorder symptoms (see CSM recommendation above), contact lenses may be stained

Suppositories, yellow, sulphasalazine 500 mg. Net price 10 = £2.88; 50 = £13.67. Label: 14, counselling, blood disorder symptoms (see CSM recommendation above), contact lenses may be stained

Retention enema, sulphasalazine 3 g in 100-mL single-dose disposable packs fitted with a nozzle. Net price 7 × 100 mL = £12.43. Label: 14, counselling, blood disorder symptoms (see CSM recommendation above), contact lenses may be stained

---

ANION-EXCHANGE RESINS

CHOLESTYRAMINE

(Colestyramine)

Indications: diarrhoea associated with Crohn's disease, ileal resection, vagotomy, diabetic vagal neuropathy, and radiation; pruritus in liver disease, and hypercholesterolaemia, see section 2.12

Cautions; Contra-indications; Side-effects: see section 2.12

Dose: diarrhoea, after initial introduction over 3–4 week period, 12–24 g daily mixed with water (or other suitable liquid), in single or up to 4 divided doses, subsequently adjusted as required; max. 36 g daily

CHILD 6–12 years, see data sheet

COUNSELLING. Other drugs should be taken at least 1 hour before or 4–6 hours after cholestyramine to reduce possible interference with absorption

Preparations

Section 2.12

CORTICOSTEROIDS

BUDESONIDE

Indications: induction of remission in mild to moderate Crohn's disease affecting the ileum or ascending colon

Cautions; Contra-indications; Side-effects: see section 6.3.2

Dose: see under Preparations

PoM **Entocort® CR** (Astra)

Capsules, e/c, m/r, grey/pink, budesonide 3 mg. Net price 100-cap pack = £90.00. Label: 5, 10 steroid card, 22, 25

Note. Dispense in original container (contains desiccant)

Dose: 9 mg once daily in the morning before breakfast for up to 8 weeks; reduce dose for the last 2–4 weeks of treatment. See also section 6.3.2

CHILD not recommended

HYDROCORTISONE

Indications: ulcerative colitis, proctitis, proctosig-moiditis

Cautions; Contra-indications; Side-effects: systemic absorption may occur, see section 6.3.2; local irritation may also occur; prolonged use should be avoided; avoid use of enemas and rectal foams in obstruction, bowel perforation, and extensive fistulas; contra-indicated in untreated infection

Dose: rectal, see under Preparations

PoM Colifoam® (Stafford-Miller)
Foam in aerosol pack, hydrocortisone acetate 10%. Net price 20.8 g (14 applications) with applicator = £7.07
Dose: initially 1 metered application (125 mg hydrocortisone acetate) inserted into the rectum once or twice daily for 2–3 weeks, then once on alternate days

PREDNISOLONE

Indications: ulcerative colitis, and Crohn's disease; other indications, see section 6.3.2, see also preparations

Cautions; Contra-indications; Side-effects: see under Hydrocortisone and section 6.3.2

Dose: by mouth, initial dose 40 mg daily, in single or divided doses, until remission occurs, followed by reducing doses

By rectum, see under Preparations

Oral preparations, see section 6.3.2

Rectal preparations
PoM Predenema® (Pharmax)
Retention enema, prednisolone 20 mg (as sodium metasulphobenzoate) in 100-mL single-dose disposable pack. Net price 1 (standard tube) = 80p, 1 (long tube) = £1.35
Dose: ulcerative colitis, initially 1 enema at bedtime for 2–4 weeks, extending course if good response obtained; CHILD not recommended
PoM Predfoam® (Pharmax)
Foam in aerosol pack, prednisolone 20 mg (as metasulphobenzoate sodium)/metered application. Net price 25 g (14 applications) with disposable applicators = £7.06
Dose: proctitis and distal ulcerative colitis, 1 metered application (containing 20 mg prednisolone) inserted into the rectum once or twice daily for 2 weeks, continued for further 2 weeks if good response; CHILD not recommended
PoM Predsol® (Evans)
Retention enema, prednisolone 20 mg (as sodium phosphate) in 100-mL single-dose disposable packs fitted with a nozzle. Net price 7 = £5.24
Dose: rectal and rectosigmoidal ulcerative colitis and Crohn's disease, initially 1 enema at bedtime for 2–4 weeks, extending course if good response obtained; CHILD not recommended
Suppositories, prednisolone 5 mg (as sodium phosphate). Net price 10 = £1.00
Dose: ADULT and CHILD proctitis and rectal complications of Crohn's disease, 1 suppository inserted night and morning after a bowel movement

CROMOGLYCATE

SODIUM CROMOGLYCATE
(Sodium cromoglicate)

Indications: food allergy (in conjunction with dietary restriction); asthma, section 3.3; allergic conjunctivitis, section 11.4.2; allergic rhinitis, section 12.2.1

Side-effects: occasional nausea, rashes, and joint pain

Dose: 200 mg 4 times daily before meals; CHILD 2–14 years 100 mg; capsules may be swallowed whole or the contents dissolved in hot water and diluted with cold water before taking. May be increased if necessary after 2–3 weeks to a max. of 40 mg/kg daily and then reduced according to the response

PoM Nalcrom® (Fisons)
Capsules, sodium cromoglycate 100 mg. Net price 100 = £31.82. Label: 22, counselling, see dose above

1.6   Laxatives

1.6.1   Bulk-forming laxatives
1.6.2   Stimulant laxatives
1.6.3   Faecal softeners
1.6.4   Osmotic laxatives
1.6.5   Bowel cleansing solutions

Before prescribing laxatives it is important to be sure that the patient *is* constipated and that the constipation is *not* secondary to an underlying undiagnosed complaint.

It is also important for those who complain of constipation to understand that bowel habit can vary considerably in frequency without doing harm. Some people tend to consider themselves constipated if they do not have a bowel movement each day. A useful definition of constipation is the passage of hard stools less frequently than the patient's own normal pattern and this can be explained to the patient.

Misconceptions about bowel habits have led to excessive laxative use. Abuse may lead to hypokalaemia and an atonic non-functioning colon.

Thus, laxatives should generally be **avoided** except where straining will exacerbate a condition (such as angina) or increase the risk of rectal bleeding as in haemorrhoids. Laxatives are also of value in *drug-induced constipation,* for the expulsion of *parasites* after anthelmintic treatment, and to clear the alimentary tract before *surgery and radiological procedures.* Prolonged treatment of constipation is seldom necessary except occasionally in the elderly.

CHILDREN. The use of laxatives in children is undesirable and the introduction of fruit purée into the diet may be sufficient to regulate bowel action. In infants constipation is often remedied by adjustment of the diet.

The laxatives that follow have been divided into 4 main groups (sections 1.6.1–1.6.4). This simple classification disguises the fact that some laxatives have a complex action.

1.6.1 Bulk-forming laxatives

Bulk-forming laxatives relieve constipation by increasing faecal mass which stimulates peristalsis; the full effect may take some days to develop and patients should be told this.

Bulk-forming laxatives are of particular value in those with small hard stools, but should not be required unless fibre cannot be increased in the diet. A balanced diet, including adequate fluid intake and fibre is of value in preventing constipation.

Bulk-forming laxatives are useful in the management of patients with *colostomy, ileostomy, haemorrhoids, anal fissure, chronic diarrhoea associated with diverticular disease, irritable bowel syndrome,* and as adjuncts in *ulcerative colitis* (section 1.5). Adequate fluid intake must be maintained to avoid intestinal obstruction. Unprocessed wheat **bran**, taken with food or fruit juice, is a most effective bulk-forming preparation. Finely ground bran, though more palatable, has poorer water-retaining properties, but can be taken as bran bread or biscuits in appropriately increased quantities. Oat bran is also used.

Methylcellulose, ispaghula, and **sterculia** are useful in patients who cannot tolerate bran. Methylcellulose also acts as a faecal softener.

BRAN

Indications: see notes above

Cautions; Contra-indications; Side-effects: see under Ispaghula Husk. Avoid in gluten enteropathies and coeliac disease

Dose: see preparation below

COUNSELLING. Preparations that swell in contact with liquid should always be carefully swallowed with water and should not be taken immediately before going to bed

Trifyba® (Sanofi Winthrop)

Powder, brown, wheat fibre 80%. Net price 56 sachets containing 3.5 g = £3.28. Counselling, see below

Note. Contains gluten

Dose: 1 sachet 2–3 times daily added to food; CHILD half to one sachet 1–2 times daily added to food

COUNSELLING. At least one glass of water or other liquid should be drunk with the meal

ISPAGHULA HUSK

Indications: see notes above

Cautions: adequate fluid intake should be maintained to avoid intestinal obstruction—it may be necessary to supervise elderly or debilitated patients or those with intestinal narrowing or decreased motility

Contra-indications: difficulty in swallowing, intestinal obstruction, colonic atony, faecal impaction

Side-effects: flatulence, abdominal distension, gastro-intestinal obstruction or impaction; hypersensitivity reported

Dose: see preparations below

COUNSELLING. Preparations that swell in contact with liquid should always be carefully swallowed with water and should not be taken immediately before going to bed

Fybogel® (R&C)

Granules, buff, effervescent, sugar- and gluten-free, ispaghula husk 3.5 g/sachet (low Na$^+$). Net price 60 sachets (plain, lemon, or orange flavoured) = £4.24. Label: 13, counselling, see above

Note. Contains aspartame 50 mg/sachet (see section 9.4.1)

Dose: 1 sachet in water twice daily preferably after meals; CHILD 6–12 years ½–1 level 5-mL spoonful (children under 6 years on doctor's advice only)

Konsyl® (Eastern)

Powder, gluten-free, ispaghula husk (micronised), *Konsyl Sugar Free* (6 g/sachet), net price 30-sachet pack = £3.99; *Konsyl Dex* (3.4 g/sachet with glucose 8 g), 60-sachet pack = £3.99; *Konsyl Orange* (3.4 g/sachet), 60-sachet pack = £3.99. Label 13, counselling, see above

Dose: 1 sachet in water 1–3 times daily before or after meals; CHILD over 6 years, ½ adult dose or less (children under 6 years on doctor's advice only)

Diarrhoea (section 1.4.1), 1 sachet in water 3 times daily

Important. Each sachet of *Konsyl Sugar Free* contains almost twice as much ispaghula husk as *Konsyl Dex* or *Konsyl Orange*

Isogel® (Pfizer Consumer)

Granules, brown, sugar- and gluten-free, ispaghula husk 90%. Net price 300 g = £2.94. Label: 13, counselling, see above

Dose: constipation, 2 teaspoonfuls in water once or twice daily, preferably at mealtimes; CHILD 1 teaspoonful

Diarrhoea (section 1.4.1), 1 teaspoonful 3 times daily

Regulan® (Procter & Gamble)

Powder, beige, effervescent, gluten-free, ispaghula husk 3.6 g/6.4-g sachet (original flavour) or 3.4 g/5.85-g sachet (orange or lemon/lime flavour). Net price 30 sachets = £2.12. Label: 13, counselling, see above

Note. The original-flavour version contains potassium 6.4 mmol/sachet; the orange and the lemon/lime-flavour versions contain potassium <1 mmol/sachet and are sugar-free (contain aspartame)

Dose: 1 sachet in 150 mL water 1–3 times daily; CHILD 6–12 years 2.5–5 mL

METHYLCELLULOSE

Indications: see notes above; obesity, see section 4.5.1

Cautions; Contra-indications; Side-effects: see under Ispaghula Husk

Dose: see preparations below

COUNSELLING. Preparations that swell in contact with liquid should always be carefully swallowed with water and should not be taken immediately before going to bed

Celevac® (Monmouth)

Tablets, pink, scored, methylcellulose '450' 500 mg. Net price 112-tab pack = £2.69. Counselling, see above and dose

Dose: 3–6 tablets twice daily. In constipation the dose should be taken with at least 300 mL of water. In diarrhoea, ileostomy, and colostomy control, minimise liquid intake for 30 minutes before and after the dose

STERCULIA

Indications: see notes above

Cautions; Contra-indications; Side-effects: see under Ispaghula Husk

COUNSELLING. Preparations that swell in contact with liquid should always be carefully swallowed with water and should not be taken immediately before going to bed

Normacol® (Norgine)

Granules, coated, gluten-free, sterculia 62%. Net price 500 g = £5.53; 60 × 7-g sachets = £4.65. Label: 25, 27, counselling, see above

Dose: 1–2 heaped 5-mL spoonfuls, or the contents of 1–2 sachets, washed down without chewing with plenty of liquid once or twice daily after meals; CHILD 6–12 years half adult dose

Normacol Plus® (Norgine)

Granules, brown, coated, gluten-free, sterculia 62%, frangula (standardised) 8%. Net price 500 g = £5.92; 60 × 7 g sachets = £4.98. Label: 25, 27, counselling, see above

Dose: constipation and after haemorrhoidectomy, 1–2 heaped 5-mL spoonfuls or the contents of 1–2 sachets washed down without chewing with plenty of liquid once or twice daily after meals

Prefil®

See section 4.5.1

1.6.2   Stimulant laxatives

The recognised stimulant laxatives include **bisacodyl** and members of the **anthraquinone** group, e.g. senna. **Docusate** sodium probably acts both as a stimulant and as a softening agent. **Danthron** has limited indications (see below) because *rodent* studies indicate potential carcinogenic risk. Powerful stimulants such as **cascara** and **castor oil** are obsolete.

Stimulant laxatives increase intestinal motility and often cause abdominal cramp. They should not be used in intestinal obstruction, and prolonged use can precipitate the onset of an atonic non-functioning colon and hypokalaemia. They should preferably be avoided in children.

Glycerol suppositories act as a rectal stimulant by virtue of the mildly irritant action of glycerol.

Soft soap is a more severe irritant; the use of soft soap enema should be **avoided**, especially in pregnancy, as it may inflame the colonic mucosa.

The **parasympathomimetics** bethanechol, distigmine, neostigmine, and pyridostigmine (see sections 7.4.1 and 10.2.1) enhance parasympathetic activity in the gut and increase intestinal motility.

They are rarely used for their gastro-intestinal effects. Organic obstruction of the gut must first be excluded and they should not be used shortly after bowel anastomosis.

Oxyphenisatin is indicated for diagnostic procedures or surgery only, since it causes hepatitis in chronic use.

BISACODYL

Indications: see under Dose; tablets act in 10–12 hours; suppositories act in 20–60 minutes

Cautions; Contra-indications; Side-effects: see notes on stimulant laxatives; tablets, griping; suppositories, local irritation

Dose: by mouth for constipation, 5–10 mg at night; occasionally necessary to increase to 15–20 mg; CHILD under 10 years 5 mg

By rectum in suppositories for constipation, 10 mg in the morning; CHILD under 10 years 5 mg

Before radiological procedures and surgery, 10 mg by mouth at bedtime for 2 days before examination and, if necessary, a 10-mg suppository 1 hour before examination; CHILD half adult dose.

Bisacodyl (Non-proprietary)

Tablets, e/c, bisacodyl 5 mg. Net generic prescription price 20 = 22p. Label: 5, 25

Suppositories, bisacodyl 10 mg. Net generic prescription price 12 = 84p

Paediatric suppositories, bisacodyl 5 mg. Net generic prescription price 5 = 81p

Note. The brand name ₦₭₷ Dulco-lax® (Windsor) is used for bisacodyl tablets, net price 20-tab pack = £1.00; suppositories (10 mg), 10 = £1.39; paediatric suppositories (5 mg), 5 = 81p
The brand name Dulco-lax® Liquid is used for sodium picosulphate elixir

DANTHRON

(Dantron)

Indications: only for: constipation in geriatric practice; prophylaxis and treatment of analgesic-induced constipation in terminally ill patients of all ages; constipation in cardiac failure and coronary thrombosis (conditions in which bowel movement must be free of strain); acts within 6–12 hours

Cautions; Contra-indications; Side-effects: see notes on stimulant laxatives; urine may be coloured red; avoid prolonged contact with skin (as in incontinent patients) since irritation and excoriation may occur; avoid in pregnancy and breast-feeding; *rodent* studies indicate potential carcinogenic risk

Dose: see under preparations

With poloxamer '188' (as co-danthramer)

Note. Co-danthramer suspension 5 mL = one co-danthramer capsule, **but** strong co-danthramer suspension 5 mL = two strong co-danthramer capsules

PoM **Co-danthramer** (Non-proprietary)

Capsules, co-danthramer 25/200 (danthron 25 mg, poloxamer '188' 200 mg). Net generic prescription price 60-cap pack = £12.86. Label: 14 (urine red)

Dose: 1–2 capsules at bedtime; CHILD 1 capsule at bedtime (restricted indications, see notes above)
Available from Napp

Strong capsules, co-danthramer 37.5/500 (danthron 37.5 mg, poloxamer '188' 500 mg). Net generic prescription price 60-cap pack = £15.55. Label: 14 (urine red)

Dose: 1–2 capsules at bedtime (restricted indications, see notes above); CHILD under 12 years not recommended
Available from Napp

Suspension, co-danthramer 25/200 in 5 mL (danthron 25 mg, poloxamer '188' 200 mg/5 mL). Net generic prescription price 300 mL = £11.20, 1 litre = £37.53. Label: 14 (urine red)

Dose: 5–10 mL at night; CHILD 2.5–5 mL (restricted indications, see notes above)
Available from Galen (Ailax®), Hillcross, Napp (NHS Codalax®)

Strong suspension, co-danthramer 75/1000 in 5 mL (danthron 75 mg, poloxamer '188' 1 g/ 5 mL). Net generic prescription price 300 mL = £30.12, 1 litre = £100.36. Label: 14 (urine red)

Dose: 5 mL at night (restricted indications, see notes above); CHILD under 12 years not recommended
Available from Napp (NHS Codalax Forte®)

With docusate sodium (as co-danthrusate)

PoM **Co-danthrusate** (Non-proprietary)

Capsules, co-danthrusate 50/60 (danthron 50 mg, docusate sodium 60 mg). Net generic prescription price 63-cap pack = £13.46. Label: 14 (urine red)
Dose: 1–3 capsules, usually at night; CHILD 6–12 years 1 capsule (restricted indications, see notes above)
Available from Evans (NHS Normax®), Galen (Capsuvac®), Hillcross

Suspension, yellow, co-danthrusate 50/60 (danthron 50 mg, docusate sodium 60 mg/5 mL). Net generic prescription price 200 mL = £6.40. Label: 14 (urine red)

Dose: 5–15 mL at night; CHILD 6–12 years 5 mL at night (restricted indications, see notes above)
Available from Evans (NHS Normax®)

DOCUSATE SODIUM

(Dioctyl Sodium Sulphosuccinate)

Indications: constipation (oral preparations act within 1–2 days); adjunct in abdominal radiological procedures

Cautions; Contra-indications; Side-effects: see notes on stimulant laxatives; do not give with liquid paraffin; rectal preparations not indicated if haemorrhoids or anal fissure

Dose: by mouth, constipation, up to 500 mg daily in divided doses; CHILD over 6 months 12.5 mg 3 times daily; 2–12 years 12.5–25 mg 3 times daily (use paediatric oral solution only)

With barium meal, 400 mg

Dioctyl® (Schwarz)

Capsules, yellow/white, docusate sodium 100 mg. Net price 100-cap pack = £4.65

[1] *Adult solution*, sugar-free, docusate sodium 50 mg/5 mL. Net price 300-mL pack = £2.48

1. Formerly Dioctyl® Oral Solution 1%

Paediatric solution, sugar-free, docusate sodium 12.5 mg/5 mL. Net price 125-mL pack = 97p

Rectal preparations
Fletchers' Enemette® (Pharmax)

Enema, docusate sodium 90 mg, glycerol 3.78 g/ 5 mL with macrogol and sorbic acid. Net price 5-mL unit = 32p

Dose: ADULT and CHILD over 3 years, 5-mL unit when required

Norgalax Micro-enema® (Norgine)

Enema, docusate sodium 120 mg in 10-g single-dose disposable packs. Net price 10-g unit = 64p

Dose: ADULT and CHILD over 12 years, 10-g unit

GLYCEROL

(Glycerin)

Indications: constipation
Dose: see below

Glycerol Suppositories, BP

(Glycerin Suppositories)

Suppositories, gelatin 140 mg, glycerol 700 mg, purified water to 1 g. Net price 12 = 51p (infant), 54p (child), 51p (adult)

Dose: 1 suppository moistened with water before use. The usual sizes are for *infants* small (1-g mould), *children* medium (2-g mould), *adults* large (4-g mould)

OXYPHENISATIN

(Oxyphenisatine)

Indications: see under Dose

Cautions; Contra-indications; Side-effects: see notes on stimulant laxatives; avoid repeated use owing to liver toxicity; **important:** consider general warnings relating to bowel cleansing solutions on p. 52

Veripaque® (Sanofi Winthrop)

Enema, powder for reconstitution, oxyphenisatin 50 mg in 3 g. Net price 1 vial = £2.03

Dose: by rectum before diagnostic procedures or surgery, oxyphenisatin 50 mg dissolved in 2 litres of water given over 5–8 minutes

Adjuvant to barium enema, oxyphenisatin 50 mg mixed thoroughly with 2 litres of barium sulphate enema

---

SENNA

Indications: constipation; acts in 8–12 hours
Cautions; Contra-indications; Side-effects: see notes on stimulant laxatives

Senna Tablets, total sennosides (calculated as sennoside B) 7.5 mg. Net price 20 = 30p

Dose: 2–4 tablets, usually at night; initial dose should be low then gradually increased; CHILD over 6 years, half adult dose (on doctor's advice only)
Note. The brand name NHS Senokot® (see below) is used for Senna tablets; for those on sale to the public lower dose recommended

---

Manevac® (Galen)

Granules, coated, senna fruit 12.4%, ispaghula 54.2%. Net price 250 g = £3.78, 400 g = £5.53, 56 × 4-g sachets = £3.80. Label: 25, 27, counselling, see Ispaghula Husk

Dose: 1–2 level 5-mL spoonfuls (or sachets) with water or warm drink after supper and, if necessary, before breakfast *or* every 6 hours in resistant cases for 1–3 days; CHILD 5–12 years 1 level 5-mL spoonful (or sachet) daily

Note. One level 5-mL spoonful is equivalent to one 4-g sachet

Senokot® (R&C)

NHS *Tablets*, see above

Granules, brown, total sennosides (calculated as sennoside B) 15 mg/5 mL or 5.5 mg/g (one 5-mL spoonful = 2.7 g). Net price 100 g = £2.25

Dose: 5–10 mL, usually at bedtime; CHILD over 6 years 2.5–5 mL in the morning

Note. Lower dose on packs on sale to the public

Syrup, brown, total sennosides (calculated as sennoside B) 7.5 mg/5 mL. Net price 100 mL pack = £1.58

Dose: 10–20 mL, usually at bedtime; CHILD 2–6 years 2.5–5 mL in the morning (doctor's advice only), over 6 years 5–10 mL

Note. Lower dose on packs on sale to the public

SODIUM PICOSULPHATE

(Sodium Picosulfate)

Indications: constipation; bowel evacuation before abdominal radiological procedures, endoscopy, and surgery (section 1.6.5)

Cautions; Contra-indications; Side-effects: see notes on stimulant laxatives

Dose: see below

Sodium Picosulphate Elixir, sodium picosulphate 5 mg/5 mL. Acts within 10–14 hours. Net price 100 mL = £1.47

Dose: 5–15 mL at night; CHILD 2–5 years 2.5 mL, 5–10 years 2.5–5 mL

Note. The brand names NHS Laxoberal® and Dulcolax® Liquid (both Windsor) are used for sodium picosulphate elixir 5 mg/5 mL

The brand name Dulco-lax® is also used for bisacodyl tablets and suppositories

Before radiography, endoscopy or surgery
See section 1.6.5

OTHER STIMULANT LAXATIVES

Unstandardised preparations of cascara, frangula, rhubarb, and senna should be **avoided** as their laxative action is unpredictable. Aloes, colocynth, and jalap should be **avoided** as they have a drastic purgative action.

Phenolphthalein can cause rashes. It may colour alkaline urine pink.

Stimulant laxative preparations on sale to the public (not prescribable on the NHS) together with their significant ingredients:

Agarol® (agar, liquid paraffin, phenolphthalein), **Alophen®** (aloin, phenolphthalein)
Beechams Pills® (aloin), **Bonomint®** (phenolphthalein), **Boots Compound Laxative®** (fig, senna), **Brooklax®** (phenolphthalein)
Califig® (fig, senna), **Calsalettes®** (aloin), **Carters Little Pills®** (aloin, phenolphthalein)
Delax® (liquid paraffin, phenolphthalein)
Ex-lax® (phenolphthalein)
Fam-lax® (phenolphthalein, rhubarb)
Juno Junipah Salts® (juniper berry oil, sodium bicarbonate, sodium phosphate, sodium sulphate), **Juno Junipah Tablets®** (juniper berry oil, phenolphthalein, sodium chloride, sodium phosphate, sodium sulphate)
Kest® (magnesium sulphate, phenolphthalein)
Nylax® (bisacodyl, phenolphthalein, senna)
Potter's Cleansing Herb® (aloes, cascara, senna)
Reguletts® (phenolphthalein), **Rhuaka®** (cascara, rhubarb, senna)
Senlax® (senna), **Sure-Lax®** (phenolphthalein)

1.6.3 Faecal softeners

Liquid paraffin, the classical lubricant, has disadvantages (see below). Bulk laxatives (section 1.6.1) and non-ionic surfactant 'wetting' agents e.g. docusate sodium (section 1.6.2) also have softening properties. Such drugs are useful for oral administration in the management of haemorrhoids and anal fissure; glycerol suppositories (section 1.6.2) are useful for rectal use.

Enemas containing **arachis oil** (ground-nut oil, peanut oil) lubricate and soften impacted faeces and promote a bowel movement.

ARACHIS OIL

Indications: see notes above
Dose: see below

Fletchers' Arachis Oil Retention Enema®
(Pharmax)

Enema, arachis oil in 130-mL single-dose disposable packs. Net price 130 mL = £1.07

Dose: to soften impacted faeces, 130 mL; the enema should be warmed before use; CHILD under 3 years not recommended; over 3 years reduce adult dose in proportion to body-weight (medical supervision only)

LIQUID PARAFFIN

Indications: constipation
Cautions: CSM recommends avoid prolonged use, and has contra-indicated in children less than 3 years of age
Side-effects: anal seepage of paraffin and consequent anal irritation after prolonged use, granulomatous reactions caused by absorption of small quantities of liquid paraffin (especially from the emulsion), lipoid pneumonia, and interference with the absorption of fat-soluble vitamins
Dose: see under preparation

Liquid Paraffin Oral Emulsion, BP

Oral emulsion, liquid paraffin 5 mL, vanillin 5 mg, chloroform 0.025 mL, benzoic acid solution 0.2 mL, methylcellulose-20 200 mg, saccharin sodium 500 micrograms, water to 10 mL

Dose: 10–30 mL at night when required

COUNSELLING. Should not be taken immediately before going to bed

With phenolphthalein, see Other Stimulant Laxatives

1.6.4   Osmotic laxatives

These act by retaining fluid in the bowel by osmosis or by changing the pattern of water distribution in the faeces.

Saline purgatives such as **magnesium hydroxide** are commonly abused but are satisfactory for occasional use; adequate fluid intake should be maintained. **Magnesium salts** are useful where rapid bowel evacuation is required. **Sodium salts** should be avoided as they may give rise to sodium and water retention in susceptible individuals. **Phosphate enemas** are useful in bowel clearance before radiology, endoscopy, and surgery.

Lactulose is a semi-synthetic disaccharide which is not absorbed from the gastro-intestinal tract. It produces an osmotic diarrhoea of low faecal pH, and discourages the proliferation of ammonia-producing organisms. It is therefore useful in the treatment of *hepatic encephalopathy*. **Lactitol** is a similar disaccharide.

LACTITOL

Indications; Contra-indications; Side-effects: see under Lactulose

Dose: constipation, initially 20 g daily in a single dose with morning or evening meal, subsequently adjusted to produce one stool daily (dose of 10 g daily may be sufficient); CHILD 1–6 years 2.5–5 g, 6–12 years 5–10 g, 12–16 years 10–20 g daily, subsequently adjusted to produce one stool daily

Hepatic encephalopathy, 500–700 mg/kg daily in 3 divided doses with meals, subsequently adjusted to produce 2 soft stools daily

By nasogastric administration, as a 40% solution (200 g/500 mL), 1–2 mL/kg body-weight daily

COUNSELLING. Powder should be mixed with food or liquid and one to two glasses of liquid should be drunk with the meal

Lactitol (Non-proprietary)

Powder, lactitol 10 g/sachet. Net price 10-sachet pack = £1.00. Counselling, see above

Available from Zyma

LACTULOSE

Indications: constipation (may take up to 48 hours to act), hepatic encephalopathy (portal systemic encephalopathy)

Contra-indications: galactosaemia, intestinal obstruction

Side-effects: flatulence, cramps, and abdominal discomfort

Dose: see under preparations below

COUNSELLING. Powder can be placed on tongue and washed down with water or other liquid *or* sprinkled on food *or* mixed with water or other liquid before swallowing

Lactulose (Non-proprietary)

Solution, lactulose 3.1–3.7 g/5 mL with other ketoses. Net generic prescription price 200-mL pack = £1.03

Dose: constipation, initially 15 mL twice daily, adjusted according to patient's needs; CHILD under 1 year 2.5 mL, 1–5 years 5 mL, 5–10 years 10 mL twice daily

Hepatic encephalopathy, 30–50 mL 3 times daily, subsequently adjusted to produce 2–3 soft stools daily

Available from APS, Ashbourne (Osmolax®), Berk (Laxose®), Cox, CP, Galen (Lactugal®), Norton, Sandoz (Regulose®), Solvay (NHS Duphalac®)

Note. A proprietary brand of lactulose 3.3 g/5 mL (Regulose®) is on sale to the public

Powder, lactulose 10 g/sachet, with other ketoses. Net price 30-sachet pack = £3.00. Counselling, see above

Dose: constipation, 10 g twice daily, adjusted according to patient's needs; CHILD 5–10 years 5 g twice daily, under 5 years lactulose solution recommended

Hepatic encephalopathy, 20–30 g 3 times daily, subsequently adjusted to produce 2–3 soft stools daily

Available from Solvay (Lactulose Dry, Duphalac Dry®)

MACROGOLS

(Polyethylene glycols)

Indications; Dose: see under preparation below

Cautions: pregnancy and breast-feeding

Contra-indications: intestinal perforation or obstruction, paralytic ileus, severe inflammatory conditions of the intestinal tract (such as Crohn's disease, ulcerative colitis, and toxic megacolon)

Side-effects: abdominal distension and pain, nausea

Movicol® (Norgine)

Oral powder, macrogol 3350 (polyethylene glycol 3350) 13.125 g, sodium bicarbonate 178.5 mg, sodium chloride 350.7 mg, potassium chloride 46.6 mg/sachet. Net price 20-sachet pack = £9.85. Label: 13

Dose: short-term treatment of chronic constipation, 2–3 sachets daily in divided doses; each sachet dissolved in 125 mL of water and drunk immediately; ELDERLY initially 1 sachet daily; CHILD not recommended

MAGNESIUM SALTS

Indications; Dose: see under preparations

Cautions: renal impairment (risk of magnesium accumulation); hepatic impairment (see Appendix 2); elderly and debilitated; see also notes above; **interactions:** Appendix 1 (magnesium salts)

Contra-indications: acute gastro-intestinal conditions

Side-effects: colic

Cautionary label wordings, see inside back cover

Magnesium hydroxide
Magnesium Hydroxide Mixture, BP
(Cream of Magnesia)
  Aqueous suspension containing about 8% hydrated magnesium oxide. Do not store in cold place
  Dose: constipation, 25–50 mL when required

Magnesium hydroxide with liquid paraffin
Liquid Paraffin and Magnesium Hydroxide Emulsion, BP
  Oral emulsion, 25% liquid paraffin in aqueous suspension containing 6% hydrated magnesium oxide
  Dose: constipation, 5–20 mL when required
  Note. Liquid paraffin and magnesium hydroxide preparations on sale to the public include: N̶H̶S̶ Cremaffin® and N̶H̶S̶ Milpar®

Magnesium sulphate
Magnesium Sulphate. Label: 13, 23
  Dose: rapid bowel evacuation (acts in 2–4 hours) 5–10 g in a tumblerful of water preferably before breakfast
  Note. Magnesium sulphate is on sale to the public as Epsom Salts; N̶H̶S̶ Andrews Liver Salts® (citric acid, magnesium sulphate, sodium bicarbonate) is also on sale to the public

For bowel evacuation before radiography and surgery
  See section 1.6.5

PHOSPHATES (RECTAL)
  Indications: rectal use in constipation; bowel evacuation before abdominal radiological procedures, endoscopy, and surgery
  Cautions: elderly and debilitated; see also notes above
  Contra-indications: acute gastro-intestinal conditions
  Side-effects: local irritation
  Dose: see below

Carbalax® (Pharmax)
  Suppositories, sodium acid phosphate 1.69 g (as anhydrous salt) in an effervescent basis. Net price 12 = £2.24
  Dose: constipation, 1 suppository, inserted 30 minutes before evacuation is required; moisten with water before use; CHILD, not recommended

Fleet® Ready-to-use Enema (De Witt)
  Enema, sodium acid phosphate 21.4 g, sodium phosphate 9.4 g/118 mL. Net price single-dose pack (standard tube) = 46p
  Dose: ADULT and CHILD over 12 years, 118 mL; CHILD 3–12 years, on doctor's advice only (under 3 years not recommended)

Fletchers' Phosphate Enema® (Pharmax)
  Enema, sodium acid phosphate 12.8 g, sodium phosphate 10.24 g, purified water, freshly boiled and cooled, to 128 mL (corresponds to Phosphates Enema Formula B). Net price 128 mL with standard tube = 46p, with long rectal tube = 64p
  Dose: 128 mL; CHILD, over 3 years, reduced according to body weight (under 3 years not recommended)

SODIUM CITRATE (RECTAL)
  Indications: rectal use in constipation
  Cautions: elderly and debilitated; see also notes above
  Contra-indications: acute gastro-intestinal conditions
  Dose: see below

Fleet® Micro-enema (De Witt)
  Enema, sodium citrate 450 mg, sodium lauryl sulphoacetate 45 mg, together with glycerol, sorbitol, propylene glycol, and carbopol, in 5-mL single-dose disposable packs with nozzle. Net price 5 mL = 45p
  Dose: ADULT and CHILD over 3 years, 5 mL

Micolette Micro-enema® (Dominion)
  Enema, sodium citrate 450 mg, sodium lauryl sulphoacetate 45 mg, glycerol 625 mg, together with citric acid, potassium sorbate, and sorbitol in a viscous solution, in 5-mL single-dose disposable packs with nozzle. Net price 5 mL = 32p
  Dose: ADULT and CHILD over 3 years, 5–10 mL

Micralax Micro-enema® (Evans)
  Enema, sodium citrate 450 mg, sodium alkylsulphoacetate 45 mg, sorbic acid 5 mg, together with glycerol and sorbitol in a viscous solution in 5-mL single-dose disposable packs with nozzle. Net price 5 mL = 45p
  Dose: ADULT and CHILD over 3 years, 5 mL

Relaxit Micro-enema® (Crawford)
  Enema, sodium citrate 450 mg, sodium lauryl sulphate 75 mg, sorbic acid 5 mg, together with glycerol and sorbitol in a viscous solution in 5-mL single-dose disposable packs with nozzle. Net price 5 mL = 31p
  Dose: ADULT and CHILD over 3 years, 5 mL

1.6.5   Bowel cleansing solutions

Bowel cleansing solutions are used before colonic surgery, colonoscopy, or radiological examination to ensure the bowel is free of solid contents. They are **not** treatments for constipation.

BOWEL CLEANSING SOLUTIONS
  Indications: see above
  Cautions: pregnancy; ulcerative colitis; diabetes mellitus; reflux oesophagitis; impaired gag reflex; unconscious or semiconscious or possibility of regurgitation or aspiration
  Contra-indications: gastro-intestinal obstruction, gastric retention, gastro-intestinal ulceration, perforated bowel; toxic colitis, toxic megacolon or ileus
  Side-effects: nausea and bloating; less frequently abdominal cramps (usually transient—reduced by taking more slowly); vomiting

Citramag® (Bioglan)
  Powder, effervescent, providing when dissolved in water magnesium citrate 17.7 g/sachet. Net price 10-sachet pack = £11.41. Label 10, patient information leaflet, 13, counselling, see below

---

Dose: bowel evacuation before radiological examination and surgery, 1 sachet dissolved in 200 mL water and taken at 8 a.m. on day before procedure; CHILD 5–9 years one-third adult dose; over 10 years one-half adult dose

COUNSELLING. The patient information leaflet advises that hot water is needed to make the solution and provides guidance on reconstitution; it also mentions need for high fluid, low residue diet beforehand (according to hospital advice), and explains that only clear fluids can be taken after Citramag® until procedure completed

Fleet Phospho-soda® (De Witt)

Oral solution, sugar-free, sodium dihydrogen phosphate dihydrate 24.4 g, disodium phosphate dodecahydrate 10.8 g/45 mL. Net price 2 × 45-mL bottles = £4.79. Label: 10 patient information leaflet, counselling

Dose: by mouth

First dose, in the morning (7.00 a.m.) on the day before the procedure, 45 mL diluted with half a glass (120 mL) of cool water, followed by one full glass (240 mL) of cool water

At mid-day, follow with at least 3 full glasses (720 mL) of water or clear liquids

Second dose, in the evening (7.00 p.m.) on the day before the procedure, 45 mL diluted with half a glass (120 mL) of cool water, followed by one full glass (240 mL) of cool water

Additional clear liquids may be taken up until midnight if necessary

CHILD not recommended

Note. No solid foods may be taken for breakfast, lunch or evening meal on the day of taking the preparation

Klean-Prep® (Norgine)

Oral powder, macrogol 3350 (polyethylene glycol 3350) 59 g, anhydrous sodium sulphate 5.685 g, sodium bicarbonate 1.685 g, sodium chloride 1.465 g, potassium chloride 743 mg/sachet. Contains aspartame (see section 9.4.1). Net price 4 sachets = £8.39. Label: 10 patient information leaflet, counselling

Four sachets when reconstituted with water to 4 litres provides an iso-osmotic solution for bowel cleansing before surgery, colonoscopy or radiological procedures

Dose: by mouth, 250 mL (1 tumblerful) of reconstituted solution every 10–15 minutes, or by nasogastric tube 20–30 mL/minute, until 4 litres have been consumed or watery stools are free of solid matter; CHILD not recommended

The solution from all 4 sachets should be drunk within 4–6 hours (250 mL drunk rapidly every 10–15 minutes); flavouring such as clear fruit cordials may be added if required; to facilitate gastric emptying domperidone or metoclopramide may be given 30 minutes before starting.

Alternatively the administration may be divided into two, e.g. taking the solutions from 2 sachets on the evening before examination and the remaining 2 on the morning of the examination

After reconstitution the solution should be kept in a refrigerator and discarded if unused after 24 hours

Note. Contra-indicated in patients under 20 kg body-weight; allergic reactions reported

Picolax® (Nordic)

Oral powder, sugar-free, sodium picosulphate 10 mg/sachet, with magnesium citrate (for bowel evacuation before radiological procedures, endoscopy, and surgery). Net price 2 sachets = 59p. Label: 10, patient information leaflet, 13, counselling, see below

Dose: ADULT and CHILD over 9 years, 1 sachet in water in morning (before 8 a.m.) and a second in afternoon (between 2 and 4 p.m.) of day preceding procedures; CHILD 1–2 years quarter sachet morning and afternoon, 2–4 years half sachet morning and afternoon, 4–9 years 1 sachet morning and half sachet afternoon

Acts within 3 hours of first dose

Note. Low residue diet recomended for 2 days before examination and copious intake of water or other clear fluids recommended during treatment

COUNSELLING. Patients should be warned that heat is generated on addition to water; for this reason the powder should be added initially to 30 mL (2 tablespoonfuls) of water; after 5 minutes (when reaction complete) the solution should be further diluted to 150 mL (about a tumblerful)

1.7 Preparations for haemorrhoids

1.7.1 Soothing haemorrhoidal preparations
1.7.2 Compound haemorrhoidal preparations with corticosteroids
1.7.3 Rectal sclerosants

Anal and perianal pruritus, soreness, and excoriation are best treated by application of bland ointments and suppositories (section 1.7.1). These conditions occur commonly in patients suffering from haemorrhoids, fistulas, and proctitis. Careful local toilet with attention to any minor faecal soiling, adjustment of the diet to avoid hard stools, the use of bulk-forming materials such as bran (section 1.6.1) and a high residue diet are helpful. In proctitis these measures may supplement treatment with corticosteroids or sulphasalazine (see section 1.5).

When necessary topical preparations containing **local anaesthetics** (section 1.7.1) or **corticosteroids** (section 1.7.2) are used provided perianal thrush has been excluded. Perianal thrush is best treated with **nystatin** by mouth and by local application (see sections 5.2, 7.2.2, and 13.10.2).

1.7.1 Soothing haemorrhoidal preparations

Soothing preparations containing mild astringents such as bismuth subgallate, zinc oxide, and hamamelis may give symptomatic relief in haemorrhoids. Many proprietary preparations also contain lubricants, vasoconstrictors, or mild antiseptics.

Local anaesthetics are used to relieve pain associated with *haemorrhoids,* and *pruritus ani* but good evidence is lacking. Lignocaine ointment (see section 15.2) is used before emptying the bowel to relieve pain associated with *anal fissure.* Alternative local anaesthetics include amethocaine, cinchocaine, and pramoxine, but they are more irritant. Local anaesthetic ointments can be absorbed through the rectal mucosa therefore excessive application should be **avoided**, particularly in infants and children. They should be used for short periods only (no longer than a few days) since they may cause sensitisation of the anal skin.

Soothing haemorrhoidal preparations on sale to the public together with their significant ingredients include:

Anacal® (heparinoid, laureth '9'), **Anodesyn®** (allantoin, lignocaine), **Anusol® cream** (bismuth oxide, Peru balsam, zinc oxide), **Anusol® ointment** and **suppositories** (bismuth oxide, bismuth subgallate, Peru balsam, zinc oxide)
Germoloids® (lignocaine, zinc oxide)
Hemocane® (benzoic acid, bismuth oxide, cinnamic acid, lignocaine, zinc oxide)
Lanacane® cream (benzocaine, chlorothymol, resorcinol)
Nupercainal® (cinchocaine)
Preparation H® (shark liver oil, yeast cell extract)

1.7.2   Compound haemorrhoidal preparations with corticosteroids

Corticosteroids are often combined with local anaesthetics and soothing agents in preparations for haemorrhoids. They are suitable for occasional short-term use after exclusion of infections, such as herpes simplex; see section 13.4 for general comments on topical corticosteroids and section 1.7.1 for comment on local anaesthetics.

PoM **Anugesic-HC®** (P-D)

Cream, benzyl benzoate 1.2%, bismuth oxide 0.875%, hydrocortisone acetate 0.5%, Peru balsam 1.85%, pramoxine hydrochloride 1%, zinc oxide 12.35%. Net price 30 g (with rectal nozzle) = £3.09

Apply night and morning and after a bowel movement; do not use for longer than 7 days; CHILD not recommended

Suppositories, buff, benzyl benzoate 33 mg, bismuth oxide 24 mg, bismuth subgallate 59 mg, hydrocortisone acetate 5 mg, Peru balsam 49 mg, pramoxine hydrochloride 27 mg, zinc oxide 296 mg. Net price 12 = £2.24

Insert 1 suppository night and morning and after a bowel movement; do not use for longer than 7 days; CHILD not recommended

PoM **Anusol-HC®** (P-D)

Ointment, benzyl benzoate 1.25%, bismuth oxide 0.875%, bismuth subgallate 2.25%, hydrocortisone acetate 0.25%, Peru balsam 1.875%, zinc oxide 10.75%. Net price 30 g (with rectal nozzle) = £2.90

Apply night and morning and after a bowel movement; do not use for longer than 7 days; CHILD not recommended
Note. A proprietary brand (Anusol Plus HC® ointment) is on sale to the public

Suppositories, benzyl benzoate 33 mg, bismuth oxide 24 mg, bismuth subgallate 59 mg, hydrocortisone acetate 10 mg, Peru balsam 49 mg, zinc oxide 296 mg. Net price 12 = £2.24

Additives: include tartrazine lake

Insert 1 suppository night and morning and after a bowel movement; do not use for longer than 7 days; CHILD not recommended
Note. A proprietary brand (Anusol Plus HC® suppositories) is on sale to the public

PoM **Betnovate®** (Glaxo)

Rectal ointment, betamethasone valerate 0.05%, lignocaine hydrochloride 2.5%, phenylephrine hydrochloride 0.1%. Net price 30 g (with applicator) = £1.50

Apply 2–3 times daily until inflammation subsides then once daily, externally or by rectum; do not use for longer than 7 days; CHILD under 1 year not recommended

Perinal® (Dermal)

Spray application, hydrocortisone 0.2%, lignocaine hydrochloride 1%. Net price 30-mL pack = £6.31

Spray twice over the affected area up to 3 times daily; do not use for longer than 1–2 weeks; CHILD under 14 years not recommended

PoM **Proctofoam HC®** (Stafford-Miller)

Foam in aerosol pack, hydrocortisone acetate 1%, pramoxine hydrochloride 1%. Net price 21.2-g pack (approx. 40 applications) with applicator = £4.71

Dose: haemorrhoids and proctitis, 1 applicatorful (4–6 mg hydrocortisone acetate, 4–6 mg pramoxine hydrochloride) by rectum 2–3 times daily and after a bowel movement (max. 4 times daily); do not use for longer than 7 days; CHILD not recommended

PoM **Proctosedyl®** (Roussel)

Ointment, cinchocaine (dibucaine) hydrochloride 0.5%, hydrocortisone 0.5%. Net price 30 g = £6.48 (with cannula)

Apply morning and night and after a bowel movement, externally or by rectum; do not use for longer than 7 days

Suppositories, cinchocaine (dibucaine) hydrochloride 5 mg, hydrocortisone 5 mg. Net price 12 = £2.93

Insert 1 suppository night and morning and after a bowel movement; do not use for longer than 7 days

PoM **Scheriproct®** (Schering Health)

Ointment, cinchocaine (dibucaine) hydrochloride 0.5%, prednisolone hexanoate 0.19%. Net price 30 g = £4.41

Apply twice daily for 5–7 days (3–4 times daily on 1st day if necessary), then once daily for a few days after symptoms have cleared

Suppositories, cinchocaine (dibucaine) hydrochloride 1 mg, prednisolone hexanoate 1.3 mg. Net price 12 = £2.08

Insert 1 suppository daily after a bowel movement, for 5–7 days (in severe cases initially 2–3 times daily)

PoM **Ultraproct®** (Schering Health)

Ointment, cinchocaine (dibucaine) hydrochloride 0.5%, fluocortolone hexanoate 0.095%, fluocortolone pivalate 0.092%. Net price 30 g (with rectal nozzle) = £4.57

Apply twice daily for 5–7 days (3–4 times daily on 1st day if necessary), then once daily for few days after symptoms have cleared

Suppositories, cinchocaine (dibucaine) hydrochloride 1 mg, fluocortolone hexanoate 630 micrograms, fluocortolone pivalate 610 micrograms. Net price 12 = £2.15

Insert 1 suppository daily after a bowel movement, for 5–7 days (in severe cases initially 2–3 times daily) then 1 suppository every other day for 1 week

PoM **Uniroid-HC®** (Unigreg)

Ointment, cinchocaine (dibucaine) hydrochloride 0.5%, hydrocortisone 0.5%. Net price 30 g (with applicator) = £4.43

Apply twice daily and after a bowel movement, externally or by rectum; do not use for longer than 7 days; CHILD under 12 years not recommended

Suppositories, cinchocaine (dibucaine) hydrochloride 5 mg, hydrocortisone 5 mg. Net price 12 = £2.00

Insert 1 suppository twice daily and after a bowel movement; do not use for longer than 7 days; CHILD under 12 years not recommended

PoM **Xyloproct®** (Astra)

Ointment (water-miscible), aluminium acetate 3.5%, hydrocortisone acetate 0.275%, lignocaine 5%, zinc oxide 18%. Net price 30 g (with applicator) = £3.39

Apply several times daily; short-term use only

Suppositories, aluminium acetate 50 mg, hydrocortisone acetate 5 mg, lignocaine 60 mg, zinc oxide 400 mg. Net price 10 = £1.59

Insert 1 suppository at night and after a bowel movement; short-term use only

1.7.3 Rectal sclerosants

Oily phenol injection is used to inject haemorrhoids particularly when unprolapsed.

PHENOL

Indications: see notes above
Side-effects: irritation, tissue necrosis

PoM **Oily Phenol Injection, BP,** phenol 5% in a suitable fixed oil. Net price 5-mL amp = £4.16

Dose: 2–3 mL into the submucosal layer at the base of the pile; several injections may be given at different sites, max. total injected 10 mL at any one time
Available from Evans

1.8 Stoma care

Prescribing for patients with stoma calls for special care. The following is a brief account of some of the main points to be borne in mind.

Enteric-coated and *modified-release* preparations are **unsuitable**, particularly in patients with ileostomies, as there may not be sufficient release of the active ingredient.

Laxatives. Enemas and washouts should **not** be prescribed for patients with ileostomies as they may cause rapid and severe dehydration.

Colostomy patients may suffer from constipation and whenever possible should be treated by increasing fluid intake or dietary fibre. **Bulk-forming drugs** (section 1.6.1) should be tried. If they are insufficient, as small a dose as possible of senna (section 1.6.2) should be used.

Antidiarrhoeals. Drugs such as **loperamide, codeine phosphate,** or **co-phenotrope** (diphenoxylate with atropine) are effective. Bulk-forming drugs (section 1.6.1) may be tried but it is often difficult to adjust the dose appropriately.

Antibiotics should **not** be given for an episode of acute diarrhoea.

Antacids. The tendency to diarrhoea from magnesium salts or constipation from aluminium salts may be increased in these patients.

Diuretics should be used with caution in patients with ileostomies as they may become excessively dehydrated and potassium depletion may easily occur. It is usually advisable to use a **potassium-sparing** diuretic (see section 2.2.3).

Digoxin. Patients with a stoma are particularly susceptible to hypokalaemia if on digoxin therapy and potassium supplements or a potassium-sparing diuretic may be advisable (for comment see section 9.2.1.1).

Potassium supplements. Liquid formulations are preferred to modified-release formulations (see above).

Analgesics. Opioid analgesics (see section 4.7.2) may cause troublesome constipation in colostomy patients. When a non-opioid analgesic is required **paracetamol** is usually suitable but anti-inflammatory analgesics may cause gastric irritation and bleeding.

Iron preparations may cause loose stools and sore skin in these patients. If this is troublesome and if iron is definitely indicated an intramuscular iron preparation (see section 9.1.1.2) should be used. Modified-release preparations should be **avoided** for the reasons given above.

Patients are usually given advice about the use of *cleansing agents*, *protective creams*, *lotions*, *deodorants*, or *sealants* whilst in hospital, either by the surgeon or by the health authority stoma care nurses. Voluntary organisations offer help and support to patients with stoma.

For details of **stoma appliances and associated products**, see Appendix 8.

1.9 Drugs affecting intestinal secretions

1.9.1 Drugs acting on the gall bladder

The use of laproscopic cholecystectomy and of endoscopic biliary techniques has limited the place of the bile acids **chenodeoxycholic acid** and **ursodeoxycholic acid** in gallstone disease. They are suitable for patients not treatable by other means who have mild symptoms, unimpaired gall bladder function, and small or medium sized radiolucent stones; they are not suitable for radio-opaque stones, which are unlikely to be dissolved. Patients should preferably be supervised in hospital because radiological monitoring is required. Long-term prophylaxis may be needed after complete dissolution of the gallstones has been confirmed (preferably with cholecystograms and ultrasound on two separate occasions) as gallstones may recur in up to 25% of patients within one year of stopping treatment.

Ursodeoxycholic acid is also used in primary biliary cirrhosis and in primary sclerosing cholangitis [unlicensed indications].

CHENODEOXYCHOLIC ACID

Indications; Cautions: see notes above

Contra-indications: do not use when stones are radio-opaque, in pregnancy (see Appendix 4; non-hormonal contraceptive measures should be taken in women of childbearing age), in non-functioning gall bladders, in chronic liver disease, and inflammatory diseases of the small intestine and colon

Side-effects: diarrhoea particularly initially with high dosage (reduce dose for few days), pruritus, minor hepatic abnormalities and transient rise in serum transaminases

Dose: 10–15 mg/kg daily as a single dose at bedtime *or* in divided doses for 3–24 months, depending on size of stone; treatment is continued for at least 3 months after stones dissolve

PoM **Chendol 125®** (CP)

Capsules, orange/white, chenodeoxycholic acid 125 mg. Net price 224-cap pack = £47.50

PoM **Chenofalk®** (Thames)

Capsules, chenodeoxycholic acid 250 mg. Net price 60 = £25.20

Additives: include gluten

With ursodeoxycholic acid

PoM **Combidol®** (CP)

Tablets, f/c, chenodeoxycholic acid 125 mg, ursodeoxycholic acid 125 mg. Net price 60-tab pack = £40.00

Dose: 3 tablets (patients greater than 120% of ideal body weight, 6 tablets) daily as a single dose at bedtime or in divided doses; treatment continued for approx. 3 months after stones dissolve; CHILD not recommended

PoM **Lithofalk®** (Thames)

Tablets, scored, chenodeoxycholic acid 250 mg, ursodeoxycholic acid 250 mg. Net price 60-tab pack = £57.14

Dose: 2 tablets (patients greater than 80 kg, 3 tablets) daily as a single dose at bedtime; treatment continued for up to 3 months after stones have dissolved; CHILD not recommended

URSODEOXYCHOLIC ACID

Indications; Cautions; Contra-indications: see under Chenodeoxycholic Acid

Side-effects: see under Chenodeoxycholic Acid; diarrhoea occurs rarely; liver changes have not been reported

Dose: 8–12 mg/kg (obese patients up to 15 mg/kg) daily in two divided doses, for up to 2 years; treatment is continued for 3–4 months after stones dissolve

PoM **Destolit®** (Merrell)

Tablets, scored, ursodeoxycholic acid 150 mg. Net price 60 = £18.92. Label: 21

PoM **Ursofalk®** (Thames)

Capsules, ursodeoxycholic acid 250 mg. Net price 60 = £31.50. Label: 21

Additives: include gluten

With chenodeoxycholic acid

See under Chenodeoxycholic acid

OTHER PREPARATIONS FOR BILIARY DISORDERS

A **terpene** mixture (Rowachol®) raises biliary cholesterol solubility. It is not considered to be a useful adjunct.

PoM **Rowachol®** (Monmouth)

Capsules, green, e/c, borneol 5 mg, camphene 5 mg, cineole 2 mg, menthol 32 mg, menthone 6 mg, pinene 17 mg in olive oil. Net price 50-cap pack = £7.35. Label: 22

Dose: 1–2 capsules 3 times daily before food (but see notes above)

Interactions: Appendix 1 (*Rowachol®*)

1.9.2   Drugs which increase gastric acidity

Muripsin®, which contained glutamic acid hydrochloride, was formerly used in achlorhydria and hypochlorhydria but was of uncertain value. It has now been discontinued.

1.9.3   Aprotinin

See section 2.11.

1.9.4   Pancreatin

Supplements of pancreatin are given by mouth to compensate for reduced or absent exocrine secretion in cystic fibrosis, and following pancreatectomy, total gastrectomy, or chronic pancreatitis. They assist the digestion of starch, fat, and protein.

Pancreatin is inactivated by gastric acid therefore pancreatin preparations are best taken with food (or immediately before or after food). Gastric acid secretion may be reduced by giving cimetidine or ranitidine an hour beforehand (section 1.3). Concurrent use of antacids also reduces gastric acidity. The newer enteric-coated preparations such as Creon®, Nutrizym GR®, and Pancrease® deliver a higher enzyme concentration in the duodenum (provided the granules are swallowed whole without chewing). Higher-strength versions are now also available (**important:** CSM advice on p. 57).

Since pancreatin is also inactivated by heat, excessive heat should be avoided if preparations are mixed with liquids or food; the resulting mixtures should not be kept for more than one hour.

Dosage is adjusted according to size, number, and consistency of stools, so that the patient thrives; extra allowance may be needed if snacks are taken between meals.

Pancreatin can irritate the perioral skin and buccal mucosa if retained in the mouth, and excessive doses can cause perianal irritation. The most frequent side-effects are gastro-intestinal including nausea, vomiting, and abdominal discomfort; hyperuricaemia and hyperuricosuria have been associated with very high doses. Hypersensitivity reactions occur occasionally and may affect those handling the powder.

PANCREATIN

Note. The pancreatin preparations which follow are all of porcine origin

Indications; Cautions; Side-effects: see above and (for higher-strength preparations) see below

▼ PoM **Creon**® (Solvay)

Capsules, brown/yellow, enclosing buff-coloured e/c granules of pancreatin, providing: protease 210 units, lipase 8000 units, amylase 9000 units. Net price 100 = £13.33. Counselling, see dose

Dose: ADULT and CHILD initially 1–2 capsules with meals either taken whole or contents mixed with fluid or soft food (then swallowed immediately without chewing); higher doses may be required according to response

Granules, brown, e/c, pancreatin, providing: protease 1 125 units, lipase 20 000 units, amylase 22 500 units/ sachet. Net price 40-sachet pack = £13.33. Counselling, see dose

Dose: ADULT and CHILD initially 1 sachet with meals either washed down or sprinkled on soft food (then swallowed immediately without chewing); higher doses may be required according to response

Note. One sachet of Creon granules contains the equivalent of 2½ Creon capsules

Nutrizym GR® (Merck)

Capsules, green/orange, enclosing e/c pellets of pancreatin, providing minimum of: protease 650 units, lipase 10 000 units, amylase 10 000 units. Net price 100 = £13.15. Counselling, see dose

Dose: ADULT and CHILD 1–2 capsules with meals swallowed whole or contents sprinkled on soft food (then swallowed immediately without chewing); higher doses may be required according to response

Nutrizym 10® (Merck)

Capsules, red/yellow, enclosing e/c minitablets of pancreatin providing minimum of: protease 500 units, lipase 10 000 units, amylase 9000 units. Net price 100 = £13.15. Counselling, see dose

Dose: ADULT and CHILD 1–2 capsules with meals and 1 capsule with snacks, swallowed whole or contents taken with water or sprinkled on soft food (then swallowed immediately without chewing); higher doses may be required according to response

Pancrease® (Cilag)

Capsules, enclosing e/c beads of pancrelipase USP, providing minimum of: protease 330 units, lipase 5000 units, amylase 2900 units. Net price 100 = £17.07. Counselling, see dose

Dose: ADULT and CHILD 1–2 (occasionally 3) capsules during each meal and 1 capsule with snacks swallowed whole or contents sprinkled on liquid or soft food (then swallowed immediately without chewing); higher doses may be required according to response

Pancrex® (Paines & Byrne)

Granules, pancreatin, providing minimum of: protease 300 units, lipase 5000 units, amylase 4000 units/g. Net price 300 g = £20.39. Label: 25, counselling, see dose

Dose: ADULT and CHILD 5–10 g just before meals washed down or mixed with liquid

Pancrex V® (Paines & Byrne)

Capsules, pancreatin, providing minimum of: protease 430 units, lipase 8000 units, amylase 9000 units. Net price 300-cap pack = £15.80. Counselling, see dose

Dose: ADULT and CHILD over 1 year 2–6 capsules with meals, swallowed whole or sprinkled on food; CHILD up to 1 year 1–2 capsules mixed with feeds

Capsules '125', pancreatin, providing minimum of: protease 160 units, lipase 2950 units, amylase 3300 units. Net price 300-cap pack = £9.72. Counselling, see dose

Dose: NEONATE 1–2 capsules with feeds

Tablets, e/c, s/c, pancreatin, providing minimum of: protease 110 units, lipase 1900 units, amylase 1700 units. Net price 300-tab pack = £4.51. Label: 5, 25, counselling, see dose

Dose: ADULT and CHILD 5–15 tablets before meals

Tablets forte, e/c, s/c, pancreatin, providing minimum of: protease 330 units, lipase 5600 units, amylase 5000 units. Net price 300-tab pack = £13.74. Label: 5, 25, counselling, see dose

Dose: ADULT and CHILD 6–10 tablets before meals

Powder, pancreatin, providing minimum of: protease 1400 units, lipase 25 000 units, amylase 30 000 units/ g. Net price 300 g = £24.28. Counselling, see dose

Dose: ADULT and CHILD 0.5–2 g with meals washed down or mixed with liquid; NEONATE 250–500 mg with each feed

Higher-strength preparations

The **CSM** has advised of data associating the high-strength pancreatin preparations Nutrizym 22® and Pancreatin HL® with the development of large bowel strictures (fibrosing colonopathy) in children with cystic fibrosis aged between 2 and 13 years. There was only minimal use of Panzytrat® 25 000 during the study period but an identical preparation has been implicated in Denmark. No association was found with Creon® 25 000. The following was recommended:

— Pancrease HL®, Nutrizym 22®, Panzytrat® 25 000 [now discontinued] should not be used in children aged 15 years or less with cystic fibrosis;

— the total dose of pancreatic enzyme supplements used in patients with cystic fibrosis should not usually exceed 10 000 units of lipase per kg body-weight daily;

— if a patient on any pancreatin preparation develops new abdominal symptoms (or any change in existing abdominal symptoms) the patient should be reviewed to exclude the possibility of colonic damage.

Possible risk factors are gender (boys at greater risk than girls), more severe cystic fibrosis, and concomitant use of laxatives. The peak age for developing fibrosing colonopathy is between 2 and 8 years.

COUNSELLING. It is important to ensure adequate hydration at all times in patients receiving higher-strength pancreatin preparations.

▼ PoM **Creon**® **25 000** (Solvay)

Capsules, orange/yellow, enclosing brown-coloured e/c pellets of pancreatin, providing: protease (total) 1000 units, lipase 25 000 units, amylase 18 000 units. Net price 50-cap pack = £19.50. Counselling, see above and under dose

Dose: ADULT and CHILD initially 1 capsule with meals either taken whole or contents mixed with fluid or soft food (then swallowed immediately without chewing)

▼ PoM **Nutrizym 22**® (Merck)

Capsules, red/yellow, enclosing e/c minitablets of pancreatin, providing minimum of: protease 1100 units, lipase 22 000 units, amylase 19 800 units. Net price 100-cap pack = £30.30. Counselling, see above and under dose

Dose: 1–2 capsules with meals and 1 capsule with snacks, swallowed whole or contents taken with water or sprinkled on soft food (then swallowed immediately without chewing)

CHILD under 15 years not recommended

▼ PoM **Pancrease HL**® (Cilag)

Capsules, enclosing light brown e/c minitablets of pancreatin, providing minimum of: protease 1250 units, lipase 25 000 units, amylase 22 500 units. Net price 100 = £36.18. Counselling, see above and under dose

Dose: 1–2 capsules during each meal and 1 capsule with snacks swallowed whole or contents sprinkled on liquid or soft food (then swallowed immediately without chewing)

CHILD under 15 years not recommended

2: Drugs used in the treatment of diseases of the
CARDIOVASCULAR SYSTEM

In this chapter, drug treatment is discussed under the following headings:

2.1   Positive inotropic drugs

2.1.1   Cardiac glycosides
2.1.2   Phosphodiesterase inhibitors

Positive inotropic drugs increase the force of contraction of the myocardium; for sympathomimetics with inotropic activity see section 2.7.1.

2.1.1 Cardiac glycosides

The principal actions of the cardiac glycosides are an increase in the force of myocardial contraction and a reduction in the conductivity of the heart. They are most useful in the treatment of *supraventricular tachycardias*, especially for controlling ventricular response in atrial fibrillation. *Heart failure* may also be improved, even in patients in sinus rhythm, because of changes in the availability of intracellular calcium; this action is relatively unimportant, however, compared with the effects that can be achieved with diuretics and ACE inhibitors (see section 2.5.5). Except when needed to maintain satisfactory rhythm, cardiac glycosides can often be withdrawn from patients with heart failure that is well controlled, without clinical deterioration. In the elderly who are particularly susceptible to digitalis toxicity, cardiac glycosides should be used with special care in the management of heart failure without atrial fibrillation.

Loss of appetite, nausea, and vomiting are common toxic effects; sinus bradycardia, atrioventricular block, ventricular extrasystoles, and sometimes ventricular tachycardia or atrial tachycardia with block also occur—especially in the presence of underlying conducting system defects or myocardial disease. These unwanted effects depend both on the plasma concentrations of the drugs and on the sensitivity of the conducting system or myocardium, which is often increased in heart disease. Thus, no one plasma concentration can indicate toxicity reliably but the likelihood increases progressively through the range 1.5 to 3 micrograms/litre for digoxin; higher steady-state concentrations must certainly be avoided. Measurements of plasma concentration are not necessary, however, unless problems occur during maintenance treatment. Hypokalaemia predisposes to toxicity, therefore diuretics used with digoxin should either be potassium sparing or should be given with potassium supplements.

Renal function is the most important determinant of digoxin dosage, whereas elimination of digitoxin depends on metabolism by the liver. Toxicity can often be managed by discontinuing therapy and correcting hypokalaemia if appropriate; serious manifestations require urgent specialist management. Digoxin-specific antibody fragments are available for reversal of life-threatening overdosage (see next page).

Digoxin is the glycoside most commonly used. In patients with *mild failure* a loading dose is not required, and a satisfactory plasma concentration can be achieved over a period of about a week, using a dose of 125 to 250 micrograms twice a day which may then be reduced having special regard to renal function. Because it has a long half-life maintenance doses need only be given once daily (but higher doses should be divided to avoid nausea). For management of *atrial fibrillation* the maintenance dose can usually be governed by ventricular response which should not be allowed to fall below 60 beats per minute except in special and recognised circumstances, e.g. with the concomitant administration of beta-blockers.

When *rapid control* is needed, digoxin may be given intravenously in a digitalising dose of 0.75 to 1 mg, preferably as an infusion (suggested volume 50 mL) over two or more hours (too rapid a rate of administration is associated with nausea and risk of arrhythmias); this is followed by normal maintenance therapy. The intramuscular route is not recommended.

Digitoxin has a long half-life and maintenance doses need only be given once daily or on alternate days.

CHILDREN. The dose is based on body-weight; they require a relatively larger dose of digoxin than adults.

DIGOXIN

Indications: heart failure, supraventricular arrhythmias (particularly atrial fibrillation)
Cautions: recent infarction; sick sinus syndrome; thyroid disease; reduce dose in the elderly and in renal impairment; avoid hypokalaemia; avoid rapid intravenous administration (nausea and risk of arrhythmias); pregnancy (see also Appendix 4); **interactions:** Appendix 1 (cardiac glycosides)

Contra-indications: intermittent complete heart block, second degree AV block; supraventricular arrhythmias caused by Wolff-Parkinson-White syndrome; hypertrophic obstructive cardiomyopathy (unless concomitant atrial fibrillation and heart failure — but with caution)

Side-effects: usually associated with excessive dosage, include: anorexia, nausea, vomiting, diarrhoea, abdominal pain; visual disturbances, headache, fatigue, drowsiness, confusion, delirium, hallucinations; arrhythmias, heart block; see also notes above

Dose: by mouth, rapid digitalisation, 1–1.5 mg in divided doses over 24 hours; less urgent digitalisation, 250–500 micrograms daily (higher dose divided)

Maintenance, 62.5–500 micrograms daily (higher dose divided) according to renal function and, in atrial fibrillation, on heart-rate response; usual range, 125–250 micrograms daily (elderly 125 micrograms)

Emergency loading dose *by intravenous infusion*, 250–500 micrograms over 10–20 minutes (see also Cautions), followed by further fractions at intervals of 4–8 hours (depending on the response), to a total loading dose of 0.5–1 mg (see notes above for an alternative regimen)

Note. The above doses may need to be reduced if digoxin (or another cardiac glycoside) has been given in the preceding 2 weeks. For plasma concentration monitoring blood should ideally be taken at least 6 hours after a dose

PoM Digoxin (Non-proprietary)
Tablets, digoxin 62.5 micrograms, net price 20 = 9p; 125 micrograms, 20 = 6p; 250 micrograms, 20 = 9p
Injection, digoxin 250 micrograms/mL, see Lanoxin®
Paediatric injection, digoxin 100 micrograms/mL (hosp. only, available from Boots)

PoM Lanoxin® (Wellcome)
Tablets, digoxin 125 micrograms, net price 20 = 32p; 250 micrograms (scored), 20 = 32p
Injection, digoxin 250 micrograms/mL. Net price 2-mL amp = 65p

PoM Lanoxin-PG® (Wellcome)
Tablets, blue, digoxin 62.5 micrograms. Net price 20 = 32p
Elixir, yellow, digoxin 50 micrograms/mL. Do not dilute, measure with pipette. Net price 60 mL = £5.23. Counselling, use of pipette

DIGITOXIN

Indications: heart failure, supraventricular arrhythmias (particularly atrial fibrillation)
Cautions; Contra-indications; Side-effects: see under Digoxin
Dose: maintenance, 100 micrograms daily *or* on alternate days; may be increased to 200 micrograms daily if necessary

PoM Digitoxin (Non-proprietary)
Tablets, digitoxin 100 micrograms, net price 20 = £2.75

DIGOXIN-SPECIFIC ANTIBODY

Digoxin-specific antibody fragments are indicated for the treatment of known or strongly suspected digoxin or digitoxin overdosage, where measures beyond the withdrawal of the cardiac glycoside and correction of any electrolyte abnormality are felt to be necessary (see also notes above).

PoM Digibind® (Wellcome)
Injection, powder for preparation of infusion, digoxin-specific antibody fragments (F(ab)) 38 mg. Net price per vial = £87.44 (hosp. and poisons centres only)
Dose: see data sheet

2.1.2 Phosphodiesterase inhibitors

Enoximone and **milrinone** are selective phosphodiesterase inhibitors which exert most of their effect on the myocardium. Sustained haemodynamic benefit has been observed after administration, but as yet there is no conclusive evidence of any beneficial effect on survival.

ENOXIMONE

Indications: congestive heart failure where cardiac output reduced and filling pressures increased

Cautions: heart failure associated with hypertrophic cardiomyopathy, stenotic or obstructive valvular disease or other outlet obstruction; monitor blood pressure, heart rate, ECG, central venous pressure, fluid and electrolyte status, platelet count, hepatic enzymes; reduce dose in renal impairment; avoid extravasation; pregnancy and breast-feeding

Side-effects: ectopic beats; less frequently ventricular tachycardia or supraventricular arrhythmias (more likely in patients with pre-existing arrhythmias); hypotension; also headache, insomnia, nausea and vomiting, diarrhoea; occasionally, chills, oliguria, fever, urinary retention; upper and lower limb pain

Dose: by slow intravenous injection (rate not exceeding 12.5 mg/minute), diluted before use, initially 0.5–1 mg/kg, then 500 micrograms/kg every 30 minutes until satisfactory response or total of 3 mg/kg given; maintenance, initial dose of up to 3 mg/kg may be repeated every 3–6 hours as required

By intravenous infusion, initially 90 micrograms/kg/minute over 10–30 minutes, followed by continuous or intermittent infusion of 5–20 micrograms/kg/minute

Total dose over 24 hours should not normally exceed 24 mg/kg

PoM Perfan® (Merrell)
Injection, enoximone 5 mg/mL. For dilution before use. Net price 20-mL amp = £15.02
Note. Plastic apparatus should be used; crystal formation if glass used

MILRINONE

Indications: short-term treatment of severe congestive heart failure unresponsive to conventional maintenance therapy (not immediately after myocardial infarction); acute heart failure, including low output states, following heart surgery

Cautions; Side-effects: see under Enoximone; also correct hypokalaemia, monitor renal function, chest pain reported

Dose: by slow intravenous injection (over 10 minutes), diluted before use, 50 micrograms/kg followed by *intravenous infusion* at a rate of 375–750 nanograms/kg/minute, usually for up to 12 hours following surgery or for 48–72 hours in congestive heart failure; max. daily dose 1.13 mg/kg

PoM **Primacor**® (Sanofi Winthrop)
Injection, milrinone (as lactate) 1 mg/mL. For dilution before use. Net price 10-mL amp = £17.39

2.2   Diuretics

2.2.1	Thiazides and related diuretics
2.2.2	Loop diuretics
2.2.3	Potassium-sparing diuretics
2.2.4	Potassium-sparing diuretics with other diuretics
2.2.5	Osmotic diuretics
2.2.6	Mercurial diuretics
2.2.7	Carbonic anhydrase inhibitors
2.2.8	Diuretics with potassium

Thiazides (section 2.2.1) are used to relieve oedema due to *heart failure* and, in lower doses, to reduce *blood pressure*.

Loop diuretics (section 2.2.2) are used in pulmonary oedema due to *left ventricular failure* and in patients with *longstanding heart failure* who no longer respond to thiazides.

Combination diuretic therapy may be effective in patients with *oedema resistant to treatment with one diuretic*. For example, a loop diuretic may be combined with a potassium-sparing diuretic (section 2.2.3).

The combination of a thiazide with a potassium-sparing diuretic is of value in *less severe heart failure* when hypokalaemia is difficult to counter or when any degree of hypokalaemia should be avoided, as in patients with a continuing tendency to life-threatening ventricular arrhythmias.

THE ELDERLY. Diuretics are overprescribed in old age and the elderly are particularly susceptible to many of their side-effects. Lower initial doses should be used, and subsequently adjusted according to renal function. They should not be used on a long-term basis to treat simple gravitational oedema (which will usually respond to increased movement, raising the legs, and support stockings).

POTASSIUM LOSS. Hypokalaemia may occur with both thiazide and loop diuretics; the risk of hypokalaemia depends more on duration of action than

on potency and is thus greater with thiazides than with loop diuretics.

Hypokalaemia is dangerous in severe coronary artery disease and in patients also being treated with cardiac glycosides. Often the use of potassium-sparing diuretics (section 2.2.3) avoids the need to take potassium supplements.

In hepatic failure hypokalaemia caused by diuretics can precipitate encephalopathy, particularly in alcoholic cirrhosis; diuretics may also increase the risk of hypomagnesaemia in alcoholic cirrhosis, leading to arrhythmias.

Potassium supplements are seldom necessary when thiazides are used in the routine treatment of hypertension. For further comment see section 9.2.1.1.

2.2.1   Thiazides and related diuretics

Thiazides and related compounds are moderately potent diuretics; they inhibit sodium reabsorption at the beginning of the distal convoluted tubule. They act within 1 to 2 hours of oral administration and most have a duration of action of 12 to 24 hours; they are usually administered early in the day so that the diuresis does not interfere with sleep.

In the management of *hypertension* a low dose of a thiazide, e.g. bendrofluazide 2.5 mg daily, produces a maximal or near-maximal blood pressure lowering effect, with very little biochemical disturbance. Higher doses cause more marked changes in plasma potassium, uric acid, glucose, and lipids, with no advantage in blood pressure control, and should not be used. Optimum doses for the control of *heart failure* may be larger, and long-term effects are of less importance.

Bendrofluazide is widely used for mild or moderate heart failure when the patient is not desperately ill and severe pulmonary oedema is not present. It is also used for hypertension—alone in the treatment of mild hypertension or with other drugs in more severe hypertension.

Chlorthalidone, a thiazide-related compound, has a longer duration of action than the thiazides and may be given on alternate days to control oedema. It is also useful if acute retention is liable to be precipitated by a more rapid diuresis or if patients dislike the altered pattern of micturition promoted by diuretics.

Other thiazides do not offer any significant advantage over those mentioned above, and newer ones are more expensive than the longer-established thiazides.

Metolazone is particularly effective when combined with a loop diuretic (even in renal failure); profound diuresis may occur therefore the patient should be monitored carefully.

Xipamide resembles chlorthalidone structurally, and is more potent than the other thiazides.

Indapamide is also chemically related to chlorthalidone. It is claimed to lower blood pressure with less metabolic disturbance, particularly less aggravation of diabetes mellitus.

BENDROFLUAZIDE
(Bendroflumethiazide)

Indications: oedema, hypertension (see also notes above)

Cautions: may cause hypokalaemia, aggravates diabetes and gout; may exacerbate systemic lupus erythematosus; elderly (see notes above); pregnancy (see also Appendix 4) and breast-feeding; hepatic and renal impairment (avoid if severe, see Appendixes 2 and 3); see also notes above; porphyria (see section 9.8.2); **interactions:** Appendix 1 (diuretics)

Contra-indications: refractory hypokalaemia, hyponatraemia, hypercalcaemia; severe renal and hepatic impairment; symptomatic hyperuricaemia; Addison's disease

Side-effects: postural hypotension and mild gastro-intestinal effects; impotence (reversible on withdrawal of treatment); hypokalaemia (see also notes above), hypomagnesaemia, hyponatraemia, hypercalcaemia, hypochloraemic alkalosis, hyperuricaemia, gout, hyperglycaemia, and increases in plasma cholesterol concentration; less commonly rashes, photosensitivity; blood disorders (including neutropenia and thrombocytopenia — when given in late pregnancy neonatal thrombocytopenia has been reported); pancreatitis, intrahepatic cholestasis, and hypersensitivity reactions (including pneumonitis, pulmonary oedema, severe skin reactions) also reported

Dose: oedema, initially 5–10 mg in the morning, daily *or* on alternate days; maintenance 5–10 mg 1–3 times weekly

Hypertension, 2.5 mg in the morning; higher doses rarely necessary (see notes above)

PoM Bendrofluazide (Non-proprietary)
Tablets, bendrofluazide 2.5 mg, net price 20 = 10p; 5 mg, 20 = 7p
Available from APS, Ashbourne (Neo-Bendromax®), Berk (Berkozide®), Cox, Goldshield (Neo-NaClex®, 5 mg only), Hillcross, Knoll (Aprinox®), Norton

BENZTHIAZIDE
Cautions; Contra-indications; Side-effects: see under Bendrofluazide

Preparation
Ingredient of Dytide® (section 2.2.4)

CHLOROTHIAZIDE
Indications: oedema, hypertension (see also notes above)
Cautions; Contra-indications; Side-effects: see under Bendrofluazide
Dose: oedema, usually 0.25–1 g daily in 1–2 divided doses; maintenance dose may be given daily, on alternate days, or less frequently; max. 1 g daily
Hypertension, initially 250 mg daily; max. 500 mg daily in single or divided doses (but see also notes above)

PoM Saluric® (MSD)
Tablets, scored, chlorothiazide 500 mg. Net price 20 = 68p

CHLORTHALIDONE
(Chlortalidone)

Indications: oedema, hypertension (see also notes above); diabetes insipidus (see section 6.5.2)
Cautions; Contra-indications; Side-effects: see under Bendrofluazide
Dose: oedema, initially 50 mg in the morning *or* 100–200 mg on alternate days, reduced for maintenance if possible
Hypertension, 25 mg, increased to 50 mg if necessary, in the morning (see also notes above)

PoM Hygroton® (Geigy)
Tablets, yellow, scored, chlorthalidone 50 mg, net price 28-tab pack = £1.37

CLOPAMIDE
Cautions; Contra-indications; Side-effects: see under Bendrofluazide

Preparation
Ingredient of Viskaldix® (see under Pindolol, section 2.4)

CYCLOPENTHIAZIDE
Indications: oedema, hypertension (see also notes above)
Cautions; Contra-indications; Side-effects: see under Bendrofluazide
Dose: oedema, 250–500 micrograms daily in the morning; in heart failure may be increased to 1 mg daily (reduce to lowest effective dose for maintenance)
Hypertension, initially 250 micrograms daily in the morning, increased if necessary to 500 micrograms daily (see also notes above)

PoM Navidrex® (Ciba)
Tablets, scored, cyclopenthiazide 500 micrograms. Net price 100-tab pack = £1.77
Additives: include gluten

HYDROCHLOROTHIAZIDE
Indications: oedema, hypertension (see also notes above)
Cautions; Contra-indications; Side-effects: see under Bendrofluazide
Dose: oedema, initially 25–50 mg daily, reduced for maintenance if possible; severe oedema in patients unable to tolerate loop diuretics, initially 75 mg daily
Hypertension, 25 mg daily, increased to 50 mg daily if necessary (see also notes above)
ELDERLY. In some patients (especially the elderly) an initial dose of 12.5 mg daily may be sufficient

PoM HydroSaluric® (MSD)
Tablets, both scored, hydrochlorothiazide 25 mg, net price 20 = 29p; 50 mg, 20 = 54p

---

HYDROFLUMETHIAZIDE

Indications: oedema, hypertension (see also notes above)

Cautions; Contra-indications; Side-effects: see under Bendrofluazide

Dose: oedema, initially 50–200 mg in the morning; maintenance 25–50 mg on alternate days
Hypertension, 25–50 mg daily (see also notes above)

PoM Hydrenox® (Knoll)
Tablets, hydroflumethiazide 50 mg. Net price 20 = 44p

INDAPAMIDE

Indications: essential hypertension

Cautions: renal impairment (stop if deterioration); monitor plasma potassium and urate concentrations in elderly, hyperaldosteronism, gout, or with concomitant cardiac glycosides; hyperparathyroidism (discontinue if hypercalcaemia); pregnancy and breast-feeding; **interactions:** Appendix 1 (diuretics)

Contra-indications: recent cerebrovascular accident, severe hepatic impairment

Side-effects: hypokalaemia, headache, dizziness, fatigue, muscular cramps, nausea, anorexia, diarrhoea, constipation, dyspepsia, rashes (erythema multiforme, epidermal necrolysis reported); rarely orthostatic hypotension, palpitations, increase in liver enzymes, blood disorders (including thrombocytopenia), hyponatraemia, metabolic alkalosis, hyperglycaemia, increased plasma urate concentrations, paraesthesia, photosensitivity, impotence, renal impairment, reversible acute myopia; diuresis with doses above 2.5 mg daily

Dose: 2.5 mg daily in the morning

PoM Indapamide (Non-proprietary)
Tablets, s/c, indapamide 2.5 mg. Net price 60-tab pack = £6.87
Available from APS, Ashbourne (Nindaxa 2.5®), Cox, Hillcross, Opus (Opumide®), Trinity (Natramid®)

PoM Natrilix® (Servier)
Tablets, f/c, indapamide 2.5 mg. Net price 30-tab pack = £3.89, 60-tab pack = £7.63

MEFRUSIDE

Indications: oedema, hypertension (see also notes above)

Cautions; Contra-indications; Side-effects: see under Bendrofluazide

Dose: initially 25–50 mg in the morning, increased to 75–100 mg for oedema; maintenance 25 mg daily *or* on alternate days (see also notes above)

PoM Baycaron® (Bayer)
Tablets, scored, mefruside 25 mg. Net price 20 = £1.41

METOLAZONE

Indications: oedema, hypertension (see also notes above)

Cautions; Contra-indications; Side-effects: see under Bendrofluazide; also profound diuresis on concomitant administration with frusemide (monitor patient carefully)

Dose: see preparations below

PoM Metenix 5® (Hoechst)
Tablets, blue, metolazone 5 mg. Net price 100-tab pack = £8.53
Dose: oedema, 5–10 mg in the morning, increased if necessary to 20 mg daily in resistant oedema, max. 80 mg daily
Hypertension, initially 5 mg in the morning; maintenance 5 mg on alternate days

Low dose formulation
Note. Xuret® brand of metolazone has a much lower dose than other brands of metolazone. It must therefore be prescribed by brand name and is not interchangeable with other brands of metolazone

PoM Xuret® (Galen)
Tablets, metolazone 500 micrograms. Net price 56-tab pack = £7.36
Dose: mild to moderate hypertension, 1 tablet daily in the morning; increased if necessary to 2 tablets daily

POLYTHIAZIDE

Indications: oedema, hypertension (see also notes above)

Cautions; Contra-indications; Side-effects: see under Bendrofluazide

Dose: usually 1–4 mg daily; in hypertension 500 micrograms daily may be adequate

PoM Nephril® (Pfizer)
Tablets, scored, polythiazide 1 mg. Net price 28-tab pack = 79p

XIPAMIDE

Indications: oedema, hypertension (see also notes above)

Cautions; Contra-indications: see under Bendrofluazide

Side-effects: gastro-intestinal disturbances; mild dizziness; hypokalaemia, more rarely other electrolyte disturbances such as hyponatraemia

Dose: oedema, initially 40 mg in the morning, increased to 80 mg in resistant cases; maintenance 20 mg in the morning
Hypertension, 20 mg in the morning

PoM Diurexan® (ASTA Medica)
Tablets, scored, xipamide 20 mg. Net price 14-tab pack = £2.19

2.2.2   Loop diuretics

Loop diuretics are used in pulmonary oedema due to *left ventricular failure* and in patients with *long-standing heart failure* who no longer respond to thiazides. These drugs inhibit resorption from the ascending loop of Henle in the renal tubule and are powerful diuretics. Hypokalaemia may develop, and care is needed to avoid hypotension. If there is an enlarged prostate, urinary retention may occur; this is less likely if small doses and less potent diuretics are used initially.

Frusemide and **bumetanide** are similar in activity; both act within 1 hour of oral administration and diuresis is complete within 6 hours so that, if necessary, they can be given twice in one day without interfering with sleep. Following intravenous administration they have a peak effect within 30 minutes. The diuresis associated with these drugs is dose related. In patients with impaired renal function very large doses may occasionally be needed; in such doses both drugs can cause deafness and bumetanide can cause myalgia.

Ethacrynic acid has a similar onset and duration of action. Gastro-intestinal side-effects are more severe and deafness may occur in renal failure, especially when given intravenously.

Piretanide has properties similar to those of frusemide and bumetanide, but is promoted for the treatment of hypertension. **Torasemide** also has properties similar to those of frusemide and bumetanide, and has been introduced recently for oedema and for hypertension.

FRUSEMIDE
(Furosemide)

Indications: oedema, oliguria due to renal failure

Cautions: pregnancy (see also Appendix 4) and breast-feeding; may cause hypokalaemia and hyponatraemia; aggravates diabetes mellitus and gout; liver failure, prostatic enlargement; porphyria (see section 9.8.2); **interactions:** Appendix 1 (diuretics)

Contra-indications: precomatose states associated with liver cirrhosis; renal failure with anuria

Side-effects: hyponatraemia, hypokalaemia, and hypomagnesaemia (see also section 2.2), hypochloraemic alkalosis, increased calcium excretion, hypotension; less commonly nausea, gastro-intestinal disturbances, hyperuricaemia and gout; hyperglycaemia (less common than with thiazides); temporary increase in plasma cholesterol and triglyceride concentrations; rarely rashes, photosensitivity and bone marrow depression (withdraw treatment), pancreatitis (with large parenteral doses), tinnitus and deafness (usually with large parenteral doses and rapid administration and in renal impairment)

Dose: by mouth, oedema, initially 40 mg in the morning; maintenance 20 mg daily *or* 40 mg on alternate days, increased in resistant oedema to 80 mg daily; CHILD 1–3 mg/kg daily
Oliguria, initially 250 mg daily; if necessary larger doses, increasing in steps of 250 mg, may be given every 4–6 hours to a max. of a single dose of 2 g (rarely used)
By intramuscular injection or slow intravenous injection (rate not exceeding 4 mg/minute), initially 20–50 mg; CHILD 0.5–1.5 mg/kg to a max. daily dose of 20 mg

By intravenous infusion (by syringe pump if necessary), in oliguria, initially 250 mg over 1 hour (rate not exceeding 4 mg/minute), if satisfactory urine output not obtained in the subsequent hour further 500 mg over 2 hours, then if no satisfactory response within subsequent hour, further 1 g over 4 hours, if no response obtained dialysis probably required; effective dose (up to 1 g) can be repeated every 24 hours

PoM Frusemide (Non-proprietary)
Tablets, frusemide 20 mg, net price 20 = 21p; 40 mg, 20 = 14p; 500 mg, 20 = £5.99
Various strengths available from APS, Ashbourne (Froop®), Berk (Dryptal®), Cox, CP (including Rusyde®), Hillcross, Norton
Oral solutions, sugar-free, frusemide 1 mg/mL available as Lasix® paediatric liquid; frusemide 4 mg, 8 mg, and 10 mg/mL available from Rosemont (special order)
Injection, frusemide 10 mg/mL, net price 2-mL amp = 23p
Available from Antigen, Evans, Phoenix (all also 5-mL amp)

PoM Lasix® (Hoechst)
Tablets, all scored, frusemide 20 mg, net price 28-tab pack = 82p; 40 mg, 28-tab pack = £1.19; 500 mg (yellow), 20 = £11.44
Paediatric liquid, sugar-free, frusemide 1 mg/mL when reconstituted with purified water, freshly boiled and cooled, net price 150 mL = £1.10
Injection, frusemide 10 mg/mL, net price 2-mL amp = 25p; 5-mL amp = 53p; 25-mL amp = £2.21
Note. Large volume frusemide injections also available from Antigen, IMS (Min-I-Jet®)

BUMETANIDE

Indications: oedema, oliguria due to renal failure
Cautions; Contra-indications: see under Frusemide (but has been used in porphyria, see section 9.8.2)
Side-effects: see under Frusemide; also myalgia (see notes above)
Dose: by mouth, 1 mg in the morning, repeated after 6–8 hours if necessary; severe cases, increased up to 5 mg or more daily
ELDERLY, 500 micrograms daily may be sufficient
By intravenous injection, 1–2 mg, repeated after 20 minutes; when *intramuscular injection* considered necessary, 1 mg initially then adjusted according to response
By intravenous infusion, 2–5 mg over 30–60 minutes

PoM Burinex® (Leo)
Tablets, both scored, bumetanide 1 mg, net price 28-tab pack = £1.72; 5 mg, 20 = £7.81
Liquid, green, sugar-free, bumetanide 1 mg/5 mL. Net price 150 mL = £3.32
Injection, bumetanide 500 micrograms/mL. Net price 2-mL amp = 40p; 4-mL amp = 69p; 10-mL amp = £1.46

ETHACRYNIC ACID
(Etacrynic Acid)

Indications: oedema, oliguria due to renal failure

Cautions; Contra-indications; Side-effects: see under Frusemide and notes above; also contra-indicated in breast-feeding; gastro-intestinal disturbances more severe; also pain on injection

Dose: by mouth, initially 50 mg daily after breakfast; effective initial range of 50–150 mg daily (max. 400 mg) can often be reduced for maintenance and given on alternate days (daily doses above 50 mg divided)

By slow intravenous injection or infusion, 50 mg, increased to 100 mg if necessary

PoM **Edecrin**® (MSD)

Tablets, scored, ethacrynic acid 50 mg. Net price 20 = £1.20. Label: 21

Injection, powder for reconstitution, ethacrynic acid (as sodium salt). Net price 50-mg vial = £1.26

PIRETANIDE

Indications: hypertension

Cautions; Contra-indications; Side-effects: see under Frusemide; side-effects less marked at dosage level used for hypertension

Dose: 6–12 mg in the morning with food

PoM **Arelix**® (Hoechst)

Capsules, m/r, green/orange, enclosing yellow pellets, piretanide 6 mg. Net price 28-cap pack = £3.61. Label: 21

TORASEMIDE

Indications: oedema, hypertension

Cautions; Contra-indications; Side-effects: see under Frusemide; avoid in pregnancy and breast-feeding

Dose: by mouth, oedema, 5 mg once daily, preferably in the morning, increased if required to 20 mg once daily; usual max. 40 mg daily

Hypertension, 2.5 mg daily, increased if necessary to 5 mg once daily

By slow intravenous injection at a rate of 4 mg/minute, 10 mg daily, increased if necessary to 20 mg daily (20 mg initially in acute conditions such as pulmonary oedema); usual max. 40 mg daily (higher doses, up to 200 mg daily, may be required particularly in oedema of renal origin)

▼ PoM **Torem**® (Boehringer Mannheim)

Tablets, torasemide 2.5 mg, net price 28-tab pack = £4.25; 5 mg (scored), 28-tab pack = £6.23; 10 mg (scored), 28-tab pack = £9.16

Injection, torasemide 5 mg/mL, net price 2-mL amp = 40p, 4-mL amp = 74p

2.2.3   Potassium-sparing diuretics

Amiloride and **triamterene** on their own are weak diuretics. They cause retention of potassium and are therefore used as a more effective alternative to giving potassium supplements with thiazide or loop diuretics. (See section 2.2.4 for compound preparations with thiazides or loop diuretics.)

Spironolactone is also a potassium-sparing diuretic, and potentiates thiazide or loop diuretics by antagonising aldosterone. It is of value in the treatment of the oedema of cirrhosis of the liver and is effective in oedema of heart failure, particularly when congestion has caused hepatic engorgement.

Spironolactone is also used in primary hyperaldosteronism (Conn's syndrome).

Potassium canrenoate has similar uses to spironolactone, but can be given parenterally. It is metabolised to canrenone, which is also a metabolite of spironolactone.

Potassium supplements must **not** be given with potassium-sparing diuretics. It is also important to bear in mind that administration of a potassium-sparing diuretic to a patient receiving an ACE inhibitor can cause severe hyperkalaemia.

AMILORIDE HYDROCHLORIDE

Indications: oedema, potassium conservation with thiazide and loop diuretics

Cautions: pregnancy and breast-feeding; monitor in renal impairment (avoid if moderate to severe, see also Appendix 3); diabetes mellitus; elderly; **interactions:** Appendix 1 (diuretics)

Contra-indications: hyperkalaemia, renal failure

Side-effects: include gastro-intestinal disturbances, dry mouth, rashes, confusion, orthostatic hypotension, hyperkalaemia, hyponatraemia

Dose: used alone, initially 10 mg daily *or* 5 mg twice daily, adjusted according to response; max. 20 mg daily

With other diuretics, congestive heart failure and hypertension, initially 5–10 mg daily; cirrhosis with ascites, initially 5 mg daily

PoM **Amiloride** (Non-proprietary)

Tablets, amiloride hydrochloride 5 mg, net price 20 = 42p

Available from APS, Ashbourne (Amilospare®), Berk (Berkamil®), Cox, CP, Hillcross, Norton

Oral solution, sugar-free, amiloride hydrochloride 5 mg/5 mL, net price 125 mL = £27.35

Available from Rosemont (Amilamont®)

PoM **Midamor**® (Morson)

Tablets, yellow, amiloride hydrochloride 5 mg. Net price 100-tab pack = £1.95

Compound preparations with thiazide or loop diuretics, see section 2.2.4

TRIAMTERENE

Indications: oedema, potassium conservation with thiazide and loop diuretics

Cautions; Contra-indications: see under Amiloride Hydrochloride; may cause blue fluorescence of urine

Side-effects: include gastro-intestinal disturbances, dry mouth, rashes; slight decrease in blood pressure, hyperkalaemia, hyponatraemia; photosensitivity and blood disorders also reported; triamterene found in kidney stones

Dose: initially 150–250 mg daily, reducing to alternate days after 1 week; taken in divided doses after breakfast and lunch; lower initial dose when given with other diuretics

COUNSELLING. Urine may look slightly blue in some lights

PoM Dytac® (Pharmark)

Capsules, maroon, triamterene 50 mg. Net price 30-cap pack = £6.98. Label: 14 (see above), 21

Compound preparations with thiazides or loop diuretics, see section 2.2.4

ALDOSTERONE ANTAGONISTS

POTASSIUM CANRENOATE

Indications: oedema associated with secondary hyperaldosteronism, liver failure, chronic decompensated heart disease

Cautions; Contra-indications; Side-effects: see under Spironolactone; nausea and vomiting may occur, particularly after high doses; pain and irritation at injection site

Dose: by slow intravenous injection or intravenous infusion, 200–400 mg daily (exceptionally 800 mg)

PoM Spiroctan-M® (Boehringer Mannheim)

Injection, potassium canrenoate 20 mg/mL. Net price 10-mL amp = 71p

---

SPIRONOLACTONE

Indications: oedema and ascites in cirrhosis of the liver, malignant ascites, nephrotic syndrome, congestive heart failure; primary hyperaldosteronism

Cautions: potential human metabolic products carcinogenic in *rodents*; elderly; hepatic impairment; renal impairment (avoid if moderate to severe); monitor electrolytes (discontinue if hyperkalaemia occurs); porphyria (see section 9.8.2); **interactions:** Appendix 1 (diuretics)

Contra-indications: hyperkalaemia, hyponatraemia, severe renal impairment; pregnancy and breast-feeding; Addison's disease

Side-effects: gastro-intestinal disturbances; impotence, gynaecomastia; menstrual irregularities; lethargy, headache, confusion; rashes; hyperkalaemia (see also Cautions); hyponatraemia; hepatotoxicity, osteomalacia, and blood disorders reported

Dose: 100–200 mg daily, increased to 400 mg if required; CHILD initially 3 mg/kg daily in divided doses

PoM Spironolactone (Non-proprietary)

Tablets, spironolactone 25 mg, net price 20 = 54p; 50 mg, 20 = £1.54; 100 mg, 20 = £1.79

Available from APS, Ashbourne (Spirospare®), Berk (Spirolone®), Cox, Hillcross, Lagap (Laractone®), Norton

Oral suspensions, sugar-free, spironolactone 5 mg, 10 mg, 25 mg, and 50 mg/5 mL available from Rosemont (special order)

PoM Aldactone® (Searle)

Tablets, all f/c, spironolactone 25 mg (buff), net price 100-tab pack = £9.88; 50 mg (off-white), 100-tab pack = £19.76; 100 mg (buff), 28-tab pack = £11.07

PoM Spiroctan® (Boehringer Mannheim)

Tablets, both s/c, spironolactone 25 mg (blue, contains tartrazine), net price 100-tab pack = £7.22; 50 mg (green), 100-tab pack = £13.85

Capsules, green, spironolactone 100 mg. Net price 28-cap pack = £7.56

Compound preparations with thiazides or loop diuretics, see section 2.2.4

2.2.4 Potassium-sparing diuretics with other diuretics

Although it is preferable to prescribe thiazides (section 2.2.1) and potassium-sparing diuretics (section 2.2.3) separately, the use of fixed combinations may be justified if compliance is a problem. Potassium-sparing diuretics are not usually necessary in the routine treatment of hypertension, unless hypokalaemia develops. For **interactions**, see Appendix 1 (diuretics).

Amiloride with thiazides

PoM Co-amilozide (Non-proprietary)

Tablets, co-amilozide 2.5/25 (amiloride hydrochloride 2.5 mg, hydrochlorothiazide 25 mg). Net price 28-tab pack = £1.94

Available from CP, Du Pont (Moduret 25®), Lagap

Dose: hypertension, oedema, 1–4 tablets, increased if necessary to a max. of 8, daily

Tablets, co-amilozide 5/50 (amiloride hydrochloride 5 mg, hydrochlorothiazide 50 mg). Net price 20 = 78p

Available from APS, Ashbourne (Amilmaxco 5/50®), Baker Norton (Amil-Co®), Berk (Delvas®), Cox, CP, Du Pont (Moduretic®), Hillcross, Lagap, Norton

Dose: hypertension, oedema, 1–2 tablets, increased if necessary to max. of 4, daily

Oral solution, co-amilozide 5/50 (amiloride hydrochloride 5 mg, hydrochlorothiazide 50 mg)/5 mL. Net price 200 mL = £4.61

Available from Du Pont (Moduretic®)

Dose: as for co-amilozide 5 /50 tablets above (5 mL = 1 tablet)

PoM Navispare® (Ciba)

Tablets, f/c, orange, amiloride hydrochloride 2.5 mg, cyclopenthiazide 250 micrograms. Net price 28-tab pack = £2.06

Additives: include gluten

Dose: hypertension, 1–2 tablets in the morning

Amiloride with loop diuretics

PoM Co-amilofruse (Non-proprietary)

Tablets, co-amilofruse 2.5/20 (amiloride hydrochloride 2.5 mg, frusemide 20 mg). Net price 28-tab pack = £3.17, 56-tab pack = £6.21

Available from CP (Aridil®), Hillcross, Rhône-Poulenc Rorer (Frumil LS®)

Dose: oedema, 1 tablet in the morning

Tablets, co-amilofruse 5/40 (amiloride hydrochloride 5 mg, frusemide 40 mg). Net price 28-tab pack = £3.12

Available from Baker Norton (Fru-Co®), Hoechst (Lasoride®), Rhône-Poulenc Rorer (Frumil®)

Dose: oedema, 1–2 tablets in the morning

Tablets, co-amilofruse 10/80 (amiloride hydrochloride 10 mg, frusemide 80 mg). Net price 28-tab pack = £7.20, 56-tab pack = £14.11

Available from CP (Aridil®), Rhône-Poulenc Rorer (Frumil Forte®)

Dose: oedema, 1 tablet in the morning

PoM Burinex A® (Leo)

Tablets, ivory, scored, amiloride hydrochloride 5 mg, bumetanide 1 mg. Net price 28-tab pack = £3.20

Dose: oedema, 1–2 tablets daily

Triamterene with thiazides

COUNSELLING. Urine may look slightly blue in some lights

PoM Dyazide® (SK&F)

Tablets, peach, scored, co-triamterzide 50/25 (triamterene 50 mg, hydrochlorothiazide 25 mg). Net price 30-tab pack = £2.41. Label: 14 (see above), 21

Dose: hypertension, 1 tablet daily after breakfast; oedema, 2 tablets daily (1 after breakfast and 1 after midday meal) increased to 3 daily if necessary (2 after breakfast and 1 after midday meal); usual maintenance, 1 daily or 2 on alternate days; max. 4 daily

Note. Tablets containing co-triamterzide 50/25 (triamterene 50 mg and hydrochlorothiazide 25 mg) are also available from Ashbourne (TriamaxCo®), Baker Norton (Triam-Co®)

PoM Dytide® (Pharmark)

Capsules, clear/maroon, triamterene 50 mg, benzthiazide 25 mg. Net price 30-cap pack = £6.97. Label: 14 (see above), 21

Dose: oedema, initially 3 capsules daily (2 after breakfast and 1 after midday meal) for 1 week then 1 or 2 on alternate days

PoM Kalspare® (Dominion)

Tablets, orange, f/c, scored, triamterene 50 mg, chlorthalidone 50 mg. Net price 28-tab pack = £3.19. Label: 14 (see above), 21

Dose: hypertension, oedema, 1–2 tablets in the morning

Triamterene with loop diuretics

COUNSELLING. Urine may look slightly blue in some lights

PoM Frusene® (Fisons)

Tablets, yellow, scored, triamterene 50 mg, frusemide 40 mg. Net price 56-tab pack = £5.94. Label: 14 (see above), 21

Dose: oedema, ½–2 tablets daily in the morning

Spironolactone with thiazides

PoM Co-flumactone (Non-proprietary)

Tablets, co-flumactone 25/25 (hydroflumethiazide 25 mg, spironolactone 25 mg). Net price 100-tab pack = £16.86

Available from Baker Norton (Spiro-Co®), Searle (Aldactide 25®)

Dose: congestive heart failure, initially 4 tablets daily; range 1–8 daily

Tablets, co-flumactone 50/50 (hydroflumethiazide 50 mg, spironolactone 50 mg). Net price 28-tab pack = £8.92

Available from Baker Norton (Spiro-Co 50®), Searle (Aldactide 50®)

Dose: congestive heart failure, initially 2 tablets daily; range 1–4 daily

Spironolactone with loop diuretics

PoM Lasilactone® (Hoechst)

Capsules, blue/white, spironolactone 50 mg, frusemide 20 mg. Net price 28-cap pack = £4.91

Dose: resistant oedema, 1–4 capsules daily

2.2.5   Osmotic diuretics

Osmotic diuretics are rarely used in heart failure as they may acutely expand the blood volume. **Mannitol** is used in cerebral oedema—a typical dose is 1 g/kg as a 20% solution given by rapid intravenous infusion.

MANNITOL

Indications: see notes above

Cautions: extravasation causes inflammation and thrombophlebitis

Contra-indications: congestive cardiac failure, pulmonary oedema

Side-effects: chills, fever

Dose: by intravenous infusion, diuresis, 50–200 g over 24 hours, preceded by a test dose of 200 mg/kg by slow intravenous injection

Cerebral oedema, see notes above

PoM Mannitol (Non-proprietary)

Intravenous infusion, mannitol 10%, 20%, and 25%

Available from Baxter (10% and 20%) and IMS (Min-I-Jet® Mannitol 25%)

2.2.6   Mercurial diuretics

They are effective diuretics but are now almost never used because of their nephrotoxicity. Mersalyl **must** be given by intramuscular injection; intravenous use may cause severe hypotension and sudden death.

MERSALYL

Indications: oedema unresponsive to other diuretics (but see notes above)

Cautions: recent myocardial infarction, treatment with cardiac glycosides, frequent extrasystoles

Contra-indications: renal impairment; pregnancy; porphyria (see section 9.8.2)

Side-effects: gastro-intestinal disturbances, allergic reactions; see also notes above

PoM Mersalyl Injection, mersalyl sodium 100 mg, theophylline 50 mg/mL

Dose: by deep intramuscular injection, 0.5–2 mL

2.2.7   Carbonic anhydrase inhibitors

Acetazolamide and dichlorphenamide are weak diuretics, and are little used for their diuretic effect. They inhibit the formation of aqueous fluid, and are used in glaucoma (see section 11.6). Although acetazolamide is used as a prophylactic measure for mountain sickness it is not a substitute for acclimatisation.

2.2.8   Diuretics with potassium

Many patients on diuretics do not need potassium supplements (see section 9.2.1.1). For many of those who do, the amount of potassium ion in combined preparations may not be enough, and for this reason their use is to be discouraged.

Diuretics with potassium and potassium-sparing diuretics should **not** usually be given together.

COUNSELLING. Modified-release potassium tablets should be swallowed whole with plenty of fluid during meals while sitting or standing

PoM **Burinex K**® (Leo)
Tablets, bumetanide 500 micrograms, potassium 7.7 mmol for modified release. Net price 20 = 81p. Label: 25, 27, counselling, see above

PoM **Diumide-K Continus**® (ASTA Medica)
Tablets, f/c, white/orange, frusemide 40 mg, potassium 8 mmol for modified release. Net price 30-tab pack = £3.13. Label: 25, 27, counselling, see above

PoM **Lasikal**® (Hoechst)
Tablets, white/yellow, f/c, frusemide 20 mg, potassium 10 mmol for modified release. Net price 100-tab pack = £5.31. Label: 25, 27, counselling, see above

PoM **Lasix+K**® (Hoechst)
Calendar pack, 30 white scored tablets, frusemide 40 mg; 60 m/r yellow tablets, potassium chloride (potassium 10 mmol). Net price = £2.97. Label: 25, 27, counselling, see above

PoM **Neo-NaClex-K**® (Goldshield)
Tablets, pink/white, f/c, bendrofluazide 2.5 mg, potassium 8.4 mmol for modified release. Net price 20 = £1.18. Label: 25, 27, counselling, see above

2.3   Anti-arrhythmic drugs

2.3.1   Management of arrhythmias
2.3.2   Drugs for arrhythmias

2.3.1   Management of arrhythmias

Management of an arrhythmia, apart from the treatment of associated heart failure, requires precise diagnosis of the type of arrhythmia, and electrocardiography is essential.

ECTOPIC BEATS. If spontaneous with a normal heart, these rarely require treatment beyond reassurance. If they are particularly troublesome, beta-blockers are sometimes effective and may be safer than other suppressant drugs.

ATRIAL FIBRILLATION. The ventricular rate can usually be controlled with digoxin. If adequate control at rest or during exercise cannot be achieved readily, a beta-blocker or verapamil may be added if ventricular function is adequate. In some cases other classes of drugs may be appropriate. Anticoagulants may be indicated especially in valvular or myocardial disease, and in the elderly (aspirin is less effective at preventing emboli and should only be considered if the risk is low).

ATRIAL FLUTTER. The ventricular rate can often be controlled with digoxin. Reversion to sinus rhythm (if indicated) is best achieved by appropriately synchronised d.c. shock, rather than by drug therapy. If the arrhythmia is long-standing a period of treatment with anticoagulants should be considered before cardioversion to avoid the complication of emboli.

PAROXYSMAL SUPRAVENTRICULAR TACHYCARDIA. In most patients this remits spontaneously or can be returned to sinus rhythm by reflex vagal stimulation with respiratory manoeuvres, prompt squatting, or pressure over one carotid sinus (**important:** pressure over carotid sinus should be restricted to monitored patients—it can be dangerous in recent ischaemia, digitalis toxicity, or the elderly).

If vagal stimulation fails, intravenous administration of adenosine is usually the treatment of choice; digitalisation or intravenous administration of a beta-blocker may also be effective. Intravenous administration of verapamil is useful for patients without myocardial or valvular disease (**important:** never in patients recently treated with beta-blockers, see p. 98). For arrhythmias that are poorly tolerated, synchronised d.c. shock usually provides rapid relief.

In cases of paroxysmal supraventricular tachycardia with block, digitalis toxicity should be suspected. In addition to stopping administration of the cardiac glycoside and giving potassium supplements, intravenous administration of a beta-blocker may be useful. Specific digoxin antibody is available if the toxicity is considered life-threatening (section 2.1.1).

ARRHYTHMIAS AFTER MYOCARDIAL INFARCTION. It is best to do nothing in patients with a paroxysmal tachycardia or rapid irregularity of the pulse until an ECG record is obtainable. If the condition of the patient is such that death due to the arrhythmia seems possible lignocaine should be given intravenously (see p. 72). Bradycardia, particularly if complicated by hypotension, should be treated with atropine sulphate, given intravenously in a dose of 0.3 to 1 mg, repeated if the initial dose is effective.

VENTRICULAR TACHYCARDIA. Drug treatment is used both for the treatment of ventricular tachycardia and for prophylaxis of recurrent attacks that merit suppression. Ventricular tachycardia requires treatment most commonly in the acute stage of myocardial infarction, but the likelihood of this and other life-threatening arrhythmias diminishes sharply over the first 24 hours after the attack, especially in patients without heart failure or shock. Lignocaine is the preferred drug for emergency use. Other drugs are best administered under specialist supervision. Very rapid ventricular tachycardia causes profound circulatory collapse and should be treated urgently with d.c. shock.

Torsades de pointes is a special form of ventricular tachycardia which tends to occur in the presence of a long QT interval (usually drug induced, but hypokalaemia, severe bradycardia, and genetic predisposition may also be implicated). The episodes are usually self-limiting, but are frequently recurrent and may cause impairment (or loss) of consciousness. If not controlled, the arrhythmia may progress to ventricular fibrillation. Intravenous infusion of magnesium sulphate (see section 9.5.1.3) is usually effective. Anti-arrhythmics (including lignocaine) may further prolong the QT interval, thus worsening the condition.

2.3.2   Drugs for arrhythmias

Anti-arrhythmic drugs can be classified clinically into those that act on supraventricular arrhythmias (e.g. verapamil), those that act on both supraventricular and ventricular arrhythmias (e.g. disopyramide), and those that act on ventricular arrhythmias (e.g. lignocaine).

They can also be classified according to their effects on the electrical behaviour of myocardial cells during activity (termed 'action potential'):

Class Ia, b, c: membrane stabilising drugs (e.g. quinidine, lignocaine, flecainide respectively)

Class II: beta-blockers

Class III: amiodarone, bretylium, and sotalol (also Class II)

Class IV: calcium-channel blockers (includes verapamil but not the nifedipine group)

This latter classification (the Vaughan Williams classification) is of less clinical significance.

CAUTIONS. The negative inotropic effects of anti-arrhythmic drugs tend to be additive therefore special care should be taken if two or more are used, especially in impaired myocardial function. Most or all drugs that are effective in countering arrhythmias can also provoke them in some circumstances; moreover, hypokalaemia enhances the arrhythmogenic (pro-arrhythmic) effect of many drugs.

SUPRAVENTRICULAR ARRHYTHMIAS

Adenosine is usually the treatment of choice for terminating paroxysmal supraventricular tachycardia. As it has a very short duration of action (half-life only about 8 to 10 seconds, except in those taking dipyridamole—see below), most side-effects are short lived. Unlike verapamil, adenosine may be used after a beta-blocker. Verapamil may be preferable to adenosine in asthma.

Oral administration of a **cardiac glycoside** (such as digoxin, section 2.1.1) is the treatment of choice in slowing ventricular response in cases of atrial fibrillation and atrial flutter. Intravenous digoxin, preferably infused slowly, is occasionally required if the ventricular rate needs rapid control. Ouabain acts more quickly but may be difficult to obtain since it is not on the UK market.

Verapamil (section 2.6.2) is usually effective for supraventricular tachycardias. An initial intravenous dose (**important**: serious beta-blocker interaction hazard, see p. 98) may be followed by oral treatment; hypotension may occur with larger doses. It should not be used for tachyarrhythmias where the QRS complex is wide (i.e. broad complex) unless a supraventricular origin has been established beyond reasonable doubt. It is also contra-indicated in atrial fibrillation with pre-excitation (e.g. Wolff-Parkinson-White syndrome). It should not be used in children with arrhythmias without specialist advice; some supraventricular arrhythmias in childhood can be accelerated by verapamil with dangerous consequences.

Drugs for both supraventricular and ventricular arrhythmias include **amiodarone**, **beta-blockers**, **disopyramide**, **flecainide**, **procainamide**, **propafenone** and **quinidine**, see below under Supraventricular and Ventricular Arrhythmias.

ADENOSINE

Indications: rapid reversion to sinus rhythm of paroxysmal supraventricular tachycardias, including those associated with accessory pathways (e.g. Wolff-Parkinson-White syndrome); aid to diagnosis of broad or narrow complex supraventricular tachycardias

Cautions: atrial fibrillation or flutter with accessory pathway (increased conduction down anomalous pathway may develop); heart transplant (see below); **interactions:** Appendix 1 (adenosine)—**important:** interaction with dipyridamole liable to be serious

Contra-indications: second- or third-degree AV block and sick sinus syndrome (unless pacemaker fitted); asthma

Side-effects: include transient facial flush, chest pain, dyspnoea, bronchospasm, choking sensation, nausea, light-headedness; severe bradycardia reported (requiring temporary pacing); ECG may show transient rhythm disturbances

Dose: by rapid intravenous injection into central or large peripheral vein, 3 mg over 2 seconds with cardiac monitoring; if necessary followed by 6 mg after 1–2 minutes, and then by 12 mg after a further 1–2 minutes; increments should not be given if high level AV block develops at any particular dose

Note. 3-mg dose ineffective in a number of patients, therefore higher initial dose used in some circumstances but patients with *heart transplant* are **very sensitive** to effects of adenosine, and should **not** receive higher initial dose. Also if essential to give with dipyridamole (see also Cautions) reduce initial dose to 0.5–1 mg.

▼ PoM **Adenocor**® (Sanofi Winthrop)
Injection, adenosine 3 mg/mL in physiological saline. Net price 2-mL vial = £4.05 (hosp. only)
Note. Intravenous infusion of adenosine (Adenoscan®, Sanofi Winthrop) may be used in conjunction with radionuclide myocardial perfusion imaging in patients who cannot exercise adequately or for whom exercise is inappropriate—consult manufacturer's literature

---

CARDIAC GLYCOSIDES
Section 2.1.1

VERAPAMIL
Section 2.6.2

SUPRAVENTRICULAR AND VENTRICULAR ARRHYTHMIAS

Amiodarone is used in the treatment of tachycardia associated with the Wolff-Parkinson-White syndrome. It may only be used for the treatment of other arrhythmias when other drugs are ineffective or contra-indicated and should be initiated only under hospital or specialist supervision. These include paroxysmal supraventricular, nodal and ventricular tachycardias, atrial fibrillation and flutter, and ventricular fibrillation. It may be given by intravenous infusion as well as by mouth, and has the advantage of causing little or no myocardial depression. Unlike oral amiodarone, intravenous amiodarone may act relatively rapidly.

Amiodarone has a very long half-life (extending to several weeks) and only needs to be given once daily (but high doses may cause nausea unless divided). Many weeks or months may be required to achieve steady-state plasma concentrations; this is particularly important when interactions with amiodarone are considered (see also Appendix 1).

Most patients taking amiodarone develop corneal microdeposits (reversible on withdrawal of treatment); these rarely interfere with vision, but drivers may be dazzled by headlights at night. Because of the possibility of phototoxic reactions, patients should be advised to shield the skin from light and to use a wide-spectrum sunscreen such as RoC Total Sunblock® (section 13.8.1) to protect against both long ultraviolet and visible light.

Amiodarone contains iodine and can cause disorders of thyroid function; both hypothyroidism and hyperthyroidism may occur. Clinical assessment is unreliable, and laboratory tests should be performed every 6 months. Thyroxine (T4) may be raised in the absence of hyperthyroidism; therefore tri-iodothyronine (T3), T4, and thyroid-stimulating hormone (thyrotrophin, TSH) should all be measured. A raised T3 and T4 with a very low or undetectable TSH concentration suggests the development of thyrotoxicosis. The thyrotoxicosis may be very refractory, and amiodarone should usually be withdrawn at least temporarily to help achieve control. Hypothyroidism can be treated with replacement therapy without withdrawing amiodarone if it is essential.

Pneumonitis should always be suspected if new or progressive shortness of breath or cough develops in a patient taking amiodarone. Fresh neurological symptoms should raise the possibility of peripheral neuropathy.

Beta-blockers act as anti-arrhythmic drugs principally by attenuating the effects of the sympathetic system on automaticity and conductivity within the heart, for details see section 2.4. For special reference to the role of **sotalol** in ventricular arrhythmias, see also p. 75.

Disopyramide may be given by intravenous injection to control arrhythmias after myocardial infarction (including those not responding to lignocaine), but it impairs cardiac contractility. Oral administration of disopyramide is useful but it has an antimuscarinic effect which limits its use in patients with glaucoma or prostatic hypertrophy.

Flecainide belongs to the same general class as lignocaine. It may be of value for serious symptomatic ventricular arrhythmias. It may also be indicated for junctional re-entry tachycardias. Preliminary results with paroxysmal atrial fibrillation are promising. As with quinidine it may precipitate serious arrhythmias in a small minority of patients (including those with otherwise normal hearts).

Procainamide can be given by intravenous injection to control ventricular arrhythmias, but prolonged oral use can cause a syndrome resembling systemic lupus erythematosus.

Propafenone is used for the prophylaxis and treatment of ventricular arrhythmias and also for some supraventricular arrhythmias. It has complex mechanisms of action, including weak beta-blocking activity (therefore great caution is needed in obstructive airways disease—contra-indicated if severe).

Quinidine may be effective in suppressing supraventricular and ventricular arrhythmias. It may itself precipitate rhythm disorders, and is best used on specialist advice; it can cause hypersensitivity reactions and gastro-intestinal upsets.

Drugs for supraventricular arrhythmias include **adenosine**, **cardiac glycosides** and **verapamil**, see above under Supraventricular Arrhythmias. Drugs for ventricular arrhythmias include **bretylium**, **lignocaine**, **mexiletine**, **moracizine**, **phenytoin**, and **tocainide**, see below under Ventricular Arrhythmias.

AMIODARONE HYDROCHLORIDE

Indications: see notes above (should be initiated in hospital or under specialist supervision)

Cautions: liver-function and thyroid-function tests required in long-term therapy (but interferes with tests of thyroid function, see notes above); heart failure; renal impairment; elderly; severe bradycardia and conduction disturbances in excessive dosage; intravenous use may cause moderate and transient fall in blood pressure (circulatory collapse precipitated by rapid administration or overdosage); porphyria (see section 9.8.2); **interactions:** Appendix 1 (amiodarone)

Contra-indications: sinus bradycardia, sino-atrial heart block; unless pacemaker fitted avoid in severe conduction disturbances or sinus node disease; thyroid dysfunction; pregnancy and breast-feeding (see also Appendixes 4 and 5); iodine sensitivity; avoid *intravenous use* in severe respiratory failure, circulatory collapse, severe arterial hypotension, congestive heart failure

Side-effects: reversible corneal microdeposits (sometimes with night glare), rarely impaired vision due to optic neuritis; peripheral neuropathy and myopathy (usually reversible on withdrawal); bradycardia and conduction disturbances (see Cautions); phototoxicity and rarely persistent slate-grey skin discoloration (see also notes); hypothyroidism, hyperthyroidism, diffuse pulmonary alveolitis and fibrosis, hepatitis; rarely nausea, vomiting, metallic taste, tremor, nightmares, vertigo, headache, sleeplessness, fatigue, benign raised intracranial pressure, epididymitis; ataxia, rashes (including exfoliative dermatitis), vasculitis, alopecia, thrombocytopenia, increased prothrombin time reported; anaphylaxis on rapid injection, also bronchospasm or apnoea in respiratory failure

Dose: by mouth, 200 mg 3 times daily for 1 week reduced to 200 mg twice daily for a further week; maintenance, usually 200 mg daily or the minimum required to control the arrhythmia

By intravenous infusion via caval catheter, 5 mg/kg over 20–120 minutes with ECG monitoring; max. 1.2 g in 24 hours

PoM Amiodarone Hydrochloride (Non-proprietary)

Tablets, amiodarone hydrochloride 100 mg, net price 28-tab pack = £4.52; 200 mg, 28-tab pack = £6.97. Label: 11
Available from APS, Cox, Generics, Hillcross, Norton

PoM Cordarone X® (Sanofi Winthrop)

Tablets, both scored, amiodarone hydrochloride 100 mg, net price 28-tab pack = £5.00; 200 mg, 28-tab pack = £8.19. Label: 11

Injection, amiodarone hydrochloride 50 mg/mL. Net price 3-mL amp = £1.50. For dilution and use as an infusion

DISOYRAMIDE

Indications: ventricular arrhythmias, especially after myocardial infarction; supraventricular arrhythmias

Cautions: glaucoma; heart failure (avoid if severe); prostatic enlargement; hepatic and renal impairment; elderly; pregnancy and breast-feeding; **interactions:** Appendix 1 (disopyramide)

Contra-indications: second- and third-degree heart block and sinus node dysfunction (unless pacemaker fitted); cardiogenic shock; severe uncompensated heart failure

Side-effects: gastro-intestinal irritation; myocardial depression, hypotension, atrioventricular block; antimuscarinic effects include dry mouth, blurred vision, urinary retention; psychosis, cholestatic jaundice, hypoglycaemia also reported

Dose: by mouth, 300–800 mg daily in divided doses

By slow intravenous injection, 2 mg/kg over at least 5 minutes to a max. of 150 mg, with ECG monitoring, followed immediately *either* by 200 mg *by mouth,* then 200 mg every 8 hours for 24 hours *or* 400 micrograms/kg/hour *by intravenous infusion;* max. 300 mg in first hour and 800 mg daily

PoM Disopyramide (Non-proprietary)

Capsules, disopyramide (as phosphate) 100 mg, net price 20 = £1.31; 150 mg, 20 = £2.31
Available from APS, Hillcross, Lagap (100 mg), Monmouth (Isomide® 100 mg), Norton (100 mg)

PoM Rythmodan® (Roussel)

Capsules, disopyramide 100 mg (green/beige), net price 84-cap pack = £7.53; 150 mg, 84-cap pack = £10.99

Injection, disopyramide (as phosphate) 10 mg/mL, net price 5-mL amp = 68p

Modified release

PoM Dirythmin SA® (Astra)

Durules® (= tablets, m/r), f/c, disopyramide (as phosphate) 150 mg. Net price 20 = £2.47. Label: 25
Dose: 300 mg every 12 hours; max. 750 mg daily

PoM Rythmodan Retard® (Roussel)

Tablets, m/r, scored, f/c, disopyramide (as phosphate) 250 mg. Net price 56-tab pack = £16.24. Label: 25
Dose: 250–375 mg every 12 hours
Note. Modified-release capsules containing disopyramide (as phosphate) 250 mg also available from Monmouth (Isomide® CR)

FLECAINIDE ACETATE

Indications: (should be initiated in hospital)
Tablets and injection: AV nodal reciprocating tachycardia, arrhythmias associated with Wolff-Parkinson-White syndrome and similar conditions with accessory pathways, paroxysmal atrial fibrillation in patients with disabling symptoms (arrhythmias of recent onset will respond more readily)

Tablets only: symptomatic sustained ventricular tachycardia, premature ventricular contractions and/or non-sustained ventricular tachycardia causing disabling symptoms in patients resistant to or intolerant of other therapy

Injection only: ventricular tachyarrhythmias resistant to other treatment

Cautions: patients with pacemakers (especially those who may be pacemaker dependent because stimulation threshold may rise appreciably); avoid in sinus node dysfunction, atrial conduction defects, second-degree or greater AV block, bundle branch block or distal block unless pacing rescue available; atrial fibrillation following heart surgery; elderly (see Dose); hepatic and renal impairment (see Appendixes 2 and 3); pregnancy (toxicity in *animal* studies) and breast-feeding; **interactions:** Appendix 1 (flecainide)

Contra-indications: heart failure; history of myocardial infarction and either asymptomatic ventricular ectopics or asymptomatic non-sustained ventricular tachycardia; long-standing atrial fibrillation where no attempt has been made to convert to sinus rhythm; haemodynamically significant valvular heart disease

Side-effects: dizziness, visual disturbances (corneal deposits reported); arrhythmogenic (pro-arrhythmic) effect; rarely nausea and vomiting, photosensitivity; reversible increases in liver enzymes, jaundice; ataxia, peripheral neuropathy, pulmonary fibrosis, pneumonitis also reported

Dose: by mouth, ventricular arrhythmias, 100 mg twice daily; max. 400 mg daily (usually reserved for rapid control or in heavily built patients), reduced after 3–5 days if possible

Supraventricular arrhythmias, 50 mg twice daily, increased if required to max. 300 mg daily

ELDERLY. Rate of elimination may be reduced—care on dose adjustment

By slow intravenous injection, 2 mg/kg over 10–30 minutes, max. 150 mg, with ECG monitoring; followed if required by *infusion* at a rate of 1.5 mg/kg/hour for 1 hour, subsequently reduced to 100–250 micrograms/kg/hour for up to 24 hours; max. cumulative dose in first 24 hours, 600 mg; transfer to *oral* treatment, as above

PoM **Tambocor**® (3M)

Tablets, flecainide acetate 50 mg, net price 60-tab pack = £16.28; 100 mg (scored), 60-tab pack = £23.26

Injection, flecainide acetate 10 mg/mL. Net price 15-mL amp = £4.95

PROCAINAMIDE HYDROCHLORIDE

Indications: ventricular arrhythmias, especially after myocardial infarction; atrial tachycardia

Cautions: elderly; hepatic and renal impairment, asthma, myasthenia gravis; pregnancy; **interactions:** Appendix 1 (procainamide)

Contra-indications: heart block, heart failure, hypotension; systemic lupus erythematosus; not indicated for torsades de pointes (can exacerbate); breast-feeding

Side-effects: nausea, diarrhoea, rashes, fever, myocardial depression, heart failure, lupus erythematosus-like syndrome, agranulocytosis after prolonged treatment; psychosis and angioedema also reported

Dose: by mouth, ventricular arrhythmias, up to 50 mg/kg daily in divided doses, preferably controlled by measurement of plasma concentration (dosage intervals can range from 3–6 hours); atrial arrhythmias, higher doses may be required

By slow intravenous injection, rate not exceeding 50 mg/minute, 100 mg with ECG monitoring, repeated at 5-minute intervals until arrhythmia controlled; max. 1 g

By intravenous infusion, 500–600 mg over 25–30 minutes with ECG monitoring, followed by maintenance at rate of 2–6 mg/minute, then if necessary oral treatment as above, starting 3–4 hours after infusion

PoM **Pronestyl**® (Squibb)

Tablets, scored, procainamide hydrochloride 250 mg. Net price 100-tab pack = £4.70

Injection, procainamide hydrochloride 100 mg/mL. Net price 10-mL vial = £1.90

PROPAFENONE HYDROCHLORIDE

Indications: ventricular arrhythmias; paroxysmal supraventricular tachyarrhythmias which include paroxysmal atrial flutter or fibrillation and paroxysmal re-entrant tachycardias involving the AV node or accessory pathway, where standard therapy ineffective or contra-indicated

Cautions: heart failure; hepatic and renal impairment; elderly; pacemaker patients; pregnancy and breast-feeding (see Appendixes 4 and 5); great caution in obstructive airways disease owing to beta-blocking activity (contra-indicated if severe); **interactions:** Appendix 1 (propafenone)

Contra-indications: uncontrolled congestive heart failure, cardiogenic shock (except arrhythmia induced), severe bradycardia, uncontrolled electrolyte disturbances, severe obstructive pulmonary disease, marked hypotension; myasthenia gravis; unless adequately paced avoid in sinus node dysfunction, atrial conduction defects, second degree or greater AV block, bundle branch block or distal block

Side-effects: constipation, blurred vision, dry mouth (due to antimuscarinic action); dizziness, nausea and vomiting, fatigue, bitter taste, diarrhoea, headache, and allergic skin reactions reported; postural hypotension, particularly in elderly; bradycardia, sino-atrial, atrioventricular, or intraventricular blocks; arrhythmogenic (pro-arrhythmic) effect; rarely hypersensitivity reactions (cholestasis, blood disorders, lupus syndrome); seizures; myoclonus also reported

Dose: 70 kg and over, initially 150 mg 3 times daily after food under direct hospital supervision with ECG monitoring and blood pressure control (if QRS interval prolonged by more than 20%, reduce dose or discontinue until ECG returns to normal limits); may be increased at intervals of at least 3 days to 300 mg twice daily and, if necessary, to max. 300 mg 3 times daily; under 70 kg, reduce dose

ELDERLY may respond to lower doses

PoM **Arythmol**® (Knoll)

Tablets, both f/c, propafenone hydrochloride 150 mg, net price 90-tab pack = £19.48; 300 mg (scored), 60-tab pack = £19.48. Label: 21, 25

QUINIDINE

Indications: suppression of supraventricular tachycardias and ventricular arrhythmias (see notes above)

Cautions: 200-mg test dose to detect hypersensitivity reactions; **interactions:** Appendix 1 (quinidine)

Contra-indications: heart block

Side-effects: see under Procainamide Hydrochloride; also ventricular arrhythmias, thrombocytopenia, haemolytic anaemia; rarely granulomatous hepatitis; also cinchonism (see Quinine, section 5.4.1)

Dose: by mouth, quinidine sulphate 200–400 mg 3–4 times daily

Note. Quinidine sulphate 200 mg ≡ quinidine bisulphate 250 mg

PoM **Quinidine Sulphate** (Non-proprietary)

Tablets, quinidine sulphate 200 mg; 300 mg

Note. May be difficult to obtain

Modified release

PoM Kinidin Durules® (Astra)

Tablets, m/r, f/c, quinidine bisulphate 250 mg. Net price 100-tab pack = £11.05. Label: 25

Dose: 500 mg every 12 hours, adjusted as required

VENTRICULAR ARRHYTHMIAS

Bretylium is only used as an anti-arrhythmic drug in resuscitation. It is given both intramuscularly and intravenously but can cause severe hypotension, particularly after intravenous administration; nausea and vomiting can occur with either route. The intravenous route should only be used in emergency when there is doubt about absorption because of inadequate circulation.

Lignocaine is relatively safe when used by slow intravenous injection and should be considered first for emergency use. Though effective in suppressing ventricular tachycardia and reducing the risk of ventricular fibrillation following myocardial infarction, it has not been shown to reduce mortality when used prophylactically in this condition. In patients with cardiac or hepatic failure doses may need to be reduced to avoid convulsions, depression of the central nervous system, or depression of the cardiovascular system.

Mexiletine may be given as a slow intravenous injection if lignocaine is ineffective; it has a similar action. Adverse cardiovascular and central nervous system effects may limit the dose tolerated; nausea and vomiting may prevent an effective dose being given by mouth.

Moracizine is a newer drug for the prophylaxis and treatment of serious and life-threatening ventricular arrhythmias. In common with other anti-arrhythmic drugs it may aggravate arrhythmias and exacerbate congestive heart failure.

Phenytoin by slow intravenous injection was formerly used in ventricular arrhythmias particularly those caused by cardiac glycosides, but this use is now obsolete.

Tocainide is an analogue of lignocaine; because of a high incidence of blood disorders its use is limited to treatment of life-threatening symptomatic ventricular tachyarrhythmias associated with severely compromised left ventricular function in patients who do not respond to other therapy or for whom other therapy is contra-indicated.

Drugs for both supraventricular and ventricular arrhythmias include **amiodarone, beta-blockers, disopyramide, flecainide, procainamide, propafenone** and **quinidine**, see above under Supraventricular and Ventricular Arrhythmias.

BRETYLIUM TOSYLATE
(Bretylium Tosilate)

Indications: ventricular arrhythmias resistant to other treatment

Cautions: do not give noradrenaline or other sympathomimetic amines; may exacerbate ventricular arrhythmias due to cardiac glycosides; **interactions:** Appendix 1 (adrenergic neurone blockers)

Contra-indications: phaeochromocytoma

Side-effects: hypotension, nausea and vomiting; tissue necrosis reported after intramuscular injection (rotate sites)

Dose: *by slow intravenous injection,* 5–10 mg/kg over 8–10 minutes (preferably 15–30 minutes) with blood pressure and ECG monitoring; may be repeated after 1–2 hours to a total dosage of 30 mg/kg (intravenous dose being diluted to 10 mg/mL in glucose 5% or sodium chloride intravenous infusion)

Maintenance 5–10 mg/kg *by intramuscular injection, by intravenous infusion* (over 15–30 minutes) every 6–8 hours, *or* 1–2 mg/minute *by continuous intravenous infusion*

PoM Bretylate® (Wellcome)

Injection, bretylium tosylate 50 mg/mL. Net price 10-mL amp = £19.81

PoM Min-I-Jet® Bretylium Tosylate (IMS)

Injection, bretylium tosylate 50 mg/mL. Net price 10-mL disposable syringe = £19.75

LIGNOCAINE HYDROCHLORIDE
(Lidocaine Hydrochloride)

Indications: ventricular arrhythmias, especially after myocardial infarction

Cautions: lower doses in congestive cardiac failure, in hepatic failure, and following cardiac surgery; elderly; **interactions:** Appendix 1 (lignocaine)

Contra-indications: sino-atrial disorders, all grades of atrioventricular block, severe myocardial depression; porphyria (see section 9.8.2)

Side-effects: dizziness, paraesthesia, or drowsiness (particularly if injection too rapid); other CNS effects include confusion, respiratory depression and convulsions; hypotension and bradycardia (may lead to cardiac arrest); hypersensitivity reported

Dose: *by intravenous injection,* in patients without gross circulatory impairment, 100 mg as a bolus over a few minutes (50 mg in lighter patients or those whose circulation is severely impaired), followed immediately by *infusion* of 4 mg/minute for 30 minutes, 2 mg/minute for 2 hours, then 1 mg/minute; reduce concentration further if infusion continued beyond 24 hours (ECG monitoring and specialist advice for infusion)

IMPORTANT. Following intravenous injection lignocaine has a short duration of action (lasting for 15–20 minutes). If an *intravenous infusion* is not immediately available the initial *intravenous injection* of 50–100 mg can be repeated if necessary once or twice at intervals of not less than 10 minutes

PoM Lignocaine in Glucose Infusion (Non-proprietary)

Infusion, lignocaine hydrochloride 0.1% (1 mg/mL) and 0.2% (2 mg/mL) in glucose intravenous infusion 5%. 500-mL containers

Available from Baxter

PoM Min-I-Jet® Lignocaine (IMS)

Injection, lignocaine hydrochloride 1% (10 mg/mL), net price 10-mL disposable syringe = £3.39; 2% (20 mg/mL), 5-mL disposable syringe = £3.07

PoM **Xylocard**® (Astra)

Injection 100 mg, lignocaine hydrochloride (anhydrous) 20 mg/mL. Net price 5-mL syringe = £1.61

MEXILETINE HYDROCHLORIDE

Indications: ventricular arrhythmias, especially after myocardial infarction

Cautions: hepatic impairment; close monitoring on initiation of therapy (including ECG, blood pressure, etc.); **interactions:** Appendix 1 (mexiletine)

Contra-indications: bradycardia, cardiogenic shock; high degree AV block (unless pacemaker fitted)

Side-effects: nausea, vomiting, constipation; bradycardia, hypotension, atrial fibrillation, palpitations, conduction defects, exacerbation of arrhythmias, torsades de pointes; drowsiness, confusion, convulsions, psychiatric disorders, dysarthria, ataxia, paraesthesia, nystagmus, tremor; jaundice, hepatitis, and blood disorders reported; see also notes above

Dose: by mouth, initial dose 400 mg (may be increased to 600 mg if opioid analgesics also given), followed after 2 hours by 200–250 mg 3–4 times daily

By intravenous injection, 100–250 mg at a rate of 25 mg/minute with ECG monitoring followed by *infusion* of 250 mg as a 0.1% solution over 1 hour, 125 mg/hour for 2 hours, then 500 micrograms/minute

PoM **Mexitil**® (Boehringer Ingelheim)

Capsules, mexiletine hydrochloride 50 mg (purple/red), net price 100-cap pack = £4.95; 200 mg (red), 100-cap pack = £11.87

Injection, mexiletine hydrochloride 25 mg/mL. Net price 10-mL amp = £1.49

Modified release
PoM **Mexitil PL**® (Boehringer Ingelheim)

Perlongets® (= capsules, m/r, each enclosing 5 miniature tablets), turquoise/scarlet, mexiletine hydrochloride 360 mg. Net price 56-cap pack = £11.97. Label: 25

Dose: 1 capsule twice daily

MORACIZINE HYDROCHLORIDE

Indications: ventricular arrhythmias in patients with underlying cardiac disease and history of ventricular fibrillation or sustained ventricular tachycardia, or of symptomatic non-sustained ventricular tachycardia, or of disabling symptoms due to premature ventricular contraction

Cautions: sick sinus syndrome; pre-existing conduction abnormalities; congestive heart failure; hepatic and renal impairment; pregnancy and breast-feeding; **interactions:** Appendix 1 (moracizine)

Contra-indications: second-degree or greater AV block (unless paced); cardiogenic shock

Side-effects: include gastro-intestinal disturbances; dizziness, headache, fatigue, palpitations, dyspnoea; arrhythmogenic (pro-arrhythmic effect); chest pain; congestive heart failure; reversible increases in liver enzymes, jaundice; thrombocytopenia

Dose: (initiated in hospital) usually 600–900 mg daily in 3 divided doses, adjusted by steps of 150 mg daily at intervals of 3 days; max. recommended daily dose 900 mg; rapid control, initially 400–500 mg, then 200 mg every 8 hours

Note. Patients well controlled on 3 divided doses daily may be given same total daily dosage in 2 divided doses (every 12 hours)

▼ PoM **Ethmozine**® (Monmouth)

Tablets, all f/c, moracizine hydrochloride 200 mg, net price 100-tab pack = £47.93; 250 mg, 100-tab pack = £59.36; 300 mg, 100-tab pack = £71.60

PHENYTOIN SODIUM

Indications: arrhythmias (but see notes above); for use in epilepsy, see section 4.8.1

Cautions; Contra-indications; Side-effects: see section 4.8.2

Dose: arrhythmias, *by intravenous injection* via caval catheter, 3.5–5 mg/kg at a rate not exceeding 50 mg/minute, with blood pressure and ECG monitoring; repeat once if necessary (rarely used, see notes above)

Preparations
See section 4.8.2

TOCAINIDE HYDROCHLORIDE

Indications: ventricular arrhythmias (restricted use—see notes above)

Cautions: weekly blood counts essential for first 12 weeks, then monthly; correct hypokalaemia; advise patients to report pulmonary symptoms; severe hepatic or renal impairment; elderly; uncompensated heart failure, bradycardia and hypotension; pregnancy (toxicity in *animal* studies); **interactions:** Appendix 1 (tocainide)

Contra-indications: second-degree or greater AV block (unless paced)

Side-effects: CNS effects including tremor, dizziness, confusion, visual hallucinations, convulsions, paraesthesia; gastro-intestinal effects including nausea and vomiting; abnormal liver-function tests (hepatitis and jaundice reported); fever and rash (including Stevens-Johnson syndrome and exfoliative dermatitis); lupus erythematosus-like syndrome; pulmonary fibrosis, interstitial pneumonitis, fibrosing alveolitis; agranulocytosis, aplastic anaemia, and thrombocytopenia—see also notes above; arrhythmogenic (pro-arrhythmic) effect

Dose: 1.2 g daily in 3 divided doses; max. 2.4 g daily

PoM **Tonocard**® (Astra)

Tablets, yellow, f/c, tocainide hydrochloride 400 mg, net price 20 = £3.27

2.4   Beta-adrenoceptor blocking drugs

CSM ADVICE. Beta-blockers, even those with apparent cardioselectivity, should **not** be used in patients with asthma or a history of obstructive airways disease, unless no alternative treatment is available. In such cases the risk of inducing bronchospasm should be appreciated and appropriate precautions taken.

Beta-adrenoceptor blocking drugs (beta-blockers) block the beta-adrenoreceptors in the heart, peripheral vasculature, bronchi, pancreas, and liver.

Many beta-blockers are now available and in general they are all equally effective. There are, however, differences between them which may affect choice in treating particular diseases or individual patients.

Intrinsic sympathomimetic activity (ISA, partial agonist activity) represents the capacity of beta-blockers to stimulate as well as to block adrenergic receptors. **Oxprenolol, pindolol**, and **acebutolol** have intrinsic sympathomimetic activity; the newer **celiprolol** also has intrinsic sympathomimetic activity (see also below); they tend to cause less bradycardia than the other beta-blockers and may also cause less coldness of the extremities.

Some beta-blockers are *lipid soluble* and some are *water soluble*. **Atenolol, celiprolol, nadolol,** and **sotalol** are the most water-soluble; they are less likely to enter the brain, and may therefore cause less sleep disturbance and nightmares. Water-soluble beta-blockers are excreted by the kidneys; they accumulate in renal impairment and dosage reduction is therefore often necessary.

Some beta-blockers have a *relatively short duration of action* and have to be given twice or three times daily. Many of these are, however, available in modified-release formulations so that in general it is not necessary to give beta-blockers more often than once daily for hypertension. For angina twice-daily treatment may sometimes be needed even with a modified-release formulation.

All beta-blockers *slow the heart* and may induce myocardial depression and precipitate heart failure. They should not therefore be given to patients who have incipient cardiac failure or those with second- or third-degree AV block; they may, however, be used with caution in patients whose heart failure is well controlled. **Sotalol** may prolong the QT interval, and has occasionally caused life-threatening ventricular arrhythmias (**important:** particular care should be taken to avoid hypokalaemia in patients taking sotalol).

Labetalol, celiprolol, and **carvedilol** are beta-blockers which have in addition an arteriolar vasodilating action, by diverse mechanisms, and thus lower peripheral resistance. There is no evidence that these drugs have important advantages over other beta-blockers in the treatment of hypertension.

Beta-blockers may *precipitate asthma* and this effect can be dangerous. Some, such as **atenolol, betaxolol, bisoprolol, metoprolol**, and (to a lesser extent) **acebutolol**, have less effect on the beta$_2$ (bronchial) receptors and are, therefore, relatively *cardioselective*, but they are **not** *cardiospecific*. They have a lesser effect on airways resistance but are **not** free of this side-effect. **Important:** see also **CSM** advice below.

Beta-blockers are also associated with *fatigue, coldness of the extremities* (may be less common with those with ISA, see above), and *sleep disturbances with nightmares* (may be less common with the water-soluble ones, see above).

Beta-blockers can lead to a small deterioration of *glucose tolerance* in diabetics; they also interfere with metabolic and autonomic responses to hypoglycaemia. Their use is not contra-indicated in diabetics, but cardioselective beta-blockers (see above) may be preferable and they should be avoided altogether in those with frequent episodes of hypoglycaemia.

HYPERTENSION. Beta-blockers are effective *antihypertensives* but their mode of action is not understood; they reduce cardiac output, alter baroceptor reflex sensitivity, and block peripheral adrenoceptors. Some beta-blockers depress plasma renin secretion. It is possible that a central effect may also explain their mode of action. Blood pressure can usually be controlled with relatively few side-effects. In general the dose of beta-blocker does not have to be as high as originally thought. The maximum dose of **oxprenolol** and **propranolol** necessary is probably 320 mg daily. **Atenolol** can usually be given in a dose of 50 mg daily and it is no longer considered necessary to increase to 100 mg.

Combined thiazide/beta-blocker preparations may help compliance but combined preparations should only be used when blood pressure is not adequately controlled by a thiazide or a beta-blocker alone. Beta-blockers reduce, but do not abolish, the tendency for diuretics to cause hypokalaemia.

Beta-blockers can be used to control the pulse rate in patients with *phaeochromocytoma*. However, they should never be used alone as beta-blockade without concurrent alpha-blockade may lead to a hypertensive crisis. For this reason phenoxybenzamine should always be used together with the beta-blocker.

ANGINA. Beta-blockers improve exercise tolerance and relieve symptoms in patients with *angina*; this effect is caused by their reduction of cardiac work. As with hypertension there is no good evidence of the superiority of any one drug, although occasionally a patient will respond better to one beta-blocker than to another. There is some evidence that sudden withdrawal may cause an exacerbation of angina therefore gradual reduction of dose is preferable when beta-blockers are to be stopped. There is a risk of precipitating heart failure when beta-blockers and verapamil are used together in established ischaemic heart disease (**important**: see p. 98.)

MYOCARDIAL INFARCTION. Several studies have shown that some beta-blockers can cause a reduction in the recurrence rate of *myocardial infarction*. However, pre-existing heart failure, hypotension, bradyarrhythmias, and obstructive airways disease render this group of drugs unsuitable in some patients who have recovered from a myocardial infarction. **Atenolol** and **metoprolol** may reduce early mortality after intravenous and subsequent oral administration in the acute phase, while **timolol** and **propranolol** have protective value when started in the early convalescent phase. The evidence relating to other beta-blockers is less convincing; some have not been tested in trials of secondary protection. It is also not known whether the protective effect of beta-blockers continues after two years; it is possible that sudden cessation may cause a rebound worsening of myocardial ischaemia.

ARRHYTHMIAS. Beta-blockers act as *anti-arrhythmic drugs* principally by attenuating the effects of the sympathetic system on automaticity and conductivity within the heart. They may be used in conjunction with digoxin to control the ventricular response in atrial fibrillation, especially in patients with thyrotoxicosis. Beta-blockers are also useful in the management of supraventricular tachycardias, and are used to control those following myocardial infarction, see above.

Esmolol is a relatively cardioselective beta-blocker with a very short duration of action, used intravenously for the short-term treatment of supraventricular arrhythmias, sinus tachycardia, or hypertension, particularly in the peri-operative period. It may also be used in other situations, such as acute myocardial infarction, where sustained beta blockade might be hazardous.

Sotalol, a non-cardioselective beta-blocker with additional class III anti-arrhythmic activity, is used for prophylaxis in paroxysmal supraventricular arrhythmias. It also suppresses ventricular ectopic beats and non-sustained ventricular tachycardia. It has been shown to be more effective than lignocaine in the termination of spontaneous sustained ventricular tachycardia due to coronary disease or cardiomyopathy. However, it may induce torsades de pointes in susceptible patients.

THYROTOXICOSIS. Beta-blockers are used in preoperative preparation for thyroidectomy. Administration of propranolol can reverse clinical symptoms of *thyrotoxicosis* within 4 days. Routine tests of increased thyroid function remain unaltered. The thyroid gland is rendered less vascular thus making surgery easier (see section 6.2.2).

OTHER USES. Beta-blockers have been used to alleviate some symptoms of *anxiety*; probably patients with palpitations, tremor, and tachycardia respond best (see also sections 4.1.2 and 4.9.3). Beta-blockers are also used in the *prophylaxis of migraine* (see section 4.7.4.2). Beta-blockers are used topically in *glaucoma* (see section 11.6).

PROPRANOLOL HYDROCHLORIDE

Indications: see under Dose

Cautions: late pregnancy and breast-feeding (see also Appendixes 4 and 5); avoid abrupt withdrawal in angina; reduce oral dose of propranolol in liver disease; liver function deteriorates in portal hypertension; reduce initial dose in renal impairment; diabetes; myasthenia gravis; in anaphylaxis, reduced response to adrenaline (see also p. 143); see also notes above; **interactions:** Appendix 1 (beta-blockers), **important:** verapamil interaction, see also p. 98

Contra-indications: asthma or history of obstructive airways disease (**important:** see CSM advice below), uncontrolled heart failure, marked bradycardia, sick sinus syndrome, second or third degree AV block, cardiogenic shock; phaeochromocytoma (apart from specific use with alpha-blockers, see also notes above)

CSM ADVICE. Beta-blockers, even those with apparent cardioselectivity, should **not** be used in patients with asthma or a history of obstructive airways disease, unless no alternative treatment is available. In such cases the risk of inducing bronchospasm should be appreciated and appropriate precautions taken.

Side-effects: bradycardia, heart failure, conduction disorders, bronchospasm, peripheral vasoconstriction, gastro-intestinal disturbances, fatigue, sleep disturbances; rare reports of rashes and dry eyes (reversible on withdrawal), exacerbation of psoriasis; overdosage: see Emergency Treatment of Poisoning, p. 22

Dose: by mouth, hypertension, initially 80 mg twice daily, increased at weekly intervals as required; maintenance 160–320 mg daily

Portal hypertension, initially 40 mg twice daily, increased to 80 mg twice daily according to heart-rate; max. 160 mg twice daily

Phaeochromocytoma (only with an alpha-blocker), 60 mg daily for 3 days before surgery *or* 30 mg daily in patients unsuitable for surgery

Angina, initially 40 mg 2–3 times daily; maintenance 120–240 mg daily

Arrhythmias, hypertrophic obstructive cardiomyopathy, anxiety tachycardia, and thyrotoxicosis (adjunct), 10–40 mg 3–4 times daily

Anxiety with symptoms such as palpitations, sweating, tremor, 40 mg twice daily, increased to 3 times daily if necessary

Prophylaxis after myocardial infarction, 40 mg 4 times daily for 2–3 days, then 80 mg twice daily, beginning 5 to 21 days after infarction

Migraine prophylaxis and essential tremor, initially 40 mg 2–3 times daily; maintenance 80–160 mg daily

By intravenous injection, arrhythmias and thyrotoxic crisis, 1 mg over 1 minute; if necessary repeat at 2-minute intervals; max. 10 mg (5 mg in anaesthesia)

Note. Excessive bradycardia can be countered with intravenous injection of atropine sulphate 0.6–2.4 mg in divided doses of 600 micrograms; for overdosage see Emergency Treatment of Poisoning, p. 22

PoM Propranolol (Non-proprietary)

Tablets, propranolol hydrochloride 10 mg, net price 20 = 5p; 40 mg, 20 = 7p; 80 mg, 20 = 14p; 160 mg, 20 = 28p. Label: 8

Available from APS (Apsolol®), Ashbourne (Propanix®), Berk (Berkolol®), Cox, CP (Cardinol®), DDSA (Angilol®), Hillcross

Oral solution (syrup), propranolol hydrochloride 5 mg/5 mL, 10 mg/5 mL and 50 mg/5 mL available from Rosemont (special order)

PoM Inderal® (Zeneca)

Tablets, all pink, f/c, propranolol hydrochloride 10 mg, net price 100-tab pack = 89p; 40 mg, 100-tab pack = £2.40; 80 mg, 60-tab pack = £2.35. Label: 8

Injection, propranolol hydrochloride 1 mg/mL, net price 1-mL amp = 21p

Modified release

PoM Half-Inderal LA® (Zeneca)

Capsules, m/r, lavender/pink, propranolol hydrochloride 80 mg. Net price 28-cap pack = £5.40. Label: 8, 25

Note. Modified-release capsules containing propranolol hydrochloride 80 mg also available from APS, CP, Norton (Half Beta-Prograne®)

PoM Inderal-LA® (Zeneca)

Capsules, m/r, lavender/pink, propranolol hydrochloride 160 mg. Net price 28-cap pack = £6.67. Label: 8, 25

Note. Modified-release capsules containing propranolol hydrochloride 160 mg also available from APS, Ashbourne (Propanix SR®), Hillcross, Lagap (Bedranol SR®), Norton (Beta-Prograne®), Opus (Lopranol LA®), Trinity (Probeta LA®)

With diuretic

PoM Inderetic® (Zeneca)

Capsules, propranolol hydrochloride 80 mg, bendrofluazide 2.5 mg. Net price 100-cap pack = £9.74. Label: 8

Dose: hypertension, 1 capsule twice daily

PoM Inderex® (Zeneca)

Capsules, pink/grey, propranolol hydrochloride 160 mg (m/r), bendrofluazide 5 mg. Net price 28-cap pack = £7.45. Label: 8, 25

Dose: hypertension, 1 capsule daily

ACEBUTOLOL

Indications: see under Dose

Cautions; Contra-indications; Side-effects: see under Propranolol Hydrochloride

Dose: hypertension, initially 400 mg once daily *or* 200 mg twice daily, increased after 2 weeks to 400 mg twice daily if necessary

Angina, initially 400 mg once daily *or* 200 mg twice daily; 300 mg 3 times daily in severe angina; up to 1.2 g daily has been used

Arrhythmias, 0.4–1.2 g daily in 2–3 divided doses

PoM Sectral® (Rhône-Poulenc Rorer)

Capsules, acebutolol (as hydrochloride) 100 mg (buff/white), net price 84-cap pack = £7.66; 200 mg (buff/pink), 56-cap pack = £9.82. Label: 8

Tablets, f/c, acebutolol 400 mg (as hydrochloride). Net price 28-tab pack = £9.53. Label: 8

With diuretic

PoM Secadrex® (Rhône-Poulenc Rorer)

Tablets, f/c, acebutolol 200 mg (as hydrochloride), hydrochlorothiazide 12.5 mg. Net price 28-tab pack = £9.00. Label: 8

Dose: hypertension, 1 tablet daily, increased to 2 daily as a single dose if necessary

ATENOLOL

Indications: see under Dose

Cautions; Contra-indications; Side-effects: see under Propranolol Hydrochloride; reduce dose in renal impairment (25-mg tablets available)

Dose: by mouth,

Hypertension, 50 mg daily (higher doses no longer considered necessary)

Angina, 100 mg daily in 1 or 2 doses

Arrhythmias, 50–100 mg daily

By intravenous injection, arrhythmias, 2.5 mg at a rate of 1 mg/minute, repeated at 5-minute intervals to a max. of 10 mg

Note. Excessive bradycardia can be countered with intravenous injection of atropine sulphate 0.6–2.4 mg in divided doses of 600 micrograms; for overdosage see Emergency Treatment of Poisoning, p. 22

By intravenous infusion, arrhythmias, 150 micrograms/kg over 20 minutes, repeated every 12 hours if required

Early intervention within 12 hours of infarction, 5–10 mg *by slow intravenous injection,* then *by mouth* 50 mg after 15 minutes, 50 mg after 12 hours, then 100 mg daily

PoM Atenolol (Non-proprietary)

Tablets, atenolol 25 mg, net price 28-tab pack = £2.33; 50 mg, 28-tab pack = £1.01; 100 mg, 28-tab pack = £1.38. Label: 8

Various strengths available from Antigen, APS, Ashbourne (Atenix®), Berk (Antipressan®), Cox, CP (Totamol®), Hillcross, Lagap, Norton

PoM Tenormin® (Stuart)

'25' tablets, f/c, atenolol 25 mg. Net price 28-tab pack = £4.62. Label: 8

LS tablets, orange, f/c, scored, atenolol 50 mg. Net price 28-tab pack = £5.35. Label: 8

Tablets, orange, f/c, scored, atenolol 100 mg. Net price 28-tab pack = £6.81. Label: 8

Syrup, sugar-free, atenolol 25 mg/5mL. Net price 300 mL = £8.14. Label: 8

Injection, atenolol 500 micrograms/mL. Net price 10-mL amp = £1.00 (hosp. only)

With diuretic

PoM Co-tenidone (Non-proprietary)

Tablets, co-tenidone 50/12.5 (atenolol 50 mg, chlorthalidone 12.5 mg), net price 28-tab pack = £5.48; co-tenidone 100/25 (atenolol 100 mg, chlorthalidone 25 mg), 28-tab pack = £8.16. Label: 8

Available from APS, Ashbourne (AtenixCo®), Berk (Tenchlor®), Bioglan, Cox, CP (Totaretic®), Hillcross, Norton

Dose: hypertension, 1 tablet daily (but see also under Dose above)

PoM **Kalten**® (Stuart)

Capsules, red/ivory, atenolol 50 mg, co-amilozide 2.5/25 (anhydrous amiloride hydrochloride 2.5 mg, hydrochlorothiazide 25 mg). Net price 28-cap pack = £8.39. Label: 8

Dose: hypertension, 1 capsule daily

PoM **Tenoret 50**® (Stuart)

Tablets, brown, f/c, co-tenidone 50/12.5 (atenolol 50 mg, chlorthalidone 12.5 mg). Net price 28-tab pack = £5.70. Label: 8

Dose: hypertension, 1 tablet daily

PoM **Tenoretic**® (Stuart)

Tablets, brown, f/c, co-tenidone 100/25 (atenolol 100 mg, chlorthalidone 25 mg). Net price 28-tab pack = £8.12. Label: 8

Dose: hypertension, 1 tablet daily (but see also under Dose above)

With calcium-channel blocker

Note. Only indicated when calcium-channel blocker or beta-blocker alone proves inadequate

PoM **Beta-Adalat**® (Bayer)

Capsules, reddish-brown, atenolol 50 mg, nifedipine 20 mg (m/r). Net price 28-cap pack = £10.90. Label: 8, 25

Dose: hypertension, 1 capsule daily, increased if necessary to twice daily; elderly, 1 daily

Angina, 1 capsule twice daily

PoM **Tenif**® (Stuart)

Capsules, reddish-brown, atenolol 50 mg, nifedipine 20 mg (m/r). Net price 28-cap pack = £10.63. Label: 8, 25

Dose: hypertension, 1 capsule daily, increased if necessary to twice daily; elderly, 1 daily

Angina, 1 capsule twice daily

BETAXOLOL HYDROCHLORIDE

Indications: hypertension; glaucoma, see section 11.6

Cautions; Contra-indications; Side-effects: see under Propranolol Hydrochloride; reduce dose in renal impairment

Dose: 20 mg daily (elderly patients 10 mg), increased to 40 mg if required

PoM **Kerlone**® (Lorex)

Tablets, f/c, scored, betaxolol hydrochloride 20 mg. Net price 28-tab pack = £7.51. Label: 8

BISOPROLOL FUMARATE

Indications: hypertension, angina

Cautions; Contra-indications; Side-effects: see under Propranolol Hydrochloride; reduce dose in hepatic and renal impairment

Dose: usual dose 10 mg daily (5 mg may be adequate in some patients); max. recommended dose 20 mg daily

PoM **Emcor**® (Merck)

LS Tablets, yellow, f/c, scored, bisoprolol fumarate 5 mg. Net price 28-tab pack = £7.78. Label: 8

Tablets, orange, f/c, scored, bisoprolol fumarate 10 mg. Net price 28-tab pack = £8.74. Label: 8

PoM **Monocor**® (Lederle)

Tablets, both f/c, bisoprolol fumarate 5 mg (pink), net price 28-tab pack = £7.78; 10 mg, 28-tab pack £8.74. Label: 8

With diuretic

PoM **Monozide 10**® (Lederle)

Tablets, f/c, bisoprolol fumarate 10 mg, hydrochlorothiazide 6.25 mg. Net price 28-tab pack = £11.20. Label: 8

Dose: hypertension, 1 tablet daily

CARTEOLOL

See section 11.6

CARVEDILOL

Indications: hypertension

Cautions; Contra-indications: as for Propranolol Hydrochloride; also hepatic impairment

Side-effects: postural hypotension, dizziness, headache, fatigue, gastro- intestinal disturbances, bradycardia; occasionally diminished peripheral circulation, dry eyes, influenza-like symptoms; rarely angina, A-V block, exacerbation of intermittent claudication; allergic skin reactions, nasal stuffiness, wheezing, depressed mood, sleep disturbances, paraesthesia, heart failure, changes in liver enzymes, thrombocytopenia, leucopenia also reported

Dose: initially 12.5 mg daily, increased after 2 days to usual dose of 25 mg once daily; if necessary may be further increased at intervals of at least 2 weeks to max. 50 mg daily in single or divided doses; ELDERLY initial dose of 12.5 mg may provide satisfactory control

▼ PoM **Eucardic**® (Boehringer Mannheim)

Tablets, both scored, carvedilol 12.5 mg (peach), net price 28-tab pack = £9.56; 25 mg, 28-tab pack = £11.95. Label: 8

CELIPROLOL HYDROCHLORIDE

Indications: mild to moderate hypertension

Cautions; Contra-indications: as for Propranolol Hydrochloride; also avoid in severe renal impairment

Side-effects: headache, dizziness, fatigue, nausea and somnolence; also bradycardia, bronchospasm

Dose: 200 mg once daily in the morning, increased to 400 mg once daily if necessary

PoM **Celectol**® (Rhône-Poulenc Rorer)

Tablets, both f/c, scored, celiprolol hydrochloride 200 mg (yellow), net price 28-tab pack = £9.08; 400 mg, 28-tab pack = £17.15. Label: 8, 22

ESMOLOL HYDROCHLORIDE

Indications: short-term treatment of supraventricular arrhythmias (including atrial fibrillation, atrial flutter, sinus tachycardia); tachycardia and hypertension in peri-operative period

Cautions; Contra-indications; Side-effects: see under Propranolol Hydrochloride
Dose: by intravenous infusion, usually within range 50–200 micrograms/kg/minute (consult data sheet for details of dose titration)

PoM **Brevibloc®** (Gensia)
Injection, esmolol hydrochloride 10 mg/mL, net price 10-mL vial = £5.90
Injection concentrate, esmolol hydrochloride 250 mg/mL (for dilution before infusion), 10-mL amp = £65.90

LABETALOL HYDROCHLORIDE
Indications: hypertension (including hypertension in pregnancy, hypertension with angina, and hypertension following acute myocardial infarction); hypertensive crisis (but see section 2.5); controlled hypotension in anaesthesia
Cautions; Contra-indications: as for Propranolol Hydrochloride; interferes with laboratory tests for catecholamines; liver damage (see below)
LIVER DAMAGE. Severe hepatocellular damage reported after both short-term and long-term treatment. Appropriate laboratory testing needed at first symptom of liver dysfunction and if laboratory evidence of damage (or if jaundice) labetalol should be stopped and not restarted
Side-effects: postural hypotension (avoid upright position during and for 3 hours after intravenous administration), tiredness, weakness, headache, rashes, scalp tingling, difficulty in micturition, epigastric pain, nausea, vomiting; liver damage (see above); rarely lichenoid rash
Dose: by mouth, initially 100 mg (50 mg in elderly) twice daily with food, increased at intervals of 14 days to usual dose of 200 mg twice daily; up to 800 mg daily in 2 divided doses (3–4 divided doses if higher); max. 2.4 g daily
By intravenous injection, 50 mg over at least 1 minute, repeated after 5 minutes if necessary; max. 200 mg
Note. Excessive bradycardia can be countered with intravenous injection of atropine sulphate 0.6–2.4 mg in divided doses of 600 micrograms; for overdosage see Emergency Treatment of Poisoning, p. 22
By intravenous infusion, 2 mg/minute; usual range 50–200 mg, higher doses in phaeochromocytoma
Hypertension of pregnancy, 20 mg/hour, doubled every 30 minutes; usual max. 160 mg/hour
Hypertension following infarction, 15 mg/hour, gradually increased to max. 120 mg/hour

PoM **Labetalol Hydrochloride** (Non-proprietary)
Tablets, all f/c, labetalol hydrochloride 100 mg, net price 20 = £1.42; 200 mg, 20 = £2.03; 400 mg, 20 = £3.64. Label: 8, 21
Available from APS, Cox, Hillcross, Norton
PoM **Trandate®** (Evans)
Tablets, all orange, f/c, labetalol hydrochloride 50 mg, net price 56-tab pack. £5.05; 100 mg, 56-tab pack = £5.56; 200 mg, 56-tab pack = £9.02; 400 mg, 50-tab pack = £11.21. Label: 8, 21
Injection, labetalol hydrochloride 5 mg/mL. Net price 20-mL amp = £2.83

LEVOBUNOLOL HYDROCHLORIDE
See section 11.6

METIPRANOLOL
See section 11.6

METOPROLOL TARTRATE
Indications: see under Dose
Cautions; Contra-indications; Side-effects: see under Propranolol Hydrochloride; reduce dose in hepatic impairment
Dose: by mouth, hypertension, initially 100 mg daily, maintenance 100–200 mg daily in 1–2 doses
Angina, 50–100 mg 2–3 times daily
Arrhythmias, usually 50 mg 2–3 times daily; up to 300 mg daily in divided doses if necessary
Migraine prophylaxis, 100–200 mg daily in divided doses
Thyrotoxicosis (adjunct), 50 mg 4 times daily
By intravenous injection, arrhythmias, up to 5 mg at rate 1–2 mg/minute, repeated after 5 minutes if necessary, total dose 10–15 mg
Note. Excessive bradycardia can be countered with intravenous injection of atropine sulphate 0.6–2.4 mg in divided doses of 600 micrograms; for overdosage see Emergency Treatment of Poisoning, p. 22
In surgery, 2–4 mg *by slow intravenous injection* at induction or to control arrhythmias developing during anaesthesia; 2-mg doses may be repeated to a max. of 10 mg
Early intervention within 12 hours of infarction, 5 mg *by intravenous injection* every 2 minutes to a max. of 15 mg, followed after 15 minutes by 50 mg *by mouth* every 6 hours for 48 hours; maintenance 200 mg daily in divided doses

PoM **Metoprolol Tartrate** (Non-proprietary)
Tablets, metoprolol tartrate 50 mg, net price 20 = 70p; 100 mg, 20 = £1.33. Label: 8
Available from APS, Ashbourne (Mepranix®), Berk (Arbralene®), Cox, Hillcross, Norton
PoM **Betaloc®** (Astra)
Tablets, both scored, metoprolol tartrate 50 mg, net price 100-tab pack = £3.30; 100 mg, 100-tab pack = £6.13. Label: 8
Injection, metoprolol tartrate 1 mg/mL. Net price 5-mL amp = 44p
PoM **Lopresor®** (Geigy)
Tablets, both f/c, scored, metoprolol tartrate 50 mg (pink), net price 56-tab pack = £5.13; 100 mg (blue), 56-tab pack = £9.54. Label: 8

Modified release
PoM **Betaloc-SA®** (Astra)
Durules® (= tablets, m/r), metoprolol tartrate 200 mg. Net price 28-tab pack = £4.56. Label: 8, 25
Dose: hypertension, angina, 200–400 mg daily; migraine prophylaxis, 200 mg daily
PoM **Lopresor SR®** (Geigy)
Tablets, m/r, yellow, f/c, metoprolol tartrate 200 mg. Net price 28-tab pack = £8.98. Label: 8, 25
Dose: hypertension, 200 mg daily; angina, 200–400 mg daily; migraine prophylaxis, 200 mg daily

With diuretic

PoM Co-Betaloc® (Astra)

Tablets, scored, metoprolol tartrate 100 mg, hydrochlorothiazide 12.5 mg. Net price 28-tab pack = £4.66. Label: 8

Dose: hypertension, 1–3 tablets daily in single or divided doses

PoM Co-Betaloc SA® (Astra)

Tablets, yellow, f/c, metoprolol tartrate (m/r) 200 mg, hydrochlorothiazide 25 mg. Net price 28-tab pack = £5.74. Label: 8, 25

Dose: hypertension, 1 tablet daily

NADOLOL

Indications: see under Dose

Cautions; Contra-indications; Side-effects: see under Propranolol Hydrochloride; reduce dose in renal impairment

Dose: hypertension, 80 mg daily, increased at weekly intervals if required; max. 240 mg daily

Angina, 40 mg daily, increased at weekly intervals if required; usual max. 160 mg daily

Arrhythmias, initially 40 mg daily, increased to 160 mg if required; reduce to 40 mg if bradycardia occurs

Migraine prophylaxis, initially 40 mg daily, increased by 40 mg at weekly intervals; usual maintenance dose 80–160 mg daily

Thyrotoxicosis (adjunct), 80–160 mg daily

PoM Corgard® (Sanofi Winthrop)

Tablets, both blue, nadolol 40 mg, net price 28-tab pack = £3.76; 80 mg, 28-tab pack = £5.45. Label: 8

With diuretic

PoM Corgaretic 40® (Sanofi Winthrop)

Tablets, scored, nadolol 40 mg, bendrofluazide 5 mg. Net price 28-tab pack = £5.92. Label: 8

Dose: hypertension, 1–2 tablets daily

PoM Corgaretic 80® (Sanofi Winthrop)

Tablets, scored, nadolol 80 mg, bendrofluazide 5 mg. Net price 28-tab pack = £8.47. Label: 8

Dose: hypertension, 1–2 tablets daily

OXPRENOLOL HYDROCHLORIDE

Indications: see under Dose

Cautions; Contra-indications; Side-effects: see under Propranolol Hydrochloride

Dose: hypertension, 80–160 mg daily in 2–3 divided doses, increased as required at 1–2 week intervals; max. 480 mg daily

Angina, 40–160 mg 3 times daily

Arrhythmias, initially 20–40 mg 3 times daily, increased as necessary

Anxiety symptoms (short-term use), initially 40 mg twice daily, increased if necessary to 160 mg daily in divided doses

PoM Oxprenolol (Non-proprietary)

Tablets, all coated, oxprenolol hydrochloride 20 mg, net price 20 = 33p; 40 mg, 20 = 44p; 80 mg, 20 = 69p; 160 mg, 20 = £1.16. Label: 8

Available from APS (Apsolox®, 80-mg tablets contain tartrazine), Cox, Hillcross, Norton

PoM Trasicor® (Ciba)

Tablets, all f/c, oxprenolol hydrochloride 20 mg (contain gluten), net price 100-tab pack = £2.31; 40 mg (contain gluten), 100-tab pack = £4.62; 80 mg (yellow), 56-tab pack = £5.17. Label: 8

Modified release

PoM Slow-Trasicor® (Ciba)

Tablets, m/r, f/c, oxprenolol hydrochloride 160 mg. Net price 28-tab pack = £6.08. Label: 8, 25

Dose: hypertension, angina, initially 160 mg daily in the morning; if necessary may be increased to max. 480 mg daily in 1–2 divided doses

Note. Modified-release tablets containing oxprenolol hydrochloride 160 mg also available from Norton

With diuretic

PoM Trasidrex® (Ciba)

Tablets, red, s/c, co-prenozide 160/0.25 (oxprenolol hydrochloride 160 mg (m/r), cyclopenthiazide 250 micrograms). Net price 28-tab pack = £7.40. Label: 8, 25

Dose: hypertension, 1 tablet daily, increased if necessary to 2 daily as a single dose

PINDOLOL

Indications: see under Dose

Cautions; Contra-indications; Side-effects: see under Propranolol Hydrochloride; reduce dose in renal impairment

Dose: hypertension, initially 5 mg 2–3 times daily *or* 15 mg once daily, increased as required at weekly intervals; usual maintenance 15–30 mg daily; max. 45 mg daily

Angina, 2.5–5 mg up to 3 times daily

PoM Visken® (Sandoz)

Tablets, both scored, pindolol 5 mg, net price 100-tab pack = £7.27; 15 mg, 30-tab pack = £6.54. Label: 8

With diuretic

PoM Viskaldix® (Sandoz)

Tablets, scored, pindolol 10 mg, clopamide 5 mg. Net price 28-tab pack = £5.58. Label: 8

Dose: hypertension, 1 tablet daily in the morning, increased if necessary to 2 daily; max. 3 daily

SOTALOL HYDROCHLORIDE

Indications:

Tablets and injection: life-threatening arrhythmias including ventricular tachyarrhythmias, symptomatic non-sustained ventricular tachyarrhythmias

Tablets only: prophylaxis of paroxysmal atrial tachycardia or fibrillation, paroxysmal AV re-entrant tachycardias (both nodal and involving accessory pathways), paroxysmal supraventricular tachycardia after cardiac surgery, maintenance of sinus rhythm following cardioversion of atrial fibrillation or flutter

Injection only: electrophysiological study of inducible ventricular and supraventricular arrhythmias; temporary substitution for tablets

Cautions: see under Propranolol Hydrochloride; reduce dose in renal impairment (avoid if severe); correct hypokalaemia, hypomagnesaemia, or other electrolyte disturbances; severe or prolonged diarrhoea; **interactions:** Appendix 1 (beta-blockers), **important:** verapamil interaction see also p. 98

Contra-indications: see under Propranolol Hydrochloride; congenital or acquired long QT syndrome; torsades de pointes; renal failure

Side-effects: see under Propranolol Hydrochloride; arrhythmogenic (pro-arrhythmic) effect (torsades de pointes—increased risk in women)

Dose: by mouth with ECG monitoring and measurement of corrected QT interval, arrhythmias, initially 80 mg daily in 1–2 divided doses increased gradually at intervals of 2–3 days to usual dose of 160–320 mg daily in 2 divided doses; higher doses of 480–640 mg daily for life-threatening ventricular arrhythmias under specialist supervision

By intravenous injection over 10 minutes, acute arrhythmias, 20–120 mg with ECG monitoring, repeated if necessary with 6-hour intervals between injections

Diagnostic use, see manufacturer's literature

Note. Excessive bradycardia can be countered with intravenous injection of atropine sulphate 0.6–2.4 mg in divided doses of 600 micrograms; for overdosage see Emergency Treatment of Poisoning, p. 22

PoM **Beta-Cardone®** (Evans)

Tablets, all scored, sotalol hydrochloride 40 mg (green), net price 100-tab pack = £3.96; 80 mg (pink), 100-tab pack = £5.87; 200 mg, 30-tab pack = £4.15. Label: 8

PoM **Sotacor®** (Bristol-Myers)

Tablets, sotalol hydrochloride 80 mg, net price 28-tab pack = £3.49; 160 mg, 28-tab pack = £6.89. Label: 8

Injection, sotalol hydrochloride 10 mg/mL. Net price 4-mL amp = £1.76

TIMOLOL MALEATE

Indications: see under Dose

Cautions; Contra-indications; Side-effects: see under Propranolol Hydrochloride

Dose: hypertension, initially 5 mg twice daily *or* 10 mg once daily; gradually increased if necessary to max. 60 mg daily (given in divided doses above 20 mg daily)

Angina, initially 5 mg 2–3 times daily, usual maintenance 35–45 mg daily (range 15–45 mg daily)

Prophylaxis after infarction, initially 5 mg twice daily, increased after 2 days to 10 mg twice daily, starting 7 to 28 days after infarction

Migraine prophylaxis, 10–20 mg once daily

Glaucoma, see section 11.6

PoM **Betim®** (Leo)

Tablets, scored, timolol maleate 10 mg. Net price 100-tab pack = £8.55. Label: 8

PoM **Blocadren®** (MSD)

Tablets, blue, scored, timolol maleate 10 mg. Net price 100-tab pack = £8.55. Label: 8

With diuretic

PoM **Moducren®** (Morson)

Tablets, blue, scored, timolol maleate 10 mg, co-amilozide 2.5/25 (amiloride hydrochloride 2.5 mg, hydrochlorothiazide 25 mg). Net price 28-tab pack = £8.00. Label: 8

Dose: hypertension, 1–2 tablets daily as a single dose

PoM **Prestim®** (Leo)

Tablets, scored, timolol maleate 10 mg, bendrofluazide 2.5 mg. Net price 100-tab pack = £14.32. Label: 8

Dose: hypertension, 1–2 tablets daily; max. 4 daily

PoM **Prestim Forte®** (Leo)

Tablets, scored, timolol maleate 20 mg, bendrofluazide 5 mg. Net price 100-tab pack = £28.65. Label: 8

Dose: hypertension, ½–2 tablets daily in single or divided doses

---

2.5   Drugs affecting the renin-angiotensin system and some other antihypertensive drugs

2.5.1	Vasodilator antihypertensive drugs
2.5.2	Centrally acting antihypertensive drugs
2.5.3	Adrenergic neurone blocking drugs
2.5.4	Alpha-adrenoceptor blocking drugs
2.5.5	Drugs affecting the renin-angiotensin system
2.5.6	Ganglion-blocking drugs
2.5.7	Tyrosine hydroxylase inhibitors

Antihypertensive therapy has improved the outlook for patients with high blood pressure by decreasing the frequency of stroke, heart failure, and renal failure: treatment also reduces the incidence of coronary events.

All patients should be given advice on non-pharmacological measures to reduce high blood pressure, including achieving ideal body weight, avoiding high alcohol intake and high sodium intake, and taking regular exercise. Cigarette smoking has a powerful adverse effect on cardiovascular risk in hypertensive subjects, and the importance of stopping should be emphasised.

The recommendations of the British Hypertension Society are that specific antihypertensive treatment is indicated:

Where the initial blood pressure is *systolic ≥ 200 mmHg or diastolic ≥ 110 mmHg, treat* if these values are confirmed on 3 separate occasions over 1-2 weeks (**important:** if very severe or in presence of associated conditions such as heart failure, immediate treatment needed—see also below);

Where the initial blood pressure is *systolic 160–199 mmHg or diastolic 90–109 mmHg* (or when higher initial values fall to this range) take one of the following courses of action:

- if *vascular complications or end-organ damage* (e.g. left ventricular hypertrophy, renal impairment) *or diabetes* present, **treat** if *systolic ≥ 160 mmHg or diastolic ≥ 90 mmHg* confirmed on at least 3 separate occasions;
- if *no vascular complications, no end-organ damage and no diabetes* repeat blood pressure measurements at monthly intervals for 3–6 months and **treat** if the average value during this period is *systolic ≥ 160 mmHg or diastolic ≥ 100 mmHg*;
- if the average value is *systolic <160 mmHg and diastolic 90–99 mmHg* treatment may be withheld but continue to monitor; however **consider treatment** if sustained in this range in older patients (over 60 years), and in those with a particularly high risk of cardiovascular complications (e.g. strong family history).

The usual aim should be to reduce the systolic pressure to below 160 mmHg and the diastolic pressure to below 90 mmHg.

Malignant (or accelerated) hypertension or very severe hypertension (diastolic blood pressure > 140 mmHg) requires urgent treatment in hospital but is not an indication for parenteral antihypertensive therapy. Normally treatment should be by mouth with a beta-blocker (atenolol or labetalol) or a calcium-channel blocker (nifedipine). Within the first 24 hours the diastolic blood pressure should be reduced to 100–110 mmHg. Over the next two or three days blood pressure should be normalised by using beta-blockers, calcium-channel blockers, diuretics, vasodilators, or angiotensin-converting enzyme inhibitors. Very rapid falls in blood pressure can cause reduced cerebral perfusion leading to cerebral infarction and blindness, a reduction in renal perfusion causing a deterioration in renal function, and myocardial ischaemia. Parenteral antihypertensive drugs are, therefore, hardly ever necessary. (On the rare occasions when a parenteral antihypertensive is necessary, sodium nitroprusside by infusion is the drug of choice.)

In moderate to severe hypertension (diastolic blood pressure > 110 mmHg) or in patients with vascular complications, drugs are best added 'stepwise' until control has been achieved; an attempt can then be made to 'step down' treatment under supervision. In uncomplicated mild hypertension (diastolic blood pressure < 110 mmHg), drugs may be substituted rather than added. Whenever the blood pressure is consistently well below the target level it is reasonable to try stepping down treatment cautiously, by gradually decreasing the dose or number of drugs, under close supervision. In some patients, usually those with mild hypertension and no end organ damage, it may even be possible to withdraw treatment completely; any subsequent rise in blood pressure may be delayed for several months, therefore blood pressure should be monitored indefinitely.

The strategy for reducing blood pressure is probably best as follows:

1. *Non-drug treatment*—obesity, high alcohol intake, high salt intake, and lack of regular exercise, may elevate blood pressure and these should be corrected.

2. *Diuretic therapy.* The optimum dose of a thiazide (section 2.2.1) used to treat hypertension is the lowest possible dose; higher doses do not have a major additional antihypertensive effect, but do cause more metabolic side-effects. Potassium supplements or potassium-sparing diuretics are usually not necessary in the routine treatment of hypertension, but plasma potassium concentration should be checked 3 to 4 weeks after starting treatment.

3. *Beta-adrenoceptor blocking drugs* (section 2.4) are used with a thiazide where they are not effective alone.

4(a). *ACE inhibitors* (section 2.5.5.1) may cause a precipitate drop in blood pressure in patients with renal impairment and/or receiving diuretic therapy; they should be given in low initial doses and where possible diuretic therapy should be omitted for a few days before starting.

4(b). *Calcium-channel blockers* have antihypertensive efficacy broadly similar to that of thiazides or beta-blockers. Their safety during long-term treatment is less well established; they should therefore be considered for hypertension only when thiazides and beta-blockers are contra-indicated, not tolerated, or fail to control blood pressure (and should usually be avoided in heart failure). There are **important** differences between calcium-channel blockers (see section 2.6.2).

5. *Other drugs*—vasodilators (hydralazine, minoxidil), alpha-blockers (prazosin, terazosin, doxazosin), and centrally acting drugs (methyldopa) are generally reserved for patients whose blood pressure is not controlled by, or who have contra-indications to, the drugs already mentioned.

Systolic hypertension. Isolated systolic hypertension (systolic blood pressure > 160 mmHg, diastolic < 90 mmHg) is associated with an increased risk of stroke and coronary events, particularly in those over 60 years. Systolic blood pressure averaging 160 mmHg or higher over 3 to 6 months (despite appropriate non-drug treatment) should be lowered in those over 60 years, even if diastolic hypertension is absent. Patients with severe postural hypotension should not receive blood pressure lowering drugs. The regimen proven effective is a low dose of a thiazide, with addition of a beta-blocker when necessary. Isolated systolic hypertension is uncommon in younger patients but by extrapolation it seems reasonable to recommend that a threshold pressure of 160 mmHg should also be an indication for treatment.

Hypertension in pregnancy. It is important to control blood pressure in pregnancy. High blood pressure may be due to pre-existing essential hypertension or to pre-eclampsia. Oral methyldopa is safe in pregnancy. Beta-blockers are effective and safe in the third trimester but may cause intra-uterine growth retardation when used from earlier in pregnancy. Hydralazine by intravenous injection can be used to control hypertensive crises. For use of magnesium sulphate in eclampsia, see section 9.5.1.3.

HYPERTENSION IN THE ELDERLY. Antihypertensive therapy reduces the incidence of cardiovascular complications substantially in elderly hypertensive subjects. The benefit is evident up to at least 85 years of age, and it is probably inappropriate to apply a strict age limit when coming to a decision on drug therapy. Elderly subjects who have a good outlook for longevity from other points of view should have their blood pressure lowered if they are hypertensive. The criteria for treatment are diastolic blood pressure averaging 90 mmHg or higher *or* systolic averaging 160 mmHg or higher over 3 to 6 months observation (despite appropriate non-drug treatment). A low dose of a thiazide is the clear drug of first choice, with addition of a beta-blocker when necessary.

2.5.1   Vasodilator antihypertensive drugs

These are potent drugs, especially when used in combination with a beta-blocker and a thiazide. **Important:** for a warning on the hazards of a very rapid fall in blood pressure, see section 2.5.

Diazoxide is used by intravenous injection in hypertensive emergencies.

Hydralazine given by mouth is a useful adjunct to other treatment, but when used alone causes tachycardia and fluid retention. Side-effects can be few if the dose is kept below 100 mg daily, but systemic lupus erythematosus should be suspected if there is unexplained weight loss, arthritis, or any other unexplained ill health.

Sodium nitroprusside is given by intravenous infusion to control severe hypertensive crises.

Minoxidil should be reserved for the treatment of severe hypertension resistant to other drugs. Vasodilatation is accompanied by increased cardiac output and tachycardia and the patients develop fluid retention. For this reason a beta-blocker and a diuretic (usually frusemide, in high dosage) are mandatory. Hypertrichosis is troublesome and renders this drug unsuitable for women.

Prazosin, doxazosin, and **terazosin** (section 2.5.4) have alpha-blocking and vasodilator properties.

DIAZOXIDE

Indications: acute treatment of severe hypertension associated with renal disease (but see section 2.5); hypoglycaemia, see section 6.1.4

Cautions: ischaemic heart disease, pregnancy, labour, impaired renal function; **interactions:** Appendix 1 (diazoxide)

Side-effects: tachycardia, hyperglycaemia, sodium and water retention

Dose: by rapid intravenous injection (less than 30 seconds), 1–3 mg/kg to max. single dose of 150 mg (see below); may be repeated after 5–15 minutes if required

Note. Single doses of 300 mg have been associated with angina and with myocardial and cerebral infarction

PoM Eudemine® (Link)
Injection, diazoxide 15 mg/mL. Net price 20-mL amp = £18.90

HYDRALAZINE HYDROCHLORIDE

Indications: moderate to severe hypertension, with beta-blocker and thiazide; hypertensive crisis (but see section 2.5)

Cautions: reduce initial dose in renal impairment; coronary artery disease (may provoke angina, avoid after myocardial infarction until stabilised), cerebrovascular disease; over-rapid blood pressure reduction is occasionally encountered even with low parenteral doses; pregnancy (see also Appendix 4), breast-feeding; **interactions:** Appendix 1 (hydralazine)

Contra-indications: idiopathic systemic lupus erythematosus, severe tachycardia, high output heart failure, myocardial insufficiency due to mechanical obstruction, cor pulmonale, dissecting aortic aneurysm; porphyria (see section 9.8.2)

Side-effects: tachycardia, fluid retention, nausea, and vomiting; headache; systemic lupus erythematosus-like syndrome after long-term therapy with over 100 mg daily (or less in women) (see also notes above); rarely rashes, fever, changes in blood count, peripheral neuritis; blood disorders reported (including haemolytic anaemia)

Dose: by mouth, 25 mg twice daily, increased to a max. of 50 mg twice daily (see notes above)

By slow intravenous injection, 5–10 mg over 20 minutes; may be repeated after 20–30 minutes (see Cautions)

By intravenous infusion, initially 200–300 micrograms/minute; maintenance usually 50–150 micrograms/minute

PoM Hydralazine (Non-proprietary)
Tablets, hydralazine hydrochloride 25 mg, net price 20 = 22p; 50 mg, 20 = 44p
PoM Apresoline® (Ciba)
Tablets, both s/c, hydralazine hydrochloride 25 mg (yellow), net price 100-tab pack = £1.97; 50 mg (violet), 100-tab pack = £3.87
Additives: include gluten
Injection, powder for reconstitution, hydralazine hydrochloride. Net price 20-mg amp = 35p

MINOXIDIL

Indications: severe hypertension, in addition to a diuretic and a beta-blocker

Cautions: see notes above; angina; after myocardial infarction (until stabilised); lower doses in dialysis patients; pregnancy; porphyria (see section 9.8.2); **interactions:** Appendix 1 (minoxidil)

Contra-indications: phaeochromocytoma

Side-effects: sodium and water retention; weight gain, peripheral oedema, tachycardia, hypertrichosis; reversible rise in creatinine and blood urea nitrogen; occasionally, gastro-intestinal disturbances, breast tenderness, rashes

Dose: initially 5 mg (elderly, 2.5 mg) daily, in 1–2 doses, increased by 5–10 mg every 3 or more days; max. usually 50 mg daily

PoM Loniten® (Upjohn)
Tablets, all scored, minoxidil 2.5 mg, net price 100-tab pack = £12.34; 5 mg, 100-tab pack = £21.98; 10 mg, 100-tab pack = £42.62

SODIUM NITROPRUSSIDE

Indications: hypertensive crisis (but see section 2.5); controlled hypotension in anaesthesia; acute or chronic heart failure

Cautions: hypothyroidism, severe renal impairment, ischaemic heart disease, impaired cerebral circulation, elderly; monitor blood pressure and plasma-cyanide concentration; pregnancy and breast-feeding; **interactions:** Appendix 1 (nitroprusside)

WITHDRAWAL. Normal duration of treatment should not exceed 72 hours (terminate over at least 10–30 minutes to avoid rebound)

Contra-indications: severe hepatic impairment; vitamin B_{12} deficiency; Leber's optic atrophy; compensatory hypertension

Side-effects: associated with over rapid reduction in blood pressure (reduce infusion rate): headache, dizziness, nausea, retching, abdominal pain, perspiration, palpitations, apprehension, retrosternal discomfort; occasionally reduced platelet count, acute transient phlebitis

CYANIDE. Side-effects caused by excessive plasma concentration of the cyanide metabolite include tachycardia, sweating, hyperventilation, arrhythmias, marked metabolic acidosis (discontinue and give antidote, see p. 24)

Dose: hypertensive crisis, in patients not already receiving antihypertensives, *by intravenous infusion,* 0.3 micrograms/kg/minute initially, then adjusted; usual range 0.5–6 micrograms/kg/minute (20–400 micrograms/minute); max. 8 micrograms/kg/minute—stop if not marked response in 10 minutes (if response obtained give for few hours only to avoid cyanide risk); lower doses for patients already being treated with antihypertensives

Lower doses should also be employed for controlled hypotension in surgery (max. 1.5 micrograms/kg/minute)

Heart failure, *by intravenous infusion,* initially 10–15 micrograms/minute, increased every 5–10 minutes as necessary; usual range 10–200 micrograms/minute; max. 280 micrograms/minute (4 micrograms/kg/minute)

PoM **Sodium Nitroprusside** (Non-proprietary)
Intravenous solution, sodium nitroprusside 10 mg/mL. For dilution and use as an infusion. 5-mL vial available from David Bull

2.5.2 Centrally acting antihypertensive drugs

This group includes **methyldopa**, which has the advantage of being safe in asthmatics, in heart failure, and in pregnancy. Side-effects are minimised if the daily dose is kept below 1 g.

Clonidine has the disadvantage that sudden withdrawal may cause a hypertensive crisis. Reserpine and rauwolfia are no longer used in Britain.

Moxonidine, a centrally acting drug, has been introduced recently for mild to moderate essential hypertension.

CLONIDINE HYDROCHLORIDE

Indications: hypertension (for use in migraine, see section 4.7.4.2)

Cautions: must be withdrawn gradually to avoid hypertensive crisis; Raynaud's syndrome or other occlusive peripheral vascular disease; history of depression; avoid in porphyria (see section 9.8.2); **interactions:** Appendix 1 (clonidine)

DRIVING. Drowsiness may affect performance of skilled tasks (e.g. driving); effects of alcohol may be enhanced

Side-effects: dry mouth, sedation, depression, fluid retention, bradycardia, Raynaud's phenomenon, headache, dizziness, euphoria, nocturnal unrest, rash, nausea, constipation, rarely impotence

Dose: by mouth, 50–100 micrograms 3 times daily, increased every second or third day; max. daily dose usually 1.2 mg

By slow intravenous injection, 150–300 micrograms; max. 750 micrograms in 24 hours

PoM **Catapres®** (Boehringer Ingelheim)
Tablets, both scored, clonidine hydrochloride 100 micrograms, net price 100-tab pack = £7.00; 300 micrograms, 100-tab pack = £16.30. Label: 3, 8
Injection, clonidine hydrochloride 150 micrograms/mL. Net price 1-mL amp = 29p

PoM **Dixarit®** (migraine), see section 4.7.4.2

Modified release
PoM **Catapres® Perlongets** (Boehringer Ingelheim)
Capsules, m/r, red/yellow, clonidine hydrochloride 250 micrograms. Net price 56-cap pack = £13.89. Label: 3, 8, 25
Dose: usually 1 capsule in the evening; 2–3 capsules daily (1 morning and 1–2 evening) if necessary

METHYLDOPA

Indications: hypertension, in conjunction with diuretic; hypertensive crisis when immediate effect not necessary

Cautions: positive direct Coombs' test in up to 20% of patients (may affect blood cross-matching); interference with laboratory tests; reduce initial dose in renal impairment; blood counts and liver-function tests advised; history of depression; **interactions:** Appendix 1 (methyldopa)

DRIVING. Drowsiness may affect performance of skilled tasks (e.g. driving); effects of alcohol may be enhanced

Contra-indications: depression, active liver disease, phaeochromocytoma; porphyria (see section 9.8.2)

Side-effects: dry mouth, sedation, depression, drowsiness, diarrhoea, fluid retention, failure of ejaculation, liver damage, haemolytic anaemia, lupus erythematosus-like syndrome, parkinsonism, rashes, nasal stuffiness

Dose: by mouth, 250 mg 2–3 times daily, gradually increased at intervals of 2 or more days; max. daily dose 3 g; ELDERLY 125 mg twice daily initially, gradually increased; max. daily dose 2 g (see also notes above)

By intravenous infusion, methyldopate hydrochloride 250–500 mg, repeated after 6 hours if required

PoM **Methyldopa** (Non-proprietary)
Tablets, coated, methyldopa (anhydrous) 125 mg, net price 20 = 41p; 250 mg, 20 = 59p; 500 mg, 20 = £1.23. Label: 3, 8
Available from APS, Berk (Dopamet®), Cox, CP, Hillcross, Norton

PoM **Aldomet®** (MSD)
Tablets, all yellow, f/c, methyldopa (anhydrous) 125 mg, net price 20 = 34p; 250 mg, 20 = 63p; 500 mg, 20 = £1.27. Label: 3, 8
Suspension, methyldopa 250 mg/5mL. Net price 200 mL = £3.96. Label: 3, 8
Injection, methyldopate hydrochloride 50 mg/mL. Net price 5-mL amp = £2.31

With diuretic
PoM **Hydromet**® (MSD)
Tablets, pink, f/c, methyldopa (anhydrous) 250 mg, hydrochlorothiazide 15 mg. Net price 20 = £1.52. Label: 3, 8

MOXONIDINE

Indications: mild to moderate essential hypertension
Cautions: renal impairment (see Appendix 3); avoid abrupt withdrawal (if concomitant treatment with beta-blocker has to be stopped, discontinue beta-blocker first, then moxonidine after few days); **interactions:** see Appendix 1 (moxonidine)
Contra-indications: history of angioedema; conduction disorders (sick sinus syndrome, sino-atrial block, second or third degree AV block); bradycardia; life-threatening arrhythmia; severe heart failure; severe coronary artery disease, unstable angina; severe liver disease or renal impairment; also on theoretical grounds: Raynaud's syndrome, intermittent claudication, epilepsy, depression, Parkinson's disease, glaucoma; pregnancy and breast-feeding
Side-effects: dry mouth; headache, fatigue, sedation, dizziness, nausea, sleep disturbance, vasodilatation
Dose: 200 micrograms once daily in the morning, increased if necessary after 3 weeks to 400 micrograms daily in 1–2 divided doses; max. 600 micrograms daily in 2 divided doses

▼ PoM **Physiotens**® (Solvay)
Tablets, f/c, moxonidine 200 micrograms (pink), net price 28-tab pack = £10.45; 400 micrograms (red), 28-tab pack = £14.26. Label: 3

2.5.3   Adrenergic neurone blocking drugs

These drugs prevent the release of noradrenaline from postganglionic adrenergic neurones. Guanethidine also depletes the nerve endings of noradrenaline. These drugs do not control supine blood pressure and may cause postural hypotension. For this reason they have largely fallen from use, but may be necessary with other therapy in resistant hypertension.

GUANETHIDINE MONOSULPHATE

Indications: moderate to severe hypertension that has failed to respond adequately to other antihypertensives, in conjunction with a diuretic or a vasodilator antihypertensive
Cautions: postural hypotension may cause falls in elderly; coronary or cerebral arteriosclerosis, asthma, history of peptic ulceration; pregnancy;   **interactions:** Appendix 1 (adrenergic neurone blockers)
Contra-indications: phaeochromocytoma, renal failure, heart failure
Side-effects: postural hypotension, failure of ejaculation, fluid retention, nasal congestion, headache, diarrhoea, drowsiness
Dose: by mouth, 10 mg daily, increased by 10 mg at weekly intervals; usual daily dose 25–50 mg
By intramuscular injection, 10–20 mg, repeated after 3 hours if required

PoM **Ismelin**® (Ciba)
Tablets, guanethidine monosulphate 10 mg, net price 20 = 46p; 25 mg (pink), 28-tab pack = £1.44
Additives: include gluten
Injection, guanethidine monosulphate 10 mg/mL. Net price 1-mL amp = 23p

BETHANIDINE SULPHATE

Indications; Cautions; Contra-indications; Side-effects: see under Guanethidine Monosulphate (except diarrhoea)
Dose: 10 mg (elderly 5 mg) 3 times daily after food, increased by 5 mg at intervals; max. daily dose 200 mg

PoM **Bendogen**® (Lagap)
Tablets, scored, bethanidine sulphate 10 mg, net price 100-tab pack = £15.14. Label: 21

BRETYLIUM TOSYLATE
Section 2.3.2

DEBRISOQUINE

Indications; Cautions; Contra-indications; Side-effects: see under Guanethidine Monosulphate (except diarrhoea)
Dose: 10 mg 1–2 times daily, increased by 10 mg every 3 days; usual range 20–60 mg daily (120 mg or higher in severe hypertension)

PoM ¹**Debrisoquine** (Cambridge)
Tablets, scored, debrisoquine (as sulphate) 10 mg, net price 100-tab pack = £12.91
1. Former brand name Declinax®

2.5.4   Alpha-adrenoceptor blocking drugs

Prazosin has post-synaptic alpha-blocking and vasodilator properties and rarely causes tachycardia. It may, however, cause a rapid reduction in blood pressure after the first dose and should be introduced with caution. **Doxazosin** and **terazosin** have properties similar to those of prazosin.

Indoramin is also an effective alpha-blocker but has many side-effects.

PROSTATIC HYPERPLASIA. Prazosin, doxazosin, indoramin and terazosin are also indicated for benign prostatic hyperplasia (see section 7.4.1).

ALFUZOSIN
See section 7.4.1

DOXAZOSIN

Indications: hypertension, usually in conjunction with thiazide or beta-blocker; benign prostatic hyperplasia, see section 7.4.1
Cautions: care with initial dose (postural hypotension); pregnancy and breast-feeding (see Appendixes 4 and 5); **interactions:** Appendix 1 (alpha-blockers)
Side-effects: postural hypotension (rarely associated with fainting); dizziness, vertigo, headache, fatigue, asthenia, oedema, somnolence, nausea, rhinitis, urinary incontinence reported
Dose: hypertension, 1 mg daily, increased after 1–2 weeks to 2 mg daily, and thereafter to 4 mg daily, if necessary; max. 16 mg daily
Benign prostatic hyperplasia, see section 7.4.1

PoM Cardura® (Invicta)

Tablets, doxazosin (as mesylate) 1 mg, net price 28-tab pack = £10.56; 2 mg, 28-tab pack = £14.08; 4 mg, 28-tab pack = £17.60

INDORAMIN

Indications: hypertension, usually in conjunction with thiazide or beta-blocker; benign prostatic hyperplasia, see section 7.4.1

Cautions: avoid alcohol (enhances rate and extent of absorption); control incipient heart failure with diuretics and digoxin; hepatic or renal impairment; elderly patients; Parkinson's disease; epilepsy (convulsions in *animal* studies); history of depression; **interactions:** Appendix 1 (alpha-blockers)

DRIVING. Drowsiness may affect performance of skilled tasks (e.g. driving); effects of alcohol may be enhanced

Contra-indications: established heart failure; patients receiving MAOIs

Side-effects: sedation; also dizziness, depression, failure of ejaculation, dry mouth, nasal congestion, extrapyramidal effects, weight gain

Dose: hypertension, initially 25 mg twice daily, increased by 25–50 mg daily at intervals of 2 weeks; max. daily dose 200 mg in 2–3 divided doses

Benign prostatic hyperplasia, see section 7.4.1

PoM Baratol® (Monmouth)

Tablets, both f/c, indoramin (as hydrochloride) 25 mg (blue), net price 100-tab pack = £23.00; 50 mg (green, scored), 100-tab pack = £40.79. Label: 2

Prostatic hyperplasia
PoM Doralese®: see section 7.4.1

PRAZOSIN HYDROCHLORIDE

Indications: see under Dose

Cautions: first dose may cause collapse due to hypotension (therefore should be taken on retiring to bed); elderly; reduce initial dose in renal impairment; pregnancy and breast-feeding; **interactions:** Appendix 1 (alpha-blockers)

Contra-indications: not recommended for congestive heart failure due to mechanical obstruction (e.g. aortic stenosis)

Side-effects: postural hypotension, drowsiness, weakness, dizziness, headache, lack of energy, nausea, palpitations; urinary frequency, incontinence reported

Dose: hypertension, 500 micrograms 2–3 times daily, the initial dose on retiring to bed at night (to avoid collapse, see Cautions); increased to 1 mg 2–3 times daily after 3–7 days; further increased if necessary to max. 20 mg daily

Congestive heart failure, 500 micrograms 2–4 times daily (initial dose at bedtime, see above), increasing to 4 mg daily in divided doses; maintenance 4–20 mg daily (but rarely used)

Raynaud's syndrome, initially 500 micrograms twice daily (initial dose at bedtime, see above); maintenance 1–2 mg twice daily

Benign prostatic hyperplasia, see section 7.4.1

PoM Prazosin (Non-proprietary)

Tablets, prazosin hydrochloride 500 micrograms, net price 100-tab pack = £3.93; 1 mg, 100-tab pack = £4.96; 2 mg, 100-tab pack = £6.73; 5 mg, 100-tab pack = £14.53. Label: 3, counselling, see dose above

Available from APS, Ashbourne (Alphavase®), Cox, Hillcross, Norton

PoM Hypovase® (Invicta)

Tablets, prazosin hydrochloride 500 micrograms, net price 56-tab pack = £2.09; 1 mg (orange, scored), 56-tab pack = £2.69; 2 mg (scored), 56-tab pack = £3.66; starter pack of 8 × 500-microgram tabs with 32 × 1-mg tabs = £2.52. Label: 3, counselling, see dose above

Note. Hypovase® (Benign Prostatic Hypertrophy), see section 7.4.1

TAMSULOSIN HYDROCHLORIDE

See section 7.4.1

TERAZOSIN

Indications: mild to moderate hypertension; benign prostatic hyperplasia, see section 7.4.1

Cautions: first dose may cause collapse due to hypotension (within 30–90 minutes, therefore should be taken on retiring to bed) (may also occur with rapid dose increase); **interactions:** Appendix 1 (alpha-blockers)

Side-effects: dizziness, lack of energy, peripheral oedema; urinary frequency reported

Dose: hypertension, 1 mg at bedtime (compliance with bedtime dose important, see Cautions); dose doubled after 7 days if necessary; usual maintenance dose 2–10 mg once daily; more than 20 mg daily rarely improves efficacy

Benign prostatic hyperplasia, see section 7.4.1

PoM Hytrin® (Abbott)

Tablets, terazosin (as hydrochloride) 2 mg (yellow), net price 28-tab pack = £12.55; 5 mg (tan), 28-tab pack = £18.89; 10 mg (blue), 28-tab pack = £26.59: starter pack of 7 × 1-mg tabs with 21 × 2-mg tabs = £13.00. Label: 3, counselling, see dose above

Note. Hytrin BPH® (for benign prostatic hyperplasia), see section 7.4.1

PHAEOCHROMOCYTOMA

Phenoxybenzamine is a powerful alpha-blocker with many side-effects. It is used with a beta-blocker in the short-term management of severe hypertensive episodes associated with phaeochromocytoma; it is also used in the management of severe shock unresponsive to conventional therapy.

Phentolamine is a short-acting alpha-blocker used rarely as a suppression test for phaeochromocytoma.

PHENOXYBENZAMINE HYDROCHLORIDE

Indications: phaeochromocytoma (see notes above)

Cautions: elderly; congestive heart failure; severe heart disease (see also Contra-indications); cerebrovascular disease (avoid if history of cerebrovascular accident); renal impairment; carcinogenic in *animals*; pregnancy; avoid in porphyria (see section 9.8.2); avoid infusion in hypovolaemia; avoid extravasation (irritant to tissues)

Contra-indications: history of cerebrovascular accident; during recovery period after myocardial infarction (usually 3–4 weeks)

Side-effects: postural hypotension with dizziness and marked compensatory tachycardia, lassitude, nasal congestion, miosis, inhibition of ejaculation; rarely gastro-intestinal disturbances; decreased sweating and dry mouth after intravenous infusion; idiosyncratic profound hypotension within few minutes of starting infusion

Dose: by mouth, phaeochromocytoma, 10 mg daily, increased by 10 mg daily; usual dose 1–2 mg/kg daily in 2 divided doses

PoM **Dibenyline®** (Forley)

Capsules, red/white, phenoxybenzamine hydrochloride 10 mg. Net price 30-cap pack = £20.22

Injection concentrate, phenoxybenzamine hydrochloride 50 mg/mL. To be diluted before use. Net price 3 × 2-mL amp = £43.88 (hosp. only)

Dose: by intravenous infusion (preferably through large vein), phaeochromocytoma and adjunct in severe shock, 1 mg/kg daily in 200 mL physiological saline over at least 2 hours; do not repeat within 24 hours (intensive care facilities needed)

CAUTION: Owing to risk of contact sensitisation doctors, nurses, and other health workers should avoid contamination of hands

PHENTOLAMINE MESYLATE

Indications: hypertensive episodes due to phaeochromocytoma e.g. during surgery; diagnosis of phaeochromocytoma

Cautions: monitor blood pressure (avoid in hypotension), heart rate; renal impairment; gastritis, peptic ulcer; elderly; **interactions:** Appendix 1 (alpha-blockers)

ASTHMA. Presence of sulphites in ampoules may (especially in patients with asthma) lead to hypersensitivity (with bronchospasm and shock)

Contra-indications: hypotension; history of myocardial infarction; coronary insufficiency, angina, or other evidence of coronary artery disease

Side-effects: postural hypotension, tachycardia, dizziness; nausea and vomiting, diarrhoea, nasal congestion; also acute or prolonged hypotension, angina, chest pain, arrhythmias

Dose: hypertensive episodes, *by intravenous injection,* 2–5 mg repeated if necessary
Diagnosis of phaeochromocytoma, consult data sheet

PoM **Rogitine®** (Ciba)

Injection, phentolamine mesylate 10 mg/mL. Net price 1-mL amp = 27p

2.5.5   Drugs affecting the renin-angiotensin system

2.5.5.1   Angiotensin-converting enzyme inhibitors
2.5.5.2   Angiotensin-II receptor antagonists

2.5.5.1 ANGIOTENSIN-CONVERTING ENZYME INHIBITORS

Angiotensin-converting enzyme inhibitors (ACE inhibitors) inhibit the conversion of angiotensin I to angiotensin II. They are effective and generally well tolerated.

HYPERTENSION. ACE inhibitors should be considered for hypertension when thiazides and beta-blockers are contra-indicated, not tolerated, or fail to control blood pressure; they are particularly indicated for hypertension in insulin-dependent diabetics with nephropathy (see also section 6.1.5), and possibly for hypertension in all diabetics. ACE inhibitors may cause *very rapid falls of blood pressure* in some patients. Therefore where possible any diuretic therapy should be stopped for a few days before initiating therapy and the first dose should preferably be given at bedtime.

DIABETIC NEPHROPATHY. For comment on the role of ACE inhibitors in the management of diabetic nephropathy, see section 6.1.5.

HEART FAILURE. ACE inhibitors have a valuable role in all grades of heart failure, combined when appropriate with diuretic and digoxin treatment. They improve prognosis substantially, and in this respect are superior to regimens such as modified-release nitrates with hydralazine. ACE inhibitor treatment is indicated in any patient with heart failure who has no contra-indications. To avoid *dangerous hyperkalaemia,* any potassium-sparing diuretic should be omitted from the diuretic regimen before introducing an ACE inhibitor, changing to the loop diuretic alone; potassium supplements should also be discontinued. *Profound first-dose hypotension* may occur when ACE inhibitors are introduced to patients with heart failure who are already taking a high dose of a loop diuretic (e.g. frusemide 80 mg daily or higher). Temporary withdrawal of the loop diuretic reduces the risk, but may cause severe rebound pulmonary oedema. The ACE inhibitor should therefore be started at very low dosage (e.g. captopril 6.25 mg), with the patient recumbent and under close medical supervision, and with facilities to treat profound hypotension. In these circumstances and in other special risk groups (see below) the patient should be admitted to hospital for initiation.

MYOCARDIAL INFARCTION. ACE inhibitors also improve the prognosis of patients who have left ventricular failure, even transiently, after acute myocardial infarction, and of patients with asymptomatic left ventricular dysfunction. Treatment in clinically stable patients should generally be initiated 3 to 10 days after the myocardial infarction.

INITIATION IN HOSPITAL. ACE inhibitor therapy for heart failure should be initiated under close medical supervision (in hospital *in severe heart failure*). Initiation in hospital is also recommended for patients with *mild to moderate heart failure*:

receiving multiple or high-dose diuretic therapy (e.g. more than 80 mg of frusemide daily or its equivalent);

with hypovolaemia;

with hyponatraemia (plasma sodium below 130 mmol/litre);

with pre-existing hypotension (systolic blood pressure below 90 mmHg);

with unstable heart failure;

with renal impairment (plasma creatinine above 150 micromol/litre);

receiving high-dose vasodilator therapy;

aged 70 years or more.

RENAL EFFECTS. In patients with *severe bilateral renal artery stenosis* (or severe stenosis of the artery supplying a single functioning kidney), ACE inhibitors reduce or abolish glomerular filtration and are likely to cause severe and progressive renal failure. They are thus **contra-indicated** in patients known to have these forms of critical renovascular disease.

ACE inhibitor treatment is unlikely to have an adverse effect on overall renal function in patients with *severe unilateral renal artery stenosis* and a *normal contralateral kidney*, but glomerular filtration is likely to be reduced (or even abolished) in the affected kidney and the long-term consequences are unknown.

In general, ACE inhibitors are therefore best avoided in **all** patients with *known or suspected renovascular disease*, unless the blood pressure cannot be controlled by other drugs. If they are used in these circumstances renal function needs to be monitored with great care.

ACE inhibitors should also be used with particular caution in patients who may have *undiagnosed and clinically silent* renovascular disease. This includes patients with peripheral vascular disease or with severe generalised atherosclerosis.

Renal function and electrolytes should be checked before starting ACE inhibitors and monitored during treatment (more frequently if features mentioned above present). Although ACE inhibitors now have a specialised role in some forms of renal disease they also occasionally cause *impairment of renal function* which may progress and become severe in other circumstances (at particular risk are the elderly).

Concomitant treatment with *NSAIDs* increases the risk of renal damage, and *potassium-sparing diuretics* (or *potassium-containing salt substitutes*) increase the risk of hyperkalaemia.

PREGNANCY. ACE inhibitors are contra-indicated in pregnancy, and should be avoided in patients who may become pregnant.

COMBINATION PRODUCTS. A number of products incorporating an ACE inhibitor with a thiazide diuretic are now available. Use of these combination products should be reserved for patients whose blood pressure has not responded to a thiazide diuretic or an ACE inhibitor alone (see also comments above).

CAPTOPRIL

Indications: mild to moderate hypertension alone or with thiazide therapy and severe hypertension resistant to other treatment (but see cautions and notes above); congestive heart failure (adjunct); following myocardial infarction, see dose; diabetic nephropathy (microalbuminuria greater than 30 mg/day) in insulin-dependent diabetes

Cautions: diuretics (**important:** see notes above); first doses may cause hypotension especially in patients taking diuretics, on a low-sodium diet, on dialysis, or dehydrated; peripheral vascular disease or generalised atherosclerosis owing to risk of clinically silent renovascular disease (see also notes above); monitor renal function before and during treatment, and **reduce dose** in renal impairment (see also notes above); possible increased risk of agranulocytosis in collagen vascular disease (blood counts recommended); anaphylactoid reactions (see below); breast-feeding (see Appendix 5); may potentiate hypoglycaemic effects of insulin or oral antidiabetic drugs; **interactions:** Appendix 1 (ACE inhibitors)

ANAPHYLACTOID REACTIONS. To prevent anaphylactoid reactions, ACE inhibitors should be avoided during dialysis with high-flux polyacrylonitrile membranes and during low-density lipoprotein apheresis with dextran sulphate; they should also be withheld before desensitisation with wasp or bee venom

Contra-indications: hypersensitivity to ACE inhibitors (including angioedema); known or suspected renovascular disease (see also notes above), aortic stenosis or outflow tract obstruction; pregnancy (see notes above and Appendix 4); porphyria (see section 9.8.2)

Side-effects: hypotension (see Cautions); dizziness, headache, fatigue, asthenia, nausea (occasionally vomiting), diarrhoea (occasionally constipation), muscle cramps, persistent dry cough, throat discomfort, voice changes, taste alteration (may be associated with weight loss), stomatitis, dyspepsia, abdominal pain; renal impairment (see Cautions and notes above); hyperkalaemia (more common in renal impairment, see notes above); angioedema, urticaria, rashes (erythema multiforme and toxic epidermal necrolysis reported), and hypersensitivity reactions (see below for Symptom Complex), blood disorders (including thrombocytopenia, neutropenia, agranulocytosis, and aplastic anaemia); other side-effects reported include upper respiratory tract symptoms, hyponatraemia, tachycardia, palpitations, arrhythmias, myocardial infarction and cerebrovascular accident (possibly associated with severe hypotension), back pain, flushing, jaundice (hepatocellular or cholestatic), pancreatitis, sleep disturbances, nervousness, mood changes, paraesthesia, impotence, onycholysis, alopecia

SYMPTOM COMPLEX. A symptom complex has been reported for ACE inhibitors which may include fever, serositis, vasculitis, myalgia, arthralgia, positive antinuclear antibody, raised erythrocyte sedimentation rate, eosinophilia, leucocytosis; rash, photosensitivity or other skin reactions may occur.

Dose: hypertension, used alone, initially 12.5 mg twice daily; if used in addition to diuretic (see notes), in elderly, or in renal impairment, initially 6.25 mg twice daily (first dose at bedtime); usual maintenance dose 25 mg twice daily; max. 50 mg twice daily (rarely 3 times daily in severe hypertension)

Heart failure (adjunct), initially 6.25–12.5 mg under close medical supervision (see notes above); usual maintenance dose 25 mg 2–3 times daily; usual max. 150 mg daily

Prophylaxis after infarction in clinically stable patients with asymptomatic or symptomatic left ventricular dysfunction (radionuclide ventriculography or echocardiography undertaken before initiation), initially 6.25 mg, starting as early as 3 days after infarction, then increased over several weeks to 150 mg daily (if tolerated) in divided doses

Diabetic nephropathy, 75–100 mg daily in divided doses; if further blood pressure reduction required, other antihypertensives may be used in conjunction with captopril; in severe renal impairment, initially 12.5 mg twice daily (if concomitant diuretic therapy required, loop diuretic rather than thiazide should be chosen)

PoM Capoten® (Squibb)
Tablets, captopril 12.5 mg (scored), net price 100 = £18.86; 25 mg, 56-tab pack = £12.03, 100-tab pack = £21.49; 50 mg (scored), 56-tab pack = £20.50, 100-tab pack = £36.61 (also available as Acepril®)

With diuretic
Note. For mild to moderate hypertension in patients stabilised on the individual components in the same proportions

PoM Capozide® (Squibb)
LS tablets, scored, captopril 25 mg, hydrochlorothiazide 12.5 mg. Net price 28-tab pack = £11.25
Tablets, scored, captopril 50 mg, hydrochlorothiazide 25 mg. Net price 28-tab pack = £14.14 (also available as Acezide®)

CILAZAPRIL

Indications: hypertension (but see cautions and notes above); congestive heart failure (adjunct)
Cautions; Contra-indications; Side-effects: see under Captopril and notes above
Dose: hypertension, initially 1 mg once daily; if used in those receiving a diuretic (see notes), in elderly, or in renal impairment, initially 500 micrograms once daily; in renovascular hypertension (see notes), liver cirrhosis, initially 250–500 micrograms once daily; usual maintenance dose 1–2.5 mg once daily; max. 5 mg daily
Note. Discontinue diuretic for 2–3 days beforehand (see also notes above)
Heart failure (adjunct), initially 500 micrograms once daily under close medical supervision (see notes above), increased to 1 mg once daily; usual maintenance dose 1–2.5 mg daily; max. 5 mg daily

PoM Vascace® (Roche)
Tablets, all f/c, cilazapril 250 micrograms (pink), net price 28-tab pack = £3.87; 500 micrograms (white), 28-tab pack = £4.10; 1 mg (yellow), 28-tab pack = £7.06; 2.5 mg (pink), 28-tab pack = £10.67; 5 mg (brown), 28-tab pack = £14.95

ENALAPRIL MALEATE

Indications: all grades of hypertension (but see cautions and notes above); treatment of congestive heart failure (adjunct); prevention of symptomatic heart failure and prevention of coronary ischaemic events in patients with left ventricular dysfunction
Cautions; Contra-indications; Side-effects: see under Captopril and notes above
Dose: hypertension, used alone, initially 5 mg once daily; if used in addition to diuretic (see notes), in elderly patients, or in renal impairment, initially 2.5 mg daily; usual maintenance dose 10–20 mg once daily; in severe hypertension may be increased to max. 40 mg once daily
Heart failure (adjunct), asymptomatic left ventricular dysfunction, initially 2.5 mg daily under close medical supervision (see notes above); usual maintenance 20 mg daily in 1–2 divided doses

PoM Innovace® (MSD)
Tablets, enalapril maleate 2.5 mg, net price 50 = £10.00; 5 mg (scored), 28-tab pack = £7.86, 50 = £14.03; 10 mg (red), 28-tab pack = £11.03, 50 = £19.69; 20 mg (peach), 28-tab pack = £13.10, 50 = £23.40; titration pack of 11 × 2.5-mg tabs and 14 × 5-mg tabs = £6.12

With diuretic
Note. For mild to moderate hypertension in patients stabilised on the individual components in the same proportions
PoM Innozide® (MSD)
Tablets, yellow, scored, enalapril maleate 20 mg, hydrochlorothiazide 12.5 mg. Net price 28-tab pack = £14.56

FOSINOPRIL

Indications: hypertension (but see cautions and notes above); congestive heart failure (adjunct)
Cautions; Contra-indications; Side-effects: see under Captopril and notes above
Dose: hypertension, initially and usual maintenance 10 mg daily; max. 40 mg once daily
Note. In hypertension, if used in addition to diuretic, discontinue diuretic several days before and resume after about 4 weeks if blood pressure inadequately controlled (if diuretic therapy cannot be stopped careful medical supervision for several hours)
Heart failure (adjunct), initially 10 mg daily under close medical supervision (see notes above); if initial dose well tolerated, may be increased to up to 40 mg once daily

PoM Staril® (Squibb)
Tablets, fosinopril sodium 10 mg, net price 28-tab pack = £12.04; 20 mg, 28-tab pack = £13.00

LISINOPRIL

Indications: all grades of hypertension (but see cautions and notes above); congestive heart failure (adjunct); following myocardial infarction in haemodynamically stable patients

Cautions; Contra-indications; Side-effects: see under Captopril and notes above

Dose: hypertension, initially 2.5 mg daily; usual maintenance dose 10–20 mg daily; max. 40 mg daily

Note. In hypertension discontinue diuretic for 2–3 days beforehand and resume later if required (see also notes above)

Heart failure (adjunct), initially 2.5 mg daily under close medical supervision (see notes above); usual maintenance dose 5–20 mg daily

Prophylaxis after myocardial infarction, systolic blood pressure >120 mmHg, 5 mg within 24 hours, followed by further 5 mg 24 hours later, then 10 mg after a further 24 hours, and continuing with 10 mg once daily for 6 weeks (or continued if heart failure); systolic blood pressure 100-120 mmHg, initially 2.5 mg, increasing to maintenance dose of 5 mg once daily

Note. Should not be started if systolic blood pressure <100 mmHg; temporarily reduce maintenance dose to 2.5 mg daily if systolic blood pressure ≤ 100 mmHg during treatment; withdraw if prolonged hypotension occurs (systolic blood pressure < 90 mmHg for more than 1 hour)

PoM **Carace**® (Du Pont)
Tablets, lisinopril 2.5 mg (blue), net price 28-tab pack = £7.64; 5 mg (scored), 28-tab pack = £9.58; 10 mg (yellow, scored), 28-tab pack = £11.83; 20 mg (orange, scored), 28-tab pack = £13.38

PoM **Zestril**® (Zeneca)
Tablets, lisinopril (as dihydrate) 2.5 mg, net price 28-tab pack = £7.64; 5 mg (pink, scored), 28-tab pack = £9.58; 10 mg (pink), 28-tab pack = £11.83; 20 mg (red), 28-tab pack = £13.38

With diuretic
Note. For mild to moderate hypertension in patients stabilised on the individual components in the same proportions

PoM **Carace Plus**® (Du Pont)
Carace 10 Plus tablets, blue, lisinopril 10 mg, hydrochlorothiazide 12.5 mg. Net price 28-tab pack = £11.83

¹*Carace 20 Plus tablets,* yellow, scored, lisinopril 20 mg, hydrochlorothiazide 12.5 mg. Net price 28-tab pack = £13.38
1. Formerly called Carace Plus®

PoM **Zestoretic**® (Zeneca)
Zestoretic 10 tablets, peach, lisinopril (as dihydrate) 10 mg, hydrochlorothiazide 12.5 mg. Net price 28-tab pack = £11.83

¹*Zestoretic 20 tablets,* lisinopril (as dihydrate) 20 mg, hydrochlorothiazide 12.5 mg. Net price 28-tab pack = £13.38
1. Formerly called Zestoretic®

MOEXIPRIL HYDROCHLORIDE

Indications: hypertension (but see cautions and notes above)

Cautions; Contra-indications; Side-effects: see under Captopril and notes above

Dose: used alone, initially 7.5 mg once daily; if used in addition to diuretic (see notes), with calcium-channel blocker (e.g. nifedipine), in elderly, in renal or hepatic impairment, initially 3.75 mg once daily; usual range 15–30 mg once daily; doses above 30 mg daily not shown to increase efficacy

Note. If possible discontinue diuretic 2–3 days beforehand (see also notes above); if diuretic cannot be stopped, careful medical supervision for at least 2 hours and until blood pressure stabilised for at least an additional hour

▼ PoM **Perdix**® (Schwarz)
Tablets, f/c, both pink, scored, moexipril hydrochloride 7.5 mg, net price 28-tab pack = £8.50; 15 mg, 28-tab pack = £9.80

PERINDOPRIL

Indications: hypertension (but see cautions and notes above); congestive heart failure (adjunct)

Cautions; Contra-indications; Side-effects: see under Captopril and notes above

Dose: hypertension, initially 2 mg daily; usual maintenance dose 4 mg once daily; max. 8 mg daily

Note. In hypertension discontinue diuretic 2–3 days beforehand and resume later if required (see also notes above)

Heart failure (adjunct), initial dose 2 mg in the morning under close medical supervision (see notes above); usual maintenance 4 mg daily

PoM **Coversyl**® (Servier)
Tablets, perindopril erbumine (= tert-butylamine) 2 mg, net price 30-tab pack = £9.45; 4 mg (scored), 30-tab pack = £13.65. Label: 22

QUINAPRIL

Indications: all grades of essential hypertension (but see cautions and notes above); congestive heart failure (adjunct)

Cautions; Contra-indications; Side-effects: see under Captopril and notes above

Dose: hypertension, initially 10 mg once daily; with a diuretic, in elderly, or in renal impairment initially 2.5 mg daily; usual maintenance dose 20–40 mg daily in single or 2 divided doses; up to 80 mg daily has been given

Heart failure (adjunct), initial dose 2.5 mg under close medical supervision (see notes above); usual maintenance 10–20 mg daily in 2 divided doses; up to 40 mg daily has been given

PoM **Accupro**® (P-D)
Tablets, all brown, f/c, quinapril 5 mg, net price 28-tab pack = £10.30; 10 mg, 28-tab pack = £10.07; 20 mg, 28-tab pack = £9.79; 40 mg, 28-tab pack = £9.75

With diuretic
Note. For hypertension in patients stabilised on the individual components in the same proportions

PoM **Accuretic**® (P-D)
Tablets, pink, f/c, scored, quinapril 10 mg, hydrochlorothiazide 12.5 mg. Net price 28-tab pack = £9.79

RAMIPRIL

Indications: mild to moderate hypertension (but see cautions and notes above); congestive heart failure (adjunct); following myocardial infarction in patients with clinical evidence of heart failure

Cautions; Contra-indications; Side-effects: see under Captopril and notes above

Dose: hypertension, initially 1.25 mg daily, increased at intervals of 1–2 weeks; usual range 2.5–5 mg once daily; max. 10 mg daily

Note. In hypertension, discontinue diuretic for 2–3 days beforehand and resume later if required (see also notes above); patients with renal impairment or congestive heart failure require initiation under close medical supervision in hospital; close medical supervision is also required for patients with hepatic impairment

Heart failure (adjunct), initially 1.25 mg once daily under close medical supervision (see notes above), increased if necessary at intervals of 1–2 weeks; max. 10 mg daily (daily doses of 2.5 mg or more may be taken in 1–2 divided doses)

Note. In heart failure, reduce dose of any high dose diuretic beforehand

Prophylaxis after myocardial infarction (started in hospital 3 to 10 days after infarction), initially 2.5 mg twice daily, increased after 2 days to 5 mg twice daily; maintenance 2.5–5 mg twice daily

Note. If initial 2.5–mg dose not tolerated, give 1.25 mg twice daily for 2 days before increasing to 2.5 mg twice daily, then 5 mg twice daily; withdraw if 2.5 mg twice daily not tolerated

PoM Tritace® (Hoechst)

Capsules, ramipril 1.25 mg (yellow/white), net price 28-cap pack = £5.30; 2.5 mg (orange/white), 28-cap pack = £7.51; 5 mg (red/white), 28-cap pack = £9.55

TRANDOLAPRIL

Indications: mild to moderate hypertension (but see cautions and notes above)

Cautions; Contra-indications; Side-effects: see under Captopril and notes above

Dose: initially 500 micrograms once daily, increased at intervals of 2–4 weeks; usual range 1–2 mg once daily; max. 4 mg daily

Note. If used in addition to diuretic, discontinue diuretic 2–3 days beforehand and resume later if required; patients with renal or hepatic impairment or congestive heart failure require initiation under close medical supervision

▼ PoM Gopten® (Knoll)

Capsules, trandolapril 500 micrograms (red/yellow), net price 14-cap pack = £4.09; 1 mg (red/orange), 28-cap pack = £10.33; 2 mg (red/red), 28-cap pack = £12.28

Additives: include gluten

▼ PoM Odrik® (Roussel)

Capsules, trandolapril 500 micrograms (red/yellow), net price 28-cap pack = £8.19; 1 mg (red/orange), 28-cap pack = £10.34; 2 mg (red/red), 28-cap pack = £12.29

2.5.5.2 ANGIOTENSIN-II RECEPTOR ANTAGONISTS

Losartan is a specific angiotensin-II receptor antagonist which has properties similar to those of the ACE inhibitors. However, unlike ACE inhibitors, it does not inhibit the breakdown of bradykinin and other kinins, and thus does not appear to cause the persistent dry cough which commonly complicates ACE inhibitor therapy. It may therefore be an alternative for patients who have to discontinue an ACE inhibitor because of persistent cough. Beyond this its role in the management of hypertension remains to be established.

LOSARTAN POTASSIUM

Indications: hypertension

Cautions: hepatic impairment (consider reducing initial dose); renal impairment (see under Dose); renal artery stenosis (see also Renal Effects, p. 87); monitor plasma potassium, particularly in elderly and in renal impairment; intravascular volume depletion (e.g. patients taking high-dose diuretics); **interactions:** Appendix 1 (as for ACE inhibitors)

Contra-indications: pregnancy and breast-feeding

Side-effects: dizziness; orthostatic hypotension, hyperkalaemia, rash, taste disturbance, liver function changes also reported

Dose: initially and usual maintenance 50 mg once daily (elderly over 75 years, moderate to severe renal impairment, intravascular volume depletion, initially 25 mg once daily); if necessary increased after several weeks to 100 mg once daily

▼ PoM Cozaar® (MSD)

Tablets, both f/c, losartan potassium 25 mg (Half Strength), net price 7-tab pack = £4.31; 50 mg (scored), 28-tab pack = £17.23

2.5.6 Ganglion-blocking drugs

TRIMETAPHAN CAMSYLATE

(Trimetaphan Camsilate)

Indications: controlled hypotension in surgery

Cautions: hepatic or renal impairment, diabetes mellitus, elderly, cerebral or coronary vascular disease, adrenal insufficiency, Addison's disease, CNS degenerative disease

Contra-indications: severe arteriosclerosis, severe cardiac disease, pyloric stenosis, pregnancy

Side-effects: tachycardia and respiratory depression (particularly with muscle relaxants); constipation, increased intra-ocular pressure, pupillary dilatation

Dose: by intravenous infusion, 3–4 mg/minute initially, then adjusted according to response

PoM ¹Trimetaphan Camsylate (Cambridge)

Injection, trimetaphan camsylate 50 mg/mL. Net price 5-mL amp = £8.30. For dilution and use as an infusion

1. Former brand name Arfonad®

2.5.7   Tyrosine hydroxylase inhibitors

Metirosine inhibits the enzyme tyrosine hydroxylase, and hence the synthesis of catecholamines. It is used in the pre-operative management of phaeochromocytoma, and long term in patients unsuitable for surgery; an alpha-adrenoceptor blocking drug (e.g. phenoxybenzamine) may also be required. Metirosine should **not** be used to treat essential hypertension.

METIROSINE

Indications: see notes above
Cautions: maintain high fluid intake and adequate blood volume; may impair ability to drive or operate machinery; **interactions:** Appendix 1 (metirosine)
Side-effects: sedation; extrapyramidal symptoms; diarrhoea (may be severe); hypersensitivity reactions
Dose: initially 250 mg 4 times daily, increased to max. of 4 g daily in divided doses; doses of 2–3 g daily should be given for 5–7 days before surgery

PoM Demser® (MSD)
Capsules, blue, metirosine 250 mg (hosp. only). Label: 2

2.6   Nitrates, calcium-channel blockers, and potassium-channel activators

2.6.1	Nitrates
2.6.2	Calcium-channel blockers
2.6.3	Potassium-channel activators
2.6.4	Peripheral and cerebral vasodilators
2.6.5	Flosequinan

Most patients with *angina pectoris* are treated with beta-blockers (section 2.4) or calcium-channel blockers (section 2.6.2). However, short-acting nitrates (section 2.6.1) retain an important role in for prophylactic use before exertion and for chest pain occurring at rest. Nitrates are sometimes used as sole therapy, especially in elderly patients with infrequent symptoms.

Vasodilators are known to act in *heart failure* either by:

arteriolar dilatation which reduces both peripheral vascular resistance and left ventricular pressure at systole and results in improved cardiac output, *or* venous dilatation which results in dilatation of capacitance vessels, increase of venous pooling, and diminution of venous return to the heart (decreasing left ventricular end-diastolic pressure).

2.6.1   Nitrates

Sublingual **glyceryl trinitrate** is one of the most effective drugs for providing rapid symptomatic relief of angina, but its effect lasts only for 20 to 30 minutes. Though a potent coronary vasodilator, its principal benefit follows from a reduction in venous return which reduces left ventricular work. Unwanted effects such as flushing, headache, and

postural hypotension may limit therapy, especially when angina is severe or when patients are unusually sensitive to the effects of nitrates; the 300-microgram tablet is often appropriate when glyceryl trinitrate is first used. Duration of action may be prolonged by *modified-release* preparations. The *aerosol spray* provides an alternative method of rapid relief of symptoms for those who find difficulty in dissolving sublingual preparations. The *percutaneous* preparations may be useful in the prophylaxis of angina for patients who suffer attacks at rest, especially at night.

Isosorbide dinitrate is active *sublingually* and is a more stable preparation for those who only require nitrates infrequently. It is also effective by mouth for prophylaxis; although the effect is slower in onset, it may persist for several hours. Duration of action of up to 12 hours is claimed for *modified-release* preparations. The activity of isosorbide dinitrate may depend on the production of active metabolites, the most important of which is isosorbide mononitrate. **Isosorbide mononitrate** itself is also available for angina prophylaxis, though the advantages over isosorbide dinitrate have not yet been firmly established.

Glyceryl trinitrate or isosorbide dinitrate may be tried by *intravenous injection* when the sublingual form is ineffective in patients with chest pain due to myocardial infarction or severe ischaemia. Intravenous injections are also useful in the treatment of acute left ventricular failure.

TOLERANCE. Some patients on long-acting or transdermal nitrates rapidly develop tolerance (with reduced therapeutic effects). Reduction of blood-nitrate concentrations to low levels for 4 to 8 hours each day usually maintains effectiveness in such patients. If tolerance is suspected after the use of transdermal patches they should be removed for several consecutive hours in each 24 hours; in the case of modified-release tablets of isosorbide dinitrate (and conventional formulations of isosorbide mononitrate), the second of the two daily doses can be given after about 8 hours rather than after 12 hours. Conventional formulations of isosorbide mononitrate should not usually be given more than twice daily unless small doses are used; modified-release formulations of isosorbide mononitrate should only be given once daily.

GLYCERYL TRINITRATE

Indications: prophylaxis and treatment of angina; left ventricular failure
Cautions: severe hepatic or renal impairment; hypothyroidism, malnutrition, or hypothermia; recent history of myocardial infarction; metal-containing transdermal systems should be removed before cardioversion or diathermy; tolerance (see notes above); **interactions:** Appendix 1 (glyceryl trinitrate)
Contra-indications: hypersensitivity to nitrates; hypotensive conditions and hypovolaemia; hypertrophic obstructive cardiomyopathy, aortic stenosis, cardiac tamponade, constrictive pericarditis, mitral stenosis; marked anaemia, head trauma, cerebral haemorrhage, closed-angle glaucoma

---

Side-effects: throbbing headache, flushing, dizziness, postural hypotension, tachycardia (but paradoxical bradycardia has occurred)

INJECTION. Specific side-effects following injection (particularly if given too rapidly) include severe hypotension, nausea and retching, diaphoresis, apprehension, restlessness, muscle twitching, retrosternal discomfort, palpitations, abdominal pain, syncope; prolonged administration has been associated with methaemoglobinaemia

Dose: sublingually, 0.3–1 mg, repeated as required

By mouth, 2.6–6.4 mg as modified-release tablets, 2–3 times daily; severe angina, 10 mg 3 times daily

By intravenous infusion, 10–200 micrograms/minute

Short-acting tablets and sprays

Glyceryl Trinitrate (Non-proprietary)

Sublingual tablets, glyceryl trinitrate 300 micrograms, net price 100 = £2.84; 500 micrograms, 100 = 32p; 600 micrograms, 100 = 62p. Label: 16

Note. Glyceryl trinitrate tablets should be supplied in glass containers of not more than 100 tablets, closed with a foil-lined cap, and containing no cotton wool wadding; they should be discarded after 8 weeks in use

Coro-Nitro Pump Spray® (Boehringer Mannheim)

Aerosol spray, glyceryl trinitrate 400 micrograms/metered dose. Net price 200-dose unit = £3.28

Dose: treatment or prophylaxis of angina, spray 1–2 doses under tongue and then close mouth

Glytrin Spray® (Sterwin)

Aerosol spray, glyceryl trinitrate 400 micrograms/metered dose. Net price 200-dose unit = £3.28. Label: 10 patient information leaflet

Dose: treatment or prophylaxis of angina, spray 1–2 doses under tongue and then close mouth

Caution: flammable

GTN 300 mcg (Martindale)

Sublingual tablets, glyceryl trinitrate 300 micrograms. Net price 100 = £2.84. Label: 16

Nitrolingual Pumpspray® (Lipha)

Aerosol spray, glyceryl trinitrate 400 micrograms/metered dose. Net price 200-dose unit = £4.10

Dose: treatment or prophylaxis of angina, spray 1–2 doses under tongue and then close mouth

Modified-release tablets

Nitrocontin Continus® (ASTA Medica)

Tablets, m/r, pink, glyceryl trinitrate 6.4 mg, net price 100-tab pack = £4.28. Label: 25

Suscard® (Pharmax)

Buccal tablets, m/r, glyceryl trinitrate 1 mg, net price 20 = £1.96; 2 mg, 20 = £2.84; 3 mg, 20 = £4.10; 5 mg, 20 = £5.58. Counselling, see administration below

Dose: treatment of angina, 2 mg as required (1 mg in sensitive patients), increased to 3 mg if necessary; prophylaxis 1–3 mg 3 times daily; 5 mg in severe angina

Unstable angina (adjunct), up to 5 mg with ECG monitoring

Congestive heart failure, 5 mg 3 times daily, increased to 10 mg 3 times daily in severe cases

Acute heart failure, 5 mg repeated until symptoms abate

ADMINISTRATION. Tablets are placed between upper lip and gum, and left to dissolve; vary site to reduce risk of dental caries

Sustac® (Pharmax)

Tablets, m/r, all pink, glyceryl trinitrate 2.6 mg, net price 20 = £1.19; 6.4 mg, 20 = £1.72; 10 mg, 20 = £2.39. Label: 25

Parenteral preparations

Note. Glass or polyethylene apparatus is preferable; loss of potency will occur if PVC is used

PoM **Glyceryl Trinitrate** (Non-proprietary)

Injection, glyceryl trinitrate 5 mg/mL. To be diluted before use. Net price 5-mL amp = £6.49; 10-mL amp = £12.98

Available from David Bull

PoM **Nitrocine®** (Schwarz)

Injection, glyceryl trinitrate 1 mg/mL. To be diluted before use or given undiluted with syringe pump. Net price 10-mL amp = £8.27; 50-mL bottle = £19.38

PoM **Nitronal®** (Lipha)

Injection, glyceryl trinitrate 1 mg/mL. To be diluted before use or given undiluted with syringe pump. Net price 5-mL vial = £2.16; 50-mL vial = £17.64

PoM **Tridil®** (Du Pont)

Injection, to be diluted before use, glyceryl trinitrate 500 micrograms/mL, net price 10-mL amp = £4.39; 5 mg/mL, 10-mL amp = £21.33

Transdermal preparations

Deponit® (Schwarz)

Patches, self-adhesive, transparent, glyceryl trinitrate, '5' patch (releasing approx. 5 mg/24 hours when in contact with skin), net price 30 = £19.25; '10' patch (releasing approx. 10 mg/24 hours), 30 = £21.19

ADMINISTRATION: prophylaxis of angina, apply one '5' or one '10' patch to lateral chest wall, upper arm, or shoulder; replace every 24 hours, siting replacement patch on different area; see also notes above

Minitran® (3M)

Patches, self-adhesive, transparent, glyceryl trinitrate, '5' patch (releasing approx. 5 mg/24 hours when in contact with skin), net price 30 = £13.08; '10' patch (releasing approx. 10 mg/24 hours), 30 = £14.49; '15' patch (releasing approx. 15 mg/24 hours), 30 = £15.98

ADMINISTRATION: prophylaxis of angina, apply one '5' patch to chest or upper arm; replace every 24 hours, siting replacement patch on different area; adjust dose according to response; see also notes above

Maintenance of venous patency ('5' patch only), see literature

Nitro-Dur® (Schering-Plough)

Patches, self-adhesive, buff, glyceryl trinitrate, '0.1 mg/h' patch (releasing approx. 2.5 mg/24 hours when in contact with skin), net price 28 = £11.85; '0.2 mg/h' patch (releasing approx. 5 mg/24 hours), 28 = £13.15; '0.4 mg/h' patch (releasing approx. 10 mg/24 hours), 28 = £14.56; '0.6 mg/h' patch (releasing approx. 15 mg/24 hours), 28 = £16.02

ADMINISTRATION: prophylaxis of angina, apply one '0.2 mg/h' patch to chest or outer upper arm; replace every 24 hours, siting replacement patch on different area; adjust dose according to response; see also notes above

Percutol® (Dominion)

Ointment, glyceryl trinitrate 2%. Net price 60 g = £9.55. Counselling, see administration below

Additives: include wool fat

ADMINISTRATION: prophylaxis of angina, usual dose 1–2 inches of ointment measured on to *Applirule*, and applied (usually to chest, abdomen, or thigh) without rubbing in and secured with surgical tape, every 3–4 hours as required; to determine dose, ½ inch on first day then increased by ½ inch/day until headache occurs, then reduced by ½ inch

Note. 1 inch of ointment contains glyceryl trinitrate 16.64 mg

Transiderm-Nitro® (Geigy)

Patches, self-adhesive, pink, glyceryl trinitrate, '5' *patch* (releasing approx. 5 mg/24 hours when in contact with skin), net price 30 = £18.97; '10' *patch* (releasing approx. 10 mg/24 hours), 30 = £20.86

ADMINISTRATION: prophylaxis of angina, apply one '5' or one '10' patch to lateral chest wall; replace every 24 hours, siting replacement patch on different area; max. two '10' patches daily; see also notes above

Prophylaxis of phlebitis and extravasation ('5' patch only), see literature

ISOSORBIDE DINITRATE

Indications: prophylaxis and treatment of angina; left ventricular failure

Cautions; Contra-indications; Side-effects: see under Glyceryl Trinitrate

Dose: sublingually, 5–10 mg

By mouth, daily in divided doses, angina 30–120 mg, left ventricular failure 40–160 mg, up to 240 mg if required

By intravenous infusion, 2–10 mg/hour; higher doses up to 20 mg/hour may be required

Short-acting tablets and sprays

Isosorbide Dinitrate (Non-proprietary)

Tablets, isosorbide dinitrate 10 mg, net price 20 = 24p; 20 mg, 20 = 42p

Available from APS, Berk, Cox, Hillcross, Norton

Imtack Spray® (Astra)

Aerosol spray, isosorbide dinitrate 1.25 mg/metered dose. Net price 200-dose unit = £4.28

Dose: treatment or prophylaxis of angina, spray 1–3 doses under tongue and then close mouth

Caution: flammable

Isordil® (Monmouth)

Tablets (sublingual), pink, isosorbide dinitrate 5 mg. Net price 100-tab pack = £1.43. Label: 26

Tablets, both scored, isosorbide dinitrate 10 mg, net price 100-tab pack = £1.45; 30 mg, 100-tab pack = £3.45

Sorbichew® (Stuart)

Tablets (chewable), green, scored, isosorbide dinitrate 5 mg. Net price 100-tab pack = £1.51. Label: 24

Sorbitrate® (Stuart)

Tablets, both scored, isosorbide dinitrate 10 mg (yellow), net price 100-tab pack = £1.51; 20 mg (blue), 100-tab pack = £2.10

Modified-release preparations

Cedocard Retard® (Pharmacia)

Retard-20 tablets, m/r, yellow, scored, isosorbide dinitrate 20 mg. Net price 60-tab pack = £5.71. Label: 25

Dose: prophylaxis of angina, 1 tablet every 12 hours

Retard-40 tablets, m/r, orange-red, scored, isosorbide dinitrate 40 mg. Net price 60-tab pack = £11.09. Label: 25

Dose: prophylaxis of angina, 1–2 tablets every 12 hours

Isoket Retard® (Schwarz)

Retard-20 tablets, m/r, yellow, scored, isosorbide dinitrate 20 mg. Net price 50-tab pack = £3.24. Label: 25

Retard-40 tablets, m/r, orange, scored, isosorbide dinitrate 40 mg. Net price 50-tab pack = £7.99. Label: 25

Dose: prophylaxis of angina, 20–40 mg every 12 hours

Isordil Tembids® (Monmouth)

Capsules, m/r, blue/clear, isosorbide dinitrate 40 mg. Net price 100-cap pack = £15.54. Label: 25

Dose: prophylaxis of angina, 1 capsule 2–3 times daily

Soni-Slo® (Lipha)

Capsules, m/r, pink/clear, enclosing off-white pellets, isosorbide dinitrate 20 mg. Net price 20 = £1.19. Label: 25

Capsules, m/r, yellow/clear, enclosing off-white pellets, isosorbide dinitrate 40 mg. Net price 20 = £1.40. Label: 25

Dose: prophylaxis of angina, 40–120 mg daily in divided doses

Sorbid SA® (Stuart)

Sorbid-20 SA capsules, m/r, red/yellow, isosorbide dinitrate 20 mg. Net price 56-cap pack = £3.50. Label: 25

Dose: prophylaxis of angina, 1–2 capsules twice daily

Sorbid-40 SA capsules, m/r, red/clear, isosorbide dinitrate 40 mg. Net price 56-cap pack = £5.00. Label: 25

Dose: prophylaxis of angina, 1–2 capsules twice daily

Parenteral preparations

PoM **Isoket®** (Schwarz)

Injection 0.05%, isosorbide dinitrate 500 micrograms/mL. To be diluted before use or given undiluted with syringe pump. Net price 50-mL bottle = £10.06

Injection 0.1%, isosorbide dinitrate 1 mg/mL. To be diluted before use. Net price 10-mL amp = £3.79; 50-mL bottle = £18.81; 100-mL bottle = £25.98

Note. Glass or polyethylene infusion apparatus is preferable; loss of potency if PVC used

ISOSORBIDE MONONITRATE

Indications: prophylaxis and treatment of angina; adjunct in congestive heart failure

Cautions; Contra-indications; Side-effects: see under Glyceryl Trinitrate

Dose: initially 20 mg 2–3 times daily *or* 40 mg twice daily (10 mg twice daily in those who have not previously received nitrates); up to 120 mg daily in divided doses if required

---

Isosorbide Mononitrate (Non-proprietary)

Tablets, isosorbide mononitrate 10 mg, net price 20 = 82p; 20 mg, 20 = 87p; 40 mg, 20 = £2.26. Label: 25

Various strengths available from APS, Ashbourne (Isib®), Berk, Cox, CP, Dominion, Hillcross, Lagap, Norton, Opus (Angeze®)

Elantan® (Schwarz)

Elantan 10 tablets, scored, isosorbide mononitrate 10 mg. Net price 50 = £3.33. Label: 25

PoM *Elantan 20 tablets*, scored, isosorbide mononitrate 20 mg. Net price 50 = £4.11. Label: 25

PoM *Elantan 40 tablets*, scored, isosorbide mononitrate 40 mg. Net price 50 = £7.07. Label: 25

Ismo® (Boehringer Mannheim)

Ismo 10 tablets, isosorbide mononitrate 10 mg. Net price 60-tab pack = £3.39. Label: 25

Ismo 20 tablets, isosorbide mononitrate 20 mg. Net price 60-tab pack = £4.97. Label: 25

Starter pack, 8 tablets, isosorbide mononitrate 10 mg; 60 tablets, scored, isosorbide mononitrate 20 mg. Net price = £5.38. Label: 25

Ismo 40 tablets, isosorbide mononitrate 40 mg. Net price 100-tab pack = £13.61. Label: 25

Isotrate® (Bioglan)

Tablets, isosorbide mononitrate 20 mg. Net price 60-tab pack = £7.09. Label: 25

Monit® (Lorex)

LS Tablets, isosorbide mononitrate 10 mg. Net price 56-tab pack = £3.37. Label: 25

Tablets, scored, isosorbide mononitrate 20 mg. Net price 56-tab pack = £4.30. Label: 25

Mono-Cedocard® (Pharmacia)

Mono-Cedocard 10 tablets, orange, scored, isosorbide mononitrate 10 mg. Net price 60-tab pack = £3.68. Label: 25

Mono-Cedocard 20 tablets, scored, isosorbide mononitrate 20 mg. Net price 100-tab pack = £6.83. Label: 25

Mono-Cedocard 40 tablets, scored, isosorbide mononitrate 40 mg. Net price 60-tab pack = £9.12. Label: 25

Modified release

Elantan LA® (Schwarz)

Elantan LA 25 capsules, m/r, brown/white, enclosing white micropellets, isosorbide mononitrate 25 mg. Net price 28-cap pack = £7.00. Label: 25
Dose: prophylaxis of angina, 1 capsule in the morning, increased if necessary to 2 capsules

Elantan LA 50 capsules, m/r, brown/pink, enclosing white micropellets, isosorbide mononitrate 50 mg. Net price 28-cap pack = £11.30. Label: 25
Dose: prophylaxis of angina, 1 capsule daily in the morning, increased if necessary to 2 capsules

PoM **Imdur®** (Astra)

Durules® (= tablets m/r), yellow, f/c, scored, isosorbide mononitrate 60 mg. Net price 28-tab pack = £11.14. Label: 25
Dose: prophylaxis of angina, 1 tablet in the morning (half a tablet if headache occurs), increased to 2 tablets if required

Isib 60XL® (Ashbourne)

Tablets, m/r, scored, ivory, isosorbide mononitrate 60 mg. Net price 28-tab pack = £10.02. Label: 25
Dose: prophylaxis of angina, 1 tablet in the morning (half a tablet for 2–4 days if headache occurs), increased if necessary to 2 tablets

Ismo Retard® (Boehringer Mannheim)

Tablets, m/r, s/c, isosorbide mononitrate 40 mg. Net price 28-tab pack = £10.24. Label: 25
Dose: prophylaxis of angina, 1 tablet daily in morning

¹MCR-50® (Pharmacia)

Capsules, m/r, containing white micropellets, isosorbide mononitrate 50 mg. Net price 28-cap pack = £11.02. Label: 25
Dose: prophylaxis of angina, 1 capsule in morning increased to 2 capsules if required
1. Full product name Mono Cedocard Retard-50®

Monit SR® (Lorex)

Tablets, m/r, s/c, isosorbide mononitrate 40 mg. Net price 28-tab pack = £10.24. Label: 25
Dose: prophylaxis of angina, 1 tablet daily in morning

Monomax SR® (Trinity)

Capsules, m/r, isosorbide mononitrate 40 mg, net price 28-cap pack = £8.70; 60 mg, 28-cap pack = £9.46. Label: 25
Dose: prophylaxis of angina, 40 mg once daily increased if necessary to 60 mg daily

---

PENTAERYTHRITOL TETRANITRATE
(Pentaerithrityl Tetranitrate)

Indications: prophylaxis of angina
Cautions; Contra-indications; Side-effects: see under Glyceryl Trinitrate

Mycardol® (Sanofi Winthrop)

Tablets, scored, pentaerythritol tetranitrate 30 mg. Net price 20 = 96p. Label: 22
Dose: 2 tablets 3–4 times daily

2.6.2   Calcium-channel blockers

Calcium-channel blockers (less correctly called 'calcium-antagonists') interfere with the inward displacement of calcium ions through the slow channels of active cell membranes. They influence the myocardial cells, the cells within the specialised conducting system of the heart, and the cells of vascular smooth muscle. Thus, myocardial contractility may be reduced, the formation and propagation of electrical impulses within the heart may be depressed, and coronary or systemic vascular tone may be diminished. They should usually be **avoided** in *heart failure* because they may further depress cardiac function and cause clinically significant deterioration.

Calcium-channel blockers differ in their predeliction for the various possible sites of action therefore their therapeutic effects are disparate, with much greater variation than those of beta-blockers. There are important differences between verapamil and the dihydropyridine calcium-channel blockers, such as nifedipine, nicardipine and isradipine.

Verapamil is used for the treatment of *angina, hypertension,* and *arrhythmias* (section 2.3.2). It reduces cardiac output, slows the heart rate, and may impair atrioventricular conduction. It may precipitate heart failure, exacerbate conduction disor-

---

ders, and cause hypotension at high doses and should **not** be used with beta-blockers (see p. 98). Constipation is the most common side-effect.

Nifedipine relaxes vascular smooth muscle and dilates coronary and peripheral arteries. It has more influence on vessels and less on the myocardium than does verapamil, and unlike verapamil has no anti-arrhythmic activity. It rarely precipitates heart failure because any negative inotropic effect is offset by a reduction in left ventricular work. **Nicardipine** has similar effects to those of nifedipine and may produce less reduction of myocardial contractility. **Amlodipine** and **felodipine** also resemble nifedipine and nicardipine in their effects and do not reduce myocardial contractility. They have a longer duration of action and can be given once daily. Nifedipine, nicardipine, and amlodipine are used for the treatment of angina or hypertension. All are valuable in forms of *angina associated with coronary vasospasm*; they are useful as adjuncts to beta-blockers for patients with severe symptoms, and as alternative treatment for those who are intolerant of beta-blockers. Side-effects associated with vasodilatation such as flushing and headache (which become less obtrusive after a few days), and ankle swelling (which does not respond to diuretics) are common.

Isradipine and **lacidipine** have similar effects to those of nifedipine and nicardipine; they are only indicated for *hypertension*.

Nimodipine is related to nifedipine but the smooth muscle relaxant effect preferentially acts on cerebral arteries. Its use is confined to prevention of *vascular spasm following subarachnoid haemorrhage*.

Diltiazem is effective in most forms of *angina*; the longer-acting formulation is also used for *hypertension*. It may be used in patients for whom beta-blockers are contra-indicated or ineffective. It has a less negative inotropic effect than verapamil and significant myocardial depression occurs rarely. Nevertheless because of the risk of bradycardia it should be used with caution in association with beta-blockers.

UNSTABLE ANGINA. Calcium-channel blockers do not reduce the risk of myocardial infarction in unstable angina. Their use should be reserved for patients resistant to treatment with beta-blockers, nitrates, and anticoagulation with aspirin and intravenous heparin.

WITHDRAWAL. There is some evidence that sudden withdrawal of calcium-channel blockers may be associated with an exacerbation of angina.

AMLODIPINE BESYLATE

Indications: hypertension, prophylaxis of angina

Cautions: pregnancy and breast-feeding; hepatic impairment; **interactions:** Appendix 1 (calcium-channel blockers)

Side-effects: headache, oedema, fatigue, nausea, flushing, dizziness; gum hyperplasia, erythema multiforme reported

Dose: hypertension or angina, initially 5 mg once daily; max. 10 mg once daily

PoM Istin® (Pfizer)

Tablets, amlodipine (as besylate) 5 mg. Net price 28-tab pack = £11.85; 10 mg, 28-tab pack = £17.70

DILTIAZEM HYDROCHLORIDE

Indications: prophylaxis and treatment of angina; hypertension

Cautions: reduce dose in hepatic and renal impairment; heart failure or significantly impaired left ventricular function, mild bradycardia (avoid if severe), first degree AV block, or prolonged PR interval; **interactions:** Appendix 1 (calcium-channel blockers)

Contra-indications: severe bradycardia, left ventricular failure, second- or third-degree AV block (unless pacemaker fitted), sick sinus syndrome; pregnancy and breast-feeding (see Appendixes 4 and 5)

Side-effects: bradycardia, sino-atrial block, atrioventricular block, hypotension, malaise, headache, hot flushes, gastro-intestinal disturbances, oedema (notably of ankles); rarely rashes (erythema multiforme reported); altered liver function tests; hepatitis and depression reported

Dose: angina, 60 mg 3 times daily (elderly initially twice daily); increased if necessary to 360 mg daily

Longer-acting formulations, see under preparations below

Standard formulations

Note. These formulations are licensed as generics and there is no requirement for brand name dispensing. Although their means of formulation has called for the strict designation 'modified-release' their duration of action corresponds to that of tablets requiring administration 3 times daily

PoM Diltiazem (Non-proprietary)

Tablets, m/r (but see note above), diltiazem hydrochloride 60 mg. Net price 100 = £6.44. Label: 25

Available from APS, Ashbourne (Angiozem®), Berk, Cox, Hillcross, Lagap, Norton, Thames (Britiazim®)

PoM Adizem-60® (Napp)

Tablets, m/r (but see note above), f/c, diltiazem hydrochloride 60 mg. Net price 100-tab pack = £15.38. Label: 25

PoM Tildiem® (Lorex)

Tablets, m/r (but see note above), off-white, diltiazem hydrochloride 60 mg. Net price 100-tab pack = £13.25. Label: 25

Longer-acting formulations

Note. To avoid confusion between these different formulations of diltiazem, prescribers should specify the brand to be dispensed

PoM Adizem-SR® (Napp)

Capsules, m/r, diltiazem hydrochloride 90 mg (white), net price 56-cap pack = £11.06; 120 mg (brown/white), 56-cap pack = £12.29; 180 mg (brown/white), 56-cap pack = £18.43. Label: 25

Dose: see next page

Tablets, m/r, f/c, scored, diltiazem hydrochloride 120 mg. Net price 56-tab pack = £18.14. Label: 25

Dose: mild to moderate hypertension, usually 120 mg twice daily (dose form not appropriate for initial dose titration)

Angina, initially 90 mg twice daily (elderly, dose form not appropriate for initial dose titration); increased to 180 mg twice daily if required

PoM Adizem-XL® (Napp)

Capsules, m/r, diltiazem hydrochloride 120 mg (pink/blue), net price 30-cap pack = £11.49; 180 mg (dark pink/blue), 30-cap pack = £13.03; 240 mg (red/blue), 30-cap pack = £14.48; 300 mg (maroon/blue), 30-cap pack = £11.49. Label: 25

Dose: angina and mild to moderate hypertension, initially 240 mg once daily, increased if necessary to 300 mg once daily; in elderly and in hepatic or renal impairment, initially 120 mg daily

PoM Angitil SR® (Trinity)

Capsules, m/r, diltiazem hydrochloride 90 mg (white), net price 56-cap pack = £8.85; 120 mg (brown), 56-cap pack = £9.83; 180 mg (brown), 56-cap pack = £14.74. Label: 25

Dose: angina and mild to moderate hypertension, initially 90 mg twice daily (elderly and in hepatic and renal impairment, dose form not appropriate for initial dose titration); increased if necessary to 120 mg or 180 mg twice daily

PoM Calcicard CR® (Norton)

Tablets, m/r, both f/c, diltiazem hydrochloride 90 mg, net price 56-tab pack = £11.06; 120 mg, 56-tab pack = £12.29. Label: 25

Dose: mild to moderate hypertension, initially 90 mg or 120 mg twice daily; up to 360 mg daily may be required: ELDERLY and in hepatic and renal impairment, initially 120 mg once daily; up to 240 mg daily may be required

Angina, initially 90 mg or 120 mg twice daily; up to 480 mg daily in divided doses may be required; ELDERLY and in hepatic and renal impairment, dose form not appropriate for initial dose titration; up to 240 mg daily may be required

PoM Dilzem SR® (Elan)

Capsules, m/r, all beige, diltiazem hydrochloride 60 mg, net price 100-cap pack = £13.50; 90 mg, 60-cap pack = £10.94; 120 mg, 60-cap pack = £12.15. Label: 25

Dose: angina and mild to moderate hypertension, initially 90 mg twice daily (elderly 60 mg twice daily); up to 180 mg twice daily may be required

PoM Dilzem XL® (Elan)

Capsules, m/r, diltiazem hydrochloride 120 mg, net price 30-cap pack = £8.10; 180 mg, 30-cap pack = £11.10; 240 mg, 30-cap pack = £11.40. Label: 25

Dose: angina and mild to moderate hypertension, initially 180 mg once daily (elderly and in hepatic and renal impairment, 120 mg once daily); if necessary may be increased to 360 mg once daily

PoM Slozem® (Lipha)

Capsules, m/r, diltiazem hydrochloride 120 mg (pink/clear), net price 28-cap pack = £7.00; 180 mg (pink/clear), 28-cap pack = £9.24; 240 mg (red/clear), 28-cap pack = £9.80. Label: 25

Dose: angina and mild to moderate hypertension, initially 240 mg once daily (elderly and in hepatic and renal impairment, 120 mg once daily); if necessary may be increased to 360 mg once daily

PoM Tildiem LA® (Lorex)

Capsules, m/r, diltiazem hydrochloride 200 mg (pink/grey, containing white pellets), net price 28-cap pack = £11.10; 300 mg (white/yellow, containing white pellets), 28-cap pack = £11.80. Label: 25

Dose: angina and mild to moderate hypertension, initially 300 mg once daily before or with food, increased to 400 mg daily, and if necessary to 500 mg daily; ELDERLY and in hepatic or renal impairment, initially 200 mg daily, increased if necessary to 300 mg daily

PoM Tildiem Retard® (Lorex)

Tablets, m/r, diltiazem hydrochloride 90 mg, net price 56-tab pack = £11.06; 120 mg, 56-tab pack = £12.29. Label: 25

COUNSELLING. Tablet membrane may pass through gastro-intestinal tract unchanged, but being porous has no effect on efficacy

Dose: mild to moderate hypertension, initially 90 mg or 120 mg twice daily (elderly once daily); up to 360 mg daily may be required (elderly up to 240 mg daily)

Angina, initially 90 mg or 120 mg twice daily (elderly, dose form not appropriate for initial dose titration); up to 480 mg daily in divided doses may be required (elderly up to 240 mg daily)

With diuretic

PoM Adizem-XL Plus® (Napp)

Capsules, m/r, blue/white, diltiazem hydrochloride 150 mg, hydrochlorothiazide 12.5 mg. Net price 30-cap pack = £11.49. Label: 25

Dose: mild to moderate hypertension in patients stabilised on the individual components in the same proportions, usually 2 capsules daily in the morning

FELODIPINE

Indications: hypertension, angina

Cautions: withdraw if ischaemic pain occurs; hepatic impairment; breast-feeding; **interactions:** Appendix 1 (calcium-channel blockers)

Contra-indications: pregnancy

Side-effects: flushing, headache, palpitations, dizziness, fatigue, gravitational oedema, rash and pruritus, gum hyperplasia

Dose: hypertension, initially 5 mg daily in the morning; usual maintenance 5–10 mg once daily; doses above 20 mg daily rarely needed

Angina, initially 5 mg daily in the morning, increased if necessary to 10 mg once daily

PoM Plendil® (Schwarz)

Tablets, m/r, f/c, felodipine 5 mg, net price 28-tab pack = £8.12; 10 mg, 28-tab pack = £10.92. Label: 25

ISRADIPINE

Indications: hypertension

Cautions: tight aortic stenosis; sick sinus syndrome (if pacemaker not fitted); reduce dose in hepatic or renal impairment; pregnancy (may prolong labour); **interactions:** Appendix 1 (calcium-channel blockers)

Side-effects: headache, flushing, dizziness, tachycardia and palpitations, localised peripheral oedema; hypotension uncommon; rarely weight gain, fatigue, abdominal discomfort, rashes

Dose: 2.5 mg twice daily (1.25 mg twice daily in elderly, hepatic or renal impairment); increased if necessary after 3–4 weeks to 5 mg twice daily (exceptionally up to 10 mg twice daily); maintenance 2.5 or 5 mg once daily may be sufficient

PoM **Prescal**® (Ciba)

Tablets, yellow, scored, isradipine 2.5 mg. Net price 56-tab pack = £12.53

LACIDIPINE

Indications: hypertension

Cautions: cardiac conduction abnormalities; poor cardiac reserve; hepatic impairment; withdraw if ischaemic pain occurs shortly after initiating treatment; breast-feeding; **interactions:** Appendix 1 (calcium-channel blockers)

Contra-indications: pregnancy

Side-effects: headache, flushing, oedema, dizziness, palpitations; also asthenia, rash (including pruritus and erythema), gastro-intestinal disturbances, polyuria, chest pain (see Cautions), gingival hyperplasia

Dose: 4 mg as a single daily dose, increased if necessary after 3–4 weeks to 6 mg daily; in hepatic impairment, initially 2 mg daily; ELDERLY, initially 2 mg daily, increased if necessary to 4 mg after 4 weeks

PoM **Motens**® (Boehringer Ingelheim)

Tablets, both f/c, lacidipine 2 mg, net price 28-tab pack = £10.66; 4 mg (scored), 28-tab pack = £14.50. Label: 21

NICARDIPINE HYDROCHLORIDE

Indications: prophylaxis and treatment of angina; mild to moderate hypertension

Cautions: withdraw if ischaemic pain occurs or existing pain worsens within 30 minutes of initiating treatment or increasing dose; congestive heart failure or significantly impaired left ventricular function; elderly; hepatic or renal impairment; **interactions:** Appendix 1 (calcium-channel blockers)

Contra-indications: advanced aortic stenosis; pregnancy

Side-effects: dizziness, headache, peripheral oedema, flushing, palpitations, nausea; also gastro-intestinal disturbances, drowsiness, insomnia, tinnitus, hypotension, rashes, salivation, frequency of micturition; thrombocytopenia reported

Dose: initially 20 mg 3 times daily, increased to 30 mg 3 times daily (usual range 50–120 mg daily); patients with hypertension controlled on 20–30 mg 3 times daily can be given 30–40 mg twice daily

PoM **Cardene**® (Roche)

Capsules, nicardipine hydrochloride 20 mg (blue/white), net price 100-cap pack = £15.98; 30 mg (blue/pale blue), 56-cap pack = £10.39

Modified release
PoM **Cardene SR**® (Roch

Capsules, m/r, nicardipin
net price 56-cap pack = £
cap pack = £14.35. Label:
Dose: mild to moderate hy
twice daily; usual effective
(range 30–60 mg twice daily)

NIFEDIPINE

Indications: prophylaxis and treatment of angina; hypertension; Raynaud's phenomenon

Cautions: withdraw if ischaemic pain occurs or existing pain worsens shortly after initiating treatment; poor cardiac reserve; heart failure or significantly impaired left ventricular function (heart failure deterioration observed); severe hypotension; reduce dose in hepatic impairment; diabetes mellitus; may inhibit labour; breast-feeding (see Appendix 5); **interactions:** Appendix 1 (calcium-channel blockers)

Contra-indications: cardiogenic shock; advanced aortic stenosis; pregnancy (toxicity in *animal* studies); porphyria (see section 9.8.2)

Side-effects: headache, flushing, dizziness, lethargy; tachycardia, palpitations: also gravitational oedema, rash (erythema multiforme reported), nausea, increased frequency of micturition, eye pain, gum hyperplasia; depression reported; telangiectasia reported

Dose: see preparations below

PoM **Adalat**® (Bayer)

Capsules, both orange, nifedipine 5 mg, net price 20 = £1.42; 10 mg, 20 = £1.80. Label: 21, counselling, see dose
Dose: angina and Raynaud's phenomenon, initially 10 mg (elderly and hepatic impairment, 5 mg) 3 times daily with or after food; usual maintenance 5–20 mg 3 times daily; for immediate effect in angina bite into capsule and swallow liquid
Hypertension, not recommended therefore no dose stated
Note. Nifedipine capsules also available from APS, Ashbourne (Angiopine®), Berk, Cox, Hillcross, Norton

Modified release
Note. To avoid confusion between these different formulations of nifedipine, prescribers should specify the brand to be dispensed
PoM **Adalat**® **LA** (Bayer)

LA 30 tablets, m/r, pink, nifedipine 30 mg. Net price 28-tab pack = £10.36. Label: 25
LA 60 tablets, m/r, pink, nifedipine 60 mg. Net price 28-tab pack = £15.40. Label: 25
COUNSELLING. Tablet membrane may pass through gastro-intestinal tract unchanged, but being porous has no effect on efficacy
Dose: mild to moderate hypertension and angina prophylaxis, 30 mg once daily, increased if necessary; max. 90 mg once daily
Caution: dose form not appropriate for use in hepatic impairment or where there is a history of oesophageal or gastro-intestinal obstruction, decreased lumen diameter of the gastro-intestinal tract, or inflammatory bowel disease (including Crohn's disease)

...at® Retard (Bayer)

...10 tablets, m/r, pink, nifedipine 10 mg. Net
...ce 56-tab pack = £8.66. Label: 21, 25

...etard 20 tablets, m/r, pink, nifedipine 20 mg. Net
price 56-tab pack = £10.81. Label: 21, 25

Dose: hypertension and angina prophylaxis, 20 mg
twice daily with or after food (initial titration 10 mg
twice daily); usual maintenance 10–40 mg twice daily

PoM Adipine® MR (Trinity)

Tablets, m/r, nifedipine 10 mg (apricot), net price
56-tab pack = £6.93; 20 mg (pink), 56-tab pack =
£8.65. Label: 25

Dose: hypertension and angina prophylaxis, 20 mg
twice daily after food (initial titration 10 mg twice
daily); max. 40 mg twice daily

PoM Angiopine MR® (Ashbourne)

Tablets, m/r, brown, nifedipine 20 mg. Net price
56-tab pack = £8.65. Label: 25

Dose: hypertension and angina prophylaxis, 20 mg
twice daily (dose form not appropriate for initial dose
titration in hepatic impairment); max. 80 mg daily

PoM Cardilate MR® (Norton)

Tablets, m/r, brown, nifedipine 20 mg. Net price
100-tab pack = £18.35. Label: 25

Dose: hypertension and angina prophylaxis, 20 mg
twice daily (dose form not appropriate for initial dose
titration in hepatic impairment); max. 80 mg daily

PoM Coracten® (Evans)

Capsules, m/r, nifedipine 10 mg (grey/pink,
enclosing yellow pellets), net price 60-cap pack =
£7.15; 20 mg (pink/brown, enclosing yellow pellets), 60-cap pack = £9.97. Label: 25

Dose: hypertension and angina prophylaxis, one 20-mg
capsule every 12 hours, adjusted within range 10–40 mg
every 12 hours

PoM Hypolar® Retard 20 (Lagap)

Tablets, m/r, red, f/c, nifedipine 20 mg. Net price
56-tab pack = £10.60. Label: 25

Dose: hypertension and angina prophylaxis, 20 mg
twice daily, increased if necessary to 40 mg twice daily

PoM Nifelease® (Lennon)

Tablets, m/r, scored, pink, nifedipine 20 mg. Net
price 100-tab pack = £18.99. Label: 25

Dose: hypertension and angina prophylaxis, 20 mg
twice daily, increased if necessary to 40 mg twice daily

PoM Nifensar XL® (Rhône-Poulenc Rorer)

Tablets, m/r, yellow, nifedipine 20 mg. Net price
28-tab pack = £7.37. Label: 21, 25

Dose: mild to moderate hypertension, initially 40 mg
once daily (initially 20 mg in elderly not previously
treated with nifedipine, or in renal impairment); usual
maintenance dose 20–40 mg daily; max. 100 mg daily

PoM Unipine XL® (Ethical Generics Ltd)

Tablets, m/r, nifedipine 30 mg. Net price 28-tab
pack = £10.08. Label: 23, 25

Dose: mild to moderate hypertension, 30 mg once daily,
preferably in the morning, increased if necessary to
60 mg once daily

With atenolol
Section 2.4

NIMODIPINE

Indications: prevention and treatment of
ischaemic neurological deficits following subarachnoid haemorrhage

Cautions: cerebral oedema or severely raised
intracranial pressure; avoid concomitant administration of nimodipine tablets and infusion, other
calcium-channel blockers, or beta-blockers;
impaired renal function or nephrotoxic drugs;
pregnancy; **interactions:** Appendix 1 (calcium-
channel blockers)

Side-effects: hypotension, variation in heart-rate,
flushing, headache, gastro-intestinal disorders,
nausea, and feeling of warmth; thrombocytopenia
and ileus reported; transient increase in liver
enzymes after intravenous administration

Dose: prevention, *by mouth*, 60 mg every 4 hours
(total daily dose 360 mg), starting within 4 days
of subarachnoid haemorrhage and continued for
21 days

Treatment, *by intravenous infusion* via central
catheter, 1 mg/hour initially, increased after 2
hours to 2 mg/hour, providing no severe decrease
in blood pressure; patients with unstable blood
pressure or weighing less than 70 kg,
500 micrograms/hour initially or less if necessary;
treatment should start as soon as possible and
should continue for at least 5 days (max. 14
days); in the event of surgical intervention during
treatment continue for at least 5 days after

PoM Nimotop® (Bayer)

Tablets, yellow, f/c, nimodipine 30 mg. Net price
100-tab pack = £38.85

Intravenous infusion, nimodipine 200 micrograms/
mL; also contains ethanol 20% and macrogol
'400' 17%. Net price 50-mL vial (with polyethylene infusion catheter) = £13.24; 250-mL bottle =
£66.20

Note. Polyethylene or polypropylene apparatus should
be used; PVC should be avoided

VERAPAMIL HYDROCHLORIDE

Indications: see under Dose

Cautions: first-degree AV block; acute phase of
myocardial infarction (avoid if bradycardia,
hypotension, left ventricular failure); patients taking beta-blockers (**important:** see below); reduce
dose in hepatic impairment; children, specialist
advice only (see section 2.3.2); pregnancy and
breast-feeding; **interactions:** Appendix 1 (calcium-channel blockers)

VERAPAMIL AND BETA-BLOCKERS. **Verapamil** should not
be injected into patients recently treated with beta-
blockers because of the risk of hypotension and asystole.
It has been suggested that when verapamil injection has
been given first, an interval of 30 minutes before giving
a beta-blocker is sufficient but this too is open to doubt.
It may even be hazardous to give verapamil and a beta-
blocker together by mouth (should only be contemplated
if myocardial function well preserved).

Contra-indications: hypotension, bradycardia,
second- and third-degree AV block, sick sinus
syndrome, cardiogenic shock, sino-atrial block;
history of heart failure or significantly impaired
left ventricular function, even if controlled by
therapy; atrial flutter or fibrillation complicating
Wolff-Parkinson-White syndrome; porphyria (see
section 9.8.2)

Side-effects: constipation; less commonly nausea, vomiting, flushing, headache, dizziness, fatigue, ankle oedema; rarely reversible impairment of liver function, allergic reactions (erythema, pruritus); rarely gynaecomastia and gingival hyperplasia after long-term treatment; after intravenous administration, hypotension, bradycardia, heart block, and asystole

Dose: by mouth, supraventricular arrhythmias (but see also Contra-indications), 40–120 mg 3 times daily

Angina, 80–120 mg 3 times daily

Hypertension, 240–480 mg daily in 2–3 divided doses

By slow intravenous injection over 2 minutes (3 minutes in elderly), 5–10 mg (preferably with ECG monitoring); in paroxysmal tachyarrhythmias a further 5 mg after 5–10 minutes if required

PoM **Verapamil** (Non-proprietary)

Tablets, coated, verapamil hydrochloride 40 mg, net price 20 = 19p; 80 mg, 20 = 38p; 120 mg, 20 = 59p; 160 mg, 20 = £1.07

Various strengths available from APS, Berk (Berkatens®), Cox, Hillcross, Lagap, Norton

Oral solution, sugar-free, verapamil hydrochloride 40 mg/5 mL available from Rosemont (special order)

PoM **Cordilox**® (Baker Norton)

Tablets, all yellow, f/c, verapamil hydrochloride 40 mg, net price 100-tab pack = £4.57; 80 mg, 100-tab pack = £9.15; 120 mg, 100-tab pack = £13.70; 160 mg, 56-tab pack = £12.77

Injection, verapamil hydrochloride 2.5 mg/mL, net price 2-mL amp = £1.11

PoM **Securon**® (Knoll)

Tablets, f/c, verapamil hydrochloride 40 mg, net price 100 = £4.57; 80 mg (scored), 100 = £9.14; 120 mg (scored), 60-tab pack = £7.67, 100 = £13.69

Injection, verapamil hydrochloride 2.5 mg/mL. Net price 2-mL amp = £1.08

Modified release

PoM **Half Securon SR**® (Knoll)

Tablets, m/r, f/c, verapamil hydrochloride 120 mg. Net price 28-tab pack = £6.82. Label: 25

Dose: hypertension, 1 tablet daily, increased if necessary to max. 4 tablets daily (doses above 2 tablets daily as 2 divided doses)

Angina, see Securon SR® (may be used for dose titration)

PoM **Securon SR**® (Knoll)

Tablets, m/r, pale green, f/c, verapamil hydrochloride 240 mg. Net price 28-tab pack = £10.64. Label: 25

Dose: hypertension, 1 tablet daily, increased to twice daily if necessary (new patients, initial dose ½ tablet); angina, 1 tablet twice daily (may sometimes be reduced to once daily)

PoM **Univer**® (Rhône-Poulenc Rorer)

Capsules, m/r, verapamil hydrochloride 120 mg (yellow/dark blue), net price 28-cap pack = £6.83; 180 mg (yellow), 56-cap pack = £16.50; 240 mg (yellow/dark blue), 28-cap pack = £11.13. Label: 25

Dose: hypertension, 240 mg daily, max. 480 mg daily (new patients, initial dose 120 mg); angina, 360 mg daily, max. 480 mg daily

2.6.3 Potassium-channel activators

Nicorandil is a member of a new class of drugs termed potassium-channel activators. It has both arterial and venous vasodilating properties and is indicated for the prevention and long-term treatment of angina pectoris. Its current place in therapy is uncertain.

NICORANDIL

Indications: prophylaxis and treatment of angina

Cautions: hypovolaemia; low systolic blood pressure; acute pulmonary oedema; acute myocardial infarction with acute left ventricular failure and low filling pressures; pregnancy and breast-feeding; **interactions:** Appendix 1 (nicorandil)

DRIVING. Patients should be warned not to drive or operate machinery until it is established that their performance is unimpaired

Contra-indications: cardiogenic shock; left ventricular failure with low filling pressures; hypotension

Side-effects: headache (especially on initiation, usually transitory); cutaneous vasodilatation with flushing; nausea, vomiting, dizziness, weakness also reported; at high dosage, reduction in blood pressure and/or increase in heart rate

Dose: initially 10 mg twice daily (if susceptible to headache 5 mg twice daily); usual dose 10–20 mg twice daily; up to 30 mg twice daily may be used

▼ PoM **Ikorel**® (Rhône-Poulenc Rorer)

Tablets, both scored, nicorandil 10 mg, net price 60-tab pack = £11.66; 20 mg, 60-tab pack = £19.88

2.6.4 Peripheral and cerebral vasodilators

2.6.4.1 Peripheral vasodilators and related drugs
2.6.4.2 Cerebral vasodilators

2.6.4.1 PERIPHERAL VASODILATORS AND RELATED DRUGS

Most serious peripheral disorders, such as *intermittent claudication,* are now known to be due to occlusion of vessels, either by spasm or sclerotic plaques; use of vasodilators may increase blood flow at rest, but the few controlled studies carried out have shown little improvement in walking distance. Rest pain is rarely affected.

Management of *Raynaud's syndrome* includes avoidance of exposure to cold and stopping smoking. More severe symptoms may require vasodilator treatment, which is most often successful in primary Raynaud's syndrome. Nifedipine (section 2.6.2), prazosin (section 2.5.4) and thymoxamine have all been shown to be beneficial; cinnarizine, naftidrofuryl, nicotinic acid derivatives, and oxpentifylline are not established as being effective.

Vasodilator therapy is not established as being effective for *chilblains* (see section 13.14).

CINNARIZINE

Indications: peripheral vascular disease, Raynaud's syndrome
Cautions; Side-effects: see section 4.6
Dose: initially, 75 mg 3 times daily; maintenance, 75 mg 2–3 times daily

Stugeron Forte® (Janssen)
Capsules, orange/ivory, cinnarizine 75 mg. Net price 100-cap pack = £7.85. Label: 2
Stugeron®: see section 4.6

NAFTIDROFURYL OXALATE

Indications: see under Dose
Side-effects: nausea, epigastric pain, rash, hepatitis, hepatic failure
Dose: peripheral vascular disease, 100–200 mg 3 times daily; cerebral vascular disease, 100 mg 3 times daily

PoM **Praxilene®** (Lipha)
Capsules, pink, naftidrofuryl oxalate 100 mg. Net price 84-cap pack = £8.60. Label: 25, 27

NICOTINIC ACID DERIVATIVES

Indications: peripheral vascular disease (for hyperlipidaemia, see section 2.12)
Side-effects: flushing, dizziness, nausea, vomiting, hypotension (more frequent with nicotinic acid than derivatives); occasional diabetogenic effect reported with nicotinic acid and nicotinyl alcohol; rarely associated with nodular changes to liver (monitor on prolonged high dosage)

Hexopal® (Sanofi Winthrop)
Tablets, scored, inositol nicotinate 500 mg. Net price 20 = £4.07
　Dose: 1 g 3 times daily, increased to 4 g daily if required
Tablets forte, scored, inositol nicotinate 750 mg. Net price 112-tab pack = £34.02
　Dose: 1.5 g twice daily
Suspension, sugar-free, inositol nicotinate 1 g/5 mL. Net price 300 mL = £20.85
　Dose: as for tablets (above)
Ronicol® (Tillomed)
Tablets, scored, nicotinyl alcohol 25 mg (as tartrate). Net price 100-tab pack = £5.55
　Dose: 25–50 mg 4 times daily
Timespan® (= tablets m/r), red, s/c, nicotinyl alcohol 150 mg (as tartrate). Net price 100-tab pack = £23.70. Label: 25
　Dose: 150–300 mg twice daily

OXPENTIFYLLINE

(Pentoxifylline)
Indications: peripheral vascular disease
Cautions: hypotension, coronary artery disease; avoid in porphyria (see section 9.8.2); **interactions:** Appendix 1 (oxpentifylline)

Contra-indications: cerebral haemorrhage, extensive retinal haemorrhage, acute myocardial infarction
Side-effects: gastro-intestinal disturbances, dizziness, headache; rarely flushing, tachycardia
Dose: 400 mg 2–3 times daily

PoM **Trental®** (Hoechst)
Tablets, m/r, pink, s/c, oxpentifylline 400 mg. Net price 90-tab pack = £15.11; also 250-tab pack (hosp. only). Label: 21, 25

THYMOXAMINE

(Moxisylyte)
Indications: primary Raynaud's syndrome (short-term treatment)
Cautions: diabetes mellitus
Contra-indications: active liver disease
Side-effects: nausea, diarrhoea, flushing, headache, dizziness; hepatic reactions including cholestatic jaundice and hepatitis reported to CSM
Dose: initially 40 mg 4 times daily, increased to 80 mg 4 times daily if poor initial response; discontinue after 2 weeks if no response

PoM **Opilon®** (P-D)
Tablets, yellow, f/c, thymoxamine 40 mg (as hydrochloride). Net price 120-tab pack = £28.00. Label: 21

OTHER PREPARATION USED IN PERIPHERAL VASCULAR DISEASE

Rutosides (oxerutins, Paroven®) are not vasodilators and are not generally regarded as effective preparations as capillary sealants or for the treatment of cramps; side-effects include headache, flushing, rashes, mild gastro-intestinal disturbances.

Paroven® (Zyma)
Capsules, yellow, oxerutins 250 mg. Net price 120-cap pack = £13.67
Dose: For relief of symptoms of oedema associated with chronic venous insufficiency, 500 mg twice daily

2.6.4.2 CEREBRAL VASODILATORS

These drugs are claimed to improve mental function. Some improvements in performance of psychological tests have been reported but the drugs have not been shown clinically to be of much benefit in dementia.

CO-DERGOCRINE MESYLATE

A mixture in equal proportions of dihydroergocornine mesylate, dihydroergocristine mesylate, and (in the ratio 2 : 1) α- and β-dihydroergocryptine mesylates
Indications: adjunct in elderly patients with mild to moderate dementia
Cautions: severe bradycardia
Side-effects: gastro-intestinal disturbances, flushing, headache, rash, nasal congestion; dizziness and postural hypotension in hypertensive patients
Dose: 1.5 mg 3 times daily before meals *or* 4.5 mg once daily before a meal

PoM **Hydergine®** (Sandoz)
Tablets, co-dergocrine mesylate 1.5 mg (scored), net price 100-tab pack = £10.78; 4.5 mg, 28-tab pack = £10.78. Label: 22

2.6.5 Flosequinan

Flosequinan is a direct-acting vasodilator, producing both arterial and venous vasodilatation. Its use was restricted to patients with *congestive heart failure* who were not responsive to, or were intolerant of, diuretics, ACE inhibitors, and digoxin (where appropriate). It has now been withdrawn.

2.7 Sympathomimetics

2.7.1	Inotropic sympathomimetics
2.7.2	Vasoconstrictor sympathomimetics
2.7.3	Cardiopulmonary resuscitation

The properties of sympathomimetics vary according to whether they act on alpha or on beta adrenergic receptors. Adrenaline (section 2.7.3) acts on both alpha and beta receptors and increases both heart rate and contractility ($beta_1$ effects); it can cause peripheral vasodilation (a $beta_2$ effect) or vasoconstriction (an alpha effect).

2.7.1 Inotropic sympathomimetics

The cardiac stimulants **dobutamine** and **dopamine** act on $beta_1$ receptors in cardiac muscle, and increase contractility with little effect on rate; they are used in cardiogenic shock. Dosage of dopamine is critical since although low doses induce vasodilatation and increase renal perfusion, higher doses (more than 5 micrograms per kg per minute) lead to vasoconstriction and may exacerbate heart failure.

Xamoterol also acts on $beta_1$ receptors but being a partial agonist it provokes only a modest stimulatory response at rest. **Important:** restricted to **mild heart failure only**, owing to deterioration in patients with moderate to severe heart failure, see p. 102.

Dopexamine acts on $beta_2$ receptors in cardiac muscle to produce its positive inotropic effect; and on peripheral dopamine receptors to increase renal perfusion; it is reported not to induce vasoconstriction.

Isoprenaline is less selective and increases both heart rate and contractility; it may prevent Stokes-Adams attacks, but insertion of a pacemaker is preferable. It is now only used as a short-term emergency treatment of heart block or severe bradycardia.

Arbutamine is used in the Genesa® system for pharmacological stress testing, which simulates the effects of physical exercise on the heart, and thus provides an alternative in patients unable to perform exercise tests adequately.

DOBUTAMINE

Indications: inotropic support in infarction, cardiac surgery, cardiomyopathies, septic shock, and cardiogenic shock

Cautions: severe hypotension complicating cardiogenic shock; **interactions:** Appendix 1 (sympathomimetics)

Side-effects: tachycardia and marked increase in systolic blood pressure indicate overdosage

Dose: by intravenous infusion, 2.5–10 micrograms/kg/minute, adjusted according to response

PoM Dobutrex® (Lilly)

Strong sterile solution, dobutamine (as hydrochloride) 12.5 mg/mL. For dilution and use as an intravenous infusion. Net price 20-mL vial = £8.35

Note. Strong sterile solution containing dobutamine (as hydrochloride) 12.5 mg/mL also available in 20-mL amps from David Bull, Phoenix

PoM Posiject® (Boehringer Ingelheim)

Strong sterile solution, dobutamine (as hydrochloride) 50 mg/mL. For dilution and use as an intravenous infusion. Net price 5-mL amp = £5.50

DOPAMINE HYDROCHLORIDE

Indications: cardiogenic shock in infarction or cardiac surgery

Cautions: correct hypovolaemia; low dose in shock due to acute myocardial infarction—see notes above; **interactions:** Appendix 1 (sympathomimetics)

Contra-indications: tachyarrhythmia, phaeochromocytoma

Side-effects: nausea and vomiting, peripheral vasoconstriction, hypotension, hypertension, tachycardia

Dose: by intravenous infusion, 2–5 micrograms/kg/minute initially (see notes above)

PoM Dopamine Hydrochloride (Non-proprietary)

Strong sterile solution, dopamine hydrochloride 40 mg/mL; 160 mg/mL, 5-mL amps. For dilution and use as an intravenous infusion

Available from Antigen, David Bull

PoM Dopamine Hydrochloride in Dextrose (Glucose) Injection (Abbott)

Intravenous infusion, dopamine hydrochloride 1.6 mg/mL in glucose 5% intravenous infusion, net price 250-mL container (400 mg) = £11.69; 3.2 mg/mL, 250-mL container (800 mg) = £22.93 (both hosp. only)

PoM Intropin® (Du Pont)

Strong sterile solution, dopamine hydrochloride 40 mg/mL, net price 5-mL amp or syringe = £4.68. For dilution and use as an intravenous infusion

PoM Select-A-Jet® Dopamine (IMS)

Strong sterile solution, dopamine hydrochloride 40 mg/mL. Net price 5-mL vial = £4.14; 10-mL vial = £6.65; 20-mL vial = £11.86. For dilution and use as an intravenous infusion

DOPEXAMINE HYDROCHLORIDE

Indications: inotropic support and vasodilator in heart failure associated with cardiac surgery

Cautions: myocardial infarction, recent angina, hypokalaemia, hyperglycaemia; correct hypovolaemia before starting, monitor blood pressure, pulse, plasma potassium, blood glucose; avoid abrupt withdrawal; **interactions:** Appendix 1 (sympathomimetics)

Contra-indications: left ventricular outlet obstruction such as hypertrophic cardiomyopathy or aortic stenosis; phaeochromocytoma, thrombocytopenia

Side-effects: increased heart rate (occasionally excessive tachycardia, particularly in atrial fibrillation), ventricular ectopic beats; also reported: nausea, vomiting, anginal pain, tremor

Dose: by intravenous infusion via caval catheter, 500 nanograms/kg/minute, may be increased to 1 microgram/kg/minute and further increased up to 6 micrograms/kg/minute in increments of 1 microgram/kg/minute at intervals of 10–15 minutes

PoM Dopacard® (Speywood)
Strong sterile solution, dopexamine hydrochloride 10 mg/mL (1%). For dilution and use as an intravenous infusion. Net price 5-mL amp = £21.00
Note. Contact with metal in infusion apparatus should be minimised

---

ISOPRENALINE HYDROCHLORIDE

Indications: heart block, severe bradycardia
Cautions: ischaemic heart disease, diabetes mellitus, hyperthyroidism; **interactions:** Appendix 1 (sympathomimetics)
Side-effects: tachycardia, arrhythmias, hypotension, sweating, tremor, headache
Dose: by mouth, initially 30 mg every 6 hours, range 90–840 mg daily (but oral route rarely used)
By intravenous infusion, 0.5–10 micrograms/ minute

PoM Min-I-Jet® Isoprenaline (IMS)
Injection, isoprenaline hydrochloride 20 micrograms/mL. Net price 10-mL disposable syringe = £4.05
PoM Saventrine® (Pharmax)
Tablets, isoprenaline hydrochloride 30 mg. Net price 20 = £1.67
PoM Saventrine IV® (Pharmax)
Strong sterile solution, isoprenaline hydrochloride 1 mg/mL. For dilution and use as an intravenous infusion. Net price 2-mL amp = 44p

---

XAMOTEROL

Indications: chronic mild heart failure (in patients not breathless at rest but limited by symptoms on exertion)
Cautions: withdraw if heart failure deteriorates; cardiac outflow obstruction, arrhythmias (maintain concurrent digoxin in atrial fibrillation), obstructive airways disease (withdraw if worsening, and reverse bronchospasm with inhaled bronchodilator such as salbutamol), reduce dose in renal impairment; pregnancy (toxicity in *animal* studies); **interactions:** Appendix 1 (xamoterol)

Contra-indications: moderate to severe heart failure; breast-feeding
HEART FAILURE. Patients in whom xamoterol is contra-indicated are those:
who are short of breath or fatigued at rest or limited on minimal exercise;
with resting tachycardia (>90 beats per minute) or hypotension (systolic BP <100 mmHg);
with peripheral oedema, raised jugular venous pressure, enlarged liver, or third heart sound;
with (or with history of) acute pulmonary oedema;
who require treatment with frusemide in dose in excess of 40 mg daily (or equivalent);
who require ACE inhibitor treatment
Side-effects: gastro-intestinal disturbances, headache, dizziness, bronchospasm, hypotension; also reported: chest pain, palpitations, muscle cramp, rashes
Dose: 200 mg daily for 1 week, then 200 mg twice daily
IMPORTANT. Treatment should be started in hospital after full assessment of severity of heart failure by exercise test

PoM Corwin® (Stuart)
Tablets, yellow, f/c, xamoterol (as fumarate) 200 mg. Net price 56-tab pack = £25.94

2.7.2 Vasoconstrictor sympathomimetics

Vasoconstrictor sympathomimetics raise blood pressure transiently by acting on alpha-adrenergic receptors to constrict peripheral vessels. They are sometimes used as an emergency method of elevating blood pressure, notably in spinal anaesthesia.

The danger of vasoconstrictors is that although they raise blood pressure they do so at the expense of perfusion of vital organs such as the kidney. Further, in many patients with shock the peripheral resistance is already high, and to raise it further is unhelpful. Thus the use of vasoconstrictors in the treatment of shock is to be generally **deprecated**. The use of plasma substitutes, or of inotropic agents such as dopamine or dobutamine (section 2.7.1) is more appropriate. Treatment of the underlying condition is obviously important.

Spinal and epidural anaesthesia may result in sympathetic block with resultant hypotension. Management may include intravenous fluids (which are usually given prophylactically), oxygen, elevation of the legs, and injection of a pressor drug such as ephedrine or methoxamine. As well as constricting peripheral vessels **ephedrine** also accelerates the heart rate (by acting on beta receptors). Use is made of this dual action of ephedrine to manage associated bradycardia (although intravenous injection of atropine sulphate 400 to 600 micrograms may also be required if bradycardia persists). When the hypotension occurs in association with tachycardia the pure alpha-adrenergic stimulant action of **methoxamine** is more appropriate.

EPHEDRINE HYDROCHLORIDE

Indications: see under Dose

Cautions: hyperthyroidism, diabetes mellitus, ischaemic heart disease, hypertension, elderly; may cause acute retention in prostatic hypertrophy; **interactions:** Appendix 1 (sympathomimetics)

Side-effects: tachycardia, anxiety, restlessness, insomnia; also tremor, arrhythmias, dry mouth, cold extremities; acute retention in prostatic hypertrophy

Dose: reversal of hypotension from spinal or epidural anaesthesia, *by slow intravenous injection* of a solution containing ephedrine hydrochloride 3 mg/mL, 3–6 mg (max. 9 mg) repeated every 3–4 minutes to max. 30 mg

PoM **Ephedrine Hydrochloride** (Non-proprietary)

Injection, ephedrine hydrochloride 30 mg/mL. For dilution before intravenous administration. 1-mL amp [unlicensed]

METARAMINOL

Indications: acute hypotension (see notes above)

Cautions; Contra-indications; Side-effects: see under Noradrenaline Acid Tartrate; metaraminol has a longer duration of action than noradrenaline, see also warning below; also tachycardia; fatal ventricular arrhythmia reported in Laennec's cirrhosis

HYPERTENSIVE RESPONSE. Since metaraminol has a longer duration of action than noradrenaline, an excessive vasopressor response may cause a prolonged rise in blood pressure

Dose: by intravenous infusion, 15–100 mg in 500 mL, adjusted according to response

PoM **Aramine®** (MSD)

Injection, metaraminol 10 mg (as tartrate)/mL. Net price 1-mL amp = 57p

METHOXAMINE HYDROCHLORIDE

Indications: acute hypotension (see notes above)

Cautions; Contra-indications; Side-effects: see under Noradrenaline Acid Tartrate; methoxamine has a longer duration of action than noradrenaline, see also warning below

HYPERTENSIVE RESPONSE. Since methoxamine has a longer duration of action than noradrenaline, an excessive vasopressor response may cause a prolonged rise in blood pressure

Dose: by intramuscular injection, 5–20 mg

By slow intravenous injection, 5–10 mg (rate 1 mg/minute)

PoM **Vasoxine®** (Wellcome)

Injection, methoxamine hydrochloride 20 mg/mL. Net price 1-mL amp = 52p

NORADRENALINE ACID TARTRATE

(Norepinephrine Bitartrate)

Indications: see under preparations

Cautions: coronary, mesenteric, or peripheral vascular thrombosis; following myocardial infarction, Prinzmetal's variant angina, thyroid disease, diabetes mellitus; hypoxia or hypercapnia; appropriate blood volume replacement required; elderly; extravasation at injection site may cause necrosis; **interactions:** Appendix 1 (sympathomimetics)

Contra-indications: hypertension (monitor blood pressure and rate of flow frequently), pregnancy

Side-effects: hypertension, headache, bradycardia, arrhythmias, peripheral ischaemia

Dose: see under preparations

PoM **Levophed®** (Sanofi Winthrop)

Strong sterile solution, noradrenaline acid tartrate 2 mg/mL (equivalent to noradrenaline base 1 mg/mL). For dilution and use as an intravenous infusion. Net price 2-mL amp = £1.01; 4-mL amp = £1.50; 20-mL amp = £6.35

Dose: acute hypotension, *by intravenous infusion,* via central venous catheter, of a solution containing noradrenaline acid tartrate 80 micrograms/mL (equivalent to noradrenaline base 40 micrograms/mL) at an initial rate of 0.16–0.33 mL/minute, adjusted according to response

PoM **Levophed Special®** (Sanofi Winthrop)

Injection, noradrenaline acid tartrate 200 micrograms/mL (equivalent to noradrenaline base 100 micrograms/mL). Net price 2-mL amp = 98p

Dose: cardiac arrest, *by rapid intravenous or intracardiac injection,* 0.5 to 0.75 mL of a solution containing noradrenaline acid tartrate 200 micrograms/mL (equivalent to noradrenaline base 100 micrograms/mL)

PHENYLEPHRINE HYDROCHLORIDE

Indications: acute hypotension (see notes above)

Cautions; Contra-indications; Side-effects: see under Noradrenaline Acid Tartrate; phenylephrine has a longer duration of action than noradrenaline, see also warning below; since phenylephrine induces tachycardia or reflex bradycardia it should also be avoided in severe coronary disease, bradycardia, and hyperthyroidism

HYPERTENSIVE RESPONSE. Since phenylephrine has a longer duration of action than noradrenaline, an excessive vasopressor response may cause a prolonged rise in blood pressure

Dose: by subcutaneous or intramuscular injection, 5 mg

By slow intravenous injection, 100–500 micrograms

By intravenous infusion, 10 mg in 500 mL, adjusted according to response

PoM **Phenylephrine Injection 1%** (Knoll)

Injection, phenylephrine hydrochloride 10 mg/mL. For dilution before intravenous injection or infusion. Net price 1-mL amp = £2.40

ADVANCED CARDIAC LIFE SUPPORT

Responsive? No **Breathing?** No **Pulse?** No **Start CPR** 2:15

Call for help

Including
- defibrillator
- airway adjuncts
- oxygen
- emergency kit

Consider 2 rescuer CPR
1:5

and **mouth-to-mask** ventilation

Precordial thump

Place paddles correctly

If flat trace, check switches, connections and gain.

Give oxygen

Intubate

Cannulate large vein

Continue CPR

EMD
QRS without palpable pulse

VF

PULSELESS VT

ASYSTOLE

Think of, and if indicated, give specific treatment for:

hypovolaemia
tension pneumothorax
cardiac tamponade
pulmonary embolism
drug overdose/intoxication
hypothermia
electrolyte imbalance

Precordial thump

DC shock 200 J ①

DC shock 200 J ②

DC shock 360 J ③

If not already
- intubate
- iv access

Adrenaline 1mg iv

10 CPR sequences of 1:5 ventilation/compression

DC shock 360 J ④

DC shock 360 J ⑤

DC shock 360 J ⑥

Precordial thump

VF excluded? → yes

no

DC shock 200 J

DC shock 200 J

DC shock 360 J

If not already:
- intubate
- iv access

Adrenaline 1mg iv

10 CPR sequences of 1:5 ventilation/compression

(Atropine 3 mg iv *once only*)

no → Electrical activity evident?

yes

Pace

If not already
- intubate
- iv access

Adrenaline 1mg iv

10 CPR sequences of 1:5 ventilation/compression

Consider
- pressor agents
- calcium
- alkalising agents
- adrenaline 5 mg iv

Notes:
I. The interval between shocks 3 and 4 should not be > 2 mins.
II. Adrenaline given during loop approx. every 2-3 mins.
III. Continue loops for as long as defibrillation is indicated.
IV. After 3 loops consider • alkalising agents • antiarrhythmic agents

Note:
If no response after 3 cycles, consider high dose adrenaline 5 mg iv.

If an IV line cannot be established, consider giving double or triple doses of adrenaline or atropine via an endotracheal tube.

PROLONGED RESUSCITATION:

Consider alkalising agents, e.g. 50 mmol sodium bicarbonate (50ml of 8.4%) or according to blood gas results.

POST RESUSCITATION CARE

Check
- arterial blood gases
- electrolytes
- chest x-ray
Observe monitor and treat patient in an intensive care area.

European Resuscitation Council
in co-operation with
Resuscitation Council (UK)

© Copyright ERC 1992

Available from

LAERDAL MEDICAL LTD.
Laerdal House, Orpington, Kent BR6 OHX.
Tel. 0689 876634, Fax 0689 873800

6314-P

2.7.3   Cardiopulmonary resuscitation

In *cardiac arrest* adrenaline 1 in 10 000 (1 mg per 10 mL) is recommended in a dose of 10 mL by central intravenous injection. The procedure for cardiopulmonary resuscitation is given in the algorithm (see next page) which reflects the recommendations of the European Resuscitation Council and the Resuscitation Council (UK).

For *acute anaphylaxis* see p. 143.

ADRENALINE
(Epinephrine)

Indications; Dose: see notes above
Cautions: ischaemic heart disease, diabetes mellitus, hyperthyroidism, hypertension; **interactions:** Appendix 1 (sympathomimetics)
Side-effects: anxiety, tremor, tachycardia, headache, cold extremities; in overdosage arrhythmias, cerebral haemorrhage, pulmonary oedema

PoM **Adrenaline Injection,** adrenaline   1   in 10 000 (adrenaline 100 micrograms/mL as acid tartrate). 10-mL amp.

Available from Martindale (special order); also from IMS (Min-I-Jet® Adrenaline 3- and 10-mL disposable syringes)
Note. Adrenaline Injection BP is 1 in 1000 (adrenaline 1 mg/mL, as acid tartrate), see p. 143

ATROPINE SULPHATE
See section 15.1.3

CALCIUM SALTS
See section 9.5.1.1

2.8   Anticoagulants and protamine

2.8.1   Parenteral anticoagulants
2.8.2   Oral anticoagulants
2.8.3   Protamine sulphate

The main use of anticoagulants is to prevent thrombus formation or extension of an existing thrombus in the slower-moving venous side of the circulation, where the thrombus consists of a fibrin web enmeshed with platelets and red cells. They are therefore widely used in the prevention and treatment of *deep-vein thrombosis in the legs.*

Anticoagulants are of less use in preventing thrombus formation in arteries, for in faster-flowing vessels thrombi are composed mainly of platelets with little fibrin. They are used to prevent thrombi forming on *prosthetic heart valves.*

2.8.1   Parenteral anticoagulants

HEPARIN

Heparin initiates anticoagulation rapidly but has a short duration of action. It is now often referred to as being **standard** or **unfractionated heparin** to distinguish it from the **low molecular weight heparins** (see next page), which have a longer duration of action.

TREATMENT. For the initial treatment of *deep-vein thrombosis and pulmonary embolism* heparin is given as an *intravenous loading dose,* followed by *continuous intravenous infusion* (using an infusion pump) or by *intermittent subcutaneous injection;* the use of *intermittent intravenous injection* is no longer recommended. An oral anticoagulant (usually warfarin, see section 2.8.2) is started at the same time as the heparin (which needs to be continued for at least 3 days, until the oral anticoagulant has taken effect). Laboratory monitoring is essential—preferably on a daily basis, determination of the APTT (activated partial thromboplastin time) being the most widely used technique. Heparin is also used in regimens for the management of *myocardial infarction* (see also section 2.10), the management of *unstable angina pectoris,* and the management of *acute peripheral arterial occlusion.*

PROPHYLAXIS. In patients undergoing *general surgery,* low-dose heparin by subcutaneous injection is widely advocated to *prevent postoperative deep-vein thrombosis and pulmonary embolism* in 'high risk' patients (i.e. those with obesity, malignant disease, history of deep-vein thrombosis or pulmonary embolism, patients over 40, or those with an established thrombophilic disorder or who are undergoing large or complicated surgical procedures); laboratory monitoring is not required with this *standard prophylactic regimen.*

To combat the increased risk in *major orthopaedic surgery* an *adjusted dose regimen* may be used (with monitoring) or *low molecular weight heparin* (see next page) may be selected.

EXTRACORPOREAL CIRCUITS. Heparin is also used in the maintenance of extracorporeal circuits in *cardiopulmonary bypass* and *haemodialysis.*

HAEMORRHAGE. If haemorrhage occurs it is usually sufficient to withdraw heparin, but if rapid reversal of the effects of heparin is required, protamine sulphate (section 2.8.3) is a specific antidote (but only partially reverses the effects of low molecular weight heparins).

HEPARIN

Indications: see under Dose
Cautions: hepatic and renal impairment (avoid if severe); pregnancy; **interactions:** Appendix 1 (heparin)
THROMBOCYTOPENIA. Clinically important thrombocytopenia is immune-mediated, and does not usually develop until after 6 to 10 days; it may be complicated by thrombosis. The CSM has recommended platelet counts for patients receiving heparin for longer than 5 days (and that heparin should be stopped immediately in those who develop thrombocytopenia). Alternatives for patients requiring continued anticoagulation are low molecular weight heparins (but cross reactivity may occur), a heparinoid (such as danaparoid), warfarin, or epoprostenol

Contra-indications: haemophilia and other haemorrhagic disorders, thrombocytopenia, peptic ulcer, recent cerebral haemorrhage, severe hypertension, severe liver disease (including oesophageal varices), renal failure, after major trauma or recent surgery (especially to eye or nervous system), hypersensitivity to heparin

Side-effects: haemorrhage (see notes above), skin necrosis, thrombocytopenia (see Cautions), hypersensitivity reactions (including urticaria, angioedema, and anaphylaxis); osteoporosis after prolonged use (and rarely alopecia)

Dose:

Treatment of deep-vein thrombosis and pulmonary embolism, *by intravenous injection,* loading dose of 5000 units (10 000 units in severe pulmonary embolism) followed by continuous *infusion* of 1000–2000 units/hour *or by subcutaneous injection* of 15 000 units every 12 hours (laboratory monitoring essential—preferably on a daily basis)

SMALL ADULT OR CHILD, lower loading dose *then,* 15–25 units/kg/hour *by intravenous infusion, or* 250 units/kg every 12 hours by *subcutaneous injection*

Unstable angina, acute peripheral arterial occlusion, as intravenous regimen for deep-vein thrombosis and pulmonary embolism, above

Prophylaxis in orthopaedic surgery, see notes above

Prophylaxis in general surgery (see notes above), *by subcutaneous injection,* 5000 units 2 hours before surgery, then every 8–12 hours for 7 days or until patient is ambulant (monitoring not needed); during pregnancy (with monitoring), 5000–10 000 units every 12 hours (**important:** not intended to cover prevention of prosthetic heart valve thrombosis in pregnancy which calls for separate specialist management)

MYOCARDIAL INFARCTION. For the prevention of *coronary re-occlusion after thrombolysis* heparin is used in a variety of regimens according to locally agreed protocols

For the prevention of *mural thrombosis* heparin is considered effective when given by *subcutaneous injection* of 12 500 units every 12 hours for at least 10 days

Note. Doses above reflect the guidelines of the British Society for Haematology; for doses of the low molecular weight heparins, see pp. 106–7

PoM Heparin Injection (heparin sodium)
1000 units/mL, net price 1-mL amp = 18p; 5-mL amp = 54p; 5-mL vial = 46p

5000 units/mL, net price 1-mL amp = 36p; 5-mL amp = 95p; 5-mL vial = 92p

25 000 units/mL, net price 1-mL amp = 97p; 5-mL vial = £3.44

PoM Calciparine® (Sanofi Winthrop)
Injection (subcutaneous only), heparin calcium 25 000 units/mL. Net price 0.2-mL syringe = 68p; 0.5-mL syringe = £1.46; 0.8-mL syringe = £1.76

PoM Minihep® (Leo)
Injection (subcutaneous only), heparin sodium 25 000 units/mL. Net price 0.2-mL amp = 67p

PoM Minihep Calcium® (Leo)
Injection (subcutaneous only), heparin calcium 25 000 units/mL. Net price 0.2-mL amp = 67p

PoM Monoparin® (CP)
Injection, heparin sodium (mucous) 1000 units/mL, net price 1-mL amp = 18p; 5-mL amp = 54p; 10-mL amp = 72p; 20-mL = £1.38; 5000 units/mL, 1-mL amp = 36p; 5-mL amp = 95p; 25 000 units/mL, 0.2-mL amp = 44p, 1-mL amp = 97p

PoM Monoparin Calcium® (CP)
Injection, heparin calcium 25 000 units/mL. Net price 0.2-mL amp = 47p

PoM Multiparin® (CP)
Injection, heparin sodium (mucous) 1000 units/mL, net price 5-mL vial = 46p; 5000 units/mL, 5-mL vial = 92p; 25 000 units/mL, 5-mL vial = £3.44

PoM Pump-Hep® (Leo)
Injection, heparin sodium (mucous) 1000 units/mL. Net price 5-mL amp = 39p; 10-mL amp = 64p; 20-mL amp = 95p

PoM Unihep® (Leo)
Injection, heparin sodium (mucous) 1000 units/mL, net price 1-mL amp = 13p; 5000 units/mL, 1-mL amp = 27p; 10 000 units/mL, 1-mL amp = 44p; 25 000 units/mL, 1-mL amp = £1.04

PoM Uniparin Calcium® (CP)
Injection (subcutaneous only), heparin calcium 25 000 units/mL. Net price 0.5-mL syringe = £1.50

PoM Uniparin Forte® (CP)
Injection (subcutaneous only), heparin sodium 25 000 units/mL. Net price 0.4-mL syringe = £1.53

LOW MOLECULAR WEIGHT HEPARINS

There is evidence that the low molecular weight heparins, **certoparin**, **dalteparin**, **enoxaparin**, and **tinzaparin**, are as effective and as safe as unfractionated heparin in the prevention of venous thrombo-embolism; in orthopaedic practice they are probably more effective. They have a longer duration of action than unfractionated heparin; *once-daily subcutaneous* dosage means that they are convenient to use. The standard prophylactic regimen does not require monitoring.

Some low molecular weight heparins are also used in the treatment of deep-vein thrombosis and for the prevention of clotting in extracorporeal circuits.

HAEMORRHAGE. See under Heparin.

CERTOPARIN

Indications: see notes above and under preparations

Cautions; Contra-indications; Side-effects: see under Heparin

▼ **PoM Alphaparin®** (Alpha)
Injection, certoparin sodium 3000 units/0.3-mL syringe, net price 1 syringe = £3.00; 3000 units/0.5-mL amp = £2.75
Dose: prophylaxis of deep-vein thrombosis, *by subcutaneous injection,* 3000 units 1–2 hours before surgery, then 3000 units every 24 hours for 7–10 days (or until the patient is mobile)

DALTEPARIN

Indications: see notes above and under preparations

Cautions; Contra-indications; Side-effects: see under Heparin

PoM Fragmin® (Pharmacia)

Injection (syringe), dalteparin sodium 12 500 units/mL, 0.2-mL syringe (2500 units) = £1.95; 25 000 units/mL, 0.2-mL syringe (5000 units) = £2.96

Dose: prophylaxis of deep-vein thrombosis, *by subcutaneous injection*, moderate risk, 2500 units 1-2 hours before surgery then 2500 units every 24 hours for 5 days; high risk, 2500 units 1-2 hours before surgery, then 2500 units 12 hours later, then 5000 units every 24 hours for 5 days

Injection (ampoule), 2500 units/mL, net price 4-mL amp (10 000 units) = £5.36; 10 000 units/mL, 1-mL amp (10 000 units) = £5.36; 12 500 units/mL, 0.2-mL syringe (2500 units) = £1.95; 25 000 units/mL, 0.2-mL syringe (5000 units) = £2.96

Dose: treatment of deep-vein thrombosis, *by subcutaneous injection*, 200 units/kg as a single daily dose (max. 18 000 units daily); patients with increased risk of haemorrhage, 100 units/kg twice daily

Note. Monitoring not required with once daily treatment regimen, and not generally necessary with twice daily regimen; if monitoring required, blood should be taken 3–4 hours after a dose (recommended plasma concentration 0.5–1 unit/mL)

Prevention of clotting in extracorporeal circuits, consult manufacturer's literature

ENOXAPARIN

Indications: see notes above and under preparations

Cautions; Contra-indications; Side-effects: see under Heparin

PoM Clexane® (Rhône-Poulenc Rorer)

Injection, enoxaparin 100 mg/mL. Net price 0.2-mL syringe (20 mg, 2000 units) = £3.55; 0.4-mL syringe (40 mg, 4000 units) = £4.73

Dose: prophylaxis of deep-vein thrombosis, *by subcutaneous injection*, moderate risk, 20 mg (2000 units) 1-2 hours before surgery then 20 mg (2000 units) every 24 hours for 7–10 days; high risk, 40 mg (4000 units) 12 hours before surgery then 40 mg (4000 units) every 24 hours for 7–10 days

Prevention of clotting in extracorporeal circuits, consult manufacturer's literature

TINZAPARIN

Indications: see notes above and under preparations

Cautions; Contra-indications; Side-effects: see under Heparin

ASTHMA. Presence of sulphites in ampoules may (especially in patients with asthma) lead to hypersensitivity (with bronchospasm and shock)

PoM Innohep® (Leo)

Injection, tinzaparin 3500 units/0.3-mL syringe, net price 1 syringe = £3.12; 5000 units/0.5-mL ampoule, 1 amp = £2.97

Dose: prophylaxis of deep-vein thrombosis, *by subcutaneous injection*, general surgery, 3500 units 2 hours before surgery, then 3500 units every 24 hours for 7–10 days; orthopaedic surgery (high risk), 50 units/kg 2 hours before surgery, then 50 units/kg every 24 hours for 7–10 days

▼*Injection,* tinzaparin sodium 20 000 units/mL, 2-mL vial = £38.50

Dose: treatment of deep-vein thrombosis, *by subcutaneous injection*, 175 units/kg once daily for at least 6 days (and until adequate oral anticoagulation established)

Note. This treatment regimen does not require monitoring

▼*Injection,* tinzaparin sodium 1000 units/mL, net price 5-mL amp = £4.20

Dose: for prevention of clotting in extracorporeal circuits, consult manufacturer's literature

HEPARINOIDS

Danaparoid is a heparinoid used for prophylaxis of deep-vein thrombosis in patients undergoing general or orthopaedic surgery. Providing there is no evidence of cross-sensitivity, it may also have a role in patients who develop thrombocytopenia in association with heparin.

DANAPAROID SODIUM

Indications: prophylaxis of deep vein thrombosis in general and orthopaedic surgery

Cautions: hepatic and renal impairment (avoid if severe); pregnancy and breast-feeding

ASTHMA. Presence of sulphite in ampoules may (especially in patients with asthma) lead to hypersensitivity (with bronchospasm and shock)

Contra-indications: see under Heparin; cross-reactivity to heparin-induced thrombocytopenia

Side-effects: haemorrhage (see notes above); thrombocytopenia (may be cross-reactivity with heparin); hypersensitivity reactions (including rash); liver enzyme changes; osteoporosis with excessive dosage; bruising or pain at injection site

Dose: *by subcutaneous injection,* 750 units 1–4 hours before surgery, then twice daily for 7–10 days

Note. If patient cannot be operated on immediately (e.g. after hip fracture), twice daily administration may be initiated, providing the last pre-operative dose is given not later than 1 hour before surgery

▼ **PoM Orgaran®** (Durbin)

Injection, danaparoid sodium 1250 units/mL, net price 0.6-mL amp (750 units) = £12.50

HEPARIN FLUSHES

For maintaining catheter patency sodium chloride injection 0.9% is as effective as heparin flushes for up to 48 hours, and is therefore recommended for cannulas intended to be in place for 48 hours or less. Heparin flushes are recommended for cannulas intended to be in place for longer than 48 hours.

PoM **Canusal**® (CP)
Solution, heparin sodium 100 units/mL. Net price 2-mL amp = 29p. To maintain patency of catheters, cannulas, etc., 200 units flushed through every 4 hours or as required. Not for therapeutic use

PoM **Hep-Flush**® (Leo)
Solution, heparin sodium 100 units/mL. Net price 2-mL amp = 25p; 10-mL vial = £1.27. To maintain patency of catheters, cannulas, etc., 200 units flushed through every 4–8 hours. Not for therapeutic use .

PoM **Heplok**® (Leo)
Solution, heparin sodium 10 units/mL. Net price 5-mL amp = 29p. To maintain patency of catheters, cannulas, etc., 10–50 units flushed through every 4 hours. Not for therapeutic use

PoM **Hepsal**® (CP)
Solution, heparin sodium 10 units/mL. Net price 5-mL amp = 25p (glass), 30p (polypropylene). To maintain patency of catheters, cannulas, etc., 50 units flushed through every 4 hours or as required. Not for therapeutic use

---

EPOPROSTENOL

Epoprostenol (prostacyclin) can be given to inhibit platelet aggregation during renal dialysis either alone or with heparin. Since its half-life is only about 3 minutes it must be given by continuous intravenous infusion. It is a potent vasodilator and therefore its side-effects include flushing, headache, and hypotension.

EPOPROSTENOL

Indications: see notes above
Cautions: anticoagulant monitoring required when given with heparin
Side-effects: see notes above; also bradycardia, pallor, sweating with higher doses
Dose: see manufacturer's literature

PoM **Flolan**® (Wellcome)
Infusion, powder for reconstitution, epoprostenol (as sodium salt). Net price 500-microgram vial (with diluent) = £103.86

2.8.2   Oral anticoagulants

Oral anticoagulants antagonise the effects of vitamin K, and take at least 48 to 72 hours for the anticoagulant effect to develop fully; if an immediate effect is required, heparin must be given concomitantly.

USES. The main indication for oral anticoagulant therapy is *deep-vein thrombosis*. Patients with *pulmonary embolism* should also be treated, as should those with *atrial fibrillation who are at risk of embolisation*, and those with *prosthetic heart valves* (to prevent emboli developing on the valves); antiplatelet drugs may also be useful in these patients.

Oral anticoagulants should not be used in cerebral thrombosis or peripheral arterial occlusion, but may be of value in patients with *transient brain ischaemic attacks* whether due to carotid or vertebrobasilar arterial disease; if these patients also have severe hypertension anticoagulants are contraindicated, and antiplatelet drugs are an alternative (section 2.9).

Warfarin is the drug of choice; **nicoumalone** and **phenindione** are seldom used.

DOSE. Whenever possible, the base-line prothrombin time should be determined before the initial dose is given.

The usual adult induction dose of warfarin is 10 mg[1] daily for 2 days (higher doses no longer recommended). The subsequent maintenance dose depends upon the prothrombin time (reported as INR); the currently recommended therapeutic ranges are:

INR 2–2.5 for prophylaxis of deep-vein thrombosis including surgery on high-risk patients;

INR 2–3 for prophylaxis in hip surgery and fractured femur operations, for treatment of deep-vein thrombosis, pulmonary embolism, systemic embolism, prevention of venous thrombo-embolism in myocardial infarction, mitral stenosis with embolism, transient ischaemic attacks, atrial fibrillation, and tissue prosthetic heart valves;

INR 3–4.5 for recurrent deep-vein thrombosis and pulmonary embolism, arterial disease including myocardial infarction, and mechanical prosthetic heart valves.

It is essential that the INR be determined:

daily or on alternate days in early days of treatment, *then* at longer intervals (depending on response[2]) *then* up to every 8 weeks

The daily maintenance dose of warfarin is usually 3 to 9 mg (taken at the **same time** each day).

HAEMORRHAGE. The main adverse effect of all oral anticoagulants is haemorrhage. Omission of dosage with checking of the INR is essential. The following recommendations of the British Society for Haematology are based on the result of the INR and the clinical state:

Life-threatening haemorrhage—immediately give phytomenadione (vitamin K_1) 5 mg by slow intravenous injection and a concentrate of factors II, IX, X (with factor VII concentrate if available). If no concentrate is available, fresh frozen plasma should be infused (approximately 1 litre for an adult) but this may not be as effective

Less severe haemorrhage e.g. haematuria and epistaxis—withhold warfarin for one or more days and consider giving phytomenadione (vitamin K_1) 0.5–2 mg[3] by slow intravenous injection

INR 4.5–7 without haemorrhage—withhold warfarin for 1 or 2 days then review

INR >7 without haemorrhage—withhold warfarin and consider giving phytomenadione (vitamin K_1) 500 micrograms by slow intravenous injection

Unexpected bleeding at therapeutic levels[4]—investigate possibility of underlying cause e.g. unsuspected renal or alimentary tract pathology

---

1. Less than 10 mg if base-line prothrombin time prolonged, if liver-function tests abnormal, or if patient in cardiac failure, on parenteral feeding, less than average body weight, or over 80 years of age.

2. Change in patient's clinical condition, particularly associated with liver disease, intercurrent illness, or drug administration, necessitates more frequent testing. See also **interactions**, Appendix 1 (warfarin). Major changes in diet (especially involving vegetables) and in alcohol consumption may also affect warfarin control.

3. Usually 1 mg adequate and should be given if INR greater than desired; higher doses will prevent oral anticoagulants from acting for several days or even weeks.

4. Should always be investigated regardless of INR since even if patients over-anticoagulated bleeding generally has an additional underlying cause.

PREGNANCY. Oral anticoagulants are teratogenic and should not be given in the first trimester of pregnancy. Women at risk of pregnancy should be warned of this danger since stopping warfarin before the sixth week of gestation may largely avoid the risk of fetal abnormality. Oral anticoagulants cross the placenta with risk of placental or fetal haemorrhage, especially during the last few weeks of pregnancy and at delivery. Therefore, if at all possible, oral anticoagulants should be avoided in pregnancy, especially in the first and third trimesters. Difficult decisions may have to be made, particularly in women with prosthetic heart valves or with a history of recurrent venous thrombosis or pulmonary embolism.

TREATMENT BOOKLETS. Anticoagulant treatment booklets should be issued to patients, and are available for distribution to local healthcare professionals from Health Authorities and also from:

England:	Scottish Office
HMSO	Health Department
Broadway	Room 64
Chadderton	St. Andrew's House
Oldham	Edinburgh EH1 3DH
Lancs OL9 6QH	

Wales:	Northern Ireland Office
Room 106	Central Services Agency
Royal Pharmaceutical	27 Adelaide St
Society of Great Britain	Belfast BT2 8FH

These booklets include advice for patients on anticoagulant treatment.

WARFARIN SODIUM

Indications: prophylaxis of embolisation in rheumatic heart disease and atrial fibrillation; prophylaxis after insertion of prosthetic heart valve; prophylaxis and treatment of venous thrombosis and pulmonary embolism; transient ischaemic attacks

Cautions: hepatic or renal disease, recent surgery; **interactions:** Appendix 1 (warfarin)

Contra-indications: pregnancy (see notes above), peptic ulcer, severe hypertension, bacterial endocarditis

Side-effects: haemorrhage—see notes above for British Society for Haematology recommendations; other side-effects reported include hypersensitivity, rash, alopecia, diarrhoea, unexplained drop in haematocrit, 'purple toes', skin necrosis, jaundice, hepatic dysfunction; also nausea, vomiting, and pancreatitis

Dose: see notes above

PoM **Warfarin** (Non-proprietary)

Tablets, all scored, warfarin 1 mg (brown), net price 20 = 16p; 3 mg (blue), 20 = 20p; 5 mg (pink), 20 = 29p. Label: 10 anticoagulant card

Available from APS, Cox, Goldshield (Marevan®), Hillcross, Lagap, Norton

NICOUMALONE

(Acenocoumarol)

Indications; Cautions; Contra-indications; Side-effects: see under Warfarin Sodium; avoid breast-feeding

Dose: 8–12 mg on 1st day; 4–8 mg on 2nd day; maintenance dose usually 1–8 mg daily

PoM **Sinthrome®** (Geigy)

Tablets, nicoumalone 1 mg. Net price 20 = 49p. Label: 10 anticoagulant card

PHENINDIONE

Indications: prophylaxis of embolisation in rheumatic heart disease and atrial fibrillation; prophylaxis after insertion of prosthetic heart valve; prophylaxis and treatment of venous thrombosis and pulmonary embolism

Cautions; Contra-indications; Side-effects: see under Warfarin Sodium; also hypersensitivity reactions including rashes, fever, leucopenia, agranulocytosis, diarrhoea, renal and hepatic damage; urine coloured pink; avoid breast-feeding; **interactions:** Appendix 1 (phenindione)

Dose: 200 mg on 1st day; 100 mg on 2nd day; maintenance dose usually 50–150 mg daily

PoM **Dindevan®** (Goldshield)

Tablets, phenindione 10 mg, net price 20 = 91p; 25 mg (green), 20 = £1.25; 50 mg, 20 = £1.61. Label: 10 anticoagulant card, 14 (urine pink)

2.8.3 Protamine sulphate

Although protamine sulphate is used to counteract overdosage with heparin, if used in excess it has an anticoagulant effect.

PROTAMINE SULPHATE

(Protamine Sulfate)

Indications; Cautions: see above; also if increased risk of allergic reaction to protamine (includes previous treatment with protamine insulin, allergy to fish, men who are infertile or who have had a vasectomy)

Side-effects: flushing, hypotension, bradycardia, dyspnoea

Dose: by slow intravenous injection, 1 mg neutralises 100 units heparin (mucous) or 80 units heparin (lung) when given within 15 minutes; if longer time, less protamine required as heparin rapidly excreted; max. 50 mg

PoM **Protamine Sulphate** (Non-proprietary)

Injection, protamine sulphate 10 mg/mL. Net price 5-mL amp = 98p

Available from Evans, Knoll

PoM **Prosulf®** (CP)

Injection, protamine sulphate 10 mg/mL. Net price 5-mL amp = 98p (glass), £1.20 (polypropylene)

2.9   Antiplatelet drugs

By decreasing platelet aggregation, these drugs may inhibit thrombus formation on the arterial side of the circulation, where thrombi are formed by platelet aggregation and anticoagulants have little effect.

Encouraging results have been obtained using **aspirin** 75–300 mg daily for the *secondary* prevention of thrombotic cerebrovascular or cardiovascular disease. Aspirin 150–300 mg daily is used to reduce mortality after myocardial infarction. Low doses of aspirin (such as 75 or 100 mg daily) are also given following bypass surgery.

Dipyridamole is used by mouth as an adjunct to oral anticoagulation for prophylaxis of thromboembolism associated with prosthetic heart valves.

Abciximab (ReoPro®, Lilly) is a monoclonal antibody which inhibits platelet aggregation and thrombus formation. It is indicated for use by experienced physicians as an adjunct to heparin and aspirin for the prevention of ischaemic complications in high-risk patients undergoing percutaneous transluminal coronary angioplasty. Abciximab should be used once only.

For use of epoprostenol, see section 2.8.1.

ASPIRIN (antiplatelet)
(Acetylsalicylic Acid)

Indications: prophylaxis of cerebrovascular disease or myocardial infarction (see notes above)
Cautions: asthma; uncontrolled hypertension; pregnancy (but see Appendix 4); **interactions:** Appendix 1 (aspirin)
Contra-indications: children under 12 years and in breast-feeding (Reye's syndrome, see section 4.7.1); active peptic ulceration; haemophilia and other bleeding disorders
Side-effects: bronchospasm; gastro-intestinal haemorrhage (occasionally major), also other haemorrhage (e.g. subconjunctival)
Dose: see notes above

Aspirin (Non-proprietary)
Dispersible tablets, aspirin 75 mg, net price 20 = 5p; 300 mg, see section 4.7.1. Label: 13, 21, 32
Angettes 75® (Bristol-Myers)
Tablets, aspirin 75 mg. Net price 56-tab pack = £1.88. Label: 32
Caprin® (Sinclair)
Tablets, e/c, pink, aspirin 75 mg, net price 56-tab pack = £3.08; 300 mg, see section 4.7.1. Label: 5, 25, 32
Disprin CV® (R&C)
Tablets, both m/r, aspirin 100 mg, net price 28-tab pack = £1.68; 300 mg, 28-tab pack = £1.99. Label: 25, 32
Nu-Seals® Aspirin (Lilly)
Tablets, e/c, aspirin 75 mg, net price 56-tab pack = £3.09; 300 mg, see section 4.7.1. Label: 5, 25, 32
Note. Tablets may be chewed at diagnosis for rapid absorption
Aspirin enteric-coated tablets also available from Ashbourne (postMI 75EC®)

DIPYRIDAMOLE

Indications: see notes above
Cautions: rapidly worsening angina, aortic stenosis, recent myocardial infarction; may exacerbate migraine, hypotension; **interactions:** Appendix 1 (dipyridamole)—**important:** interaction with adenosine liable to be serious
Side-effects: nausea, diarrhoea, throbbing headache, hypotension
Dose: by mouth, 300–600 mg daily in 3–4 divided doses before food
By intravenous injection, diagnostic only, see manufacturer's literature

PoM **Dipyridamole** (Non-proprietary)
Tablets, coated, dipyridamole 25 mg, net price 20 = 38p; 100 mg, 20 = £1.06. Label: 22
Available from APS, Ashbourne (Cerebrovase®), Berk (Modaplate®), Cox, Hillcross, Lagap, Norton
PoM **Persantin®** (Boehringer Ingelheim)
Tablets, both s/c, dipyridamole 25 mg (orange), net price 84-tab pack = £1.78; 100 mg, 84-tab pack = £4.95. Label: 22
Injection, dipyridamole 5 mg/mL. Net price 2-mL amp = 11p

2.10   Fibrinolytic drugs

Fibrinolytic drugs act as thrombolytics by activating plasminogen to form plasmin, which degrades fibrin and so breaks up thrombi.

Streptokinase is used in the treatment of *life-threatening venous thrombosis*, and in *pulmonary embolism*, but treatment must be started rapidly.

Urokinase is currently used for *thrombolysis in the eye* and in *arteriovenous shunts*. It has the advantage of being non-immunogenic.

The value of thrombolytic drugs for the treatment of *myocardial infarction* has been established. **Streptokinase, alteplase,** and **anistreplase** have all been shown to reduce mortality when given by the intravenous route with comparable efficacy. The potential for benefit lessens as the delay from the onset of major symptoms increases, but the value of treatment within the first 12 hours is reasonably well established. Knowledge of the role of adjuvant therapy is also incomplete, but in the case of streptokinase the reduction in mortality by aspirin has been shown to be additive whilst immediate heparin is necessary to obtain full efficacy from alteplase. Thrombolytic drugs are indicated for any patient with acute myocardial infarction for whom the benefit is believed to outweigh the risk of treatment. Trials have shown that the benefit is greatest in those with ECG changes that include ST segment elevation and in those with anterior infarction. Patients should not be excluded on account of age alone because mortality in this group is high and the percentage reduction in mortality is the same as in younger patients.

CAUTIONS. Risk of bleeding from venepuncture or invasive procedures, any external chest compression, pregnancy (see Appendix 4), possibility of pre-existing thrombus as in abdominal aneurysm or enlarged left atrium with atrial fibrillation (risk of

---

dissolution of clot and subsequent embolisation), diabetic retinopathy, recent or concurrent anticoagulant therapy.

CONTRA-INDICATIONS.   Recent   haemorrhage, trauma, or surgery (including dental extraction), coagulation defects, bleeding diatheses, aortic dissection, coma, history of cerebrovascular disease especially recent events or with any residual disability, recent symptoms of possible peptic ulceration, heavy vaginal bleeding, severe hypertension, pulmonary disease with cavitation, acute pancreatitis, severe liver disease, oesophageal varices; also in the case of streptokinase or anistreplase, previous allergic reactions to either drug.

Prolonged persistence of antibodies to streptokinase and anistreplase may reduce the effectiveness of subsequent treatment, therefore neither drug should be repeated beyond 4 days of first administration.

SIDE-EFFECTS.   Side-effects of thrombolytics are mainly nausea and vomiting and bleeding. Back pain has been reported. Bleeding is usually limited to the site of injection, but intracerebral haemorrhage or bleeding from other sites may occur. Serious bleeding calls for discontinuation of the thrombolytic and may require administration of coagulation factors and antifibrinolytic drugs (aprotinin or tranexamic acid). Streptokinase and anistreplase may cause allergic reactions and anaphylaxis has been reported (for details of management see Allergic Emergencies, section 3.4.3). Guillain-Barré syndrome has been reported rarely after streptokinase treatment.

ALTEPLASE
(rt-PA, tissue-type plasminogen activator)

Indications: acute myocardial infarction (see notes above); pulmonary embolism

Cautions; Contra-indications; Side-effects: see notes above

Dose: myocardial infarction, initiated within 6 hours, 15 mg by *intravenous injection*, followed by *intravenous infusion* of 50 mg over 30 minutes, then 35 mg over 60 minutes (total dose 100 mg over 90 minutes); for administration more than 6 hours after infarction, consult product literature

Pulmonary embolism, 10 mg by *intravenous injection* over 1–2 minutes followed by *intravenous infusion* of 90 mg over 2 hours

Patients less than 65 kg require lower doses

PoM **Actilyse®** (Boehringer Ingelheim)
Injection, powder for reconstitution, alteplase 20 mg (11.6 mega units)/vial, net price per vial (with diluent and transfer device) = £200.00; 50 mg (29 mega units)/vial, pack of 2 vials (with diluent, transfer device, and infusion bag) = £750.00

ANISTREPLASE
(APSAC)

Indications: acute myocardial infarction (see notes above)

Cautions; Contra-indications; Side-effects: see notes above

Dose: by intravenous injection, 30 units over 4–5 minutes; treatment should be initiated as soon as possible and preferably within 6 hours

PoM **Eminase®** (Monmouth)
Injection, powder for reconstitution, anistreplase. Net price 30-unit vial = £495.00 (also available in injection pack with 5-mL amp water for injections and disposable syringe and needle)

STREPTOKINASE

Indications: deep-vein thrombosis, pulmonary embolism, acute arterial thromboembolism, thrombosed arteriovenous shunts; acute myocardial infarction (see notes above); topical use, see section 13.11.7

Cautions; Contra-indications; Side-effects: see notes above

Dose: by intravenous infusion, 250 000 units over 30 minutes, then 100 000 units every hour for up to 24–72 hours according to condition (see data sheet)

Myocardial infarction, 1 500 000 units over 60 minutes followed by aspirin 150 mg daily *by mouth* for at least 4 weeks (see data sheet)

PoM **Kabikinase®** (Pharmacia)
Injection, powder for reconstitution, streptokinase; net price 250 000-unit vial = £15.00; 750 000-unit vial = £40.00; 1.5 million-unit vial = £85.00

PoM **Streptase®** (Hoechst)
Injection, powder for reconstitution, streptokinase; net price 250 000-unit vial = £15.36; 750 000-unit vial = £40.26; 1.5 million-unit vial = £80.52 (hosp. only)

UROKINASE

Indications: thrombosed arteriovenous shunts and intravenous cannulas; thrombolysis in the eye; deep-vein thrombosis, pulmonary embolism, peripheral vascular occlusion

Cautions; Contra-indications; Side-effects: see notes above

Dose: by instillation into arteriovenous shunt, 5000–25 500 International units in 2–3 mL sodium chloride injection 0.9%

By intravenous infusion 4400 International units/kg over 10 minutes, then 4400 units/kg/hour for 12 hours in pulmonary embolism or 12–24 hours in deep-vein thrombosis; for bolus injection for pulmonary embolism consult data sheet

Peripheral vascular occlusion, consult data sheet

Intra-ocular administration, 5000 International units in 2 mL sodium chloride injection 0.9%

PoM **Urokinase** (Non-proprietary)

Injection, powder for reconstitution, urokinase; net price 5000 International unit vial = £9.75; 25 000 International unit vial = £27.79; 100 000 International unit vial = £60.00

Available from Leo, Serono (Ukidan®)

2.11   Antifibrinolytic drugs and haemostatics

Fibrin dissolution can be impaired by the administration of **tranexamic acid**, which inhibits plasminogen activation and fibrinolysis. It may be useful when haemorrhage cannot be staunched (e.g. in prostatectomy and dental extraction in haemophilia) and can be particularly useful in menorrhagia (see section 6.4.1.2). Tranexamic acid may also be used in hereditary angioedema and in streptokinase overdose.

Desmopressin (see section 6.5.2) is used in the management of mild to moderate haemophilia.

Aprotinin is a proteolytic enzyme inhibitor acting on plasmin and kallidinogenase (kallikrein). It is indicated for patients at high risk of major blood loss during and after open heart surgery with extracorporeal circulation and for patients in whom optimal blood conservation during open heart surgery is an absolute priority; it is also indicated for the treatment of life-threatening haemorrhage due to hyperplasminaemia (occasionally observed during the mobilisation and dissection of malignant tumours, in acute promyelocytic leukaemia, and following thrombolytic therapy).

Ethamsylate reduces capillary bleeding in the presence of a normal number of platelets. It does not act by fibrin stabilisation, but probably by correcting abnormal platelet adhesion.

APROTININ

Indications: see notes above

Side-effects: occasionally hypersensitivity reactions and localised thrombophlebitis

Dose: by slow intravenous injection or infusion

Open heart surgery, loading dose, 2 000 000 units (200 mL) after induction of anaesthesia and before sternotomy—initial 50 000 units (5 mL) *by slow intravenous injection* over several minutes (to detect allergy), remainder *by intravenous infusion* over 20 minutes; maintenance dose, *by intravenous infusion* 500 000 units (50 mL) every hour until end of operation (or early postoperative period in septic endocarditis); pump prime, 2 000 000 units (200 mL) in priming volume of extracorporeal circuit; in septic endocarditis 3 000 000 units (300 mL) added to pump prime

Hyperplasminaemia, *by slow intravenous injection or by infusion* initially, 500 000 units (50 mL) to 1 000 000 units (100 mL) at max. rate 10 mL/min; followed if necessary by 200 000 units (20 mL) every hour until bleeding stops

PoM **Trasylol**® (Bayer)

Injection, aprotinin 10 000 kallikrein inactivator units/mL. Net price 50-mL vial = £20.53

Note. Aprotinin injection containing 10 000 kallikrein inactivator units/mL also available from Paines & Byrne

ETHAMSYLATE
(Etamsylate)

Indications: see under preparations

Contra-indications: porphyria (see section 9.8.2)

Side-effects: nausea, headache, rashes

Dose: see below

PoM **Dicynene**® (Delandale)

Tablets, scored, ethamsylate 500 mg, net price 100-tab pack = £22.13

Dose: short-term treatment of blood loss in menorrhagia, 500 mg 4 times daily during menstruation

Injection, ethamsylate 125 mg/mL. Net price 2-mL amp = 82p

Dose: prophylaxis and treatment of periventricular haemorrhage in low birth-weight infants, by intramuscular or intravenous injection, 12.5 mg/kg every 6 hours

IMPORTANT. The ampoules currently available contain a total of 250 mg in 2 mL volume therefore **small fraction only** required for neonatal use

TRANEXAMIC ACID

Indications: see notes above

Cautions: reduce dose in renal impairment; massive haematuria (avoid if risk of ureteric obstruction); regular eye examinations and liver function tests in long-term treatment of hereditary angioedema

Note. Requirement for regular eye examinations during long-term treatment is based on unsatisfactory evidence

Contra-indications: thromboembolic disease

Side-effects: nausea, vomiting, diarrhoea (reduce dose); giddiness on rapid intravenous injection

Dose: by mouth, 1–1.5 g 2–4 times daily

By slow intravenous injection, 0.5–1 g 3 times daily

PoM **Cyklokapron**® (Pharmacia)

Tablets, f/c, scored, tranexamic acid 500 mg. Net price 60-tab pack = £14.97

Syrup, tranexamic acid 500 mg/5 mL. Net price 300 mL = £15.60

Injection, tranexamic acid 100 mg/mL. Net price 5-mL amp = £1.35

BLOOD PRODUCTS

FACTOR VIIa (RECOMBINANT)

Recombinant factor VIIa is used in patients with inhibitors to factors VIII and IX

Available from Novo Nordisk (▼NovoSeven®)

FACTOR VIII FRACTION, DRIED
(Human Antihaemophilic Fraction, Dried)

Dried factor VIII fraction is prepared from human plasma by a suitable fractionation technique

Indications: control of haemorrhage in haemophilia A

Cautions: intravascular haemolysis after large or frequently repeated doses in patients with blood groups A, B, or AB—less likely with high potency concentrates

Side-effects: allergic reactions including chills, fever; hyperfibrinogenaemia occurred after massive doses with earlier products but less likely since fibrinogen content has now been substantially reduced

Available from Alpha (Alpha VIII), Armour (Monoclate-P®), BPL (8SM®, 8Y®), SNBTS (High Potency Factor VIII Concentrate)

Note. Preparation of recombinant human antihaemophilic factor VIII (octocog alfa) available from Bayer (▼Kogenate®), Baxter (▼Recombinate®)

FACTOR VIII INHIBITOR BYPASSING FRACTION

Preparations with factor VIII inhibitor bypassing activity are prepared from human plasma

Human Factor VIII Inhibitor Bypassing Fraction (*FEIBA*, Immuno) is used in patients with factor VIII inhibitors

Note. A porcine preparation of antihaemophilic factor for patients with inhibitors to human factor VIII is available from Speywood (Hyate C®)

FACTOR IX FRACTION, DRIED

Dried factor IX fraction is prepared from human plasma by a suitable fractionation technique; it may also contain clotting factors II, VII, and X.

Indications: congenital factor IX deficiency (haemophilia B)

Cautions: risk of thrombosis—principally with former low purity products

Contra-indications: disseminated intravascular coagulation

Side-effects: allergic reactions, including chills, fever

Available from Alpha (Alphanine®), Armour (▼Mononine®), BPL (Dried Factor IX Fraction, Heat-Treated; ▼Replenine®), SNBTS (Human Factor IX Concentrate, Heat Treated)

FRESH FROZEN PLASMA

Fresh frozen plasma is prepared from the supernatant liquid obtained by centrifugation of one donation of whole blood

Indications: to replace coagulation factors or other plasma proteins where their concentration or functional activity is critically reduced, e.g. to reverse warfarin effect

Cautions: avoid in circulatory overload; need for compatibility

Side-effects: allergic reactions including chills, fever, bronchospasm; adult respiratory distress syndrome

Available from Regional Blood Transfusion Services and BPL

2.12 Lipid-lowering drugs

There are a number of common conditions, some familial, in which there are very high plasma concentrations of cholesterol, or triglycerides, or both. There is evidence that therapy which lowers low density lipoprotein (LDL) cholesterol and raises high density lipoprotein (HDL) cholesterol reduces the progression of coronary atherosclerosis and may even induce regression. There is also evidence that lowering LDL-cholesterol by 25 to 35% is effective in both the primary and secondary prevention of clinical manifestations of coronary heart disease.

Treatment with lipid-lowering drugs should be considered in patients with coronary heart disease and those at high risk of developing coronary heart disease on account of multiple risk factors or severe hyperlipidaemia inadequately controlled by a modified fat diet. Any drug therapy must be combined with strict adherence to diet, maintenance of near-ideal body weight and, if appropriate, reduction of blood pressure and cessation of smoking.

Severe hyperlipidaemia often requires combinations of lipid-lowering drugs such as an anion-exchange resin with a fibrate, an HMG CoA reductase inhibitor, or nicotinic acid. Combinations of HMG CoA reductase inhibitors with nicotinic acid or a fibrate carry an increased risk of side-effects (including rhabdomyolysis) and should be used with great caution.

CSM advice. The CSM has advised that rhabdomyolysis associated with lipid-lowering drugs such as the fibrates and statins appears to be rare (approx. 1 case in every 100 000 treatment years) but may be increased in those with renal impairment and possibly in those with hypothyroidism. Concomitant treatment with cyclosporin may increase plasma-statin concentrations and the risk of muscle toxicity, and concomitant treatment with a fibrate and a statin may also be associated with an increased risk of serious muscle toxicity.

ANION-EXCHANGE RESINS

Cholestyramine and **colestipol** are anion-exchange resins used in the management of hypercholesterolaemia. They act by binding bile acids, preventing their reabsorption; this promotes hepatic conversion of cholesterol into bile acids; the resultant increased LDL-receptor activity of liver cells increases the breakdown of LDL-cholesterol. Thus both compounds effectively reduce LDL-cholesterol but can aggravate hypertriglyceridaemia.

COUNSELLING. Other drugs should be taken at least 1 hour before or 4–6 hours after cholestyramine or colestipol to reduce possible interference with absorption.

CHOLESTYRAMINE
(Colestyramine)

Indications: hyperlipidaemias, particularly type IIa, in patients who have not responded adequately to diet and other appropriate measures; primary prevention of coronary heart disease in men aged 35–59 years with primary hypercholesterolaemia who have not responded to diet and other appropriate measures; pruritus associated with partial biliary obstruction and primary biliary cirrhosis; diarrhoeal disorders, see section 1.5

Cautions: supplements of fat-soluble vitamins and of folic acid may be required with high doses, particularly in children; pregnancy and breast-feeding; **interactions:** Appendix 1 (cholestyramine and colestipol)

Contra-indications: complete biliary obstruction (not likely to be effective)

Side-effects: nausea and vomiting, constipation or diarrhoea, heartburn, flatulence, abdominal discomfort; on prolonged use, increased bleeding tendency (due to hypoprothrombinaemia associated with vitamin K deficiency); hyperchloraemic acidosis reported on prolonged use of anion-exchange resins

Dose: lipid reduction (after initial introduction over 3–4 weeks) 8–24 g daily in water (or other suitable liquid) in single or up to 4 divided doses; up to 36 g daily if necessary

Pruritus, 4–8 g daily in water (or other suitable liquid)

Diarrhoeal disorders, see section 1.5

CHILD 6–12 years, see data sheet

PoM **Questran®** (Bristol-Myers)
Powder, orange, cholestyramine (anhydrous) 4 g/sachet. Net price 60-sachet pack = £21.06, 180-sachet pack = £63.19. Label: 13, counselling, avoid other drugs at same time (see notes above)

PoM [1] **Questran Light®** (Bristol-Myers)
Powder, orange, cholestyramine (anhydrous) 4 g/sachet, with aspartame. Net price 60-sachet pack = £22.11, 180-sachet pack = £66.34. Label: 13, counselling, avoid other drugs at same time (see notes above)

1. Formerly Questran A

COLESTIPOL HYDROCHLORIDE

Indications: hyperlipidaemias, particularly type IIa, in patients who have not responded adequately to diet and other appropriate measures

Cautions; Contra-indications; Side-effects: see under Cholestyramine

Dose: 5 g 1–2 times daily in liquid increased if necessary at intervals of 1–2 months to max. of 30 g daily (in single or 2 divided doses)

PoM **Colestid®** (Upjohn)
Granules, yellow, colestipol hydrochloride 5 g/sachet. Net price 30 sachets = £12.54. Label: 13, counselling, avoid other drugs at same time (see notes above)

Colestid Orange, granules, yellow/orange, colestipol hydrochloride 5 g/sachet, with aspartame. Net price 30 sachets = £12.54. Label: 13, counselling, avoid other drugs at same time (see notes above)

CLOFIBRATE GROUP

Clofibrate, bezafibrate, ciprofibrate, fenofibrate, and **gemfibrozil** can be regarded as broad-spectrum lipid-modulating agents in that although their main action is to decrease serum triglycerides they also tend to reduce LDL-cholesterol and to raise HDL-cholesterol.

All can cause a myositis-like syndrome (see also CSM advice above), especially in patients with impaired renal function. In addition, clofibrate predisposes to gallstones by increasing biliary cholesterol excretion; it is therefore only indicated in patients who have had a cholecystectomy.

BEZAFIBRATE

Indications: hyperlipidaemias of types IIa, IIb, III, IV and V in patients who have not responded adequately to diet and other appropriate measures

Cautions: renal impairment (avoid if severe — see also under Myotoxicity below); **interactions:** Appendix 1 (clofibrate group)

MYOTOXICITY. Special care needed in patients with renal disease, as progressive increases in serum creatinine concentration or failure to follow dosage guidelines may result in myotoxicity (rhabdomyolysis)

Contra-indications: severe renal or hepatic impairment, hypoalbuminaemia, primary biliary cirrhosis, gall bladder disease, nephrotic syndrome, pregnancy and breast-feeding

Side-effects: gastro-intestinal (e.g. nausea, anorexia, gastric pain), pruritus, urticaria, impotence; also headache, dizziness, vertigo, fatigue, hair loss; myotoxicity (with myasthenia or myalgia)—special risk in renal impairment (see under Cautions)

Dose: see preparations below

PoM **Bezalip®** (Boehringer Mannheim)
Tablets, f/c, bezafibrate 200 mg. Net price 100-tab pack = £10.30. Label: 21
Dose: 200 mg 3 times daily with or after food; may be reduced to 200 mg twice daily in hypertriglyceridaemia

PoM **Bezalip-Mono®** (Boehringer Mannheim)
Tablets, m/r, f/c, bezafibrate 400 mg. Net price 28-tab pack = £8.50. Label: 21, 25
Dose: 1 tablet daily after food (dose form not appropriate in renal impairment)

CIPROFIBRATE

Indications: hyperlipidaemias of types IIa, IIb, III, and IV in patients who have not responded adequately to diet

Cautions; Contra-indications; Side-effects: see under Bezafibrate

Dose: 100 mg daily

PoM **Modalim®** (Sanofi Winthrop)
Tablets, scored, ciprofibrate 100 mg. Net price 28-tab pack = £13.38

CLOFIBRATE

Indications: hyperlipidaemias of types IIb, III, IV and V in patients who have not responded adequately to diet and other appropriate measures (but see also notes above)

Cautions; Contra-indications: see under Bezafibrate and notes above

Side-effects: see under Bezafibrate; also cholesterol cholelithiasis

Dose: over 65 kg, 2 g daily (50–65 kg, 1.5 g daily) in 2 or 3 divided doses

PoM Atromid-S® (Zeneca)

Capsules, red, clofibrate 500 mg. Net price 100-cap pack = £4.08. Label: 21

FENOFIBRATE

Indications: hyperlipidaemias of types IIa, IIb, III, IV, and V in patients who have not responded adequately to diet and other appropriate measures

Cautions: see under Bezafibrate

Contra-indications: severe renal or hepatic impairment; existing gall bladder disease; pregnancy and breast-feeding

Side-effects: see under Bezafibrate

Dose: see preparations below

PoM Lipantil® (Fournier)

Capsules, fenofibrate 100 mg. Net price 84-cap pack = £19.80. Label: 21

Dose: initially 300 mg daily in divided doses with food, adjusted according to response within range 200–400 mg daily; CHILD 5 mg/kg daily

Lipantil Micro capsules, orange, fenofibrate (micronised) 200 mg. Net price 30-cap pack = £24.40. Label: 21

Dose: initially 1 capsule daily with food (dose form not appropriate for children or in renal impairment)

Note. Improved bioavailability of micronised fenofibrate may allow a lower total daily dose than with conventional formulation

GEMFIBROZIL

Indications: hyperlipidaemias of types IIa, IIb, III, IV and V in patients who have not responded adequately to diet and other appropriate measures; primary prevention of coronary heart disease in men aged 40–55 years with hyperlipidaemias that have not responded to diet and other appropriate measures

Cautions: lipid profile, blood counts, and liver-function tests before initiating long-term treatment; renal impairment; **interactions:** Appendix 1 (clofibrate group)

Contra-indications: alcoholism, hepatic impairment, gallstones; pregnancy and breast-feeding

Side-effects: gastro-intestinal disturbances; also rash, dermatitis, pruritus, urticaria, impotence, headache, dizziness, blurred vision, cholestatic jaundice, angioedema, laryngeal oedema, atrial fibrillation, pancreatitis, myasthenia, myopathy, rhabdomyolysis, painful extremities, myalgia accompanied by increases in creatine kinase

Dose: 1.2 g daily, usually in 2 divided doses; range 0.9–1.5 g daily

PoM Lopid® (P-D)

'300' capsules, white/maroon, gemfibrozil 300 mg. Net price 112-cap pack = £29.64

'600' tablets, f/c, gemfibrozil 600 mg. Net price 56-tab pack = £29.64

STATINS

Simvastatin, pravastatin and **fluvastatin** belong to a class of drugs which competitively inhibit 3-hydroxy-3-methylglutaryl coenzyme A (HMG CoA) reductase, an enzyme that catalyses a step in cholesterol synthesis, especially in the liver. They are more potent than anion-exchange resins in lowering LDL-cholesterol but less effective than the clofibrate group in reducing triglycerides and raising HDL-cholesterol. They are unlikely to be of benefit in the homozygous form of familial hypercholesterolaemia.

There is evidence that statins produce important reductions in coronary events, in all cardiovascular events, and in total mortality in patients aged up to 70 years with coronary heart disease (history of angina or acute myocardial infarction) and with plasma cholesterol of 5.5–8 mmol/litre. They also have a role in primary prevention of coronary heart disease in some patients with hypercholesterolaemia and increased risk of coronary events.

The main side-effect is reversible myositis (see also CSM advice, p. 113), which is rare except in patients also receiving cyclosporin, nicotinic acid, or gemfibrozil (careful monitoring of liver function and creatine phosphokinase should be performed if these drugs are used with an HMG CoA reductase inhibitor).

COUNSELLING. Advise patient to report promptly unexplained muscle pain, tenderness, weakness.

FLUVASTATIN

Indications: primary hypercholesterolaemia (hyperlipidaemia type IIa) in patients with cholesterol concentration of 6.5 mmol/litre or greater who have not responded adequately to dietary control

Cautions; Contra-indications; Side-effects: see under Simvastatin; also avoid in severe renal impairment; **interactions:** Appendix 1 (statins)

Dose: initially 20 mg daily in the evening; usual range 20–40 mg daily in the evening, adjusted at intervals of 4 weeks; up to 40 mg twice daily may be required

▼ **PoM Lescol®** (Sandoz)

Capsules, fluvastatin (as sodium salt) 20 mg (brown/yellow), net price 28-cap pack = £14.90; 40 mg (brown/orange), 28-cap pack = £15.90, 56-cap pack = £29.80. Counselling, muscle effects, see notes above

PRAVASTATIN

Indications: primary hypercholesterolaemia (hyperlipidaemia type IIa), in patients with cholesterol concentration of 6.5 mmol/litre or greater who have not responded adequately to dietary control; adjunct to diet to slow progressive course of coronary atherosclerosis and reduce incidence of clinical cardiac events in patients with hypercholesterolaemia and documented atherosclerotic coronary artery disease

Cautions; Contra-indications; Side-effects: see under Simvastatin; **interactions**: Appendix 1 (statins)

Dose: usual range 10–40 mg once daily at night, adjusted at intervals of not less than 4 weeks

PoM Lipostat® (Squibb)

Tablets, both pink, pravastatin sodium 10 mg, net price 28-tab pack = £16.18; 20 mg, 28-tab pack = £31.09. Counselling, muscle effects, see notes above

---

SIMVASTATIN

Indications: primary hypercholesterolaemia (hyperlipidaemia type IIa) in patients who have not responded adequately to diet and other appropriate measures; to reduce incidence of clinical coronary events and slow progression of coronary atherosclerosis in patients with coronary heart disease and cholesterol concentration of 5.5 mmol/litre or greater

Cautions: monitor liver function (see below); history of liver disease (avoid if active); high alcohol intake; avoid pregnancy during and for 1 month after treatment; advise patients to report unexplained muscle pain (see also Muscle Effects below); **interactions:** Appendix 1 (statins)

LIVER FUNCTION. Tests required before and during treatment—more frequently if raised serum transaminase concentrations develop and progress; discontinue treatment if serum transaminase concentrations rise to and persist at 3 times upper limit of normal

Contra-indications: active liver disease; pregnancy (adequate contraception in women of childbearing age) and breast-feeding (see Appendixes 4 and 5); porphyria (see section 9.8.2)

Side-effects: muscle effects (see below); gastro-intestinal effects (including nausea, constipation or diarrhoea); headache, fatigue, insomnia, rash, rhabdomyolysis, hepatitis, pancreatitis reported; raised creatine phosphokinase concentrations (discontinue if markedly raised or myopathy diagnosed); hypersensitivity syndrome (including angioedema) reported

MUSCLE EFFECTS. Myalgia, myositis and myopathy reported with statins; if creatine phosphokinase concentration markedly elevated (> 10 times upper limit of normal), and myopathy suspected or diagnosed, discontinue treatment. Increased incidence of myopathy if statins given with a fibrate, lipid-lowering doses of nicotinic acid, or immunosuppressants such as cyclosporin. Rhabdomyolysis with acute renal impairment secondary to myoglobinuria also reported

Dose: hypercholesterolaemia, 10 mg daily at night, adjusted at intervals of not less than 4 weeks; usual range 10–40 mg once daily at night
Coronary heart disease, initially 20 mg once daily at night

PoM Zocor® (MSD)

Tablets, all f/c, simvastatin 10 mg (peach), net price 28-tab pack = £18.29; 20 mg (tan), 28-tab pack = £31.09; 40 mg (red), 28-tab pack = £47.04. Counselling, muscle effects, see notes above

---

NICOTINIC ACID GROUP

The value of **nicotinic acid** is limited by its side-effects, especially vasodilatation. In doses of 1.5 to 3 g daily it lowers both cholesterol and triglyceride concentrations by inhibiting synthesis; it also increases HDL-cholesterol. **Acipimox** seems to have fewer side-effects but may be less effective in its lipid-modulating capabilities.

ACIPIMOX

Indications: hyperlipidaemias of types IIa, IIb, and IV in patients who have not responded adequately to diet and other appropriate measures

Cautions: renal impairment

Contra-indications: peptic ulcer; pregnancy

Side-effects: vasodilatation, flushing, itching, rashes, erythema; occasionally, heartburn, epigastric pain, nausea, diarrhoea, headache, malaise

Dose: usually 500–750 mg daily in divided doses

PoM Olbetam® (Pharmacia)

Capsules, brown/pink, acipimox 250 mg. Net price 90-cap pack = £38.61. Label: 21

NICOTINIC ACID

Indications: see notes above

Cautions: diabetes mellitus, gout, liver disease, peptic ulcer; **interactions:** Appendix 1 (nicotinic acid)

Contra-indications: pregnancy, breast-feeding

Side-effects: flushing, dizziness, headache, palpitations, pruritus (prostaglandin-mediated symptoms can be reduced by low initial doses taken with meals, or by taking aspirin 75 mg 30 minutes before the dose); nausea, vomiting; rarely impaired liver function and rashes

Dose: initially 100–200 mg 3 times daily (see above), gradually increased over 2–4 weeks to 1–2 g 3 times daily

PoM [1]Nicotinic Acid Tablets, nicotinic acid 50 mg, net price 100 = £7.90. Label: 21

1. If max. daily dose exceeds 600 mg or if intended for treatment of hyperlipidaemia

---

FISH OILS

A fish-oil preparation (Maxepa®), rich in omega-3 marine triglycerides, is useful in the treatment of severe hypertriglyceridaemia; however, it can sometimes aggravate hypercholesterolaemia.

OMEGA-3 MARINE TRIGLYCERIDES

Indications: reduction of plasma triglycerides in patients with severe hypertriglyceridaemia judged to be at special risk of ischaemic heart disease and/or pancreatitis, in conjunction with dietary and other methods (see notes above)

Side-effects: occasional nausea and belching

Dose: see under preparations below

Maxepa® (Innovex)

Capsules, 1 g (approx. 1.1 mL) concentrated fish oils containing, as percentage of total fatty acid composition, eicosapentaenoic acid 18%, docosahexaenoic acid 12%. Vitamin A content less than 100 units/g, vitamin D content less than 10 units/g. Net price 200-cap pack = £28.57. Label: 21
Dose: 5 capsules twice daily with food

Emulsion, cream-coloured, concentrated fish oils containing, as percentage of total fatty acid composition, eicosapentaenoic acid 9%, docosahexaenoic acid 6%. Vitamin A content less than 100 units/g, vitamin D content less than 10 units/g. Net price 150 mL = £11.79. Label: 21
Dose: 10 mL twice daily with food

Liquid, golden-coloured, concentrated fish oils containing, as percentage of total fatty acid composition, eicosapentaenoic acid 18% w/w, docosahexaenoic acid 12% w/w. Vitamin A content less than 100 units/g, vitamin D content less than 10 units/g. Net price 150 mL = £21.43. Label: 21
Dose: 5 mL twice daily with food

OTHER DRUGS

Probucol decreases both LDL- and HDL-cholesterol; despite the latter effect it appears to promote resolution of xanthomata. Moreover, its antioxidant properties may decrease the atherogenicity of LDL.

PROBUCOL

Indications: see notes above
Cautions: ECG before treatment in patients with recent myocardial damage, ventricular arrhythmias; avoid pregnancy during and for 6 months after stopping treatment
Contra-indications: pregnancy and breast-feeding
Side-effects: generally mild and transient and mainly consist of gastro-intestinal effects such as nausea, vomiting, flatulence, diarrhoea, abdominal pain; ventricular arrhythmias and angioedema rarely reported
Dose: 500 mg twice daily with food

PoM **Lurselle®** (Merrell)
Tablets, scored, probucol 250 mg. Net price 120-tab pack = £13.07. Label: 21

2.13 Local sclerosants

Ethanolamine oleate and sodium tetradecyl sulphate are used in sclerotherapy of varicose veins, and phenol is used in haemorrhoids (see section 1.7.3).

ETHANOLAMINE OLEATE
(Monoethanolamine Oleate)
Indications: sclerotherapy of varicose veins
Cautions: extravasation may cause necrosis of tissues
Contra-indications: inability to walk, acute phlebitis, oral contraceptive use, obese legs
Side-effects: allergic reactions (including anaphylaxis)

PoM **Ethanolamine Oleate Injection**, ethanolamine oleate 5%. Net price 5-mL amp = £2.05
Available from Evans
Dose: by slow injection into empty isolated segment of vein, 2–5 mL divided between 3–4 sites; repeated at weekly intervals

SODIUM TETRADECYL SULPHATE
Indications: sclerotherapy of varicose veins
Cautions; Contra-indications; Side-effects: see under Ethanolamine Oleate

PoM **Fibro-Vein®** (STD Pharmaceutical)
Injection, sodium tetradecyl sulphate 0.2%, net price 5-mL amp = £2.20; 0.5%, 2-mL amp = £1.35; 1%, 2-mL amp = £1.46; 3%, 2-mL amp = £1.64, 5-mL vial = £3.15
Dose: by slow injection into empty isolated segment of vein, 0.1–1 mL according to site and condition being treated (consult manufacturer's literature)

3: Drugs used in the treatment of diseases of the
RESPIRATORY SYSTEM

In this chapter, drug treatment is described under the following headings:

3.1 Bronchodilators
3.2 Corticosteroids
3.3 Cromoglycate and related therapy
3.4 Antihistamines, hyposensitisation, and allergic emergencies
3.5 Respiratory stimulants and pulmonary surfactants
3.6 Oxygen
3.7 Mucolytics
3.8 Aromatic inhalations
3.9 Cough preparations
3.10 Systemic nasal decongestants

The initial treatment of exacerbations of chronic bronchitis and bacterial pneumonia is indicated in section 5.1 (table 1) and the treatment of tuberculosis is discussed in section 5.1.9.

3.1 Bronchodilators

3.1.1 Adrenoceptor stimulants
3.1.2 Antimuscarinic bronchodilators
3.1.3 Theophylline
3.1.4 Compound bronchodilator preparations
3.1.5 Peak flow meters, inhaler devices and nebulisers

3.1.1 Adrenoceptor stimulants
(Sympathomimetics)

The selective beta$_2$-adrenoceptor stimulants (selective beta$_2$-stimulants, selective beta$_2$-agonists) (section 3.1.1.1) such as salbutamol or terbutaline (preferably given by aerosol inhalation) are the safest and most effective beta-stimulants for asthma. They are recommended over the less selective beta-adrenoceptor stimulants such as isoprenaline or orciprenaline (section 3.1.1.2), which should be avoided whenever possible.

Adrenaline (see also section 2.7.3) (which has both alpha- and beta-adrenoceptor stimulant properties) is used in the emergency management of allergic and anaphylactic reactions (see section 3.4.3).

3.1.1.1 SELECTIVE BETA$_2$-ADRENOCEPTOR STIMULANTS

Most *mild to moderate* attacks of asthma respond rapidly to aerosol administration of a selective beta$_2$-adrenoceptor stimulant such as salbutamol or terbutaline. If beta$_2$-adrenoceptor stimulant inhalation is needed *more than once daily* prophylactic treatment should be considered, using a stepped approach as outlined on p. 120. However in *more severe attacks* a short course of an oral corticosteroid may be necessary to bring the asthma under control (section 3.2). Treatment of patients with *severe acute asthma* or airways obstruction (see

also below) is safer in hospital where oxygen and resuscitation facilities are immediately available (see also Acute Severe Asthma table, p. 121).

Patients with *chronic bronchitis* and *emphysema* are often described as having irreversible airways obstruction, but they usually respond partially to the beta$_2$-adrenoceptor stimulant drugs or to the antimuscarinic drugs ipratropium or oxitropium (section 3.1.2).

There is some evidence that patients who use beta$_2$-adrenoceptor stimulants on an 'as required' basis show a greater improvement in their asthma than those using them on a regular basis. For patients who require beta$_2$-adrenoceptor stimulants more than once daily, prophylactic treatment with an inhaled corticosteroid, cromoglycate, or nedocromil, should be tried.

There are some differences between the various selective beta$_2$-adrenoceptor stimulant drugs. **Salbutamol** and **terbutaline** are available in the widest range of formulations. **Rimiterol** has a shorter duration of action than salbutamol, terbutaline and fenoterol. **Fenoterol** may be less beta$_2$-selective than salbutamol.

Salmeterol is a longer-acting beta$_2$-adrenoceptor stimulant for twice daily administration; it is **not** suitable for the relief of an acute attack (a short-acting beta$_2$-stimulant such as salbutamol should be used). Salmeterol should be added to existing corticosteroid therapy and **not** replace it.

Eformoterol is a long-acting beta$_2$-adrenoceptor stimulant that has been introduced recently. It is reported to be similar in action to salmeterol but to have a more rapid onset of action.

Chronic Asthma table, see p. 120
Acute Severe Asthma table, see p. 121

INHALATION. *Pressurised (aerosol) inhalation*[1] is an effective and convenient method of administration for *mild to moderate* airways obstruction. The duration of action of an aerosol inhalation depends on the drug that it contains and the dose administered. With recommended doses rimiterol will usually last for 1 to 2 hours, salbutamol, terbutaline and fenoterol for 3 to 5 hours, and salmeterol for around 12 hours. Aerosol inhalation is preferred because it provides relief more rapidly and causes fewer side-effects (such as tremor and nervous tension) than tablets; this is because the drug is delivered directly to the bronchi and is therefore effective in smaller doses.

Patients should be given careful instruction on the use of their pressurised (aerosol) inhalers and it is important to check that they continue to use them

1. The British Medical Association has recommended that, where safety and efficacy will not be compromised, doctors should prescribe alternatives to pressurised metered dose inhalers containing chlorofluorocarbons (CFCs); see also CSM advice on p. 123.

correctly as inadequate technique may be mistaken for drug failure. In particular, it should be emphasised that they must inhale slowly and hold their breath for 10 seconds after inhalation. Most patients can be successfully taught to use pressurised (aerosol) inhalers but some patients, particularly the elderly, the arthritic, and small children are unable to use them; some patients are unable to synchronise their breathing with the administration of aerosol. For such patients a variety of *breath-actuated aerosol inhalers* and *spacing devices* (see section 3.1.5) is now available. Alternatively *dry powder inhalers*, activated by the patient's inspiration, are of value; some occasionally cause coughing.

The **dose** should be stated **explicitly** in terms of the number of inhalations at one time, the frequency, and the maximum number of inhalations allowed in 24 hours. High doses of beta$_2$-stimulants can be dangerous in some patients. Excessive use is usually an indication of **inadequately treated** asthma and should be treated with preventative medication such as an inhaled corticosteroid. Patients should be advised to seek medical advice when they fail to obtain their usual degree of symptomatic relief as this usually indicates a worsening of the asthma and may require alternative medication. When patients with asthma **are not adequately controlled** with inhalation of a beta$_2$-stimulant once or twice daily, **addition of a prophylactic drug** such as a corticosteroid inhalation should be considered (see Chronic Asthma table, p. 121); this is more convenient for the patient than higher doses of beta$_2$-stimulants and usually provides better overall control.

Respirator (or *nebuliser*) *solutions* of salbutamol and terbutaline are used for the treatment of *acute asthma* both in hospital and in general practice. They are administered over a period of about 15 minutes from a nebuliser, usually driven by oxygen in hospital. An electrical compressor is most suitable for domiciliary use but these are costly and not currently prescribable under the NHS. Patients with a severe attack of asthma should have oxygen if possible during nebulisation since beta-adrenoceptor stimulants can cause an increase in arterial hypoxaemia. For patients with *chronic bronchitis and hypercapnia*, however, oxygen can be dangerous, and the nebuliser should be driven by air. The dose prescribed by nebuliser is substantially higher than that prescribed by metered dose inhaler. For example, a 2.5-mL Ventolin Nebule® contains 2.5 mg of salbutamol, which is equivalent to 25 puffs from the aerosol inhaler. Patients should therefore be warned that it is dangerous to exceed the stated dose and that if they fail to respond to the usual dose of their respirator solution they should call for help. See also guidelines in section 3.1.5.

ORAL. *Oral preparations* are available for patients who cannot manage the inhaled route. They are sometimes used for children, though the inhaled route is better and most children can use one or other of the inhalation devices available. They have a slower onset but a slightly more prolonged action than the aerosol inhalers. The *modified-release* preparations may be of value in patients with *nocturnal asthma* as an alternative to the modified-release theophylline preparations (section 3.1.3).

PARENTERAL. *Intravenous*, and occasionally *subcutaneous*, injections of salbutamol and terbutaline are given for severe bronchospasm.

CHILDREN. Selective beta$_2$-adrenoceptor stimulants are useful even in children under the age of 18 months. They are most effective by the *inhaled route*, but an inhalation device may be needed (with the technique carefully checked). They are also effective *by mouth*. In severe attacks *nebulisation* using a selective beta$_2$-adrenoceptor stimulant or ipratropium is advisable (see also Asthma tables, pp. 120–21).

PREGNANCY AND BREAST-FEEDING. It is particularly important that asthma should be well-controlled during pregnancy; where this is achieved asthma has no important effects on pregnancy, labour, or the fetus.

Inhalation has particular advantages as a means of drug administration during pregnancy because the therapeutic action can be achieved without the need for plasma concentrations liable to have a pharmacological effect on the fetus.

Severe exacerbations of asthma can have an adverse effect on pregnancy and should be treated promptly with conventional therapy, including oral or parenteral administration of corticosteroids and nebulisation of a selective beta$_2$-adrenoceptor stimulant; prednisolone is the preferred corticosteroid for oral administration since placental transfer is slower than with some others.

Although theophylline has been given without adverse effects during pregnancy or breast-feeding there have been occasional reports of toxicity in the fetus and neonate.

SEVERE ACUTE ASTHMA

Severe asthma can be fatal and **must** be treated promptly and energetically. It is characterised by persistent dyspnoea poorly relieved by bronchodilators, exhaustion, a high pulse rate (usually over 110/minute), and a very low peak expiratory flow. The respiration is so shallow that wheezing may be absent. Such patients should be given oxygen (if available) and a large dose of a **corticosteroid** (see section 6.3.4)—for adults hydrocortisone 200 mg (preferably as sodium succinate) intravenously or prednisolone 40 mg by mouth, children half these doses. They should also be given **salbutamol** or **terbutaline** by nebuliser with oxygen if available. For a table outlining the management of acute severe asthma, see p. 121.

If there is little response the following additional treatment should be considered: **ipratropium** by nebuliser (section 3.1.2), **aminophylline** by slow intravenous injection, if the patient has not already been receiving theophylline (section 3.1.3), or change of administration of the beta$_2$-selective adrenoceptor stimulant to the intravenous route.

Start at **step most appropriate** to initial severity; **'rescue'** course of prednisolone at **any time** and **any step**

Adult step 1

Inhaled short-acting beta$_2$ stimulant as required (up to once daily)

Note. Move to step 2 if needed more than once daily (or night-time symptoms)

Adult step 2

Inhaled short-acting beta$_2$ stimulant as required
  plus
Regular standard-dose inhaled corticosteroid
  or try
Regular cromoglycate or nedocromil (but change to inhaled corticosteroid if control not achieved)

Note. Higher dose of inhaled corticosteroid may be required to gain initial control; some adults benefit from doubling for short period to cover an exacerbation

Adult step 3

Inhaled short-acting beta$_2$ stimulant as required
  plus
Regular high-dose inhaled corticosteroid (large-volume spacer)

Note. In few who have problems with high-dose inhaled corticosteroid continue with standard-dose inhaled corticosteroid *and add* regular inhaled long-acting beta$_2$ stimulant *or* regular modified-release oral theophylline *or* may *try* regular cromoglycate or nedocromil
In few with disproportionately prominent night-time symptoms (despite otherwise good control with standard-dose or high-dose corticosteroid inhalations), a modified-release oral theophylline *or* a long-acting inhaled beta$_2$ stimulant *or* a modified-release oral beta$_2$ stimulant, may be considered for administration at night

Adult step 4

Inhaled short-acting beta$_2$ stimulant as required
  with
Regular high-dose inhaled corticosteroid (large-volume spacer)
  plus sequential therapeutic trial of one or more of
Inhaled long-acting beta$_2$ stimulant
Modified-release oral theophylline
Inhaled ipratropium or oxitropium
Modified-release oral beta$_2$ stimulant
High-dose inhaled bronchodilators
Cromoglycate or nedocromil

Note. High doses of inhaled bronchodilators should only be considered if the patient does not respond to standard doses; beta$_2$ stimulants and ipratropium (or oxitropium) can be given using a nebuliser (or by multiple actuations of a metered dose inhaler with a large-volume spacer); for requirements before and when prescribing nebulisers, see p. 130

Adult step 5

Inhaled short-acting beta$_2$ stimulant as required
  with
Regular high-dose inhaled corticosteroid (large-volume spacer) *and with* one or more long-acting bronchodilators (see step 4)
  plus
Regular prednisolone tablets (as single daily dose)

Note. In addition to regular prednisolone tablets, continue high-dose inhaled corticosteroid (in exceptional cases doses exceeding those licensed may be used); these patients should normally be referred to a hospital asthma clinic

Stepping adult down

Review treatment every 3–6 months; if control achieved stepwise reduction may be possible; in patients whose treatment was started recently at step 4 or 5 (or contained corticosteroid tablets) reduction may take place after short interval; in chronic asthma a 3–6 month period of stability should be shown before slow stepwise reduction is undertaken

Child step 1

Short-acting beta$_2$ stimulant as required (not more than once daily)

Note. Whenever possible inhaled (less effective and more side-effects when given by mouth)

Child step 2

Inhaled short-acting beta$_2$ stimulant as required
  plus
Regular inhaled cromoglycate (powder or large-volume spacer)

Note. Try cromoglycate for 4–6 weeks before going to step 3 (supply peak flow meter where appropriate)

Child step 3

Inhaled short-acting beta$_2$ stimulant as required
  plus
Regular inhaled corticosteroid in standard paediatric dose (large-volume spacer)
  Consider for stabilisation
  Soluble tablets prednisolone 1–2 mg/kg daily for 1–5 days (max. 40 mg daily)
  or temporary doubling of dose of inhaled corticosteroid

Note. After 1 month assess effect on peak flow and/or symptoms and adjust dose; if control not adequate consider doubling dose of inhaled corticosteroid for 1 month (alternatively give short course of soluble prednisolone tablets by mouth or consider introducing other treatments)

Child step 4

Inhaled short-acting beta$_2$ stimulant as required
  plus
Regular inhaled corticosteroid in high paediatric dose (large-volume spacer or dry powder device)
  Consider
  Soluble prednisolone tablets 1–2 mg/kg daily for 1–5 days (max. 40 mg daily)
  Regular inhaled long-acting beta$_2$ stimulant

Note. Long-acting beta$_2$ stimulant should probably be reserved for supplementing treatment in child already receiving cromoglycate or a corticosteroid

Child step 5a

Inhaled short-acting beta$_2$ stimulant as required
  with
Regular inhaled corticosteroid in high paediatric dose (large-volume spacer or dry powder device)
As in step 4, consider soluble tablets prednisolone *with* regular inhaled long-acting beta$_2$ stimulant
  plus
  Regular modified-release oral theophylline *or* nebulised beta$_2$ stimulant

Note. Modified-release oral theophylline may be helpful (particularly for nocturnal symptoms), but has appreciable side-effects in up to one-third of children (plasma or salivary-concentration monitoring recommended); similar clinical improvements, with fewer side-effects, have been shown with modified-release oral salbutamol

Child step 5b

As step 5a
  plus
Prednisolone 5–10 mg on alternate days
  Consider
  Regular inhaled ipratropium *or* subcutaneous infusion of short-acting beta$_2$ stimulant

Stepping child down

Regularly review need for treatment; in older child use peak flow record to assess speed of withdrawal; stop cromoglycate or corticosteroid after 6–12 months of few or no symptoms (if symptoms seasonal consider stopping at end of season).

Based on tables in: British Thoracic Society, the British Paediatric Association and others. Guidelines on the Management of Asthma. *Thorax* 1993; **48** (suppl); S1–S24. Reproduced with permission of BMJ Specialist Journals

MANAGEMENT OF ACUTE SEVERE ASTHMA IN GENERAL PRACTICE

Uncontrolled asthma in adults

— Speech normal
— Pulse <110 beats/minute
— Respiration <25 breaths/minute
— Peak flow >50% of predicted or best

Treat at home but response to treatment **must** be assessed before doctor leaves

Treatment:
Nebulised salbutamol 5 mg or nebulised terbutaline 10 mg
Monitor response 15–30 minutes after nebulisation

If peak flow 50–75% of predicted or best give:
Oral prednisolone 30–60 mg
and step up usual treatment
Alternatively if peak flow >75% of predicted or best:
Step up usual treatment

Follow up
Monitor symptoms and peak flow
Set up self management plan
Review in surgery within 48 hours
Modify treatment at review according to guidelines for chronic asthma (see opposite page)

Important: regard each emergency consultation as being for **acute severe asthma** until shown otherwise.

Acute severe asthma in adults

— Cannot complete sentences
— Pulse ≥110 beats/minute
— Respiration ≥25 breaths/minute
— Peak flow <50% of predicted or best
Seriously consider hospital admission if more than one of above features present

Treatment:
Oxygen 40–60% if available
Nebulised salbutamol 5 mg or nebulised terbutaline 10 mg
Oral prednisolone 30–60 mg or i/v hydrocortisone 200 mg
Monitor response 15–30 minutes after nebulisation

If any signs of acute asthma persist:
Arrange hospital admission
While awaiting ambulance repeat nebulised beta$_2$ stimulant and give with nebulised ipratropium 500 micrograms
or give subcutaneous terbutaline
or give slow intravenous aminophylline 250 mg (**important:** not if taking an oral theophylline)
Alternatively if symptoms have improved, respiration and pulse settling, and peak flow >50% of predicted or best:
Step up usual treatment *and* continue prednisolone

Follow up
Monitor symptoms and peak flow
Set up self management plan
Review in surgery within 24 hours
Modify treatment at review (see opposite page)

Life-threatening asthma in adults

— Silent chest
— Cyanosis
— Bradycardia or exhaustion
— Peak flow <33% of predicted or best
Arrange IMMEDIATE hospital admission

Treatment:
Oral prednisolone 30–60 mg or i/v hydrocortisone 200 mg (immediately)
Oxygen-driven nebuliser in ambulance
Nebulised[1] beta$_2$ stimulant with nebulised ipratropium or subcutaneous terbutaline
or slow intravenous aminophylline 250 mg (**important:** not if taking an oral theophylline)
STAY WITH PATIENT UNTIL AMBULANCE ARRIVES
1. If no nebuliser available give 2 puffs of beta$_2$ stimulant using large-volume spacer and repeat 10 – 20 times

Important: do not give bolus aminophylline to patient already taking an oral theophylline.

Important: patients with severe or life-threatening attacks may not be distressed and may not have all these abnormalities; the presence of any should alert doctor.

Signs of acute asthma in children

Acute severe asthma:
— too breathless to talk
— too breathless to feed
— respiration ≥50 breaths/minute
— pulse ≥140 beats/minute
— peak flow <50% of predicted or best

Life-threatening features:
— peak flow <33% of predicted or best
— cyanosis, silent chest, or poor respiratory effort
— fatigue or exhaustion
— agitation or reduced level of consciousness

Important: failure to respond adequately at **any time** requires immediate referral to hospital.

Features of treatment of acute asthma in children

— short-acting beta$_2$ stimulant from metered dose inhaler using large-volume spacer device may be as effective as use of nebuliser; dose is one puff every few seconds until improvement occurs (max. 20 puffs), using face mask in very young child
— terbutaline may be given subcutaneously in severe episodes
— oxygen is of benefit

— a child requiring high-dose inhaled bronchodilators should also receive soluble tablets prednisolone 1–2 mg/kg (max. 40 mg) once daily for up to 5 days if necessary; child needs immediate referral to hospital if failure to respond
— aminophylline should no longer be used in children at home

Further treatment of these patients is safer in hospital where resuscitation facilities are immediately available. Treatment should **never** be delayed for investigations, patients should **never** be sedated, and the possibility of a pneumothorax should also be remembered.

If the patient deteriorates despite appropriate pharmacological treatment, intermittent positive pressure ventilation may be needed temporarily.

SALBUTAMOL

Indications: asthma and other conditions associated with reversible airways obstruction; premature labour, see section 7.1.3

Cautions: hyperthyroidism, myocardial insufficiency, arrhythmias, susceptibility to QT-interval prolongation, hypertension, pregnancy and breast-feeding (but appropriate to use, see notes above); diabetes—especially intravenous administration to diabetics (monitor blood glucose; ketoacidosis reported); see also notes above; **interactions:** Appendix 1 (sympathomimetics, beta₂)

HYPOKALAEMIA. The CSM has advised that potentially serious hypokalaemia may result from beta₂-adrenoceptor stimulant therapy. Particular caution is required in severe asthma, as this effect may be potentiated by concomitant treatment with theophylline and its derivatives, corticosteroids, and diuretics, and by hypoxia. Plasma-potassium concentrations should therefore be monitored in severe asthma.

Side-effects: fine tremor (usually hands), nervous tension, headache, peripheral vasodilatation, palpitations, tachycardia (seldom troublesome when given by aerosol inhalation); rarely muscle cramps; hypokalaemia after high doses (for **CSM** advice see under Cautions above); hypersensitivity reactions including paradoxical bronchospasm, urticaria, and angioedema reported; slight pain on intramuscular injection

Dose: by mouth, 4 mg (elderly and sensitive patients initially 2 mg) 3–4 times daily; max. single dose 8 mg (but unlikely to provide much extra benefit or to be tolerated); CHILD under 2 years 100 micrograms/kg 4 times daily; 2–6 years 1–2 mg 3–4 times daily, 6–12 years 2 mg

By subcutaneous or intramuscular injection, 500 micrograms, repeated every 4 hours if necessary

By slow intravenous injection, 250 micrograms, repeated if necessary

By intravenous infusion, initially 5 micrograms/minute, adjusted according to response and heart-rate usually in range 3–20 micrograms/minute, or more if necessary

By aerosol inhalation, 100–200 micrograms (1–2 puffs); for persistent symptoms up to 3–4 times daily (but see also Chronic asthma table); CHILD 100 micrograms (1 puff), increased to 200 micrograms (2 puffs) if necessary

Prophylaxis in exercise-induced bronchospasm, 200 micrograms (2 puffs); CHILD 100 micrograms (1 puff)

By inhalation of a powder (Rotacaps®, Ventodisks®; for Accuhaler® dose see under preparation), 200–400 micrograms; for persistent symptoms up to 3–4 times daily (but see also Chronic Asthma table); CHILD 200 micrograms

Prophylaxis in exercise-induced bronchospasm (*powder*), 400 micrograms; CHILD 200 micrograms

Note. Bioavailability appears to be lower, so recommended doses for dry powder inhalers are twice those in a metered inhaler

By inhalation of nebulised solution, chronic bronchospasm unresponsive to conventional therapy and severe acute asthma, ADULT and CHILD over 18 months 2.5 mg, repeated up to 4 times daily; may be increased to 5 mg if necessary, but medical assessment should be considered since alternative therapy may be indicated; CHILD under 18 months, clinical efficacy uncertain (transient hypoxaemia may occur—consider supplemental oxygen)

Oral

PoM Salbutamol (Non-proprietary)

Tablets, salbutamol (as sulphate) 2 mg, net price 20 = 14p; 4 mg, 20 = 27p

Available from A&H (Ventolin®), APS, Berk (Asmaven®), Cox, Hillcross, Norton

PoM Ventolin® (A&H)

Tablets, both pink, scored, salbutamol (as sulphate), 2 mg, net price 20 = 22p; 4 mg, 20 = 43p

Syrup, sugar-free, salbutamol 2 mg (as sulphate)/ 5 mL. Net price 150 mL = 71p

PoM Volmax® (DF)

Tablets, m/r, salbutamol (as sulphate) 4 mg, net price 56-tab pack = £10.55; 8 mg, 56-tab pack = £12.66. Label: 25

Dose: 8 mg twice daily; CHILD 3–12 years 4 mg twice daily

Parenteral

PoM Ventolin® (A&H)

Injection, salbutamol 50 micrograms (as sulphate)/ mL. Net price 5-mL amp = 57p

Injection, salbutamol 500 micrograms (as sulphate)/mL. Net price 1-mL amp = 43p

Solution for intravenous infusion, salbutamol 1 mg (as sulphate)/mL. Dilute before use. Net price 5-mL amp = £3.08

Inhalation

COUNSELLING. Advise patients not to exceed prescribed dose and to follow manufacturer's directions; if a previously effective dose of inhaled salbutamol fails to provide at least 3 hours relief, a doctor's advice should be obtained as soon as possible

PoM Salbutamol (Non-proprietary)

Aerosol inhalation, salbutamol 100 micrograms/ metered inhalation, net price 200-dose unit = £1.71. Counselling, dose

Available from A&H (Ventolin®), APS, Ashbourne (Maxivent®), Baker Norton (Salamol®), Berk (Asmaven®), Cox, CP, 3M (Salbulin®), Norton

Note. Vortex-based aerosol inhalers releasing salbutamol 100 micrograms/metered inhalation also available from Evans (Salbutamol Spacehaler®)

Additives: include CFC propellants

PoM **Aerolin® Autohaler** (3M)

Aerosol inhalation, salbutamol 100 micrograms (as sulphate)/metered inhalation. Net price 200-dose breath-actuated unit = £10.51; also 100-dose unit = £5.26 (hosp. only). Counselling, dose

Additives: include CFC propellants

Note. Breath-actuated aerosol inhalers containing salbutamol 100 micrograms/metered inhalation also available from Baker Norton (Salamol Easi-Breathe®)

▼ PoM **Airomir®** (3M)

Aerosol inhalation, salbutamol (as sulphate) 100 micrograms/metered inhalation. Net price 200-dose unit = £2.06. Counselling, dose

Additives: include HFA-134a (a non-CFC propellant)

Note. Can only be supplied against a generic prescription when prescription has been written for 'salbutamol sulphate inhaler', salbutamol sulphate inhaler CFC free', or 'salbutamol inhaler CFC free'

PoM **Steri-Neb Salamol®** (Baker Norton)

Nebuliser solution, salbutamol 0.1% (1 mg/mL, as sulphate), net price 20 × 2.5 mL (2.5 mg) = £3.06; 0.2% (2 mg/mL), 20 × 2.5 mL (5 mg) = £6.14. May be diluted with sterile sodium chloride 0.9% if administration time in excess of 10 minutes is required

GLAUCOMA. For warning of *acute angle closure glaucoma* in patients receiving nebulised ipratropium and salbutamol, see p. 127

PoM **Ventodisks®** (A&H)

Dry powder for inhalation, disks containing 8 blisters of salbutamol (as sulphate) 200 micrograms/blister, net price 14 disks with Diskhaler® device = £7.11; 14-disk refill = £6.54; 400 micrograms/blister, 14 disks with Diskhaler® device = £12.02; 14-disk refill = £11.45. Counselling, dose

PoM **Ventolin®** (A&H)

Accuhaler® (dry powder for inhalation), disk containing 60 blisters of salbutamol (as sulphate) 200 micrograms/blister with *Accuhaler®* device, net price = £5.00. Counselling, dose

Dose: by inhalation of powder, 200 micrograms; for persistant symptoms up to 4 times daily (but see also Chronic Asthma table); CHILD 200 micrograms

Prophylaxis in allergen- or exercise-induced bronchospasm, 200 micrograms

Aerosol inhalation, salbutamol 100 micrograms/metered inhalation. Net price 200-dose unit = £2.30. Counselling, dose

Additives: include CFC propellants

Nebules® (for use with nebuliser), salbutamol 0.1% (1 mg/mL, as sulphate), net price 2.5 mL (2.5 mg) = 19p; 0.2% (2 mg/mL), 2.5 mL (5 mg) = 38p. May be diluted with sterile sodium chloride 0.9% if administration time in excess of 10 minutes is required

GLAUCOMA. For warning of *acute angle closure glaucoma* in patients receiving nebulised ipratropium and salbutamol, see p. 127

Respirator solution (for use with a nebuliser or ventilator), salbutamol 0.5% (5 mg/mL, as sulphate). Net price 20 mL = £2.71 (hosp. only). May be diluted with sterile sodium chloride 0.9%

GLAUCOMA. For warning of *acute angle closure glaucoma* in patients receiving nebulised ipratropium and salbutamol, see p. 127

Rotacaps® (dry powder for inhalation; for use with Ventolin Rotahaler®), salbutamol (as sulphate), 200 micrograms (light-blue/clear), net price 112-cap pack = £5.92; 400 micrograms (dark-blue/clear), 112-cap pack = £10.01. Counselling, dose

Compound preparations

For some **compound preparations** containing salbutamol, see section 3.1.4

Inhaler devices
See section 3.1.5

> **CSM advice.** Chlorofluorocarbons (CFCs) are gradually being replaced by hydrofluoroalkanes (HFAs) as the propellants used in pressurised (aerosol) inhalations for asthma.
> The CSM has requested doctors to report any adverse reaction to the new HFA-containing inhalers and to include the brand name of the inhaler on the yellow card.

TERBUTALINE SULPHATE

Indications; Cautions; Side-effects: see under Salbutamol; premature labour, see section 7.1.3

Dose: by mouth, 2.5 mg 3 times daily for 1–2 weeks, then up to 5 mg 3 times daily; CHILD 75 micrograms/kg 3 times daily; 7–15 years 2.5 mg 2–3 times daily

By subcutaneous, intramuscular, or slow intravenous injection, 250–500 micrograms up to 4 times daily; CHILD 2–15 years 10 micrograms/kg to a max. of 300 micrograms

By continuous intravenous infusion as a solution containing 3–5 micrograms/mL, 1.5–5 micrograms/minute for 8–10 hours; reduce dose for children

By aerosol inhalation, adults and children 250–500 micrograms (1–2 puffs); for persistent symptoms up to 3–4 times daily (but see also Chronic Asthma table)

By inhalation of powder (Turbohaler®), 500 micrograms (1 inhalation); for persistent symptoms up to 4 times daily (but see also Chronic Asthma table)

By inhalation of nebulised solution, 5–10 mg 2–4 times daily; additional doses may be necessary in severe acute asthma; CHILD, up to 3 years 2 mg, 3–6 years 3 mg; 6–8 years 4 mg, over 8 years 5 mg, 2–4 times daily

Oral and parenteral
PoM **Bricanyl®** (Astra)

Tablets, scored, terbutaline sulphate 5 mg. Net price 20 = 74p

Syrup, sugar-free, terbutaline sulphate 1.5 mg/5 mL. Net price 300 mL = £2.36

Injection, terbutaline sulphate 500 micrograms/mL. Net price 1-mL amp = 27p; 5-mL amp = £1.27

PoM **Bricanyl SA®** (Astra)

Tablets, m/r, terbutaline sulphate 7.5 mg. Net price 20 = £1.55. Label: 25

Dose: 7.5 mg twice daily

PoM **Monovent®** (Lagap)

Syrup, terbutaline sulphate 1.5 mg/5 mL. Net price 300 mL = £2.25

Inhalation

COUNSELLING. Advise patients not to exceed prescribed dose and to follow manufacturer's directions; if a previously effective dose of inhaled terbutaline fails to provide at least 3 hours relief, a doctor's advice should be obtained as soon as possible; little sensation associated with use of Turbohaler®

PoM **Bricanyl**® (Astra)

Aerosol inhalation, terbutaline sulphate 250 micrograms/metered inhalation. Net price 400-dose unit = £5.31; 400-dose unit with Spacer device (collapsible extended mouthpiece) = £7.21; 400-dose refill canister for use with Nebuhaler or Spacer inhaler = £5.21. Counselling, dose
Additives: include CFC propellants

Turbohaler® (= dry powder inhaler), terbutaline sulphate 500 micrograms/inhalation. Net price 100-dose unit = £7.96. Counselling, dose

Respules® (= single-dose units for nebulisation), terbutaline sulphate 2.5 mg/mL. Net price 20 × 2-mL units = £3.67

Respirator solution (for use with a nebuliser or ventilator), terbutaline sulphate 10 mg/mL. Net price 10 mL = £1.32. Before use dilute with sterile sodium chloride 0.9%

Inhaler devices
See section 3.1.5

Chronic Asthma table, see p. 120?
Acute Severe Asthma table, see p. 121

BAMBUTEROL HYDROCHLORIDE

Note. Bambuterol is a pro-drug of terbutaline

Indications: asthma and other conditions associated with reversible airways obstruction

Cautions; Side-effects: see under Salbutamol; reduce dose in renal impairment; avoid in cirrhosis, severe hepatic impairment; manufacturer advises avoid in pregnancy

Dose: 20 mg once daily at bedtime if patient has previously tolerated beta$_2$-adrenoceptor stimulants; other patients, initially 10 mg once daily at bedtime, increased if necessary after 1–2 weeks to 20 mg once daily; CHILD not recommended

▼ PoM **Bambec**® (Novex)

Tablets, both scored, bambuterol hydrochloride 10 mg, net price 28-tab pack = £10.95; 20 mg, 28-tab pack = £13.14

EFORMOTEROL FUMARATE

Indications: reversible airways obstruction (including nocturnal asthma and prevention of exercise-induced bronchospasm) in patients requiring long-term regular bronchodilator therapy, who should normally also be receiving regular and adequate doses of inhaled anti-inflammatory drugs (e.g. corticosteroids and/or sodium cromoglycate) or oral corticosteroids; see also Chronic Asthma table, p. 120

Note. Eformoterol is not for immediate relief of acute attacks and existing corticosteroid therapy should not be reduced or withdrawn

Cautions; Side-effects: see under Salbutamol and notes above; oropharyngeal irritation, conjunctival irritation and eyelid oedema, taste disturbances, rash, insomnia, nausea and pruritus also reported; manufacturer advises avoid in pregnancy (unless no more-established alternative) and breast-feeding; **important:** potential for paradoxical bronchospasm (calling for discontinuation and alternative therapy)

Dose: by inhalation of a powder, ADULT over 18 years 12–24 micrograms twice daily; CHILD under 18 years not recommended

▼ PoM **Foradil**® (Geigy)

Dry powder for inhalation, eformoterol fumarate 12 micrograms/capsule, net price 56-dose unit (with inhaler device) = £24.00, 14-dose unit (with inhaler device) = £6.00 (hosp. only). Counselling, dose
COUNSELLING. Advise patients that eformoterol should not be used for relief of acute attacks, not to exceed prescribed dose, and to follow manufacturer's directions; if a previously effective dose of inhaled eformoterol fails to provide at least 2 hours relief, a doctor's advice should be obtained as soon as possible

FENOTEROL HYDROBROMIDE

Indications: reversible airways obstruction
Cautions; Side-effects: see under Salbutamol
Dose: by aerosol inhalation, 200 micrograms (2 puffs Berotec '100') 1–3 times daily, and see also Berotec '200' below (but see also Chronic asthma table); CHILD 6–12 years 100 micrograms (1 puff Berotec '100')

Persistent bronchospasm not adequately controlled by Berotec '100', *by aerosol inhalation,* 200–400 micrograms (1–2 puffs Berotec '200') 1–3 times daily; not more than 400 micrograms (2 puffs Berotec '200') every 6 hours; max. 1.6 mg daily (**important:** see also Chronic asthma table); CHILD under 16 years, not recommended

PoM **Berotec**® (Boehringer Ingelheim)

'100' aerosol inhalation, fenoterol hydrobromide 100 micrograms/metered inhalation. Net price 200-dose unit = £2.36. Counselling, dose
Additives: include CFC propellants

'200' aerosol inhalation, fenoterol hydrobromide 200 micrograms/metered inhalation. Net price 200-dose unit = £2.78. Counselling, dose
Additives: include CFC propellants

Note. Only for persistent bronchospasm inadequately controlled by Berotec '100'
COUNSELLING. Advise patients not to exceed prescribed dose and to follow manufacturer's directions; if a previously effective dose of inhaled fenoterol fails to provide at least 3 hours relief, a doctor's advice should be obtained as soon as possible

Compound preparations
For some **compound preparations** containing fenoterol, see section 3.1.4

PIRBUTEROL

Indications: reversible airways obstruction
Cautions; Side-effects: see under Salbutamol
Dose: by inhalation, 200–400 micrograms (1–2 puffs); persistent symptoms, up to 4 times daily (but see also Chronic Asthma table)
CHILD under 12 years not recommended

PoM **Exirel®** (3M)

Aerosol inhalation, pirbuterol 200 micrograms (as acetate)/metered inhalation. Net price 200-dose unit = £3.78. Counselling, dose

Additives: include CFC propellants

COUNSELLING. Advise patients not to exceed prescribed dose and to follow manufacturer's directions; if a previously effective dose of inhaled pirbuterol fails to provide at least 3 hours relief, a doctor's advice should be obtained as soon as possible

REPROTEROL HYDROCHLORIDE

Indications: reversible airways obstruction

Cautions; Side-effects: see under Salbutamol

Dose: by aerosol inhalation, 0.5–1 mg (1–2 puffs); persistent symptoms, up to 3 times daily (but see also Chronic Asthma table); CHILD 6–12 years 500 micrograms (1 puff)

PoM **Bronchodil®** (ASTA Medica)

Aerosol inhalation, reproterol hydrochloride 500 micrograms/metered inhalation. Net price 400-dose unit = £7.34. Counselling, dose

Additives: include CFC propellants

COUNSELLING. Advise patients not to exceed prescribed dose and to follow manufacturer's directions; if a previously effective dose of inhaled reproterol fails to provide at least 3 hours relief, a doctor's advice should be obtained as soon as possible

RIMITEROL HYDROBROMIDE

Indications: reversible airways obstruction

Cautions; Side-effects: see under Salbutamol

Dose: by aerosol inhalation, adults and children 200–600 micrograms (1–3 puffs); should not be repeated in less than 30 minutes; max. 8 doses daily (but see also Chronic Asthma table)

PoM **Pulmadil®** (3M)

Aerosol inhalation, rimiterol hydrobromide 200 micrograms/metered inhalation. Net price 300-dose unit = £5.06. Counselling, dose

Additives: include CFC propellants

COUNSELLING. Advise patients not to exceed prescribed dose and to follow manufacturer's directions; if a previously effective dose of inhaled rimiterol fails to provide at least 1–2 hours relief, a doctor's advice should be obtained as soon as possible

SALMETEROL

Indications: reversible airways obstruction (including nocturnal asthma and prevention of exercise-induced bronchospasm) in patients requiring long-term regular bronchodilator therapy, who should normally also be receiving regular and adequate doses of inhaled anti-inflammatory drugs (e.g. corticosteroids and/or, in children, sodium cromoglycate) or oral corticosteroids; see also Chronic Asthma table, p. 120

Note. CSM has emphasised that salmeterol is not for immediate relief of acute attacks and that existing corticosteroid therapy should not be reduced or withdrawn

Cautions; Side-effects: see under Salbutamol and notes above; **important:** significant incidence of paradoxical bronchospasm, which may be clinically important in severe or deteriorating asthma

Dose: by inhalation, 50 micrograms (2 puffs or 1 blister) twice daily; up to 100 micrograms (4 puffs or 2 blisters) twice daily in more severe airways obstruction; CHILD under 4 years not recommended, over 4 years, 50 micrograms (2 puffs or 1 blister) twice daily

PoM **Serevent®** (A&H)

Accuhaler® (dry powder for inhalation), disk containing 60 blisters of salmeterol (as xinafoate (= hydroxynaphthoate)) 50 micrograms/blister with *Accuhaler®* device, net price = £29.97. Counselling, dose

Aerosol inhalation, salmeterol (as xinafoate (= hydroxynaphthoate)) 25 micrograms/metered inhalation, net price 120-inhalation unit = £28.60. Counselling, dose

Additives: include CFC propellants

Diskhaler® (dry powder for inhalation), disks containing 4 blisters of salmeterol (as xinafoate (= hydroxynaphthoate)) 50 micrograms/blister, net price 14 disks with Diskhaler® device = £29.97; 14-disk refill = £29.40. Counselling, dose

COUNSELLING. Advise patients that salmeterol should **not** be used for relief of acute attacks, not to exceed prescribed dose, and to follow manufacturer's directions; if a previously effective dose of inhaled salmeterol fails to provide at least 12 hours relief, a doctor's advice should be obtained as soon as possible

TULOBUTEROL HYDROCHLORIDE

Indications: reversible airways obstruction

Cautions: see under Salbutamol; also mild renal impairment (avoid if severe); pregnancy (manufacturer states not yet established)

Contra-indications: moderate to severe renal impairment; acute liver failure, chronic liver disease

Side-effects: see under Salbutamol

Dose: 2 mg twice daily; increased if necessary to 2 mg 3 times daily; CHILD 6–10 years 0.5–1 mg twice daily; over 10 years, 1–2 mg twice daily

PoM **Respacal®** (UCB Pharma)

Tablets, f/c, scored, tulobuterol hydrochloride 2 mg. Net price 60-tab pack = £12.54

Syrup, sugar-free, tulobuterol hydrochloride 1 mg/ 5 mL. Net price 150 mL = £4.48

3.1.1.2 OTHER ADRENOCEPTOR STIMULANTS

These preparations (including the partially selective orciprenaline) are now regarded as less suitable and less safe for use as bronchodilators than the selective beta$_2$-adrenoceptor stimulants, as they are more likely to cause arrhythmias and other side-effects. They should be avoided whenever possible.

Adrenaline injection (1 in 1000) is used in the emergency treatment of acute allergic and anaphylactic reactions (section 3.4.3).

EPHEDRINE HYDROCHLORIDE

Indications: reversible airways obstruction, but see notes above

Cautions: hyperthyroidism, diabetes mellitus, ischaemic heart disease, hypertension, renal impairment, elderly; may cause acute retention in prostatic hypertrophy; interaction with MAOIs a disadvantage; **interactions:** Appendix 1 (sympathomimetics)

Side-effects: tachycardia, anxiety, restlessness, insomnia common; also tremor, arrhythmias, dry mouth, cold extremities

Dose: 3 times daily, 15–60 mg; CHILD 3 times daily, up to 1 year 7.5 mg, 1–5 years 15 mg, 6–12 years 30 mg (not recommended, see above)

PoM ¹ **Ephedrine Hydrochloride** (Non-proprietary)
Tablets, ephedrine hydrochloride 15 mg, net price 20 = 44p; 30 mg, 20 = 50p; 60 mg, 20 = £1.11
Elixir, ephedrine hydrochloride 15 mg/5 mL in a suitable flavoured vehicle, containing alcohol 12%. Net price 100 mL = 81p
1. For exemptions see *Medicines, Ethics and Practice,* No. 16, London, Pharmaceutical Press, 1996 (and subsequent editions as available)
For a list of **cough and decongestant preparations on sale to the public**, including those containing ephedrine, see section 3.9.2

ISOPRENALINE SULPHATE

Indications: reversible airways obstruction, but see notes above

Cautions; Side-effects: see under Salbutamol (section 3.1.1.1) and notes above; **interactions:** Appendix 1 (sympathomimetics)
COUNSELLING. Advise patients not to exceed prescribed dose and to follow manufacturer's directions; if a previously effective dose of inhaled isoprenaline fails to provide at least 3 hours relief, a doctor's advice should be obtained as soon as possible

PoM **Medihaler-iso®** (3M)
Aerosol inhalation, isoprenaline sulphate 80 micrograms/metered inhalation. Net price 400-dose vial = £2.43
Additives: include CFC propellants
Note. Not recommended therefore no dose stated
PoM **Medihaler-iso® Forte** (3M)
Aerosol inhalation, isoprenaline sulphate 400 micrograms/metered inhalation. Net price 400-dose vial = £2.82
Additives: include CFC propellants
Note. Not recommended therefore no dose stated

ORCIPRENALINE SULPHATE

Indications: reversible airways obstruction, but see notes above

Cautions; Side-effects: see under Salbutamol (section 3.1.1.1) and notes above; **interactions:** Appendix 1 (sympathomimetics)

Dose: by mouth, 20 mg 4 times daily; CHILD up to 1 year 5–10 mg 3 times daily, 1–3 years 5–10 mg 4 times daily, 3–12 years 40–60 mg daily in divided doses (but not recommended, see above)

By aerosol inhalation, 750–1500 micrograms (1–2 puffs) repeated if necessary after not less than 30 minutes to a max. of 9 mg (12 puffs) daily; CHILD up to 6 years 750 micrograms (1 puff) up to 4 times daily, 6–12 years 750–1500 micrograms (1–2 puffs) up to 4 times daily (but not recommended, see notes above)

PoM **Alupent®** (Boehringer Ingelheim)
Tablets, scored, orciprenaline sulphate 20 mg. Net price 100-tab pack = £3.80
Syrup, sugar-free, orciprenaline sulphate 10 mg/5 mL. Net price 100 mL = 75p

Aerosol inhalation, orciprenaline sulphate 750 micrograms/metered inhalation. Net price 300-dose vial with mouthpiece = £3.22; refill vial = £2.66. Counselling, dose
Additives: include CFC propellants
COUNSELLING. Advise patients not to exceed prescribed dose and to follow manufacturer's directions; if a previously effective dose of inhaled orciprenaline fails to provide at least 3 hours relief, a doctor's advice should be obtained as soon as possible

PSEUDOEPHEDRINE HYDROCHLORIDE

Cautions; Side-effects: see under Ephedrine Hydrochloride

Preparations
See section 3.10

3.1.2   Antimuscarinic bronchodilators

These drugs have traditionally been regarded as more effective in relieving bronchoconstriction associated with chronic bronchitis. **Ipratropium** may provide some bronchodilation in patients with chronic bronchitis who fail to respond to the selective beta$_2$-adrenoceptor stimulants (section 3.1.1.1). Unlike the older antimuscarinic drugs, side-effects are rare and it does not increase sputum viscosity or affect mucociliary clearance of sputum. The aerosol inhalation has a maximum effect 30–60 minutes after use; its duration of action is 3 to 6 hours and bronchodilatation can usually be maintained with treatment three times a day.

Oxitropium has a similar action to that of ipratropium.

IPRATROPIUM BROMIDE

Indications: reversible airways obstruction, particularly in chronic bronchitis
Cautions: glaucoma (standard doses unlikely to be harmful but see also under nebuliser, below); prostatic hypertrophy; pregnancy
Side-effects: dry mouth occasionally reported; rarely urinary retention, constipation
Dose: see below

PoM **Atrovent®** (Boehringer Ingelheim)
COUNSELLING. Advise patient not to exceed prescribed dose and to follow manufacturer's directions
Aerocaps® (dry powder for inhalation; for use with Atrovent Aerohaler®), green, ipratropium bromide 40 micrograms. Net price pack of 100 caps with Aerohaler® = £14.53; 100 caps = £10.53. Counselling, dose
Dose: by inhalation of powder, 40 micrograms (1 Aerocap®) 3–4 times daily (may be doubled in less responsive patients); CHILD under 12 years, not recommended
Note. One Atrovent Aerocap® is equivalent to 2 puffs of Atrovent® metered aerosol inhalation *or* 1 puff of Atrovent Forte® metered aerosol inhalation
Aerosol inhalation, ipratropium bromide 20 micrograms/metered inhalation. Net price 200-dose unit = £4.21. Counselling, dose
Additives: include CFC propellants
Dose: by aerosol inhalation, 20–40 micrograms (1–2 puffs), in early treatment up to 80 micrograms (4 puffs) at a time, 3–4 times daily; CHILD up to 6 years 20 micrograms (1 puff) 3 times daily, 6–12 years 20–40 micrograms (1–2 puffs) 3 times daily

---

Autohaler® (= breath-actuated aerosol inhalation), ipratropium bromide 20 micrograms/metered inhalation. Net price 200-dose unit = £10.43. Counselling, dose
Additives: include CFC propellants
Dose: by aerosol inhalation, 20–40 micrograms (1–2 puffs), in early treatment up to 80 micrograms (4 puffs) at a time, 3–4 times daily; CHILD up to 6 years 20 micrograms (1 puff) 3 times daily, 6–12 years 20–40 micrograms (1–2 puffs) 3 times daily

Forte aerosol inhalation, ipratropium bromide 40 micrograms/metered inhalation. Net price 200-dose unit = £5.65. Counselling, dose
Additives: include CFC propellants
Dose: by aerosol inhalation 40 micrograms (1 puff), in early treatment 80 micrograms (2 puffs), 3–4 times daily; CHILD 6–12 years 40 micrograms (1 puff) 3 times daily

Nebuliser solution, isotonic, ipratropium bromide 250 micrograms/mL (0.025%); net price 20 × 1-mL unit-dose vials (preservative-free) = £6.82; 20 × 2-mL vials = £8.00. If dilution is necessary use only sterile sodium chloride solution 0.9%
Dose: reversible airways obstruction, *by inhalation of nebulised solution*, 100–500 micrograms (0.4–2 mL of a 0.025% solution) up to 4 times daily; CHILD 3–14 years 100–500 micrograms up to 3 times daily. Dilution of solution is adjusted according to equipment and length of administration. Because paradoxical bronchospasm has occurred, *first dose* should be inhaled under medical supervision
GLAUCOMA. *Acute angle closure glaucoma* has been reported in patients given nebulised ipratropium, particularly when used in association with nebulised salbutamol. Special caution is needed and care should be taken to **avoid** escape from mask to patient's eyes

PoM **Steri-Neb Ipratropium**® (Baker Norton)
Nebuliser solution unit, isotonic, ipratropium bromide 0.025% (250 micrograms/mL), net price 20 × 1-mL (250 micrograms) unit-dose vials (preservative free) = £6.14; 20 × 2-mL (500 micrograms) = £7.20. If dilution is necessary use only sterile sodium chloride 0.9%
Dose (and cautions relating to paradoxical bronchospasm and glaucoma): see under Atrovent Nebuliser Solution, above

For some **compound preparations** containing ipratropium, see section 3.1.4

OXITROPIUM BROMIDE

Indications: reversible airways obstruction, particularly in chronic bronchitis
Cautions; Side-effects: see under Ipratropium Bromide; rarely blurring of vision
Dose: by aerosol inhalation, 200 micrograms (2 puffs) 2–3 times daily; CHILD not recommended

PoM **Oxivent**® (Boehringer Ingelheim)
Aerosol inhalation, oxitropium bromide 100 micrograms/metered inhalation. Net price 200-dose unit = £12.98. Counselling, dose
Additives: include CFC propellants
Autohaler® (= breath-actuated aerosol inhalation), oxitropium bromide 100 micrograms/metered inhalation. Net price 200-dose unit = £19.65. Counselling, dose
Additives: include CFC propellants
COUNSELLING. Advise patient not to exceed prescribed dose and to follow manufacturer's directions

3.1.3 Theophylline

Theophylline is used for the relief of *bronchospasm*. It may have an additive effect when used in conjunction with small doses of beta$_2$-adrenoceptor stimulants; the combination may increase the risk of side-effects, including hypokalaemia (for CSM advice see p. 122).

Theophylline is metabolised in the liver and there is considerable variation in its half-life in healthy non-smokers, which is even more marked in smokers, in patients with hepatic impairment or heart failure, or if other drugs are taken concurrently. The half-life is *increased* in heart failure, cirrhosis, viral infections, and by drugs such as cimetidine, ciprofloxacin, erythromycin, fluvoxamine, and oral contraceptives. The half-life is *decreased* in smokers and in heavy drinkers, and by drugs such as phenytoin, carbamazepine, rifampicin, and barbiturates. For other interactions of theophylline see Appendix 1.

These differences in half-life are important because theophylline has a narrow margin between the therapeutic and toxic dose. In most subjects *plasma concentrations* of between 10 and 20 mg/ litre are required for satisfactory bronchodilatation. Side-effects can occur with concentrations below 20 mg/litre and are common at concentrations above 30–40 mg/litre.

Theophylline modified-release preparations are usually able to produce adequate plasma concentrations for up to 12 hours. When given as a single dose at night they have a useful role in controlling *nocturnal asthma* and *early morning wheezing*. There is no evidence that **choline theophyllinate** (a derivative of theophylline) is better tolerated than the modified-release preparations. The use of *rapid-release* oral theophylline preparations has declined because of the high incidence of side-effects associated with rapid absorption.

Theophylline is given by injection as **aminophylline**, a mixture of theophylline with ethylenediamine, which is 20 times more soluble than theophylline alone. Aminophylline may be given by **very slow** intravenous injection (over at least 20 minutes); it is too irritant for intramuscular use.

Intravenous aminophylline has a role in the treatment of *severe attacks of asthma* that do not respond rapidly to a nebulised beta$_2$-adrenoceptor stimulant (see also Acute Severe Asthma table, p. 121). Measurement of *plasma concentrations* may be helpful, and is **essential** if aminophylline is to be given to patients who have been taking oral theophylline preparations, as serious side-effects such as convulsions and arrhythmias can occasionally occur before the appearance of other symptoms of toxicity.

Aminophylline injection was formerly also used in the treatment of left ventricular failure but has been superseded for this purpose by diuretics (see sections 2.2.1 and 2.2.2) and the opioid analgesics (see section 4.7.2). However, it may have a role in patients with heart failure who are also suffering from asthma and bronchitis, where opioids are contra-indicated, though care is needed in those with increased myocardial excitability.

Aminophylline was formerly available for *rectal administration* as suppositories but these caused proctitis and the response was unpredictable; there was a particular risk of toxicity in children.

THEOPHYLLINE

Indications: reversible airways obstruction, severe acute asthma; for guidelines see also Asthma tables (pp. 120–21)

Cautions: cardiac disease, hypertension, hyperthyroidism, peptic ulcer, hepatic impairment (reduce dose), epilepsy, pregnancy and breastfeeding, elderly, fever; **CSM** advice on hypokalaemia risk, p. 120; avoid in porphyria (see section 9.8.2); **interactions:** Appendix 1 (theophylline) and notes above—**important**, see also below

FLUVOXAMINE INTERACTION. **CSM** advises that fluvoxamine seriously increases plasma-theophylline concentration and recommends that concomitant use should usually be avoided (or where not possible halve theophylline dose and monitor plasma-theophylline concentrations closely)—for other major interactions see Appendix 1 and notes above

Side-effects: tachycardia, palpitations, nausea, gastro-intestinal disturbances, headache, insomnia, arrhythmias, and convulsions especially if given rapidly by intravenous injection; overdosage: see Emergency Treatment of Poisoning, p. 20

Dose: see below

Note. Plasma theophylline concentration for optimum response 10–20 mg/litre (55–110 micromol/litre); narrow margin between therapeutic and toxic dose, see also notes above

Nuelin® (3M)

Tablets, scored, theophylline 125 mg. Net price 90-tab pack = £3.44. Label: 21

Dose: 125 mg 3–4 times daily after food, increased to 250 mg if required; CHILD 7–12 years 62.5–125 mg 3–4 times daily

Liquid, brown, theophylline hydrate 60 mg (as sodium glycinate)/5 mL. Net price 300 mL = £3.07. Label: 21

Dose: 120–240 mg 3–4 times daily after food; CHILD 2–6 years 60–90 mg, 7–12 years 90–120 mg, 3–4 times daily

Modified release

Note. The Council of the Royal Pharmaceutical Society of Great Britain advises pharmacists that if a general practitioner prescribes a modified-release, oral theophylline preparation without specifying a brand name, the pharmacist should contact the prescriber and agree the brand to be dispensed. Additionally, it is essential that a patient discharged from hospital should be maintained on the brand on which that patient was stabilised as an in-patient.

Lasma® (Pharmax)

Tablets, m/r, scored, theophylline 300 mg. Net price 20 = £1.89. Label: 25

Dose: 300 mg every 12 hours (increased after 1 week to 450 mg every 12 hours in patients over 70 kg); adjust dose by 150-mg increments as required

Total daily dose may be given as single dose at night when nocturnal symptoms predominate (daytime symptoms then controlled with inhaled bronchodilators)

Nuelin SA® (3M)

SA tablets, m/r, theophylline 175 mg. Net price 60-tab pack = £3.59. Label: 25

Dose: 175–350 mg every 12 hours; CHILD over 6 years 175 mg every 12 hours

SA 250 tablets, m/r, scored, theophylline 250 mg. Net price 60-tab pack = £5.03. Label: 25

Dose: 250–500 mg every 12 hours; CHILD over 6 years 125–250 mg every 12 hours

Slo-Phyllin® (Lipha)

Capsules, all m/r, theophylline 60 mg (white/clear, enclosing white pellets), net price 56-cap pack = £1.92; 125 mg (brown/clear, enclosing white pellets), 56-cap pack = £2.42; 250 mg (blue/clear, enclosing white pellets), 56-cap pack = £3.02. Label: 25 *or* counselling, see below

Dose: 250–500 mg every 12 hours; CHILD, every 12 hours, 2–6 years 60–120 mg, 7–12 years 125–250 mg

COUNSELLING. Swallow whole with fluid *or* swallow enclosed granules with soft food (e.g. yoghurt)

Theo-Dur® (Astra)

Tablets, m/r, both scored, theophylline 200 mg, net price 20 = £1.21; 300 mg, 20 = £1.75. Label: 25

Dose: 300 mg every 12 hours, adjust dose by 100–150-mg steps as required; CHILD up to 35 kg 100 mg, over 35 kg 200 mg, every 12 hours

For nocturnal asthma, total daily requirement may be given as single evening dose

Uniphyllin Continus® (Napp)

Tablets, m/r, all scored, theophylline 200 mg, net price 56-tab pack = £4.05; 300 mg, 56-tab pack = £6.17; 400 mg, 56-tab pack = £7.32. Label: 25

Dose: 200 mg every 12 hours increased after 1 week to 300 mg every 12 hours; over 70 kg 200–300 mg every 12 hours increased after 1 week to 400 mg every 12 hours

May be appropriate to give larger evening or morning dose to achieve optimum therapeutic effect when symptoms most severe; in patients whose night- or daytime symptoms persist despite other therapy, who are not currently receiving theophylline, total daily requirement may be added as single evening or morning dose

CHILD over 7 years, 9 mg/kg twice daily; some children with chronic asthma may require 10–16 mg/kg every 12 hours

For a list of **cough and decongestant preparations on sale to the public**, including those containing theophylline, see section 3.9.2

AMINOPHYLLINE

Note. Aminophylline is a stable mixture or combination of theophylline and ethylenediamine; the ethylenediamine confers greater solubility in water

Indications: reversible airways obstruction, severe acute asthma

Cautions; Side-effects: see under Theophylline; also allergy to ethylenediamine can cause urticaria, erythema, and exfoliative dermatitis

Dose: see below

Note. Plasma theophylline concentration for optimum response 10–20 mg/litre (55–110 micromol/litre); narrow margin between therapeutic and toxic dose, see also notes above

Aminophylline (Non-proprietary)

Tablets, aminophylline 100 mg, net price 20 = 20p. Label: 21

Dose: by mouth, 100–300 mg, 3–4 times daily, after food

PoM *Injection*, aminophylline 25 mg/mL, net price 10-mL amp = 72p

Available from Antigen, Evans, IMS (Min-I-Jet®), Phoenix

Dose: by slow intravenous injection (over 20 minutes), 250–500 mg (5 mg/kg); maintenance, if required, in patients not previously treated with theophylline, 500 micrograms/kg/hour *by slow intravenous infusion* CHILD, *by slow intravenous injection* (over 20 minutes), 5 mg/kg; maintenance, if required, in patients not previously treated with theophylline, 6 months–9 years 1 mg/kg/hour, 10–16 years 800 micrograms/kg/hour *by slow intravenous infusion*

Modified release
See advice on p. 128

Pecram® (Zyma)

Tablets, m/r, yellow, aminophylline hydrate 225 mg. Net price 20 = 99p. Label: 25

Dose: 1 tablet twice daily initially, increased if necessary to 2 tablets twice daily (steady-state concentrations usually reached after 3–4 days); CHILD not recommended

Phyllocontin Continus® (Napp)

Tablets, m/r, yellow, f/c, aminophylline hydrate 225 mg. Net price 60-tab pack = £3.52. Label: 25

Dose: 1 tablet twice daily initially, increased after 1 week to 2 tablets twice daily

Forte tablets, m/r, yellow, f/c, aminophylline hydrate 350 mg. Net price 60-tab pack = £5.85. Label: 25

Note. Forte tablets are for smokers and other patients with decreased theophylline half-life (see notes above)

Paediatric tablets, m/r, peach, aminophylline hydrate 100 mg. Net price 50-tab pack = £1.89. Label: 25

Dose: CHILD over 3 years, 6 mg/kg twice daily initially, increased after 1 week to 12 mg/kg twice daily; some children with chronic asthma may require 13–20 mg/kg every 12 hours

Note. Modified-release tablets containing aminophylline 225 mg and 350 mg also available from Ashbourne (Amnivent®), Norton (Norphyllin® SR)

CHOLINE THEOPHYLLINATE

Indications: reversible airways obstruction
Cautions; Side-effects: see under Theophylline
Dose: *by mouth*, CHILD 3–6 years 62.5–125 mg 3 times daily (at intervals of not less than 6 hours)

Note. Plasma theophylline concentration for optimum response 10–20 mg/litre (55–110 micromol /litre); narrow margin between therapeutic and toxic dose, see also notes above

Choledyl® (P-D)

Syrup, yellow, choline theophyllinate 62.5 mg/5 mL. Net price 200 mL = £2.57

3.1.4 Compound bronchodilator preparations

Most compound bronchodilator preparations have no place in the management of patients with airways obstruction.

In general, patients are best treated with single-ingredient preparations, such as a selective beta₂-adrenoceptor stimulant (section 3.1.1.1) or ipratropium bromide (section 3.1.2), so that the dose of each drug can be adjusted. This flexibility is lost with combinations, although those in which both components are effective may occasionally have a role when compliance is a problem.

For **cautions, contra-indications** and **side-effects** see under individual monographs.

PoM **Combivent®** (Boehringer Ingelheim)

Aerosol inhalation, ipratropium bromide 20 micrograms, salbutamol 100 micrograms (as sulphate)/metered inhalation. Net price 200-dose unit = £6.00. Counselling, dose

Additives: include CFC propellants

Dose: 2 puffs 4 times daily; CHILD under 12 years not recommended

Nebuliser solution, isotonic, ipratropium bromide 500 micrograms, salbutamol 2.5 mg (as sulphate)/2.5-mL vial, net price 60 unit-dose vials (preservative-free) = £33.00

Dose: by inhalation of nebulised solution, 1 vial 3–4 times daily; CHILD under 12 years not recommended

GLAUCOMA. In addition to other potential side-effects acute angle glaucoma has been reported with nebulised ipratropium—for details, see p. 127

PoM **Duovent®** (Boehringer Ingelheim)

Aerosol inhalation, fenoterol hydrobromide 100 micrograms, ipratropium bromide 40 micrograms/metered inhalation. Net price 200-dose unit with mouthpiece = £5.76 (extension tube also available). Counselling, dose

Additives: include CFC propellants

Dose: 1–2 puffs 3–4 times daily; CHILD over 6 years 1 puff 3 times daily

Autohaler® (= breath-actuated aerosol inhalation), fenoterol hydrobromide 100 micrograms, ipratropium bromide 40 micrograms/metered inhalation. Net price 200-dose unit = £11.57. Counselling, dose

Additives: include CFC propellants

Dose: 1–2 puffs 3–4 times daily; CHILD over 6 years 1 puff 3 times daily

Nebuliser solution, isotonic, fenoterol hydrobromide 1.25 mg, ipratropium bromide 500 micrograms/4-mL vial, net price 20 unit-dose vials = £10.00

Dose: acute severe asthma or acute exacerbation of chronic asthma, *by inhalation of nebulised solution*, 1 vial (4 mL); may be repeated up to max. 4 vials in 24 hours; CHILD under 14 years, not recommended

GLAUCOMA. In addition to other potential side-effects acute angle-closure glaucoma has been reported with nebulised ipratropium—for details, see p. 127

Preparations on sale to the public

For **compound bronchodilator preparations** on sale to the public, see p. 149

3.1.5 Peak flow meters, inhaler devices and nebulisers

PEAK FLOW METERS

Measurement of peak flow is particularly helpful for patients who are 'poor perceivers' and hence slow to detect deterioration in their asthma, and for those with moderate or severe asthma. Patients must be given clear guidelines as to the action they should take if their peak flow falls below a certain level. Patients can be encouraged to adjust some of their own treatment (within specified limits) according to changes in peak flow rate.

Ferraris Pocketpeak® (Ferraris)

Peak flow meter, standard (90–710 litres/minute), net price = £6.42, low range (40–370 litres/minute) = £6.42, replacement mouthpiece = 38p (for adult or child)

Mini-Wright® (Clement Clarke)

Peak flow meter, standard (60 to 800 litres/minute), net price = £6.51, low range (30 to 400 litres/minute) = £6.51, replacement mouthpiece = 38p (for adult or child)

Vitalograph® (Vitalograph)

Peak flow meter, standard (50 to 750 litres/minute), now called Asmaplan®, net price = £6.65, low range (25 to 280 litres/minute) = £6.65, replacement mouthpiece = 40p (for adult or child)

INHALER DEVICES

A variety of *spacing devices* is now available for use with *pressurised (aerosol) inhalers*. By providing a space between inhaler and mouth, they reduce the velocity of the aerosol and subsequent impaction on the oropharynx; in addition they allow more time for evaporation of the propellant so that a larger proportion of the particles can be inhaled and deposited in the lungs; also co-ordination of inspiration with actuation of the aerosol is less important. They range from the Bricanyl Spacer® (for terbutaline), a collapsible extended mouthpiece, to larger spacing devices with a one-way valve (Nebuhaler®, Volumatic®). Spacing devices are particularly useful for patients with poor inhalation technique, for children, for patients requiring higher doses, for nocturnal asthma, and for patients prone to develop candidiasis with inhaled corticosteroids.

Alternatively *dry powder inhalers*, activated by the patient's inspiration, are of value; some occasionally cause coughing.

Accuhaler® (A&H)
Breath-actuated device for use with Flixotide, Serevent and Ventolin

AeroChamber® (3M)
Spacer device, large-volume device. For use with Airomir® inhaler, net price standard device (blue) = £8.00, with mask (blue) = £16.00; child device (yellow) with mask = £14.36; infant device (orange) with mask = £14.36

Aerohaler® (Boehringer Ingelheim)
Breath-actuated device for use with Atrovent Aerocaps

NHS Babyhaler® (A&H)
Spacer device for paediatric use with Becotide 50 and Ventolin inhalers. Net price = £11.34

Diskhaler® (A&H)
Breath-actuated device for use with Becodisks, Becloforte, Flixotide, Serevent, and Ventodisks

Fisonair® (Fisons)
Large volume spacer device for use with Intal, see p. 136

NHS Haleraid® (Glaxo)
Device to place over standard inhalers as aid to operation by patients with impaired strength in hands (e.g. with arthritis). Available as Haleraid-120 for 120-dose inhalers and Haleraid-200 for 200-dose inhalers. Net price = 80p

Nebuhaler® (Astra)
Spacer inhaler, large-volume device. For use with Bricanyl and Pulmicort refill canisters, net price = £4.28; with paediatric mask = £4.28

Rotahaler® (A&H)
Breath-actuated device for use with Rotacaps. Available as Becotide Rotahaler, Ventolin Rotahaler, and Ventide Rotahaler. Net price = 78p

Spinhaler® (Fisons)
Breath-actuated device for use with Intal Spincaps, see p. 136

Syncroner® (Fisons)
Spacer device for use with Aerocrom, Intal, and Tilade

Volumatic® (A&H)
Spacer inhaler, large-volume device. For use with Becloforte, Becotide, Flixotide, Serevent, Ventide, and Ventolin inhalers, net price = £2.75; with paediatric mask = £2.75

NEBULISERS

In England and Wales nebulisers and compressors are not available on the NHS (but they are free of VAT); some nebulisers (but not compressors) are available on form GP10A in Scotland (for details consult Scottish Drug Tariff).

Nebulisers convert a solution of a drug into an aerosol for inhalation. They are used to deliver higher doses of drug to the airways than is usual with standard inhalers. The main indications for use of a nebuliser are:

to deliver a beta-adrenoceptor stimulant or ipratropium to a patient with an *acute exacerbation* of asthma or of chronic airway obstruction;

to deliver a beta-adrenoceptor stimulant or ipratropium on a *regular basis* to a patient with severe asthma or reversible airways obstruction who has been shown to benefit from regular treatment with higher doses;

to deliver *prophylactic medication* such as cromoglycate or a corticosteroid to a patient unable to use other inhalational devices (particularly a young child);

to deliver an *antibiotic* (such as colistin) to a patient with chronic purulent infection (as in cystic fibrosis or bronchiectasis);

to deliver *pentamidine* for the prophylaxis and treatment of *Pneumocystis pneumonia* to a patient with AIDS.

The proportion of a nebuliser solution that reaches the lungs depends on the type of nebuliser and although it can be as high as 30% it is more frequently close to 10% and sometimes below 10%. The remaining solution is left in the nebuliser as residual volume or it is deposited in the mouthpiece and tubing. The extent to which the nebulised solution is deposited in the airways or alveoli depends on particle size. Particles with a mass median diameter of 1–5 microns are deposited in the airways and are therefore appropriate for asthma whereas a particle size of 1–2 microns is needed for alveolar deposition of pentamidine to combat pneumocystis infection. The type of nebuliser is therefore chosen according to the deposition required and according to the viscosity of the solution (antibiotic solutions usually being more viscous).

Some jet nebulisers are able to increase drug output during inspiration and hence increase efficiency.

The patient should be aware that the dose of a bronchodilator given by nebulisation is usually **much higher** than that from an aerosol inhaler; see below for British Thoracic Society guidelines.

The following are the British Thoracic Society guidelines for giving regular nebulised bronchodilators:

diagnosis should be reviewed and confirmed;

other methods of administration should be explored;

patients should be complying with corticosteroid or cromoglycate (or nedocromil) prophylaxis;

increased bronchodilatation should be obtained without unacceptable side-effects;

an initial 3-week home trial should be undertaken (with peak flow monitoring);

If prescribed:

- oral and written instructions should be given to patient on method and frequency of use, action to be taken in event of asthma worsening, and when to attend for follow-up;
- supervision should normally entail attendance at asthma clinic or home visits by trained asthma nurse or physiotherapist;
- supervision should include evaluation of peak flow, monitoring of prescriptions, and twice yearly servicing of compressor (see also recommendations for individual compressors).

Jet nebulisers

Jet nebulisers utilise the Venturi principle for nebulisation; they are more widely used than ultrasonic nebulisers. Most jet nebulisers require an optimum gas flow rate of 6–8 litres/minute and in hospital can be driven by piped air or oxygen. Domiciliary oxygen cylinders do not provide an adequate flow rate therefore for domiciliary use an electrical compressor is used.

For patients with *chronic bronchitis and hypercapnia*, oxygen can be dangerous and the nebuliser should be driven by air (see also p. 119).

> **Important:** the Department of Health has reminded users of the need to use the correct grade of tubing when connecting a nebuliser to a medical gas supply or compressor.

NHS Medix All Nebuliser® (Medix)

Jet nebuliser, disposable; for use with bronchodilators, antimuscarinics, corticosteroids, and antibiotics, replacement recommended every 2–3 months if used 4 times a day. Compatible with **NHS AC 2000 Hi Flo®**, **NHS World Traveller Hi Flo®**, and **NHS Econoneb®**. Net price 5 = £7.50

NHS Medix Antibiotic Circuit® (Medix)

Jet nebuliser, closed-system; for use with antibiotics and other respiratory drugs. Compatible with **NHS AC 2000 Hi Flo®**, **NHS Econoneb®**, and **NHS Turboneb®**. Net price 1 = £7.30

NHS Medix System® (Medix)

Jet nebuliser, consisting of mouthpiece, tubing, and nebuliser chamber. Net price 1 = £2.80; mask kits with tubing and nebuliser chamber also available, net price 1 (adult) = £2.90; 1 (child) = £2.90

NHS Pari LC Plus Filter® (Pari)

Jet nebuliser, closed system, non-disposable, for hospital or home use with low flow compressors; supplied with filter/valve set. Compatible with **NHS Pari TurboBoy®** and **NHS Pari JuniorBoy®** compressors. Net price 1 = £19.90, replacement filters 100 = £33.30

NHS Pari LC Plus® (Pari)

Jet nebuliser, non-disposable, for hospital or home use with low flow compressors; for use with bronchodilators, antibiotics, and corticosteroids, replacement recommended yearly if used 4 times a day. Compatible with **NHS Pari TurboBoy®**, **NHS Pari JuniorBoy®** and **NHS Pari WalkBoy®** compressors. Net price 1 = £13.90

NHS Pari Baby® (Pari)

Jet nebuliser, non-disposable, for hospital or home use with low flow compressors; for use with bronchodilators, antibiotics and corticosteroids; replacement recommended yearly if used 4 times a day. Compatible with **NHS Pari TurboBoy®**, **NHS Pari JuniorBoy®**, **NHS Pari WalkBoy®** compressors. Available separately for children aged less than 1 year, 1–4 years or 4–7 years. Net price 1 (with connection hose) = £25.00

NHS Sidestream Durable® (Medic-Aid)

Jet nebuliser, non-disposable, for home use; for use with bronchodilators; yearly replacement recommended if 4 six-minute treatments used per day. Compatible with **NHS CR50®**, **NHS Freeway Lite®** and **NHS Porta-Neb 50®** (depending on nebulising solution). Net price 10 pack = £94.50; patient pack with **NHS CR50®** compressor = £98.50. **NHS Disposable Sidestream®** nebuliser also available

Note. This has been developed to replace the **NHS System 22 Acorn®**

NHS Ventstream® (Medic-Aid)

Jet nebuliser, closed-system, for use with low flow compressors, compatible with **NHS CR50®**, **NHS Porta-Neb 50®** and **NHS Freeway Lite®** compressors; for use with antibiotics, bronchodilators, and corticosteroids, replacement recommended yearly if used 3 times a day. Net price 1 with filter = £27.00; 10-pack with filter = £250.00; 1 without filter = £23.00; 10-pack without filter = £215.00; patient pack with **NHS CR 50®** compressor = £119.95

Home compressors with nebulisers

NHS AC 2000 HI FLO® (Medix)

Portable, home use, containing 1 **NHS Jet Nebuliser®** set with mouthpiece, 1 adult or 1 child mask, 1 spare inlet filter, filter spanner. Mains operated. Nebulises bronchodilators and antibiotics. Net price 1 = £99.00; carrying case available

NHS Aquilon® (Henleys)

Portable, home use, with 1 adult or 1 child mask and tubing. Mains operated. Net price = £81.30

NHS Atmolette Si® (Sinclair)

Hospital, clinic and home use, with mask or mouthpiece. Mains operated. Net price = £150.00

NHS Econoneb® (Medix)

Home, clinic and hospital use, used with 1 **NHS Jet Nebuliser®** set with mouthpiece, 1 adult or 1 child mask, 1 spare inlet filter, filter spanner. Compatible with all types of jet nebuliser sets and also the **NHS Micro Cirrus®** nebuliser (recommended for alveolar deposition). Nebulises bronchodilators, corticosteroids, and antibiotics. Mains operated. Net price 1 = £90.00

NHS Freeway Lite® (Medic-Aid)

Portable, containing 1 **NHS Sidestream Durable®** reusable nebuliser, 1 adult or 1 child mask, 1 mouthpiece, 1 Coiled Duratube®, 2 filters. Net price 1 = £149.00 with carrying case. **NHS Freeway Lite Luxury®** contains additional battery. Net price 1 = £198.00

Also compatible with **NHS Ventstream®** closed system nebuliser

NHS M-Flo® (Medix)

Portable, home use, containing 1 **NHS Jet Nebuliser®** set with mouthpiece, spare inlet filter, filter spanner. Mains operated. Nebulises bronchodilators and corticosteroids. Net price 1 = £85.00

NHS Medi-Neb® (Timesco)

Range of compressors all supplied with adult and child mask, vapourising chamber, and PVC tubing, including: **NHS Medi-Neb Elite®**, *home use*. Mains operated. Net price 1 = £79.95. **NHS Medi-Neb Companion®**, *portable*. Mains/car battery operated. Net price 1 = £94.95 (includes car battery adaptor and carrying case). **NHS Medi-Neb Companion Plus®**, *portable*. Mains/battery operated. Net price 1 = £139.95 (includes rechargeable battery, car battery adaptor, and carrying case). **NHS Medi-Neb Tempest®**, *home/hospital use*. Mains operated. Net price 1 = £89.95

All used for nebulising antibiotics and bronchodilators

NHS Pari TurboBoy® (Pari)

Portable, for hospital or home use, containing **NHS Pari LC Plus** with connection tube and mains cable. Filter replacement recommended every 12 months or 550 hours of use. Compatible with **NHS Pari LC Plus®**,

NHS Pari LC Plus Filter®, and **NHS Pari Baby®** nebulisers. Net price = £109.00

NHS Pari JuniorBoy® (Pari)

Portable, for hospital or home use, containing **NHS Pari LC Plus** with connection tube and mains cable. Filter replacement recommended every 12 months or 550 hours of use. Compatible with **NHS Pari LC Plus®**, **NHS Pari LC Plus Filter®**, and **NHS Pari Baby®** nebulisers. Net price = £119.00

NHS Pari WalkBoy® (Pari)

Portable, containing 1 **NHS Pari LC Plus®** nebuliser with connection tube, mains cable, rechargeable battery and carrying bag. Compatible with **NHS Pari LC Plus®** and **NHS Pari Baby®** nebulisers. Net price 1 = £219.00; car cigarette lighter adapter = £63.00

NHS Porta-Neb® (Medic-Aid)

Portable, containing 1 **NHS Sidestream Durable®** reusable nebuliser, 1 angled flow-through mouthpiece, 1 adult or 1 child mask, 1 Duratube® supply tubing, 4 spare filters. Mains operated; for use with bronchodilators. Net price 1 = £109.50; carrying case available

Also compatible with **NHS Ventstream®** closed-system nebuliser; for use with antibiotics, bronchodilators, and corticosteroids

NHS Pulmo-Aide® (De Vilbiss)

Home, clinic use, containing disposable nebuliser set, mouthpiece, mask, mains lead, tubing, thumb-valve. For use with bronchodilators. Net price 1 = £99.50. **NHS Pulmo-Aide Escort®**, *portable*, containing disposable nebuliser set, transformer, rechargeable battery, AC to DC adapter charger, DC lead with car adapter, and carrying case. For use with bronchodilators. Net price 1 = £198.50. **NHS Pulmo-Aide AP50®**, *home, clinic, hospital use*. Net price 1 = £180.00, 1 with antipollution kit = £188.50. **NHS Pulmo-Aide Sunmist®**, *home use*, containing nebuliser set, mouthpiece, face mask, mains lead. Net price 1 = £84.25

NHS SunMist® (De Vilbiss)

Home, clinic and hospital use, with mouthpiece. Mains operated. Net price = £89.50. **NHS SunMist Plus®**, *home, clinic and hospital use*, with mouthpiece, higher flow rate. Mains operated. Net price = £102.25.

NHS Tourer® (Henleys)

Portable, home use. Mains/car battery operated; for use with antibiotics and bronchodilators. Net price = £131.50, rechargeable battery pack = £52.06

NHS World Traveller HI FLO® (Medix)

Portable, containing 1 **NHS Jet Nebuliser®** set with mouthpiece, 1 adult or 1 child mask, 1 spare inlet filter, filter spanner. Battery/mains operated; rechargeable battery pack available. Nebulises bronchodilators, corticosteroids, and antibiotics. Net price 1 excluding battery = £135.00; 1 with battery = £180.00; carrying case available

Compressors

NHS System 22 CR50® (Medic-Aid)

Home, clinic and hospital use. Mains operated. Net price 1 = £89.50. Also compatible with **NHS Ventstream®**, and **NHS Sidestream Durable®**

NHS System 22 CR60® (Medic-Aid)

Hospital use, high flow compressor. Mains operated. Net price = £199.90. Also compatible with **NHS System 22 Antibiotic Tee®** for nebulisation of high viscosity drugs such as antibiotics

NHS Turboneb® (Medix)

Hospital use, high flow compressor. Mains operated. Net price 1 = £115.00. Also compatible with **NHS Medix Antibiotic Circuit®** for nebulisation of respiratory drugs in particular viscous antibiotics

Ultrasonic nebulisers

Ultrasonic nebulisers produce an aerosol by ultrasonic vibration of the drug solution and therefore do not require a gas flow

NHS AeroSonic® (De Vilbiss)

Portable, containing 1 controlling unit, chamber assembly, carrying case, AC to DC adapter/charger, DC lead, 1 mouthpiece with check valve and adapter. Net price 1 = £250.00

NHS Omron U1 MicroAir® (Hutchings)

Portable. Battery operated/mains adaptor. Net price = £325.00

NHS Omron NE U07® (Hutchings)

Portable. Mains operated or rechargeable battery pack. Net price = £166.00 (mains version), £253.00 (rechargeable version)

NHS Sonix 2000® (Medix)

Portable, delivery rate adjustable to suit user. Supplied with carrying case and DC lead. Mains/car battery operated; rechargeable battery pack available. Net price 1 excluding battery = £150.00, 1 with battery = £215.00

NHS Ultra Neb 2000® (De Vilbiss)

Hospital, clinic and home use, delivery rate adjustable. Supplied with stand. Net price = £1125.50

NEBULISER DILUENT

Nebulisation may be carried out using an undiluted nebuliser solution or it may require dilution beforehand. The usual diluent is sodium chloride 0.9% (physiological saline).

PoM Steri-Neb Saline® (Baker Norton)

Solution, sodium chloride 0.9% in single-dose units of 2.5 mL. Net price 20 = £3.66

3.2   Corticosteroids

Corticosteroids have been used in *asthma* for many years. Their mode of action is not fully understood but they reduce bronchial mucosal inflammation (and hence reduce oedema and secretion of mucus into the airway).

Corticosteroids are usually of no benefit in patients with *chronic bronchitis* and *emphysema*; some patients with asthma, however, may be clinically indistinguishable from those with chronic bronchitis except that they will respond to a trial course of corticosteroids.

INHALATION. The use of inhaled corticosteroids has increased so that they are now recommended for prophylactic treatment when patients are using a beta$_2$-stimulant more than once daily (see Chronic Asthma table). They have many fewer side-effects than those associated with systemic administration (see section 6.3.2), but nevertheless these need to be borne in mind, including the potential of higher inhaled doses to induce *adrenal suppression* and to have *effects on bone metabolism* (for further details see below). The *growth retardation in children* associated with oral corticosteroid therapy does not appear to be a significant problem with inhaled therapy although it remains a wise policy to monitor linear growth.

Corticosteroid *aerosol inhalations* must be used regularly to obtain maximum benefit; alleviation of symptoms usually occurs 3 to 7 days after initiation. **Beclomethasone dipropionate**, **budesonide** and **fluticasone propionate** appear to be equally effective; fluticasone achieves the same effect as the other two with half the dose. If a beta$_2$-adrenoceptor stimulant is to be used at the same time as an inhaled corticosteroid it should be used first to help increase the penetration of the inhaled corticosteroid.

Patients who have been taking long-term oral corticosteroids can often be transferred to an inhaled corticosteroid but the transfer must be done slowly, with gradual reduction in dose of oral corticosteroid, and at a time when the asthma is well controlled.

High-dose aerosol inhalations are available for patients who only have a partial response to standard inhalers. The maximum doses for high-dose corticosteroid inhalations are associated with some *adrenal suppression* (see section 6.3.2), therefore patients on high doses should be given a 'steroid card' and may need corticosteroid cover during an episode of stress (e.g. an operation). Systemic therapy may also be necessary during episodes of infection or increased bronchoconstriction where higher doses are needed and access of inhaled drug to small airways may be reduced; patients may need a reserve supply of tablets.

Inhaled corticosteroids have considerably fewer systemic effects than oral corticosteroids, but effects on bone metabolism can be detected following inhalation of higher doses of beclomethasone, budesonide and fluticasone. Although there is no firm evidence that this may lead to increased osteoporosis in the future, it is sensible to ensure that the dose of inhaled corticosteroid is no higher than necessary to keep a patient's asthma under good control. The dose may therefore be reduced cautiously when the asthma has been well controlled for a few weeks as long as the patient knows that it is necessary to reinstate it should the asthma deteriorate or the peak flow rate fall.

Corticosteroids are preferably inhaled from aerosol inhalers using *'spacer devices'* (see section 3.1.5). These increase airway deposition and reduce oropharyngeal deposition, resulting in a marked reduction in the incidence of candidiasis; these devices are bulky, but most patients only need to use them morning and night. *Dry powder inhalers* are actuated by the patient's inhalation and are particularly useful for patients who are unable to use the aerosol inhalers.

Budesonide is available as a *suspension for nebulisation* (Pulmicort Respules®).

ORAL. *Acute attacks* of asthma should be treated with short courses of oral corticosteroids starting with a high dose, e.g. prednisolone 30 to 60 mg (30 to 40 mg usually adequate) daily for a few days, gradually reducing once the attack has been controlled. Patients whose asthma has deteriorated rapidly usually respond quickly to corticosteroids, which can then be tailed down over a few days; more gradual reduction is necessary in those whose asthma has deteriorated gradually. For use of corticosteroids in the emergency treatment of *severe acute asthma* see table on p. 121.

In *chronic continuing asthma*, when the response to other anti-asthma drugs has been relatively small, continued administration of oral corticosteroids may be necessary; in such cases high doses of inhaled corticosteroids should be continued so that oral requirements are reduced to a minimum. Oral corticosteroids should normally be taken as a single dose in the morning to reduce the disturbance to circadian cortisol secretion. Dosage should always be titrated to the lowest dose which controls symptoms. Regular peak flow measurements often help both patient and doctor to adjust the dose optimally. Prednisolone is available as tablets of 1 mg as well as 5 mg, and the smaller tablets may conveniently be used to adjust the maintenance dosage to the minimum necessary.

Alternate-day administration has not been very successful in the management of asthma in adults as they tend to deteriorate during the second 24 hours. If an attempt is made to introduce this, pulmonary function should be monitored carefully over the 48 hours.

PARENTERAL. For the use of hydrocortisone injection in the emergency treatment of *severe acute asthma*, see Acute Severe Asthma table, p. 121.

BECLOMETHASONE DIPROPIONATE
(Beclometasone Dipropionate)

Indications: prophylaxis of asthma especially if not fully controlled by bronchodilators or cromoglycate

Cautions: see notes above; also active or quiescent tuberculosis; may need to reinstate systemic therapy during periods of stress or when airways obstruction or mucus prevent drug access to smaller airways

PARADOXICAL BRONCHOSPASM. The potential for paradoxical bronchospasm (calling for discontinuation and alternative therapy) should be borne in mind—if mild it may be prevented by inhalation of a beta$_2$-adrenoceptor stimulant (or by transfer from an aerosol inhalation to a dry powder inhalation)

Side-effects: see notes above; also hoarseness and candidiasis of mouth or throat (usually only with large doses); rarely rash

CANDIDIASIS. Candidiasis can be reduced by using spacer, see notes above, and responds to antifungal lozenges, see section 12.3.2, without discontinuation of therapy—rinsing the mouth with water (or cleaning child's teeth) after inhalation of a dose may also be helpful

Dose: see preparations below

Standard-dose inhalers

PoM **AeroBec®** (3M)

AeroBec 50 Autohaler® (breath-actuated aerosol inhalation), beclomethasone dipropionate 50 micrograms/metered inhalation, net price 200-dose unit = £11.00. Label: 8, counselling, dose
Additives: include CFC propellants

AeroBec 100 Autohaler® (breath-actuated aerosol inhalation), beclomethasone dipropionate 100 micrograms/metered inhalation, net price 200-dose unit = £13.50. Label: 8, counselling, dose
Additives: include CFC propellants

Dose: by aerosol inhalation, 200 micrograms twice daily *or* 100 micrograms 3–4 times daily (in more severe cases initially 600–800 micrograms daily); CHILD 50–100 micrograms 2–4 times daily

Note. Breath-actuated aerosol inhalers containing beclomethasone dipropionate 50 micrograms/metered inhalation and 100 micrograms/metered inhalation also available from Baker Norton (Beclazone Easi-Breathe®)

PoM **Becodisks®** (A&H)

Dry powder for inhalation, disks containing 8 blisters of beclomethasone dipropionate 100 micrograms/blister, net price 14 disks with Diskhaler® device = £10.99, 14-disk refill = £10.42;
200 micrograms/blister, 14 disks with Diskhaler® device = £20.90, 14-disk refill = £20.33;
400 micrograms/blister, 7 disks with Diskhaler® device = £20.90, 7-disk refill = £20.33. Label: 8, counselling, dose

Dose: by inhalation of powder, 400 micrograms twice daily *or* 200 micrograms 3–4 times daily; CHILD 100 micrograms 2–4 times daily *or* 200 micrograms twice daily

PoM **Becotide Inhaler®** (A&H)

Becotide-50 aerosol inhalation, beclomethasone dipropionate 50 micrograms/metered inhalation. Net price 200-dose unit = £5.43. Label: 8, counselling, dose

Becotide-100 aerosol inhalation, beclomethasone dipropionate 100 micrograms/metered inhalation. Net price 200-dose unit = £10.32. Label: 8, counselling, dose

Becotide-200 aerosol inhalation, beclomethasone dipropionate 200 micrograms/metered inhalation. Net price 200-dose unit = £19.61. Label: 8, counselling, dose

Note. Becotide-200 not indicated for children

Dose: by aerosol inhalation, 200 micrograms twice daily *or* 100 micrograms 3–4 times daily (in more severe cases initially 600–800 micrograms daily); CHILD 50–100 micrograms 2–4 times daily *or* 100–200 micrograms twice daily

Note. Aerosol inhalers containing beclomethasone dipropionate 50 micrograms/metered inhalation and 100 micrograms/metered inhalation also available from Baker Norton (Beclazone®) and 3M (Filair®); vortex-based aerosol inhalers releasing beclomethasone dipropionate 50 micrograms/metered inhalation and 100 micrograms/metered inhalation available from Evans (BDP Spacehaler®)

Additives: all include CFC propellants

PoM **Becotide Rotacaps®** (A&H)

Rotacaps® (dry powder for inhalation; for use with Becotide Rotahaler®), beclomethasone dipropionate 100 micrograms (buff/clear), net price 112-cap pack = £8.47; 200 micrograms (brown/clear), 112-cap pack = £16.09; 400 micrograms (dark brown/clear), 112-cap pack = £30.54. Label: 8, counselling, dose

Dose: by inhalation of powder, 200 micrograms 3–4 times daily or 400 micrograms twice daily; CHILD 100 micrograms 2–4 times daily *or* 200 micrograms twice daily

Chronic Asthma table, see p. 120
Acute Severe Asthma table, see p. 121

High-dose inhalers
Note. High-dose inhalers not indicated for children

PoM **AeroBec Forte®** (3M)

Aerosol inhalation, beclomethasone dipropionate 250 micrograms/metered inhalation, net price 200-inhalation breath-actuated unit (Autohaler®) = £25.10. Label: 8, counselling, dose, 10 steroid card

Additives: include CFC propellants
Dose: by aerosol inhalation, 500 micrograms twice daily *or* 250 micrograms 4 times daily; if necessary may be increased to 500 micrograms 4 times daily
Note. Breath-actuated aerosol inhalers containing beclomethasone dipropionate 250 micrograms/metered inhalation also available from Baker Norton (Beclazone Easi-Breathe®)

PoM **Becloforte®** (A&H)

Aerosol inhalation, beclomethasone dipropionate 250 micrograms/metered inhalation. Net price 200-dose unit = £23.10; net price Becloforte® VM (2 Becloforte® inhalers with Volumatic®) = £46.20; 200-puff unit with spacer device (Becloforte Integra®) = £23.10; 200-dose refill for use with Becloforte Integra® = £18.02. Label: 8, counselling, dose, 10 steroid card
Dose: by aerosol inhalation, 500 micrograms (2 puffs) twice daily *or* 250 micrograms (1 puff) 4 times daily; if necessary may be increased to 500 micrograms 3–4 times daily
Note. Aerosol inhalers containing beclomethasone dipropionate 250 micrograms/metered inhalation also available from Baker Norton (Beclazone®) and 3M (Filair Forte®); vortex-based aerosol inhalers releasing beclomethasone dipropionate 250 micrograms/metered inhalation available from Evans (BDP Spacehaler®)
Additives: all include CFC propellants

Dry powder for inhalation, disks containing 8 blisters of beclomethasone dipropionate 400 micrograms/blister, net price 14 disks with Diskhaler® device = £39.70; 14-disk refill = £39.13. Label: 8, counselling, dose, 10 steroid card
Dose: by inhalation of powder, 400 micrograms twice daily; if necessary may be increased to 800 micrograms twice daily

Compound preparations
(Not recommended)
PoM **Ventide®** (A&H)

Aerosol inhalation, beclomethasone dipropionate 50 micrograms, salbutamol 100 micrograms/metered inhalation. Net price 200-dose unit = £6.02. Label: 8, counselling, dose
Additives: include CFC propellants
Dose: maintenance, 2 puffs 3–4 times daily; CHILD 1–2 puffs 2–4 times daily
Paediatric Rotacaps® (dry powder for inhalation; for use with Ventide Rotahaler®), light grey/clear, beclomethasone dipropionate 100 micrograms, salbutamol (as sulphate) 200 micrograms. Net price 112-cap pack = £14.10. Label: 8, counselling, dose
Dose: by inhalation of powder, 1 Paediatric Rotacap® 2–4 times daily
Rotacaps® (dry powder for inhalation; for use with Ventide Rotahaler), dark grey/clear, beclomethasone dipropionate 200 micrograms, salbutamol (as sulphate) 400 micrograms. Net price 112-cap pack = £25.57. Label: 8, counselling, dose
Dose: by inhalation of powder, 1 Rotacap® 3–4 times daily

Inhaler devices
See section 3.1.5

BUDESONIDE

Indications; Cautions; Side-effects: see under Beclomethasone Dipropionate
Dose: see preparations below

PoM **Pulmicort Inhaler®** (Astra)

LS aerosol inhalation, budesonide 50 micrograms/metered inhalation. Net price 200-dose unit with standard or Spacer inhaler = £6.66; 200-dose refill for use with Nebuhaler or Spacer inhaler = £4.54. Label: 8, counselling, dose
Additives: include CFC propellants

Aerosol inhalation, budesonide 200 micrograms/metered inhalation. Net price 200-dose unit with standard or Spacer inhaler = £19.00; 200-dose refill for use with Nebuhaler or Spacer inhaler = £17.00; 100-dose unit with standard and Spacer inhaler = £7.96 (hosp. only). Label: 8, counselling, dose, 10 steroid card
Additives: include CFC propellants

Dose: by aerosol inhalation, 200 micrograms twice daily; may be reduced in well-controlled asthma to not less than 200 micrograms daily; in severe asthma dose may be increased to 1.6 mg daily; CHILD 50–400 micrograms twice daily; in severe asthma may be increased to 800 micrograms daily

PoM **Pulmicort Turbohaler®** (Astra)

Turbohaler® (= dry powder inhaler), budesonide 100 micrograms/inhalation, net price 200-dose unit = £18.50; 200 micrograms/inhalation, 100-dose unit = £18.50; 400 micrograms/inhalation, 50-dose unit = £18.50. Label: 8, counselling, dose, 10 steroid card
Note. Little sensation associated with use

Dose: by inhalation of powder, when starting treatment, during periods of severe asthma, and while reducing or discontinuing oral corticosteroids, 0.2–1.6 mg daily in divided doses; in less severe cases 200–800 micrograms daily; patients already controlled on an inhaled corticosteroid administered twice daily may be transferred to once-daily dosing (each evening) at the same equivalent total daily dose (up to 800 micrograms once daily); CHILD 200–800 micrograms daily in divided doses (800 micrograms daily in severe asthma)

PoM **Pulmicort Respules®** (Astra)

Respules® (= single-dose units for nebulisation), budesonide 250 micrograms/mL, net price 20 × 2-mL (500 micrograms) unit = £32.00; 500 micrograms/mL, 20 × 2-mL (1 mg) unit = £44.64. May be diluted up to 50% with sterile sodium chloride 0.9%. Label: 8, counselling, dose, 10 steroid card

Dose: by inhalation of nebulised suspension, when starting treatment, during periods of severe asthma, and while reducing or discontinuing oral corticosteroids, 1–2 mg twice daily (may be increased further in very severe asthma); CHILD 3 months–12 years, 0.5–1 mg twice daily
Maintenance, usually half above doses
Croup, 2 mg as a single dose (*or* as two 1-mg doses separated by 30 minutes)

Inhaler devices
See section 3.1.5

FLUTICASONE PROPIONATE

Indications; Cautions; Side-effects: see under Beclomethasone Dipropionate
Dose: see preparations below

PoM **Flixotide®** (A&H)

Accuhaler® (dry powder for inhalation), disk containing 60 blisters of fluticasone propionate 50 micrograms/blister with Accuhaler® device, net price = £8.23; 100 micrograms/blister with Accuhaler® device = £12.80; 250 micrograms/blister with Accuhaler® device = £24.23; 500 micrograms/blister with Accuhaler® device = £40.23. Label: 8, counselling, dose; 250- and 500-microgram strengths also label 10 steroid card
Note. Flixotide Accuhaler® 250 micrograms and 500 micrograms are not indicated for children

Dose: by inhalation of powder, ADULT and CHILD over 16 years, 100–250 micrograms twice daily, increased according to severity of asthma to 1 mg twice daily; CHILD under 4 years not recommended, 4–16 years, 50–100 micrograms twice daily adjusted as necessary

Aerosol inhalation, fluticasone propionate 25 micrograms/metered inhalation, net price 120-dose unit = £6.86; 50 micrograms/metered inhalation, 120-dose unit = £11.43; 125 micrograms/metered inhalation, 120-dose unit = £22.86; 250 micrograms/metered inhalation, 120-dose unit = £38.86. Label: 8, counselling, dose; 250-microgram strength also label 10 steroid card
Additives: include CFC propellants
Note. Flixotide 125 micrograms and 250 micrograms inhalers not indicated for children

Dose: by aerosol inhalation, ADULT and CHILD over 16 years, 100–250 micrograms twice daily, increased according to severity of asthma to 1 mg twice daily; CHILD 4–16 years, 50–100 micrograms twice daily adjusted as necessary

Diskhaler® (dry powder for inhalation), fluticasone propionate
50 micrograms/blister, net price 14 disks of 4 blisters with Diskhaler® device = £8.23, 14-disk refill = £7.66;
100 micrograms/blister, 14 disks of 4 blisters with Diskhaler® device = £12.80, 14-disk refill = £12.23;
250 micrograms/blister, 14 disks of 4 blisters with Diskhaler® device = £24.23, 14-disk refill = £23.66;
500 micrograms/blister, 14 disks of 4 blisters with Diskhaler® device = £40.23, 14-disk refill = £39.66. Label: 8, counselling, dose; 250- and 500-microgram strengths also label 10 steroid card
Note. Flixotide Diskhaler® 250 micrograms and 500 micrograms are not indicated for children

Dose: by inhalation of powder, ADULT and CHILD over 16 years, 100–250 micrograms twice daily, increased according to severity of asthma to 1 mg twice daily; CHILD 4–16 years, 50–100 micrograms twice daily adjusted as necessary

3.3   Cromoglycate and related therapy

Regular inhalation of sodium cromoglycate can reduce the incidence of attacks of asthma and allow dosage reduction of bronchodilators and oral corticosteroids. In general, prophylaxis with sodium cromoglycate is less effective in adults than prophylaxis with corticosteroid inhalations (see Chronic asthma table) but the fact that in the long term corticosteroid inhalations may be associated with more side-effects needs to be borne in mind. Sodium cromoglycate is of no value in the treatment of acute attacks of asthma.

Sodium cromoglycate is of value in the prevention of exercise-induced asthma, a single dose being inhaled half-an-hour beforehand.

The mode of action of sodium cromoglycate is not completely understood. It may be of value in asthma with an allergic basis, but, in practice, it is difficult to predict who will benefit, therefore it is reasonable to try it for a period of 4 to 6 weeks. Children seem to respond better than adults. Dose frequency is adjusted according to response but is usually 3 to 4 times a day initially; this may subsequently be reduced.

If inhalation of the dry powder form of sodium cromoglycate causes bronchospasm a selective beta$_2$-adrenoceptor stimulant such as salbutamol or terbutaline should be inhaled a few minutes beforehand. The nebuliser solution is useful for young children who cannot manage the dry powder inhaler or the aerosol.

Nedocromil has a pharmacological action similar to that of sodium cromoglycate.

> Chronic Asthma table, see p. 120
> Acute Severe Asthma table, see p. 121

SODIUM CROMOGLYCATE

(Sodium Cromoglicate)

Indications: prophylaxis of asthma; food allergy, section 1.5

Side-effects: coughing, transient bronchospasm, and throat irritation due to inhalation of powder (see also notes above)

Dose: see preparations below

COUNSELLING. Regular use is necessary

PoM Intal® (Fisons)

Aerosol inhalation, sodium cromoglycate 5 mg/metered inhalation. Net price 112-puff unit = £17.35; 2 × 112-puff unit with spacer device (Syncroner®) = £34.52; also available with large volume spacer inhaler (Fisonair®), complete unit = £20.05. Label: 8

Additives: include CFC propellants

Dose: by aerosol inhalation, adults and children, 10 mg (2 puffs) 4 times daily initially, increased in severe cases or during periods of risk to 6–8 times daily; additional doses may also be taken before exercise; maintenance 5 mg (1 puff) 4 times daily

Note. Sodium cromoglycate 5 mg/metered inhalation also available from Baker Norton (Cromogen®, contains CFC propellants)

Spincaps®, yellow/clear, sodium cromoglycate 20 mg. Net price 112-cap pack = £13.72. Label: 8

Dose: by inhalation of powder, adults and children, 20 mg 4 times daily, increased in severe cases to 8 times daily

Spinhaler insufflator® (for use with Intal Spincaps). Net price = £1.89

Nebuliser solution, sodium cromoglycate 10 mg/mL. Net price 2-mL amp = 31p. For use with power-operated nebuliser

Dose: by inhalation of nebulised solution, adults and children, 20 mg 4 times daily, increased in severe cases to 6 times daily

Note. Sodium cromoglycate 10 mg/mL also available for nebulisation in 2-mL unit doses as Steri-Neb Cromogen® (Baker Norton)

Compound preparations

Note. The compound inhalation of sodium cromoglycate with a beta-adrenoceptor stimulant is not recommended as the inhalation is liable to be used inappropriately for relief of bronchospasm rather than for its prophylactic effect

PoM Aerocrom® (Fisons)

Aerosol inhalation, sodium cromoglycate 1 mg, salbutamol (as sulphate) 100 micrograms/metered inhalation, net price 200-puff unit = £16.38; 200-puff unit with spacer device (Syncroner®) = £16.38. Label: 8

Additives: include CFC propellants

Dose: by aerosol inhalation, 2 inhalations 4 times daily; CHILD, not recommended

NEDOCROMIL SODIUM

Indications: prophylaxis of asthma

Side-effects: see under Sodium Cromoglycate; also headache, nausea, vomiting, dyspepsia, abdominal pain (mild and transient); bitter taste (masked by mint flavour)

Dose: by aerosol inhalation, ADULT and CHILD over 6 years 4 mg (2 puffs) 4 times daily, when control achieved may be possible to reduce to twice daily

COUNSELLING. Regular use is necessary

PoM Tilade® (Fisons)

Aerosol inhalation, nedocromil sodium 2 mg/metered inhalation. Net price 2 × 56-puff mint-flavoured units = £20.58; 2 × 112-puff unit with spacer device (Syncroner®) = £41.14. Label: 8

Additives: include CFC propellants

RELATED THERAPY

Antihistamines are of no value in the treatment of bronchial asthma. **Ketotifen** is an antihistamine with an action said to resemble that of sodium cromoglycate, but it has proved disappointing.

KETOTIFEN

Indications: see notes above

Cautions: previous anti-asthmatic treatment should be continued for a minimum of 2 weeks after initiation of ketotifen treatment; pregnancy and breast-feeding (see appendixes 4 and 5); **interactions:** Appendix 1 (antihistamines)—also, manufacturer advises avoid with oral antidiabetics (fall in thrombocyte count reported)

DRIVING. Drowsiness may affect performance of skilled tasks (e.g. driving); effects of alcohol enhanced

Side-effects: drowsiness, dry mouth, slight dizziness; CNS stimulation, weight gain also reported

Dose: 1 mg twice daily with food increased if necessary to 2 mg twice daily; initial treatment in readily sedated patients 0.5–1 mg at night; CHILD over 2 years 1 mg twice daily

PoM Zaditen® (Sandoz)

Capsules, ketotifen 1 mg (as hydrogen fumarate). Net price 60-cap pack = £8.14. Label: 2, 8, 21

Tablets, scored, ketotifen 1 mg (as hydrogen fumarate). Net price 60-tab pack = £8.14. Label: 2, 8, 21

Elixir, ketotifen 1 mg (as hydrogen fumarate)/ 5 mL. Net price 150 mL = £4.82. Label: 2, 8, 21

3.4 Antihistamines, hyposensitisation, and allergic emergencies

3.4.1 Antihistamines
3.4.2 Hyposensitisation
3.4.3 Allergic emergencies

3.4.1 Antihistamines

All antihistamines are of potential value in the treatment of *nasal allergies*, particularly seasonal (hay fever), and may be of some value in *vasomotor rhinitis*. They reduce rhinorrhoea and sneezing but are usually less effective for nasal congestion.

Oral antihistamines are also of some value in preventing *urticaria* and are used to treat *urticarial rashes, pruritus,* and *insect bites and stings*; they are also used in *drug allergies*. Injections of chlorpheniramine or promethazine are used as an adjunct to adrenaline in the emergency treatment of *anaphylaxis* and *angioedema* (section 3.4.3). For the use of antihistamines in *nausea and vomiting*, see section 4.6.

There is no evidence that any one of the older, sedative antihistamines is superior to any other and patients vary widely in their responses. They differ somewhat in duration of action and incidence of side-effects (drowsiness and antimuscarinic effects). Most are relatively short-acting but some, (e.g. promethazine) act for up to 12 hours. They all cause sedation but **promethazine**, **trimeprazine**, and **dimenhydrinate** may be more sedating whereas **chlorpheniramine**, **cyclizine**, and **mequitazine** may be less so.

Acrivastine, **astemizole**, **cetirizine**, **loratadine**, and **terfenadine** are newer antihistamines; they are a very major advance over the older antihistamines. They cause less sedation and psychomotor impairment because they only penetrate the blood brain barrier to a slight extent (and for this reason do not alleviate pruritus of non-allergic origin). Astemizole has a relatively slow onset of action and is more appropriate for use on a regular basis than when symptoms occur.

DISADVANTAGES OF ANTIHISTAMINES. Drowsiness is a particular disadvantage with most of the older antihistamines (although paradoxical stimulation may rarely occur, especially in high dosage or in children); drowsiness is considerably less of a problem with the newer ones (see also notes above).

Other side-effects that are more common with the older antihistamines include headache, psychomotor impairment, antimuscarinic effects such as urinary retention, dry mouth, blurred vision, and gastro-intestinal disturbances.

Other side-effects of antihistamines reported include rashes and photosensitivity reactions, palpitations and arrhythmias (**important**: see especially risks associated with *astemizole* and *terfenadine*, see below and p. 138), hypersensitivity reactions (including bronchospasm, angioedema, and anaphylaxis), convulsions, sweating, myalgia, paraesthesia, blood disorders, extrapyramidal effects, tremor, liver dysfunction, sleep disturbances, depression, hypotension, and hair loss.

Antihistamines should be used with caution in epilepsy, prostatic hypertrophy, urinary retention, glaucoma, and hepatic disease (astemizole and terfenadine in particular should be avoided if significant impairment). Most antihistamines should be avoided in **porphyria**, but chlorpheniramine and cyclizine have been used (see section 9.8.2). **Interactions:** Appendix 1 (antihistamines; **important**: special problems with *astemizole* and *terfenadine*). **Pregnancy** and **breast-feeding**: Appendixes 4 and 5 (antihistamines).

NON-SEDATIVE ANTIHISTAMINES

DRIVING. Although drowsiness is rare, nevertheless patients should be advised that it can occur and may affect performance of skilled tasks (e.g. driving); excess alcohol should be avoided.

ACRIVASTINE

Indications: symptomatic relief of allergy such as hay fever, urticaria

Cautions; Contra-indications: see notes above; pending specific studies avoid in renal impairment

Side-effects: see notes above; incidence of sedation and antimuscarinic effects low

Dose: 8 mg 3 times daily; CHILD under 12 years, not recommended; ELDERLY not recommended

PoM Semprex® (Wellcome)

Capsules, acrivastine 8 mg. Net price 84-cap pack = £5.04. Counselling, driving

ASTEMIZOLE

Indications: symptomatic relief of allergy such as hay fever, urticaria

Cautions; Contra-indications: see Terfenadine and notes above; pregnancy and breast-feeding (see below); **important:** see also Arrhythmias, below

PREGNANCY AND BREAST-FEEDING. Manufacturer advises avoid in pregnancy (toxicity at high doses in *animals*) and advises that women of childbearing potential should use contraception while taking astemizole and (owing to long half-life) for several weeks after stopping. Manufacturer also advises avoid in breast-feeding

ARRHYTHMIAS. Rare hazardous arrhythmias are associated with astemizole and terfenadine particularly in association with increased blood concentrations—these two antihistamines should *not* be taken concomitantly (and the long half-life of astemizole should be borne in mind).

Recommendations are: *not to exceed* recommended dose, *to avoid* in significant hepatic impairment, and *to avoid* concomitant administration of *ketoconazole, itraconazole and other imidazole antifungals* and of *erythromycin and clarithromycin, to avoid* if hypokalaemia (or other electrolyte imbalance) or prolonged QT interval known or suspected and *to avoid* concomitant administration of potentially arrhythmogenic drugs such as *anti-arrhythmics, antipsychotics, tricyclic antidepressants, quinine,* and of drugs liable to produce electrolyte imbalance such as *diuretics.*

If syncope occurs the antihistamine should be discontinued and patient evaluated for potential arrhythmias

Side-effects: see notes above; weight gain occurs infrequently; incidence of sedation and antimuscarinic effects low; **important**: ventricular arrhythmias (including torsades de pointes) have followed excessive dosage, for recommendations see also Arrhythmias above

Dose: 10 mg daily (must **not** be exceeded); CHILD under 6 years not recommended, 6–12 years 5 mg daily (must **not** be exceeded)

PoM ¹**Hismanal**® (Janssen)

Tablets, scored, astemizole 10 mg. Net price 30-tab pack = £5.70. Counselling, driving

Suspension, sugar-free, astemizole 5 mg/5 mL. Net price 200 mL = £5.80. Counselling, driving

1. Tablets can be sold to the public for the treatment of hay fever in adults and children over 12 years; another brand on sale to the public is Pollon-eze®

CETIRIZINE

Indications: symptomatic relief of allergy such as hay fever, urticaria

Cautions; Contra-indications: see notes above; halve dose in renal impairment; incidence of sedation and antimuscarinic effects low

Side-effects: see notes above

Dose: ADULT and CHILD over 6 years, 10 mg daily *or* 5 mg twice daily; CHILD 2–6 years, hayfever, 5 mg daily *or* 2.5 mg twice daily

PoM ¹**Zirtek**® (UCB Pharma)

Tablets, f/c, scored, cetirizine hydrochloride 10 mg. Net price 30-tab pack = £8.73. Counselling, driving

Oral solution, sugar-free, cetirizine hydrochloride 5 mg/5 mL. Net price 200 mL = £14.95. Counselling, driving

1. Tablets can be sold to the public for adults and children over 12 years provided packs do not contain more than 10 days' supply

LORATADINE

Indications: symptomatic relief of allergy such as hay fever, urticaria

Cautions; Contra-indications; Side-effects: see notes above; incidence of sedation and antimuscarinic effects low; pregnancy (toxicity at high doses in *animals*) and breast-feeding (see also appendixes 4 and 5)

Dose: 10 mg daily; CHILD 2–12 years, under 30 kg 5 mg daily, over 30 kg 10 mg daily

PoM ¹**Clarityn**® (Schering-Plough)

Tablets, scored, loratadine 10 mg. Net price 30-tab pack = £7.57. Counselling, driving

Syrup, yellow, loratadine 5 mg/5 mL. Net price 100 mL = £7.57. Counselling, driving

1. Tablets can be sold to the public for adults and children over 12 years provided packs do not contain more than 10 days' supply

TERFENADINE

Indications: symptomatic relief of allergy such as hay fever, urticaria

Cautions; Contra-indications: see notes above; **important**, see also Arrhythmias, below

ARRHYTHMIAS. Rare hazardous arrhythmias are associated with astemizole and terfenadine particularly in association with increased blood concentrations—these two antihistamines should *not* be taken concomitantly (and the long half-life of astemizole should be borne in mind).

Recommendations are: *not to exceed* recommended dose, *to avoid* in significant hepatic impairment, and *to avoid* concomitant administration of *ketoconazole, itraconazole and other imidazole antifungals* and of *erythromycin and clarithromycin, to avoid* if hypokalaemia (or other electrolyte imbalance) or prolonged QT interval known or suspected and *to avoid* concomitant administration of potentially arrhythmogenic drugs such as *anti-arrhythmics, antipsychotics, tricyclic antidepressants* and of drugs liable to produce electrolyte imbalance such as *diuretics.*

If syncope occurs the antihistamine should be discontinued and patient evaluated for potential arrhythmias

Side-effects: see notes above; incidence of sedation and antimuscarinic effects low; **important:** ventricular arrhythmias (including torsades de pointes) have followed excessive dosage, see also Arrhythmias above

Dose: hay fever, allergic rhinitis, 60 mg daily increased if necessary to 120 mg daily, in single or 2 divided doses;

Allergic skin conditions, 120 mg daily in single or 2 divided doses;

CHILD (hay fever, allergic rhinitis or allergic skin conditions) 3–6 years 15 mg twice daily; 6–12 years 30 mg twice daily

PoM ¹**Triludan**® (Merrell)

Tablets, scored, terfenadine 60 mg. Net price 60-tab pack = £5.40. Counselling, driving

Forte tablets, terfenadine 120 mg. Net price 7-tab pack = £2.21; 30-tab pack = £5.40. Counselling, driving

Suspension, sugar-free, terfenadine 30 mg/5 mL. Net price 200 mL = £4.13. Counselling, driving

1. Tablets can be sold to the public for adults and children over 6 years provided packs do not contain more than 10 days' supply; other brands on sale to the public include Aller-Eze Clear® (terfenadine 60 mg), Boots Antihistamine Tablets® (terfenadine 60 mg), Boots One-a-Day Antihistamine Tablets® (terfenadine 120 mg), Histafen® (terfenadine 60 mg), Seldane® (terfenadine 120 mg), Terfenor® (terfenadine 30 mg, 60 mg, 120 mg), Terfex® (terfenadine 60 mg); terfenadine 60-mg tablets also available from APS, Ashbourne (Terfinax® 60), Cox, Hillcross, and Norton

SEDATIVE ANTIHISTAMINES

DRIVING. Drowsiness may affect performance of skilled tasks (e.g. driving); effects of alcohol enhanced.

AZATADINE MALEATE

Indications: symptomatic relief of allergy such as hay fever, urticaria
Cautions; Contra-indications; Side-effects: see notes above
Dose: 1 mg, increased if necessary to 2 mg, twice daily; CHILD under 1 year not recommended, 1–6 years 250 micrograms twice daily, 6–12 years 0.5–1 mg twice daily

Optimine® (Schering-Plough)
Tablets, scored, azatadine maleate 1 mg. Net price 56-tab pack = £2.80. Label: 2
Syrup, azatadine maleate 500 micrograms/5 mL. Net price 120 mL = £1.39. Label: 2

BROMPHENIRAMINE MALEATE

Indications: symptomatic relief of allergy such as hay fever, urticaria
Cautions; Contra-indications; Side-effects: see notes above
Dose: 4–8 mg 3–4 times daily; CHILD up to 3 years 0.4–1 mg/kg daily in 4 divided doses, 3–6 years 2 mg 3–4 times daily, 6–12 years 2–4 mg 3–4 times daily

Dimotane® (Wyeth)
Tablets, peach, scored, brompheniramine maleate 4 mg. Net price 20 = 59p. Label: 2
Elixir, yellow-green, brompheniramine maleate 2 mg/5 mL. Net price 100 mL = 71p. Label: 2
Dimotane LA® (Wyeth)
Tablets, m/r, peach, s/c, brompheniramine maleate 12 mg. Net price 20 = 89p. Label: 2, 25
 Dose: 12–24 mg twice daily; CHILD 6–12 years 12 mg at bedtime, increased if necessary to 12 mg twice daily
For a list of **cough and decongestant preparations on sale to the public**, including those containing brompheniramine, see section 3.9.2.
For compound preparations containing brompheniramine and pseudoephedrine, see also section 3.10

BUCLIZINE

Ingredient of Migraleve® (see Analgesics with Antiemetics, section 4.7.4.1)

CHLORPHENIRAMINE MALEATE

(Chlorphenamine Maleate)
Indications: symptomatic relief of allergy such as hay fever, urticaria; emergency treatment of ana-phylactic reactions (section 3.4.3)
Cautions; Contra-indications; Side-effects: see notes above. Injections may be irritant and cause transitory hypotension or CNS stimulation

Dose: by mouth, 4 mg every 4–6 hours, max. 24 mg daily; CHILD under 1 year not recommended, 1–2 years 1 mg twice daily, 2–5 years 1 mg every 4–6 hours, max. 6 mg daily, 6–12 years 2 mg every 4–6 hours, max. 12 mg daily
By subcutaneous or intramuscular injection, 10–20 mg, repeated if required; max. 40 mg in 24 hours
By slow intravenous injection over 1 minute, 10–20 mg

Piriton® (A&H)
Tablets, ivory, chlorpheniramine maleate 4 mg. Net price 20 = 19p. Label: 2
Syrup, chlorpheniramine maleate 2 mg/5 mL. Net price 150 mL = £1.42. Label: 2
PoM *Injection,* chlorpheniramine maleate 10 mg/mL. Net price 1-mL amp = 12p
 Note. In addition to Piriton®, proprietary brands of chlorpheniramine maleate tablets on sale to the public include Calimal®; chlorpheniramine maleate 4 mg tablets are also available from Cox and Hillcross
For a list of **cough and decongestant preparations on sale to the public**, including those containing chlorphenir-amine, see section 3.9.2

CINNARIZINE
See section 4.6

CLEMASTINE

Indications: symptomatic relief of allergy such as hay fever, urticaria
Cautions; Contra-indications; Side-effects: see notes above
Dose: 1 mg twice daily; CHILD under 1 year not recommended, 1–3 years 250–500 micrograms twice daily; 3–6 years 500 micrograms twice daily; 6–12 years 0.5–1 mg twice daily

Tavegil® (Sandoz)
Tablets, scored, clemastine 1 mg (as hydrogen fumarate). Net price 50-tab pack = £2.05. Label: 2
Elixir, sugar-free, clemastine 500 micrograms (as hydrogen fumarate)/5 mL. Net price 150 mL = 96p. Label: 2
Note. In addition to Tavegil®, proprietary brands of clem-astine hydrogen fumarate on sale to the public include Aller-eze®; it is also on sale to the public combined with phenylpropanolamine (Aller-eze Plus®)

CYCLIZINE
See section 4.6

CYPROHEPTADINE HYDROCHLORIDE

Indications: symptomatic relief of allergy such as hay fever, urticaria; migraine
Cautions; Contra-indications; Side-effects: see notes above; may cause weight gain
Dose: allergy, usual dose 4 mg 3–4 times daily; usual range 4–20 mg daily, max. 32 mg daily; CHILD under 2 years not recommended, 2–6 years 2 mg 2–3 times daily, max. 12 mg daily; 7–14 years 4 mg 2–3 times daily, max. 16 mg daily
Migraine, 4 mg with a further 4 mg after 30 min-utes if necessary; maintenance, 4 mg every 4–6 hours

Periactin® (MSD)

Tablets, scored, cyproheptadine hydrochloride 4 mg. Net price 20 = 57p. Label: 2

DIMENHYDRINATE

See section 4.6

DIPHENHYDRAMINE HYDROCHLORIDE

Indications: see under Preparations

Cautions; Contra-indications; Side-effects: see notes above

Preparations

Proprietary brands of diphenhydramine hydrochloride on sale to the public to aid relief of temporary sleep disturbance in adults include Medinex® (diphenhydramine hydrochloride 10 mg/5 mL and Nytol® (diphenhydramine hydrochloride tablets 25 mg and 50 mg)

For a list of **cough and decongestant preparations on sale to the public**, including those containing diphenhydramine, see section 3.9.2

DIPHENYLPYRALINE HYDROCHLORIDE

Cautions; Contra-indications; Side-effects: see notes above

Preparations

For a list of **cough and decongestant preparations on sale to the public**, including those containing diphenylpyraline, see section 3.9.2

DOXYLAMINE

Cautions; Contra-indications; Side-effects: see notes above

Preparations

Ingredient of **cough and decongestant preparations** (section 3.9.2.) and of **compound analgesics** (section 4.7.1.) on sale to the public

HYDROXYZINE HYDROCHLORIDE

Indications: pruritus, anxiety (short-term)

Cautions; Contra-indications; Side-effects: see notes above

Dose: pruritus, initially 25 mg at night increased if necessary to 25 mg 3–4 times daily; CHILD 6 months–6 years initially 5–15 mg daily increased if necessary to 50 mg daily in divided doses; over 6 years initially 15–25 mg daily increased if necessary to 50–100 mg daily in divided doses

Anxiety (adults only), 50–100 mg 4 times daily

PoM Atarax® (Pfizer)

Tablets, both s/c, hydroxyzine hydrochloride 10 mg (orange), net price 84-tab pack = £1.52; 25 mg (green), 28-tab pack = £1.02. Label: 2

Syrup, hydroxyzine hydrochloride 10 mg/5 mL. Net price 150-mL pack = 85p. Label: 2

PoM Ucerax® (UCB Pharma)

Tablets, f/c, scored, hydroxyzine hydrochloride 25 mg, net price 25-tab pack = £1.73. Label: 2

Syrup, hydroxyzine hydrochloride 10 mg/5 mL. Net price 200-mL pack = £1.91. Label: 2

KETOTIFEN

See section 3.3

MEQUITAZINE

Indications: symptomatic relief of allergy such as hay fever, urticaria

Cautions; Contra-indications; Side-effects: see notes above

Dose: 5 mg twice daily; CHILD under 12 years, not recommended

PoM Primalan® (Rhône-Poulenc Rorer)

Tablets, mequitazine 5 mg. Net price 56-tab pack = £2.80. Label: 2

PHENINDAMINE TARTRATE

Indications: symptomatic relief of allergy such as hay fever, urticaria

Cautions; Contra-indications; Side-effects: see notes above; may cause mild CNS stimulation

Dose: 25–50 mg 1–3 times daily; CHILD over 10 years 25 mg 1–3 times daily

Thephorin® (Sinclair)

Tablets, s/c, phenindamine tartrate 25 mg. Net price 50-tab pack = £1.66. Label: 2

PHENIRAMINE MALEATE

Indications: symptomatic relief of allergy such as hay fever, urticaria

Cautions; Contra-indications; Side-effects: see notes above

Daneral SA® (Hoechst)

Tablets, m/r, pink, s/c, pheniramine maleate 75 mg. Net price 30-tab pack = £2.54. Label: 2, 25

Dose: 75–150 mg at night or 75 mg night and morning

For a list of **cough and decongestant preparations on sale to the public**, including those containing pheniramine, see section 3.9.2

PROMETHAZINE HYDROCHLORIDE

Indications: symptomatic relief of allergy such as hay fever, urticaria; emergency treatment of anaphylactic reactions (section 3.4.3)

For use in premedication, see section 15.1.4.1; sedation, see section 4.1.1; motion sickness see section 4.6

Cautions; Contra-indications; Side-effects: see notes above; intramuscular injection may be painful

Dose: by mouth, 25 mg at night increased to 50 mg if necessary *or* 10–20 mg 2–3 times daily; CHILD under 2 years not recommended, 2–5 years 5–15 mg daily, 5–10 years 10–25 mg daily

By deep intramuscular injection, 25–50 mg; max. 100 mg; CHILD 5–10 years 6.25–12.5 mg

By slow intravenous injection in emergencies, 25–50 mg, max. 100 mg, as a solution containing 2.5 mg/mL in water for injections

---

Phenergan® (Rhône-Poulenc Rorer)

Tablets, both blue, f/c, promethazine hydrochloride 10 mg, net price 56-tab pack = £1.00; 25 mg, 56-tab pack = £1.49. Label: 2

Elixir, golden, promethazine hydrochloride 5 mg/ 5 mL. Net price 100 mL = £1.12. Label: 2

PoM *Injection*, promethazine hydrochloride 25 mg/ mL. Net price 1-mL amp = 34p

Promethazine hydrochloride injection 25 mg/mL (1-mL and 2-mL ampoules) also available from Antigen

Note. Proprietary brands of promethazine hydrochloride on sale to the public include Phenergan Nightime® (promethazine hydrochloride tablets 25 mg, for occasional insomnia in adults), Sominex® (promethazine hydrochloride tablets 20 mg, for occasional insomnia in adults) and Q-Mazine® (promethazine hydrochloride 5 mg/5 mL for urticaria and other skin conditions in children)

For a list of **cough and decongestant preparations on sale to the public**, including those containing promethazine, see section 3.9.2

PROMETHAZINE THEOCLATE
See section 4.6

TRIMEPRAZINE TARTRATE
(Alimemazine Tartrate)

Indications: urticaria and pruritus; premedication, see section 15.1.4.1

Cautions; Contra-indications; Side-effects: see notes above; see also under Chlorpromazine Hydrochloride, section 4.2.1

Dose: 10 mg 2–3 times daily, in severe cases up to max. 100 mg daily has been used; ELDERLY 10 mg 1–2 times daily; CHILD under 2 years not recommended; over 2 years 2.5–5 mg 3–4 times daily

PoM Vallergan® (Rhône-Poulenc Rorer)

Tablets, blue, f/c, trimeprazine tartrate 10 mg. Net price 28-tab pack = £1.03. Label: 2

Syrup, straw coloured, trimeprazine tartrate 7.5 mg /5 mL. Net price 100 mL = £1.17. Label: 2

Syrup forte, trimeprazine tartrate 30 mg/5 mL. Net price 100 mL = £2.42. Label: 2

Note. For use of Forte Syrup see section 15.1.4.1

TRIPROLIDINE HYDROCHLORIDE

Cautions; Contra-indications; Side-effects: see notes above

Preparations

For a list of **cough and decongestant preparations on sale to the public**, including those containing triprolidine, see section 3.9.2

3.4.2   Hyposensitisation

Except for wasp and bee sting allergy the value of specific hyposensitisation is uncertain; administration of allergen extract desensitising vaccines is associated with a significant risk of anaphylaxis, see CSM advice below. Most atopic (allergic) patients are sensitive to a wide range of allergens hence hyposensitisation with an extract of a single allergen is usually no more than partially successful.

Diagnostic skin tests are unreliable and can only be used in conjunction with a detailed history of allergen exposure.

CSM advice. After re-examination of the efficacy and safety of desensitising vaccines, the CSM has concluded that they should only be used for the following indications:

—Seasonal allergic hay fever (which has not responded to anti-allergy drugs) caused by pollens, using licensed products only—patients with *asthma* should not be treated with desensitising vaccines as they are more likely to develop severe adverse reactions.

—Hypersensitivity to wasp and bee venoms—since reactions can be life-threatening, *asthma* is not an absolute contra-indication. There is inadequate evidence of benefit from other allergens such as house dust, house dust mite, animal danders and foods and they are *not* recommended. Desensitising vaccines should be avoided in pregnant women, in children under five years old, and in those taking beta-blockers.

Recent experience indicates that bronchospasm usually develops within 1 hour and anaphylaxis within 30 minutes of injection. Therefore patients need to be monitored for 1 hour after injection. If symptoms or signs of hypersensitivity **develop** (e.g. rash, urticaria, bronchospasm, faintness), **even when mild**, the patient should be observed until these have **completely resolved**.

For details of the management of anaphylactic shock, see section 3.4.3.

ALLERGEN EXTRACT VACCINES

Each set usually contains vials for the administration of graded amounts to patients undergoing hyposensitisation. Maintenance sets containing vials at the highest strength are also available. Manufacturer's literature must be consulted for details of allergens, vial strengths, and administration

Indications: hypersensitivity to one or more common allergens (see notes above)

Cautions: see notes above including CSM advice; manufacturers recommend that patients should be warned not to eat a heavy meal before the injection

CSM advice. The CSM has advised that facilities for cardiopulmonary resuscitation must be immediately available and patients monitored closely for one hour after each injection, for full details see above.

Contra-indications: pregnancy, febrile conditions, acute asthma

Side-effects: allergic reactions, especially in small children

Dose: by subcutaneous injection, see manufacturer's literature

---

Wasp and bee venom allergy preparations

PoM Pharmalgen® (ALK)

Bee venom extract (*Apis mellifera*) or wasp venom extract (*Vespula* spp.). Net price initial treatment set = £62.59 (bee), £76.73 (wasp); maintenance treatment set = £72.82 (bee), £93.67 (wasp)

3.4.3   Allergic emergencies

Adrenaline provides physiological reversal of the immediate symptoms (such as laryngeal oedema, bronchospasm, and hypotension) associated with hypersensitivity reactions such as *anaphylaxis* and *angioedema*. See below for full details of *adrenaline administration* and for *adjunctive treatment*.

ANAPHYLAXIS

Anaphylactic shock requires prompt energetic treatment of *laryngeal oedema, bronchospasm,* and *hypotension.* Atopic individuals are particularly susceptible. *Insect bites* are a recognised risk (in particular *wasp* and *bee stings*). Certain foods, including *eggs, fish, cow's milk protein, peanuts,* and *nuts* may also precipitate anaphylaxis. Medicinal products particularly associated with anaphylaxis include *blood products, vaccines, hyposensitising (allergen) preparations, antibiotics, aspirin and other NSAIDs, iron injections, heparin,* and *neuromuscular blocking drugs.* In the case of drugs, anaphylaxis is more likely after parenteral administration; resuscitation facilities must always be available for injections associated with special risk. Anaphylactic reactions may also be associated with *additives and excipients* in foods and medicines; some oils, such as arachis (peanut) oil, may be contaminated with allergenic proteins from their original source—it is wise to check the full formula of preparations which may contain *allergenic fats or oils* (including those for topical application, particularly if they are intended for use in the mouth or for application to the nasal mucosa).

First-line treatment includes securing the airway, restoration of blood pressure (laying the patient flat, raising the feet), and administration of **adrenaline** injection. This is given **intramuscularly** in a dose of 0.5–1 mg (0.5–1 mL adrenaline injection 1 in 1000); a dose of 300 micrograms (0.3 mL adrenaline injection 1 in 1000) may be appropriate for *immediate self-administration.* The dose is repeated every 10 minutes, according to blood pressure and pulse, until improvement occurs [important: possible need for *intravenous route* using *dilute solution,* see below]. **Oxygen** administration is also of primary importance. An antihistamine (e.g. **chlorpheniramine,** given by slow intravenous injection in a dose of 10–20 mg, see p. 139) is a useful adjunctive treatment, given after adrenaline injection and continued for 24 to 48 hours to prevent relapse. In patients on non-cardioselective beta-blockers severe anaphylaxis may not respond to adrenaline injection, calling for addition of **salbutamol** by intravenous injection.

Continuing deterioration requires further treatment including intravenous fluids (see section 9.2.2), intravenous aminophylline (see p. 129) or a nebulised beta$_2$-adrenoceptor stimulant (such as salbutamol or terbutaline, see p. 122 and p. 123); in addition to oxygen, assisted respiration and possibly emergency tracheotomy may be necessary.

An intravenous corticosteroid e.g. **hydrocortisone** (as sodium succinate) in a dose of 100–300 mg is of secondary value in the initial management of anaphylactic shock as the onset of action is delayed for several hours, but should be given *to prevent further deterioration* in severely affected patients.

When a patient is so ill that there is *doubt as to the adequacy of the circulation,* the initial injection of adrenaline may need to be given as a *dilute solution by the intravenous route,* for details of *cau-*

tions, dose and *strength,* see under Intravenous Adrenaline, below.

Some patients with severe allergy to insect stings or foods are encouraged to carry pre-filled adrenaline syringes (e.g. *EpiPen®*) for *self-administration* during periods of risk; adrenaline inhalations (*Medihaler-epi®*) are much less effective, but may be useful for the individual without other symptoms who is beginning to develop angioedema and laryngeal oedema (**important:** for patients with previous very serious reactions *adrenaline injection is always the first line of treatment*).

ANGIOEDEMA

Angioedema is dangerous if *laryngeal oedema* is present. In this circumstance adrenaline injection and oxygen should be given as described under Anaphylaxis (see above); antihistamines and corticosteroids should also be given (see again above). Tracheal intubation and other measures may be necessary.

The administration of C_1 esterase inhibitor (in fresh frozen plasma or in partially purified form) may terminate acute attacks of *hereditary angioedema,* but is not practical for long-term prophylaxis.

INTRAMUSCULAR (OR SUBCUTANEOUS) ADRENALINE

The *intramuscular route* is the *first choice route* for the administration of adrenaline in the management of anaphylactic shock. Adrenaline has a rapid onset of action after intramuscular administration and in the shocked patient its absorption from the intramuscular site may be faster and more reliable than from the subcutaneous site (the intravenous route should be reserved for extreme emergency when there is doubt as to the adequacy of the circulation, for details of *cautions, dose* and *strength* see under Intravenous Adrenaline, below).

Patients with severe allergy should ideally be instructed in the self-administration of adrenaline by intramuscular injection (for details see under Self-administration of Adrenaline, below).

Prompt injection of adrenaline is of paramount importance and the recommendations in the following table avoid the need for complex dosage calculations in children.

Volume of adrenaline injection **1 in 1000** (1 mg/mL) for **intramuscular** injection (or alternatively **subcutaneous** injection) in anaphylactic shock

Age	Volume of adrenaline 1 in 1000
Under 1 year	0.05 mL
1 year	0.1 mL
2 years	0.2 mL[1]
3–4 years	0.3 mL[1]
5 years	0.4 mL[1]
6–12 years	0.5 mL[1]
Adult	0.5–1 mL

These doses may be repeated every 10 minutes, according to blood pressure and pulse, until improvement occurs (may be repeated several times).
1. Suitable for robust children in these age groups; for underweight children use half these doses.

INTRAVENOUS ADRENALINE

Where the patient is severely ill and there is real doubt about adequacy of the circulation and absorption from the intramuscular injection site, adrenaline may be given by *slow intravenous injection* in a dose of 500 micrograms (5 mL of the dilute 1 in 10 000 adrenaline injection) given at a rate of 100 micrograms (1 mL of the dilute 1 in 10 000 adrenaline injection) per minute, *stopping when a response has been obtained*; children can be given a dose of 10 micrograms/kg (0.1 mL/kg of the dilute 1 in 10 000 adrenaline injection) by *slow intravenous injection* over several minutes. *Constant vigilance* is needed to ensure that the *correct strength* is used; anaphylactic shock kits need to make a *very clear distinction* between the 1 in 10 000 strength and the 1 in 1000 strength. It is *also* important that, where intramuscular injection might still succeed, time should *not be wasted* seeking intravenous access.

For reference to the use of the intravenous route for *cardiac resuscitation*, see section 2.7.3.

SELF-ADMINISTRATION OF ADRENALINE

Individuals who are at considerable risk of anaphylaxis need to carry adrenaline with them at all times and need to be *instructed in advance* how to inject it. In addition, the packs need to be labelled so that in the case of rapid collapse someone else is able to administer the adrenaline. It is important to ensure that an adequate supply is provided to treat symptoms until medical assistance is available.

Some patients may best be able to cope with a pre-assembled syringe fitted with a needle suitable for very rapid administration (if necessary by a bystander). *EpiPen*® consists of a fully assembled syringe and needle delivering a dose of 300 micrograms of adrenaline by *intramuscular injection*; a 150-microgram version (*EpiPen*® Jr) is also available for use in children. Other products for the immediate treatment of individuals at risk of anaphylaxis are available but are not licensed for use in the UK. *Anapen*® *Adult* is a fully assembled device that delivers 300 micrograms of adrenaline by *intramuscular injection*; a 150-microgram version (*Anapen*® *Junior*) is also available. *Anapen*® is available on a named-patient basis from Allerayde. *Ana-Guard*® is a pre-filled syringe that delivers two 300-microgram doses of adrenaline by *subcutaneous or intramuscular injection*; it can be adjusted to administer smaller doses for children. *Ana-Kit*® includes a similar pre-filled adrenaline syringe, chewable tablets of chlorpheniramine maleate 2 mg, 2 sterile pads impregnated with 70% isopropyl alcohol, and a tourniquet. *Ana-Guard*® and *Ana-Kit*® are available on a named-patient basis from IDIS.

INHALATION OF ADRENALINE

Adrenaline inhalation (Medihaler-epi®) is also available, but the ability to inhale during an attack may be limited. Nevertheless, it may be useful for the individual without other symptoms who is beginning to develop angioedema and laryngeal oedema (**important**: for those with previous very severe reactions *adrenaline injection* needs to remain the *first line of treatment*).

ADRENALINE
(Epinephrine)

Indications: emergency treatment of acute anaphylaxis; angioedema; cardiopulmonary resuscitation, section 2.7.3

Cautions: hyperthyroidism, diabetes mellitus, ischaemic heart disease, hypertension, elderly patients

INTERACTIONS. Severe anaphylaxis in patients on non-cardioselective beta-blockers may not respond to adrenaline injection calling for *intravenous injection of salbutamol* (see p. 122). Patients on tricyclic antidepressants are considerably more susceptible to arrhythmias calling for a *much reduced* dose of adrenaline. Other **interactions**, see Appendix 1 (sympathomimetics).

Side-effects: anxiety, tremor, tachycardia, arrhythmias, cold extremities; also hypertension (risk of cerebral haemorrhage) and pulmonary oedema (on excessive dosage or extreme sensitivity); nausea, vomiting, sweating, weakness, and dizziness also reported

Dose: acute anaphylaxis, *by intramuscular (or subcutaneous) injection* see notes and table above

Acute anaphylaxis when there is doubt as to the adequacy of the circulation, *by intravenous injection* (dilute, extreme caution), see notes above

IMPORTANT. Intravenous route should be used with **extreme care**, see notes above

Intramuscular or subcutaneous
PoM Adrenaline Injection, BP, 1 in 1000 (Non-proprietary)

Injection, adrenaline (as acid tartrate) 1 mg/mL, net price 0.5-mL amp = 42p; 1-mL amp = 32p

Available from Antigen, Boots, Evans, Hillcross, Martindale, Phoenix

PoM Min-I-Jet® Adrenaline (IMS)

Injection, adrenaline 1 in 1000 (1 mg/mL as hydrochloride). Net price 1 mL (with 25 gauge × 0.25 inch needle for subcutaneous injection) = £7.37, 1 mL (with 21 gauge × 1.5 inch needle for intramuscular injection) = £3.91 (both disposable syringes)

Intravenous
Extreme caution, see notes above
PoM Adrenaline Injection, 1 in 10 000 (Non-proprietary)

Injection, adrenaline (as acid tartrate) 100 micrograms/mL. 10-mL amp.

Available from Martindale (special order); also from IMS (Min-I-Jet® Adrenaline 3- and 10-mL disposable syringes)

Cautionary label wordings, see inside back cover

Prices are **net**, see p.1

Intramuscular injection for self-administration

PoM **EpiPen®** (ALK)

Epipen® Auto-injector, adrenaline 1 mg/mL (adrenaline 1 in 1000), net price 2-mL *Auto-injector* delivering a single dose of 300 micrograms = £23.50

Note. 1.7 mL of the solution remains in the *Auto-injector* after use

Dose: by intramuscular injection, ADULT and CHILD over 30 kg, 300 micrograms repeated after 15 minutes as necessary

Epipen® Jr Auto-injector, adrenaline 500 micrograms/mL (adrenaline 1 in 2000), net price 2-mL *Auto-injector* delivering a single dose of 150 micrograms = £23.50

Note. 1.7 mL of the solution remains in the *Auto-injector* after use

Dose: by intramuscular injection, CHILD 15–30 kg, 10 micrograms/kg repeated after 10 minutes as necessary

Inhalation

PoM **Medihaler-epi®** (3M)

Aerosol inhalation, adrenaline acid tartrate 280 micrograms/metered inhalation. Net price 400-inhalation unit = £2.43

Additives: include CFC propellants

Dose: by aerosol inhalation, adjunct to anaphylaxis treatment only (see notes above), min. of 20 puffs; CHILD 10–15 puffs under adult supervision

3.5   Respiratory stimulants and pulmonary surfactants

3.5.1   Respiratory stimulants
3.5.2   Pulmonary surfactants

3.5.1   Respiratory stimulants

Respiratory stimulants (analeptic drugs) have a limited place in the treatment of ventilatory failure in patients with chronic obstructive airways disease. They are effective only when given by intravenous injection or infusion and have a short duration of action. Their use has largely been replaced by ventilatory support. However, occasionally when the latter is contra-indicated and in patients with hypercapnic respiratory failure who are becoming drowsy or comatose, respiratory stimulants in the short term may arouse patients sufficiently to co-operate and clear their secretions.

Respiratory stimulants may be harmful in respiratory failure since they stimulate non-respiratory as well as respiratory muscles. They should only be given under **expert supervision** in hospital and must be combined with active physiotherapy. There is at present no oral respiratory stimulant available for long-term use in chronic respiratory failure.

Doxapram (see section 15.1.7) is given by continuous intravenous infusion. Frequent arterial blood gas studies and pH measurements are necessary during treatment to ensure the correct dosage (for full details see section 15.1.7).

Nikethamide (now discontinued by most suppliers) and ethamivan (now discontinued) were formerly used as respiratory stimulants but are no longer recommended; the effective doses were close to those causing toxic effects, especially convulsions.

DOXAPRAM HYDROCHLORIDE

See section 15.1.7

3.5.2   Pulmonary surfactants

A number of pulmonary surfactants have recently been developed for the management of respiratory distress syndrome (hyaline membrane disease) in preterm infants.

BERACTANT

Indications: treatment of respiratory distress syndrome in preterm infants who are intubated and receiving mechanical ventilation, whose heart rate and arterial oxygenation are continuously monitored

Cautions: continuous monitoring required to avoid hyperoxaemia (due to rapid improvement in arterial oxygen concentration)

Side-effects: pulmonary haemorrhage reported

Dose: by endotracheal tube, phospholipid 100 mg/kg equivalent to a volume of 4 mL/kg, preferably within 8 hours of birth; may be repeated within 48 hours at intervals of at least 6 hours for up to 4 doses

PoM **Survanta®** (Abbott)

Suspension, beractant (bovine lung extract) providing phospholipid 25 mg/mL, with lipids and proteins, Net price 8-mL vial = £306.43

COLFOSCERIL PALMITATE

Indications: as for Beractant (also prophylaxis of respiratory distress syndrome)

Cautions; Side-effects: as for Beractant; may increase incidence of pulmonary haemorrhage; obstruction of endotracheal tube by mucous secretions

Dose: by endotracheal tube, treatment, 67.5 mg/kg; if still intubated, may be repeated after 12 hours; prophylaxis, first dose soon after birth, if still intubated may be repeated 12 and 24 hours later

PoM **Exosurf Neonatal®** (Wellcome)

Suspension, colfosceril palmitate 108 mg for reconstitution with 8 mL water for injections (when reconstituted, contains 67.5 mg/5 mL). Net price per vial (with endotracheal tube connectors) = £306.43

PORACTANT ALFA

Indications: as for Beractant

Cautions; Side-effects: as for Beractant; also transient depression of cerebro-electrical activity; data sheet reports no evidence of increased risk of pulmonary haemorrhage

Dose: by endotracheal tube, 100–200 mg/kg as soon as possible after diagnosing respiratory distress syndrome; if still intubated, further doses of 100 mg/kg may be repeated after 12 and 24 hours if required; max. total dose 300–400 mg/kg

PoM **Curosurf®** (Serono)

Suspension, poractant alfa (porcine lung phospholipid fraction) 80 mg/mL. Net price 1.5-mL vial = £400.00; 3-mL vial = £800.00

PUMACTANT

Indications: as for Beractant (also prophylaxis of respiratory distress syndrome)
Cautions: as for Beractant
Side-effects: obstruction of endotracheal tube
Dose: by endotracheal tube, 100 mg as soon as possible after intubation; if still intubated may be repeated after 1 hour and again at 24 hours after intubation

▼ PoM **Alec**® (Britannia)
Suspension, pumactant 100 mg (human lung phospholipid fraction) for reconstitution with 2 mL sterile sodium chloride 0.9%. Net price per vial (with syringe and catheter) = £150.00

3.6 Oxygen

Oxygen should be regarded as a drug. It is prescribed for hypoxaemic patients to increase alveolar oxygen tension and decrease the work of breathing necessary to maintain a given arterial oxygen tension. The concentration depends on the condition being treated; an inappropriate concentration may have serious or even lethal effects.

High concentration oxygen therapy, with concentrations of up to 60% for short periods, is safe in conditions such as pneumonia, pulmonary thromboembolism, and fibrosing alveolitis. In such conditions low arterial oxygen (P_aO_2) is usually associated with low or normal arterial carbon dioxide (P_aCO_2), therefore there is little risk of hypoventilation and carbon dioxide retention.

In severe acute asthma, the arterial carbon dioxide (P_aCO_2) is usually subnormal but as asthma deteriorates may rise steeply (particularly in children). These patients usually require high concentrations of oxygen and if the arterial carbon dioxide (P_aCO_2) remains high despite other treatment intermittent positive pressure ventilation needs to be considered urgently. Where facilities for blood gas measurements are not immediately available, for example while transferring the patient to hospital, 35% to 50% oxygen delivered through a conventional mask is recommended. Exceptionally, asthma is diagnosed in patients with a long history of chronic bronchitis and probable respiratory failure; in these patients a lower concentration (24% to 28%) may be needed to limit oxygen-induced reduction of respiratory drive.

Low concentration oxygen therapy (controlled oxygen therapy) is reserved for patients with ventilatory failure due to chronic obstructive airways disease or other causes. The concentration should not exceed 28% and in some patients a concentration above 24% may be excessive. The aim is to provide the patient with just enough oxygen to improve hypoxaemia without worsening pre-existing carbon dioxide retention and respiratory acidosis. Treatment should be initiated in hospital as repeated blood gas measurements are required to estimate the correct concentration.

DOMICILIARY OXYGEN. Oxygen should only be prescribed for patients in the home after careful evaluation in hospital by respiratory experts; it should never be prescribed on a placebo basis.

Patients should be **advised of the fire risks** when receiving oxygen therapy.

OXYGEN CYLINDERS

Oxygen is occasionally prescribed for intermittent use for episodes of hypoxaemia of short duration, for example asthma. It is important, however, that the patient does not rely on oxygen instead of obtaining medical help or taking more specific treatment.

Alternatively, intermittent oxygen may be prescribed for patients with advanced irreversible respiratory disorders to increase mobility and capacity for exercise and to ease discomfort, for example in chronic obstructive bronchitis, emphysema, widespread fibrosis, and primary or thromboembolic pulmonary hypertension. Appropriate patients may be prescribed portable equipment through the hospital service, refillable from cylinders in the home.

Under the NHS oxygen may be supplied by pharmacy contractors as cylinders. Oxygen flow can be adjusted as the cylinders are equipped with an oxygen flow meter with 'medium' (2 litres/minute) and 'high' (4 litres/minute) settings. The Health Authorities have lists of pharmacy contractors who provide domiciliary oxygen services.

Patients are supplied with either constant or variable performance masks. The Intersurgical 010 28% or Ventimask Mk IV 28% are constant performance masks and provide a nearly constant supply of oxygen (28%) over a wide range irrespective of the patient's breathing pattern. The variable performance masks include the Intersurgical 005 Mask and the Venticaire Mask; the concentration of oxygen supplied to the patient varies with the rate of flow of oxygen and also with the patient's breathing pattern.

PORTABLE OXYGEN CYLINDERS. Portable oxygen sets are not prescribable on the NHS since the fitting is not compatible with the Drug Tariff oxygen equipment. However, Medigas and BOC supply a portable oxygen cylinder called a 'PD oxygen cylinder', which has the same bull-nose fitting as the normal domiciliary headsets (Prescriptions must therefore specify 'PD oxygen cylinder'). The PD oxygen cylinder holds about 300 litres of oxygen which will last approximately 2 hours at a standard flow rate of 2 litres/minute.

OXYGEN CONCENTRATORS

Long-term administration of oxygen (at least 15 hours daily) may prolong survival in patients with severe chronic obstructive airways disease with cor pulmonale.

Department of Health guidelines suggest that this treatment should be provided for patients who fulfil the following criteria:

$P_aO_2 < 7.3$ kPa; $P_aCO_2 > 6$ kPa;
$FEV_1 < 1.5$ litre and FVC < 2 litre

The measurements should be stable on two occasions at least three weeks apart after the patient has received appropriate bronchodilator therapy.

Less information is available on long-term oxygen in patients with a similar degree of hypoxaemia and airflow obstruction but no hypercapnia; the Department of Health suggests that these patients should not be denied this form of treatment but the effects of long-term therapy have not yet been assessed completely.

Increased respiratory depression is seldom a problem in patients with stable respiratory failure treated with low concentrations of oxygen although it may occur during exacerbations; patients and relatives should be warned to call for medical help if drowsiness or confusion occur.

Oxygen concentrators are more economical for patients requiring oxygen for long periods, and in England and Wales are now prescribable on the NHS on a regional tendering basis (see below). A concentrator was formerly only provided for a patient who required oxygen for 15 hours a day but it has been found to be cost-effective to provide one for a patient requiring it for 8 hours a day (or 21 cylinders per month).

PRESCRIBING ARRANGEMENTS FOR OXYGEN CONCENTRATORS

Prescribe concentrator and accessories (face mask, nasal cannula, and humidifier) on form FP10. Specify amount of oxygen required (hours per day) and flow rate. If required, prescribe back-up oxygen set and cylinder at same time. Inform patient that the supplier will be in contact to make arrangements and that the prescription form is to be given to the person who installs the concentrator.

Inform supplier by telephone (see table below) that a concentrator has been prescribed. The supplier will send written confirmation of the order to the prescriber, the patient, and the Health Authority.

Follow the same procedure if a back-up oxygen set and cylinder are required later.

Health Authority regional group	Supplier
Eastern	De Vilbiss Health Care UK Ltd
North Western London North North Wales West Midlands	to order: Dial 0800 020202
London South (includes Kent, Surrey, and Sussex)	Omnicare Group Ltd to order: Dial 0500 823773
Central and South Wales Northern South Western Yorkshire (South and West) and Humberside	Oxygen Therapy Co Ltd to order: Dial 0800 373580

In **Scotland** refer the patient for assessment by a respiratory consultant. If the need for a concentrator is confirmed the consultant will arrange for the provision of a concentrator through the Common Services Agency.

3.7   Mucolytics

Mucolytics are often prescribed to facilitate expectoration by reducing sputum viscosity in chronic asthma and bronchitis. Few patients, however, have been shown to derive much benefit from them although they do render sputum less viscid. Steam inhalation with postural drainage, is good expectorant therapy in bronchiectasis and some chronic bronchitics.

For reference to the newly introduced dornase alfa, see below.

CARBOCISTEINE

Indications: reduction of sputum viscosity
Contra-indications: active peptic ulceration
Side-effects: occasional gastro-intestinal irritation, rashes
Dose: 750 mg 3 times daily initially, then 1.5 g daily in divided doses; CHILD 2–5 years 62.5–125 mg 4 times daily, 6–12 years 250 mg 3 times daily

NHS PoM * Carbocisteine Capsules (Non-proprietary)
Capsules, carbocisteine 375 mg. Net price 30-cap pack = £3.70
NHS PoM * Carbocisteine Syrup (Non-proprietary)
Oral liquid, carbocisteine 125 mg/5 mL, net price 300 mL = £4.05; 250 mg/5 mL, 300 mL = £5.19
* except, for patients under the age of 18 years, any condition which, through damage or disease, affects the airways and has required a tracheostomy and endorsed 'SLS' ('S2B' in Scotland)
Note. The brand name **NHS** Mucodyne® (Rhône-Poulenc Rorer) is used for carbocisteine preparations; capsules and 250 mg/5 mL strength of syrup contain tartrazine

METHYL CYSTEINE HYDROCHLORIDE
(Mecysteine Hydrochloride)
Indications: reduction of sputum viscosity
Dose: 100–200 mg 3–4 times daily before meals reduced to 200 mg twice daily after 6 weeks; CHILD over 5 years 100 mg 3 times daily
Prophylaxis, 100–200 mg 2–3 times every other day during winter months

NHS Visclair® (Sinclair)
Tablets, yellow, s/c, e/c, methyl cysteine hydrochloride 100 mg. Net price 20 = £3.66. Label: 5, 22, 25

DORNASE ALFA

Dornase alfa is a genetically engineered version of a naturally occurring human enzyme which cleaves extracellular deoxyribonucleic acid (DNA). It is administered by inhalation using a jet nebuliser (see section 3.1.5).

DORNASE ALFA

Phosphorylated glycosylated recombinant human deoxyribonuclease 1 (rhDNase)

Indications: management of cystic fibrosis patients with a forced vital capacity (FVC) of greater than 40% of predicted to improve pulmonary function

Cautions: pregnancy and breast-feeding (manufacturers do not recommend)

Side-effects: pharyngitis, voice changes, laryngitis, rashes, urticaria

Dose: by inhalation of nebulised solution (by jet nebuliser), 2500 units (2.5 mg) once daily (patients over 21 years may benefit from twice daily dosage); CHILD under 5 years not recommended

▼ PoM **Pulmozyme®** (Roche)
Nebuliser solution, dornase alfa 1000 units (1 mg)/mL. Net price 2.5-mL (2500 units) vial = £20.39
Note. For use undiluted with jet nebulisers only; ultrasonic nebulisers are unsuitable

3.8   Aromatic inhalations

Inhalations containing volatile substances such as eucalyptus oil are traditionally used and although the vapour may contain little of the additive it encourages deliberate inspiration of warm moist air which is often comforting in bronchitis; boiling water should not be used owing to the risk of scalding. Inhalations are also used for the relief of nasal obstruction in acute rhinitis or sinusitis.

CHILDREN. The use of strong aromatic decongestants (applied as rubs or to pillows) is not advised for infants under the age of 3 months. Mothers with young infants in whom nasal obstruction with mucus is a problem can readily be taught appropriate techniques of suction aspiration.

Benzoin Tincture, Compound, BP

(Friars' Balsam)

Tincture, balsamic acids approx. 4.5%. Label: 15
Directions for use: add one teaspoonful to a pint of hot, **not** boiling, water and inhale the vapour

Menthol and Eucalyptus Inhalation, BP 1980

Inhalation, racementhol or levomenthol 2 g, eucalyptus oil 10 mL, light magnesium carbonate 7 g, water to 100 mL
Directions for use: add one teaspoonful to a pint of hot, **not** boiling, water and inhale the vapour

NHS **Karvol®** (Crookes)

Inhalation capsules, menthol 35.55 mg, with chlorbutol, pine oils, terpineol, and thymol. Net price 10-cap pack = £1.12
Directions for use: inhale vapour from contents of 1 capsule expressed into handkerchief or a pint of hot, **not** boiling, water; avoid in infants under 3 months

3.9   Cough preparations

3.9.1   Cough suppressants

The drawbacks of prescribing cough suppressants are rarely outweighed by the benefits of treatment and only occasionally are they useful, as, for example, if sleep is disturbed by a dry cough. Cough suppressants may cause sputum retention and this may be harmful in patients with chronic bronchitis and bronchiectasis.

Opioid cough suppressants such as codeine, dextromethorphan, and pholcodine are seldom sufficiently potent to be effective in severe cough; all tend to cause constipation.

Sedative antihistamines, such as diphenhydramine, are used as the cough suppressant component of many compound cough preparations on sale to the public; all tend to cause drowsiness which may reflect their main mode of action.

CHILDREN. The use of cough suppressants containing codeine or similar opioid analgesics is not generally recommended in children and should be avoided altogether in those under 1 year of age.

CODEINE PHOSPHATE

Indications: dry or painful cough

Cautions: asthma; hepatic and renal impairment; history of drug abuse; see also notes above and section 4.7.2; **interactions:** Appendix 1 (opioid analgesics)

Contra-indications: liver disease, ventilatory failure

Side-effects: constipation, respiratory depression in sensitive patients or if given large doses

PoM ¹ **Codeine Linctus, BP**
Linctus, codeine phosphate 15 mg/5 mL. Net price 100 mL = 30p (diabetic, 68p)
Dose: 5–10 mL 3–4 times daily; CHILD 5–12 years, 2.5–5 mL
Available from APS, Galen (Galcodine®, sugar-free), Norton
Note. BP 1993 directs that when Diabetic Codeine Linctus is prescribed, Codeine Linctus formulated with a vehicle appropriate for administration to diabetics, whether or not labelled 'Diabetic Codeine Linctus', shall be dispensed or supplied
1. Can be sold to the public provided the maximum single dose does not exceed 5 mL

Codeine Linctus, Paediatric, BP

Linctus, codeine phosphate 3 mg/5 mL. Net price 100 mL = 19p
Dose: CHILD 1–5 years 5 mL 3–4 times daily
Available from Evans, Galen (Galcodine® Paediatric, sugar-free)
Note. BP 1993 directs that Paediatric Codeine Linctus may be prepared extemporaneously by diluting Codeine Linctus with a suitable vehicle in accordance with the manufacturer's instructions
For a list of **cough and decongestant preparations on sale to the public,** including those containing codeine, see section 3.9.2

PHOLCODINE

Indications: dry or painful cough

Cautions; Contra-indications; Side-effects: see under Codeine Phosphate

Pholcodine Linctus, BP

Linctus, pholcodine 5 mg/5 mL in a suitable flavoured vehicle, containing citric acid monohydrate 1%. Net price 100 mL = 25p
Dose: 5–10 mL 3–4 times daily; CHILD 5–12 years 2.5–5 mL
Available from APS, Boehringer Ingelheim (Pavacol-D®, sugar-free), Galen (Galenphol®, sugar-free), Norton

Pholcodine Linctus, Strong, BP

Linctus, pholcodine 10 mg/5 mL in a suitable flavoured vehicle, containing citric acid monohydrate 2%. Net price 100 mL = 36p
   Dose: 5 mL 3–4 times daily
   Available from APS (sugar-free), Norton

Galenphol® (Galen)

Paediatric linctus, orange, sugar-free, pholcodine 2 mg/
5 mL. Net price 90-mL pack = £1.11
   Dose: CHILD 1–5 years 5 mL 3 times daily; 6–12 years
   5–10 mL

For a list of **cough and decongestant preparations on
sale to the public**, including those containing pholcodine,
see section 3.9.2

PALLIATIVE CARE

Diamorphine and methadone are available in linctuses to control distressful cough in terminal lung
cancer although morphine is now preferred (see
Palliative Care, p. 12). In other circumstances they
are contra-indicated because they induce sputum
retention and ventilatory failure as well as causing
opioid dependence.

DIAMORPHINE HYDROCHLORIDE

Indications: cough in terminal disease

Cautions; Contra-indications; Side-effects: see
   notes in section 4.7.2; more potent than morphine

Dose: see below

CD Diamorphine Linctus, BPC 1973

Linctus, diamorphine hydrochloride 3 mg, oxymel
1.25 mL, glycerol 1.25 mL, compound tartrazine
solution 0.06 mL, syrup to 5 mL. It should be
recently prepared. Label: 2
   Dose: 2.5–10 mL every 4 hours

METHADONE HYDROCHLORIDE

Indications: cough in terminal disease

Cautions; Contra-indications; Side-effects: see
   notes in section 4.7.2; longer-acting than morphine therefore effects may be cumulative

Dose: see below

CD Methadone Linctus

Linctus, methadone hydrochloride 2 mg/5 mL in a
suitable vehicle with a tolu flavour. Label: 2
   Dose: 2.5–5 mL every 4–6 hours, reduced to twice daily
   on prolonged use

MORPHINE HYDROCHLORIDE

Indications: cough in terminal disease (see also
   p. 12)

Cautions; Contra-indications; Side-effects: see
   notes in section 4.7.2

Dose: initially 5 mg every 4 hours

Preparations

See section 4.7.2

3.9.2   Expectorant and demulcent cough preparations

Expectorants are claimed to promote expulsion of
bronchial secretions but there is no evidence that
any drug can specifically facilitate expectoration.
The assumption that sub-emetic doses of expectorants, such as ammonium chloride, ipecacuanha,
and squill promote expectoration is a myth. However, a simple expectorant mixture may serve a useful placebo function and has the advantage of being
inexpensive.

Demulcent cough preparations contain soothing substances such as syrup or glycerol and certainly some patients believe that such preparations
relieve a dry irritating cough. Preparations such as
simple linctus have the advantage of being harmless and inexpensive; **paediatric simple linctus** is
particularly useful in children and sugar-free versions are available.

Compound cough preparations are on sale to
the public; the rationale for some is dubious.

CHILDREN. The use of cough suppressants containing codeine or similar opioid analgesics is not generally recommended in children and should be
avoided altogether in those under 1 year of age.

Ammonia and Ipecacuanha Mixture, BP

Mixture, ammonium bicarbonate 200 mg, liquorice
liquid extract 0.5 mL, ipecacuanha tincture 0.3 mL,
concentrated camphor water 0.1 mL, concentrated
anise water 0.05 mL, double-strength chloroform
water 5 mL, water to 10 mL. It should be recently
prepared
   Dose: 10–20 mL 3–4 times daily

Simple Linctus, BP

Linctus, citric acid monohydrate 2.5% in a suitable
vehicle with an anise flavour. Net price 100 mL =
17p
   Dose: 5 mL 3–4 times daily
   A sugar-free version is available from Pinewood and
   various wholesalers.

Simple Linctus, Paediatric, BP

Linctus, citric acid monohydrate 0.625% in a suitable
vehicle with an anise flavour. Net price 100 mL =
16p
   Dose: CHILD, 5–10 mL 3–4 times daily
   A sugar-free version is available from Pinewood and
   various wholesalers.

3.10   Systemic nasal decongestants

These preparations are of doubtful value but unlike
the preparations for local application (see section
12.2.2) they do not give rise to rebound nasal congestion. They contain sympathomimetics, and
should therefore be **avoided** in patients with hypertension, hyperthyroidism, coronary heart disease, or
diabetes, and in patients taking monoamine-oxidase
inhibitors; **interactions:** Appendix 1 (sympathomimetics). Many of the preparations also contain
antihistamines which may cause drowsiness and
affect ability to drive or operate machinery.

For a list of cough and decongestant preparations
on sale to the public, including those containing
systemic nasal decongestants, see section 3.9.2
above.

PSEUDOEPHEDRINE HYDROCHLORIDE

Indications; Dose: see notes above and under preparations

Cautions; Side-effects: see under Ephedrine Hydrochloride (section 3.1.1.2)

Galpseud® (Galen)

Tablets, pseudoephedrine hydrochloride 60 mg. Net price 20 = 87p

Dose: 1 tablet 3 times daily

Linctus, orange, sugar-free, pseudoephedrine hydrochloride 30 mg/5 mL. Net price 140 mL = 96p

Dose: 10 mL 3 times daily; CHILD 2–6 years 2.5 mL, 6–12 years 5 mL

Sudafed® (Warner Wellcome)

Tablets, red, f/c, pseudoephedrine hydrochloride 60 mg. Net price 20 = £1.15

Dose: 1 tablet every 4–6 hours (up to 4 times daily)

Elixir, red, pseudoephedrine hydrochloride 30 mg/5 mL. Net price 100 mL = 93p

Dose: 10 mL every 4–6 hours (up to 4 times daily); CHILD 2–5 years 2.5 mL, 6–12 years 5 mL

Preparations on sale to the public

For a list of **cough and decongestant preparations on sale to the public**, including those containing pseudoephedrine, see below

---

Systemic cough and decongestant preparations on sale to the public, together with their significant ingredients.

Important: in overdose contact **Poisons Information Services** (p. 18) for full details of the ingredients.

Actifed® (pseudoephedrine, triprolidine), **Actifed Compound Linctus®** (dextromethorphan, pseudoephedrine, triprolidine), **Actifed Expectorant®** (guaiphenesin, pseudoephedrine, triprolidine), **Actifed Junior Cough Relief®** (dextromethorphan, triprolidine), **Anestan®** (ephedrine, theophylline), **Anidox Spansules®** (diphenylpyraline, phenylpropanolamine)

Baby Meltus® (dilute acetic acid), **Balm of Gilead Cough Mixture®** (Gilead extract, squill, lobelia), **Barum Cold Relief with Decongestant®** (paracetamol, phenylephrine), **Beechams All-In-One®** (guaiphenesin, paracetamol, phenylephrine), **Beechams Hot Lemon®**, **Hot Lemon and Honey®**, **Hot Blackcurrant®**, **Beechams Powders Capsules®** with Decongestant (paracetamol, phenylephrine), **Benylin Chesty Cough®** (ammonium chloride, diphenhydramine, menthol), **Benylin Childrens Cough®** (diphenhydramine, menthol), **Benylin with Codeine®** (codeine, diphenhydramine, menthol), **Benylin Cough and Congestion®** (dextromethorphan, diphenhydramine, menthol, pseudoephedrine), **Benylin Dry Cough®** (dextromethorphan, diphenhydramine, menthol), **Benylin Four Flu®** (diphenhydramine, paracetamol, pseudoephedrine), **Benylin Non-drowsy for Chesty Coughs®** (guaiphenesin, menthol), **Benylin Non-drowsy for Dry Coughs®** (dextromethorphan), **Benylin Sugar-free for Children®** (diphenhydramine, menthol), **Benylin Day and Night Cold and Flu Relief®** (*day tablets,* paracetamol, phenylpropanolamine, *night tablets,* paracetamol, diphenhydramine), **Boots Bronchial Cough Mixture®** (ammonium carbonate, ammonium chloride, guaiphenesin), **Boots Catarrh Syrup for Children®** (diphenhydramine, pseudoephedrine), **Boots Catarrh Cough Syrup®** (codeine, creosote), **Boots Cold Capsules®** (diphenylpyraline, phenylpropanolamine), **Boots Cold and Influenza Mixture®** (squill, ammonium acetate), **Boots Cold Relief Tablets®** (paracetamol, phenylephrine), **Boots Cough Linctus for Children®** (ephedrine, ipecacuanha), **Boots Cough Relief for Children®** (diphenhydramine, pholcodine), **Boots Day Cold Comfort®** (paracetamol, pholcodine, pseudoephedrine), **Boots Day-time Cough Relief®** (pholcodine), **Boots Decongestant Tablets®** (pseudoephedrine), **Boots Night-Cold Comfort®** (diphenhydramine, paracetamol, pholcodine, pseudoephedrine), **Boots Night-time Cough Relief®** (diphenhydramine, pholcodine), **Bronal®** (dextromethorphan), **Bronalin Dry Cough®** (dextromethorphan, pseudoephedrine), **Bronalin Expectorant®** (ammonium chloride, diphenhydramine), **Bronalin Paediatric®** (diphenhydramine), **Buttercup Syrup Traditional®** (squill), **Buttercup Honey and Lemon®** and **Blackcurrant®** (ipecacuanha, menthol)

Cabdrivers® and **Cabdrivers Sugar-free®** (dextromethorphan, menthol), **Cabdrivers Junior®** (ephedrine), **CAM®** (ephedrine), **Catarrh-Ex®** (paracetamol, pseudoephedrine), **Coldrex Blackcurrant Powders®**, **Hot Lemon Powders®** and **Tablets®** (paracetamol, phenylephrine), **Contac 400®** (phenylpropanolamine, chlorpheniramine), **Contac CoughCaps®** (dextromethorphan), **Covonia®** (dextromethorphan, menthol), **Covonia for Children®** (dextromethorphan, menthol), **Cupal Baby Cough®** (dilute acetic acid)

Davenol® (carbinoxamine, ephedrine, pholcodine), **Day Nurse®**, **Day Nurse Hot®** (dextromethorphan, paracetamol, phenylpropanolamine), **Dimotane Elixir®**, **Tablets®** and **Dimotane LA®** (brompheniramine), **Dimotane Expectorant®** (brompheniramine, guaiphenesin, pseudoephedrine), **Dimotane Co®** and **Dimotane Co Paediatric®** (brompheniramine, codeine, pseudoephedrine), **Dimotane Plus®** and **Dimotane Plus Paediatric®** (brompheniramine, pseudoephedrine), **Dimotapp®**, **Dimotapp Paediatric®**, and **Dimotapp LA®** (brompheniramine, phenylephrine, phenylpropanolamine), **Do-Do Expectorant®** (guaiphenesin), **Do-Do Chesteze®** (ephedrine, theophylline), **Dristan Tablets®** (aspirin, chlorpheniramine, phenylephrine)

Ecdylin® (ammonium chloride, diphenhydramine), **ES Bronchial®** (ammonium bicarbonate, ipecacuanha, senna, squill), **Eskornade®** (diphenylpyraline, phenylpropanolamine), **Evacode®** (codeine), **Evaphol®** (pholcodine), **Expulin®** (chlorpheniramine, menthol, pholcodine, pseudoephedrine), **Expulin Decongestant for Babies and Children®** (chlorpheniramine, ephedrine, menthol), **Expulin Dry®** (menthol, pholcodine), **Expulin Paediatric®** chlorpheniramine, menthol, pholcodine)

Famel® (pholcodine), **Famel Expectorant®** (guaiphenesin), **Famel Original®** (codeine, creosote), **Fennings Little Healers®** (ipecacuanha), **Fisherman's Friend Honey Cough Syrup®** (cineole, menthol, squill), **Flurex Bedtime®** (diphenhydramine, paracetamol, pseudoephedrine), **Flurex Capsules®** and **Tablets®** (paracetamol, phenylephrine), **Franol®** and **Franol Plus®** (both ephedrine, theophylline), **Franolyn Chesty®** (ephedrine, guaiphenesin, theophylline), **Franolyn Dry®** (dextromethorphan)

Galcodine® (codeine), **Galcodine Paediatric®** (codeine), **Galenphol®** (pholcodine), **Galenphol Paediatric®** (pholcodine), **Galenphol Strong®** (pholcodine), **Galloway's®** (ipecacuanha, squill), **Galpseud®** (pseudoephedrine), **Galpseud Plus®** (chlorpheniramine, pseudoephedrine), **Gee's Linctus®** (opium, squill, tolu), **Guanor Expectorant®** (ammonium chloride, diphenhydramine, menthol)

Haymine® (chlorpheniramine, ephedrine), **Hill's Balsam Adult Expectorant®** (ipecacuanha, pholcodine), **Hill's Balsam Cough Suppressant®** (pholcodine), **Histalix®** (ammonium chloride, diphenhydramine, menthol)

Jackson's All Fours® (guaiphenesin), **Junior Lemsip®** (paracetamol, phenylephrine), **Junior Meltus Dry Cough®** (dextromethorphan, pseudoephedrine), **Junior Meltus Expectorant®** (guaiphenesin), **Junior Mucron®** (ipecacuanha, phenylpropanolamine)

Lem-Plus Capsules® (paracetamol, phenylephrine), **Lemsip Cold Relief® Capsules with Decongestant, Lemsip Flu Strength®, Lemsip Lemon®** or **Blackcurrant®, Lemsip Junior®, Lemsip Menthol Extra®** (all paracetamol, phenylephrine), **Lemsip Chesty Cough®** (guaiphenesin), **Lemsip Expectorant®** (ammonium chloride, diphenhydramine), **Lemsip Flu Strength Nighttime®** (chlorpheniramine, dextromethorphan, paracetamol, phenylpropanolamine), **Liqufruta Honey and Lemon®, Blackcurrant®** (ipecacuanha, menthol), **Liqufruta Garlic®** (guaiphenesin)

Medised® (paracetamol, promethazine), **Melo®** (ipecacuanha), **Meltus Baby®** (dilute acetic acid), **Meltus Cough Control®** (dextromethorphan), **Meltus Dry Cough®** (dextromethorphan, pseudoephedrine), **Meltus Expectorant®, Meltus Honey and Lemon®** (guaiphenesin), **Mu-Cron Tablets®** (paracetamol, phenylpropanolamine)

Night Nurse® (dextromethorphan, paracetamol, promethazine), **Nirolex®** (ephedrine, guaiphenesin, menthol), **Nirolex for Children®** (guaiphenesin), **Numark Cold Relief Capsules® With Decongestant** (paracetamol, phenylephrine), **Numark Cold Relief Powders®** (paracetamol), **Nurofen Cold and Flu®** (ibuprofen, pseudoephedrine), **Nurse Sykes Balsam®** (guaiphenesin)

Owbridges® (dilute acetic acid, guaiphenesin, ammonium acetate)

Pavacol D® (pholcodine), **Phensedyl Plus®** (promethazine, pholcodine, pseudoephedrine), **Procol®** (pseudoephedrine), **Pulmo Bailly®** (codeine, guaiacol)

Robitussin Chesty Cough® (guaiphenesin), **Robitussin Chesty Cough with Congestion®** (guaiphenesin, pseudoephedrine), **Robitussin Dry Cough®** (dextromethorphan), **Robitussin Junior Persistant Cough®** (dextromethorphan)

Secron® (ephedrine, vinegar of ipecacuanha), **Sinutab®** (paracetamol, phenylpropanolamine), **Sinutab Nightime®** (paracetamol, phenylpropanolamine, phenyltoloxamine), **SP Cold Relief Capsules®** (paracetamol, phenylephrine), **Sudafed®** (pseudoephedrine), **Sudafed Co®** (paracetamol, pseudoephedrine), **Sudafed Expectorant®** (guaiphenesin, pseudoephedrine), **Sudafed Linctus®** (dextromethorphan, pseudoephedrine), **Sudafed Plus®** (pseudoephedrine, triprolidine)

Tancolin® (dextromethorphan), **Terpoin®** (cineole, codeine, menthol), **Throaties Family Cough Linctus®** (ipecacuanha), **Tixylix Catarrh®** (diphenhydramine, menthol), **Tixylix Chesty Cough** (guaiphenesin), **Tixylix Cough and Cold®** (chlorpheniramine, pholcodine, pseudoephedrine), **Tixylix Daytime®** (pholcodine), **Tixylix Nighttime®** (pholcodine, promethazine), **Triogesic®** (paracetamol, phenylpropanolamine), **Triominic®** (pheniramine, phenylpropanolamine)

Uniflu with Gregovite C® (codeine, diphenhydramine, paracetamol, phenylephrine)

Venos for Dry Coughs®, Venos Expectorant® (guaiphenesin), **Venos Honey and Lemon®, Vicks Action®** (ibuprofen, pseudoephedrine), **Vicks Children's Vaposyrup Dry Cough®** (dextromethorphan), **Vicks Coldcare®** (paracetamol, dextromethorphan, phenylpropanolamine), **Vicks Expectorant Cough Syrup®** (guaiphenesin), **Vicks Medinite®** (dextromethorphan, doxylamine, ephedrine, paracetamol), **Vicks Original Formula®** (honey, menthol), **Vicks Vaposyrup Chesty Cough®** (guaiphenesin), **Vicks Vaposyrup Dry Cough®** (dextromethorphan), **Vicks Vaposyrup Chesty Coughs and Nasal Congestion®** (guaiphenesin, phenylpropanolamine), **Vicks Vaposyrup Dry Coughs and Nasal Congestion®** (dextromethorphan, phenylpropanolamine)

4: Drugs acting on the
CENTRAL NERVOUS SYSTEM

In this chapter, drug treatments are discussed under the following headings:

4.1 Hypnotics and anxiolytics

Most anxiolytics ('sedatives') will induce sleep when given at night and most hypnotics will sedate when given during the day. Prescribing of these drugs is widespread but dependence (both physical and psychological) and tolerance occurs. This may lead to difficulty in withdrawing the drug after the patient has been taking it regularly for more than a few weeks (see Dependence and Withdrawal, below). Hypnotics and anxiolytics should therefore be reserved for short courses to alleviate acute conditions after causal factors have been established.

Benzodiazepines are the most commonly used anxiolytics and hypnotics; they act at benzodiazepine receptors which are associated with gamma-aminobutyric acid (GABA) receptors. Older drugs such as meprobamate and barbiturates (section 4.1.3) are **not** recommended—they have more side-effects and interactions than benzodiazepines and are much more dangerous in overdosage.

PARADOXICAL EFFECTS. A paradoxical increase in hostility and aggression may be reported by patients taking benzodiazepines. The effects range from talkativeness and excitement, to aggressive and antisocial acts. Adjustment of the dose (up or down) usually attenuates the impulses. Increased anxiety and perceptual disorders are other paradoxical effects. Increased hostility and aggression after barbiturates and alcohol usually indicates intoxication.

DRIVING. Hypnotics and anxiolytics may impair judgement and increase reaction time, and so affect ability to drive or operate machinery; they increase the effects of alcohol. Moreover the hangover effects of a night dose may impair driving on the following day.

DEPENDENCE AND WITHDRAWAL. Withdrawal of a benzodiazepine *should be gradual* as abrupt withdrawal may produce confusion, toxic psychosis, convulsions, or a condition resembling delirium tremens. Abrupt withdrawal of an older drug, such as a barbiturate (section 4.1.3), may be even more likely to have serious effects.

The *benzodiazepine withdrawal syndrome* may not develop until up to 3 weeks after stopping a long-acting benzodiazepine, but may occur within a few hours in the case of a short-acting one. It is characterised by insomnia, anxiety, loss of appetite and body weight, tremor, perspiration, tinnitus, and perceptual disturbances. These symptoms may be similar to the original complaint and encourage further prescribing; some symptoms may continue for weeks or months after stopping benzodiazepines entirely.

A benzodiazepine *can be withdrawn* in steps of about one-eighth (range one-tenth to one-quarter) of the daily dose every fortnight. A suggested withdrawal protocol for patients who have difficulty is as follows:

1. Transfer patient to equivalent daily dose of diazepam[1] preferably taken at night
2. Reduce diazepam dose in fortnightly steps of 2 or 2.5 mg; if withdrawal symptoms occur, maintain this dose until symptoms improve
3. Reduce dose further, if necessary in smaller fortnightly steps[2]; it is better to reduce too slowly rather than too quickly
4. Stop completely; time needed for withdrawal can vary from about 4 weeks to a year or more

Counselling may help; beta-blockers should **only** be tried if other measures fail; antidepressants should **only** be used if clinical depression present; **avoid** antipsychotics (which may aggravate withdrawal symptoms)

> **CSM advice**
>
> 1. Benzodiazepines are indicated for the short-term relief (two to four weeks only) of anxiety that is severe, disabling or subjecting the individual to unacceptable distress, occurring alone or in association with insomnia or short-term psychosomatic, organic or psychotic illness.
> 2. The use of benzodiazepines to treat short-term 'mild' anxiety is inappropriate and unsuitable.
> 3. Benzodiazepines should be used to treat insomnia only when it is severe, disabling, or subjecting the individual to extreme distress.

1. Approximate equivalent doses, diazepam 5 mg
   ≡ chlordiazepoxide 15 mg
   ≡ loprazolam 0.5–1 mg
   ≡ lorazepam 500 micrograms
   ≡ lormetazepam 0.5–1 mg
   ≡ nitrazepam 5 mg
   ≡ oxazepam 15 mg
   ≡ temazepam 10 mg
2. Steps may be adjusted according to initial dose and duration of treatment and can range from diazepam 500 micrograms (one-quarter of a 2-mg tablet) to 2.5 mg

Prices are **net**, see p. 1

4.1.1 Hypnotics

Before a hypnotic is prescribed the cause of the insomnia should be established and, where possible, underlying factors should be treated. However, it should be noted that some patients have unrealistic sleep expectations, and others understate their alcohol consumption which is often the cause of the insomnia.

Transient insomnia may occur in those who normally sleep well and may be due to extraneous factors such as noise, shift work, and jet lag. If a hypnotic is indicated one that is rapidly eliminated should be chosen, and only one or two doses should be given.

Short-term insomnia is usually related to an emotional problem or serious medical illness. It may last for a few weeks, and may recur; a hypnotic can be useful but should not be given for more than three weeks (preferably only one week). Intermittent use is desirable with omission of some doses. A rapidly eliminated drug is generally appropriate.

Chronic insomnia is rarely benefited by hypnotics and is more often due to mild dependence caused by injudicious prescribing. Psychiatric disorders such as anxiety, depression, and abuse of drugs and alcohol are common causes. Sleep disturbance is very common in depressive illness and early wakening is often a useful pointer. The underlying psychiatric complaint should be treated, adapting the drug regimen to alleviate insomnia. For example, amitriptyline, prescribed for depression, will also help to promote sleep if it is taken at night. Other causes of insomnia include daytime cat-napping and physical causes such as pain, pruritus, and dyspnoea.

Hypnotics should **not** be prescribed indiscriminately and routine prescribing is undesirable. Ideally, they should be reserved for short courses in the acutely distressed. Tolerance to their effects develops within 3 to 14 days of continuous use and long-term efficacy cannot be assured. A major drawback of long-term use is that withdrawal causes rebound insomnia and precipitates a withdrawal syndrome (section 4.1).

Where prolonged administration is unavoidable hypnotics should be discontinued as soon as feasible and the patient warned that sleep may be disturbed for a few days before normal rhythm is re-established; broken sleep with vivid dreams and increased REM (rapid eye movement) may persist for several weeks.

CHILDREN. The prescribing of hypnotics to children, except for occasional use such as for night terrors and somnambulism (sleep-walking), is not justified.

ELDERLY. Hypnotics should be avoided in the elderly, who are at risk of becoming ataxic and confused and so liable to fall and injure themselves.

BENZODIAZEPINES

Benzodiazepines used as hypnotics include **nitrazepam**, **flunitrazepam**, and **flurazepam** which have a prolonged action and may give rise to residual effects on the following day; repeated doses tend to be cumulative.

Loprazolam, **lormetazepam**, and **temazepam** act for a shorter time and they have little or no hangover effect. Withdrawal phenomena however are more common with the short-acting benzodiazepines.

Benzodiazepine anxiolytics such as **diazepam** given as a single dose at night may also be used as hypnotics.

For general guidelines on benzodiazepine prescribing see section 4.1.2 and for benzodiazepine withdrawal see section 4.1.

NITRAZEPAM

Indications: insomnia (short-term use)

Cautions: respiratory disease, muscle weakness, history of drug or alcohol abuse, marked personality disorder, pregnancy and breast-feeding (see Appendixes 4 and 5); reduce dose in elderly and debilitated, and in hepatic (avoid if severe) and renal impairment (see Appendixes 2 and 3); avoid prolonged use (and abrupt withdrawal thereafter); porphyria (see section 9.8.2); **interactions:** Appendix 1 (anxiolytics and hypnotics)

DRIVING. Drowsiness may persist the next day and affect performance of skilled tasks (e.g. driving); effects of alcohol enhanced

Contra-indications: respiratory depression; acute pulmonary insufficiency; severe hepatic impairment, myasthenia gravis, sleep apnoea syndrome; not for phobic or obsessional states and not for use alone to treat depression (or anxiety associated with depression) or chronic psychosis

Side-effects: drowsiness and lightheadedness the next day; confusion and ataxia (especially in the elderly); amnesia may occur; dependence; see also under Diazepam (section 4.1.2); overdosage: see Emergency Treatment of Poisoning, p. 23

Dose: 5–10 mg at bedtime; ELDERLY (or debilitated) 2.5–5 mg; CHILD not recommended

PoM **Nitrazepam** (Non-proprietary)

Tablets, nitrazepam 5 mg, net price 20 = 13p. Label: 19

Available from APS, Berk, Cox, CP, DDSA (NHS Remnos®), Norton, Roche (NHS Mogadon®), Unigreg (NHS Unisomnia®)

Oral suspension, nitrazepam 2.5 mg/5 mL. Net price 150 mL = £4.35. Label: 19

Available from Norgine (NHS Somnite®)

FLUNITRAZEPAM

Indications: insomnia (short-term use)

Cautions; Contra-indications; Side-effects: see under Nitrazepam

Dose: 0.5–1 mg at bedtime; max. 2 mg; ELDERLY (or debilitated) 500 micrograms (max. 1 mg); CHILD not recommended

NHS PoM **Rohypnol**® (Roche)

Tablets, purple, f/c, scored, flunitrazepam 1 mg. Net price 30-tab pack = £4.08. Label: 19

FLURAZEPAM

Indications: insomnia (short-term use)

Cautions; Contra-indications; Side-effects: see under Nitrazepam

Dose: 15–30 mg at bedtime; ELDERLY (or debilitated) 15 mg; CHILD not recommended

NHS PoM **Dalmane**® (Roche)

Capsules, flurazepam (as hydrochloride), 15 mg (grey/yellow), net price 30-cap pack = £2.70; 30 mg (black/grey), 30-cap pack = £3.47. Label: 19

LOPRAZOLAM

Indications: insomnia (short-term use)

Cautions; Contra-indications; Side-effects: see under Nitrazepam

Dose: 1 mg at bedtime, increased to 1.5 or 2 mg if required; ELDERLY (or debilitated) 0.5–1 mg; CHILD not recommended

PoM **Loprazolam** (Non-proprietary)

Tablets, loprazolam 1 mg (as mesylate). Net price 28-tab pack = £1.30. Label: 19

Available from Roussel (previously NHS Dormonoct®)

LORMETAZEPAM

Indications: insomnia (short-term use)

Cautions; Contra-indications; Side-effects: see under Nitrazepam; shorter acting

Dose: 0.5–1.5 mg at bedtime; ELDERLY (or debilitated) 500 micrograms; CHILD not recommended

PoM **Lormetazepam** (Non-proprietary)

Tablets, lormetazepam 500 micrograms, net price 20 = 53p; 1 mg, 20 = 98p. Label: 19

Available from APS, Cox, Norton, Wyeth

TEMAZEPAM

Indications: insomnia (short-term use); see also section 15.1.4.1 for peri-operative use

Cautions; Contra-indications; Side-effects: see under Nitrazepam; shorter acting

Dose: 10–20 mg at bedtime, exceptional circumstances 30–40 mg; ELDERLY (or debilitated) 10 mg at bedtime, exceptional circumstances 20 mg; CHILD not recommended

CD ¹**Temazepam** (Non-proprietary)

NHS *Gel-filled capsules* (soft gelatin), temazepam 10 mg, net price 20 = 37p; 15 mg, 20 = 62p; 20 mg, 20 = 60p; 30 mg, 20 = £1.24. Label: 19

Note. The name NHS Temazepam Gelthix® is used for some gel-filled capsules

WARNING. Gel-filled capsules may be particularly subject to abuse; gangrene has followed abuse by injection

Tablets, temazepam 10 mg, net price 20 = 63p; 20 mg, 20 = £1.08. Label: 19

Oral solution, temazepam 10 mg/5 mL, net price 300 mL = £9.95. Label: 19

1. See p. 7 for prescribing requirements for temazepam

ZOLPIDEM AND ZOPICLONE

Zopiclone is a cyclopyrrolone and **zolpidem** is an imidazopyridine. Although neither are benzodiazepines both act on the same receptors (or receptor sub-types) as benzodiazepines. Both have a short duration of action with little or no hangover effect, but as with other hypnotics they should not be used for long-term treatment.

ZOLPIDEM TARTRATE

Indications: insomnia (short-term use)

Cautions: depression, history of drug or alcohol abuse, hepatic impairment (reduce dose, avoid if severe); renal impairment; avoid prolonged use (and abrupt withdrawal thereafter); **interactions:** Appendix 1 (anxiolytics and hypnotics)

DRIVING. Drowsiness may persist the next day and affect performance of skilled tasks (e.g. driving); effects of alcohol enhanced

Contra-indications: obstructive sleep apnoea, acute pulmonary insufficiency, respiratory depression, myasthenia gravis, severe hepatic impairment, pregnancy and breast-feeding

Side-effects: diarrhoea, nausea, vomiting, vertigo, dizziness, headache, daytime drowsiness, asthenia; memory disturbances, nightmares, nocturnal restlessness, depression, confusion, perceptual disturbances or diplopia, tremor, ataxia, falls reported

Dose: 10 mg at bedtime; ELDERLY (or debilitated) 5 mg; CHILD not recommended

▼ PoM **Stilnoct**® (Lorex)

Tablets, f/c, zolpidem tartrate 5 mg. Net price 28-tab pack = £3.36. Label: 19

ZOPICLONE

Indications: insomnia (short-term use)

Cautions: hepatic (avoid if severe) and renal impairment (see also Appendixes 2 and 3); elderly; history of drug abuse, psychiatric illness; avoid prolonged use (and abrupt withdrawal thereafter); **interactions:** Appendix 1 (anxiolytics and hypnotics)

DRIVING. Drowsiness may persist the next day and affect performance of skilled tasks (e.g. driving); effects of alcohol enhanced

Contra-indications: myasthenia gravis, respiratory failure, severe sleep apnoea syndrome, severe hepatic impairment; pregnancy and breast-feeding

Side-effects: bitter or metallic taste; gastro-intestinal disturbances including nausea and vomiting, dry mouth; irritability, confusion, depressed mood; drowsiness, dizziness, lightheadedness, and incoordination, headache; dependence; hypersensitivity reactions reported (including urticaria and rashes); hallucinations, nightmares, amnesia, and behavioural disturbances (including aggression) reported

Dose: 7.5 mg at bedtime; ELDERLY initially 3.75 mg at bedtime increased if necessary; CHILD not recommended

PoM **Zimovane**® (Rhône-Poulenc Rorer)

Tablets, f/c, scored, zopiclone 7.5 mg. Net price 28-tab pack = £4.48. Label: 19

CHLORAL AND DERIVATIVES

Chloral hydrate and derivatives were formerly popular hypnotics for children (but the use of hypnotics in children is not usually justified). There is no convincing evidence that they are particularly useful in the elderly and their role as hypnotics is now very limited. **Triclofos** causes fewer gastro-intestinal upsets than chloral hydrate.

CHLORAL HYDRATE

Indications: insomnia (short-term use)

Cautions: respiratory disease, history of drug or alcohol abuse; marked personality disorder; reduce dose in elderly and debilitated; avoid prolonged use (and abrupt withdrawal thereafter); avoid contact with skin and mucous membranes; **interactions:** Appendix 1 (anxiolytics and hypnotics)

DRIVING. Drowsiness may persist the next day and affect performance of skilled tasks (e.g. driving); effects of alcohol enhanced

Contra-indications: cardiac disease, gastritis, hepatic or renal impairment; pregnancy and breast-feeding; not recommended in porphyria

Side-effects: gastric irritation (nausea and vomiting reported), abdominal distention and flatulence; also vertigo, ataxia, staggering gait, rashes, headache, light headedness, malaise, ketonuria, excitement, nightmares, delirium (especially in the elderly), eosinophilia, reduction in white cell count; dependence (may be associated with gastritis and renal damage) on prolonged use

Dose: insomnia, 0.5–1 g (max. 2 g) with plenty of water at bedtime; CHILD 30–50 mg/kg up to a max. single dose of 1 g

PoM **Chloral Mixture, BP**
(Chloral Oral Solution)

Mixture, chloral hydrate 10% in a suitable vehicle. Extemporaneous preparations should be recently prepared according to the following formula: chloral hydrate 1 g, syrup 2 mL, water to 10 mL. Net price 100 mL = 36p. Label: 19, 27

Dose: 5–20 mL; CHILD 1–5 years 2.5–5 mL, 6–12 years 5–10 mL, taken well diluted with water at bedtime

Important. This preparation differs from Chloral Syrup BPC 1968 which contains 20% (1 g in 5 mL); dose: 2.5–10 mL, taken well diluted with water at bedtime)

PoM **Chloral Elixir, Paediatric, BP**
(Chloral Oral Solution, Paediatric)

Elixir, chloral hydrate 4% in a suitable vehicle with a blackcurrant flavour. Extemporaneous preparations should be recently prepared according to the following formula: chloral hydrate 200 mg, water 0.1 mL, blackcurrant syrup 1 mL, syrup to 5 mL. Net price 100 mL = 99p. Label: 1, 27

Dose: up to 1 year 5 mL, taken well diluted with water at bedtime

PoM **Noctec**® (Squibb)

Capsules, red, chloral hydrate 500 mg. Net price 56-cap pack = £2.13. Label: 19, 27

Dose: 1–2 capsules with plenty of water at bedtime (max. 4 capsules); CHILD not recommended

PoM **Welldorm**® (S&N Hlth.)

Tablets, blue-purple, f/c, chloral betaine 707 mg (≡chloral hydrate 414 mg). Net price 30-tab pack = £2.54. Label: 19, 27

Dose: 1–2 tablets with water or milk at bedtime, max. 5 tablets (2 g chloral hydrate) daily

Elixir, red, chloral hydrate 143 mg/5 mL. Net price 150-mL pack = £2.15. Label: 19, 27

Dose: 15–45 mL (0.4–1.3 g chloral hydrate) with water or milk, at bedtime, max. 70 mL (2 g chloral hydrate) daily; CHILD 1–1.75 mL/kg (30–50 mg/kg chloral hydrate), max. 35 mL (1 g chloral hydrate) daily

TRICLOFOS SODIUM

Indications: insomnia (short-term use)

Cautions; Contra-indications; Side-effects: see under Chloral Hydrate; less gastric irritation

Dose: see under preparation below

PoM **Triclofos Oral Solution, BP**
(Triclofos Elixir)

Oral solution, triclofos sodium 500 mg/5 mL. Net price 100 mL = £3.26. Label: 19

Available from Evans

Dose: 10–20 mL (1–2 g triclofos sodium) at bedtime; CHILD up to 1 year 25–30 mg/kg, 1–5 years 2.5–5 mL (250–500 mg triclofos sodium), 6–12 years 5–10 mL (0.5–1 g triclofos sodium)

CHLORMETHIAZOLE

Chlormethiazole may be a useful hypnotic for elderly patients because of its freedom from hangover but, as with all hypnotics, routine administration is undesirable and dependence occurs. It is indicated for use as a hypnotic only in the elderly for *very short-term use* in younger adults to attenuate alcohol withdrawal symptoms, see section 4.10).

CHLORMETHIAZOLE
(Clomethiazole)

Indications: see under Dose; status epilepticus (section 4.8.2); alcohol withdrawal (section 4.10); sedation during regional anaesthesia (section 15.1.4.1); eclampsia, see data sheet

Cautions: cardiac and respiratory disease (confusional state may indicate hypoxia); history of drug abuse; marked personality disorder; excessive sedation may occur (particularly with higher doses); hepatic impairment (especially if severe since sedation can mask hepatic coma); renal impairment; avoid prolonged use (and abrupt withdrawal thereafter); see also section 4.10; **interactions:** Appendix 1 (anxiolytics and hypnotics)

DRIVING. Drowsiness may persist the next day and affect performance of skilled tasks (e.g. driving); effects of alcohol enhanced

Contra-indications: acute pulmonary insufficiency; alcohol-dependent patients who continue to drink

Side-effects: nasal congestion and irritation (increased nasopharyngeal and bronchial secretions), conjunctival irritation, headache; rarely, paradoxical excitement, confusion, dependence, gastro-intestinal disturbances, rash, urticaria, bullous eruption, anaphylaxis, alterations in liver enzymes; intravenous infusion, see section 4.10

Dose: by mouth, severe insomnia in the elderly (short-term use), 1–2 capsules (*or* 5–10 mL syrup) at bedtime; CHILD not recommended

Restlessness and agitation in the elderly, 1 capsule (*or* 5 mL syrup) 3 times daily

Note. For an equivalent therapeutic effect 1 capsule ≡ 5 mL syrup

PoM **Heminevrin**® (Astra)

Capsules, grey-brown, chlormethiazole base 192 mg in an oily basis. Net price 60-cap pack = £4.34. Label: 19

Syrup, sugar-free, chlormethiazole edisylate 250 mg/5 mL. Net price 300-mL pack = £3.63. Label: 19

Intravenous infusion 0.8%, section 4.10

ANTIHISTAMINES

Some **antihistamines** (such as diphenhydramine and promethazine) are on sale to the public for occasional insomnia, although their prolonged duration of action may often lead to drowsiness the following day.

Promethazine is also popular for use in children, but the use of hypnotics in children is not usually justified.

DIPHENHYDRAMINE HYDROCHLORIDE

See section 3.4.1

PROMETHAZINE HYDROCHLORIDE

Indications: night sedation and insomnia (short-term use); other indications, see sections 3.4.1, 4.6, 15.1.4.1

Cautions; Contra-indications; Side-effects: see section 3.4.1

Dose: by mouth, 25 mg at bedtime increased to 50 mg if necessary; CHILD under 2 years not recommended, 2–5 years 15–20 mg, 5–10 years 20–25 mg, at bedtime

Preparations

See section 3.4.1

ALCOHOL

Alcohol is a poor hypnotic as its diuretic action interferes with sleep during the latter part of the night. With chronic use, alcohol disturbs sleep patterns and causes insomnia; **interactions:** Appendix 1 (alcohol).

4.1.2 Anxiolytics

Benzodiazepine anxiolytics can be effective in alleviating definite anxiety states and they are widely prescribed. Although there has been a tendency to prescribe these drugs to almost anyone with stress-related symptoms, unhappiness, or minor physical disease, their use in many situations is unjustified. In particular, they should not be used to treat depression, phobic or obsessional states, or chronic psychosis. In bereavement, psychological adjustment may be inhibited by benzodiazepines. In children anxiolytic treatment should be used only to relieve acute anxiety (and related insomnia) caused by fear e.g. before surgery.

Anxiolytic treatment should be limited to the lowest possible dose for the shortest possible time (see CSM advice, section 4.1). Dependence is particularly likely in patients with a history of alcohol or drug abuse and in patients with marked personality disorders.

Anxiolytics, particularly the benzodiazepines, have been termed 'minor tranquillisers'. This term is misleading because not only do they differ markedly from the antipsychotic drugs ('major tranquillisers') but their use is by no means minor. Antipsychotics, in low doses, are also sometimes used in severe anxiety for their sedative action but long-term use should be avoided in view of a possible risk of tardive dyskinesia (section 4.2.1).

BENZODIAZEPINES

Benzodiazepines are indicated for the *short-term relief of severe anxiety* but long-term use should be avoided (see p. 151). Diazepam, alprazolam, bromazepam, chlordiazepoxide, clobazam, and clorazepate have a sustained action. Shorter-acting compounds such as **lorazepam** and **oxazepam** may be preferred in patients with hepatic impairment but they carry a greater risk of withdrawal symptoms.

Diazepam or lorazepam are very occasionally administered intravenously for the *control of panic attacks*. This route is the most rapid but the procedure is not without risk (section 4.8.2) and should be used only when alternative measures have failed. The intramuscular route has no advantage over the oral route.

For guidelines on benzodiazepine withdrawal, see p. 151.

DIAZEPAM

Indications: short-term use in anxiety or insomnia, adjunct in acute alcohol withdrawal; status epilepticus and febrile convulsions see sections 4.8.2 and 4.8.3; muscle spasm see section 10.2.2; peri-operative use see section 15.1.4.1

Cautions: respiratory disease, muscle weakness (special care in myasthenia gravis), history of drug or alcohol abuse, marked personality disorder, pregnancy and breast-feeding (see Appendixes 4 and 5); reduce dose in elderly and debilitated, and in hepatic (avoid if severe) and renal impairment (see Appendixes 2 and 3); avoid prolonged use (and abrupt withdrawal thereafter); special precautions for intravenous injection (section 4.8.2); porphyria (see section 9.8.2); **interactions:** Appendix 1 (anxiolytics and hypnotics)

DRIVING. Drowsiness may affect performance of skilled tasks (e.g. driving); effects of alcohol enhanced

Contra-indications: respiratory depression; acute pulmonary insufficiency; severe hepatic impairment; not for phobic or obsessional states, not for chronic psychosis; should not be used alone in depression or in anxiety with depression

Side-effects: drowsiness and lightheadedness the next day; confusion and ataxia (especially in the elderly); amnesia may occur; dependence; paradoxical increase in aggression (see also section 4.1); *occasionally:* headache, vertigo, hypotension, salivation changes, gastro-intestinal disturbances, rashes, visual disturbances, changes in libido, urinary retention; blood disorders and jaundice reported; on intravenous injection, pain, thrombophlebitis, and rarely apnoea; overdosage: see Emergency Treatment of Poisoning, p.23

Dose: by mouth, anxiety, 2 mg 3 times daily increased if necessary to 15–30 mg daily in divided doses; ELDERLY (or debilitated) half adult dose

Insomnia associated with anxiety, 5–15 mg at bedtime

CHILD night terrors and somnambulism, 1–5 mg at bedtime

By intramuscular injection or slow intravenous injection (into a large vein, at a rate of not more than 5 mg/minute), for severe acute anxiety, control of acute panic attacks, and acute alcohol withdrawal, 10 mg, repeated if necessary after not less than 4 hours

Note. Only use intramuscular route when oral and intravenous routes not possible; special precautions for intravenous injection see section 4.8.2

By intravenous infusion—section 4.8.2

By rectum as rectal solution, for acute anxiety and agitation, 10 mg (elderly 5 mg), repeated after 5 minutes if necessary

CHILD febrile convulsions, see p. 213

By rectum as suppositories for anxiety when oral route not appropriate, 10–30 mg (higher dose divided); dose form not appropriate for less than 10 mg

PoM Diazepam (Non-proprietary)

Tablets, diazepam 2 mg, net price 20 = 6p; 5 mg, 20 = 6p; 10 mg, 20 = 12p. Label: 2 *or* 19

Available from APS, Berk (NHS Atensine®), Cox, DDSA (NHS Tensium®), Norton, Rima (NHS Rimapam®), Roche (NHS Valium®)

Oral solution, diazepam 2 mg/5 mL, net price 100 mL = £1.88. Label: 2 *or* 19

Available from Cox, Lagap (NHS Dialar®), Roche (NHS Valium®)

NHS *Strong oral solution*, diazepam 5 mg/5 mL, net price 100-mL pack = £3.30. Label: 2 *or* 19

Available from Lagap (NHS Dialar®)

Injection (solution), diazepam 5 mg/mL. Do not dilute (except for intravenous infusion). Net price 2-mL amp = 25p

Available from CP, Roche (Valium®), Phoenix

Injection (emulsion), diazepam 5 mg/mL. For intravenous injection or infusion. Net price 2-mL amp = 76p

Available from Dumex (Diazemuls®)

Rectal tubes (= rectal solution), diazepam 2 mg/mL, net price 2.5-mL (5-mg) tube = £1.27; 4 mg/mL, 2.5-mL (10-mg) tube = £1.62

Available from CP (Diazepam Rectubes®), Dumex (Stesolid®), Lagap

Suppositories, diazepam 10 mg, net price 6 = £6.51. Label: 2 *or* 19

Available from Sinclair (Valclair®)

ALPRAZOLAM

Indications: anxiety (short-term use)

Cautions; Contra-indications; Side-effects: see under Diazepam

Dose: 250–500 micrograms 3 times daily (elderly or debilitated 250 micrograms 2–3 times daily) increased if necessary to a total of 3 mg daily; CHILD not recommended

NHS PoM **Xanax®** (Upjohn)

Tablets, both scored, alprazolam 250 micrograms, net price 60-tab pack = £2.75; 500 micrograms (pink) 60-tab pack = £5.27. Label: 2

BROMAZEPAM

Indications: anxiety (short-term use)

Cautions; Contra-indications; Side-effects: see under Diazepam

Dose: 3–18 mg daily in divided doses; ELDERLY (or debilitated) half adult dose; max. (in exceptional circumstances in hospitalised patients) 60 mg daily in divided doses; CHILD not recommended

NHS PoM **Lexotan®** (Roche)

Tablets, both scored, bromazepam 1.5 mg (lilac), net price 60-tab pack = £5.47; 3 mg (pink), 60-tab pack = £6.93. Label: 2

CHLORDIAZEPOXIDE

Indications: anxiety (short-term use), adjunct in acute alcohol withdrawal

Cautions; Contra-indications; Side-effects: see under Diazepam

Dose: anxiety, 10 mg 3 times daily increased if necessary to 60–100 mg daily in divided doses; ELDERLY (or debilitated) half adult dose; CHILD not recommended

Note. The doses stated above refer equally to chlordiazepoxide and to its hydrochloride

PoM Chlordiazepoxide Capsules, chlordiazepoxide hydrochloride 5 mg, net price 20 = 30p; 10 mg, 20 = 36p. Label: 2

Various strengths available from APS, Cox, DDSA (NHS Tropium®), Lagap, Roche (NHS Librium®)

PoM Chlordiazepoxide Hydrochloride Tablets, chlordiazepoxide hydrochloride 5 mg, net price 20 = 26p; 10 mg, 20 = 32p; 25 mg, 20 = 70p. Label: 2

CLOBAZAM

Section 4.8.1

CLORAZEPATE DIPOTASSIUM

Indications: anxiety (short-term use)

Cautions; Contra-indications; Side-effects: see under Diazepam

Dose: 7.5–22.5 mg daily in 2–3 divided doses *or a* single dose of 15 mg at bedtime; ELDERLY (or debilitated) half adult dose; CHILD not recommended

NHS PoM **Tranxene®** (Boehringer Ingelheim)

Capsules, clorazepate dipotassium 7.5 mg (maroon/grey), net price 20-cap pack = £2.66; 15 mg (pink/grey), 20-cap pack = £2.78. Label: 2 *or* 19

LORAZEPAM

Indications: short-term use in anxiety or insomnia; status epilepticus (section 4.8.2); peri-operative (section 15.1.4.1)

Cautions; Contra-indications; Side-effects: see under Diazepam; short acting

Dose: by mouth, anxiety, 1–4 mg daily in divided doses; ELDERLY (or debilitated) half adult dose
Insomnia associated with anxiety, 1–2 mg at bedtime; CHILD not recommended

By intramuscular or slow intravenous injection (into a large vein), acute panic attacks, 25–30 micrograms/kg, repeated every 6 hours if necessary; CHILD not recommended

Note. Only use intramuscular route when oral and intravenous routes not possible

PoM **Lorazepam** (Non-proprietary)

Tablets, lorazepam 1 mg, net price 20 = 24p; 2.5 mg, 20 = 35p. Label: 2 *or* 19

Available from APS, Cox, CP, Lagap, Norton, Wyeth (~~NHS~~ Ativan®)

Injection, lorazepam 4 mg/mL. Net price 1-mL amp = 40p

For intramuscular injection it should be diluted with an equal volume of water for injections or physiological saline (but only use when oral and intravenous routes not possible)

Available from Wyeth (Ativan®)

OXAZEPAM

Indications: anxiety (short-term use)

Cautions; Contra-indications; Side-effects: see under Diazepam; short acting

Dose: anxiety, 15–30 mg (elderly or debilitated 10–20 mg) 3–4 times daily; CHILD not recommended
Insomnia associated with anxiety, 15–25 mg (max. 50 mg) at bedtime; CHILD not recommended

PoM **Oxazepam** (Non-proprietary)

Tablets, oxazepam 10 mg, net price 20 = 22p; 15 mg, 20 = 24p; 30 mg, 20 = 32p. Label: 2

Available from most generic manufacturers

BUSPIRONE

Buspirone is thought to act at specific serotonin ($5HT_{1A}$) receptors. Response to treatment may take up to 2 weeks. It does not alleviate the symptoms of benzodiazepine withdrawal. Therefore a patient taking a benzodiazepine still needs to have the benzodiazepine withdrawn gradually; it is advisable to do this before starting buspirone. The dependence and abuse liability of buspirone has not yet been established.

BUSPIRONE HYDROCHLORIDE

Indications: anxiety (short-term use)

Cautions: does not alleviate benzodiazepine withdrawal (see notes above); history of hepatic or renal impairment; **interactions:** Appendix 1 (anxiolytics and hypnotics)

DRIVING. May affect performance of skilled tasks (e.g. driving); effects of alcohol may be enhanced

Contra-indications: epilepsy, severe hepatic or renal impairment, pregnancy and breast-feeding

Side-effects: nausea, dizziness, headache, nervousness, lightheadedness, excitement; rarely tachycardia, palpitations, chest pain, drowsiness, confusion, dry mouth, fatigue, and sweating

Dose: initially 5 mg 2–3 times daily, increased as necessary every 2–3 days; usual range 15–30 mg daily in divided doses; max. 45 mg daily; CHILD not recommended

PoM **Buspar**® (Bristol-Myers)

Tablets, buspirone hydrochloride 5 mg, net price 126-tab pack = £39.31; 10 mg, 100-tab pack = £46.80. Counselling, driving

BETA-BLOCKERS

Beta-blockers (e.g. propranolol, oxprenolol) (see section 2.4) do not affect psychological symptoms, such as worry, tension, and fear, but they do reduce autonomic symptoms, such as palpitations, and tremor; they do not reduce non-autonomic symptoms, such as muscle tension. Beta-blockers are therefore indicated for patients with predominantly somatic symptoms; this, in turn, may prevent the onset of worry and fear. Patients with predominantly psychological symptoms may obtain no benefit.

MEPROBAMATE

Meprobamate is **less effective** than the benzodiazepines, more hazardous in overdosage, and can also induce dependence. It is **not** recommended.

MEPROBAMATE

Indications: short-term use in anxiety, but see notes above

Cautions: respiratory disease, muscle weakness, epilepsy (may induce seizures), history of drug or alcohol abuse, marked personality disorder, pregnancy; elderly and debilitated; hepatic and renal impairment; avoid prolonged use, abrupt withdrawal may precipitate convulsions; **interactions:** Appendix 1 (anxiolytics and hypnotics)

DRIVING. Drowsiness may affect performance of skilled tasks (e.g. driving); effects of alcohol enhanced

Contra-indications: acute pulmonary insufficiency; respiratory depression; porphyria (see section 9.8.2); breast-feeding

Side-effects: see under Diazepam, but the incidence is greater and drowsiness is the most common side-effect. Also gastro-intestinal disturbances, hypotension, paraesthesia, weakness, CNS effects which include headache, paradoxical excitement, disturbances of vision; rarely agranulocytosis and rashes

Dose: 400 mg 3–4 times daily; elderly patients half adult dose or less; CHILD not recommended

CD **Equanil**® (Wyeth)

Tablets, meprobamate 200 mg, net price 20 = 15p; 400 mg (scored), 20 = 22p. Label: 2

CD **Equagesic**®

Section 4.7.1

ANTIHISTAMINES

The use of antihistamines for their sedative effect in anxiety is not considered to be appropriate.

HYDROXYZINE HYDROCHLORIDE
See section 3.4.1

4.1.3   Barbiturates

The intermediate-acting **barbiturates** only have a place in the treatment of severe intractable insomnia in patients **already taking** barbiturates; they should be **avoided** in the elderly. The long-acting barbiturates, phenobarbitone and methylphenobarbitone, are still sometimes of value in epilepsy (section 4.8.1) but their use as sedatives is unjustified. The very short-acting barbiturates, methohexitone and thiopentone, are used in anaesthesia (see section 15.1.1).

IMPORTANT. It is **important** to bear in mind that a barbiturate should **not** be prescribed as a hypnotic other than for patients who are **already** receiving them and who are suffering from severe intractable insomnia.

BARBITURATES

Indications: severe intractable insomnia in patients already taking barbiturates; see also notes above

Cautions: avoid use where possible; dependence and tolerance readily occur; abrupt withdrawal may precipitate a serious withdrawal syndrome (rebound insomnia, anxiety, tremor, dizziness, nausea, convulsions, delirium, and death); repeated doses are cumulative and may lead to excessive sedation; caution in respiratory disease, renal disease, hepatic impairment; **interactions:** Appendix 1 (barbiturates and primidone)

DRIVING. Drowsiness may persist the next day and affect performance of skilled tasks (e.g. driving); effects of alcohol enhanced

Contra-indications: insomnia caused by pain; porphyria (see section 9.8.2), pregnancy, breast-feeding; avoid in children, young adults, elderly and debilitated patients, also patients with a history of drug or alcohol abuse

Side-effects: include hangover with drowsiness, dizziness, ataxia, respiratory depression, hypersensitivity reactions, headache, particularly in elderly; paradoxical excitement and confusion occasionally precede sleep; overdosage: see Emergency Treatment of Poisoning, p. 23

Dose: see under preparations below

CD Amytal® (Flynn)
Tablets, amylobarbitone (amobarbital) 50 mg, net price 20 = £1.55. Label: 19
Dose: 100–200 mg at bedtime (**important:** but see also contra-indications)

CD Sodium Amytal® (Flynn)
Capsules, both blue, amylobarbitone (amobarbital) sodium 60 mg, net price 20 = £2.89; 200 mg, 20 = £5.68. Label: 19
Dose: 60–200 mg at bedtime (**important:** but see also contra-indications)
Injection, powder for reconstitution, amylobarbitone (amobarbital) sodium. Net price 500-mg vial = £26.57. For specialised use in procedures in **expert epilepsy centres only**
Dose: by deep intramuscular injection into large muscle, preferably gluteal, (max. 5 mL at any one site) or by slow intravenous injection (max. 50 mg/minute), 0.25–1 g; max. single dose, intramuscular 500 mg, intravenous 1 g

CD Soneryl® (Rhône-Poulenc Rorer)
Tablets, pink, scored, butobarbitone (butobarbital) 100 mg. Net price 56-tab pack = 71p. Label: 19
Dose: 100–200 mg at bedtime (**important:** but see also contra-indications)

Preparations containing quinalbarbitone (secobarbital)
Note. Quinalbarbitone (secobarbital) has been transferred from schedule 3 to schedule 2 of the Misuse of Drugs Regulations 1985; receipt and supply must therefore be recorded in the CD register.

CD Seconal Sodium® (Flynn)
Capsules, both orange, quinalbarbitone (secobarbital) sodium 50 mg, net price 20 = £4.93; 100 mg, 20 = £5.91. Label: 19
Dose: 100 mg at bedtime (**important:** but see also contra-indications)

CD Tuinal® (Flynn)
Capsules, orange/blue, a mixture of amylobarbitone (amobarbital) sodium 50 mg, quinalbarbitone (secobarbital) sodium 50 mg. Net price 20 = £3.26. Label: 19
Dose: 1–2 capsules at bedtime (**important:** but see also contra-indications)
Note. Prescriptions need only specify 'Tuinal capsules'

4.2   Drugs used in psychoses and related disorders

4.2.1   Antipsychotic drugs
4.2.2   Antipsychotic depot injections
4.2.3   Antimanic drugs

Advice of Royal College of Psychiatrists on doses above BNF upper limit

Unless otherwise stated, doses in the BNF are licensed doses—any higher dose is therefore **unlicensed** (for an explanation of the significance of this, see p. 2).

1. Consider alternative approaches including adjuvant therapy and newer or atypical neuroleptics such as clozapine.
2. Bear in mind risk factors, including obesity—particular caution is indicated in older patients especially those over 70.
3. Consider potential for drug interactions—see **interactions:** Appendix 1 (phenothiazines and other antipsychotics).
4. Carry out ECG to exclude untoward abnormalities such as prolonged QT interval; repeat ECG periodically and reduce dose if prolonged QT interval or other adverse abnormality develops.
5. Increase dose slowly and not more often than once weekly.
6. Carry out regular pulse, blood pressure, and temperature checks; ensure that patient maintains adequate fluid intake.
7. Consider high-dose therapy to be for limited period and review regularly; abandon if no improvement after 3 months (return to standard dosage).

Important: When prescribing an antipsychotic for administration on an emergency basis it must be borne in mind that the intramuscular dose should be **lower** than the corresponding oral dose (owing to absence of first-pass effect), particularly if the patient is very active (increased blood flow to muscle considerably increases the rate of absorption). The prescription should specify the dose in the context of **each route** and should **not** imply that the same dose can be given by mouth or by intramuscular injection. The dose should be reviewed **daily**

4.2.1 Antipsychotic drugs

Antipsychotic drugs are also known as 'neuroleptics' and (misleadingly) as 'major tranquillisers'. Antipsychotic drugs generally tranquillise without impairing consciousness and without causing paradoxical excitement but they should not be regarded merely as tranquillisers. For conditions such as schizophrenia the tranquillising effect is of secondary importance.

In the short term they are used to quieten disturbed patients whatever the underlying psychopathology, which may be brain damage, mania, toxic delirium, agitated depression, or acute behavioural disturbance.

They are used to alleviate severe anxiety but this too should be a short-term measure. Some antipsychotic drugs (e.g. chlorpromazine, thioridazine, flupenthixol) also have an antidepressant effect while others may exacerbate depression (e.g. fluphenazine, pimozide, pipothiazine).

SCHIZOPHRENIA. Antipsychotic drugs relieve florid psychotic symptoms such as thought disorder, hallucinations, and delusions, and prevent relapse. Although they are usually less effective in apathetic withdrawn patients, they sometimes appear to have an activating influence. For example, chlorpromazine may restore an acutely ill schizophrenic, who was previously withdrawn or even mute and akinetic, to normal activity and social behaviour. Patients with acute schizophrenia generally respond better than those with chronic symptoms.

Long-term treatment of a patient with a definite diagnosis of schizophrenia may be necessary even after the first episode of illness in order to prevent the manifest illness from becoming chronic. Withdrawal of drug treatment requires careful surveillance because the patient who appears well on medication may suffer a disastrous relapse if treatment is withdrawn inappropriately. In addition the need for continuation of treatment may not become immediately evident because relapse is often delayed for several weeks after cessation of treatment.

Antipsychotic drugs are considered to act by interfering with dopaminergic transmission in the brain by blocking dopamine receptors and may give rise to the extrapyramidal effects described below, and also to hyperprolactinaemia. Antipsychotic drugs also affect cholinergic, alpha-adrenergic, histaminergic, and serotonergic receptors.

SIDE-EFFECTS. Extrapyramidal symptoms are the most troublesome. They are caused most frequently by the piperazine phenothiazines (fluphenazine, perphenazine, prochlorperazine, and trifluoperazine), the butyrophenones (benperidol, droperidol, haloperidol, and trifluperidol), and the depot preparations. They are easy to recognise but cannot be accurately predicted because they depend partly on the dose and partly on the type of drug, and on patient susceptibility. They consist of *parkinsonian symptoms* (including tremor) which may occur gradually, *dystonia* (abnormal face and body movements) which may appear after only a few doses, *akathisia* (restlessness) which may resemble an exacerbation of the condition being treated, and *tardive dyskinesia* (which usually takes longer to develop).

Parkinsonian symptoms remit if the drug is withdrawn and may be suppressed by the administration of **antimuscarinic** drugs (section 4.9.2). Routine administration of such drugs is **not** justified as not all patients are affected and because tardive dyskinesia may be unmasked or worsened by them. Furthermore, these drugs are sometimes abused for their mood-altering effects. Tardive dyskinesia is of particular concern because it may be irreversible on withdrawing therapy and treatment may be ineffective. It occurs fairly frequently in patients (especially the elderly) on long-term therapy and with high dosage, and the treatment of such patients must be carefully and regularly reviewed. Tardive dyskinesia may also occur occasionally after short-term treatment with low dosage.

Hypotension and *interference with temperature regulation* are dose-related side-effects and are liable to cause dangerous falls and hypothermia in the elderly; very serious consideration should be given before prescribing these drugs for patients over 70 years of age.

Neuroleptic malignant syndrome (hyperthermia, fluctuating level of consciousness, muscular rigidity and autonomic dysfunction with pallor, tachycardia, labile blood pressure, sweating, and urinary incontinence) is a rare but potentially fatal side-effect of some drugs. Drugs for which it has been reported in the UK include haloperidol, chlorpromazine, and flupenthixol decanoate. Discontinuation of drug therapy is essential as there is no proven effective treatment but bromocriptine and dantrolene have been used. The syndrome, which usually lasts for 5–10 days after drug discontinuation, may be unduly prolonged if depot preparations have been used.

Overdosage: see Emergency Treatment of Poisoning, p. 23.

CLASSIFICATION OF ANTIPSYCHOTICS. The **phenothiazine** derivatives can be divided into 3 main groups.

Group 1: chlorpromazine, methotrimeprazine, and promazine, generally characterised by pronounced sedative effects and moderate antimuscarinic and extrapyramidal side-effects.

Group 2: pericyazine, pipothiazine, and thioridazine, generally characterised by moderate sedative effects, marked antimuscarinic effects, but fewer extrapyramidal side-effects than groups 1 or 3.

Group 3: fluphenazine, perphenazine, prochlorperazine, and trifluoperazine, generally characterised by fewer sedative effects, fewer antimuscarinic effects, but more pronounced extrapyramidal side-effects than groups 1 and 2.

Drugs of other chemical groups tend to resemble the phenothiazines of *group 3*. They include the

butyrophenones (benperidol, droperidol, and haloperidol); **diphenylbutylpiperidines** (fluspirilene and pimozide); **thioxanthenes** (flupenthixol and zuclopenthixol); **substituted benzamides** (sulpiride); **oxypertine**; and **loxapine**. **Clozapine** differs in that it is sedative with fewer extrapyramidal effects.

CHOICE. As indicated above, the various drugs differ somewhat in predominant actions and side-effects. Selection is influenced by the degree of sedation required and the patient's susceptibility to extrapyramidal side-effects. However, the differences between antipsychotic drugs are less important than the great variability in patient response; moreover, tolerance to these secondary effects usually develops.

Prescribing of more than one antipsychotic at the same time is **not** recommended; it may constitute a hazard and there is no significant evidence that side-effects are minimised.

Chlorpromazine is widely used. It has a marked sedating effect and is useful for treating violent patients without causing stupor. Agitated states in the elderly can be controlled without confusion, a dose of 10 to 25 mg once or twice daily usually being adequate.

Flupenthixol and **pimozide** (see CSM advice p. 164) are less sedating than chlorpromazine.

Sulpiride in high doses controls florid positive symptoms, but in lower doses it has an alerting effect on apathetic withdrawn schizophrenics.

Fluphenazine, haloperidol, and **trifluoperazine** are also of value but their use is limited by the high incidence of extrapyramidal symptoms. Haloperidol may be preferred for the rapid control of hyperactive psychotic states. It is less hypotensive than chlorpromazine and is therefore also popular for agitation in the elderly, despite the high incidence of extrapyramidal side-effects.

Thioridazine was formerly popular for treating the elderly as there is a reduced incidence of extrapyramidal symptoms. However, there is a high incidence of antimuscarinic effects and possibly an increased risk of cardiotoxicity.

Promazine is not sufficiently active by mouth to be used as an antipsychotic drug.

Clozapine is indicated only for the treatment of schizophrenia in patients unresponsive to, or intolerant of, conventional antipsychotic drugs. It is less likely to cause tardive dyskinesia but as it can cause agranulocytosis, its use is restricted to patients registered with the Clozaril Patient Monitoring Service (see under Clozapine, below).

Loxapine causes relatively little sedation; in overdosage it has a high potential for serious neurological and cardiac toxicity.

Risperidone, a recently introduced antipsychotic drug, is a benzisoxazole derivative. It is less likely to cause extrapyramidal effects than conventional antipsychotics.

OTHER USES. Nausea and vomiting (section 4.6), choreas, motor tics (section 4.9.3), and intractable hiccup (see under Chlorpromazine Hydrochloride

and under Haloperidol). **Benperidol** is used in deviant antisocial sexual behaviour but its value is not established.

Equivalent doses of oral antipsychotics
These equivalences are intended **only** as an approximate guide; individual dosage instructions should **also** be checked; patients should be carefully monitored after **any** change in medication

Antipsychotic	Daily dose
Chlorpromazine	100 mg
Clozapine	50 mg[1]
Haloperidol	2–3 mg[2]
Loxapine	10–20 mg
Pimozide	2 mg[3]
Risperidone	0.5–1 mg
Sulpiride	200 mg
Thioridazine	100 mg
Trifluoperazine	5 mg

1. The prescribing of clozapine needs to comply with the Sandoz Clozaril Patient Monitoring Service, see p. 162
2. In specialist psychiatric units where very high doses are required the equivalent dose of haloperidol might be up to 10 mg
3. See also the CSM warning concerning pimozide dose, p. 164

IMPORTANT. These equivalences must **not** be extrapolated beyond the max. dose for the drug.

WITHDRAWAL. Withdrawal of antipsychotic drugs after long-term therapy should always be gradual and closely monitored to avoid the risk of acute withdrawal syndromes or rapid relapse.

DOSAGE. After an initial period of stabilisation, in most patients, the long half-life of antipsychotic drugs allows the total daily oral dose to be given as a single dose. For the advice of The Royal College of Psychiatrists on doses above the BNF upper limit, see p. 158.

CHLORPROMAZINE HYDROCHLORIDE

WARNING. Owing to the risk of contact sensitisation, pharmacists, nurses, and other health workers should avoid direct contact with chlorpromazine; tablets should not be crushed and solutions should be handled with care

Indications: see under Dose; antiemetic (in terminal illness), section 4.6; peri-operative use, see section 15.1.4.1

Cautions: cardiovascular and cerebrovascular disease, respiratory disease, parkinsonism, epilepsy (possibly avoid), acute infections, pregnancy, breast-feeding, renal and hepatic impairment (avoid if severe), history of jaundice, leucopenia (blood counts if unexplained infection or fever); hypothyroidism, myasthenia gravis, prostatic hypertrophy, closed-angle glaucoma; caution in elderly particularly in very hot or very cold weather; avoid abrupt withdrawal; patients should remain supine and the blood pressure monitored for 30 minutes after intramuscular injection; **interactions:** Appendix 1 (antipsychotics)

DRIVING. Drowsiness may affect performance of skilled tasks (e.g. driving); effects of alcohol enhanced

Contra-indications: coma caused by CNS depressants; bone-marrow depression; avoid in phaeochromocytoma

Side-effects: extrapyramidal symptoms (reversed by dose reduction or antimuscarinic drugs) and, on prolonged administration, occasionally tardive dyskinesia; hypothermia (occasionally pyrexia), drowsiness, apathy, pallor, nightmares, insomnia, depression, and, more rarely, agitation, EEG changes, convulsions; nasal congestion; antimuscarinic symptoms such as dry mouth, constipation, difficulty with micturition, and blurred vision; cardiovascular symptoms such as hypotension, tachycardia, and arrhythmias; ECG changes; respiratory depression; endocrine effects such as menstrual disturbances, galactorrhoea, gynaecomastia, impotence, and weight gain; sensitivity reactions such as agranulocytosis, leucopenia, leucocytosis, and haemolytic anaemia, photosensitisation (more common with chlorpromazine than with other antipsychotics), contact sensitisation and rashes, jaundice (including cholestatic) and alterations in liver function; neuroleptic malignant syndrome; lupus erythematosus-like syndrome reported; with prolonged high dosage, corneal and lens opacities and purplish pigmentation of the skin, cornea, conjunctiva, and retina; intramuscular injection may be painful, cause hypotension and tachycardia (see Cautions), and give rise to nodule formation; overdosage: see Emergency Treatment of Poisoning, p. 23

Dose: by mouth,

Schizophrenia and other psychoses, mania, short-term adjunctive management of severe anxiety, psychomotor agitation, excitement, and violent or dangerously impulsive behaviour initially 25 mg 3 times daily (*or* 75 mg at night), adjusted according to response, to usual maintenance dose of 75–300 mg daily (but up to 1 g daily may be required in psychoses); ELDERLY (or debilitated) third to half adult dose; CHILD (childhood schizophrenia and autism) 1–5 years 500 micrograms/kg every 4–6 hours (max. 40 mg daily); 6–12 years third to half adult dose (max. 75 mg daily)

Intractable hiccup, 25–50 mg 3–4 times daily

By deep intramuscular injection, (for relief of acute symptoms but see also Cautions and Side-effects), 25–50 mg every 6–8 hours; CHILD, as dose by mouth

By rectum in suppositories as chlorpromazine base 100 mg every 6–8 hours [unlicensed]

Note. For equivalent therapeutic effect 100 mg chlorpromazine base given *rectally* as a suppository ≡ 20–25 mg chlorpromazine hydrochloride *by intramuscular injection* ≡ 40–50 mg of chlorpromazine base or hydrochloride *by mouth*

PoM **Chlorpromazine** (Non-proprietary)

Tablets, coated, chlorpromazine hydrochloride 10 mg, net price 20 = 13p; 25 mg, 20 = 15p; 50 mg, 20 = 26p; 100 mg, 20 = 43p. Label: 2, 11
Available from Antigen, APS, DDSA (Chloractil®), Hillcross, Norton

Oral solution, chlorpromazine hydrochloride 25 mg/5 mL, net price 100 mL = 58p, 100 mg/5 mL, 100 mL = £1.16. Label: 2, 11
Available from Hillcross, Rosemont

Injection, chlorpromazine hydrochloride 25 mg/mL, net price 1-mL amp = 26p; 2-mL amp = 28p
Available from Antigen

Suppositories, chlorpromazine 100 mg. Label: 2, 11
'Special order' [unlicensed] product; contact Martindale or regional hospital manufacturing unit

PoM **Largactil®** (Rhône-Poulenc Rorer)

Tablets, all off-white, f/c, chlorpromazine hydrochloride 10 mg. Net price 56-tab pack = 35p; 25 mg, 56-tab pack = 54p; 50 mg, 56-tab pack = £1.13; 100 mg, 56-tab pack = £2.10. Label: 2, 11

Syrup, brown, chlorpromazine hydrochloride 25 mg/5 mL. Net price 100-mL pack = 61p. Label: 2, 11

Suspension forte, orange, sugar-free, chlorpromazine hydrochloride 100 mg (as embonate)/5 mL. Net price 100-mL pack = £1.28. Label: 2, 11

Injection, chlorpromazine hydrochloride 25 mg/mL. Net price 2-mL amp = 34p

BENPERIDOL

Indications: control of deviant antisocial sexual behaviour (but see notes above)

Cautions; Contra-indications; Side-effects: see under Haloperidol

Dose: 0.25–1.5 mg daily in divided doses, adjusted according to the response; ELDERLY (or debilitated) initially half adult dose; CHILD not recommended

PoM **Anquil®** (Janssen)

Tablets, benperidol 250 micrograms. Net price 20 = £5.23. Label: 2

CLOZAPINE

Indications: schizophrenia in patients unresponsive to, or intolerant of, conventional antipsychotic drugs

Cautions: see under Chlorpromazine Hydrochloride; initiation must be in hospital in-patients, and leucocyte and differential blood counts must be normal before treatment and must be monitored weekly for first 18 weeks then at least fortnightly—patients who have received clozapine for a year or more and have stable blood counts may have their blood monitoring reduced to every 4 weeks; avoid drugs which depress leucopoiesis such as co-trimoxazole and carbamazepine (and taper off conventional neuroleptic before starting); withdraw treatment if leucocyte count falls below 3000/mm³ or absolute neutrophil count falls below 1500/mm³; patients should report any infections; **interactions**: Appendix 1 (clozapine)
WITHDRAWAL. On planned withdrawal reduce dose gradually over 1–2 weeks to avoid risk of rebound psychosis. If abrupt withdrawal necessary observe patient carefully

Contra-indications: severe cardiac disease; history of drug-induced neutropenia/agranulocytosis; bone marrow disorders; alcoholic and toxic psychoses; history of circulatory collapse or paralytic ileus; drug intoxication; coma or severe CNS depression; uncontrolled epilepsy; pregnancy and breast-feeding

Side-effects: see under Chlorpromazine Hydrochloride but less sedating and high incidence of antimuscarinic symptoms; extrapyramidal symptoms may occur less frequently; neutropenia and potentially fatal agranulocytosis, fever (evaluate to rule out underlying infection or agranulocytosis), headache and dizziness, hypersalivation, urinary incontinence, priapism, pericarditis and myocarditis, and delirium; hypotension—rarely circulatory collapse with cardiac and respiratory arrest (but hypertension also reported), also nausea and vomiting; hyperglycaemia reported

Dose: (close medical supervision on initiation—risk of collapse due to hypotension) 12.5 mg once or twice on first day then 25–50 mg on second day then slowly increased (if well tolerated) in steps of 25–50 mg over 14–21 days to 300 mg daily in divided doses (larger dose at night, up to 200 mg daily may be taken as a single dose at bedtime); if necessary may be further increased in steps of 50–100 mg once (preferably) or twice weekly; usual antipsychotic dose 200–450 mg daily (max. 900 mg daily); subsequent adjustment to usual maintenance of 150–300 mg; CHILD not recommended

ELDERLY AND SPECIAL RISK GROUPS. In *elderly*, 12.5 mg once on first day—subsequent adjustments restricted to 25 mg daily; in *cardiovascular disease, hepatic* or *renal impairment* or if history of *epilepsy*, 12.5 mg on first day—subsequent adjustments slowly and in small steps (if epileptic seizures (see also Cautions), suspend for 24 hours and resume at lower dose; *restarting* after *interval of more than 2 days*, 12.5 mg once or twice on first day (but may be feasible to increase more quickly than on initiation)—unless previous respiratory or cardiac arrest with initial dosing in which case extreme caution

PoM **Clozaril**® (Sandoz)
Tablets, both yellow, clozapine 25 mg (scored), net price 28-tab pack = £12.52, 84-tab pack (hosp. only) = £37.54; 100 mg, 28-tab pack = £50.05, 84-tab pack (hosp. only) = £150.15. Label: 2, 10 patient information leaflet
Note. Patient, prescriber, and supplying pharmacist must be registered with the Sandoz Clozaril Patient Monitoring Service—takes several days to do this

DROPERIDOL
Indications: see under Dose; peri-operative use, see section 15.1.4.1
Cautions; Contra-indications; Side-effects: see under Haloperidol
Dose: by mouth, tranquillisation and emergency control in mania, 5–20 mg repeated every 4–8 hours if necessary (elderly, initially half adult dose); CHILD, 0.5–1 mg daily
By intramuscular injection, up to 10 mg repeated every 4–6 hours if necessary (elderly, initially half adult dose); CHILD, 0.5–1 mg daily

By intravenous injection, 5–15 mg repeated every 4–6 hours if necessary (elderly, initially half adult dose)
Cancer chemotherapy-induced nausea and vomiting, *by intramuscular or intravenous injection* 1–10 mg 30 minutes before starting therapy, followed by *continuous intravenous infusion* of 1–3 mg/hour *or* 1–5 mg *by intramuscular or intravenous injection* every 1–6 hours as necessary; CHILD *by intramuscular or intravenous injection* 20–75 micrograms/kg

PoM **Droleptan**® (Janssen)
Tablets, yellow, scored, droperidol 10 mg. Net price 50-tab pack = £12.30. Label: 2
Oral liquid, sugar-free, droperidol 1 mg/mL. Net price 100-mL pack (with graduated cap) = £4.47 500-mL pack = £21.25. Label: 2
Injection, droperidol 5 mg/mL. Net price 2-mL amp = 90p

FLUPENTHIXOL
(Flupentixol)
Indications: schizophrenia and other psychoses particularly with apathy and withdrawal but not mania or psychomotor hyperactivity; depression section 4.3.4
Cautions; Contra-indications; Side-effects: see under Chlorpromazine Hydrochloride but less sedating; extrapyramidal symptoms more frequent (25% of patients); avoid in senile confusional states, excitable and overactive patients; porphyria (see section 9.8.2)
Dose: psychosis, initially 3–9 mg twice daily, adjusted according to the response; max. 18 mg daily; ELDERLY (or debilitated) initially quarter to half adult dose; CHILD not recommended
Depression, see section 4.3.4

PoM **Depixol**® (Lundbeck)
Tablets, yellow, s/c, flupenthixol 3 mg (as dihydrochloride). Net price 20 = £2.85. Label: 2
Depot injection (flupenthixol decanoate): section 4.2.2
PoM **Fluanxol**® (depression), see section 4.3.4

FLUPHENAZINE HYDROCHLORIDE
Indications: see under Dose
Cautions; Contra-indications; Side-effects: see under Chlorpromazine Hydrochloride, but less sedating and fewer antimuscarinic or hypotensive symptoms; extrapyramidal symptoms, particularly dystonic reactions and akathisia, are more frequent; avoid in depression
Dose: schizophrenia and other psychoses, mania, initially 2.5–10 mg daily in 2–3 divided doses, adjusted according to response to 20 mg daily; doses above 20 mg daily (10 mg in elderly) only with special caution; CHILD not recommended
Short-term adjunctive management of severe anxiety, psychomotor agitation, excitement, and violent or dangerously impulsive behaviour, initially 1 mg twice daily, increased as necessary to 2 mg twice daily; CHILD not recommended

PoM **Moditen®** (Sanofi Winthrop)

Tablets, all s/c, fluphenazine hydrochloride 1 mg (pink), net price 20 = £1.06; 2.5 mg (yellow), 20 = £1.33; 5 mg, 20 = £1.77. Label: 2

Depot injections (fluphenazine decanoate): section 4.2.2

HALOPERIDOL

Indications: see under Dose; motor tics, section 4.9.3

Cautions; Contra-indications; Side-effects: see under Chlorpromazine Hydrochloride but less sedating, and fewer antimuscarinic or hypotensive symptoms; pigmentation and photosensitivity reactions rare. Extrapyramidal symptoms, particularly dystonic reactions and akathisia are more frequent especially in thyrotoxic patients. Rarely weight loss. Avoid in basal ganglia disease

Dose: by mouth,

Schizophrenia and other psychoses, mania, short-term adjunctive management of psychomotor agitation, excitement, and violent or dangerously impulsive behaviour, initially 1.5–3 mg 2–3 times daily *or* 3–5 mg 2–3 times daily in severely affected or resistant patients; in resistant schizophrenia up to 100 mg (rarely 120 mg) daily may be needed; adjusted according to response to lowest effective maintenance dose (as low as 5–10 mg daily); ELDERLY (or debilitated) initially half adult dose; CHILD initially 25–50 micrograms/kg daily (in 2 divided doses) to a max. of 10 mg; adolescents up to 30 mg daily (exceptionally 60 mg)

Short-term adjunctive management of severe anxiety, adults 500 micrograms twice daily; CHILD not recommended

Intractable hiccup, 1.5 mg 3 times daily adjusted according to response; CHILD not recommended

By intramuscular injection, 2–10 mg, subsequent doses being given every 4–8 hours according to response (up to every hour if necessary) to total max. 60 mg; severely disturbed patients may require initial dose of up to 30 mg; CHILD not recommended

Nausea and vomiting, 1–2 mg

PoM **Haloperidol** (Non-proprietary)

Tablets, haloperidol 1.5 mg, net price 20 = 93p; 5 mg, 20 = £2.84; 10 mg, 20 = £5.20; 20 mg, 20 = £9.38. Label: 2

PoM **Dozic®** (Rosemont)

Oral liquid, sugar-free, haloperidol 1 mg/mL, net price 100-mL pack = £4.60; 2 mg/mL, 100-mL pack = £4.80. Label: 2

PoM **Haldol®** (Janssen)

Tablets, both scored, haloperidol 5 mg (blue), net price 20 = £1.65; 10 mg (yellow), 20 = £3.21. Label: 2

Oral liquid, sugar-free, haloperidol 2 mg/mL. Net price 100-mL pack (with pipette) = £5.08. Label: 2

Oral liquid concentrate, sugar-free, haloperidol 10 mg/mL. Net price 100-mL pack = £22.27. Label: 2

Diluent purified water, freshly boiled and cooled, life of diluted concentrate 14 days. Alternatively, purified water, freshly boiled and cooled, containing 0.05% of methyl hydroxybenzoate and 0.005% of propyl hydroxybenzoate, life of diluted concentrate 2 months.

Injection, haloperidol 5 mg/mL. Net price 1-mL amp = 33p; 2-mL amp = 62p

Depot injection (haloperidol decanoate): section 4.2.2

PoM **Serenace®** (Baker Norton)

Capsules, green, haloperidol 500 micrograms. Net price 20 = 65p. Label: 2

Tablets, haloperidol 1.5 mg, net price 20 = £1.16; 5 mg (pink), 20 = £3.27; 10 mg (pale pink), 20 = £5.87; 20 mg (dark pink), 20 = £10.58. Label: 2

Oral liquid, sugar-free, haloperidol 2 mg/mL. Net price 100-mL pack = £8.77. Label: 2

Injection, haloperidol 5 mg/mL, net price 1-mL amp = 59p; 10 mg/mL, 2-mL amp = £2.03

LOXAPINE

Indications: acute and chronic psychoses

Cautions; Contra-indications: see under Chlorpromazine Hydrochloride; porphyria (see section 9.8.2)

Side-effects: see under Chlorpromazine Hydrochloride; nausea and vomiting, weight gain or loss, dyspnoea, ptosis, hyperpyrexia, flushing and headache, paraesthesia, and polydipsia also reported

Dose: initially 20–50 mg daily in 2 divided doses, increased as necessary over 7–10 days to 60–100 mg daily (max. 250 mg) in 2–4 divided doses, then adjusted to usual maintenance dose of 20–100 mg daily; CHILD not recommended

PoM **Loxapac®** (Lederle)

Capsules, loxapine (as succinate) 10 mg (yellow/green), net price 100-cap pack = £9.52; 25 mg (light green/dark green), 100-cap pack = £19.05; 50 mg (blue/dark green), 100-cap pack = £34.27. Label: 2

METHOTRIMEPRAZINE

(Levomepromazine)

Indications: see under Dose

Cautions; Contra-indications; Side-effects: see under Chlorpromazine Hydrochloride but more sedating

ELDERLY. Risk of postural hypotension particularly in patients over 50 years—not recommended for ambulant patients over 50 years unless risk of hypotensive reaction has been assessed

Dose: by mouth, schizophrenia, initially 25–50 mg daily in divided doses increased as necessary; bedpatients initially 100–200 mg daily usually in 3 divided doses, increased if necessary to 1 g daily; ELDERLY, see Cautions

Adjunctive treatment in terminal care (including management of pain and associated restlessness, distress, or vomiting), 12.5–50 mg every 4–8 hours

By intramuscular injection or by intravenous injection (by intravenous injection after dilution with an equal volume of sodium chloride 0.9% injection), adjunct in terminal care, 12.5–25 mg (severe agitation up to 50 mg) every 6–8 hours if necessary

By continuous subcutaneous infusion, adjunct in palliative care (via syringe driver), 25–200 mg daily (over 24-hour period), diluted in a suitable volume of sodium chloride 0.9% injection; CHILD (experience limited), 0.35–3 mg/kg daily

PoM Nozinan® (Link)
Tablets, scored, methotrimeprazine maleate 25 mg. Net price 20 = £3.00. Label: 2
Injection, methotrimeprazine hydrochloride 25 mg/mL. Net price 1-mL amp = £1.75

OXYPERTINE
Indications: see under Dose
Cautions; Contra-indications; Side-effects: see under Chlorpromazine Hydrochloride, but extrapyramidal symptoms may occur less frequently. With low doses agitation and hyperactivity occur and with high doses sedation. Occasionally photophobia may occur
Dose: schizophrenia and other psychoses, mania, short-term adjunctive management of psychomotor agitation, excitement, and violent or dangerously impulsive behaviour, initially 80–120 mg daily in divided doses adjusted according to the response; max. 300 mg daily; CHILD not recommended
Short-term adjunctive management of severe anxiety, initially 10 mg 3–4 times daily preferably after food; max. 60 mg daily; CHILD not recommended

PoM Oxypertine (Sanofi Winthrop)
Capsules, oxypertine 10 mg. Net price 20 = £2.12. Label: 2
Tablets, scored, oxypertine 40 mg. Net price 20 = £6.64. Label: 2
Note. The brand name Integrin® was formerly used for oxypertine preparations

PERICYAZINE
Indications: see under Dose
Cautions; Contra-indications; Side-effects: see under Chlorpromazine Hydrochloride, but more sedating; hypotension commonly occurs when treatment initiated
Dose: schizophrenia and other psychoses, initially 75 mg daily in divided doses increased at weekly intervals by steps of 25 mg according to response; usual max. 300 mg daily (elderly initially 15–30 mg daily)
Short-term adjunctive management of severe anxiety, psychomotor agitation, and violent or dangerously impulsive behaviour, initially 15–30 mg (elderly 5–10 mg) daily divided into 2 doses, taking the larger dose at bedtime, adjusted according to response

CHILD (severe mental or behavioural disorders only), initially, 500 micrograms daily for 10-kg child, increased by 1 mg for each additional 5 kg to max. total daily dose of 10 mg; dose may be gradually increased according to response but maintenance should not exceed twice initial dose INFANT under 1 year not recommended

PoM Neulactil® (Rhône-Poulenc Rorer)
Tablets, all yellow, scored, pericyazine 2.5 mg, net price 84-tab pack = £2.09; 10 mg, 84-tab pack = £5.65. Label: 2
Syrup forte, brown, pericyazine 10 mg/5 mL. Net price 100-mL pack = £2.74. Label: 2

PERPHENAZINE
Indications: see under Dose; anti-emetic, section 4.6
Cautions; Contra-indications; Side-effects: see under Chlorpromazine Hydrochloride, but less sedating; extrapyramidal symptoms, especially dystonia, more frequent, particularly at high dosage; not indicated for agitation and restlessness in the elderly
Dose: schizophrenia and other psychoses, mania, short-term adjunctive management of severe anxiety, psychomotor agitation, excitement, and violent or dangerously impulsive behaviour, initially 4 mg 3 times daily adjusted according to the response; max. 24 mg daily; ELDERLY quarter to half adult dose (but see Cautions); CHILD under 14 years not recommended

PoM Fentazin® (Forley)
Tablets, both s/c, perphenazine 2 mg, net price 20 = £3.30; 4 mg, 20 = £3.90. Label: 2

PIMOZIDE
Indications: see under Dose
Cautions; Contra-indications; Side-effects: see under Chlorpromazine Hydrochloride, but less sedating; contra-indicated in breast-feeding; serious arrhythmias reported (contra-indicated if history of arrhythmias or pre-existing congenital QT prolongation); following reports of sudden unexplained death, the CSM recommends ECG before treatment in all patients, periodic ECGs at doses over 16 mg daily and review of need for pimozide if repolarisation changes or arrhythmias develop (close supervision and preferably dose reduction advised)—for additional CSM warnings see also below; concurrent cardioactive or antipsychotic drugs, or electrolyte disturbances (notably hypokalaemia) may predispose to cardiotoxicity
ADDITIONAL CSM WARNING. In addition to the advice above, the CSM now also recommends that patients on pimozide should have an annual ECG (if the QT interval is found to be prolonged treatment should be reviewed and either withdrawn or the dose reduced under close supervision) and that pimozide should **not** be given with other antipsychotic drugs (including depot preparations), tricyclic antidepressants or other drugs known to prolong the QT interval, such as certain antimalarials, anti-arrhythmic drugs and certain antihistamines (terfenadine, astemizole) and should **not** be given with drugs which cause electrolyte disturbances (especially diuretics)

Dose: schizophrenia, initially 10 mg daily in acute conditions, adjusted according to response in increments of 2–4 mg at intervals of not less than 1 week; max. 20 mg daily; prevention of relapse, initially 2 mg daily (range 2–20 mg daily); ELDERLY half usual starting dose; CHILD not recommended

Monosymptomatic hypochondriacal psychosis, paranoid psychoses, initially 4 mg daily, adjusted according to response in increments of 2–4 mg at intervals of not less than 1 week; max. 16 mg daily; ELDERLY half usual starting dose; CHILD not recommended

Mania, hypomania, short-term adjunctive management of excitement and psychomotor agitation, initially 10 mg daily adjusted according to response in increments of 2–4 mg at intervals of not less than 1 week; max. 20 mg daily; ELDERLY half usual starting dose; CHILD not recommended

PoM **Orap**® (Janssen)
Tablets, all scored, pimozide 2 mg, net price 20 = £3.17; 4 mg (green), 20 = £6.13; 10 mg, 20 = £11.76. Label: 2

PROCHLORPERAZINE
Indications: see under Dose; anti-emetic, section 4.6
Cautions; Contra-indications; Side-effects: see under Chlorpromazine Hydrochloride, but less sedating; extrapyramidal symptoms, particularly dystonic reactions, more frequent; avoid in children (but see section 4.6 for use as anti-emetic)
Dose: by mouth, schizophrenia and other psychoses, mania, prochlorperazine maleate or mesylate, 12.5 mg twice daily for 7 days adjusted at intervals of 4–7 days to usual dose of 75–100 mg daily according to response; CHILD not recommended

Short-term adjunctive management of severe anxiety, 15–20 mg daily in divided doses; max. 40 mg daily; CHILD not recommended
By deep intramuscular injection, psychoses, mania, prochlorperazine mesylate 12.5–25 mg 2–3 times daily; CHILD not recommended
By rectum in suppositories, psychoses, mania, the equivalent of prochlorperazine maleate 25 mg 2–3 times daily; CHILD not recommended

Preparations
Section 4.6

PROMAZINE HYDROCHLORIDE
Indications: see under Dose
Cautions; Contra-indications; Side-effects: see under Chlorpromazine Hydrochloride
Dose: by mouth, short-term adjunctive management of psychomotor agitation, 100–200 mg 4 times daily; CHILD not recommended
Agitation and restlessness in elderly, 25–50 mg 4 times daily
By intramuscular injection, short-term adjunctive management of psychomotor agitation, 50 mg (25 mg in elderly or debilitated), repeated if necessary after 6–8 hours; CHILD not recommended

PoM **Promazine** (Non-proprietary)
Tablets, coated, promazine hydrochloride 25 mg and 50 mg. Label: 2
Available from Biorex
Oral solution, promazine hydrochloride 25 mg/5 mL, net price 200 mL = £1.55; 50 mg/5 mL, 200 mL = £1.60. Label: 2
Available from Rosemont

PoM **Sparine**® (Wyeth)
Suspension, yellow, promazine hydrochloride 50 mg (as embonate)/5 mL. Net price 150-mL pack = £1.29. Label: 2
Note. Not recommended for children
Injection, promazine hydrochloride 50 mg/mL. Net price 1-mL amp = 26p

RISPERIDONE
Indications: acute and chronic psychoses
Cautions; Contra-indications; Side-effects: see under Chlorpromazine Hydrochloride, but agitation may occur more frequently; dyspepsia, nausea, abdominal pain, anxiety, concentration difficulties, headache, dizziness, fatigue, and rhinitis also reported
Dose: 2 mg in 1–2 divided doses on first day *then* 4 mg in 1–2 divided doses on second day *then* 6 mg in 1–2 divided doses on third day; usual range 4–8 mg daily; doses above 10 mg daily only if benefit considered to outweigh risk (max. 16 mg daily); ELDERLY (or in hepatic or renal impairment) 500 micrograms twice daily increased to 1–2 mg twice daily; CHILD under 15 years not recommended

▼ PoM **Risperdal**® (Janssen, Organon)
Tablets, all f/c, scored, risperidone 1 mg (white), net price, 6-tab starter pack = £4.15, 20-tab pack = £13.45; 2 mg (orange), 60-tab pack = £79.56; 3 mg (yellow), 60-tab pack = £117.00; 4 mg (green), 60-tab pack = £154.44. Label: 2
Liquid, risperidone 1 mg/mL, net price 100 mL = £65.00. Label: 2
Note. Liquid may be diluted with mineral water, orange juice or black coffee (should be used within 4 hours)

SULPIRIDE
Indications: schizophrenia
Cautions; Contra-indications; Side-effects: see under Chlorpromazine Hydrochloride, but less sedating; structurally distinct from chlorpromazine hence not associated with jaundice or skin reactions; porphyria (see section 9.8.2); avoid in breast-feeding; reduce dose (preferably avoid) in renal impairment
Dose: 200–400 mg twice daily; max. 800 mg daily in patients with predominantly negative symptoms, and 2.4 g daily in patients with mainly positive symptoms; ELDERLY, initially quarter to half adult dose; CHILD under 14 not recommended

PoM **Dolmatil**® (Lorex)
Tablets, both scored, sulpiride 200 mg, net price 100-tab pack = £20.03; 400 mg (f/c), 100-tab pack = £39.50. Label: 2
Note. Also available as a generic from Cox, Norton

PoM Sulparex® (Bristol-Myers)
Tablets, scored, sulpiride 200 mg. Net price 100-tab pack = £20.03. Label: 2

PoM Sulpitil® (Pharmacia)
Tablets, scored, sulpiride 200 mg. Net price 28-tab pack = £5.61; 112-tab pack = £22.43. Label: 2

THIORIDAZINE

Indications: see under Dose

Cautions; Contra-indications; Side-effects: see under Chlorpromazine Hydrochloride, but less sedating and extrapyramidal symptoms and hypothermia rarely occur; more likely to induce hypotension and possibly increased risk of cardiotoxicity and prolongation of QT interval. Pigmentary retinopathy (with reduced visual acuity, brownish colouring of vision, and impaired night vision) occurs rarely with high doses—on prolonged use examinations for eye defects are required; sexual dysfunction, particularly retrograde ejaculation, may occur; porphyria (see section 9.8.2)

Dose: schizophrenia and other psychoses, mania, 150–600 mg daily (initially in divided doses); max. 800 mg daily (hospital patients only) for up to 4 weeks

Short-term adjunctive management of psychomotor agitation, excitement, violent or dangerously impulsive behaviour, 75–200 mg daily

Short-term adjunctive management of severe anxiety, and agitation and restlessness in the elderly, 30–100 mg daily

CHILD (severe mental or behavioural problems only) 1–5 years 1 mg/kg daily, 5–12 years 75–150 mg daily (in severe cases, up to 300 mg daily)

PoM Thioridazine (Non-proprietary)
Tablets, coated, thioridazine hydrochloride 25 mg, net price 20 = 34p; 50 mg, 20 = 70p; 100 mg, 20 = £1.36. Label: 2
Available from Cox, DDSA (Rideril®), Hillcross, Norton
Oral solution, thioridazine 25 mg (as hydrochloride)/5 mL. Net price 500-mL = £2.91. Label: 2
Available from Rosemont

PoM Melleril® (Sandoz)
Tablets, all f/c, thioridazine hydrochloride 10 mg, net price 20 = 22p; 25 mg, 20 = 31p; 50 mg, 20 = 60p; 100 mg, 20 = £1.14. Label: 2
Suspension 25 mg/5 mL, thioridazine 25 mg/5 mL. Net price 500-mL = £2.98. Label: 2
Suspension 100 mg/5 mL, thioridazine 100 mg/5 mL. Net price 500-mL = £10.89. Label: 2
Note. These suspensions should not be diluted but the two preparations may be mixed with each other to provide intermediate doses
Syrup, orange, thioridazine 25 mg (as hydrochloride)/5 mL. Net price 100-mL pack = 76p. Label: 2
Note. Also available as a generic from Hillcross

TRIFLUOPERAZINE

Indications: see under Dose; anti-emetic, section 4.6

Cautions; Contra-indications; Side-effects: see under Chlorpromazine Hydrochloride but less

sedating, and hypotension, hypothermia, and antimuscarinic side-effects occur less frequently; extrapyramidal symptoms, particularly dystonic reactions and akathisia, are more frequent (particularly when the daily dose exceeds 6 mg); caution in children

Dose: by mouth (reduce initial doses in elderly by at least half)

Schizophrenia and other psychoses, short-term adjunctive management of psychomotor agitation, excitement, and violent or dangerously impulsive behaviour, initially 5 mg twice daily, *or* 10 mg daily in modified-release form, increased by 5 mg after 1 week, then at intervals of 3 days, according to the response; CHILD up to 12 years, initially up to 5 mg daily in divided doses, adjusted according to response, age, and bodyweight

Short-term adjunctive management of severe anxiety, 2–4 mg daily in divided doses *or* 2–4 mg daily in modified-release form, increased if necessary to 6 mg daily; CHILD 3–5 years up to 1 mg daily, 6–12 years up to 4 mg daily

PoM Trifluoperazine (Non-proprietary)
Tablets, coated, trifluoperazine (as hydrochloride) 1 mg, net price 20 = 35p; 5 mg, 20 = 45p. Label: 2
Available from most generic manufacturers
Oral solution, trifluoperazine 5 mg (as hydrochloride)/5 mL. Net price 200-mL = £8.25. Label: 2
Available from Rosemont (sugar-free)

PoM Stelazine® (SK&F)
Tablets, both blue, f/c, trifluoperazine (as hydrochloride) 1 mg, net price 20 = 51p; 5 mg, 20 = 72p. Label: 2
Spansules® (= capsules m/r), all clear/yellow, enclosing dark blue, light blue, and white pellets, trifluoperazine (as hydrochloride) 2 mg, net price 60-cap pack = £3.28; 10 mg, 30-cap pack = £2.14; 15 mg, 30-cap pack = £3.22. Label: 2, 25
Syrup, yellow, sugar-free, trifluoperazine 1 mg (as hydrochloride)/5 mL. Net price 200-mL pack = £2.00. Label: 2

ZUCLOPENTHIXOL ACETATE

Indications: short-term management of acute psychosis, mania, or exacerbations of chronic psychosis

Cautions; Contra-indications; Side-effects: see under Chlorpromazine Hydrochloride; porphyria (see section 9.8.2); treatment duration should not exceed 2 weeks

Dose: by deep intramuscular injection into the gluteal muscle or lateral thigh, 50–150 mg (elderly 50–100 mg), if necessary repeated after 2–3 days (1 additional dose may be needed 1–2 days after the first injection); max. cumulative dose 400 mg per course and max. 4 injections; max. duration of treatment 2 weeks—if maintenance treatment necessary change to an oral antipsychotic 2–3 days after last injection, *or* to a longer acting antipsychotic depot injection given concomitantly with last injection of zuclopenthixol acetate; CHILD not recommended

PoM Clopixol Acuphase® (Lundbeck)
Injection (oily), zuclopenthixol acetate 50 mg/mL.
Net price 1-mL amp = £4.95; 2-mL amp = £9.55

ZUCLOPENTHIXOL DIHYDROCHLORIDE

Indications: schizophrenia and other psychoses, particularly when associated with agitated, aggressive, or hostile behaviour
Cautions; Contra-indications; Side-effects: see under Chlorpromazine Hydrochloride; should not be used in apathetic or withdrawn states; porphyria (see section 9.8.2)
Dose: initially 20–30 mg daily in divided doses, increasing to a max. of 150 mg daily if necessary; usual maintenance dose 20–50 mg daily; CHILD not recommended

PoM Clopixol® (Lundbeck)
Tablets, all f/c, zuclopenthixol (as dihydrochloride) 2 mg (pink), net price 20 = 61p; 10 mg (light brown), 20 = £1.65; 25 mg (brown), 20 = £3.30. Label: 2
Depot injection (zuclopenthixol decanoate): section 4.2.2

4.2.2   Antipsychotic depot injections

For maintenance therapy, long-acting depot injections of antipsychotic drugs are used because they are more convenient than oral preparations and ensure better patient compliance. However, they may give rise to a higher incidence of extrapyramidal reactions than oral preparations.

ADMINISTRATION. Depot antipsychotics are administered by deep intramuscular injection at intervals of 1 to 4 weeks. Patients should first be given a small test-dose as undesirable side-effects are prolonged. In general not more than 2–3 mL of oily injection should be administered at any one site; correct injection technique (including the use of z-track technique) and rotation of injection sites are essential. If the dose needs to be reduced to alleviate side-effects it is important to recognise that the plasma level may not fall for some time after reducing the dose, therefore it may be a month or longer before side-effects subside.

Equivalent doses of depot antipsychotics
These equivalences are intended **only** as an approximate guide; individual dosage instructions should **also** be checked; patients should be carefully monitored after **any** change in medication

Antipsychotic	Dose (mg)	Interval
Flupenthixol decanoate	40	2 weeks
Fluphenazine decanoate	25	2 weeks
Haloperidol (as decanoate)	100	4 weeks
Pipothiazine palmitate	50	4 weeks
Zuclopenthixol decanoate	200	2 weeks

IMPORTANT. These equivalences must **not** be extrapolated beyond the max. dose for the drug

Cautionary label wordings, see inside back cover

DOSAGE. Individual responses to neuroleptic drugs are very variable and to achieve optimum effect, dosage and dosage interval must be titrated according to the patient's response. For the advice of The Royal College of Psychiatrists on doses above the BNF upper limit, see p. 158

CHOICE. There is no clear-cut division in the use of these drugs, but **zuclopenthixol** may be suitable for the treatment of agitated or aggressive patients whereas **flupenthixol** can cause over-excitement in such patients. The incidence of extrapyramidal reactions is similar for all these drugs.

CAUTIONS. Treatment requires careful monitoring for optimum effect; extrapyramidal symptoms occur frequently. When transferring from oral to depot therapy, dosage by mouth should be gradually phased out.

CONTRA-INDICATIONS. Do not use in children, confusional states, coma caused by CNS depressants, parkinsonism, intolerance to antipsychotics.

SIDE-EFFECTS. Pain may occur at injection site and occasionally erythema, swelling, and nodules. For side-effects of specific antipsychotics see under the relevant monograph.

FLUPENTHIXOL DECANOATE
(Flupentixol Decanoate)
Indications: maintenance in schizophrenia and other psychoses
Cautions; Contra-indications; Side-effects: see under Chlorpromazine Hydrochloride (section 4.2.1) and notes above, but it may have a mood elevating effect; extrapyramidal symptoms usually appear 1–3 days after administration and continue for about 5 days but may be delayed; an alternative antipsychotic may be necessary if symptoms such as aggression or agitation appear; porphyria (see section 9.8.2)
Dose: by deep intramuscular injection into the gluteal muscle, test dose 20 mg, then after at least 7 days 20–40 mg repeated at intervals of 2–4 weeks, adjusted according to response; max. 400 mg weekly; usual maintenance dose 50 mg every 4 weeks to 300 mg every 2 weeks; ELDERLY initially quarter to half adult dose; CHILD not recommended

PoM Depixol® (Lundbeck)
Injection (oily), flupenthixol decanoate 20 mg/mL. Net price 1-mL amp = £1.55; 2-mL amp = £2.60
PoM Depixol Conc.® (Lundbeck)
Injection (oily), flupenthixol decanoate 100 mg/mL. Net price 0.5-mL amp = £3.49; 1-mL amp = £6.40
PoM Depixol Low Volume® (Lundbeck)
Injection (oily), flupenthixol decanoate 200 mg/mL. Net price 1-mL amp = £19.98

FLUPHENAZINE DECANOATE

Indications: maintenance in schizophrenia and other psychoses

Cautions; Contra-indications; Side-effects: see under Chlorpromazine Hydrochloride (section 4.2.1) and notes above. Extrapyramidal symptoms usually appear a few hours after the dose has been administered and continue for about 2 days but may be delayed. Contra-indicated in severely depressed states

Dose: by deep intramuscular injection into the gluteal muscle, test dose 12.5 mg (6.25 mg in elderly), then after 4–7 days 12.5–100 mg repeated at intervals of 14–35 days, adjusted according to response; CHILD not recommended

PoM Modecate® (Sanofi Winthrop)
Injection (oily), fluphenazine decanoate 25 mg/mL. Net price 0.5-mL amp = £1.42; 1-mL amp = £2.46; 1-mL syringe = £2.72; 2-mL amp = £4.84; 2-mL syringe = £4.93; 10-mL vial = £23.45
Note. Contains sesame oil
Note. Fluphenazine decanoate injection also available from Antigen, Berk (Decazate®), David Bull, Hillcross—at least some versions contain sesame oil

PoM Modecate Concentrate® (Sanofi Winthrop)
Injection (oily), fluphenazine decanoate 100 mg/mL. Net price 0.5-mL amp = £4.87; 1-mL amp = £9.53
Note. Contains sesame oil
Note. Fluphenazine decanoate injection also available from Antigen, Berk (Decazate®), David Bull, Hillcross—at least some versions contain sesame oil

HALOPERIDOL DECANOATE

Indications: maintenance in schizophrenia and other psychoses

Cautions; Contra-indications; Side-effects: see under Haloperidol (section 4.2.1) and notes above

Dose: by deep intramuscular injection into the gluteal muscle, haloperidol (as decanoate), initially 50 mg every 4 weeks, if necessary increasing after 2 weeks by 50-mg increments to 300 mg every 4 weeks; higher doses may be needed in some patients; ELDERLY, initially 12.5–25 mg every 4 weeks; CHILD not recommended

PoM Haldol Decanoate® (Janssen)
Injection (oily), haloperidol (as decanoate) 50 mg/mL, net price 1-mL amp = £4.35; 100 mg/mL, 1-mL amp = £5.77

PIPOTHIAZINE PALMITATE
(Pipotiazine Palmitate)

Indications: maintenance in schizophrenia and other psychoses

Cautions; Contra-indications; Side-effects: see under Chlorpromazine Hydrochloride (section 4.2.1) and notes above

Dose: by deep intramuscular injection into the gluteal muscle, test dose 25 mg, then a further 25–50 mg after 4–7 days, then adjusted according to response at intervals of 4 weeks; usual maintenance range 50–100 mg (max. 200 mg) every 4 weeks; ELDERLY initially 5–10 mg; CHILD not recommended

PoM Piportil Depot® (Rhône-Poulenc Rorer)
Injection (oily), pipothiazine palmitate 50 mg/mL. Net price 1-mL amp = £6.73; 2-mL amp = £11.01

ZUCLOPENTHIXOL DECANOATE

Indications: maintenance in schizophrenia and other psychoses, particularly with aggression and agitation

Cautions; Contra-indications; Side-effects: see under Chlorpromazine Hydrochloride (section 4.2.1) and notes above, but less sedating; porphyria (see section 9.8.2)

Dose: by deep intramuscular injection into the gluteal muscle, test dose 100 mg, followed after 7–28 days by 100–200 mg or more, followed by 200–400 mg at intervals of 2–4 weeks, adjusted according to response; max. 600 mg weekly; CHILD not recommended

PoM Clopixol® (Lundbeck)
Injection (oily), zuclopenthixol decanoate 200 mg/mL. Net price 1-mL amp = £3.23
PoM Clopixol Conc.® (Lundbeck)
Injection (oily), zuclopenthixol decanoate 500 mg/mL. Net price 1-mL amp with needle = £7.61

4.2.3 Antimanic drugs

Drugs are used in mania both to control acute attacks and also to prevent their recurrence.

ANTIPSYCHOTIC DRUGS

In an acute attack of mania, treatment with an antipsychotic drug (section 4.2.1) is usually required because it may take a few days for lithium to exert its antimanic effect. Lithium may be given concurrently with the antipsychotic drug, and treatment with the antipsychotic gradually tailed off as lithium becomes effective. Alternatively, lithium therapy may be commenced once the patient's mood has been stabilised with the antipsychotic. Haloperidol may be preferred for rapid control of acute mania. However, high doses of haloperidol, fluphenazine, or flupenthixol may be hazardous when used with lithium; irreversible toxic encephalopathy has been reported.

LITHIUM

Lithium salts are used in the *prophylaxis and treatment of mania*, in the *prophylaxis of manic-depressive illness* (bipolar illness or bipolar depression) and in the *prophylaxis of recurrent depression* (unipolar illness or unipolar depression). Lithium is unsuitable for children.

The decision to give prophylactic lithium usually requires specialist advice, and must be based on careful consideration of the likelihood of recurrence in the individual patient, and the benefit weighed against the risks. In long-term use, therapeutic concentrations have been thought to cause histological and functional changes in the kidney. The significance of such changes is not clear but is of sufficient concern to discourage long-term use of lithium unless it is definitely indicated. Patients should therefore be maintained on lithium after 3–5 years only if, on assessment, benefit persists.

PLASMA CONCENTRATIONS. Lithium salts have a narrow therapeutic/toxic ratio and should therefore not be prescribed unless facilities for monitoring plasma concentrations are available. There seem few if any reasons for preferring one or other of the salts of lithium available. Doses are adjusted to achieve plasma concentrations of 0.4 to 1.0 mmol Li^+/litre (lower end of the range for maintenance therapy and elderly patients) on samples taken 12 hours after the preceding dose. It is important to determine the optimum range for each individual patient.

Overdosage, usually with plasma concentrations over 1.5 mmol Li^+/litre, may be fatal and toxic effects include tremor, ataxia, dysarthria, nystagmus, renal impairment, and convulsions. If these potentially hazardous signs occur, treatment should be stopped, plasma-lithium concentrations redetermined, and steps taken to reverse lithium toxicity. In mild cases withdrawal of lithium and administration of generous amounts of sodium and fluid will reverse the toxicity. Plasma concentrations in excess of 2.0 mmol Li^+/litre require emergency treatment as indicated under Emergency Treatment of Poisoning, p. 23. When toxic concentrations are reached there may be a delay of 1 or 2 days before maximum toxicity occurs.

INTERACTIONS. Lithium toxicity is made worse by sodium depletion, therefore concurrent use of diuretics (particularly thiazides) is hazardous and should be avoided. For other **interactions** with lithium, see Appendix 1 (lithium).

WITHDRAWAL. There is no evidence of a lithium withdrawal state nor of rebound psychosis on withdrawal. Nevertheless, to allay any concerns about relapse, if possible lithium should be withdrawn slowly over a period of weeks.

LITHIUM CARDS. A lithium treatment card available from pharmacies tells patients how to take lithium preparations, what to do if a dose is missed, and what side-effects to expect. It also explains why regular blood tests are important and warns that some medicines and illnesses can change lithium plasma concentrations.

Cards from NPA Services, 38–42 St. Peter's St, St. Albans, Herts AL1 3NP.

LITHIUM CARBONATE

Indications: treatment and prophylaxis of mania, manic-depressive illness, and recurrent depression (see also notes above); aggressive or self-mutilating behaviour

Cautions: measure plasma concentrations regularly (every 3 months on stabilised regimens), monitor thyroid function; maintain adequate sodium and fluid intake; avoid in renal impairment, cardiac disease, and conditions with sodium imbalance such as Addison's disease; reduction in dose or discontinuation may be necessary in diarrhoea, vomiting and intercurrent infection (especially when associated with profuse sweating); caution in pregnancy (see Appendix 4), breast-feeding, elderly patients (reduce dose), diuretic treatment, myasthenia gravis; surgery (see section 15.1); if possible avoid abrupt withdrawal (see notes above); **interactions:** Appendix 1 (lithium)

COUNSELLING. Patients should maintain an adequate fluid intake and should avoid dietary changes which might reduce or increase sodium intake; lithium treatment cards are available from pharmacies (see above)

Note. **Different preparations vary widely in bioavailability**; a change in the preparation used requires the same precautions as initiation of treatment

Side-effects: gastro-intestinal disturbances, fine tremor, polyuria and polydipsia; also weight gain and oedema (may respond to dose reduction). Signs of lithium intoxication are blurred vision, increasing gastro-intestinal disturbances (anorexia, vomiting, diarrhoea), muscle weakness, increasing CNS disturbances (mild drowsiness and sluggishness increasing to giddiness with ataxia, coarse tremor, lack of co-ordination, dysarthria), and require withdrawal of treatment. With severe overdosage (plasma concentrations above 2 mmol/litre) hyperreflexia and hyperextension of limbs, convulsions, toxic psychoses, syncope, oliguria, circulatory failure, coma, and occasionally, death. Goitre, raised antidiuretic hormone concentration, hypothyroidism, hypokalaemia, ECG changes, exacerbation of psoriasis, and kidney changes may also occur. See also Emergency Treatment of Poisoning, p. 23

Dose: see under preparations below, adjusted to achieve a plasma concentration of 0.4–1.0 mmol Li^+/litre 12 hours after the preceding dose on the fourth to seventh day of treatment, then every week until dosage has remained constant for 4 weeks and every 3 months thereafter; doses are initially divided throughout the day, but once daily administration is preferred when plasma concentrations stabilised

PoM **Camcolit®** (Norgine)

Camcolit 250® tablets, f/c, scored, lithium carbonate 250 mg (6.8 mmol Li^+). Net price 20 = 58p. Label: 10 lithium card, counselling, see above

Camcolit 400® tablets, m/r, f/c, scored, lithium carbonate 400 mg (10.8 mmol Li^+). Net price 20 = 77p. Label: 10 lithium card, 25, counselling, see above

Dose (plasma monitoring, see above):
Treatment, initially 1.5–2 g daily (elderly, 0.5–1 g daily); prophylaxis, initially 0.5–1.2 g daily (elderly, 0.5–1 g daily); CHILD not recommended

Camcolit 250® should be given in divided doses, whereas Camcolit 400® may be given in single or divided doses

PoM **Liskonum®** (SK&F)

Tablets, m/r, f/c, scored, lithium carbonate 450 mg (12.2 mmol Li^+). Net price 60-tab pack = £2.82. Label: 10 lithium card, 25, counselling, see above

Dose (plasma monitoring, see above):
Treatment, initially 450–675 mg twice daily (elderly, initially 225 mg twice daily); prophylaxis, initially 450 mg twice daily (elderly, 225 mg twice daily); CHILD not recommended

---

PoM Priadel® (Delandale)

Tablets, both m/r, scored, lithium carbonate 200 mg (5.4 mmol Li⁺), net price 20 = 41p; 400 mg (10.8 mmol Li⁺), 20 = 68p. Label: 10 lithium card, 25, counselling, see above

Dose (plasma monitoring, see above):

Treatment and prophylaxis, initially 0.4–1.2 g daily as a single dose or in 2 divided doses (elderly or patients less than 50 kg, 400 mg daily); CHILD not recommended

Liquid, see under Lithium Citrate, below

LITHIUM CITRATE

Indications; Cautions; Side-effects: see under Lithium Carbonate and notes above

COUNSELLING. Patients should maintain an adequate fluid intake and should avoid dietary changes which might reduce or increase sodium intake; lithium treatment cards are available from pharmacies (see previous page)

Note. **Different preparations vary widely in bioavailability**; a change in the preparation used requires the same precautions as initiation of treatment

Dose: see under preparations below, adjusted to achieve plasma concentrations of 0.4–1.0 mmol Li⁺/litre as described under Lithium Carbonate

PoM Li-Liquid® (Rosemont)

Oral solution, lithium citrate 509 mg/5 mL (5.4 mmol Li⁺/5 mL), yellow, net price 100-mL pack = £4.30; 1.018 g/5 mL (10.8 mmol Li⁺/5 mL), orange, 100-mL pack = £8.60. Label: 10 lithium card, counselling, see above

Dose (plasma monitoring, see above):

Treatment and prophylaxis, initially 1.018–3.054 g daily in 2 divided doses (elderly or patients less than 50 kg, initially 509 mg twice daily); CHILD not recommended

PoM Litarex® (Dumex)

Tablets, m/r, lithium citrate 564 mg (6 mmol Li⁺). Net price 20 = 72p. Label: 10 lithium card, 25, counselling, see above

Dose (plasma monitoring, see above):

Treatment and prophylaxis, initially 564 mg twice daily; CHILD not recommended

PoM Priadel® (Delandale)

Tablets, see under Lithium Carbonate, above

Liquid, sugar-free, lithium citrate 520 mg/5 mL (approx. 5.4 mmol Li⁺/5 mL), net price 150-mL pack = £6.58, 300-mL pack = £13.16. Label: 10 lithium card, counselling, see above

Dose (plasma monitoring, see above):

Treatment and prophylaxis, initially 1.04–3.12 g daily in 2 divided doses (elderly or patients less than 50 kg, 520 mg twice daily); CHILD not recommended

CARBAMAZEPINE

Carbamazepine may be used for the prophylaxis of manic-depressive illness in patients unresponsive to lithium; it seems to be particularly effective in patients with rapid cycling manic-depressive illness (4 or more affective episodes per year).

CARBAMAZEPINE

Indications: prophylaxis of manic-depressive illness unresponsive to lithium; for use in epilepsy see section 4.8.1

Cautions; Contra-indications; Side-effects: see section 4.8.1

Dose: initially 400 mg daily in divided doses increased until symptoms controlled; usual range 400–600 mg daily; max. 1.6 g daily

Preparations

Section 4.8.1

4.3   Antidepressant drugs

4.3.1   Tricyclic and related antidepressant drugs

4.3.2   Monoamine-oxidase inhibitors (MAOIs)

4.3.3   SSRIs and related antidepressants

4.3.4   Other antidepressant drugs

Tricyclic and related antidepressants and the more recently developed **SSRIs and related antidepressants** are preferred to **MAOIs** because they are more effective and do not show the dangerous interactions with some *foods* and have fewer of the dangerous interactions with *drugs* that are characteristic of the MAOIs.

The choice between **older tricyclics** (e.g. amitriptyline) and **related drugs within the group** (e.g. maprotiline) depends mainly on the lower incidence of antimuscarinic side-effects associated with the related ones, such as less dry mouth and constipation; the related ones may also be associated with a lower risk of cardiotoxicity in overdosage; however, some have additional side-effects (for further details see section 4.3.1).

The **SSRIs** also have fewer antimuscarinic side-effects than the **older tricyclics** and they also seem to be less cardiotoxic in overdosage. Therefore, although not more effective, they may be preferred where there is a major risk of overdosage. The SSRIs do, however, have characteristic side-effects of their own. Hence, drowsiness, dry mouth and cardiotoxicity may be less of a problem, but gastrointestinal side-effects such as nausea and vomiting may be more common.

See section 4.2.3 for references to the role of **lithium** and **carbamazepine** in depression or in manic depressive illness.

Where the depression is very severe **electroconvulsive therapy** may be indicated.

Prescribing *more than one antidepressant at the same time* is **not** recommended. It may constitute a hazard and there is no evidence that side-effects are minimised.

Compound preparations of an *antidepressant and an anxiolytic* are **not** recommended because the dosage of the individual components should be adjusted separately. Whereas antidepressants are given continuously over several months, anxiolytics are prescribed on a **short-term** basis.

It should be noted that although anxiety is often present in depressive illness and may be the presenting symptom, the use of *antipsychotics or anxiolytics* may mask the true diagnosis. They should therefore be used with caution (but are useful adjuncts in agitated depression).

CSM advice (hyponatraemia). Hyponatraemia (usually in the elderly and possibly due to inappropriate secretion of antidiuretic hormone) has been associated with all types of antidepressants and should be considered in all patients who develop drowsiness, confusion or convulsions while taking an antidepressant.

MANAGEMENT. The patient's condition must be checked frequently, especially in the early weeks of treatment, to detect any suicidal tendencies. Limited quantities of antidepressant drugs should be prescribed at any one time as they are dangerous in overdosage. Some of the newer drugs seem less dangerous in overdose than the older tricyclics.

Treatment should be continued for 2 weeks before suppression of symptoms can be expected and thereafter should be maintained at the optimum level for at least 4–6 months after the depression has resolved. Treatment should not be withdrawn prematurely, otherwise symptoms are likely to recur. The natural history of depressive illness suggests that remission usually occurs after 3 months to a year or more. In recurrent depression, prophylactic maintenance therapy with an effective dose may need to be continued for several years.

In patients who do not respond to antidepressants, the diagnosis, dosage, compliance, and possible continuation of psychosocial or physical aggravating causes should all be carefully reviewed; other drug treatment may be successful.

WITHDRAWAL. Gastro-intestinal symptoms of nausea, vomiting, and anorexia, accompanied by headache, giddiness, 'chills', and insomnia, and sometimes by hypomania, panic-anxiety, and extreme motor restlessness may occur if an antidepressant (particularly an MAOI) is stopped suddenly after regular administration for 8 weeks or more. Reduction in dosage should preferably be carried out gradually over a period of about 4 weeks. Paroxetine has been associated with a specific withdrawal syndrome (see section 4.3.3).

4.3.1 Tricyclic and related antidepressant drugs

This section covers tricyclic antidepressants and also 1-, 2-, and 4-ring structured drugs with broadly similar properties.

These drugs are most effective for treating moderate to severe *endogenous depression* associated with psychomotor and physiological changes such as loss of appetite and sleep disturbances; improvement in sleep is usually the first benefit of therapy. Since there may be an interval of 2 weeks before the antidepressant action takes place electroconvulsive treatment may be required in severe depression when delay is hazardous or intolerable.

Some tricyclic antidepressants are also effective in the management of *panic disorder*.

For reference to the role of some tricyclic antidepressants in some forms of *neuralgia*, see section 4.7.3, and in *nocturnal enuresis* in children, see section 7.4.2.

DOSAGE. About 10 to 20% of patients fail to respond to tricyclic and related antidepressant drugs and inadequate plasma concentrations may account for some of these failures. It is important to achieve plasma concentrations which are sufficiently high for effective treatment but not so high as to cause toxic effects. Low doses should be used for initial treatment in the **elderly** (see under Side-effects, below).

In most patients the long half-life of tricyclic antidepressant drugs allows **once-daily** administration, usually at night; the use of modified-release preparations is therefore unnecessary.

CHOICE. Tricyclic and related antidepressant drugs can be roughly divided into those with additional sedative properties, e.g. **amitriptyline**, and those with less, e.g. **imipramine**. Agitated and anxious patients tend to respond best to the sedative compounds whereas withdrawn and apathetic patients will often obtain most benefit from the less sedating ones. Those with **sedative** properties include *amitriptyline, clomipramine, dothiepin, doxepin, maprotiline, mianserin, trazodone,* and *trimipramine*. Those with **less sedative** properties include *amoxapine, desipramine, imipramine, lofepramine, nortriptyline,* and *viloxazine*. Protriptyline has a **stimulant** action.

Imipramine and **amitriptyline** are well established and relatively safe and effective, but nevertheless have more marked antimuscarinic or cardiac side-effects than compounds such as **doxepin, lofepramine, mianserin, trazodone,** and **viloxazine**; this may be important in individual patients. **Amoxapine** is related to the antipsychotic loxapine and its side-effects include tardive dyskinesia.

For a comparison of *tricyclic and related antidepressants* with *SSRIs and related antidepressants* and *MAOIs*, see section 4.3.

SIDE-EFFECTS. *Arrhythmias* and *heart block* occasionally follow the use of tricyclic antidepressants, particularly amitriptyline, and may be a factor in the sudden death of patients with cardiac disease. They are also sometimes associated with *convulsions* (and should be prescribed with special caution in epilepsy as they lower the convulsive threshold); maprotiline has particularly been associated with convulsions. *Hepatic* and *haematological* reactions may occur and have been particularly associated with mianserin.

Other side-effects of tricyclic and related antidepressants include *drowsiness, dry mouth, blurred vision, constipation,* and *urinary retention* (all attributed to antimuscarinic activity), and sweating. The patient should be encouraged to persist with treatment as some tolerance to these side-effects seems to develop. They are reduced if low doses are given initially and then gradually increased, but this must be balanced against the need to obtain adequate plasma concentrations as soon as possible. Gradual introduction of treatment is particularly important in the elderly, who, because of the hypotensive effects of these drugs, are prone to attacks of *dizziness* or even *syncope*. Another side-effect to which the elderly are particularly susceptible is *hyponatraemia* (see CSM advice on p. 171).

Neuroleptic malignant syndrome (section 4.2.1) may, very rarely, arise in the course of antidepressant treatment.

For advice on *overdosage* see Emergency Treatment of Poisoning, p. 22.

WITHDRAWAL. If possible tricyclic and related antidepressants should be withdrawn slowly (see also section 4.3).

INTERACTIONS. A tricyclic or related antidepressant (or an SSRI or related antidepressant) should not be started until 2 weeks after stopping an MAOI. Conversely, an MAOI should not be started until at least a week after a tricyclic or related antidepressant (or an SSRI or related antidepressant) has been stopped (2 weeks in the case of paroxetine and sertraline and at least 5 weeks in the case of fluoxetine). For guidance relating to the reversible monoamine oxidase inhibitor, moclobemide, see p. 177. For other tricyclic antidepressant **interactions**, see Appendix 1 (antidepressants, tricyclic).

TRICYCLIC ANTIDEPRESSANTS

AMITRIPTYLINE HYDROCHLORIDE

Indications: depressive illness, particularly where sedation is required; nocturnal enuresis in children (see section 7.4.2)

Cautions: cardiac disease (particularly with arrhythmias, see Contra-indications below), history of epilepsy, pregnancy and breast-feeding see Appendixes 4 and 5, elderly, hepatic impairment (avoid if severe), thyroid disease, phaeochromocytoma, history of mania, psychoses (may aggravate psychotic symptoms), closed-angle glaucoma, history of urinary retention, concurrent electroconvulsive therapy; avoid abrupt withdrawal; also caution in anaesthesia (increased risk of arrhythmias and hypotension, see surgery section 15.1); porphyria (see section 9.8.2); see section 7.4.2 for additional nocturnal enuresis warnings; **interactions:** Appendix 1 (antidepressants, tricyclic)

DRIVING. Drowsiness may affect performance of skilled tasks (e.g. driving); effects of alcohol enhanced

Contra-indications: recent myocardial infarction, arrhythmias (particularly heart block), not indicated in manic phase, severe liver disease

Side-effects: dry mouth, sedation, blurred vision (disturbance of accommodation, increased intra-ocular pressure), constipation, nausea, difficulty with micturition; cardiovascular side-effects (such as ECG changes, arrhythmias, postural hypotension, tachycardia, syncope, particularly with high doses); sweating, tremor, rashes and hypersensitivity reactions (including urticaria, photosensitivity), behavioural disturbances (particularly children), hypomania or mania, confusion (particularly elderly), interference with sexual function, blood sugar changes; increased appetite and weight gain (occasionally weight loss); endocrine side-effects such as testicular

enlargement, gynaecomastia, galactorrhoea; also convulsions (see also Cautions), movement disorders and dyskinesias, fever, agranulocytosis, leucopenia, eosinophilia, purpura, thrombocytopenia, hyponatraemia (may be due to inappropriate antidiuretic hormone secretion) see CSM advice, p. 171, abnormal liver function tests (jaundice); for a general outline of side-effects see also notes above; overdosage: see Emergency Treatment of Poisoning, p. 22

Dose: by mouth, depression, initially 75 mg (elderly and adolescents 30–75 mg) daily in divided doses *or* as a single dose at bedtime increased gradually as necessary to max. 150 mg; usual maintenance 50–100 mg daily; CHILD under 16 years not recommended for depression

Nocturnal enuresis, CHILD 7–10 years 10–20 mg, 11–16 years 25–50 mg at night; max. period of treatment (including gradual withdrawal) 3 months—full physical examination before further course

By intramuscular or intravenous injection, depression, 10–20 mg 4 times daily; CHILD under 16 years not recommended

PoM **Amitriptyline** (Non-proprietary)
Tablets, coated, amitriptyline hydrochloride 10 mg, net price 20 = 13p; 25 mg, 20 = 9p; 50 mg, 20 = 34p. Label: 2
Available from Antigen, APS, Berk (Domical®), Cox, DDSA (Elavil®)
Oral solution, amitriptyline (as hydrochloride) 25 mg/5 mL, net price 200-mL = £12.24; 50 mg/5 mL, 200-mL = £13.40. Label: 2
Available from Rosemont (sugar-free)

PoM **Lentizol®** (P-D)
Capsules, m/r, both enclosing white pellets, amitriptyline hydrochloride 25 mg (pink), net price 100-cap pack = £4.61; 50 mg (pink/red), 100-cap pack = £8.56. Label: 2, 25

PoM **Tryptizol®** (Morson)
Tablets, all f/c, amitriptyline hydrochloride 10 mg (blue), net price 20 = 13p; 25 mg (yellow), 20 = 9p; 50 mg (brown), 20 = 34p. Label: 2
Mixture, pink, sugar-free, amitriptyline 10 mg (as embonate)/5 mL. Net price 200-mL pack = £1.87. Label: 2
Injection, amitriptyline hydrochloride 10 mg/mL. Net price 10-mL vial = 54p

Compound preparations
Not recommended, see notes above.

PoM **Triptafen®** (Forley)
Tablets, pink, s/c, amitriptyline hydrochloride 25 mg, perphenazine 2 mg. Net price 20 = £3.78. Label: 2
PoM **Triptafen-M®** (Forley)
Tablets, pink, s/c, amitriptyline hydrochloride 10 mg, perphenazine 2 mg. Net price 20 = £3.34. Label: 2

AMOXAPINE

Indications: depressive illness
Cautions; Contra-indications; Side-effects: see under Amitriptyline Hydrochloride; tardive dyskinesia reported; menstrual irregularities, breast enlargement, and galactorrhoea reported in women

---

Dose: initially 100–150 mg daily in divided doses *or* as a single dose at bedtime increased as necessary to max. 300 mg daily; usual maintenance 150–250 mg daily; ELDERLY initially 25 mg twice daily increased as necessary after 5–7 days to max. 50 mg 3 times daily; CHILD under 16 years not recommended

PoM **Asendis®** (Lederle)

Tablets, amoxapine 25 mg, net price 100-tab pack = £10.89; 50 mg (orange, scored), 100-tab pack = £18.16; 100 mg (blue, scored), 100-tab pack = £30.27. Label: 2

CLOMIPRAMINE HYDROCHLORIDE

Indications: depressive illness, phobic and obsessional states; adjunctive treatment of cataplexy associated with narcolepsy

Cautions; Contra-indications; Side-effects: see under Amitriptyline Hydrochloride

Dose: by mouth, initially 10 mg daily, increased gradually as necessary to 30–150 mg daily in divided doses *or* as a single dose at bedtime; max. 250 mg daily; usual maintenance 30–50 mg daily; ELDERLY initially 10 mg daily increased to 30–50 mg daily; CHILD not recommended

Phobic and obsessional states, initially 25 mg daily (elderly 10 mg daily) increased over 2 weeks to 100–150 mg daily; CHILD not recommended

Adjunctive treatment of cataplexy associated with narcolepsy, initially 10 mg daily gradually increased until satisfactory response (range 10–50 mg daily)

By intramuscular injection, initially 25–50 mg daily, increased by 25 mg daily to 100–150 mg daily; CHILD not recommended

By intravenous infusion (careful monitoring see Cautions), initially to assess tolerance, 25–50 mg, then increase by 25 mg daily to usual dose of 100 mg daily for 7–10 days—see data sheet for details; CHILD not recommended

PoM **Clomipramine** (Non-proprietary)

Capsules, clomipramine hydrochloride 10 mg, net price 20 = 57p; 25 mg, 20 = £1.13; 50 mg, 20 = £2.13. Label: 2

Available from APS, Cox, Generics, Hillcross, Norton

PoM **Anafranil®** (Geigy)

Capsules, clomipramine hydrochloride 10 mg (yellow/caramel), net price 84-cap pack = £3.23; 25 mg (orange/caramel), 84-cap pack = £6.35; 50 mg (grey/caramel), 56-cap pack = £8.06. Label: 2

Syrup, clomipramine hydrochloride 25 mg/5 mL. Net price 150-mL pack = £7.23. Label: 2

Injection, clomipramine hydrochloride 12.5 mg/mL. Net price 2-mL amp = 47p

PoM **Anafranil SR®** (Geigy)

Tablets, m/r, grey-red, f/c, clomipramine hydrochloride 75 mg. Net price 28-tab pack = £8.83. Label: 2, 25

DESIPRAMINE HYDROCHLORIDE

Indications: depressive illness

Cautions; Contra-indications; Side-effects: see under Amitriptyline Hydrochloride, but less sedating

Dose: 75 mg daily in divided doses *or* as a single dose at bedtime, increased as necessary to a usual max. of 200 mg (in resistant depression max. 300 mg daily with plasma concentration monitoring); usual maintenance, 75–100 mg daily; ELDERLY initially 25 mg daily then about half usual adult dose; ADOLESCENT about half usual adult dose; CHILD not recommended

PoM **Pertofran®** (Ciba)

Tablets, pink, s/c, desipramine hydrochloride 25 mg. Net price 84-tab pack = £2.99. Label: 2

DOTHIEPIN HYDROCHLORIDE
(Dosulepin Hydrochloride)

Indications: depressive illness, particularly where sedation is required

Cautions; Contra-indications; Side-effects: see under Amitriptyline Hydrochloride

Dose: initially 75 mg (elderly 50–75 mg) daily in divided doses *or* as a single dose at bedtime, increased gradually as necessary to 150 mg daily (elderly 75 mg may be sufficient); up to 225 mg daily in some circumstances (e.g. hospital use); CHILD not recommended

PoM **Dothiepin** (Non-proprietary)

Capsules, dothiepin hydrochloride 25 mg, net price 20 = 76p.

Available from APS, Ashbourne (Dothapax®), Berk (Prepadine®), Cox, Evans, Generics, Hillcross, Kent, Norton

Tablets, dothiepin hydrochloride 75 mg, net price 28-tab pack = £2.94. Label: 2

Available from APS, Ashbourne (Dothapax®), Berk (Prepadine®), Cox, Generics, Hillcross, Kent, Norton

PoM **Prothiaden®** (Knoll)

Capsules, red/brown, dothiepin hydrochloride 25 mg. Net price 20 = £1.00. Label: 2

Tablets, red, s/c, dothiepin hydrochloride 75 mg. Net price 28-tab pack = £4.00. Label: 2

DOXEPIN

Indications: depressive illness, particularly where sedation is required

Cautions; Contra-indications; Side-effects: see under Amitriptyline Hydrochloride; avoid in breast-feeding (see Appendix 5)

Dose: initially 75 mg daily in divided doses *or* as a single dose at bedtime, increased as necessary to max. 300 mg daily in 3 divided doses (up to 100 mg may be given as a single dose); range 30–300 mg daily; ELDERLY initially 10–50 mg daily, range of 30–50 mg daily may be adequate; CHILD not recommended

PoM **Sinequan**® (Pfizer)
Capsules, doxepin (as hydrochloride) 10 mg (orange), net price 56-cap pack = £1.21; 25 mg (orange/blue), 28-cap pack = 87p; 50 mg (blue), 28-cap pack = £1.43; 75 mg (yellow/blue), 28-cap pack = £2.26. Label: 2

IMIPRAMINE HYDROCHLORIDE

Indications: depressive illness; nocturnal enuresis in children (see section 7.4.2)

Cautions; Contra-indications; Side-effects: see under Amitriptyline Hydrochloride, but less sedating

Dose: depression, initially up to 75 mg daily in divided doses increased gradually to 150–200 mg (up to 300 mg in hospital patients); up to 150 mg may be given as a single dose at bedtime; usual maintenance 50–100 mg daily; ELDERLY initially 10 mg daily, increased gradually to 30–50 mg daily; CHILD not recommended for depression

Nocturnal enuresis, CHILD 7 years 25 mg, 8–11 years 25–50 mg, over 11 years 50–75 mg at bedtime; max. period of treatment (including gradual withdrawal) 3 months—full physical examination before further course

PoM **Imipramine** (Non-proprietary)
Tablets, coated, imipramine hydrochloride 10 mg, net price 20 = 16p; 25 mg, 20 = 11p. Label: 2
PoM **Tofranil**® (Geigy)
Tablets, both red-brown, s/c, imipramine hydrochloride 10 mg, net price 84-tab pack = £1.60; 25 mg, 84-tab pack = £3.05. Label: 2
Syrup, imipramine hydrochloride 25 mg/5 mL. Net price 150-mL pack = £3.11. Label: 2

LOFEPRAMINE

Indications: depressive illness

Cautions; Contra-indications; Side-effects: see under Amitriptyline Hydrochloride, but less sedating; hepatic disorders reported; contra-indicated in hepatic and severe renal impairment

Dose: 140–210 mg daily in divided doses; ELDERLY may respond to lower doses; CHILD not recommended

PoM **Lofepramine** (Non-proprietary)
Tablets, lofepramine 70 mg (as hydrochloride). Net price 56-tab pack = £10.02. Label: 2
Available from Cox
Oral suspension, lofepramine 70 mg/5 mL (as hydrochloride). Net price 200 mL = £24.65. Label: 2
Available from Rosemont (sugar-free)
PoM **Gamanil**® (Merck)
Tablets, f/c, brown-violet, lofepramine 70 mg (as hydrochloride). Net price 56-tab pack = £10.27. Label: 2

NORTRIPTYLINE

Indications: depressive illness; nocturnal enuresis in children (see section 7.4.2)

Cautions; Contra-indications; Side-effects: see under Amitriptyline Hydrochloride but less sedating

Dose: depression, low dose intially increased as necessary to 75–100 mg daily in divided doses or as a single dose; plasma concentration monitoring above 100 mg daily (max. 150 mg daily, in hospitalised patients); ADOLESCENT and ELDERLY 30–50 mg daily in divided doses; CHILD not recommended for depression

Nocturnal enuresis, CHILD 7 years 10 mg, 8–11 years 10–20 mg, over 11 years 25–35 mg, at night; max period of treatment (including gradual withdrawal) 3 months—full physical examination and ECG before further course

PoM **Allegron**® (Dista)
Tablets, nortriptyline (as hydrochloride) 10 mg, net price 20 = £1.01; 25 mg (orange, scored), 20 = £2.05. Label: 2

Compound preparations
Not recommended, see notes above.
PoM **Motipress**® (Sanofi Winthrop)
Tablets, yellow, s/c, fluphenazine hydrochloride 1.5 mg, nortriptyline 30 mg (as hydrochloride). Net price 28-tab pack = £2.83. Label: 2
PoM **Motival**® (Sanofi Winthrop)
Tablets, pink, s/c, fluphenazine hydrochloride 500 micrograms, nortriptyline 10 mg (as hydrochloride). Net price 20 = 69p. Label: 2

PROTRIPTYLINE HYDROCHLORIDE

Indications: depressive illness, particularly with apathy and withdrawal

Cautions; Contra-indications; Side-effects: see under Amitriptyline Hydrochloride but less sedating; anxiety, agitation, tachycardia, and hypotension more common; rashes associated with photosensitisation (avoid direct sunlight); daily dose above 20 mg in elderly (increased risk of cardiovascular side-effects)

Dose: initially 10 mg 3–4 times daily (elderly 5 mg 3 times daily initially) if insomnia, last dose not after 4 p.m.; usual range 15–60 mg daily; CHILD under 16 years not recommended

PoM **Concordin**® (MSD)
Tablets, both f/c, protriptyline hydrochloride 5 mg (pink), net price 20 = 44p; 10 mg, 20 = 65p. Label: 2, 11

TRIMIPRAMINE

Indications: depressive illness, particularly where sedation is required

Cautions; Contra-indications; Side-effects: see under Amitriptyline Hydrochloride

Dose: 50–75 mg daily as a single dose 2 hours before bedtime or as 25 mg midday and 50 mg evening, increased as necessary to max. of 300 mg daily for 4–6 weeks then reduce to usual maintenance dose 75–150 mg daily; ELDERLY 10–25 mg 3 times daily initially, half adult maintenance dose may be sufficient; CHILD not recommended

PoM **Surmontil**® (Rhône-Poulenc Rorer)
Capsules, green/white, trimipramine 50 mg (as maleate). Net price 28-cap pack = £5.19. Label: 2
Tablets, trimipramine (as maleate) 10 mg, net price 50-tab pack = £2.78; 25 mg, 50-tab pack = £4.62. Label: 2

RELATED ANTIDEPRESSANTS

MAPROTILINE HYDROCHLORIDE

Indications: depressive illness, particularly where sedation is required
Cautions; Contra-indications; Side-effects: see under Amitriptyline Hydrochloride, antimuscarinic effects may occur less frequently but rashes common and increased risk of convulsions at higher dosage; contra-indicated if history of epilepsy
Dose: initially 25–75 mg (elderly 30 mg) daily in 3 divided doses *or* as a single dose at bedtime, increased gradually as necessary to max. 150 mg daily; CHILD not recommended

PoM **Ludiomil**® (Ciba)
Tablets, all f/c, maprotiline hydrochloride 10 mg (pale yellow), net price 28-tab pack = 98p; 25 mg (greyish-red), 28-tab pack = £2.11; 50 mg (light orange), 28-tab pack = £4.18; 75 mg (brownish-orange), 28-tab pack = £6.21. Label: 2
Additives: include gluten

MIANSERIN HYDROCHLORIDE

Indications: depressive illness, particularly where sedation is required
Cautions; Contra-indications; Side-effects: see under Amitriptyline Hydrochloride; leucopenia, agranulocytosis and aplastic anaemia (particularly in the elderly); jaundice; arthritis, arthralgia; influenza-like syndrome may occur; fewer and milder antimuscarinic and cardiovascular effects; **interactions:** Appendix 1 (mianserin)
BLOOD COUNTS. A full **blood count** is recommended every 4 weeks during the first 3 months of treatment; subsequent clinical monitoring should continue and treatment should be stopped and a full blood count obtained if *fever, sore throat, stomatitis,* or other signs of infection develop.
Dose: initially 30–40 mg (elderly 30 mg) daily in divided doses *or* as a single dose at bedtime, increased gradually as necessary; usual dose range 30–90 mg; CHILD not recommended

PoM **Mianserin** (Non-proprietary)
Tablets, mianserin hydrochloride 10 mg, net price 20 = £1.00; 20 mg, 20 = £2.09; 30 mg, 20 = £2.86. Label: 2, 25

TRAZODONE HYDROCHLORIDE

Indications: depressive illness, particularly where sedation is required
Cautions; Contra-indications; Side-effects: see under Amitriptyline Hydrochloride but fewer antimuscarinic and cardiovascular effects; rarely priapism [discontinue immediately]; **interactions:** Appendix 1 (trazodone)

Dose: initially 150 mg (elderly 100 mg) daily in divided doses after food *or* as a single dose at bedtime; may be increased to 300 mg daily; hospital patients up to max. 600 mg daily in divided doses; CHILD not recommended

PoM **Molipaxin**® (Merrell)
Capsules, trazodone hydrochloride 50 mg (violet/green), net price 84-cap pack = £17.31; 100 mg (violet/fawn), 56-cap pack = £20.38. Label: 2, 21
Tablets, pink, f/c, trazodone hydrochloride 150 mg. Net price 28-tab pack = £11.62. Label: 2, 21
Liquid, sugar-free, trazodone hydrochloride 50 mg/5 mL. Net price 150-mL pack = £7.74. Label: 2, 21
CR tablets, m/r, blue, f/c, trazodone hydrochloride 150 mg. Net price 28-tab pack = £11.62. Label: 2, 21, 25
Dose: initially 1 tablet daily (elderly, dose form not appropriate for initial dose titration), increased if necessary to 2 tablets daily (up to 4 tablets daily in hospital patients); CHILD not recommended

VILOXAZINE HYDROCHLORIDE

Indications: depressive illness
Cautions; Contra-indications; Side-effects: see under Amitriptyline Hydrochloride, but less sedating and antimuscarinic and cardiovascular side-effects are fewer and milder; nausea and headache may occur; **interactions:** Appendix 1 (viloxazine)
Dose: 300 mg daily (preferably as 200 mg in the morning and 100 mg at midday), increased gradually as necessary; max. 400 mg daily; last dose not later than 6 p.m.; ELDERLY 100 mg daily initially, half adult maintenance dose may be sufficient; CHILD under 14 years not recommended

PoM **Vivalan**® (Zeneca)
Tablets, f/c, viloxazine 50 mg (as hydrochloride). Net price 20 = £1.23. Label: 2

4.3.2 Monoamine-oxidase inhibitors
(MAOIs)

Monoamine-oxidase inhibitors are used much less frequently than tricyclic and related antidepressants, or SSRIs and related antidepressants because of the dangers of dietary and drug interactions and the fact that it is easier to prescribe MAOIs when tricyclic antidepressants have been unsuccessful than vice versa. **Tranylcypromine** is the most **hazardous** of the MAOIs because of its stimulant action. The drugs of choice are **phenelzine** and **isocarboxazid** which are less stimulant and therefore safer.

Phobic patients and depressed patients with atypical, hypochondriacal, or hysterical features are said to respond best to MAOIs. However, MAOIs should be tried in any patients who are refractory to treatment with other antidepressants as there is occasionally a dramatic response. Response to treatment may be delayed for 3 weeks or more and may take an additional 1 or 2 weeks to become maximal.

WITHDRAWAL. If possible MAOIs should be withdrawn slowly (see also section 4.3).

TREATMENT CARD

Carry this card with you at all times. Show it to any doctor who may treat you other than the doctor who prescribed this medicine, and to your dentist if you require dental treatment.

INSTRUCTIONS TO PATIENTS
Please read carefully
While taking this medicine and for 14 days after your treatment finishes you must observe the following simple instructions:-

1   Do not eat CHEESE, PICKLED HERRING OR BROAD BEAN PODS.

2   Do not eat or drink BOVRIL, OXO, MARMITE or ANY SIMILAR MEAT OR YEAST EXTRACT.

3   Eat only FRESH foods and avoid food that you suspect could be stale or 'going off'.   This is especially important with meat, fish, poultry or offal. Avoid game.

4   Do not take any other MEDICINES (including tablets, capsules, nose drops, inhalations or suppositories) whether purchased by you or previously prescribed by your doctor, without first consulting your doctor or your pharmacist.

    NB *Treatment for coughs and colds, pain relievers, tonics and laxatives are medicines.*

5   Avoid alcoholic drinks and de-alcoholised (low alcohol) drinks.

Keep a careful note of any food or drink that disagrees with you, avoid it and tell your doctor.

Report any unusual or severe symptoms to your doctor and follow any other advice given by him.

M.A.O.I. Prepared by The Pharmaceutical Society and the British Medical Association on behalf of the Health Departments of the United Kingdom.

Printed in the UK for HMSO 8217411/150M/9.89/4529
Revised Sep. 1989

INTERACTIONS. MAOIs inhibit monoamine oxidase, thereby causing an accumulation of amine neurotransmitters. The metabolism of some amine drugs such as *indirect-acting sympathomimetics* (present in many cough and decongestant preparations, see section 3.10) is also inhibited and their pressor action may be potentiated; the pressor effect of tyramine (in some foods, such as mature cheese, yeast extracts and fermented soya bean products) may also be dangerously potentiated. These interactions may cause a dangerous rise in blood pressure. An early warning symptom may be a throbbing headache. The danger of interaction persists for up to 2 weeks after treatment with MAOIs is discontinued.

Other antidepressants should **not** be started for 2 weeks after treatment with MAOIs has been stopped. Some psychiatrists use selected tricyclics in conjunction with MAOIs but this is hazardous, indeed potentially lethal, except in experienced hands and there is no evidence that the combination is more effective than when either constituent is used alone. The combination of tranylcypromine with clomipramine is particularly **dangerous**.

Conversely, an MAOI should not be started until at least 1 week (phenelzine manufacturer specifies 2 weeks) after a *tricyclic or related antidepressant* or an *SSRI or related antidepressant* has been

stopped (2 weeks in the case of paroxetine and sertraline, at least 5 weeks in the case of fluoxetine).

In addition, an MAOI should not be started for at least a week (phenelzine manufacturer specifies 2 weeks) after a previous MAOI has been stopped (then started at a reduced dose).

For other interactions with MAOIs including those with opioid analgesics (notably pethidine), see Appendix 1 (MAOIs). For guidance on interactions relating to the reversible monoamine oxidase inhibitor, moclobemide, see p. 177. See also MAOI Treatment Card, opposite.

TREATMENT CARDS. Cards which list the necessary precautions to be taken by a patient receiving an MAOI are distributed by the Royal Pharmaceutical Society and given to patients at pharmacies and clinics. In Northern Ireland they can be obtained *via* Central Services Agency, 27 Adelaide St, Belfast BT2 8FH. In the case of the reversible MAOI, moclobemide, a patient information leaflet is available in the pack.

PHENELZINE

Indications: depressive illness

Cautions: diabetes mellitus, cardiovascular disease, epilepsy, blood disorders, concurrent electroconvulsive therapy; elderly (great caution); monitor blood pressure to detect hypotensive responses (postural hypotension) and hypertensive responses (discontinue if palpitations or frequent headaches); if possible avoid abrupt withdrawal; severe hypertensive reactions to certain drugs and foods (see Treatment Card); avoid in agitated patients; porphyria (see section 9.8.2); pregnancy and breast-feeding; surgery (see section 15.1); **interactions:** Appendix 1 (MAOIs)
DRIVING. Drowsiness may affect performance of skilled tasks (e.g. driving)

Contra-indications: hepatic impairment or abnormal liver function tests (see Appendix 2), cerebrovascular disease, phaeochromocytoma; not indicated in manic phase

Side-effects: adverse effects commonly associated with phenelzine and other MAOIs include postural hypotension (especially in elderly) and dizziness; other side-effects include drowsiness, insomnia, headache, weakness and fatigue, dryness of mouth, constipation and other gastrointestinal disturbances, oedema, myoclonic movement, hyperreflexia, elevated liver enzymes; agitation and tremors, nervousness, euphoria, arrhythmias, blurred vision, nystagmus, difficulty in micturition, sweating, convulsions, rashes, purpura, leucopenia, sexual disturbances, and weight gain with inappropriate appetite may also occur; psychotic episodes with hypomanic behaviour, confusion, and hallucinations, may be induced in susceptible persons; jaundice has been reported and, on rare occasions, fatal progressive hepatocellular necrosis; paraesthesia, peripheral neuritis, peripheral neuropathy may be due to pyridoxine deficiency; for CSM advice on possible hyponatraemia, see p. 171 (hypernatraemia also reported)

Dose: 15 mg 3 times daily, increased if necessary to 4 times daily after 2 weeks (hospital patients, max. 30 mg 3 times daily), then reduced gradually to lowest possible maintenance dose (15 mg on alternate days may be adequate); CHILD not recommended

PoM Nardil® (P-D)
Tablets, orange, f/c, phenelzine 15 mg (as sulphate). Net price 20 = £1.33. Label: 3, 10 MAOI card

ISOCARBOXAZID

Indications: depressive illness
Cautions; Contra-indications; Side-effects: see under Phenelzine
Dose: initially up to 30 mg daily in single or divided doses increased after 4 weeks if necessary to max. 60 mg daily for up to 6 weeks under close supervision only; then reduced to usual maintenance dose 10–20 mg daily (but up to 40 mg daily may be required); CHILD not recommended

PoM Isocarboxazid (Cambridge)
Tablets, pink, scored, isocarboxazid 10 mg. Net price 50 = £6.77. Label: 3, 10 MAOI card
Note. The brand name Marplan® was formerly used for isocarboxazid preparations

TRANYLCYPROMINE

Indications: depressive illness
Cautions; Contra-indications: see under Phenelzine; also contra-indicated in hyperthyroidism
Side-effects: see under Phenelzine; insomnia if given in evening; hypertensive crises with throbbing headache requiring discontinuation of treatment occur more frequently than with other MAOIs; liver damage occurs less frequently than with phenelzine
Dose: initially 10 mg twice daily not later than 3 p.m., increasing the second daily dose to 20 mg after 1 week if necessary; doses above 30 mg daily under close supervision only; usual maintenance dose 10 mg daily; CHILD not recommended

PoM Parnate® (SK&F)
Tablets, red, s/c, tranylcypromine 10 mg (as sulphate). Net price 20 = 91p. Label: 3, 10 MAOI card

Compound preparation
Not recommended, see notes above.
PoM Parstelin® (SK&F)
Tablets, green, s/c, tranylcypromine 10 mg (as sulphate), trifluoperazine 1 mg (as hydrochloride). Net price 20 = 93p. Label: 3, 10 MAOI card
Caution: contains MAOI

REVERSIBLE MAOIs

Moclobemide is a newly introduced antidepressant indicated for major depression only; it is reported to act by reversible inhibition of monoamine oxidase type A (it is therefore termed a RIMA).

INTERACTIONS. Moclobemide is claimed to cause less potentiation of the pressor effect of tyramine than the traditional (irreversible) MAOIs, but patients should avoid consuming large amounts of tyramine-rich food (such as mature cheese, yeast extracts and fermented soya bean products).

The risk of drug interactions is also claimed to be less but patients still need to avoid sympathomimetics such as ephedrine, pseudoephedrine, and phenylpropanolamine. In addition, moclobemide should not be given with another antidepressant. Owing to its short duration of action no treatment-free period is required after it has been stopped but it should not be started until at least a week after a tricyclic or related antidepressant or an SSRI or related antidepressant has been stopped (2 weeks in the case of paroxetine and sertraline, and at least 5 weeks in the case of fluoxetine), or for at least a week after an MAOI has been stopped. For other interactions, see Appendix 1 (moclobemide).

MOCLOBEMIDE

Indications: major depression
Cautions: avoid in agitated or excited patients (or give with sedative for up to 2–3 weeks), thyrotoxicosis, severe hepatic impairment, may provoke manic episodes in bipolar disorders, pregnancy and breast-feeding (patient information leaflet advises avoid); **interactions:** see notes above and Appendix 1 (moclobemide)
Contra-indications: acute confusional states, phaeochromocytoma
Side-effects: sleep disturbances, dizziness, nausea, headache, restlessness, agitation; confusional states reported; rarely raised liver enzymes; for CSM advice on possible hyponatraemia, see p. 171
Dose: initially 300 mg daily usually in divided doses after food, adjusted according to response; usual range 150–600 mg daily; CHILD not recommended

▼ **PoM Manerix®** (Roche)
Tablets, yellow, f/c, scored, moclobemide 150 mg, net price 30-tab pack = £10.50; 300 mg, 30-tab pack = £15.75. Label: 10 patient information leaflet, 21

4.3.3 SSRIs and related antidepressants

SSRIs

Citalopram, fluoxetine, fluvoxamine, paroxetine, and **sertraline** selectively inhibit the re-uptake of serotonin (5-hydroxytryptamine, 5-HT); they are termed selective serotonin re-uptake inhibitors (SSRIs) and appear to be effective antidepressants. They are less sedative than tricyclic antidepressants, with few antimuscarinic effects and with low cardiotoxicity. They do not cause weight gain. Gastro-intestinal side-effects (diarrhoea, nausea and vomiting) are dose-related; headache, restlessness and anxiety may also occur. As with tricyclic antidepressants caution is necessary in epilepsy. For a general comment on the comparison between *tricyclic and related antidepressants* and the *SSRIs and related antidepressants*, see section 4.3.

WITHDRAWAL. If possible SSRIs should be withdrawn slowly (see also section 4.3). See also next page for a CSM warning relating to paroxetine withdrawal.

INTERACTIONS. An SSRI or related antidepressant should not be started until 2 weeks after stopping an MAOI. Conversely, an MAOI should not be started until at least a week after an SSRI or related antidepressant has been stopped (2 weeks in the case of paroxetine and sertraline, at least 5 weeks in the case of fluoxetine). For guidance relating to the reversible monoamine oxidase inhibitor, moclobemide, see above. For other SSRI antidepressant interactions, see Appendix 1 (antidepressants, SSRI).

FLUOXETINE

Indications: see under Dose

Cautions: cardiac disease, epilepsy (avoid if poorly controlled, discontinue if convulsions develop), concurrent electroconvulsive therapy (prolonged seizures reported), history of mania, hepatic and renal impairment (see Appendixes 2 and 3), pregnancy and breast-feeding (see Appendixes 4 and 5), avoid abrupt withdrawal; **interactions:** Appendix 1 (antidepressants, SSRI)

DRIVING. May impair performance of skilled tasks (e.g. driving)

Contra-indications: not indicated in manic phase

Side-effects: gastro-intestinal (fairly common—include nausea, vomiting, dyspepsia, abdominal pain, diarrhoea, constipation, anorexia with weight loss and possible changes in blood sugar); hypersensitivity reactions (**important:** see also below); also dry mouth, nervousness, anxiety, headache, insomnia, palpitations, tremor, confusion, dizziness, hypotension, hypomania or mania, drowsiness, asthenia, convulsions (see Cautions above), fever, sexual dysfunction, sweating; movement disorders and dyskinesias, neuroleptic malignant syndrome-like event; hyponatraemia (may be due to inappropriate antidiuretic hormone secretion), see CSM warning on p. 171; abnormal liver function tests reported; also reported (no causal relationship established): abnormal bleeding, aplastic anaemia, cerebrovascular accident, ecchymoses, eosinophilic pneumonia, gastro-intestinal haemorrhage, hyperprolactinaemia, haemolytic anaemia, pancreatitis, pancytopenia, suicidal ideation, thrombocytopenia, thrombocytopenic purpura, vaginal bleeding on withdrawal, violent behaviour; hair loss also reported

HYPERSENSITIVITY. Angioedema, urticaria, pruritus, and other allergic reactions including anaphylaxis have been reported (discontinue if rash occurs, may be warning of impending serious systemic reaction, possibly associated with vasculitis); pharyngitis and rarely pulmonary inflammation or fibrosis (with dyspnoea only warning sign) also reported; other possible hypersensitivity signs include arthralgia, myalgia

Dose: depressive illness, 20 mg daily; CHILD not recommended

Bulimia nervosa, 60 mg daily; CHILD not recommended

Obsessive-compulsive disorder, initially 20 mg daily, dose increase may be considered if no response after several weeks, but may be increased potential for side-effects; max. 60 mg daily; CHILD not recommended

LONG DURATION OF ACTION. Account should be taken of the long half-life of fluoxetine when adjusting dosage (or in overdosage)

PoM Prozac® (Dista)

Capsules, fluoxetine (as hydrochloride) 20 mg (green/yellow), net price 30-cap pack = £20.77, 98-cap pack = £67.85; 60 mg (yellow), 30-cap pack = £62.31. Counselling, driving

Liquid, fluoxetine (as hydrochloride) 20 mg/5 mL. Net price 70-mL pack = £19.39. Counselling, driving

CITALOPRAM

Indications; depressive illness

Cautions; Contra-indications; Side-effects: see under Fluoxetine

Dose: 20 mg daily as a single dose in the morning or evening increased if necessary to max. 60 mg daily (ELDERLY max 40 mg daily); CHILD not recommended

▼ **PoM Cipramil®** (Lundbeck, Du Pont)

Tablets, f/c, scored, citalopram (as hydrobromide) 20 mg. Net price 28-tab pack = £21.28. Counselling, driving

FLUVOXAMINE MALEATE

Indications: depressive illness, obsessive-compulsive disorder

Cautions; Contra-indications; Side-effects: see under Fluoxetine; may cause decrease in heart rate; rarely increase in hepatic enzymes, usually with symptoms (withdrawal advised); galactorrhoea reported

CSM ADVICE. The CSM has advised that concomitant use of fluvoxamine and theophylline or aminophylline preparations should usually be avoided. Where this is not possible, patients taking this combination should have their theophylline dose halved and plasma theophylline levels monitored closely.

Dose: initially 100 mg daily increased if necessary to max. 300 mg daily (over 100 mg in divided doses); CHILD not recommended

Note. If no improvement in obsessive-compulsive disorder within 10 weeks, treatment should be reconsidered

PoM Faverin® (Solvay)

Tablets, f/c, scored, fluvoxamine maleate 50 mg, net price 60-tab pack = £19.00; 100 mg, 30-tab pack = £19.00. Counselling, driving

PAROXETINE

Indications: depressive illness, obsessive-compulsive disorder, panic disorder

Cautions; Contra-indications; Side-effects: see under Fluoxetine; consider gradual discontinuation by dose tapering or alternate day administration (dizziness, paraesthesia, anxiety, sleep disturbances, agitation, tremor, nausea, sweating and confusion reported on abrupt discontinuation—see also CSM advice below)

IMPORTANT. During initial treatment of panic disorder, there is potential for worsening of panic symptomatology

CSM ADVICE. Extrapyramidal reactions (including orofacial dystonias) and withdrawal syndrome are reported to the CSM more commonly than with other SSRIs

Dose: depressive illness, usually 20 mg each morning, if necessary increased gradually in increments of 10 mg to max. 50 mg daily (elderly, 40 mg daily); CHILD not recommended

Obsessive-compulsive disorder, initially 20 mg each morning, if necessary increased gradually in weekly increments of 10 mg to usual dose 40 mg daily (max. 60 mg daily, max. in elderly 40 mg daily); CHILD not recommended

Panic disorder, initially 10 mg each morning, if necessary increased gradually in weekly increments of 10 mg to usual dose of 40 mg daily (max. 50 mg daily, max. in elderly 40 mg daily); CHILD not recommended

PoM **Seroxat**® (SmithKline Beecham)

Tablets, both f/c, scored, paroxetine 20 mg (as hydrochloride), net price 30-tab pack = £20.77; 30 mg (blue), 30-tab pack = £31.16. Label: 21, counselling, driving

SERTRALINE

Indications: depressive illness

Cautions; Contra-indications; Side-effects: see under Fluoxetine; asymptomatic elevation in serum transaminases diminish on withdrawal

Dose: initially 50 mg daily, increased if necessary by increments of 50 mg over several weeks to max. 200 mg daily, then reduced to usual maintenance of 50 mg daily; doses of 150 mg or greater should not be used for more than 8 weeks; CHILD not recommended

PoM **Lustral**® (Invicta)

Tablets, sertraline (as hydrochloride) 50 mg, net price 28-tab pack = £26.51; 100 mg, 28-tab pack = £39.77. Counselling, driving

RELATED ANTIDEPRESSANTS

Venlafaxine is a new antidepressant which potentiates neurotransmitter activity in the central nervous system, probably by inhibiting re-uptake of serotonin and noradrenaline.

Nefazodone is another new antidepressant. It inhibits re-uptake of serotonin and also selectively blocks serotonin receptors.

NEFAZODONE HYDROCHLORIDE

Indications: depressive illness

Cautions: epilepsy, concurrent electroconvulsive therapy (no studies), history of mania or hypomania, elderly (especially female), hepatic and renal impairment (lower end of dose range), pregnancy; **interactions:** Appendix 1 (nefazodone)

DRIVING. May impair performance of skilled tasks (e.g. driving)

Contra-indications: breast-feeding

Side-effects: asthenia, dry mouth, nausea, somnolence, dizziness; less frequently, chills, fever, postural hypotension, constipation, lightheadedness, paraesthesia, confusion, ataxia, amblyopia and other minor visual disturbances; rarely syncope

Dose: initially 100 mg twice daily increased after 5–7 days to 200 mg twice daily, may be gradually increased if necessary to max. 300 mg twice daily (elderly usual max. 100–200 mg twice daily); ADOLESCENT and CHILD under 18 years not recommended

▼ PoM **Dutonin**® (Bristol-Myers)

Tablets, both scored, nefazodone hydrochloride 100 mg (white), net price 56-tab pack = £16.80; 200 mg (yellow), 56-tab pack = £16.80. Label: 3

VENLAFAXINE

Indications: depressive illness

Cautions: history of myocardial infarction or unstable heart disease, blood pressure monitoring may be advisable in patients taking more than 200 mg daily, history of epilepsy, hepatic or renal impairment (avoid if severe), history of drug abuse, avoid abrupt withdrawal (if taken for more than 1 week withdraw over a few days, if taken for more than 6 weeks withdraw over at least 1 week); **interactions:** Appendix 1 (venlafaxine)

DRIVING. May affect performance of skilled tasks (e.g. driving)

SKIN REACTIONS. Patients should be advised to contact doctor if rash, urticaria or related allergic reaction develops

Contra-indications: severe hepatic or renal impairment; pregnancy and breast-feeding

Side-effects: nausea, headache, insomnia, somnolence, dry mouth, dizziness (and occasionally hypotension), constipation, asthenia, sweating, nervousness, convulsions (discontinue); other side-effects reported include anorexia, dyspepsia, abdominal pain, anxiety, sexual dysfunction, visual disturbances, vasodilatation, vomiting, tremor, paraesthesia, chills, hypertension (see Cautions), palpitations, weight gain, agitation, rash (see Cautions); reversible increase in liver enzymes and alterations in serum cholesterol also reported

Dose: initially 75 mg daily in 2 divided doses increased if necessary after several weeks to 150 mg daily in 2 divided doses

Severely depressed or hospitalised patients, initially 150 mg daily in 2 divided doses increased if necessary in steps of up to 75 mg every 2–3 days to max. 375 mg daily then gradually reduced; ADOLESCENT and CHILD under 18 years not recommended

▼ PoM **Efexor**® (Wyeth)

Tablets, both peach, venlafaxine (as hydro-chloride) 37.5 mg, net price 56-tab pack = £23.97; 50 mg, 42-tab pack = £23.97; 75 mg, 56-tab pack = £39.97. Label: 21, counselling, driving, skin reactions

4.3.4   Other antidepressant drugs

FLUPENTHIXOL

The thioxanthene **flupenthixol** (Fluanxol®) has antidepressant properties, and low doses (1 to 3 mg daily) are given by mouth for this purpose. Its advantages over the tricyclic and related antidepressants are that, with the low doses employed, side-effects are fewer, and that overdosage is less toxic.

FLUPENTHIXOL
(Flupentixol)

Indications: depressive illness (short-term use). For use in psychoses, see section 4.2.1

Cautions: cardiovascular disease (including cardiac disorders and cerebral arteriosclerosis), senile confusional states, parkinsonism, renal and hepatic disease; avoid in excitable and overactive patients; porphyria (see section 9.8.2); **interactions**: Appendix 1 (phenothiazines and other antipsychotics)

DRIVING. Drowsiness may affect performance of skilled tasks (e.g. driving); effects of alcohol enhanced

Side-effects: restlessness, insomnia; hypomania reported; rarely dizziness, tremor, visual disturbances, headache, hyperprolactinaemia, extra-pyramidal symptoms

Dose: initially 1 mg (elderly 500 micrograms) in the morning, increased after 1 week to 2 mg (elderly 1 mg) if necessary. Max. 3 mg (elderly 2 mg) daily, doses above 2 mg (elderly 1 mg) being divided in 2 portions, second dose not after 4 p.m. Discontinue if no response after 1 week at maximum dosage; CHILD not recommended

COUNSELLING. Although drowsiness may occur, can also have an alerting effect so should not be taken in the evening

PoM **Depixol**® (psychoses), see section 4.2.1

PoM **Fluanxol**® (Lundbeck)

Tablets, both red, s/c, flupenthixol (as dihydro-chloride) 500 micrograms, net price 20 = 98p; 1 mg, 60-tab pack = £4.98. Label: 2, counselling, administration

TRYPTOPHAN

Tryptophan appears to benefit some patients with resistant depression when given as adjunctive therapy but tryptophan products were withdrawn following evidence of an association with the eosinophilia-myalgia syndrome; Optimax® (Merck) has now been re-introduced for patients for whom no alternative treatment is suitable.

TRYPTOPHAN
(L-Tryptophan)

Indications: restricted to use by hospital specialists *only* for patients with severe and disabling depressive illness of more than 2 years continuous duration, *only* after an adequate trial of standard antidepressant drug treatment, and *only* as an adjunct to other antidepressant medication

Cautions: eosinophilia-myalgia syndrome has been reported with tryptophan-containing products therefore close and regular surveillance required; monitor eosinophil count, haematological changes and muscle symptomatology pregnancy and breast-feeding; **interactions** Appendix 1 (tryptophan)

Contra-indications: history of eosinophilia-myalgia syndrome following use of tryptophan

Side-effects: drowsiness, nausea, headache, light-headedness; eosinophilia-myalgia syndrome, see Cautions

Dose: 1 g 3 times daily; max. 6 g daily; ELDERLY lower dose may be appropriate especially where renal or hepatic impairment; CHILD not recommended

▼ PoM **Optimax**® (Merck)

Tablets, scored, tryptophan 500 mg. Net price 84-tab pack = £16.30. Label: 3

Important. Patient and prescriber must be registered with the Optimax® Information and Clinical Support (OPTICS) Unit. A **safety questionnaire** is sent to the prescriber after **3** and **6 months** of treatment and **every 6 months** thereafter. The information is reviewed by the CSM—it is **important** that the questionnaires should be completed

4.4   Central nervous system stimulants

Central nervous system stimulants include the **amphetamines** (notably dexamphetamine) **and related drugs** (methylphenidate and pemoline) They have very few indications and in particular should **not** be used to treat depression, obesity senility, debility, or for relief of fatigue.

Caffeine is a weak stimulant present in tea and coffee. It is included in many analgesic preparations (section 4.7.1) but does not contribute to their analgesic or anti-inflammatory effect. Over-indulgence may lead to a state of anxiety.

The **amphetamines** have a limited field of usefulness and their use should be **discouraged** as they may cause dependence and psychotic states. They have **no place** in the management of **depression** or **obesity**.

Patients with *narcolepsy* may derive benefit from treatment with dexamphetamine.

Dexamphetamine, **methylphenidate** and **pemoline** have been advocated (under specialist supervision) for the management of *hyperactive children* beneficial effects have been described. However they must be used very selectively as they retard growth and the effect of long-term therapy has not been evaluated.

DEXAMPHETAMINE SULPHATE

Indications: narcolepsy, adjunct in the management of refractory hyperkinetic states in children (under specialist supervision)

Cautions: mild hypertension (contra-indicated if moderate or severe)—monitor blood pressure; history of epilepsy (discontinue if convulsions occur); monitor growth in children (see also below); avoid abrupt withdrawal; data on safety and efficacy of long-term use not complete; porphyria (see section 9.8.2); **interactions:** Appendix 1 (sympathomimetics)

SPECIAL CAUTIONS IN CHILDREN. Monitor height and weight as growth retardation may occur during prolonged therapy (drug free periods may allow catch-up in growth but withdraw slowly to avoid inducing depression or renewed hyperactivity). In psychotic children may exacerbate behavioural disturbances and thought disorder

Contra-indications: cardiovascular disease including moderate to severe hypertension (caution if mild), hyperexcitability or agitated states, hyperthyroidism, history of drug or alcohol abuse, glaucoma, predisposition to tics or Tourette syndrome (discontinue if tics occur), pregnancy and breast-feeding

DRIVING. May affect performance of skilled tasks (e.g. driving); effects of alcohol unpredictable

Side-effects: insomnia, restlessness, irritability and excitabilitiy, nervousness, night terrors, euphoria, tremor, dizziness, headache; convulsions (see also Cautions); dependence and tolerance, sometimes psychosis; anorexia, gastrointestinal symptoms, growth retardation in children (see also under Cautions); dry mouth, sweating, tachycardia (and anginal pain), palpitations, increased blood pressure; visual disturbances; cardiomyopathy reported with chronic use; central stimulants have provoked choreoathetoid movements, tics and Tourette syndrome in predisposed individuals (see also Contra-indications above); overdosage: see Emergency Treatment of Poisoning, p. 23

Dose: narcolepsy, 10 mg (elderly, 5 mg) daily in divided doses increased by 10 mg (elderly, 5 mg) daily at intervals of 1 week to a max. of 60 mg daily

Hyperkinesia, CHILD under 6 years not recommended, over 6 years 5–10 mg daily, increased if necessary by 5 mg at intervals of 1 week to usual max. 20 mg daily (older children have received max. 40 mg daily)

CD Dexedrine® (Evans)

Tablets, scored, dexamphetamine sulphate 5 mg. Net price 28-tab pack = 96p. Counselling, driving

METHYLPHENIDATE HYDROCHLORIDE

Indications: part of a comprehensive treatment programme for attention-deficit hyperactivity disorder when remedial measures alone prove insufficient (under specialist supervision)

Cautions; Contra-indications; Side-effects: see under Dexamphetamine Sulphate; other side-effects reported include rash, urticaria, fever, arthralgia, alopecia, exfoliative dermatitis, erythema multiforme, thrombocytopenic purpura, thrombocytopenia, leucopenia, (manufacturer recommends periodic complete and differential blood and platelet counts); **interactions:** Appendix 1 (sympathomimetics)

Dose: CHILD under 6 years not recommended, over 6 years, initially 5 mg 1–2 times daily, increased if necessary at weekly intervals by 5–10 mg daily to max. 60 mg daily in divided doses; discontinue if no response after 1 month, also discontinue periodically to assess child's condition (usually finally discontinued during or after puberty)

EVENING DOSE. If effect wears off in evening (with rebound hyperactivity) a dose at bedtime may be appropriate (establish need with trial bedtime dose)

CD Ritalin® (Ciba)

Tablets, scored, methylphenidate hydrochloride 10 mg, net price 30-tab pack = £5.57

PEMOLINE

Indications: adjunct in the management of hyperkinesia in children (under specialist supervision)

Cautions; Contra-indications; Side-effects: see under Dexamphetamine Sulphate; neutropenia, and liver enzyme abnormalities also reported (manufacturer recommends monitoring of hepatic enzyme levels before treatment)

Dose: CHILD under 6 years not recommended, over 6 years, initially 20 mg every morning increased by increments of 20 mg at intervals of 1 week to 60 mg every morning, followed, if no improvement, by gradual increase to max. 120 mg every morning

PoM **Volital®** (LAB)

Tablets, scored, pemoline 20 mg. Net price 50-tab pack = £3.06

COCAINE

Cocaine is a drug of addiction which causes central nervous stimulation. Its clinical use is mainly as a topical local anaesthetic (see sections 11.7 and 15.2). It has been included in analgesic elixirs for the relief of pain in palliative care but this use is obsolete. For management of cocaine poisoning, see p 23.

4.5 Appetite suppressants

4.5.1 Bulk-forming drugs
4.5.2 Centrally acting appetite suppressants

The development of obesity appears to be multifactorial. Aggravating factors may be depression or other psychosocial problems or drug treatment.

The main treatment of the obese patient is an appropriate diet, carefully explained to the patient, with support and encouragement from the doctor. Attendance at groups (for example 'weight-watchers') helps some individuals. Drugs can play only a limited role and should never be used as the sole element of treatment; their effects tend to be disappointing.

Thyroid hormones have no place in the treatment of obesity except in hypothyroid patients.

The use of diuretics is **not** appropriate for weight reduction.

4.5.1   Bulk-forming drugs

The most commonly used bulk-forming drug is **methylcellulose**. It is claimed to reduce intake by producing feelings of satiety but there is little evidence to support this claim.

METHYLCELLULOSE

Indications: adjunct in obesity (but see notes above); other indications, see section 1.6.1
Cautions: maintain adequate fluid intake
Contra-indications: gastro-intestinal obstruction
Side-effects: flatulence, abdominal distension, intestinal obstruction
Dose: see under preparations below
   COUNSELLING. Preparations that swell in contact with liquid should always be carefully swallowed with water and should not be taken immediately before going to bed

Celevac® (Monmouth)
Tablets, pink, methylcellulose '450' 500 mg. Net price 112-tab pack = £2.69. Counselling, see above and dose
   Dose: adjunct in obesity (but see notes above), 3 tablets, chewed or crushed, with a tumblerful of liquid half an hour before food or when hungry

STERCULIA

Indications; Cautions; Contra-indications; Side-effects: see under Methylcellulose
Dose: see under preparation below

Prefil® (Norgine)
Granules, brown, coated, sugar- and gluten-free, sterculia 80%, 7 g/sachet. Net price 30-sachet pack = £4.42. Label: 22, 27, counselling, administration
   Dose: adjunct in obesity (but see notes above), one sachet followed by a tumblerful of liquid ½–1 hour before food, lower initial dose in patients accustomed to a low-residue diet; CHILD reduced dose

4.5.2   Centrally acting appetite suppressants

Centrally acting appetite suppressants are sympathomimetics and most have a significant stimulant effect on the central nervous system. They are used as adjuncts in the treatment of severe obesity; they should **not** be used simply for cosmetic reasons (see also section 4.5).

Although **fenfluramine** is related to amphetamine, in standard doses it has a sedative rather than a stimulant effect. Nevertheless, abuse has occurred and abrupt withdrawal may induce depression. It is licensed for short-term use as an adjunct to continued dietary treatment of selected patients with severe obesity, who have not responded to an appropriate weight-reducing diet alone, for whom close support and supervision should be provided. Fenfluramine is **not licensed** for periods of treatment beyond 3 months.

Dexfenfluramine is the dextro isomer of fenfluramine and has a similar product licence.

Phentermine is licensed for short-term use as an adjunct to the treatment of selected patients with moderate to severe obesity, for whom close support and supervision should be provided. Abuse may be a problem with phentermine.

CHILDREN. These drugs should be avoided in children because of the possibility of growth suppression.

DEXFENFLURAMINE HYDROCHLORIDE

Indications: see notes above
Cautions; Contra-indications; Side-effects: see under Fenfluramine Hydrochloride; avoid in hepatic and renal impairment
Dose: 15 mg morning and evening, at mealtimes; max. period of treatment should not exceed 3 months; ELDERLY and CHILD not recommended

▼ PoM **Adifax®** (Servier)
Capsules, dexfenfluramine hydrochloride 15 mg, net price 60-cap pack = £8.08. Label: 2, counselling, exercise (see under Fenfluramine Hydrochloride)

FENFLURAMINE HYDROCHLORIDE

Indications: see notes above
Cautions: dependence reported, depression on sudden withdrawal (gradual reduction over at least a week preferable); elderly; porphyria (see section 9.8.2); **interactions:** Appendix 1 (sympathomimetics)
   DRIVING. Drowsiness may affect performance of skilled tasks (e.g. driving); effects of alcohol enhanced
   EXERCISE. Advise patient to report immediately dyspnoea or deterioration in exercise tolerance
Contra-indications: history of psychiatric illness (including anorexia nervosa and depression); drug or alcohol abuse; personality disorders; epilepsy; glaucoma; pregnancy and breast-feeding
Side-effects: diarrhoea and other gastro-intestinal disturbances; drowsiness, dizziness, and lethargy; also dry mouth, headache, nervousness, irritability, sleep disturbances, depression, visual disorders, hypotension, urinary frequency, impotence and loss of libido; rarely rashes, blood disorders, pulmonary hypertension (dyspnoea and deterioration in exercise tolerance may be symptoms—see also under Cautions), schizophrenia-like reactions; neurotoxicity reported in *animal* studies
Dose: see below

PoM **Ponderax**® (Servier)
Pacaps® (= capsules m/r), clear/blue, enclosing white pellets, fenfluramine hydrochloride 60 mg. Net price 60-cap pack = £7.08. Label: 2, 25, counselling, exercise
Dose: 1 capsule daily; max. period of treatment should not exceed 3 months (see also notes above); CHILD not recommended

PHENTERMINE

Indications: not recommended, see notes above
Cautions: mild hypertension (avoid if moderate to severe), diabetes mellitus, history of anxiety or depression; **interactions:** Appendix 1 (sympathomimetics)
DRIVING. May impair performance of skilled tasks (e.g. driving); effects of alcohol unpredictable
Contra-indications: cardiovascular disease (including moderate to severe hypertension), glaucoma, hyperthyroidism, epilepsy, unstable personality, history of psychiatric illness; history of drug or alcohol abuse; pregnancy (congenital malformations reported with related drugs) and breast-feeding
Side-effects: dry mouth, headache, rashes, euphoria and dependence; also insomnia, restlessness, nervousness, agitation, nausea, vomiting, dizziness, depression, psychosis, hallucinations, palpitations and tachycardia, hypertension, constipation, urinary frequency, facial oedema
Dose: 15–30 mg before breakfast; to reduce the risk of dependence max. continuous period of treatment should not exceed 4–8 weeks (followed by similar period without treatment); ELDERLY and CHILD not recommended

CD **Duromine**® (3M)
Capsules, both m/r, phentermine (as resin complex) 15 mg (green/grey), net price 30-cap pack = £1.14; 30 mg (maroon/grey), 30-cap pack = £1.50. Label: 25, counselling, driving
CD **Ionamin**® (Torbet)
Capsules, both m/r, phentermine (as resin complex) 15 mg (grey/yellow), net price 20 = £1.11; 30 mg (yellow), 20 = £1.38. Label: 25, counselling, driving

4.6   Drugs used in nausea and vertigo

Anti-emetics should be prescribed only when the cause of vomiting is known, particularly in children, otherwise the symptomatic relief that they produce may delay diagnosis. Anti-emetics are unnecessary and sometimes harmful when the cause can be treated, e.g. as in diabetic ketoacidosis, or in excessive digoxin or antiepileptic dosage.

If antinauseant drug treatment is indicated the choice of drug depends on the aetiology of vomiting.

VESTIBULAR DISORDERS

The most effective drug for the prevention of *motion sickness* is **hyoscine**. Adverse effects (drowsiness, blurred vision, dry mouth, urinary retention) are more frequent than with the antihistamines but are not generally prominent at the doses employed. **Antihistamines** are slightly less effective, but are generally better tolerated. There is no evidence that any one antihistamine is superior to another but

their duration of action and incidence of adverse effects (drowsiness and antimuscarinic effects) differ. If a sedative effect is desired **promethazine** and **dimenhydrinate** are useful, but generally a slightly less sedating antihistamine such as **cyclizine** or **cinnarizine** is preferred. **Metoclopramide** and the **phenothiazines** (except the antihistamine phenothiazine promethazine), which act selectively on the chemoreceptor trigger zone, are ineffective in motion sickness.

Vertigo and nausea associated with *Ménière's disease* and *middle-ear surgery* may be difficult to treat. **Hyoscine, antihistamines**, and **phenothiazines** (such as prochlorperazine) are effective in the prophylaxis and treatment of such conditions. **Cinnarizine** and **betahistine** have been promoted as specific treatments for Ménière's disease. In the acute attack **cyclizine** or **prochlorperazine** may be given rectally or by intramuscular injection.

Treatment of vertigo in its chronic forms is seldom fully effective but antihistamines (such as dimenhydrinate) or phenothiazines (such as prochlorperazine) may help.

For advice to avoid the inappropriate prescribing of drugs (notably phenothiazines) for dizziness in the elderly, see Prescribing for the Elderly, p. 16.

VOMITING OF PREGNANCY

Nausea in the first trimester of pregnancy does **not** require drug therapy. On rare occasions if vomiting is severe, an antihistamine or a phenothiazine (e.g. promethazine) may be required. If symptoms have not settled in 24 to 48 hours then a specialist opinion should be sought.

SYMPTOMATIC RELIEF OF NAUSEA FROM UNDERLYING DISEASE

The **phenothiazines** are dopamine antagonists and act centrally by blocking the chemoreceptor trigger zone. They are of considerable value for the prophylaxis and treatment of nausea and vomiting associated with diffuse neoplastic disease, radiation sickness, and the emesis caused by drugs such as opioid analgesics, general anaesthetics, and cytotoxic drugs. **Prochlorperazine, perphenazine**, and **trifluoperazine** are less sedating than **chlorpromazine** but severe dystonic reactions sometimes occur, especially in children.

Metoclopramide is an effective anti-emetic with a spectrum of activity closely resembling that of the phenothiazines but it has a peripheral action on the gut in addition to its central effect and therefore may be superior to the phenothiazines in the emesis associated with gastroduodenal, hepatic, and biliary disease. As with the phenothiazines, metoclopramide may induce acute dystonic reactions with facial and skeletal muscle spasms and oculogyric crises. These are more common in the young (especially girls and young women) and the very old, usually occur shortly after starting treatment, and subside within 24 hours of stopping the drug. Injection of an antiparkinsonian agent such as procyclidine (see section 4.9.2) will abort attacks. The high-dose preparation of metoclopramide is of value in the prevention of nausea and vomiting associated with cytotoxic drug therapy.

Domperidone is used for the relief of nausea and vomiting, especially when associated with cytotoxic drug therapy. It has the advantage over metoclopramide and the phenothiazines of being less likely to cause central effects such as sedation and dystonic reactions because it does not readily cross the blood-brain barrier. It may be given for the treatment of levodopa- and bromocriptine-induced vomiting in parkinsonism (section 4.9.1). Domperidone acts at the chemoreceptor trigger zone and so is unlikely to be effective in motion sickness and other vestibular disorders.

Antihistamines are active in most of these conditions, but are not usually drugs of choice.

Nabilone is a synthetic cannabinoid with anti-emetic properties, reported to be superior to prochlorperazine. It is beneficial in the relief of nausea and vomiting associated with cytotoxic drug therapy. Side-effects occur in most patients given standard doses.

Granisetron, **ondansetron** and **tropisetron** are specific (5HT$_3$) serotonin antagonists. They have a valuable role in the management of nausea and vomiting in patients receiving cytotoxics who are unable to tolerate, or whose nausea and vomiting is not controlled by, less expensive drugs.

CYTOTOXIC CHEMOTHERAPY. For *anti-emetic regimens* used in the management of nausea and vomiting induced by cytotoxic chemotherapy, see section 8.1.

ANTIHISTAMINES

CINNARIZINE
Indications: vestibular disorders, such as vertigo, tinnitus, nausea, and vomiting in Ménière's disease; motion sickness; vascular disease, see section 2.6.3
Cautions; Contra-indications; Side-effects: see under Cyclizine; also allergic skin reactions and fatigue; caution in hypotension (high doses); rarely, extrapyramidal symptoms in elderly on prolonged therapy; avoid in porphyria (see section 9.8.2)
Dose: vestibular disorders, 30 mg 3 times daily; CHILD 5–12 years half adult dose
Motion sickness, 30 mg 2 hours before travel then 15 mg every 8 hours during journey if necessary; CHILD 5–12 years half adult dose

Cinnarizine (Non-proprietary)
Tablets, cinnarizine 15 mg. Net price 20 = 91p. Label: 2
Available from APS, Ashbourne (Cinazière®), Cox, Hillcross, Norton
Stugeron® (Janssen)
Tablets, scored, cinnarizine 15 mg. Net price 20 = £1.07. Label: 2
Stugeron Forte®: see section 2.6.3

CYCLIZINE
Indications: nausea, vomiting, vertigo, motion sickness, labyrinthine disorders
Cautions; Contra-indications; Side-effects: drowsiness, occasional dry mouth and blurred vision; see also section 3.4.1 (Disadvantages of Antihistamines); cyclizine may aggravate severe heart failure and counteract the haemodynamic benefits of opioids; **interactions:** Appendix 1 (antihistamines)
DRIVING. Drowsiness may affect performance of skilled tasks (e.g. driving); effects of alcohol enhanced
Dose: by mouth, cyclizine hydrochloride 50 mg up to 3 times daily; CHILD 6–12 years 25 mg
By intramuscular or intravenous injection, cyclizine lactate 50 mg 3 times daily

Valoid® (Wellcome)
Tablets, scored, cyclizine hydrochloride 50 mg. Net price 20 = 99p. Label: 2
PoM *Injection,* cyclizine lactate 50 mg/mL. Net price 1-mL amp = 57p

DIMENHYDRINATE
Indications: nausea, vomiting, vertigo, motion sickness, labyrinthine disorders
Cautions; Contra-indications; Side-effects: see under Cyclizine; porphyria (see section 9.8.2)
Dose: 50–100 mg 2–3 times daily; CHILD 1–6 years 12.5–25 mg, 7–12 years 25–50 mg
Motion sickness, first dose 30 minutes before journey

Dramamine® (Searle)
Tablets, scored, dimenhydrinate 50 mg, net price 100-tab pack = £5.13. Label: 2
Note. A 10-tab pack is on sale to the public for motion sickness

MECLOZINE HYDROCHLORIDE
Indications: see under preparations
Cautions; Contra-indications; Side-effects: see under Cyclizine

Preparations
A proprietary brand of meclozine hydrochloride tablets 12.5 mg (Sea-legs®) is on sale to the public for motion sickness

PROMETHAZINE HYDROCHLORIDE
Indications: nausea, vomiting, vertigo, labyrinthine disorders, motion sickness; other indications, see sections 3.4.1, 4.1.1, 15.1.4.1
Cautions; Contra-indications; Side-effects: see under Cyclizine but more sedating; intramuscular injection may be painful; avoid in porphyria (see section 9.8.2)

Dose: motion sickness prevention (elixir), 25 mg at bedtime on night before travelling, repeat following morning if necessary; CHILD under 2 years not recommended, 2–5 years, 5 mg at night and following morning; 5–10 years, 10 mg at night and following morning

Preparations
See section 3.4.1

PROMETHAZINE THEOCLATE
(Promethazine Teoclate)

Indications: nausea, vertigo, labyrinthine disorders, motion sickness (acts longer than the hydrochloride)

Cautions; Contra-indications; Side-effects: see under Promethazine Hydrochloride

Dose: 25–75 mg, max. 100 mg, daily; CHILD 5–10 years, 12.5–37.5 mg daily
Motion sickness prevention, 25 mg at bedtime on night before travelling *or* 25 mg 1–2 hours before travelling; CHILD 5–10 years, half adult dose
For severe vomiting in pregnancy, 25 mg at bedtime, increased if necessary to a max. of 100 mg daily (but see also Vomiting of Pregnancy in notes above)

Avomine® (Rhône-Poulenc Rorer)
Tablets, scored, promethazine theoclate 25 mg. Net price 10-tab pack = 95p; 28-tab pack = 99p. Label: 2

PHENOTHIAZINES AND RELATED DRUGS

CHLORPROMAZINE HYDROCHLORIDE

Indications: nausea and vomiting of terminal illness (where other drugs have failed or are not available); other indications, see sections 4.2.1, 15.1.4.1

Cautions; Contra-indications; Side-effects: see section 4.2.1

Dose: by mouth, 10–25 mg every 4–6 hours; CHILD 500 micrograms/kg every 4–6 hours (1–5 years max. 40 mg daily, 6–12 years max. 75 mg daily)

By deep intramuscular injection 25 mg initially then 25–50 mg every 3–4 hours until vomiting stops; CHILD 500 micrograms/kg every 6–8 hours (1–5 years max. 40 mg daily, 6–12 years max. 75 mg daily)

By rectum in suppositories, chlorpromazine 100 mg every 6–8 hours [unlicensed]

Preparations
Section 4.2.1

DROPERIDOL
Section 4.2.1

HALOPERIDOL
Section 4.2.1

METHOTRIMEPRAZINE
Section 4.2.1

PERPHENAZINE

Indications: severe nausea, vomiting (see notes above); other indications, section 4.2.1

Cautions; Contra-indications; Side-effects: see section 4.2.1; extrapyramidal symptoms may occur, particularly in young adults, elderly, and debilitated

Dose: 4 mg 3 times daily, adjusted according to response; max. 24 mg daily (chemotherapy-induced); ELDERLY quarter to half adult dose; CHILD under 14 years not recommended

Preparations
Section 4.2.1

PROCHLORPERAZINE

Indications: severe nausea, vomiting, vertigo, labyrinthine disorders (see notes above); other indications, section 4.2.1

Cautions; Contra-indications: see under Chlorpromazine Hydrochloride (section 4.2.1). Oral route only for children (avoid if less than 10 kg); elderly (see notes above)

Side-effects: see under Chlorpromazine Hydrochloride; extrapyramidal symptoms may occur, particularly in children, elderly, and debilitated

Dose: by mouth, nausea and vomiting, prochlorperazine maleate or mesylate, acute attack, 20 mg initially then 10 mg after 2 hours; prevention 5–10 mg 2–3 times daily; CHILD (over 10 kg only) 250 micrograms/kg 2–3 times daily
Labyrinthine disorders, 5 mg 3 times daily, gradually increased if necessary to 30 mg daily in divided doses, then reduced after several weeks to 5–10 mg daily; CHILD not recommended

By deep intramuscular injection, nausea and vomiting, 12.5 mg when required followed if necessary after 6 hours by an oral dose, as above; CHILD not recommended

By rectum in suppositories, nausea and vomiting, 25 mg followed if necessary after 6 hours by oral dose, as above; *or* due to migraine, 5 mg 3 times daily; CHILD not recommended

PoM Prochlorperazine (Non-proprietary)
Tablets, prochlorperazine maleate 5 mg, net price 20 = 53p. Label: 2
Available from Ashbourne (Prozière®), Cox, Hillcross, Norton

PoM Stemetil® (Rhône-Poulenc Rorer)
Tablets, prochlorperazine maleate 5 mg (off-white), net price 84-tab pack = £3.16; 25 mg (scored), 56-tab pack = £5.57. Label: 2
Syrup, straw-coloured, prochlorperazine mesylate 5 mg/5 mL. Net price 100-mL pack = £1.78. Label: 2
Eff sachets, granules, effervescent, sugar-free, prochlorperazine mesylate 5 mg/sachet. Net price 21-sachet pack = £3.31. Label: 2, 13

Injection, prochlorperazine mesylate 12.5 mg/mL. Net price 1-mL amp = 35p

Suppositories, prochlorperazine maleate (as prochlorperazine), 5 mg, net price 10 = £4.47; 25 mg, 10 = £5.86. Label: 2

Buccal preparation
PoM **Buccastem**® (R&C)

Tablets (buccal), pale yellow, prochlorperazine maleate 3 mg. Net price 5 × 10-tab pack = £5.75. Label: 2, counselling, administration, see under Dose below

Dose: 1–2 tablets twice daily; tablets are placed high between upper lip and gum and left to dissolve; CHILD not recommended

TRIFLUOPERAZINE

Indications: severe nausea and vomiting (see notes above); other indications, section 4.2.1

Cautions; Contra-indications; Side-effects: see section 4.2.1; extrapyramidal symptoms may occur, particularly in children, elderly, and debilitated

Dose: by mouth, 2–4 mg daily in divided doses *or* as a single dose of a modified-release preparation; max. 6 mg daily; CHILD 3–5 years up to 1 mg daily, 6–12 years up to 4 mg daily

Preparations
See section 4.2.1

DOMPERIDONE AND METOCLOPRAMIDE

DOMPERIDONE

Indications: see under Dose
CHILDREN. Use in children is restricted to nausea and vomiting following cytotoxics or radiotherapy

Cautions: renal impairment; pregnancy and breast-feeding; not recommended for routine prophylaxis of post-operative vomiting or for chronic administration; **interactions:** Appendix 1 (domperidone)

Side-effects: raised prolactin concentrations (possible galactorrhoea and gynaecomastia), reduced libido reported; rashes and other allergic reactions; acute dystonic reactions reported

Dose: by mouth, acute nausea and vomiting, (including nausea and vomiting induced by levodopa and bromocriptine), 10–20 mg every 4–8 hours, max. period of treatment 12 weeks; CHILD, nausea and vomiting following cytotoxic therapy or radiotherapy only, 200–400 micrograms/kg every 4–8 hours

Functional dyspepsia, 10–20 mg 3 times daily before food and 10–20 mg at night; max. period of treatment 12 weeks; CHILD not recommended

By rectum in suppositories, nausea and vomiting, 30–60 mg every 4–8 hours; CHILD over 2 years (following cytotoxic therapy or radiotherapy only), body-weight 10–15 kg max. 15 mg twice daily, body-weight 15.5–25 kg max. 30 mg twice daily, body-weight 25.5–35 kg max. 30 mg 3 times daily, body-weight 35.5–45 kg max. 30 mg 4 times daily; since dose needs to be divided throughout day, suppositories may be cut in half for younger children

PoM **Motilium**® (Sanofi Winthrop)

Tablets, f/c, domperidone 10 mg (as maleate). Net price 30-tab pack = £2.46; 100-tab pack = £8.21

Suspension, sugar-free, domperidone 5 mg/5 mL. Net price 200-mL pack = £1.80

Suppositories, domperidone 30 mg. Net price 10 = £2.65

METOCLOPRAMIDE HYDROCHLORIDE

Indications: adults, nausea and vomiting, particularly in gastro-intestinal disorders and treatment with cytotoxics or radiotherapy; gastro-intestinal—section 1.2; migraine—section 4.7.4.1

PATIENTS UNDER 20 YEARS. Use restricted to severe intractable vomiting of known cause, vomiting of radiotherapy and cytotoxics, aid to gastro-intestinal intubation, pre-medication

Cautions: hepatic and renal impairment; elderly, young adults, and children (measure dose accurately, preferably with a pipette); may mask underlying disorders such as cerebral irritation; avoid for 3–4 days following gastro-intestinal surgery, may cause acute hypertensive response in phaeochromocytoma; pregnancy and breast-feeding; porphyria (see section 9.8.2); **interactions:** Appendix 1 (metoclopramide)

Side-effects: extrapyramidal effects (especially in children/young adults), hyperprolactinaemia, occasionally tardive dyskinesia on prolonged administration; also reported, drowsiness, restlessness, diarrhoea, depression, neuroleptic malignant syndrome; cardiac conduction abnormalities reported following intravenous administration

Dose: by mouth, or by intramuscular injection or by intravenous injection over 1–2 minutes, 10 mg (5 mg in young adults 15–19 years under 60 kg) 3 times daily; CHILD up to 1 year (up to 10 kg) 1 mg twice daily, 1–3 years (10–14 kg) 1 mg 2–3 times daily, 3–5 years (15–19 kg) 2 mg 2–3 times daily, 5–9 years (20–29 kg) 2.5 mg 3 times daily, 9–14 years (30 kg and over) 5 mg 3 times daily

Note. Daily dose of metoclopramide should not normally exceed 500 micrograms/kg, particularly for children and young adults (restricted use, see above)

For diagnostic procedures, as a single dose 5–10 minutes before examination, 10–20 mg (10 mg in young adults 15–19 years); CHILD under 3 years 1 mg, 3–5 years 2 mg, 5–9 years 2.5 mg, 9–14 years 5 mg

PoM **Metoclopramide** (Non-proprietary)

Tablets, metoclopramide hydrochloride 10 mg, net price 20 = 40p

Available from Antigen, APS, Ashbourne (Gastroflux®), Berk (Primperan®), Cox, CP, Lagap (Parmid®), Norton

Oral solution, metoclopramide hydrochloride 5 mg/5 mL, net price 100-mL pack = £1.03

Available from Berk (Primperan®, sugar-free), Lagap (Parmid® sugar-free), Rosemont (sugar-free)

Injection, metoclopramide hydrochloride 5 mg/mL, net price 2-mL amp = 16p

Available from Antigen, Phoenix

PoM **Maxolon**® (Monmouth)

Tablets, scored, metoclopramide hydrochloride 10 mg. Net price 21-tab pack = £2.42, 84-tab pack = £9.38

Syrup, sugar-free, metoclopramide hydrochloride 5 mg/5 mL. Net price 200-mL pack = £3.83

Paediatric liquid, sugar-free, metoclopramide hydrochloride 1 mg/mL. Net price 15-mL pack with pipette = £1.51. Counselling, use of pipette

Injection, metoclopramide hydrochloride 5 mg/mL. Net price 2-mL amp = 27p

High-dose (with cytotoxic chemotherapy only)

PoM **Maxolon High Dose**® (Monmouth)

Injection, metoclopramide hydrochloride 5 mg/mL. Net price 20-mL amp = £2.67.

For dilution and use as an intravenous infusion in nausea and vomiting associated with cytotoxic chemotherapy only

Dose: by continuous intravenous infusion (preferred method), initially (before starting chemotherapy), 2–4 mg/kg over 15–20 minutes, then 3–5 mg/kg over 8–12 hours; max. in 24 hours, 10 mg/kg

By intermittent intravenous infusion, initially (before starting chemotherapy), up to 2 mg/kg over at least 15 minutes then up to 2 mg/kg over at least 15 minutes every 2 hours; max. in 24 hours, 10 mg/kg

Note. Injection of metoclopramide hydrochloride 5 mg/mL also available in 20-mL ampoules from Phoenix

Modified-release preparations

Note. All unsuitable for patients under 20 years

PoM **Gastrobid Continus**® (Napp)

Tablets, m/r, metoclopramide hydrochloride 15 mg. Net price 56-tab pack = £10.16. Label: 25

Dose: patients over 20 years, 1 tablet twice daily

PoM **Gastromax**® (Pfizer)

Capsules, m/r, orange/yellow, enclosing white to light beige pellets, metoclopramide hydrochloride 30 mg. Net price 28-cap pack = £11.55. Label: 22, 25

Dose: patients over 20 years, 1 capsule daily

PoM **Maxolon SR**® (Monmouth)

Capsules, m/r, clear, enclosing white granules, metoclopramide hydrochloride 15 mg. Net price 56-cap pack = £10.76. Label: 25

Dose: patients over 20 years, 1 capsule twice daily

Compound preparations (for migraine), section 4.7.4.1

5HT₃ ANTAGONISTS

GRANISETRON

Indications: see under Dose

Cautions: pregnancy and breast-feeding

Side-effects: constipation, headache, rash; transient increases in liver enzymes; hypersensitivity reactions reported

Dose: nausea and vomiting induced by cytotoxic chemotherapy or radiotherapy, *by mouth*, 1–2 mg within 1 hour before start of treatment, then 2 mg daily in 1–2 divided doses during treatment; when intravenous infusion also used, max. combined total 9 mg in 24 hours; CHILD 20 micrograms/kg (max. 1 mg) within 1 hour before start of treatment, then 20 micrograms/kg (max. 1 mg) twice daily for up to 5 days during treatment

By intravenous injection (diluted in 15 mL and given over not less than 30 seconds) *or by intravenous infusion* (over 5 minutes), prevention, 3 mg before start of cytostatic therapy (up to 2 additional 3-mg doses may be given within 24 hours); treatment, as for prevention (the two additional doses must not be given less than 10 minutes apart); max. 9 mg in 24 hours; CHILD, *by intravenous infusion*, (over 5 minutes), prevention, 40 micrograms/kg (max. 3 mg) before start of cytostatic therapy; treatment, as for prevention—one additional dose of 40 micrograms/kg (max. 3 mg) may be given within 24 hours (not less than 10 minutes after initial dose)

Postoperative nausea and vomiting, *by intravenous injection* (diluted to 5 mL and given over 30 seconds), prevention, 1 mg before induction of anaesthesia; treatment, 1 mg, given as for prevention; max. 2 mg in one day; CHILD not recommended

PoM **Kytril**® (SmithKline Beecham)

Tablets, f/c, granisetron (as hydrochloride) 1 mg, net price 10-tab pack = £91.43; 2 mg, 5-tab pack = £91.43

Paediatric liquid, sugar-free, granisetron (as hydrochloride) 1 mg/5 mL, net price 30 mL = £54.86

Sterile solution, granisetron (as hydrochloride) 1 mg/mL, for dilution and use as injection or infusion, net price 1-mL vial = £12.00, 3-mL amp = £36.00

ONDANSETRON

Indications: see under Dose

Cautions: pregnancy and breast-feeding; moderate or severe hepatic impairment (max. 8 mg daily)

Side-effects: constipation; headache, sensation of warmth or flushing, hiccups; occasional alterations in liver enzymes; hypersensitivity reactions reported; occasional transient visual disturbances and dizziness following intravenous administration; involuntary movements, seizures, chest pain, arrhythmias, hypotension and bradycardia also reported

Dose: moderately emetogenic chemotherapy or radiotherapy, *by mouth*, 8 mg 1–2 hours before treatment *or, by slow intravenous injection*, 8 mg immediately before treatment, *then* 8 mg *by mouth* every 12 hours for up to 5 days

Severely emetogenic chemotherapy, *by slow intravenous injection*, 8 mg immediately before treatment, followed by 8 mg at intervals of 2–4 hours for 2 further doses (*or followed by* 1 mg/hour *by continuous intravenous infusion* for up to 24 hours) *then* 8 mg *by mouth* every 12 hours for up to 5 days

alternatively, by intravenous infusion over 15 minutes, 32 mg immediately before treatment *then* 8 mg *by mouth* every 12 hours for up to 5 days

Note. Efficacy may be enhanced by addition of a single dose of dexamethasone sodium phosphate 20 mg by intravenous injection

CHILD, *by slow intravenous injection or by intravenous infusion* over 15 minutes, 5 mg/m² immediately before chemotherapy then, 4 mg *by mouth* every 12 hours for up to 5 days

Prevention of postoperative nausea and vomiting, *by mouth*, 16 mg 1 hour before anaesthesia *or by intramuscular or slow intravenous injection*, 4 mg at induction of anaesthesia; CHILD over 2 years, *by slow intravenous injection*, 100 micrograms/kg (max. 4 mg) before, during, or after induction of anaesthesia

Treatment of postoperative nausea and vomiting, *by intramuscular or slow intravenous injection*, 4 mg; CHILD over 2 years, *by slow intravenous injection*, 100 micrograms/kg (max. 4 mg)

PoM **Zofran**® (Glaxo)

Tablets, both yellow, f/c, ondansetron (as hydrochloride) 4 mg, net price 30-tab pack = £121.50; 8 mg, 10-tab pack = £81.00

Injection, ondansetron (as hydrochloride) 2 mg/mL, net price 2-mL amp = £6.75; 4-mL amp = £13.50

TROPISETRON

Indications: nausea and vomiting induced by cytotoxic chemotherapy

Cautions: uncontrolled hypertension (has been aggravated by doses higher than recommended); pregnancy and breast-feeding

DRIVING. Dizziness or drowsiness may affect performance of skilled tasks (e.g. driving)

Side-effects: constipation, diarrhoea, abdominal pain; headache, dizziness, fatigue; hypersensitivity reactions reported (including facial flushing, urticaria, chest tightness, dyspnoea, bronchospasm and hypotension); collapse, syncope, bradycardia, cardiovascular collapse also reported (causal relationship not established)

Dose: by slow intravenous injection or by intravenous infusion, 5 mg shortly before chemotherapy, then 5 mg *by mouth* every morning at least 1 hour before food for 5 days; CHILD not recommended

PoM **Navoban**® (Sandoz)

Capsules, white/yellow, tropisetron (as hydrochloride) 5 mg, net price 5-cap pack = £63.37; 50-cap pack = £633.65. Label: 23

Injection, tropisetron (as hydrochloride), 1 mg/mL, net price 5-mL amp = £14.31

CANNABINOID

NABILONE

Indications: nausea and vomiting caused by cytotoxic chemotherapy, unresponsive to conventional anti-emetics (under close observation, preferably in in-patient setting)

Cautions: history of psychiatric disorder; elderly; hypertension; heart disease; adverse effects on mental state can persist for 48–72 hours after stopping; **interactions:** Appendix 1 (nabilone)

DRIVING. Drowsiness may affect performance of skilled tasks (e.g. driving); effects of alcohol enhanced

Contra-indications: severe hepatic impairment; pregnancy and breast-feeding

Side-effects: drowsiness, vertigo, euphoria, dry mouth, ataxia, visual disturbance, concentration difficulties, sleep disturbance, dysphoria, hypotension, headache and nausea; also confusion, disorientation, hallucinations, psychosis, depression, decreased coordination, tremors, tachycardia, decreased appetite, and abdominal pain

BEHAVIOURAL EFFECTS. Patients should be made aware of possible changes of mood and other adverse behavioural effects

Dose: patients over 18 years, initially 1 mg twice daily, increased if necessary to 2 mg twice daily, throughout each cycle of cytotoxic therapy and, if necessary, for 48 hours after the last dose of each cycle; max. 6 mg daily given in 3 divided doses. The first dose should be taken the night before initiation of cytotoxic treatment and the second dose 1–3 hours before the first dose of cytotoxic drug; ADOLESCENT and CHILD under 18 years not recommended

PoM ¹**Nabilone** (Cambridge)

Capsules, blue/white, nabilone 1 mg. Net price 20-cap pack = £96.08 (hosp. only). Label: 2, counselling, behavioural effects

1. Formerly Cesamet®

HYOSCINE

HYOSCINE HYDROBROMIDE

(Scopolamine Hydrobromide)

Indications: motion sickness; premedication, see section 15.1.3

Cautions: elderly, urinary retention, cardiovascular disease, gastro-intestinal obstruction, hepatic or renal impairment; porphyria (see section 9.8.2); pregnancy and breast-feeding; **interactions:** Appendix 1 (antimuscarinics)

DRIVING. Drowsiness may affect performance of skilled tasks (e.g. driving) and may persist for up to 24 hours or longer after removal of patch: effects of alcohol enhanced

Contra-indications: closed-angle glaucoma

Side-effects: drowsiness, dry mouth, dizziness, blurred vision, difficulty with micturition

Dose: motion sickness, *by mouth*, 300 micrograms 30 minutes before start of journey followed by 300 micrograms every 6 hours if required; max. 3 doses in 24 hours; CHILD 4–10 years 75–150 micrograms, over 10 years 150–300 micrograms

Note. Proprietary brands of hyoscine hydrobromide tablets (Joy-rides®, Kwells®) are on sale to the public for motion sickness

Injection, see section 15.1.3

PoM **Scopoderm TTS**® (Ciba)

Patch, self-adhesive, pink, releasing hyoscine approx. 500 micrograms/72 hours when in contact with skin. Net price 2 = £2.84. Label: 19, counselling, see below

Administration: motion sickness prevention, apply 1 patch to hairless area of skin behind ear 5–6 hours before journey; replace if necessary after 72 hours, siting replacement patch behind other ear; CHILD under 10 years not recommended

COUNSELLING. Explain accompanying instructions to patient and in particular emphasise advice to wash hands after handling and to wash application site after removing, and to use one at a time

OTHER DRUGS FOR MÉNIÈRE'S DISEASE

Betahistine has been promoted as a specific treatment for Ménière's disease.

BETAHISTINE HYDROCHLORIDE

Indications: vertigo, tinnitus and hearing loss associated with Ménière's disease

Cautions: asthma, history of peptic ulcer; pregnancy and breast-feeding; **interactions:** Appendix 1 (betahistine)

Contra-indications: phaeochromocytoma

Side-effects: gastro-intestinal disturbances; headache, rashes and pruritus reported

Dose: initially 16 mg 3 times daily, preferably with food; maintenance 24–48 mg daily; CHILD not recommended

PoM **Serc**® (Solvay)

Tablets, scored, betahistine hydrochloride 8 mg (Serc®-8), net price 120-tab pack = £10.04; 16 mg (Serc®-16), 84-tab pack = £18.03. Label: 21

4.7 Analgesics

4.7.1 Non-opioid analgesics
4.7.2 Opioid analgesics
4.7.3 Trigeminal neuralgia
4.7.4 Antimigraine drugs

For advice on pain relief in palliative care see Prescribing in Palliative Care, p. 12.

4.7.1 Non-opioid analgesics

The non-opioid drugs, paracetamol and aspirin (and other NSAIDs), are particularly suitable for pain in musculoskeletal conditions, whereas the opioid analgesics are more suitable for severe visceral pain.

Aspirin is indicated for headache, transient musculoskeletal pain, dysmenorrhoea and pyrexia. In inflammatory conditions, most physicians prefer anti-inflammatory treatment with another NSAID which may be better tolerated and more convenient for the patient. Aspirin is used increasingly for its antiplatelet properties (see section 2.9). Aspirin tablets or dispersible aspirin tablets are adequate for most purposes as they act rapidly.

Gastric irritation may be a problem; it is minimised by taking the dose after food. Enteric coated preparations are available, but have a slow onset of action and are therefore unsuitable for single-dose

analgesic use (though their prolonged action may be useful for night pain).

Aspirin interacts significantly with a number of other drugs and its interaction with warfarin is a **special hazard**, see **interactions:** Appendix 1 (aspirin).

Paracetamol is similar in efficacy to aspirin, but has no demonstrable anti-inflammatory activity; it is less irritant to the stomach and for that reason is now generally preferred to aspirin, particularly in the elderly. Overdosage with paracetamol is particularly dangerous as it may cause hepatic damage which is sometimes not apparent for 4 to 6 days. **Benorylate** is an aspirin–paracetamol ester.

Nefopam may have a place in the relief of persistent pain unresponsive to other non-opioid analgesics. It causes little or no respiratory depression, but sympathomimetic and antimuscarinic side-effects may be troublesome.

Anti-inflammatory analgesics (see section 10.1.1) are particularly useful for the treatment of patients with chronic disease accompanied by pain and inflammation. Some of them are also used in the short-term treatment of mild to moderate pain including transient musculoskeletal pain but paracetamol is now often preferred, particularly in the elderly (see section 10.1.1). They are also suitable for the relief of pain in *dysmenorrhoea* and to treat pain caused by *secondary bone tumours*, many of which produce lysis of bone and release prostaglandins (see Prescribing in Palliative Care, p. 12).

COMPOUND ANALGESIC PREPARATIONS

Compound analgesic preparations containing paracetamol or aspirin with a *low dose* of an opioid analgesic (e.g. 8 mg of codeine phosphate per compound tablet) are commonly used, but the advantages have not been substantiated. The low dose of the opioid may be enough to cause opioid side-effects (in particular, constipation) and can complicate the treatment of overdosage (see p. 22) yet may not provide significant additional relief of pain.

Compound analgesic preparations containing a *full dose* of the opioid component (e.g. 30 mg of codeine phosphate per compound tablet) carry the full range of opioid side-effects (including nausea, vomiting, severe constipation, drowsiness, respiratory depression, and risk of dependence on long-term administration). For details of the **side-effects, cautions** and **contra-indications** of opioid analgesics, see p. 194 (**important**: the elderly are particularly susceptible to opioid side-effects and should receive lower doses).

In general, when assessing pain, it is necessary to weigh up carefully whether there is a need for a non-opioid and an opioid analgesic to be taken simultaneously.

Caffeine is a weak stimulant that is often included, in small doses, in analgesic preparations. It is claimed that the addition of caffeine may enhance the analgesic effect, but the alerting effect, mild habit-forming effect and possible provocation of headache may not always be desirable. Moreover, in excessive dosage or on withdrawal caffeine may itself induce headache.

DYSMENORRHOEA

Use of an oral contraceptive prevents the pain of dysmenorrhoea which is generally associated with ovulatory cycles. If treatment is necessary paracetamol or an NSAID (see section 10.1.1) will generally provide adequate relief of pain. The vomiting and severe pain associated with dysmenorrhoea in women with endometriosis may call for an antiemetic (in addition to an analgesic). Antispasmodics (such as alverine citrate, see section 1.2) have been advocated for dysmenorrhoea but the antispasmodic action does not generally provide significant relief. Hyoscine butylbromide (see section 1.2) has also been advocated for its antispasmodic action despite the fact that its absorption following oral administration is extremely poor.

ASPIRIN

(Acetylsalicylic Acid)

Indications: mild to moderate pain, pyrexia (see notes above); see also section 10.1.1; antiplatelet, see section 2.9

Cautions: asthma, allergic disease, impaired renal or hepatic function (avoid if severe), dehydration, pregnancy; elderly; G6PD-deficiency (see section 9.1.5); **interactions:** Appendix 1 (aspirin)

Contra-indications: children under 12 years and in breast-feeding (Reye's syndrome, see below); gastro-intestinal ulceration, haemophilia; not for treatment of gout

HYPERSENSITIVITY. Aspirin and other NSAIDs are **contra-indicated** in patients with a history of hypersensitivity to aspirin or any other NSAID—*which includes those in whom attacks of asthma, angioedema, urticaria or rhinitis have been precipitated by aspirin or any other NSAID*

REYE'S SYNDROME. Owing to an association with Reye's syndrome the CSM has recommended that aspirin-containing preparations should no longer be given to children under the age of 12 years, unless specifically indicated, e.g. for juvenile arthritis (Still's disease). It is **important** to advise families that aspirin is not a suitable medicine for children with minor illness.

Side-effects: generally mild and infrequent but high incidence of gastro-intestinal irritation with slight asymptomatic blood loss, increased bleeding time, bronchospasm and skin reactions in hypersensitive patients. Prolonged administration, see section 10.1.1. Overdosage: see Emergency Treatment of Poisoning, p. 20

Dose: 300–900 mg every 4–6 hours when necessary; max. 4 g daily; CHILD not recommended (see notes above)

Aspirin (Non-proprietary)
Tablets, aspirin 300 mg. Net price 20 = 9p. Label: 21, 32
Available from most generic manufacturers

Dispersible tablets, aspirin 300 mg, net price 20 = 8p; 75 mg, see section 2.9. Label: 13, 21, 32
Available from most generic manufacturers
Note. BP directs that when no strength is stated the 300-mg strength should be dispensed, and that when soluble aspirin tablets are prescribed, dispersible aspirin tablets shall be dispensed.

Suppositories, aspirin 300 mg, net price 10 = £8.40. Label: 32
Dose: 2–3 suppositories inserted every 4 hours when necessary (max. 12 suppositories in 24 hours); CHILD not recommended (see above)
Available from Aurum (who also supply a 150-mg strength)

Caprin® (Sinclair)
Tablets, e/c, f/c, pink, aspirin 300 mg, net price 100-tab pack = £4.89; 75 mg, see section 2.9. Label: 5, 25, 32

Disprin CV®: see section 2.9

Nu-Seals® **Aspirin** (Lilly)
Tablets, e/c, aspirin 300 mg, net price 100-tab pack = £5.80; 75 mg, see section 2.9. Label: 5, 25, 32
Note. Aspirin enteric-coated also available from Ashbourne (postMI® 75)

With codeine phosphate 8 mg
Co-codaprin (Non-proprietary)
Tablets, co-codaprin 8/400 (codeine phosphate 8 mg, aspirin 400 mg). Net price 20 = 28p. Label: 21, 32
Dose: 1–2 tablets every 4–6 hours when necessary; max. 8 tablets daily
Dispersible tablets, co-codaprin 8/400 (codeine phosphate 8 mg, aspirin 400 mg). Net price 20 = 51p. Label: 13, 21, 32
Dose: 1–2 tablets in water every 4–6 hours; max. 8 tablets daily
Available from Cox
When co-codaprin tablets or dispersible tablets are prescribed and no strength is stated tablets, or dispersible tablets, respectively, containing codeine phosphate 8 mg and aspirin 400 mg should be dispensed

Other compound preparations
PoM **Aspav**® (Roussel)
Dispersible tablets, aspirin 500 mg, mixed opium alkaloids (anhydrous morphine (as morphine hydrochloride) 5 mg, papaverine hydrochloride 600 micrograms, codeine hydrochloride 520 micrograms). Net price 20 = £2.04. Label: 2, 13, 21, 32
Dose: 1–2 tablets in water every 4–6 hours if necessary; max. 8 tablets daily

NHS PoM **Doloxene Compound**® (Lilly)
Capsules, grey/red, dextropropoxyphene napsylate 100 mg, aspirin 375 mg, caffeine 30 mg. Net price 100-cap pack = £9.22. Label: 2, 21, 32
Dose: 1 capsule 3–4 times daily; max. 4 capsules daily

NHS CD **Equagesic**® (Wyeth)
Tablets, pink/white/yellow, ethoheptazine citrate 75 mg, meprobamate 150 mg, aspirin 250 mg. Net price 100-tab pack = £4.50. Label: 2, 21, 32
Dose: muscle pain, 1–2 tablets 3–4 times daily

NHS PoM **Robaxisal Forte**® (Shire)
Tablets, pink/white, scored, methocarbamol 400 mg, aspirin 325 mg. Net price 100-tab pack = £9.50. Label: 2, 21, 32
Dose: muscle pain, 2 tablets 4 times daily

Preparations on sale to the public
For a list of **preparations** containing aspirin and paracetamol **on sale to the public**, see p. 192.

PARACETAMOL

Indications: mild to moderate pain, pyrexia

Cautions: hepatic and renal impairment, alcohol dependence; **interactions:** Appendix 1 (paracetamol)

Side-effects: side-effects rare, but rashes, blood disorders; acute pancreatitis reported after prolonged use; **important:** liver damage (and less frequently renal damage) following overdosage, see Emergency Treatment of Poisoning, p. 20

Dose: by mouth, 0.5–1 g every 4–6 hours to a max. of 4 g daily; CHILD 2 months 60 mg for post-immunisation pyrexia; otherwise under 3 months (on doctor's advice only), 10 mg/kg (5 mg/kg if jaundiced); 3 months–1 year 60–120 mg, 1–5 years 120–250 mg, 6–12 years 250–500 mg; these doses may be repeated every 4–6 hours when necessary (max. of 4 doses in 24 hours)

For full Joint Committee on Vaccination and Immunisation recommendation on post-immunisation pyrexia, see section 14.1

Rectal route, see below

Paracetamol (Non-proprietary)

Tablets, paracetamol 500 mg. Net price 20 = 9p. Label: 29, 30

Available from APS, Cox, Evans, Norton, Sterling Health (NHS Panadol®)

Soluble Tablets (= Dispersible tablets), paracetamol 500 mg. Net price 60-tab pack = £2.26. Label: 13, 29, 30

Available from Sterling Health (NHS Panadol Soluble®)

Paediatric Soluble Tablets (= Paediatric dispersible tablets), paracetamol 120 mg. Net price 24-tab pack = 75p. Label: 13, 30

Available from R&C (NHS Disprol® Soluble Paracetamol)

Paediatric Oral Solution (= Paediatric Elixir), paracetamol 120 mg/5 mL. Net price 100 mL = 37p. Label: 30

Note. Sugar-free versions are available and can be ordered by specifying 'sugar-free' on the prescription.

Available from Berk, Evans, Norton, Rosemont (NHS Paldesic®), Wallace Mfg (NHS Salzone®)

Oral Suspension 120 mg/5 mL (= Paediatric Mixture), paracetamol 120 mg/5 mL. Net price 100 mL = 43p. Label: 30

Note. BP directs that when Paediatric Paracetamol Oral Suspension or Paediatric Paracetamol Mixture is prescribed Paracetamol Oral Suspension 120 mg/5 mL should be dispensed; sugar-free versions can be ordered by specifying 'sugar-free' on the prescription

Available from Cupal (Cupanol® Paediatric, sugar-free—now called Medinol® Paediatric), Norton, R&C (Disprol® Paediatric, sugar-free), Rosemont (Paldesic®), Sterling Health (Panadol®, sugar-free), Warner Wellcome (Calpol® Paediatric, Calpol® Paediatric sugar-free)

Oral Suspension 250 mg/5 mL (= Mixture), paracetamol 250 mg/5 mL. Net price 100 mL = 79p. Label: 30

Available from Cupal (NHS Cupanol® Over 6, sugar-free—now called Medinol® Over 6), Hillcross, Rosemont (Paldesic®), Warner Wellcome (NHS Calpol® 6 Plus)

Suppositories, paracetamol 125 mg, net price 10 = £11.50; 500 mg, 10 = £9.50. Label: 30

Dose: by rectum, ADULT and CHILD over 12 years 0.5–1 g up to 4 times daily; CHILD 1–5 years 125–250 mg, 6–12 years 250–500 mg

Available from Aurum (500 mg), Novex (Alvedon®, 125 mg)

Co-codamol 8/500

When co-codamol tablets, dispersible (or effervescent) tablets, or capsules are prescribed and **no strength is stated** tablets, dispersible (or effervescent) tablets, or capsules, respectively, containing codeine phosphate **8 mg** and paracetamol **500 mg** should be dispensed.

Co-codamol (Non-proprietary)

Tablets, co-codamol 8/500 (codeine phosphate 8 mg, paracetamol 500 mg) Net price 20 = 21p. Label: 29, 30

Dose: 1–2 tablets every 4–6 hours; max. 8 tablets daily; CHILD 6–12 years ½–1 tablet

Available from APS, Cox, CP, Galen, (NHS Parake®), Norton, Sterling Health (NHS Panadeine®)

Effervescent or dispersible tablets, co-codamol 8/500 (codeine phosphate 8 mg, paracetamol 500 mg). Net price 20 = 58p. Label: 13, 29, 30

Dose: 1–2 tablets in water every 4–6 hours, max. 8 tablets daily; CHILD 6–12 years ½–1 tablet, max 4 daily

Available from Roche Consumer Health (NHS Paracodol®), Sterwin

Note. The Drug Tariff allows tablets of co-codamol labelled 'dispersible' to be dispensed against an order for 'effervescent' and *vice versa*

Capsules, co-codamol 8/500 (codeine phosphate 8 mg, paracetamol 500 mg). Net price 30 = £2.14. Label: 29, 30

Dose: 1–2 capsules every 4 hours; max. 8 capsules daily

Available from Roche Consumer Health (NHS Paracodol®)

Co-codamol 30/500

When co-codamol tablets, dispersible (or effervescent) tablets, or capsules are prescribed and **no strength is stated** tablets, dispersible (or effervescent) tablets, or capsules, respectively, containing codeine phosphate **8 mg** and paracetamol **500 mg** should be dispensed (see preparations above).

See warnings and notes on p. 189 (**important:** special care in elderly—reduce dose)

PoM **Kapake®** (Galen)

Tablets, scored, co-codamol 30/500 (codeine phosphate 30 mg, paracetamol 500 mg). Net price 100-tab pack = £7.53. Label: 2, 29, 30

Dose: 1–2 tablets every 4 hours; max. 8 tablets daily; CHILD not recommended

PoM **Solpadol®** (Sanofi Winthrop)

Caplets (= tablets), co-codamol 30/500 (codeine phosphate 30 mg, paracetamol 500 mg). Net price 100-tab pack = £7.90. Label: 2, 29, 30

Dose: 2 tablets every 4 hours; max. 8 daily; CHILD not recommended

Effervescent tablets, co-codamol 30/500 (codeine phosphate 30 mg, paracetamol 500 mg). Contains 18.6 mmol Na+/tablet; avoid in *renal impairment.* Net price 100-tab pack = £9.50. Label: 2, 13, 29, 30

Dose: 2 tablets in water every 4 hours; max. 8 daily; CHILD not recommended

PoM **Tylex®** (Schwarz)

Capsules, co-codamol 30/500 (codeine phosphate 30 mg, paracetamol 500 mg). Net price 100-cap pack = £8.60. Label: 2, 29, 30

Dose: 1–2 capsules every 4 hours; max. 8 capsules daily; CHILD not recommended

Effervescent tablets, co-codamol 30/500 (codeine phosphate 30 mg, paracetamol 500 mg). Contains 13.6 mmol Na+/tablet; avoid in *renal impairment*. Net price 90-tab pack = £8.53. Label: 2, 13, 29, 30
Note. Contains aspartame 25 mg/tablet (see section 9.4.1)
Dose: 1–2 tablets in water every 4 hours; max. 8 tablets daily; CHILD not recommended

Co-methiamol
A mixture of methionine and paracetamol; methionine has no analgesic activity but may prevent paracetamol-induced liver toxicity if overdose taken

NHS **Pameton**® (SmithKline Beecham Healthcare)
Tablets, co-methiamol 250/500 (DL-methionine 250 mg, paracetamol 500 mg). Net price 60-tab pack = £3.02. Label: 29, 30
Dose: 2 tablets every 4–6 hours; max. 8 tablets daily; CHILD 6–12 years ½–1 tablet every 4–6 hours; max. 4 doses daily

Paradote® (Penn)
Tablets, f/c, co-methiamol 100/500 (DL-methionine 100 mg, paracetamol 500 mg). Net price 24-tab pack = £1.05, 96-tab pack = £2.64. Label: 29, 30
Dose: 2 tablets every 4–6 hours; max. 8 tablets daily

With dihydrocodeine tartrate 10 mg
See notes on p. 189

PoM **Co-dydramol** (Non-proprietary)
Tablets, scored, co-dydramol 10/500 (dihydrocodeine tartrate 10 mg, paracetamol 500 mg). Net price 20 = 27p. Label: 21, 29, 30
Dose: 1–2 tablets every 4–6 hours; max. 8 tablets daily; CHILD not recommended
Available from APS, Cox, CP, Galen (NHS Galake®), Norton, Sterwin
When co-dydramol tablets are prescribed and no strength is stated tablets containing dihydrocodeine tartrate 10 mg and paracetamol 500 mg should be dispensed.
Note. Tablets containing paracetamol 500 mg and dihydrocodeine 7.46 mg (NHS Paramol®) are on sale to the public. The name Paramol® was formerly applied to a brand of co-dydramol tablets

With dihydrocodeine tartrate 20 or 30 mg
See warnings and notes on p. 189 (**important**: special care in elderly—reduce dose)

PoM **Remedeine**® (Napp)
Tablets, paracetamol 500 mg, dihydrocodeine tartrate 20 mg. Net price 112-tab pack = £12.21. Label: 2, 21, 29, 30
Dose: 1–2 tablets every 4–6 hours; max. 8 tablets daily; CHILD not recommended
Effervescent tablets, paracetamol 500 mg, dihydrocodeine tartrate 20 mg. Contains 15.2 mmol Na+/tablet; avoid in *renal impairment*. Net price 56-tab pack = £7.39. Label: 2, 13, 21, 29, 30
Dose: 1–2 tablets every 4–6 hours; max. 8 tablets daily; CHILD not recommended
Forte tablets, paracetamol 500 mg, dihydrocodeine tartrate 30 mg. Net price 56-tab pack = £7.54. Label: 2, 21, 29, 30
Dose: 1–2 tablets every 4–6 hours; max. 8 tablets daily; CHILD not recommended
Forte effervescent tablets, paracetamol 500 mg, dihydrocodeine tartrate 30 mg. Contains 15.2 mmol Na+/tablet; avoid in *renal impairment*. Net price 56-tab pack = £9.15. Label: 2, 13, 21, 29, 30
Dose: 1–2 tablets every 4–6 hours; max. 8 tablets daily; CHILD not recommended

Other compound preparations
See warnings and notes on p. 189 (**important**: special care in elderly—reduce dose)

PoM **Co-proxamol** (Non-proprietary)
Tablets, co-proxamol 32.5/325 (dextropropoxyphene hydrochloride 32.5 mg, paracetamol 325 mg). Net price 20 = 25p. Label: 2, 10 patient information leaflet (if available), 29, 30
Dose: 2 tablets 3–4 times daily; max. 8 tablets daily CHILD not recommended
Available from APS, Berk, Cox (NHS Cosalgesic®), Dista (NHS Distalgesic®), Norton, Sterwin
When co-proxamol tablets are prescribed and no strength is stated tablets containing dextropropoxyphene hydrochloride 32.5 mg and paracetamol 325 mg should be dispensed.

NHS CD **Fortagesic**® (Sanofi Winthrop)
Tablets, pentazocine 15 mg (as hydrochloride), paracetamol 500 mg. Net price 100-tab pack = £7.00. Label: 2 21, 29, 30
Dose: 2 tablets up to 4 times daily; CHILD 7–12 years 1 tablet every 4 hours, max. 4 tablets daily

Preparations on Sale to the Public
The following is a list of preparations on sale to the public that contain **aspirin** or **paracetamol, alone** or with **other ingredients**. Other significant ingredients (such as codeine) are listed, but minor ingredients (such as caffeine) are not. For details of preparations containing ibuprofen or sale to the public, see section 10.1.1.
Important: in overdose contact **Poisons Information Services** (p. 18) for full details of the ingredients

Actron® (aspirin, paracetamol), **Alka-Seltzer**® (aspirin), **Anadin**® (aspirin, quinine), **Anadin Extra**®, **Anadin Extra Soluble**® (both aspirin, paracetamol), **Anadin Maximum Strength**® (aspirin), **Anadin Paracetamol**® (paracetamol), **Andrews Answer**® (paracetamol), **Angettes 75**® (aspirin), **Askit**® (aspirin, aloxiprin = polymeric product of aspirin), **Aspro**® (aspirin), **Aspro Clear**® (aspirin), **Aspro Paraclear Junior**®, **Aspro Paraclear**® (both paracetamol)
Barum Cold Relief with Decongestant® (paracetamol, phenylephrine), **Barum Extra Power Pain Reliever**® (aspirin, paracetamol), **Bayer Aspirin**® (aspirin), **Beechams-All-In-One**®, **Beechams Flu-Plus**®, **Beechams Hot Lemon**®, Hot Lemon and Honey®, Hot Blackcurrant® (all paracetamol, phenylephrine), **Beechams Powders**® (aspirin), **Beechams Powders Capsules**® With Decongestant (paracetamol, phenylephrine), **Beecham Aspirin**®, **Beechams Powders Tablets**® (both aspirin), **Benylin 4 Flu**® (paracetamol, diphenhydramine, pseudoephedrine), **Benylin Day and Night Cold and Flu Relief**® (*day tablets*, paracetamol, phenylpropanolamine, *night tablets*, paracetamol, diphenhydramine), **Boots Cold Relief Tablets**® (paracetamol, phenylephrine), **Boots Cold Relief for Children**®, **Boots Cold Relief Hot Blackcurrant**®, Hot Lemon® (paracetamol), **Boots Day Cold Comfort**® (paracetamol, pholcodine, pseudoephedrine), **Boots Headache and Indigestion Relief**® (paracetamol), **Boots Night-Cold Comfort**® (diphenhydramine, paracetamol, pholcodine, pseudoephedrine), **Boots Pain Relief Syrup for Children**® and **Boots Pain Relief Tablets**® (both paracetamol), **Boots Pain Relief Plus**® (codeine, paracetamol)
Cafadol® (paracetamol), **Calpol Extra For Adults**® (paracetamol, codeine), **Calpol Infant**®, **Calpol 6 Plus**®, **Calpol Paediatric**® (all paracetamol), **Caprin**® (aspirin), **Catarrh-Ex**® (paracetamol, pseudoephedrine), **Codamed**® (paracetamol, codeine), **Codanin**® (paracetamol, codeine), **Codis 500**® (aspirin, codeine), **Cold Relief Capsules (Thornton & Ross)** (paracetamol, phenylephrine), **Coldrex Blackcurrant Powders**®, Hot Lemon Powders®, and Tablets® (all paracetamol, phenylephrine), **Mrs. Cullen's**® (aspirin), **Cupanol Over 6**® **Cupanol Under 6**® (both paracetamol)

Day Nurse® (paracetamol, dextromethorphan, phenyl-propanolamine), **De Witt's Analgesic Pills**® (paracetamol), **Disprin**®, **Disprin CV**®, **Disprin Direct**® (all aspirin), **Disprin Extra**® (aspirin, paracetamol), **Disprol**®, **Disprol Soluble Paracetamol Suspension**®, **Disprol Soluble Paracetamol Tablets**®, **Disprol Paediatric**® (all paracetamol), **Doan's**® **Backache pills** (paracetamol, sodium salicylate), **Dristan Tablets**® (aspirin, chlorpheniramine, phenylephrine)

Elkamol® (paracetamol), **EP**® (paracetamol, codeine), **Fanalgic**® (paracetamol), **Femigraine**® (aspirin, cyclizine), **Feminax**® (paracetamol, codeine, hyoscine), **Fennings Children's Cooling Powders**® (paracetamol), **Flucaps**® (paracetamol, codeine), **Flurex Bedtime**® (paracetamol, diphenhydramine, pseudoephedrine), **Flurex Capsules and Tablets**® (paracetamol, phenylephrine), **Fynnon**® **Calcium Aspirin** (aspirin)

Hedex®, **Hedex Soluble**®, **Hedex Extra**® (all paracetamol), **Hedex Headcold**® (paracetamol, phenylephrine), **Hill's Balsam Flu Strength Hot Lemon Powders**® (paracetamol)

Infadrops® (paracetamol)

Lem-Plus Capsules® (paracetamol, phenylephrine), **Lem-Plus Powders**® (paracetamol), **Lemsip Cold Relief Capsules with Decongestant**, **Lemsip Cool Lemon**®, **Lemsip Flu Strength**®, **Lemsip Lemon**® or **Blackcurrant**®, **Lemsip Junior**®, **Lemsip Max Strength**®, **Lemsip Menthol Extra**® (all paracetamol, phenylephrine), **Lemsip Flu Strength Nightime**® (paracetamol, chlorpheniramine, dextromethorphan, phenylpropanolamine)

Maximum Strength Aspro Clear® (aspirin), **Medinol**® (paracetamol), **Medised**® (paracetamol, promethazine), **Medised Plain**®, **Medised 6+**® (both paracetamol), **Midrid**® (paracetamol, isometheptene mucate), **Migraleve**® (*pink tablets*, paracetamol, codeine, buclizine, *yellow tablets*, paracetamol, codeine), **Miradol**® (paracetamol), **Mu-Cron Tablets**® (paracetamol, phenylpropanolamine)

Night Nurse® (paracetamol, dextromethorphan, promethazine), **Numark Cold Relief Capsules**® **With Decongestant** (paracetamol, phenylephrine), **Numark Cold Relief Powders**® (paracetamol), **Nurse Sykes' Powders**® (aspirin, paracetamol), **Nu-Seals**® **Aspirin** (aspirin)

Paldesic® (paracetamol), **Pameton**® (paracetamol, methionine), **Panadeine**® (paracetamol, codeine), **Panadol**®, **Panadol Baby and Infant**®, **Panadol Extra**®, **Panadol Junior**® (all paracetamol), **Panadol Ultra**® (paracetamol, codeine), **Panaleve Junior**®, **Panaleve 6+**® (both paracetamol), **Panerel**® (paracetamol, codeine), **Paracets**® (paracetamol), **Paraclear Extra Strength**®, **Paraclear Junior**®, **Paraclear**® (all paracetamol), **Paracodol**® (paracetamol, codeine), **Paramin**® (paracetamol), **Paramol**® (paracetamol, dihydrocodeine), **Phensic**® (aspirin), **Placidex**® (paracetamol), **Platet**® (aspirin), **Powerin**® (aspirin, paracetamol), **Propain**® (paracetamol, codeine, diphenhydramine)

Resolve® (paracetamol), **Rimadol**® (paracetamol)

Salzone® (paracetamol), **Sinutab**® (paracetamol, phenylpropanolamine), **Sinutab Nightime**® (paracetamol, phenylpropanolamine, phenyltoloxamine), **Solpadeine**® (paracetamol, codeine), **SP Cold Relief Capsules**® (paracetamol, phenylephrine), **Sudafed-Co**® (paracetamol, pseudoephedrine), **Syndol**® (paracetamol, codeine, doxylamine)

Toptabs® (aspirin), **Tramil**® (paracetamol), **Triogesic**® (paracetamol, phenylpropanolamine)

Uniflu with Gregovite C® (paracetamol, codeine, diphenhydramine, phenylephrine)

Veganin® (aspirin, paracetamol, codeine), **Vicks**® **Coldcare** (paracetamol, dextromethorphan, phenylpropanolamine), **Vicks Medinite**® (paracetamol, dextromethorphan, doxylamine, ephedrine)

IBUPROFEN

Indications: fever and pain in children; see also section 10.1.1
Cautions; Contra-indications; Side-effects: see section 10.1.1

Dose: see section 10.1.1; CHILD, fever and pain, see below

Fever and pain in children
Junifen Sugar Free® (Crookes)
Suspension, sugar-free, ibuprofen 100 mg/5 mL, net price 150-mL pack = £2.37. Label: 21
   Dose: fever and pain in children, under 1 year not recommended, 1–12 years 20 mg/kg daily in divided doses *or* 1–2 years 2.5 mL 3–4 times daily, 3–7 years 5 mL, 8–12 years 10 mL
Other preparations: see section 10.1.1

KETOROLAC
See section 15.1.4.2

Other NSAIDs licensed for pain now appear in section 10.1.1. They include:

BENORYLATE	**FLURBIPROFEN**
DICLOFENAC	**KETOPROFEN**
SODIUM	**MEFENAMIC ACID**
DIFLUNISAL	**NAPROXEN**
FENOPROFEN	

NEFOPAM HYDROCHLORIDE
Indications: moderate pain
Cautions: hepatic or renal disease, elderly, urinary retention; pregnancy and breast-feeding; **interactions:** Appendix 1 (nefopam)
Contra-indications: convulsive disorders; not indicated for myocardial infarction
Side-effects: nausea, nervousness, urinary retention, dry mouth, lightheadedness; less frequently vomiting, blurred vision, drowsiness, sweating, insomnia, tachycardia, headache; confusion and hallucinations also reported; may colour urine (pink)
Dose: by mouth, initially 60 mg (elderly, 30 mg) 3 times daily, adjusted according to response; usual range 30–90 mg 3 times daily; CHILD not recommended
By intramuscular injection, 20 mg every 6 hours; CHILD not recommended
Note. Nefopam hydrochloride 20 mg by injection ≡ 60 mg by mouth

PoM Acupan® (3M)
Tablets, f/c, nefopam hydrochloride 30 mg. Net price 90-tab pack = £11.44. Label: 2, 14
Injection, nefopam hydrochloride 20 mg/mL. Net price 1-mL amp = 73p

4.7.2 Opioid analgesics
Opioid analgesics are used to relieve moderate to severe pain particularly of visceral origin. Repeated administration may cause dependence and tolerance, but this is no deterrent in the control of pain in terminal illness, for guidelines see Prescribing in Palliative Care, p. 12.

SIDE-EFFECTS. Opioid analgesics share many side-effects though qualitative and quantitative differences exist. The most common include nausea, vomiting, constipation, and drowsiness. Larger doses produce respiratory depression and hypotension. Overdosage, see Emergency Treatment of Poisoning, p. 22.

INTERACTIONS. See Appendix 1 (opioid analgesics) (**important**: special hazard with *pethidine and possibly other opioids* and MAOIs).

DRIVING. Drowsiness may affect performance of skilled tasks (e.g. driving); effects of alcohol enhanced.

CHOICE. **Morphine** remains the most valuable opioid analgesic for severe pain although it frequently causes nausea and vomiting. It is the standard against which other opioid analgesics are compared. In addition to relief of pain, morphine also confers a state of euphoria and mental detachment.

Morphine is the opioid of choice for the oral treatment of *severe pain in terminal care*. It is given regularly every 4 hours (or every 12 or 24 hours as modified-release preparations). For guidelines on dosage adjustment in palliative care, see p. 12.

Buprenorphine has both opioid agonist and antagonist properties and may precipitate withdrawal symptoms, including pain, in patients dependent on other opioids. It has abuse potential and may itself cause dependence. It has a much longer duration of action than morphine and sublingually is an effective analgesic for 6 to 8 hours. Vomiting may be a problem. Unlike most opioid analgesics its effects are only partially reversed by naloxone.

Codeine is effective for the relief of mild to moderate pain but is too constipating for long-term use.

Dextromoramide is less sedating than morphine and has a short duration of action.

Dipipanone used alone is less sedating than morphine but the only preparation available contains an anti-emetic and is therefore not suitable for regular regimens in palliative care (see p. 14).

Dextropropoxyphene given alone is a very mild analgesic somewhat less potent than codeine. Combinations of dextropropoxyphene with paracetamol (co-proxamol) or aspirin have little more analgesic effect than paracetamol or aspirin alone. An important disadvantage of co-proxamol is that overdosage (which may be combined with alcohol) is complicated by respiratory depression and acute heart failure due to the dextropropoxyphene and by hepatotoxicity due to the paracetamol. Rapid treatment is essential (see Emergency Treatment of Poisoning, p. 22).

Diamorphine (heroin) is a powerful opioid analgesic. It may cause less nausea and hypotension than morphine. In *palliative care* the greater solubility of diamorphine allows effective doses to be injected in smaller volumes and this is important in the emaciated patient.

Dihydrocodeine has an analgesic efficacy similar to that of codeine. The dose of dihydrocodeine by mouth is usually 30 mg every 4 hours; doubling the dose to 60 mg may provide some additional pain relief but this may be at the cost of more nausea and vomiting. A 40-mg tablet is now also available.

Fentanyl is used by injection for intra-operative analgesia (see section 15.1.4.3) and has been introduced recently in a transdermal drug delivery system as a self-adhesive patch which is changed every 72 hours.

Meptazinol is claimed to have a low incidence of respiratory depression. It has a reported length of action of 2 to 7 hours with onset within 15 minutes but there is an incidence of nausea and vomiting.

Methadone is less sedating than morphine and acts for longer periods. In prolonged use, methadone should not be administered more often than twice daily to avoid the risk of accumulation and opioid overdosage.

Nalbuphine has a similar efficacy to that of morphine for pain relief, but may have fewer side-effects and less abuse potential. Nausea and vomiting occur less than with other opioids but respiratory depression is similar to that with morphine.

Oxycodone is used as the pectinate in suppositories (special order from BCM Specials) for the control of *pain in palliative care*.

Pentazocine has both agonist and antagonist properties and precipitates withdrawal symptoms, including pain in patients dependent on other opioids. By injection it is more potent than dihydrocodeine or codeine, but hallucinations and thought disturbances may occur. It is not recommended and, in particular, should be avoided after myocardial infarction as it may increase pulmonary and aortic blood pressure as well as cardiac work.

Pethidine produces prompt but short-lasting analgesia; it is less constipating than morphine, but even in high doses is a less potent analgesic. It is not suitable for severe continuing pain. It is used for analgesia in labour, and in the neonate is associated with less respiratory depression than other opioid analgesics (probably because its action is weaker).

Phenazocine is effective in severe pain and has less tendency to increase biliary pressure than other opioid analgesics. It can be administered sublingually if nausea and vomiting are a problem.

Tramadol has been introduced recently and is claimed to produce analgesia by two mechanisms: an opioid effect and an enhancement of serotoninergic and adrenergic pathways. It is reported to have fewer of the typical opioid side-effects (notably, less respiratory depression, less constipation and less addiction potential); psychiatric reactions have been reported.

ADDICTS. Although caution is necessary addicts (and ex-addicts) may be treated with analgesics in the same way as other people when there is a real clinical need. Doctors are reminded that they do not require a special licence to prescribe opioid analgesics for addicts for relief of pain due to organic disease or injury.

MORPHINE SALTS

Indications: see notes above; acute pulmonary oedema; peri-operative analgesia see section 15.1.4.3

Cautions: hypotension, hypothyroidism, asthma (avoid during attack) and decreased respiratory reserve, prostatic hypertrophy; pregnancy and breast-feeding; may precipitate coma in hepatic impairment (reduce dose or avoid but many such patients tolerate morphine well); reduce dose or avoid in renal impairment (see also Appendix 3), elderly and debilitated (reduce dose); dependence (severe withdrawal symptoms if withdrawn abruptly); use of cough suppressants containing opioid analgesics not generally recommended in children and should be avoided altogether in those under at least 1 year; **interactions:** Appendix 1 (opioid analgesics)

PALLIATIVE CARE. In the control of pain in terminal illness these cautions should not necessarily be a deterrent to the use of opioid analgesics

Contra-indications: avoid in acute respiratory depression, acute alcoholism and where risk of paralytic ileus; not indicated for acute abdomen; also avoid in raised intracranial pressure or head injury (in addition to interfering with respiration, affect pupillary responses vital for neurological assessment); avoid injection in phaeochromocytoma (risk of pressor response to histamine release)

Side-effects: nausea and vomiting (particularly in initial stages), constipation, and drowsiness; larger doses produce respiratory depression and hypotension; other side-effects include difficulty with micturition, ureteric or biliary spasm, dry mouth, sweating, headache, facial flushing, vertigo, bradycardia, tachycardia, palpitations, postural hypotension, hypothermia, hallucinations, dysphoria, mood changes, dependence, miosis, decreased libido or potency, rashes, urticaria and pruritus; overdosage: see Emergency Treatment of Poisoning, p. 22

Dose: acute pain, *by subcutaneous or intramuscular injection,* 10 mg every 4 hours if necessary (15 mg for heavier well-muscled patients); CHILD up to 1 month 150 micrograms/kg, 1–12 months 200 micrograms/kg, 1–5 years 2.5–5 mg, 6–12 years 5–10 mg

By slow intravenous injection, quarter to half corresponding intramuscular dose

Patient controlled analgesia (PCA), consult hospital protocols

Myocardial infarction, *by slow intravenous injection* (2 mg/minute), 10 mg followed by a further 5–10 mg if necessary; elderly or frail patients, reduce dose by half

Acute pulmonary oedema, *by slow intravenous injection* (2 mg/minute) 5–10 mg

Chronic pain, *by mouth or by subcutaneous or intramuscular injection,* 5–20 mg regularly every 4 hours; dose may be increased according to needs; oral dose should be approximately double corresponding intramuscular dose and triple to quadruple corresponding intramuscular *diamorphine* dose (see also Prescribing in Palliative Care, p. 12); *by rectum,* as suppositories, 15–30 mg regularly every 4 hours

Note. The doses stated above refer equally to morphine hydrochloride, sulphate, and tartrate; see below for doses of **modified-release** preparations.

Oral solutions

Note. For advice on transfer from oral solutions of morphine to modified-release preparations of morphine, see Prescribing in Palliative Care, p. 12

PoM or CD Morphine Oral Solutions

Oral solutions of morphine can be prescribed by writing the formula:

Morphine hydrochloride 5 mg
Chloroform water to 5 mL

Note. The proportion of morphine hydrochloride may be altered when specified by the prescriber; if above 13 mg per 5 mL the solution becomes CD. For sample prescription see Controlled Drugs and Drug Dependence, p. 7. It is usual to adjust the strength so that the dose volume is 5 or 10 mL.

Oramorph® (Boehringer Ingelheim)

PoM *Oramorph® oral solution,* morphine sulphate 10 mg/5 mL. Net price 100-mL pack = £2.31; 250-mL pack = £5.36; 500-mL pack = £9.70. Label: 2

PoM *Oramorph® Unit Dose Vials 10 mg* (oral vials), sugar-free, morphine sulphate 10 mg/5-mL vial, net price 25 vials = £3.31. Label: 2

CD *Oramorph® Unit Dose Vials 30 mg* (oral vials), sugar-free, morphine sulphate 30 mg/5-mL vial, net price 25 vials = £9.30. Label: 2

CD *Oramorph® concentrated oral solution,* sugar-free, morphine sulphate 100 mg/5 mL. Net price 30-mL pack = £6.47; 120-mL pack = £24.15 (both with calibrated dropper). Label: 2

CD *Oramorph® Unit Dose Vials 100 mg* (oral vials), sugar-free, morphine sulphate 100 mg/5-mL vial, net price 25 vials = £31.00. Label: 2

Tablets

CD Sevredol® (Napp)

Tablets, all f/c, scored, morphine sulphate 10 mg (blue), net price 56-tab pack = £6.31; 20 mg (pink), 56-tab pack = £12.62; 50 mg (pale green), 56-tab pack = £31.55. Label: 2

Dose: severe pain uncontrolled by weaker opioid, 10–50 mg every 4 hours (dose adjusted according to need and tolerance); CHILD 3–5 years, 5 mg; 6–12 years, 5–10 mg

Modified release

CD MST Continus® (Napp)

Tablets, all m/r, f/c, morphine sulphate 5 mg (white), net price 60-tab pack = £4.50; 10 mg (brown), 60-tab pack = £7.51; 15 mg (green), 60-tab pack = £13.16; 30 mg (purple), 60-tab pack = £18.03; 60 mg (orange), 60-tab pack = £35.16; 100 mg (grey), 60-tab pack = £55.67; 200 mg (green), 60-tab pack = £111.35. Label: 2, 25

Suspension (= sachet of granules to mix with water), m/r, pink, morphine sulphate 20 mg/sachet, net price 30-sachet pack = £28.60; 30 mg/sachet, 30-sachet pack = £29.72; 60 mg/sachet, 30-sachet pack = £59.44; 100 mg/sachet, 30-sachet pack = £99.07; 200 mg/sachet pack, 30-sachet pack = £198.14. Label: 2, 13

Dose: (suspension or tablets) severe pain uncontrolled by weaker opioids, 30 mg every 12 hours, increased to 60 mg every 12 hours when required, then further increments of 25–50% if necessary. For lower initial doses in patients who have not received other opioids, see Prescribing in Palliative Care, p. 12

CHILD severe, intractable pain in cancer, initially 200–800 micrograms/kg every 12 hours, then further increments of 30–50% if necessary

Note. Prescriptions must also specify 'tablets' or 'suspension' (i.e. 'MST Continus tablets' or 'MST Continus suspension').

CD MXL® (Napp)

Capsules, m/r, morphine sulphate 30 mg (light blue), net price 30-cap pack = £13.16; 60 mg (brown), 30-cap pack = £18.03; 90 mg (pink), 30-cap pack = £26.59; 120 mg (green), 30-cap pack = £35.16; 150 mg (blue), 30-cap pack = £43.95; 200 mg (red-brown), 30-cap pack = £55.67. Label: 2, counselling, see below

Dose: prolonged severe pain uncontrolled by weaker opioids, 60 mg once daily increased in increments of 30–50% if necessary; in patients already receiving oral morphine substitute same total daily dose as MXL capsules once daily

CHILD severe, intractable pain in cancer, initially 0.4–1.6 mg/kg daily, then further increments of 30–50% if necessary

COUNSELLING. Swallow whole or open capsule and sprinkle contents on soft food

Note. Prescriptions must also specify 'capsules' (i.e. 'MXL capsules')

CD Oramorph® SR (Boehringer Ingelheim)

Tablets, all m/r, f/c, morphine sulphate 10 mg (buff), net price 60-tab pack = £5.75; 30 mg (violet), 60-tab pack = £13.80; 60 mg (orange), 60-tab pack = £26.89; 100 mg (grey), 60-tab pack = £42.59. Label: 2, 25

Dose: severe pain uncontrolled by weaker opioids, 30 mg every 12 hours, increased to 60 mg every 12 hours when required, then further increments of 25-50% if necessary. For lower initial doses in patients who have not received other opioids, see Prescribing in Palliative Care, p. 12

CHILD not recommended

Note. Prescriptions must also specify 'tablets' (i.e. 'Oramorph SR tablets')

Injections

CD Morphine Sulphate Injection, morphine sulphate 10, 15, 20, and 30 mg/mL, net price 1- and 2-mL amp (all) = 54–93p

CD Min-I-Jet® Morphine Sulphate (IMS)

Injection, morphine sulphate 10 mg/mL, net price 2-mL disposable syringe = £10.85

CD Morphine and Atropine Injection

See section 15.1.4.3

Injection with anti-emetic

CAUTION. In myocardial infarction cyclizine may aggravate severe heart failure and counteract the haemodynamic benefits of opioids, see section 4.6. **Not recommended** in palliative care, see p. 14

CD Cyclimorph® (Wellcome)

Cyclimorph-10® *Injection,* morphine tartrate 10 mg, cyclizine tartrate 50 mg/mL. Net price 1-mL amp = £1.28

Dose: by subcutaneous, intramuscular, or intravenous injection, 1 mL, repeated not more often than every 4 hours, with not more than 3 doses in any 24-hour period; CHILD 1–5 years 0.25–0.5 mL as a single dose, 6–12 years 0.5–1 mL as a single dose

Cyclimorph-15® *Injection,* morphine tartrate 15 mg, cyclizine tartrate 50 mg/mL. Net price 1-mL amp = £1.33

Dose: by subcutaneous, intramuscular, or intravenous injection, 1 mL, repeated not more often than every 4 hours, with not more than 3 doses in any 24-hour period

Suppositories

CD Morphine Suppositories, morphine hydrochloride or sulphate 15 mg, net price 12 = £5.71 30 mg, 12 = £8.35. Label: 2

Available from Evans, Martindale

Note. Both the strength of the suppositories and the morphine salt contained in them must be specified by the prescriber

Mixed opium alkaloids

Mixed opium alkaloids do not have any advantage over morphine alone; alcoholic solution of Nepenthe® was liable to evaporation and is **not** recommended—it has now been **discontinued**.

ALFENTANIL
See section 15.1.4.3

BUPRENORPHINE

Indications: moderate to severe pain; peri-operative analgesia, see section 15.1.4.3

Cautions; Contra-indications; Side-effects: see under Morphine Salts and notes above; can give rise to mild withdrawal symptoms in patients dependent on opioids; effects only partially reversed by naloxone; **interactions:** Appendix 1 (opioid analgesics)

Dose: by sublingual administration, initially 200–400 micrograms every 8 hours, increasing if necessary to 200–400 micrograms every 6–8 hours CHILD over 6 months, 16–25 kg, 100 micrograms 25–37.5 kg, 100–200 micrograms; 37.5–50 kg 200–300 micrograms

By intramuscular or slow intravenous injection 300–600 micrograms every 6–8 hours; CHILD over 6 months 3–6 micrograms/kg every 6–8 hours (max. 9 micrograms/kg)

CD Temgesic® (R&C)

Tablets (sublingual), buprenorphine (as hydrochloride), 200 micrograms, net price 50-tab pack = £6.00; 400 micrograms, 50-tab pack = £12.00 Label: 2, 26

Injection, buprenorphine 300 micrograms (as hydrochloride)/mL. Net price 1-mL amp = 55p

CODEINE PHOSPHATE

Indications: mild to moderate pain

Cautions; Contra-indications; Side-effects: see under Morphine Salts and notes above; use of cough suppressants containing codeine or similar opioid analgesics not generally recommended in children and should be avoided altogether in those under 1 year; **interactions:** Appendix 1 (opioid analgesics)

Dose: by mouth, 30–60 mg every 4 hours when necessary, to a max. of 240 mg daily; CHILD 1–12 years, 3 mg/kg daily in divided doses

By intramuscular injection, 30–60 mg every 4 hours when necessary

---

Codeine Phosphate (Non-proprietary)
PoM *Tablets*, codeine phosphate 15 mg, net price 20 = 35p; 30 mg, 20 = 38p; 60 mg, 20 = 97p. Label: 2
Note. As for schedule 2 controlled drugs, travellers needing to take codeine phosphate preparations abroad may require a doctor's letter explaining why they are necessary
PoM *Syrup*, codeine phosphate 25 mg/5 mL. Net price 100 mL = 85p. Label: 2
CD *Injection*, codeine phosphate 60 mg/mL. Net price 1-mL amp = £1.68
Codeine Linctuses
See section 3.9.1

Note. Codeine is an ingredient of some compound analgesic preparations, see sections 4.7.1 and 10.1.1 (Codafen Continus®)

DEXTROMORAMIDE

Indications: severe pain
Cautions; Contra-indications; Side-effects: see under Morphine Salts and notes above; only short duration of action (2–3 hours); avoid in obstetric analgesia (increased risk of neonatal depression); **interactions:** Appendix 1 (opioid analgesics)
Dose: by mouth, 5 mg increasing to 20 mg, when required
By rectum in suppositories, 10 mg when required

CD Palfium® (Boehringer Mannheim)
Tablets, both scored, dextromoramide (as tartrate) 5 mg, net price 60-tab pack = £4.66; 10 mg (peach), 60-tab pack = £9.21. Label: 2
Suppositories, dextromoramide 10 mg (as tartrate). Net price 10 = £2.29. Label: 2

DEXTROPROPOXYPHENE HYDROCHLORIDE

Indications: mild to moderate pain
Cautions; Contra-indications; Side-effects: see under Morphine Salts and notes above; occasional hepatotoxicity; porphyria (see section 9.8.2); compound preparations special hazard in overdose, see notes above; convulsions reported in overdose; contra-indicated in those who are suicidal or addiction prone; **interactions:** Appendix 1 (opioid analgesics)
Dose: 65 mg every 6–8 hours when necessary; CHILD not recommended
Note. 65 mg dextropropoxyphene hydrochloride ≡ 100 mg dextropropoxyphene napsylate

PoM **Dextropropoxyphene** (Non-proprietary)
Capsules, the equivalent of dextropropoxyphene hydrochloride 65 mg (as napsylate). Net price 20 = £1.64. Label: 2
Available from Lilly (NHS Doloxene®)
Note. Dextropropoxyphene is an ingredient of some compound analgesic preparations, see section 4.7.1

DIAMORPHINE HYDROCHLORIDE
(Heroin Hydrochloride)

Indications: see notes above; acute pulmonary oedema
Cautions; Contra-indications; Side-effects: see under Morphine Salts and notes above; **interactions:** Appendix 1 (opioid analgesics)

Dose: acute pain, *by subcutaneous or intramuscular injection*, 5 mg repeated every 4 hours if necessary (up to 10 mg for heavier well-muscled patients)
By slow intravenous injection, quarter to half corresponding intramuscular dose
Myocardial infarction, *by slow intravenous injection* (1 mg/minute), 5 mg followed by a further 2.5–5 mg if necessary; elderly or frail patients, reduce dose by half
Acute pulmonary oedema, *by slow intravenous injection* (1 mg/minute) 2.5–5 mg
Chronic pain, *by mouth or by subcutaneous or intramuscular injection*, 5–10 mg regularly every 4 hours; dose may be increased according to needs; intramuscular dose should be approximately half corresponding oral dose, and quarter to third corresponding oral *morphine* dose—see also Palliative Care, p. 15; *by subcutaneous infusion* (using syringe driver), see Palliative Care, p. 14

CD Diamorphine (Non-proprietary)
Tablets, diamorphine hydrochloride 10 mg. Net price 100-tab pack = £11.20. Label: 2
Available from Aurum
Injection, powder for reconstitution, diamorphine hydrochloride. Net price 5-mg amp = £1.16, 10-mg amp = £1.34, 30-mg amp = £1.60, 100-mg amp = £4.42, 500-mg amp = £20.68
Available from Berk (Diagesil®), CP, Evans, Hillcross
CD Diamorphine Linctus
See section 3.9.1

DIHYDROCODEINE TARTRATE

Indications: moderate to severe pain
Cautions; Contra-indications; Side-effects: see under Morphine Salts and notes above
Dose: by mouth, 30 mg every 4–6 hours when necessary (see also notes above); CHILD over 4 years 0.5–1 mg/kg every 4–6 hours
By deep subcutaneous or intramuscular injection, up to 50 mg repeated every 4–6 hours if necessary; CHILD over 4 years 0.5–1 mg/kg every 4–6 hours

Dihydrocodeine (Non-proprietary)
PoM *Tablets*, dihydrocodeine tartrate 30 mg. Net price 20 = 48p. Label: 2, 21
Available from most generic manufacturers
PoM *Elixir*, dihydrocodeine tartrate 10 mg/5 mL. Net price 150 mL = £2.40. Label: 2, 21
Available from Napp
CD *Injection*, dihydrocodeine tartrate 50 mg/mL. Net price 1-mL amp = £1.43
Available from Aurum, Napp (DF 118®)
Note. The brand name DF118® was formerly used for tablets of dihydrocodeine tartrate 30 mg
PoM **DF 118 Forte®** (Napp)
Tablets, dihydrocodeine tartrate 40 mg. Net price 100-tab pack = £12.05. Label: 2, 21
Dose: severe pain, 40–80 mg 3 times daily; max. 240 mg daily; CHILD not recommended

---

Cautionary label wordings, see inside back cover

Modified release

PoM **DHC Continus®** (Napp)

Tablets, m/r, dihydrocodeine tartrate 60 mg, net price 56-tab pack = £6.58; 90 mg, 56-tab pack = £10.36; 120 mg, 56-tab pack = £13.83. Label: 2, 25

Dose: chronic severe pain, 60–120 mg every 12 hours; CHILD not recommended

Note. Dihydrocodeine is an ingredient of some compound analgesic preparations, see section 4.7.1

DIPHENOXYLATE

See Co-phenotrope, section 1.4.2

DIPIPANONE HYDROCHLORIDE

Indications: moderate to severe pain

Cautions; Contra-indications; Side-effects: see under Morphine Salts and notes above; **interactions:** Appendix 1 (opioid analgesics)

CD Diconal® (Wellcome)

Tablets, pink, scored, dipipanone hydrochloride 10 mg, cyclizine hydrochloride 30 mg. Net price 50-tab pack = £7.59. Label: 2

Dose: 1 tablet gradually increased to 3 tablets every 6 hours; CHILD not recommended

CAUTION. **Not recommended** in palliative care, see p. 14

FENTANYL

Indications: chronic intractable pain due to cancer, see below; other indications, see section 15.1.4.3

Cautions; Contra-indications; Side-effects: see under Morphine Salts and notes above; local reactions such as rash, erythema and itching reported; **interactions:** Appendix 1 (opioid analgesics)

FEVER OR EXTERNAL HEAT. Monitor patients for increased side-effects if fever present (increased absorption possible); avoid exposing application site to external heat (may also increase absorption)

Administration: see under preparation, below

LONG DURATION OF ACTION. In view of the long duration of action, patients who have experienced severe side-effects should be monitored for up to 24 hours after patch removal

▼ **CD Durogesic®** (Janssen)

Patches, self-adhesive, transparent, fentanyl, '25' patch (releasing approx. 25 micrograms/hour for 72 hours), net price 5 = £28.97; '50' patch (releasing approx. 50 micrograms/hour for 72 hours), 5 = £54.11; '75' patch (releasing approx. 75 micrograms/hour for 72 hours), 5 = £75.43; '100' patch (releasing approx. 100 micrograms/hour for 72 hours), 5 = £92.97. Label: 2

ADMINISTRATION: apply to dry, non-irritated, non-irradiated, non-hairy skin on torso or upper arm, removing after 72 hours and siting replacement patch on a different area (avoid using the same area for several days). Patients who have not previously received a strong opioid analgesic, initial dose, one '25 micrograms/hour' patch replaced after 72 hours; patients who have received a strong opioid analgesic, initial dose based on previous 24-hour opioid requirement (oral morphine sulphate 90 mg over 24 hours ≈ one '25 micrograms/hour' patch, see data sheet for details); CHILD not recommended

Note. When starting to use Durogesic® initial evaluation of the analgesic effect should **not** be made before the system has been worn for **24 hours** (to allow for the gradual increase in plasma-fentanyl concentration)—previous analgesic therapy should be phased out gradually from time of first patch application; dose adjustment should normally be carried out in 72-hour steps of '25 micrograms/hour'. More than one patch may be used at a time for doses greater than '100 micrograms/hour' (but applied at *same time* to avoid confusion)—consider additional or alternative analgesic therapy if dose required exceeds 300 micrograms/hour (**important:** it may take 17 hours or longer for the plasma-fentanyl concentration to decrease by 50%, therefore replacement opioid therapy should be initiated at a low dose, increasing gradually).

CD Sublimaze®

See section 15.1.4.3

MEPTAZINOL

Indications: moderate to severe pain, including postoperative and obstetric pain and renal colic; peri-operative analgesia, see section 15.1.4.3

Cautions; Contra-indications; Side-effects: see under Morphine Salts and notes above; effects only partially reversed by naloxone

Dose: by mouth, 200 mg every 3–6 hours as required; CHILD not recommended

By intramuscular injection, 75–100 mg every 2–4 hours if necessary; obstetric analgesia, 100–150 mg according to patient's weight (2 mg/kg); CHILD not recommended

By slow intravenous injection, 50–100 mg every 2–4 hours if necessary; CHILD not recommended

PoM **Meptid®** (Monmouth)

Tablets, orange, f/c, meptazinol 200 mg. Net price 20 = £4.39. Label: 2

Injection, meptazinol 100 mg (as hydrochloride)/mL. Net price 1-mL amp = £1.92

METHADONE HYDROCHLORIDE

Indications: severe pain, see notes above; adjunct in treatment of opioid dependence, section 4.10

Cautions; Contra-indications; Side-effects: see under Morphine Salts and notes above; **interactions:** Appendix 1 (opioid analgesics)

Dose: by mouth or by subcutaneous or intramuscular injection, 5–10 mg every 6–8 hours, adjusted according to response; CHILD not recommended

CD Methadone (Non-proprietary)

Tablets, scored, methadone hydrochloride 5 mg. Net price 50 = £3.11. Label: 2

Available from Wellcome (Physeptone®)

Injection, methadone hydrochloride, 10 mg/mL, net price 1-mL amp = 86p, 2-mL amp = £1.63, 3.5-mL amp = £1.88, 5-mL amp = £2.02

Available from CP, Martindale, Wellcome (Physeptone®)

Linctus, see section 3.9.1

Mixture 1 mg/mL, section 4.10

NALBUPHINE HYDROCHLORIDE

Indications: moderate to severe pain; peri-operative analgesia, see section 15.1.4.3

Cautions; Contra-indications; Side-effects: see under Morphine Salts and notes above; **interactions:** Appendix 1 (opioid analgesics)

Dose: by subcutaneous, intramuscular, or intravenous injection, 10–20 mg for 70 kg patient every 3–6 hours, adjusted as required; CHILD up to 300 micrograms/kg repeated once or twice as necessary

Myocardial infarction, *by slow intravenous injection,* 10–20 mg repeated after 30 minutes if necessary

PoM Nubain® (Du Pont)

Injection, nalbuphine hydrochloride 10 mg/mL. Net price 1-mL amp = 73p; 2-mL amp = £1.13

PAPAVERETUM

See section 15.1.4.3

PENTAZOCINE

Indications: moderate to severe pain, but see notes above

Cautions; Contra-indications; Side-effects: see under Morphine Salts and notes above; occasional hallucinations; avoid in patients dependent on opioids and in arterial or pulmonary hypertension and heart failure; porphyria (see section 9.8.2); **interactions:** Appendix 1 (opioid analgesics)

Dose: by mouth, pentazocine hydrochloride 50 mg every 3–4 hours preferably after food (range 25–100 mg); CHILD 6–12 years 25 mg

By subcutaneous, intramuscular, or intravenous injection, moderate pain, pentazocine 30 mg, severe pain 45–60 mg every 3–4 hours when necessary; CHILD over 1 year, *by subcutaneous or intramuscular injection,* up to 1 mg/kg, *by intravenous injection* up to 500 micrograms/kg

By rectum in suppositories, pentazocine 50 mg up to 4 times daily; CHILD not recommended

CD Pentazocine (Non-proprietary)

Capsules, pentazocine hydrochloride 50 mg. Net price 20 = £3.34. Label: 2, 21

Tablets, pentazocine hydrochloride 25 mg. Net price 20 = £1.54. Label: 2, 21

Injection, pentazocine 30 mg (as lactate)/mL. Net price 1-mL amp = £1.18; 2-mL amp = £2.26

Suppositories, pentazocine 50 mg (as lactate). Net price 20 = £14.02. Label: 2

Note. The brand name **NHS** Fortral® (Sanofi Winthrop) is used for all the above preparations of pentazocine

PETHIDINE HYDROCHLORIDE

Indications: moderate to severe pain, obstetric analgesia; peri-operative analgesia, see section 15.1.4.3

Cautions; Contra-indications; Side-effects: see under Morphine Salts and notes above; avoid in severe renal impairment; not suitable for severe continuing pain; convulsions reported in overdosage; **interactions:** Appendix 1 (opioid analgesics)

Dose: by mouth, 50–150 mg every 4 hours; CHILD 0.5–2 mg/kg

By subcutaneous or intramuscular injection, 25–100 mg, repeated after 4 hours; CHILD, *by intramuscular injection,* 0.5–2 mg/kg

By slow intravenous injection, 25–50 mg, repeated after 4 hours

Obstetric analgesia, *by subcutaneous or intramuscular injection,* 50–100 mg, repeated 1–3 hours later if necessary; max. 400 mg in 24 hours

CD Pethidine (Non-proprietary)

Tablets, pethidine hydrochloride 50 mg, net price 20 = £1.39. Label: 2

Available from Roche

Injection, pethidine hydrochloride 50 mg/mL. Net price 1-mL amp = 31p; 2-mL amp = 32p. 10 mg/mL see section 15.1.4.3

Various strengths available from Martindale, Roche

CD Pamergan P100® (Martindale)

Injection, pethidine hydrochloride 50 mg, promethazine hydrochloride 25 mg/mL. Net price 2-mL amp = 69p

Dose: by intramuscular injection, for obstetric analgesia, 1–2 mL every 4 hours if necessary; severe pain, 1–2 mL every 4–6 hours if necessary; premedication, see section 15.1.4.3

Note. Although usually given intramuscularly, may be given intravenously after dilution to at least 10 mL with water for injections

PHENAZOCINE HYDROBROMIDE

Indications: severe pain

Cautions; Contra-indications; Side-effects: see under Morphine Salts and notes above; **interactions:** Appendix 1 (opioid analgesics)

Dose: by mouth or sublingually, 5 mg every 4–6 hours when necessary; single doses may be increased to 20 mg; CHILD not recommended

CD Narphen® (Napp)

Tablets, phenazocine hydrobromide 5 mg. Net price 100-tab pack = £28.51. Label: 2

PHENOPERIDINE

See section 15.1.4.3

TRAMADOL HYDROCHLORIDE

Indications: moderate to severe pain

Cautions; Contra-indications; Side-effects: see under Morphine Salts and notes above; in addition to hypotension, hypertension also occasionally reported; anaphylaxis, hallucinations and confusion also reported; caution if history of epilepsy (convulsions reported, usually after rapid intravenous injection); avoid in pregnancy and breast-feeding; not suitable as substitute in opioid-dependent patients; **interactions:** Appendix 1 (opioid analgesics)

GENERAL ANAESTHESIA. Not recommended for analgesia during light planes of general anaesthesia (increased operative recall reported)

Dose: by mouth, 50–100 mg not more often than every 4 hours; total of more than 400 mg daily by mouth not usually required; CHILD not recommended

By intramuscular injection or by intravenous injection (over 2–3 minutes) *or by intravenous infusion*, 50–100 mg every 4–6 hours

Postoperative pain, 100 mg initially then 50 mg every 10–20 minutes if necessary during first hour to total max. 250 mg (including initial dose) in first hour, *then* 50–100 mg every 4–6 hours; max. 600 mg daily; CHILD not recommended

▼ PoM **Tramake**® (Galen)
Capsules, green/off-white, tramadol hydrochloride 50 mg. Net price 100-cap pack = £17.71. Label: 2
▼ PoM **Zydol**® (Searle)
Capsules, green/yellow, tramadol hydrochloride 50 mg. Net price 100-cap pack = £17.71. Label: 2
Injection, tramadol hydrochloride 50 mg/mL. Net price 2-mL amp = £1.30

Modified release
▼ PoM **Zydol SR**® (Searle)
Tablets, all m/r, f/c, tramadol hydrochloride 100 mg, net price 60-tab pack = £19.12; 150 mg (beige), 60-tab pack = £28.68; 200 mg (orange), 60-tab pack = £38.24. Label: 2, 25
Dose: 100 mg twice daily increased if necessary to 150–200 mg twice daily; total of more than 400 mg daily by mouth not usually required; CHILD not recommended

4.7.3　Trigeminal neuralgia

Carbamazepine (section 4.8.1), taken during the acute stages of trigeminal neuralgia, reduces the frequency and severity of attacks. It has no effect on other forms of headache. A dose of 100 mg once or twice a day should be given initially and the dose slowly increased until the best response is obtained; most patients require 200 mg 3–4 times daily but a few may require an increased total daily dosage of up to 1.6 g. Plasma concentrations should be monitored when high doses are given. Occasionally extreme dizziness is encountered which is a further reason for starting treatment with a small dose and increasing it slowly.

Some cases of trigeminal neuralgia respond to **phenytoin** [unlicensed indication] (section 4.8.1) given alone or in conjunction with carbamazepine. A combination of phenytoin and carbamazepine is only required in very refractory cases or in those unable to tolerate high doses of carbamazepine.

Although **tricyclic antidepressants** are not indicated for true trigeminal neuralgia they are more effective than carbamazepine in *post-herpetic neuralgia* and may also be useful in *oral and facial pain*, particularly if it is associated with depression.

4.7.4　Antimigraine drugs

4.7.4.1 Treatment of the acute migraine attack
4.7.4.2 Prophylaxis of migraine

4.7.4.1 TREATMENT OF THE ACUTE MIGRAINE ATTACK

Most migraine headaches respond to analgesics such as **aspirin** or **paracetamol** (section 4.7.1) but as peristalsis is often reduced during migraine attacks the medication may not be sufficiently well absorbed to be effective; dispersible or effervescent preparations should therefore preferably be used.

Ergotamine is used in patients with migraine that does not respond to analgesics; it should not be given in hemiplegic migraine. It relieves migraine headache by constricting cranial arteries but visual and other prodromal symptoms are not affected; vomiting may be made worse (but can be relieved by the addition of an anti-emetic).

The value of ergotamine is limited by difficulties in absorption and by its side-effects, particularly *nausea, vomiting, abdominal pain*, and *muscular cramps*. The recommended doses of ergotamine preparations should **not** be exceeded and treatment should **not** be repeated at intervals of less than 4 days.

In some patients repeated administration of ergotamine may cause *habituation*, and headache *may be provoked* by chronic overdosage or by sudden withdrawal. To avoid habituation the frequency of administration should be limited to **no more than** twice a month. It should **never** be prescribed prophylactically but in the management of cluster headache a low dose is occasionally given daily for 1 to 2 weeks [unlicensed indication].

There are various ergotamine preparations designed to improve absorption and best results are obtained when the dose is given early in an attack. An aerosol form (Medihaler-Ergotamine®) is acceptable to some patients. Sublingual ergotamine (Lingraine®) probably has no advantage over oral treatment.

Sumatriptan is a 5-HT$_1$ agonist; it appears to be of considerable value in the treatment of an acute attack but experience is relatively limited.

Anti-emetics (section 4.6), such as **metoclopramide** by mouth or, if vomiting is likely, by intramuscular injection, or the phenothiazine and antihistamine anti-emetics, relieve the nausea associated with migraine attacks. Domperidone or prochlorperazine may be given rectally if vomiting is a problem. Metoclopramide has the added advantage of promoting gastric emptying and normal peristalsis. A single dose should be given at the onset of symptoms. Oral analgesic preparations containing metoclopramide are available (**important:** for warnings relating to extrapyramidal effects particularly in children and young adults, see p. 186).

ANALGESICS
Section 4.7.1

ANALGESICS WITH ANTI-EMETICS

Migraleve® (Pfizer Consumer)
Tablets, all f/c, *pink tablets*, buclizine hydrochloride 6.25 mg, paracetamol 500 mg, codeine phosphate 8 mg; *yellow tablets*, paracetamol 500 mg, codeine phosphate 8 mg. Net price 48-tab Duopack (32 pink + 16 yellow) = £5.10; 48 pink = £5.56; 48 yellow = £4.70. Label: 2 (pink tablets), 17, 30
Dose: 2 pink tablets at onset of attack, or if it is imminent, then 2 yellow tablets every 4 hours if necessary; max. in 24 hours 2 pink and 6 yellow; CHILD 10–14 years, half adult dose

PoM Migravess® (Bayer)

Tablets, effervescent, scored, metoclopramide hydrochloride 5 mg, aspirin 325 mg. Net price 30-tab pack = £3.60. Label: 13, 17, 32

Forte tablets, effervescent, scored, metoclopramide hydrochloride 5 mg, aspirin 450 mg. Net price 30-tab pack = £4.94. Label: 13, 17, 32

Dose: tablets or Forte tablets, 2 dissolved in water at onset of attack then every 4 hours when necessary; max. 6 tablets in 24 hours; CHILD 12–15 years, half adult dose

IMPORTANT. Ingredients include metoclopramide which can cause **severe extrapyramidal effects**, particularly in children and young adults (for further details, see p. 186)

PoM Paramax® (Lorex)

Tablets, scored, paracetamol 500 mg, metoclopramide hydrochloride 5 mg. Net price 42-tab pack = £3.99. Label: 17, 30

Sachets, effervescent powder, sugar-free, the contents of 1 sachet = 1 tablet; to be dissolved in ¼ tumblerful of liquid before administration. Net price 42-sachet pack = £5.27. Label: 13, 17, 30

Dose: (tablets or sachets): 2 at onset of attack then every 4 hours when necessary to max. of 6 in 24 hours (young adult 15–19 years, over 60 kg, max. of 5 in 24 hours); ADOLESCENT and YOUNG ADULT 12–19 years, 30–59 kg, 1 at onset of attack then 1 every 4 hours when necessary to max. of 3 in 24 hours

IMPORTANT. Ingredients include metoclopramide which can cause **severe extrapyramidal effects**, particularly in children and young adults (for further details, see p. 186)

ERGOTAMINE TARTRATE

Indications: acute attacks of migraine and migraine variants unresponsive to analgesics

Cautions: risk of peripheral vasospasm (see advice below); elderly; should not be used for migraine prophylaxis; **interactions:** Appendix 1 (ergotamine) and under Sumatriptan (Cautions), below

PERIPHERAL VASOSPASM. Warn patient to stop treatment immediately if numbness or tingling of extremities develops and to contact doctor.

Contra-indications: peripheral vascular disease, coronary heart disease, obliterative vascular disease and Raynaud's syndrome, hepatic or renal impairment, sepsis, severe or inadequately controlled hypertension, hyperthyroidism, pregnancy and breast-feeding, porphyria (see section 9.8.2)

Side-effects: nausea, vomiting, vertigo, abdominal pain, diarrhoea, muscle cramps, and occasionally increased headache (see also notes above); precordial pain, myocardial ischaemia, rarely myocardial infarction; repeated high dosage may cause ergotism with gangrene and confusion; pleural and peritoneal fibrosis may occur with excessive use

Dose: see under preparations below

PoM Cafergot® (Sandoz)

Tablets, ergotamine tartrate 1 mg, caffeine 100 mg. Net price 2 × 50-tab pack = £4.46. Label: 18, counselling, dosage

Dose: 1–2 tablets at onset; max. 4 tablets in 24 hours; not to be repeated at intervals of less than 4 days; max. 8 tablets in one week (but see also notes above); CHILD not recommended

Suppositories, ergotamine tartrate 2 mg, caffeine 100 mg. Net price 30 = £4.87. Label: 18, counselling, dosage

Dose: 1 suppository at onset; max. 2 in 24 hours; not to be repeated at intervals of less than 4 days; max. 4 suppositories in one week (but see also notes above); CHILD not recommended

PoM Lingraine® (Sanofi Winthrop)

Tablets (for sublingual use), green, ergotamine tartrate 2 mg. Net price 12 = £7.43. Label: 18, 26, counselling, dosage

Dose: 1 tablet at onset repeated after 30–60 minutes if necessary; max. 3 tablets in 24 hours and 6 tablets in one week (but see also notes above); CHILD not recommended

PoM Medihaler-Ergotamine® (3M)

Aerosol inhalation (oral), ergotamine tartrate 360 micrograms/metered inhalation. Net price 75-dose unit = £3.06. Label: 18, counselling, dosage

Additives: include CFC propellants

Dose: 360 micrograms (1 puff) repeated if necessary after 5 minutes; max. 6 inhalations in 24 hours and 15 inhalations in one week (but see also notes above); CHILD under 10 years not recommended

PoM Migril® (Wellcome)

Tablets, scored, ergotamine tartrate 2 mg, cyclizine hydrochloride 50 mg, caffeine hydrate 100 mg. Net price 20 = £11.67. Label: 2, 18, counselling, dosage

Dose: 1 tablet at onset, followed after 30 minutes by ½–1 tablet, repeated every 30 minutes if necessary; max. 4 tablets per attack and 6 tablets in one week (but see also notes above); CHILD not recommended

ISOMETHEPTENE MUCATE

Indications: migraine attack

Cautions: cardiovascular disease, hepatic and renal impairment, diabetes mellitus, hyperthyroidism; **interactions:** Appendix 1 (sympathomimetics)

Contra-indications: glaucoma, severe cardiac, hepatic and renal impairment, severe hypertension, pregnancy and breast-feeding; porphyria (see section 9.8.2)

Side-effects: dizziness, circulatory disturbances, rashes, blood disorders also reported

Midrid® (Shire)

Capsules, red, isometheptene mucate 65 mg, paracetamol 325 mg. Net price 20 = £2.38. Label: 30, counselling, dosage

Dose: migraine, 2 capsules at onset of attack, followed by 1 capsule every hour if necessary; max. 5 capsules in 12 hours; CHILD not recommended

SUMATRIPTAN

Indications: acute treatment of migraine attacks; cluster headache (subcutaneous injection only)

Cautions: not for prophylaxis; conditions which predispose to coronary artery disease (exclude pre-existing cardiac disease); hepatic (see Appendix 2) or renal impairment; pregnancy and breast-feeding; see also notes above; recommended as monotherapy and should **not** be taken with other acute migraine therapies—should **not** be taken until 24 hours after stopping an ergotamine-containing preparation (conversely, ergotamine-containing preparations should **not** be taken until 6 hours after sumatriptan); avoid concomitant use with MAOIs (including moclobemide), selective serotonin re-uptake inhibitors (SSRIs) or lithium; other **interactions:** Appendix 1 (sumatriptan)

DRIVING. Drowsiness may affect performance of skilled tasks (e.g. driving)

Contra-indications: ischaemic heart disease; previous myocardial infarction; Prinzmetal's angina, coronary vasospasm; uncontrolled hypertension

CSM advice. Following reports of chest pain and tightness (coronary vasoconstriction) CSM has emphasised that sumatriptan should **not** be used in ischaemic heart disease or Prinzmetal's angina, and that use with ergotamine should be **avoided** (see also Cautions).

Side-effects: chest pain and tightness (may be intense, involve throat, and mimic angina pectoris—vasospasm may result in arrhythmia, ischaemia or myocardial infarction—discontinue until appropriate investigations and also consider possibility of anaphylaxis, see also CSM advice above; sensations of tingling, heat, heaviness, pressure, or tightness in any part of body; flushing, dizziness, feeling of weakness, paraesthesia; fatigue, drowsiness, altered liver function tests, transient increase in blood pressure, hypotension, bradycardia or tachycardia, seizures reported; nausea and vomiting also reported; anaphylaxis also reported; transient pain at injection site

Dose: *by mouth,* 100 mg (50 mg effective in some patients) as soon as possible after onset (patient not responding should not take second dose for same attack); dose may be repeated if migraine recurs; max. 300 mg in 24 hours

By subcutaneous injection using auto-injector, 6 mg as soon as possible after onset (patients not responding should not take second dose for same attack); dose may be repeated once after not less than 1 hour if symptoms recur; max. 12 mg in 24 hours

ELDERLY over 65 years and CHILD not recommended

IMPORTANT. **Not** for intravenous injection which may cause coronary vasospasm and angina

▼ PoM **Imigran®** (Glaxo)

Tablets, f/c, sumatriptan (as succinate) 50 mg, net price 6-tab pack = £29.70, 12-tab pack = £56.43; 100 mg, 3-tab pack = £24.00, 6-tab pack = £48.00. Label: 3, 10 patient information leaflet

Injection, sumatriptan (as succinate) 12 mg/mL (= 6 mg/0.5-mL syringe), net price, treatment pack (2 × 0.5-mL pre-filled syringes and auto-injector) = £41.14; refill pack (2 × 0.5-mL pre-filled syringes) = £39.14. Label: 3, 10 patient information leaflet

4.7.4.2 PROPHYLAXIS OF MIGRAINE

Where migraine attacks are frequent, search should be made for provocative factors such as stress or diet (chocolate, cheese, alcohol, etc.). Benzodiazepines should be avoided because of the risk of dependence. In patients with more than one attack a month, one of three main prophylactic agents may be tried: pizotifen, beta-blockers, or tricyclic antidepressants (even when the patient is not obviously depressed). Long-term treatment with any of these prophylactic drugs is undesirable; the need for continuing therapy should be reviewed at intervals of about 6 months. Oral contraceptives may precipitate or worsen migraine; patients reporting a sharp increase in frequency of migraine or focal features should be recommended alternative contraceptive measures.

Pizotifen is an antihistamine and serotonin antagonist structurally related to the tricyclic antidepressants. It affords good prophylaxis but may cause weight gain. To avoid undue drowsiness treatment may be started at 500 micrograms at night and gradually increased to 3 mg; it is rarely necessary to exceed this dose.

The **beta-blockers** propranolol, metoprolol, nadolol, and timolol (see section 2.4) are all effective. Propranolol is the most commonly used in an initial dose of 40 mg 2 to 3 times daily. Beta-blockers may also be given as a single daily dose of a long-acting preparation. The value of beta-blockers is limited by their contra-indications (see section 2.4) and by interaction with ergotamine (see Appendix 1, beta-blockers).

Tricyclic antidepressants (section 4.3.1) may usefully be prescribed in a dose, for example, of amitriptyline 10 mg at night, increasing to a maintenance dose of 50 to 75 mg at night.

There is some evidence that the **calcium-channel blockers** (see section 2.6.2), e.g. verapamil and nifedipine may be useful in migraine prophylaxis.

Cyproheptadine (see section 3.4.1), an antihistamine with serotonin-antagonist and calcium channel-blocking properties, may also be tried in refractory cases.

Clonidine (Dixarit®) is probably little better than placebo and may aggravate depression or produce insomnia. **Methysergide** has dangerous side-effects (retroperitoneal fibrosis and fibrosis of the heart valves and pleura); **important:** it should only be administered under hospital supervision.

PIZOTIFEN

Indications: prevention of vascular headache including classical migraine, common migraine, and cluster headache

Cautions: urinary retention; closed-angle glaucoma, renal impairment; pregnancy and breast-feeding; **interactions:** Appendix 1 (pizotifen)

DRIVING. Drowsiness may affect performance of skilled tasks (e.g. driving); effects of alcohol enhanced

Side-effects: antimuscarinic effects, drowsiness, increased appetite and weight gain; occasionally nausea, dizziness; CNS stimulation may occur in children

Dose: 1.5 mg at night *or* 500 micrograms 3 times daily (but see also notes above), adjusted according to response within the usual range 0.5–3 mg daily; max. single dose 3 mg, max. daily dose 4.5 mg; CHILD up to 1.5 mg daily in divided doses; max. single dose at night 1 mg

PoM **Sanomigran®** (Sandoz)

Tablets, both ivory-yellow, s/c, pizotifen (as hydrogen malate), 500 micrograms, net price 20 = £1.56; 1.5 mg, 28-tab pack = £7.78. Label: 2

Elixir, pizotifen 250 micrograms (as hydrogen malate)/5 mL. Net price 300-mL pack = £4.12. Label: 2

CLONIDINE HYDROCHLORIDE

Indications: prevention of recurrent migraine (but see notes above), vascular headache, menopausal flushing; hypertension, see section 2.5.2

Cautions: depressive illness, concurrent antihypertensive therapy; porphyria (see section 9.8.2); **interactions:** Appendix 1 (clonidine)

Side-effects: dry mouth, sedation, dizziness, nausea, nocturnal restlessness; occasionally rashes

Dose: 50 micrograms twice daily, increased after 2 weeks to 75 micrograms twice daily if necessary; CHILD not recommended

oM **Dixarit**® (Boehringer Ingelheim)
Tablets, blue, s/c, clonidine hydrochloride 25 micrograms. Net price 112-tab pack = £6.68
oM **Catapres**® (hypertension), see section 2.5.2

METHYSERGIDE

Indications: prevention of severe recurrent migraine and cluster headache in patients who are refractory to other treatment and whose lives are seriously disrupted (**important:** hospital supervision only, see notes above)

Cautions: history of peptic ulceration; avoid abrupt withdrawal of treatment; after 6 months withdraw (gradually over 2 to 3 weeks) for reassessment for at least 1 month (see also notes above)

Contra-indications: renal, hepatic, pulmonary, and cardiovascular disease, severe hypertension, collagen disease, cellulitis, urinary-tract disorders, cachectic or septic conditions, pregnancy, breast-feeding

Side-effects: nausea, vomiting, heartburn, abdominal discomfort, drowsiness, and dizziness occur frequently in initial treatment; mental and behavioural disturbances, insomnia, oedema, weight gain, rashes, loss of scalp hair, cramps, arterial spasm (including coronary artery spasm with angina and possible myocardial infarction), paraesthesias of extremities, postural hypotension, and tachycardia also occur; retroperitoneal and other abnormal fibrotic reactions may occur on prolonged administration, requiring immediate withdrawal of treatment

Dose: 1 mg at bedtime, gradually increased to 1–2 mg 2–3 times daily with food (see notes above); CHILD not recommended
Carcinoid syndrome, usual range, 12–20 mg daily (hospital supervision); CHILD not recommended

oM **Deseril**® (Sandoz)
Tablets, s/c, methysergide 1 mg (as maleate). Net price 50-tab pack = £4.47. Label: 2, 21

4.8 Antiepileptics

4.8.1 Control of epilepsy
4.8.2 Drugs used in status epilepticus
4.8.3 Febrile convulsions

4.8.1 Control of epilepsy

The object of treatment is to prevent the occurrence of seizures by maintaining an effective plasma concentration of the drug. Careful adjustment of doses is necessary, starting with low doses and increasing gradually until seizures are controlled or there are overdose effects.

The frequency of administration is often determined by the plasma half-life, and should be kept as low as possible to encourage better patient compliance. Most antiepileptics, when used in average dosage, may be given twice daily. Phenobarbitone and sometimes phenytoin, which have long half-lives, may often be given as a daily dose at bedtime. However, with large doses, some antiepileptics may need to be administered 3 times daily to avoid adverse effects associated with high peak plasma concentrations. Young children metabolise antiepileptics more rapidly than adults and therefore require more frequent doses and a higher amount per kilogram body-weight.

COMBINATION THERAPY. Therapy with several antiepileptic drugs concurrently should generally be avoided. Patients are best controlled with one antiepileptic. Combinations of drugs have been used on the grounds that their therapeutic effects are additive while their individual toxicity was reduced but there is no evidence for this. In fact, toxicity may be enhanced with combination therapy. A second drug should only be added to the regimen if seizures continue despite side-effects. The use of more than two antiepileptics is rarely justified. Another disadvantage of multiple therapy is that drug interactions occur between the various antiepileptics (see below). Moreover, it is illogical to combine primidone and phenobarbitone as the former is largely metabolised to phenobarbitone in the liver, which is responsible for most, if not all, of its antiepileptic action.

INTERACTIONS. Interactions between antiepileptics are complex and may enhance toxicity without a corresponding increase in antiepileptic effect. Interactions are usually caused by *hepatic enzyme induction* or *hepatic enzyme inhibition*; *displacement from protein binding sites* is not usually a problem. These interactions are highly variable and unpredictable. Plasma monitoring is therefore often advisable with combination therapy.

Interactions that occur between antiepileptics themselves are as follows:

Carbamazepine
often lowers plasma concentration of *clonazepam, lamotrigine, phenytoin (but may also raise), topiramate, and valproate*
sometimes lowers plasma concentration of *ethosuximide, and primidone (but tendency for corresponding increase in phenobarbitone level)*

Ethosuximide
sometimes raises plasma concentration of *phenytoin*

Lamotrigine
sometimes raises plasma concentration of *an active metabolite of carbamazepine*

Phenobarbitone *or* Primidone
often lowers plasma concentration of *carbamazepine, clonazepam, lamotrigine, phenytoin (but may also raise), and valproate*
sometimes lowers plasma concentration of *ethosuximide*

Phenytoin
often lowers plasma concentration of *clonazepam, carbamazepine, lamotrigine, topiramate, and valproate*
often raises plasma concentration of *phenobarbitone*
sometimes lowers plasma concentration of *ethosuximide, and primidone (by increasing conversion to phenobarbitone)*

Topiramate
sometimes raises plasma concentration of *phenytoin*

Valproate
often raises plasma concentration of *an active metabolite of carbamazepine,* and of *lamotrigine, phenobarbitone, and phenytoin* (but may also lower)
sometimes raises plasma concentration of *ethosuximide, and primidone* (and tendency for significant
increase in phenobarbitone level)

Vigabatrin
often lowers plasma concentration of *phenytoin*
sometimes lowers plasma concentration of *phenobarbitone, and primidone*

For other important interactions see **Appendix 1**,
and for FPA guidelines on enzyme-inducing antiepileptics and **oral contraceptives**, see section
7.3.1.

WITHDRAWAL. Abrupt withdrawal of antiepileptics,
particularly the barbiturates and benzodiazepines,
should be avoided, as this may precipitate severe
rebound seizures. Reduction in dosage should be
carried out in stages and, in the case of the barbiturates, the withdrawal process may take months. The
changeover from one antiepileptic drug regimen to
another should be made cautiously, withdrawing the
first drug only when the new regimen has been
largely established.

The decision to withdraw all antiepileptics from a
seizure-free patient, and its timing, is often difficult
and may depend on individual patient factors. Even
in patients who have been seizure-free for several
years, there is a significant risk of seizure recurrence on drug withdrawal.

DRIVING. Patients suffering from epilepsy may
drive a motor vehicle (but not a heavy goods or
public service vehicle) provided that they have had
a seizure-free period of one year or, if subject to
attacks only while asleep, have established a three-
year period of asleep attacks without awake attacks.
Patients affected by drowsiness should not drive or
operate machinery.

PREGNANCY AND BREAST-FEEDING. During
pregnancy, total plasma concentrations of antiepileptics (particularly of phenytoin) may fall, particularly in the later stages but free plasma
concentrations may remain the same (or even rise).
There is an increased risk of teratogenicity associated with the use of antiepileptic drugs (reduced if
treatment is limited to a single drug). In view of the
increased risk of neural tube and other defects associated, in particular, with **carbamazepine, phenytoin** and **valproate** women taking antiepileptic
drugs who *may become pregnant* should be
informed of the possible consequences. Those
who *wish to become pregnant* should be referred to
an appropriate specialist for advice. Women who
become pregnant should be **counselled** and offered
antenatal screening (alpha-fetoprotein measurement and a second trimester ultrasound scan).

To counteract the risk of neural tube defects adequate folate supplements are advised for women
before and during pregnancy; in the case of antiepileptics such as carbamazepine and phenytoin,
doses of folic acid of the order of 5 mg daily are
recommended.

In view of the risk of neonatal bleeding associated
with carbamazepine, phenobarbitone and phenytoin, prophylactic vitamin K_1 is recommended for
the mother before delivery (as well as for the
neonate).

Breast-feeding is acceptable with all antiepileptic drugs, taken in normal doses, with the possible
exception of the barbiturates and ethosuximide
and also some of the more recently introduced
ones, see also Prescribing during Breast-feeding
(Appendix 5).

PARTIAL SEIZURES WITH OR WITHOUT SECONDARY GENERALISATION

Carbamazepine and **phenytoin** are the drugs of
choice for secondary generalised tonic-clonic seizures and for partial (focal) seizures; controlled trials with **sodium valproate** suggest similar efficacy.
Phenobarbitone and primidone are also effective
but are likely to be more sedating. Second-line
drugs include clonazepam, clobazam, and acetazolamide. The newer drugs **gabapentin**, **lamotrigine**
and **vigabatrin** are now available where control is
difficult to obtain and are effective in partial seizures with or without secondary generalisation.
Partial epilepsy and secondarily generalised seizures are more difficult to control than tonic-clonic
seizures as part of a syndrome of primary generalised epilepsy.

GENERALISED SEIZURES

TONIC-CLONIC SEIZURES (GRAND MAL). The drugs
of choice for *tonic-clonic seizures* occurring as part
of a syndrome of *primary generalised epilepsy* are
carbamazepine, phenytoin, and **sodium valproate. Phenobarbitone** and **primidone** are also
effective but may be more sedating. There is evidence that both **lamotrigine** and **vigabatrin** are
also effective, where control is difficult to obtain.

ABSENCE SEIZURES (PETIT MAL). **Ethosuximide** and
sodium valproate are the drugs of choice in simple
absence seizures. Sodium valproate is also highly
effective in treating the tonic-clonic seizures which
may co-exist with absence seizures in primary generalised epilepsy.

MYOCLONIC SEIZURES. Myoclonic seizures (myoclonic jerks) occur in a variety of syndromes, and
response to treatment varies considerably. **Sodium
valproate** is the drug of choice and **clonazepam,
ethosuximide,** and other antiepileptic drugs may be
used. For reference to the adjunctive use of piracetam, see section 4.9.3.

ATYPICAL ABSENCE, ATONIC, AND TONIC SEIZURES.
These seizure types are usually seen in childhood,
in specific epileptic syndromes, or associated with
cerebral damage or mental retardation. They may
respond poorly to the traditional drugs. **Phenytoin,
sodium valproate, lamotrigine, clonazepam,
ethosuximide,** and **phenobarbitone** may be tried.
Second-line antiepileptic drugs that are occasionally helpful, include **acetazolamide** and **corticosteroids**.

CARBAMAZEPINE

Carbamazepine is a drug of choice for simple and complex partial seizures and for tonic-clonic seizures regardless of whether they are primary or secondary to a focal discharge. It has a wider therapeutic index than phenytoin and the relationship between dose and plasma concentration is linear, but monitoring of plasma concentrations may be helpful in determining optimum dosage. It has generally fewer side-effects than phenytoin or the barbiturates, but reversible blurring of vision, dizziness, and unsteadiness are dose-related, and may be dose-limiting. These side-effects may be reduced by altering the timing of medication; use of modified release tablets (Tegretol Retard®) also significantly lessens the incidence of dose-related side-effects. It is essential to initiate carbamazepine therapy at a low dose (100–200 mg daily) and build this up slowly with increments of 100–200 mg every two weeks.

CARBAMAZEPINE

Indications: all forms of epilepsy except absence seizures; trigeminal neuralgia (section 4.7.3); prophylaxis in manic-depressive illness (4.2.3)

Cautions: hepatic or renal impairment; cardiac disease (see also Contra-indications); skin reactions (see also Side-effects), history of haematological reactions to other drugs; manufacturer recommends blood counts and hepatic and renal function tests (but evidence of practical value unsatisfactory); glaucoma; pregnancy (**important:** see p. 204 and Appendix 4 (neural tube screening)), breast-feeding (see p. 204); avoid sudden withdrawal; **interactions:** see p. 203 and Appendix 1 (carbamazepine)

BLOOD, HEPATIC or SKIN DISORDERS. Patients or their carers should be told how to recognise signs of blood, liver, or skin disorders, and advised to seek immediate medical attention if symptoms such as fever, sore throat, rash, mouth ulcers, bruising, or bleeding develop. Leucopenia which is severe, progressive or associated with clinical symptoms requires withdrawal (if necessary under cover of suitable alternative).

Contra-indications: AV conduction abnormalities (unless paced); history of bone marrow depression, porphyria (see section 9.8.2)

Side-effects: nausea and vomiting, dizziness, drowsiness, headache, ataxia, confusion and agitation (elderly), visual disturbances (especially double vision and often associated with peak plasma concentrations); constipation or diarrhoea, anorexia; mild transient generalised erythematous rash may occur in a large number of patients (withdraw if worsens or is accompanied by other symptoms); leucopenia and other blood disorders (including thrombocytopenia, agranulocytosis and aplastic anaemia); other side-effects include cholestatic jaundice, hepatitis and acute renal failure, Stevens-Johnson syndrome, toxic epidermal necrolysis, alopecia, thromboembolism, arthralgia, fever, proteinuria, lymph node enlargement, cardiac conduction disturbances (sometimes arrhythmias), dyskinesias, paraesthesia, depression, impotence (and impaired fertility), gynaecomastia, galactorrhoea, aggression, activation of psychosis; photosensitivity, pulmonary hypersensitivity (with dyspnoea and pneumonitis), hyponatraemia and oedema also reported; suppositories may cause occasional rectal irritation

Dose: by mouth, epilepsy, initially, 100–200 mg 1–2 times daily, increased slowly (see notes above) to usual dose of 0.8–1.2 g daily in divided doses; in some cases 1.6–2 g daily may be needed; ELDERLY reduce initial dose; CHILD daily in divided doses, up to 1 year 100–200 mg, 1–5 years 200–400 mg, 5–10 years 400–600 mg, 10–15 years 0.6–1 g

By rectum, as suppositories, see below

Note. Plasma concentration for optimum response 4–12 mg/litre (20–50 micromol/litre)

PoM Carbamazepine (Non-proprietary)

Tablets, carbamazepine 100 mg, net price 20 = 58p; 200 mg, 20 = £1.07; 400 mg, 20 = £2.11. Label: 3, counselling, blood, hepatic or skin disorder symptoms (see above), driving (see notes above)

Available from APS, Cox, Generics, Hillcross, Norton (Epimaz®)

PoM Tegretol® (Geigy)

Tablets, all scored, carbamazepine 100 mg, net price 20 = 56p; 200 mg, 20 = £1.03; 400 mg, 56-tab pack = £5.90. Label: 3, counselling, blood, hepatic or skin disorder symptoms (see above), driving (see notes above)

Chewtabs, orange, carbamazepine 100 mg, net price 56-tab pack = £2.95; 200 mg, 56-tab pack = £5.49. Label: 3, 21, 24, counselling, blood, hepatic or skin disorder symptoms (see above), driving (see notes above)

Liquid, sugar-free, carbamazepine 100 mg/5 mL. Net price 300-mL pack = £5.72. Label: 3, counselling, blood, hepatic or skin disorder symptoms (see above), driving (see notes above)

Suppositories, carbamazepine 125 mg, net price 5 = £7.50; 250 mg, 5 = £10.00. Label: 3, counselling, blood, hepatic or skin disorder symptoms (see above), driving (see notes above)

Dose: epilepsy, for short-term use (max. 7 days) when oral therapy temporarily not possible; suppositories of 125 mg may be considered to be approximately equivalent in therapeutic effect to tablets of 100 mg but final adjustment should always depend on clinical response (plasma concentration monitoring recommended); max. by rectum 1 g daily in 4 divided doses

PoM Tegretol® Retard (Geigy)

Tablets, m/r, both scored, carbamazepine 200 mg (beige-orange), net price 100-tab pack = £8.61; 400 mg (brown-orange), 100-tab pack = £16.93. Label: 3, 25, counselling, blood, hepatic or skin disorder symptoms (see above), driving (see notes above)

Dose: epilepsy (ADULT and CHILD over 5 years), as above; trigeminal neuralgia, as section 4.7.3; total daily dose given in 2 divided doses

ETHOSUXIMIDE

Ethosuximide is the drug of choice in simple absence seizures; it may also be used in myoclonic seizures and in atypical absence, atonic, and tonic seizures.

ETHOSUXIMIDE

Indications: absence seizures

Cautions: see notes above; hepatic and renal impairment; manufacturer recommends blood counts and hepatic and renal function tests (but evidence of practical value unsatisfactory); pregnancy and breast-feeding (see notes above); avoid sudden withdrawal; porphyria (see section 9.8.2); **interactions:** Appendix 1 (ethosuximide)

BLOOD DISORDERS. Patients or their carers should be told how to recognise signs of blood disorders, and advised to seek immediate medical attention if symptoms such as fever, sore throat, mouth ulcers, bruising or bleeding develop

Side-effects: gastro-intestinal disturbances, weight loss, drowsiness, dizziness, ataxia, dyskinesia, hiccup, photophobia, headache, depression, and mild euphoria. Psychotic states, rashes, hepatic and renal changes (see Cautions), and haematological disorders such as agranulocytosis and aplastic anaemia occur rarely (blood counts required if signs or symptoms of infection); systemic lupus erythematosus and erythema multiforme (Stevens-Johnson syndrome) reported; other side-effects reported include gum hypertrophy, swelling of tongue, irritability, hyperactivity, sleep disturbances, night terrors, inability to concentrate, aggressiveness, increased libido, myopia, vaginal bleeding

Dose: ADULT and CHILD over 6 years initially, 500 mg daily, increased by 250 mg at intervals of 4–7 days to usual dose of 1–1.5 g daily; occasionally up to 2 g daily may be needed; CHILD up to 6 years initially 250 mg daily, increased gradually to usual dose of 20 mg/kg daily

Note. Plasma concentration for optimum response 40–100 mg/litre (300–700 micromol/litre)

PoM Emeside® (LAB)

Capsules, orange, ethosuximide 250 mg. Net price 112-cap pack = £10.35. Counselling, blood disorder symptoms (see above), driving (see notes above)

Syrup, black currant or orange, ethosuximide 250 mg/5 mL. Net price 200-mL pack = £5.57. Counselling, blood disorder symptoms (see above), driving (see notes above)

PoM Zarontin® (P-D)

Capsules, orange, ethosuximide 250 mg. Net price 50-cap pack = £4.03. Counselling, blood disorder symptoms (see above), driving (see notes above)

Syrup, red, ethosuximide 250 mg/5 mL. Net price 300-mL pack = £5.60. Counselling, blood disorder symptoms (see above), driving (see notes above)

LAMOTRIGINE

Lamotrigine is an antiepileptic for partial seizures and secondarily generalised tonic-clonic seizures.

LAMOTRIGINE

Indications: monotherapy of partial seizures and primary and secondarily generalised tonic-clonic seizures; adjunctive treatment of partial seizure and secondarily generalised tonic-clonic seizures

Cautions: closely monitor (including hepatic renal and clotting parameters) and consider withdrawal if rash, fever, influenza-like symptoms drowsiness, or worsening of seizure control develops, especially in first month of treatment (although causal relationship not established lamotrigine given with other antiepileptics has been associated with rapidly progressive illness with status epilepticus, multi-organ dysfunction disseminated intravascular coagulation and death); avoid abrupt withdrawal (taper off over 2 weeks or longer); renal impairment; pregnancy and breast-feeding; **interactions:** see p. 203 and Appendix 1 (lamotrigine)

Contra-indications: hepatic impairment

Side-effects: commonly rashes (see also Cautions)—fever, malaise, influenza-like symptoms, drowsiness and rarely hepatic dysfunction, lymphadenopathy, leucopenia, and thrombocytopenia reported in conjunction with rash; angioedema Stevens-Johnson syndrome, toxic epidermal necrolysis and photosensitivity also reported diplopia, blurred vision, dizziness, drowsiness insomnia, headache, ataxia, tiredness, gastrointestinal disturbances, irritability, aggression tremor, agitation, confusion; headache, nausea dizziness, diplopia and ataxia in patients also taking carbamazepine usually resolve when dose of either drug reduced

Dose: IMPORTANT. Do not confuse the different combinations

Monotherapy, initially 25 mg daily for 14 days then 50 mg daily for further 14 days; usual maintenance as monotherapy, 100–200 mg daily in 1–2 divided doses (up to 500 mg daily has been required); ELDERLY not recommended

Adjunctive therapy with valproate, initially 25 mg every other day for 14 days then 25 mg daily for further 14 days; usual maintenance with valproate, 100–200 mg daily in 1–2 divided doses ELDERLY not recommended

Adjunctive therapy without valproate, initially 50 mg daily for 14 days then 50 mg twice daily for further 14 days; usual maintenance without valproate 200–400 mg daily in 2 divided doses ELDERLY not recommended

CHILD under 12 years, *monotherapy,* not recommended

CHILD 2–12 years, *adjunctive therapy with valproate,* initially 200 micrograms/kg daily for 14 days then 500 micrograms/kg daily for further 14 days (those weighing less than 25 kg may receive 5 mg on alternate days for first 14 days); usual maintenance with valproate 1–5mg/kg daily in 1–2 divided doses

CHILD 2–12 years *adjunctive therapy without valproate,* initially 2 mg/kg daily in 2 divided doses for 14 days then 5 mg/kg daily in 2 divided doses for further 14 days; usual maintenance without valproate 5–15 mg/kg daily in 2 divided doses

---

▼ PoM **Lamictal**® (Wellcome)

Tablets, all yellow, lamotrigine 25 mg, net price 21-tab pack (*'Valproate Add-on therapy' Starter Pack*) = £7.49, 42-tab pack (*'Monotherapy' Starter Pack*) = £14.97, 56-tab pack = £19.97; 50 mg, 42-tab pack (*'Non-valproate Add-on therapy' Starter Pack*) = £25.46, 56-tab pack = £33.95; 100 mg, 56-tab pack = £58.57; 200 mg, 56-tab pack = £99.56. Counselling, driving (see notes above)

Dispersible tablets, lamotrigine 5 mg (scored), net price 28-tab pack = £7.96; 25 mg, 56-tab pack = £19.97; 100 mg, 56-tab pack = £58.57. Label: 13, counselling, driving (see notes above)

PHENOBARBITONE AND OTHER BARBITURATES

Phenobarbitone is effective for tonic and partial seizures but may be sedative in adults and cause behavioural disturbances and hyperkinesia in children. It may be tried for atypical absence, atonic, and tonic seizures. Rebound seizures may be a problem on withdrawal. Monitoring plasma concentrations is less useful than with other drugs because tolerance occurs. **Methylphenobarbitone** is largely converted to phenobarbitone in the liver and has no advantages. **Primidone** is largely converted to phenobarbitone and this is probably responsible for its antiepileptic action. A small starting dose of primidone (125 mg) is essential, and the drug should be introduced over several weeks.

PHENOBARBITONE
(Phenobarbital)

Indications: all forms of epilepsy except absence seizures; status epilepticus, section 4.8.2

Cautions: elderly, debilitated, children, impaired renal or hepatic function, respiratory depression (avoid if severe), pregnancy and breast-feeding (see notes above); avoid sudden withdrawal; see also notes above; avoid in porphyria (see section 9.8.2); **interactions:** see p. 203 and Appendix 1 (barbiturates and primidone)

Side-effects: drowsiness, lethargy, mental depression, ataxia and allergic skin reactions; paradoxical excitement, restlessness and confusion in the elderly and hyperkinesia in children; megaloblastic anaemia (may be treated with folic acid); overdosage: see Emergency Treatment of Poisoning, p. 23

Dose: by mouth, 60–180 mg at night; CHILD 5–8 mg/kg daily

By intramuscular or intravenous injection, 50–200 mg, repeated after 6 hours if necessary; max. 600 mg daily; dilute injection 1 in 10 with water for injections before intravenous administration; status epilepticus, section 4.8.2

Note. For therapeutic purposes phenobarbitone and phenobarbitone sodium may be considered equivalent in effect. Plasma concentration for optimum response 15–40 mg/litre (60–180 micromol/litre)

CD [1]**Phenobarbitone Tablets,** phenobarbitone 15 mg, net price 20 = 7p; 30 mg, 20 = 6p; 60 mg, 20 = 11p. Label: 2, counselling, driving (see notes above)

CD [1]**Phenobarbitone Elixir,** phenobarbitone 15 mg/5 mL in a suitable flavoured vehicle, containing alcohol 38%. Net price 100 mL = 52p. Label: 2, counselling, driving (see notes above)

Note. Some hospitals supply alcohol-free formulations

CD [1]**Phenobarbitone Injection,** phenobarbitone sodium 200 mg/mL in propylene glycol 90% and water for injections 10%. Net price 1-mL amp = 86p

Note. Must be diluted before intravenous administration (see under Dose)

Available from Rhône-Poulenc Rorer (CD [1]Gardenal Sodium®), Martindale; other strengths also available from Martindale.

1. See p. 7 for prescribing requirements for phenobarbitone

METHYLPHENOBARBITONE
(Methylphenobarbital)

Indications; Cautions; Side-effects: see under Phenobarbitone

Dose: 100–600 mg daily

CD **Prominal**® (Sanofi Winthrop)

Tablets, methylphenobarbitone 30 mg, net price 20 = 78p; 60 mg, 20 = £1.03; 200 mg, 20 = £2.20. Label: 2, counselling, driving (see notes above)

PRIMIDONE

Indications: all forms of epilepsy except absence seizures; essential tremor (section 4.9.3)

Cautions; Side-effects: see under Phenobarbitone. Drowsiness, ataxia, nausea, visual disturbances, and rashes, particularly at first, usually reversible on continued administration; **interactions:** see p. 203 and Appendix 1 (barbiturates and primidone)

Dose: epilepsy, initially, 125 mg daily at bedtime, increased by 125 mg every 3 days to 500 mg daily in 2 divided doses then increased by 250 mg every 3 days to a max. of 1.5 g daily in divided doses; CHILD under 2 years, 250–500 mg daily in 2 divided doses; 2–5 years, 500–750 mg daily in 2 divided doses; 6–9 years 0.75–1 g daily in 2 divided doses

Note. Monitor plasma concentrations of derived phenobarbitone. Optimum range as for phenobarbitone.

PoM **Mysoline**® (Zeneca)

Tablets, scored, primidone 250 mg. Net price 100-tab pack = £1.77. Label: 2, counselling, driving (see notes above)

Oral suspension, primidone 250 mg/5 mL. Net price 250-mL pack = £1.01. Label: 2, counselling, driving (see notes above)

PHENYTOIN

Phenytoin is effective in tonic-clonic and partial seizures. It has a narrow therapeutic index and the relationship between dose and plasma concentra-

---

tion is non-linear; small dosage increases in some patients may produce large rises in plasma concentrations with acute toxic side-effects. Monitoring of plasma concentration greatly assists dosage adjustment. A few missed doses or a small change in drug absorption may result in a marked change in plasma concentration.

Phenytoin may cause coarse facies, acne, hirsutism, and gingival hyperplasia and so may be particularly undesirable in adolescent patients.

PHENYTOIN

Indications: all forms of epilepsy except absence seizures; trigeminal neuralgia (see also section 4.7.3)

Cautions: hepatic impairment (reduce dose), pregnancy (**important:** see notes above and Appendix 4), breast-feeding (see notes above); avoid sudden withdrawal; manufacturer recommends blood counts (but evidence of practical value unsatisfactory); avoid in porphyria (see section 9.8.2); see also notes above; **interactions:** see p. 203 and Appendix 1 (phenytoin)

BLOOD, OR SKIN DISORDERS. Patients or their carers should be told how to recognise signs of blood, or skin disorders, and advised to seek immediate medical attention if symptoms such as fever, sore throat, rash, mouth ulcers, bruising, or bleeding develop. Leucopenia which is severe, progressive or associated with clinical symptoms requires withdrawal (if necessary under cover of suitable alternative)

Side-effects: nausea, vomiting, mental confusion, dizziness, headache, tremor, transient nervousness, insomnia occur commonly; rarely dyskinesias, peripheral neuropathy; ataxia, slurred speech, nystagmus and blurred vision are signs of overdosage; rashes (discontinue, if mild re-introduce cautiously but discontinue immediately if recurrence), coarse facies, acne and hirsutism, fever and hepatitis; lupus erythematosus, erythema multiforme (Stevens-Johnson syndrome), toxic epidermal necrolysis, polyarteritis nodosa; lymphadenopathy; gingival hypertrophy and tenderness; rarely haematological effects, including megaloblastic anaemia (may be treated with folic acid), leucopenia, thrombocytopenia, agranulocytosis, and aplastic anaemia; plasma calcium may be lowered (rickets and osteomalacia)

Dose: by mouth, initially 3–4 mg/kg daily *or* 150–300 mg daily (as a single dose *or* in two divided doses) increased gradually as necessary (plasma monitoring, see notes above); usual dose 300–400 mg daily; max. 600 mg daily; CHILD 5–8 mg/kg daily (in 1 or 2 doses)

*By intravenous injection—*section 4.8.2

Note. Plasma concentration for optimum response 10–20 mg/litre (40–80 micromol/litre)

COUNSELLING. Take preferably with or after food

PoM **Phenytoin** (Non-proprietary)

Capsules, phenytoin sodium 50 mg, net price 20 = 40p; 100 mg, 20 = 56p. Label: 27, counselling, administration, blood or skin disorder symptoms (see above), driving (see notes above)

Tablets, coated, phenytoin sodium 50 mg, net price 20 = 26p; 100 mg, 20 = 31p. Label: 27, counsel-

ling, administration, blood or skin disorder symptoms (see above), driving (see notes above)

Available from APS, Berk (Pentran®), Cox

Note. On the basis of single dose tests there are no clinically relevant differences in bioavailability between available phenytoin sodium tablets and capsules but some clinics prefer patients to remain on the same brand whenever possible

PoM **Epanutin**® (P-D)

Capsules, phenytoin sodium 25 mg (white/purple), net price 20 = 39p; 50 mg (white/pink), 20 = 40p; 100 mg (white/orange), 20 = 56p; 300 mg (white/green), 20 = £1.69. Label: 27, counselling, administration, blood or skin disorder symptoms (see above), driving (see notes above)

Infatabs® (= tablets, chewable), yellow, scored, phenytoin 50 mg. Net price 20 = £1.10. Label: 24, counselling, blood or skin disorder symptoms (see above), driving (see notes above)

Note. Contain phenytoin 50 mg (as against phenytoin sodium) therefore care is needed on changing to capsules or tablets containing phenytoin sodium

Suspension, red, phenytoin 30 mg/5 mL. Net price 100 mL = 71p. Counselling, administration, blood or skin disorder symptoms (see above), driving (see notes above)

Note. Suspension of phenytoin 90 mg in 15 mL may be considered to be approximately equivalent in therapeutic effect to capsules or tablets containing phenytoin sodium 100 mg, but nevertheless care is needed in making changes

---

VALPROATE

Sodium valproate is effective in controlling tonic-clonic seizures, particularly in primary generalised epilepsy. It is a drug of choice in primary generalised epilepsy, generalised absences and myoclonic seizures, and may be tried in atypical absence, atonic, and tonic seizures. Controlled trials in partial epilepsy suggest that it has similar efficacy to that of carbamazepine and phenytoin, but more evidence is awaited. Plasma concentrations are not a useful index of efficacy, therefore routine monitoring is unhelpful. The drug has widespread metabolic effects, and may have dose-related side-effects. There has been concern over severe hepatic or pancreatic toxicity, although these effects are rare.

SODIUM VALPROATE

Indications: all forms of epilepsy

Cautions: monitor liver function before therapy and during first 6 months especially in patients most at risk (see also below), ensure no undue potential for bleeding before starting and before major surgery; severe renal impairment; pregnancy (**important** see notes above and Appendix 4 (neural tube screening)); breast-feeding; systemic lupus erythematosus; may give false-positive urine tests for ketones; avoid sudden withdrawal; porphyria (see section 9.8.2); see also notes above; **interactions:** see p. 203 and Appendix 1 (valproate)

LIVER TOXICITY. Liver dysfunction (including fatal hepatic failure) has occurred in association with valproate (especially in children under 3 years of age and those with metabolic or degenerative disorders, organic brain disease or severe seizure disorders associated with mental retardation) usually in the first 6 months of therapy and usually involving multiple antiepileptic therapy (monotherapy preferred). Raised liver enzymes are not uncommon during valproate treatment and are usually transient but patients should be reassessed clinically and liver function (including prothrombin time) monitored until return to normal—an abnormally prolonged prothrombin time (particularly in association with other relevant abnormalities) requires discontinuation of treatment. Any concomitant use of salicylates should be stopped.

BLOOD OR HEPATIC DISORDERS. Patients or their carers should be told how to recognise signs of blood or liver disorders, and advised to seek immediate medical attention if symptoms develop (advice is given on patient information leaflet).

Contra-indications: active liver disease, family history of severe hepatic dysfunction

Side-effects: gastric irritation, nausea, ataxia and tremor; hyperammonaemia, increased appetite and weight gain; transient hair loss (regrowth may be curly), oedema, thrombocytopenia, and inhibition of platelet aggregation; impaired hepatic function leading rarely to fatal hepatic failure (see also under Cautions—withdraw treatment immediately if vomiting, anorexia, jaundice, drowsiness, or loss of seizure control occurs); rashes; sedation reported (rarely lethargy and confusion associated with too high an initial dose) and also increased alertness (occasionally aggression, hyperactivity and behavioural disturbances); rarely pancreatitis (measure plasma amylase in acute abdominal pain), leucopenia, red cell hypoplasia, fibrinogen reduction; irregular periods and amenorrhoea also reported, also gynaecomastia

Dose: by mouth, initially, 600 mg daily given in 2 divided doses, preferably after food, increasing by 200 mg/day at 3-day intervals to a max. of 2.5 g daily in divided doses, usual maintenance 1–2 g daily (20–30 mg/kg daily); CHILD up to 20 kg, initially 20 mg/kg daily in divided doses, may be increased provided plasma concentrations monitored (above 40 mg/kg daily also monitor clinical chemistry and haematological parameters); over 20 kg, initially 400 mg daily in divided doses increased until control (usually in range of 20–30 mg/kg daily); max. 35 mg/kg daily

By *intravenous injection* (over 3–5 minutes) or *by intravenous infusion*, continuation of valproate treatment when oral therapy not possible, same as current dose by oral route

Initiation of valproate therapy (when oral valproate not possible), *by intravenous injection* (over 3–5 minutes), 400–800 mg (up to 10 mg/kg) followed by *intravenous infusion* up to max. 2.5 g daily; CHILD, usually 20–30 mg/kg daily, may be increased provided plasma concentrations monitored (above 40 mg/kg daily also monitor clinical chemistry and haematological parameters)

PoM Sodium Valproate (Non-proprietary)

Tablets, e/c, sodium valproate 200 mg, net price 20 = £1.20; 500 mg, 20 = £3.01. Label: 5, 25, counselling, blood or hepatic disorder symptoms (see above), driving (see notes above)

Available from Cox, CP (Orlept®), Hillcross, Norton

Oral solution, sodium valproate 200 mg/5 mL. Net price 100 mL = £1.80. Counselling, blood or hepatic disorder symptoms (see above), driving (see notes above)

Available from CP, (Orlept®, sugar-free), Hillcross, Norton (sugar-free)

PoM Epilim® (Sanofi Winthrop)

Tablets (crushable), scored, sodium valproate 100 mg. Net price 20 = 78p. Counselling, blood or hepatic disorder symptoms (see above), driving (see notes above)

Note. Sodium valproate crushable tablets also available from Hillcross

Tablets, both e/c, lilac, sodium valproate 200 mg, net price 20 = £1.28; 500 mg, 20 = £3.21. Label: 5, 25, counselling, blood or hepatic disorder symptoms (see above), driving (see notes above)

Liquid, red, sugar-free, sodium valproate 200 mg/5 mL. Net price 300-mL pack = £5.89. Counselling, blood or hepatic disorder symptoms (see above), driving (see notes above)

Syrup, red, sodium valproate 200 mg/5 mL. Net price 300-mL pack = £5.89. Counselling, blood or hepatic disorder symptoms (see above), driving (see notes above)

PoM Epilim Chrono® (Sanofi Winthrop)

Tablets, m/r, all lilac, sodium valproate 200 mg (as sodium valproate and valproic acid), net price 100-tab pack = £7.70; 300 mg, 100-tab pack = £11.55; 500 mg, 100-tab pack = £19.25. Label: 25, counselling, blood or hepatic disorder symptoms (see above), driving (see notes above)

Dose: ADULT and CHILD over 20 kg, as above, total daily dose given in 1–2 divided doses

PoM Epilim® Intravenous (Sanofi Winthrop)

Injection, powder for reconstitution, sodium valproate. Net price 400-mg vial (with 4-mL amp water for injections) = £8.77

Valproic acid

PoM Convulex® (Pharmacia)

Capsules, e/c, valproic acid 150 mg, net price 100-cap pack = £3.85; 300 mg, 100-cap pack = £7.70; 500 mg, 100-cap pack = £12.83. Counselling, blood or hepatic disorder symptoms (see above), driving (see notes above)

Dose: ADULT and CHILD initially 15 mg/kg daily in 2–4 divided doses, gradually increasing in steps of 5–10 mg/kg up to 30 mg/kg daily

EQUIVALENCE TO SODIUM VALPROATE. Manufacturer advises that Convulex® has a 1:1 dose relationship with products containing sodium valproate, but nevertheless care is needed in making changes.

VIGABATRIN

Vigabatrin is effective for use in chronic epilepsy not satisfactorily controlled by other antiepileptics. It is useful in tonic-clonic and partial seizures but has prominent behavioural side-effects in some patients.

VIGABATRIN

Indications: epilepsy not satisfactorily controlled by other antiepileptics, monotherapy for management of infantile spasms (West's syndrome)

Cautions: renal impairment; elderly; closely monitor neurological function; avoid sudden withdrawal (taper off over 2–4 weeks); history of psychosis or behavioural problems; **interactions:** see p. 203 and Appendix 1 (vigabatrin)

Contra-indications: pregnancy (see Appendix 4) and breast-feeding

Side-effects: drowsiness (rarely marked sedation, stupor, and confusion with non-specific slow wave EEG), fatigue, dizziness, nervousness, irritability, agitation, depression, abnormal thinking, headache, nystagmus, ataxia, tremor, paraesthesia, impaired concentration; less commonly confusion, aggression, psychosis, mania, memory disturbance, visual disturbance (e.g. diplopia); also weight gain, oedema, gastro-intestinal disturbances, alopecia, rash, urticaria; excitation and agitation in children; occasional increase in seizure frequency (especially if myoclonic), decrease in liver enzymes, slight decrease in haemoglobin; visual field defect, photophobia and retinal disorders (e.g. peripheral retinal atrophy) also reported

Dose: with current antiepileptic therapy, initially 1 g daily in single or 2 divided doses then increased according to response in steps of 500 mg; usual range 2–4 g daily—above 4 g daily (max. 6 g daily) only in exceptional circumstances with close monitoring for adverse effects; CHILD initially 40 mg/kg daily increased according to response to 80–100 mg/kg daily; *or* body-weight 10–15 kg, 0.5–1 g daily; body-weight 15–30 kg, 1–1.5 g daily; body-weight 30–50 kg, 1.5–3 g daily; body-weight over 50 kg, 2–4 g daily Infantile spasms (West's syndrome), *monotherapy,* 60–100 mg/kg daily, adjusted according to response over 7 days; up to 150 mg/kg daily used with good tolerability

PoM Sabril® (Merrell)

Tablets, f/c, scored, vigabatrin 500 mg, net price 100-tab pack = £44.85. Label: 3, counselling, driving (see notes above)

Powder, sugar-free, vigabatrin 500 mg/sachet. Net price 50-sachet pack = £24.33. Label: 3, 13, counselling, driving (see notes above)

Note. The contents of a sachet should be dissolved in water or a soft drink immediately before taking

---

BENZODIAZEPINES

Clonazepam is occasionally used in tonic-clonic or partial seizures, but its sedative side-effects may be prominent. **Clobazam** may be used as adjunctive therapy in the treatment of epilepsy (section 4.1.2), but the effectiveness of these and other **benzodiazepines** may wane considerably after weeks or months of continuous therapy.

CLOBAZAM

Indications: adjunct in epilepsy; anxiety (short-term use)

Cautions; Contra-indications; Side-effects: see under Diazepam

Dose: epilepsy, 20–30 mg daily; max. 60 mg daily; CHILD over 3 years, not more than half adult dose Anxiety, 20–30 mg daily in divided doses or as a single dose at bedtime, increased in severe anxiety (in hospital patients) to a max. of 60 mg daily in divided doses; ELDERLY (or debilitated) 10–20 mg daily

NHS¹ PoM Clobazam (Non-proprietary)

Capsules, clobazam 10 mg. Net price 30-cap pack = £3.96. Label: 2 *or* 19, counselling, driving (see notes above)

1. Except for epilepsy and endorsed 'SLS' ('S2B' in Scotland)

Note. The brand name **NHS** Frisium® (Hoechst) is used for clobazam capsules

CLONAZEPAM

Indications: all forms of epilepsy; myoclonus; status epilepticus, section 4.8.2

Cautions: see notes above; respiratory disease; hepatic and renal impairment; elderly and debilitated; pregnancy and breast-feeding (see notes above); avoid sudden withdrawal; porphyria (see section 9.8.2); **interactions:** see p. 203 and Appendix 1 (clonazepam)

DRIVING. Drowsiness may affect the performance of skilled tasks (e.g. driving); effects of alcohol enhanced

Contra-indications: respiratory depression; acute pulmonary insufficiency

Side-effects: drowsiness, fatigue, dizziness, muscle hypotonia, coordination disturbances; hypersalivation in infants, paradoxical aggression, irritability and mental changes; rarely, blood disorders, abnormal liver-function tests; overdosage: see Emergency Treatment of Poisoning, p. 23

Dose: 1 mg (elderly, 500 micrograms), initially at night for 4 nights, increased over 2–4 weeks to a usual maintenance dose of 4–8 mg daily in divided doses; CHILD up to 1 year 250 micrograms increased as above to 0.5–1 mg, 1–5 years 250 micrograms increased to 1–3 mg, 5–12 years 500 micrograms increased to 3–6 mg

PoM Rivotril® (Roche)

Tablets, both scored, clonazepam 500 micrograms (beige), net price 20 = 88p; 2 mg, 20 = £1.18. Label: 2, counselling, driving (see notes above)

Injection, section 4.8.2

OTHER DRUGS

Acetazolamide, a carbonic anhydrase inhibitor, is a second-line drug for both tonic-clonic and partial seizures. It is occasionally helpful in atypical absence, atonic, and tonic seizures.

Piracetam (section 4.9.3) has been introduced recently as adjunctive treatment for myoclonus.

Gabapentin is a new antiepileptic which can be given as adjunctive therapy in partial epilepsy with or without secondary generalisation.

Topiramate is another new antiepileptic which can be given as adjunctive therapy in partial seizures with or without secondary generalisation.

ACETAZOLAMIDE

Indications: see notes above

Cautions; Side-effects: see section 11.6

Dose: 0.25–1 g daily in divided doses; CHILD 8–30 mg/kg daily; max. 750 mg daily

Preparations
See section 11.6

GABAPENTIN

Indications: adjunctive treatment of partial seizures with or without secondary generalisation not satisfactorily controlled with other antiepileptics

Cautions: avoid sudden withdrawal (taper off over at least 1 week); mixed seizure disorders that include absence seizures (which may be exacerbated); elderly (may need to reduce dose), renal impairment (reduce dose), false positive readings with some urinary protein tests; pregnancy and breast-feeding; **interactions:** Appendix 1 (gabapentin)

Side-effects: somnolence, dizziness, ataxia, fatigue, nystagmus, headache, tremor, diplopia, nausea and vomiting, rhinitis, amblyopia; also convulsions, pharyngitis, dysarthria, weight gain, dyspepsia, amnesia, nervousness, coughing

Dose: 300 mg on first day, then 300 mg twice daily on second day, then 300 mg 3 times daily on third day, then increased according to response to 1.2 g daily (in 3 equally divided doses); if necessary may be further increased in steps of 300 mg daily (in 3 divided doses) to max. 2.4 g daily, usual range 0.9–1.2 g daily; max. period between doses should not exceed 12 hours; CHILD not recommended

▼ PoM **Neurontin**® (P-D)

Capsules, gabapentin 100 mg (white), net price 100-cap pack = £22.86; 300 mg (yellow), 100-cap pack = £53.00; 400 mg (orange), 100-cap pack = £61.33. Label: 3, 5, counselling, driving (see notes above)

PIRACETAM

Section 4.9.3

TOPIRAMATE

Indications: adjunctive treatment of partial seizures with or without secondary generalisation not satisfactorily controlled with other antiepileptics

Cautions: avoid abrupt withdrawal; ensure adequate hydration (especially if predisposition to nephrolithiasis); pregnancy (see notes above); renal impairment; **interactions:** see p. 203 and Appendix 1 (topiramate)

Contra-indications: breast-feeding

Side-effects: ataxia, impaired concentration, confusion, dizziness, fatigue, paraesthesia, somnolence, abnormal thinking, agitation, emotional lability (with abnormal behaviour), depression; nephrolithiasis (see Cautions); also amnesia, anorexia, aphasia, diplopia, nausea, nystagmus, speech disorder, taste alteration, abnormal vision, weight loss

Dose: initially 100 mg daily as a single dose for a week (lower dose may be used) *then* increased to 200 mg daily in 2 divided doses for a further week, *further dose increments* of 200 mg daily should be made at weekly intervals; usual dose 200–600 mg daily in 2 divided doses; max. 800 mg daily; CHILD not recommended

▼ PoM **Topamax**® (Janssen-Cilag)

Tablets, f/c, topiramate 50 mg (light yellow), net price 60-tab pack = £36.17; 100 mg (yellow), 60-tab pack = £64.80; 200 mg (salmon), 60-tab pack £125.83. Label: 3, counselling, driving (see notes above)

4.8.2 Drugs used in status epilepticus

Major status epilepticus should be *treated initially* with intravenous **diazepam**, used with caution because of the risk of respiratory depression; in situations where facilities for resuscitation are not immediately available, *small doses* of diazepam can be given intravenously or the drug can be administered as a rectal solution. Absorption from intramuscular injection or from suppositories is too slow for treatment of status epilepticus. When diazepam is given intravenously there may be a high risk of venous thrombophlebitis which is minimised by using an emulsion (Diazemuls®). **Clonazepam** and **lorazepam** are also used; lorazepam has the advantage of a long duration of action.

To *prevent recurrence* **phenytoin sodium** may be given by slow intravenous injection, with ECG monitoring in a dose of 15 mg/kg at a rate of not more than 50 mg/minute (in adults) followed by the maintenance dosage. Intramuscular use of phenytoin is not recommended (absorption is slow and erratic). Alternatively, **phenobarbitone sodium** (section 4.8.1) can be given by intravenous injection in a dose of 15 mg/kg at a rate of not more than 100 mg/minute. Other drugs which can be tried include **chlormethiazole edisylate**, given by intravenous infusion. Chlormethiazole has a short half-life, and the rate of infusion can be titrated against the patient's clinical condition (see **cautions** on next page).

Paraldehyde also remains a valuable drug. Given rectally (or occasionally by deep intramuscular injection) it causes little respiratory depression and is therefore useful where facilities for resuscitation are poor.

If the above measures fail to control seizures, anaesthesia with **thiopentone** or **a non-barbiturate anaesthetic** should be instituted with full intensive care support.

DIAZEPAM

Indications: status epilepticus; convulsions due to poisoning (see Emergency Treatment of Poisoning); other indications, see sections 4.1.2, 10.2.2, 15.1.4.1

Cautions; Contra-indications; Side-effects: see section 4.1.2; hypotension and apnoea may occur; when given intravenously facilities for reversing respiratory depression with mechanical ventilation must be at hand (but see also notes above); intravenous infusion, see also below

SPECIAL CAUTIONS FOR INTRAVENOUS INFUSION. Intravenous infusion of diazepam is potentially hazardous (especially if prolonged), calling for close and constant observation and best carried out in specialist centres with intensive care facilities. Special cautions required on prolonged intravenous infusion are as for Chlormethiazole, see below

Dose: by intravenous injection, 10–20 mg at a rate of 0.5 mL (2.5 mg) per 30 seconds, repeated if necessary after 30–60 minutes; may be followed by *intravenous infusion* to max. 3 mg/kg over 24 hours; CHILD 200–300 micrograms/kg *or* 1 mg per year of age

By rectum as rectal solution, ADULT and CHILD over 3 years 10 mg; CHILD 1–3 years and ELDERLY 5 mg; repeat after 5 minutes if necessary

PoM Diazepam (Non-proprietary)
Injection (solution), diazepam 5 mg/mL. See Appendix 6. Net price 2-mL amp = 25p
Available from CP, Roche (Valium®)
Injection (emulsion), diazepam 5 mg/mL (0.5%). See Appendix 6. Net price 2-mL amp = 76p
Available from Dumex (Diazemuls®)
Rectal tubes (= rectal solution), diazepam 2 mg/mL. Net price 2.5-mL (5-mg) tube = £1.27; 4 mg/mL, 2.5-mL (10-mg) tube = £1.62
Available from CP (Diazepam Rectubes®), Dumex (Stesolid®), Lagap

Oral preparations, section 4.1.2

CLONAZEPAM

Indications: status epilepticus; other forms of epilepsy, and myoclonus, section 4.8.1
Cautions; Contra-indications; Side-effects: see section 4.8.1. Hypotension and apnoea may occur and resuscitation facilities must be available; intravenous infusion, see also below

SPECIAL CAUTIONS FOR INTRAVENOUS INFUSION. Intravenous infusion of clonazepam is potentially hazardous (especially if prolonged), calling for close and constant observation and best carried out in specialist centres with intensive care facilities. Special cautions required on prolonged intravenous infusion are as for Chlormethiazole, see below

Dose: by intravenous injection into a large vein (over 30 seconds) *or by intravenous infusion,* 1 mg, repeated if necessary; CHILD all ages, 500 micrograms

PoM Rivotril® (Roche)
Injection, clonazepam 1 mg/mL in solvent, for dilution with 1 mL water for injections immediately before injection or as described in Appendix 6. Net price 1-mL amp (with 1 mL water for injections) = 71p

Oral preparations, section 4.8.1

CHLORMETHIAZOLE
(Clomethiazole)

Indications: status epilepticus; other indications, see sections 4.1.1, 4.10, 15.1.4.1; eclampsia, see data sheet
Cautions: see section 4.10 for general cautions; resuscitation facilities must be available; maintain clear airway (risk of mechanical obstruction in deep sedation); *rapid infusion* to be given only under direct medical supervision (risk of apnoea and hypotension—special care in those susceptible to cerebral or cardiac complications, e.g. the elderly); during *continuous infusion* sleep induced may lapse into deep unconsciousness and patient must be kept under close and constant observation; *prolonged infusion* may lead to accumulation and delay recovery, may also cause electrolyte imbalance (infusion contains only Na+ 32 mmol/litre and no other electrolytes); **interactions:** Appendix 1 (anxiolytics and hypnotics)
LENNOX GASTAUT SYNDROME. Paradoxical worsening of epilepsy may occur in the Lennox Gastaut syndrome
Contra-indications: acute pulmonary insufficiency
Side-effects: nasal congestion and irritation (with sneezing), conjunctival irritation, headache; localised thrombophlebitis, tachycardia and transient fall in blood pressure (apnoea and hypotension on rapid infusion, see cautions); see also section 4.10
Dose: by intravenous infusion, as a 0.8% solution of chlormethiazole edisylate, initially 5–15 mL (40–120 mg)/minute up to a max. total dose of 40–100 mL (320–800 mg); may then be continued if necessary at a reduced rate according to response (see notes above); usual rate 0.5–1 mL (4–8 mg)/minute
CHILD initially 0.01 mL (80 micrograms)/kg/minute, then dose increased every 2–4 hours if necessary until seizures controlled or drowsiness occurs; if no seizure for 2 days dose gradually reduced every 4–6 hours (if seizures recur dose increased to previous level)
IMPORTANT. See cautions for intravenous infusion under Cautions (above)

PoM Heminevrin® (Astra)
Intravenous infusion 0.8%, chlormethiazole edisylate 8 mg/mL. Net price 500-mL bottle = £5.12

Oral preparations, section 4.10

LORAZEPAM

Indications: status epilepticus; other indications, section 4.1.2
Cautions; Contra-indications; Side-effects: see section 4.1.2; hypotension and apnoea may occur and resuscitation facilities must be available
Dose: by intravenous injection (into large vein), 4 mg; CHILD 2 mg

Preparations
Section 4.1.2

PARALDEHYDE

Indications: status epilepticus

Cautions: bronchopulmonary disease, hepatic impairment; avoid intramuscular injection near sciatic nerve (causes severe causalgia)

INTRAVENOUS INFUSION. Paraldehyde has been given by intravenous infusion (diluted in physiological saline) in specialist centres with intensive care facilities but this method of administration is no longer recommended

Side-effects: rashes; pain and sterile abscess after intramuscular injection; rectal irritation after enema

Dose: by deep intramuscular injection, as a single dose, 5–10 mL; usual max. 20 mL daily with not more than 5 mL at any one site; CHILD up to 3 months 0.5 mL, 3–6 months 1 mL, 6–12 months 1.5 mL, 1–2 years 2 mL, 3–5 years 3–4 mL, 6–12 years 5–6 mL

By intravenous infusion, formerly given in a dose of up to 4–5 mL diluted to a 4% solution with sodium chloride intravenous infusion 0.9%, but **no longer recommended**

By rectum, 5–10 mL, administered as a 10% enema in physiological saline (some centres mix paraldehyde with an equal volume of arachis (peanut) oil instead); CHILD as for intramuscular dose
Note. Do not use paraldehyde if it has a brownish colour or an odour of acetic acid. Avoid contact with rubber and plastics.

PoM Paraldehyde (Non-proprietary)
Injection, sterile paraldehyde 5-mL and 10-mL amp
Note. May temporarily be unavailable

PHENYTOIN SODIUM

Indications: status epilepticus; seizures in neurosurgery; arrhythmias, see section 2.3.2

Cautions: hypotension and heart failure; resuscitation facilities must be available; injection solutions alkaline (irritant to tissues); see also section 4.8.1; **interactions:** see p. 203 and Appendix 1 (phenytoin)

Contra-indications: sinus bradycardia, sino-atrial block, and second- and third-degree heart block; Stokes-Adams syndrome; porphyria (see section 9.8.2)

Side-effects: intravenous injection may cause cardiovascular and CNS depression (particularly if injection too rapid) with arrhythmias, hypotension, and cardiovascular collapse; alterations in respiratory function (including respiratory arrest)

Dose: by slow intravenous injection or infusion (with blood pressure and ECG monitoring), status epilepticus, 15 mg/kg, at a rate not exceeding 50 mg per minute, as a loading dose (see also notes above). Maintenance doses of about 100 mg should be given thereafter at intervals of every 6–8 hours, monitored by measurement of plasma concentrations; rate and dose reduced according to weight; CHILD 15 mg/kg as a loading dose (neonate 15–20 mg/kg at rate of 1–3 mg/kg/minute)
Note. Phenytoin is now also licensed for administration by intravenous infusion (at the same rate of administra-

tion as the injection—not exceeding 50 mg/minute, for further details of the infusion, see Appendix 6). To avoid local venous irritation each injection or infusion should be both preceded and followed by an injection of sterile physiological saline through the same needle or or catheter

By intramuscular injection, not recommended (see notes above)

PoM Epanutin Ready Mixed Parenteral® (P-D)
Injection, phenytoin sodium 50 mg/mL with propylene glycol 40% and alcohol 10% in water for injections. Net price 5-mL amp = £4.07
Note. Phenytoin injection also available from Antigen, David Bull

Oral preparations, section 4.8.1

4.8.3   Febrile convulsions

Brief febrile convulsions need only simple treatment such as tepid sponging or bathing, or antipyretic medication, e.g. **paracetamol** (section 4.7.1). *Prolonged febrile convulsions* (those lasting 15 minutes or longer), *recurrent convulsions,* or those occurring in a child at known risk must be treated more actively, as there is the possibility of resulting brain damage. **Diazepam** is the drug of choice given either by slow intravenous injection in a dose of 250 micrograms/kg (section 4.8.2) or preferably rectally in solution (section 4.8.2) in a dose of 500 micrograms/kg (max. 10 mg), repeated if necessary (for full details of dose, see p. 212). The rectal route is preferred as satisfactory absorption is achieved within minutes and administration is much easier. Suppositories are not suitable because absorption is too slow.

Intermittent prophylaxis (i.e. the anticonvulsant administered at the onset of fever) is possible in only a small proportion of children. Again **diazepam** is the treatment of choice, orally or rectally.

The exact role of continuous prophylaxis in children at risk from prolonged or complex febrile convulsions is controversial. It is probably indicated in only a small proportion of children, including those whose first seizure occurred at under 14 months or who have pre-existing neurological abnormalities or who have had previous prolonged or focal convulsions. Thus long-term anticonvulsant prophylaxis is rarely indicated.

4.9   Drugs used in parkinsonism and related disorders

In idiopathic Parkinson's disease, progressive degeneration of pigment-containing cells of the substantia nigra leads to deficiency of the neurotransmitter dopamine. This, in turn, results in a neurohumoral imbalance in the basal ganglia, causing the characteristic signs and symptoms of the illness to appear. The pathogenesis of this process is still obscure and current drug therapy aims simply to correct the imbalance. Although this approach fails to prevent the progression of the disease, it greatly improves the quality and expectancy of life of most patients.

The patient should be advised at the outset of the limitations of treatment and possible side-effects. About 10 to 20% of patients are unresponsive to treatment.

ELDERLY. Antiparkinsonian drugs carry a special risk of inducing confusion in the elderly. It is particularly important to initiate treatment with low doses and to use small increments.

4.9.1   Dopaminergic drugs used in parkinsonism

Levodopa, used with a **dopa-decarboxylase inhibitor**, is the treatment of choice for patients disabled by idiopathic Parkinson's disease. It is least valuable in elderly patients and in those with long-standing disease who may not tolerate a dose large enough to overcome their deficit. It is also less valuable in patients with post-encephalitic disease who are particularly susceptible to the side-effects. Parkinsonism caused by generalised degenerative brain disease does not normally respond to levodopa. It should not be used for neuroleptic-induced parkinsonism.

Levodopa, the amino-acid precursor of dopamine, acts mainly by replenishing depleted striatal dopamine. It improves bradykinesia and rigidity more than tremor. It is generally administered in conjunction with an extracerebral dopa-decarboxylase inhibitor which prevents the peripheral degradation of levodopa to dopamine but, unlike levodopa, does not cross the blood-brain barrier. Effective brain concentrations of dopamine can thereby be achieved with lower doses of levodopa. At the same time the reduced peripheral formation of dopamine decreases peripheral side-effects such as nausea and vomiting and cardiovascular effects. There is also less delay in onset of therapeutic effect and a smoother clinical response. A disadvantage is an increased incidence of abnormal involuntary movements.

The extracerebral dopa-decarboxylase inhibitors given with levodopa are benserazide (in **co-beneldopa**) and carbidopa (in **co-careldopa**).

When co-careldopa 10/100 (10 mg of carbidopa for each 100 mg of levodopa) is used the dose of carbidopa may be insufficient to achieve full inhibition of extracerebral dopa-decarboxylase; co-careldopa 25/100 (25 mg of carbidopa for each 100 mg of levodopa) should then be used so that the daily dose of carbidopa is at least 75 mg.

Levodopa therapy should be initiated with low doses and gradually increased, by small increments, at intervals of 2 to 3 days. The final dose is usually a compromise between increased mobility and dose-limiting side-effects. Intervals between doses may be critical and should be chosen to suit the needs of the individual patient. Nausea and vomiting are rarely dose-limiting but doses should be taken after meals. Domperidone (section 4.6) may be useful in controlling vomiting. The most frequent dose-limiting side-effects of levodopa are involuntary movements and psychiatric complications. As the patient ages, the maintenance dose may need to be reduced.

During the first 6 to 18 months of levodopa therapy there may be a slow improvement in the response of the patient which is maintained for 1½ to 2 years; thereafter a slow decline may occur. Particularly troublesome is the 'on-off' effect the incidence of which increases as the treatment progresses. This is characterised by fluctuations in performance with normal performance during the 'on' period and weakness and akinesia lasting for 2 to 4 hours during the 'off' period.

'End-of-dose' deterioration may also occur where the duration of benefit after each dose becomes progressively shorter. Modified-release preparations may help with 'end-of-dose' deterioration or nocturnal immobility and rigidity.

Selegiline is a monoamine-oxidase-B inhibitor used in severe parkinsonism in conjunction with levodopa to reduce 'end-of-dose' deterioration. Early treatment with selegiline may delay the need for levodopa therapy but there is no convincing evidence that it delays disease progression. Selegiline given with levodopa may be associated with increased mortality in the longer term, but this remains to be confirmed. Selegiline need not necessarily be withdrawn from patients stabilised on treatment; sudden withdrawal of selegiline may exacerbate symptoms.

Bromocriptine acts by direct stimulation of surviving dopamine receptors. Although effective, it has no advantages over levodopa. It should be reserved for patients for whom levodopa alone is no longer adequate or who despite careful titration cannot tolerate levodopa. Its use is often limited by its side-effects and when used with levodopa, abnormal involuntary movements and confusional states are common.

Lysuride is a newly introduced drug for parkinsonism; it is similar to bromocriptine in its action.

Pergolide is another newly introduced drug; it acts mainly on dopamine D_2 receptors. Like bromocriptine and lysuride it is sometimes useful in reducing 'off' periods and in ameliorating fluctuations in the later stage of Parkinson's disease. All these dopaminergic drugs may cause serious neuropsychiatric side-effects and occasionally may cause retroperitoneal fibrosis.

Amantadine has modest antiparkinsonian effects. It improves mild bradykinetic disabilities as well as tremor and rigidity. Unfortunately only a small proportion of patients derive much benefit from this drug and tolerance to its effects occurs. However it has the advantage of being relatively free from side-effects.

Apomorphine is a potent stimulator of D_1 and D_2 receptors, which is sometimes helpful in stabilising patients experiencing unpredictable 'off' periods with levodopa treatment. It is essential to establish patients on domperidone for three days before starting apomorphine. Long-term specialist supervision is advisable throughout apomorphine treatment.

LEVODOPA

Indications: parkinsonism (but not drug-induced extrapyramidal symptoms), see notes above

Cautions: pulmonary disease, peptic ulceration, cardiovascular disease, diabetes mellitus, osteomalacia, open-angle glaucoma, skin melanoma, psychiatric illness (avoid if severe). In prolonged therapy, psychiatric, hepatic, haematological, renal, and cardiovascular surveillance is advisable. Warn patients who benefit from therapy to resume normal activities gradually; avoid abrupt withdrawal; pregnancy (toxicity in *animals*) and breast-feeding; **interactions:** Appendix 1 (levodopa)

Contra-indications: closed-angle glaucoma

Side-effects: anorexia, nausea and vomiting, insomnia, agitation, postural hypotension (rarely labile hypertension), dizziness, tachycardia, arrhythmias, reddish discoloration of urine and other body fluids, rarely hypersensitivity; abnormal involuntary movements and psychiatric symptoms which include hypomania and psychosis may be dose-limiting; depression, drowsiness, headache, flushing, sweating, gastro-intestinal bleeding, peripheral neuropathy, and liver enzyme changes also reported

Dose: initially 125–500 mg daily in divided doses after meals, increased according to response (but rarely used alone, see notes above)

PoM **Levodopa** (Cambridge)

Tablets, scored, levodopa 500 mg. Net price 20 = £3.50. Label: 14, 21

Note. The brand name Larodopa® was formerly used for levodopa tablets

CO-BENELDOPA

A mixture of benserazide hydrochloride and levodopa in mass proportions corresponding to 1 part of benserazide and 4 parts of levodopa

Indications; Cautions; Contra-indications; Side-effects: see under Levodopa and notes above

Dose: expressed as levodopa, initially 50–100 mg twice daily, adjusted according to response; usual maintenance dose 400–800 mg daily in divided doses after meals

Note. When transferring patients from levodopa, 3 capsules co-beneldopa 25/100 (Madopar 125®) should be substituted for 2 g levodopa; the levodopa should be discontinued 12 hours beforehand

PoM **Madopar®** (Roche)

Capsules 62.5, blue/grey, co-beneldopa 12.5/50 (benserazide 12.5 mg (as hydrochloride), levodopa 50 mg). Net price 100-cap pack = £7.76. Label: 14, 21

Capsules 125, blue/pink, co-beneldopa 25/100 (benserazide 25 mg (as hydrochloride), levodopa 100 mg). Net price 100-cap pack = £10.81. Label: 14, 21

Capsules 250, blue/caramel, co-beneldopa 50/200 (benserazide 50 mg (as hydrochloride), levodopa 200 mg). Net price 100-cap pack = £18.43. Label: 14, 21

Dispersible tablets 62.5, scored, co-beneldopa 12.5/50 (benserazide 12.5 mg (as hydrochloride), levodopa 50 mg). Net price 100-tab pack = £8.29. Label: 14, 21, counselling, administration, see below

Dispersible tablets 125, scored, co-beneldopa 25/100 (benserazide 25 mg (as hydrochloride) levodopa 100 mg). Net price 100-tab pack = £14.70. Label: 14, 21, counselling, administration, see below

Note. The tablets may be dispersed in water or orange squash or swallowed whole

PoM **Madopar® CR** (Roche)

Capsules 125, m/r, dark green/light blue, co-beneldopa 25/100 (benserazide 25 mg (as hydrochloride), levodopa 100 mg). Net price 100-cap pack = £17.97. Label: 5, 14, 25

Dose: Patients not receiving levodopa therapy, initially 1 capsule 3 times daily (max. initial dose 6 capsules daily)

Fluctuations in response related to plasma-levodopa concentration or to timing of dose, initially 1 capsule substituted for every 100 mg of levodopa and given at same dosage frequency, subsequently increased every 2–3 days according to response; average increase of 50% needed over previous levodopa dose and titration may take up to 4 weeks

Supplementary dose of conventional Madopar® may be needed with first morning dose; if response still poor to total daily dose of Madopar® CR plus Madopar® corresponding to 1.2 g levodopa, consider alternative therapy

CO-CARELDOPA

A mixture of carbidopa and levodopa; the proportions are expressed in the form *x/y* where *x* and *y* are the strengths in milligrams of carbidopa and levodopa respectively

Indications; Cautions; Contra-indications; Side-effects: see under Levodopa and notes above

Dose: expressed as levodopa, initially 100–125 mg 3–4 times daily adjusted according to response; usual maintenance dose 0.75–1.5 g daily in divided doses after food. See also under Sinemet-Plus®

Note. When transferring patients from levodopa, 3 tablets co-careldopa 25/250 (Sinemet-275®) should be substituted for 4 g levodopa; the levodopa should be discontinued 12 hours beforehand

PoM **Sinemet®** (Du Pont)

Tablets (Sinemet-110), blue, scored, co-careldopa 10/100 (carbidopa 10 mg (as monohydrate), levodopa 100 mg). Net price 20 = £1.71. Label: 14, 21

Tablets (Sinemet-275), blue, scored, co-careldopa 25/250 (carbidopa 25 mg (as monohydrate), levodopa 250 mg). Net price 20 = £3.57. Label: 14, 21

PoM **Sinemet LS®** (Du Pont)

Tablets, yellow, scored, co-careldopa 12.5/50 (carbidopa 12.5 mg (as monohydrate), levodopa 50 mg). Net price 84-tab pack = £6.87. Label: 14, 21

Note. 2 tablets Sinemet LS® ≡ 1 tablet Sinemet Plus®

PoM **Sinemet-Plus®** (Du Pont)

Tablets, yellow, scored, co-careldopa 25/100 (carbidopa 25 mg (as monohydrate), levodopa 100 mg). Net price 20 = £2.52. Label: 14, 21

Dose: initially 1 tablet 3 times daily, adjusted according to response to 8 tablets daily in divided doses; larger doses by gradual substitution of Sinemet® for Sinemet-Plus®

Note. The daily dose of carbidopa required to achieve full inhibition of extracerebral dopa-decarboxylase is 75 mg; co-careldopa 25/100 provides an adequate dose of carbidopa when low doses of levodopa are needed

Modified release

PoM Half Sinemet® CR (Du Pont)

Tablets, m/r, pink, co-careldopa 25/100 (carbidopa 25 mg (as monohydrate), levodopa 100 mg). Net price 56-tab pack = £18.56. Label: 14, 25

Dose: for fine adjustment of Sinemet® CR dose (see below)

PoM Sinemet® CR (Du Pont)

Tablets, m/r, peach, co-careldopa 50/200 (carbidopa 50 mg (as monohydrate), levodopa 200 mg). Net price 56-tab pack = £21.84. Label: 14, 25

Dose: initial treatment or fluctuations in response to conventional levodopa therapy, 1 Sinemet® CR tablet twice daily; both dose and interval then adjusted according to response at intervals of not less than 3 days; if transferring from existing levodopa therapy withdraw 8 hours beforehand; 1 tablet Sinemet® CR twice daily can be substituted for a daily dose of levodopa 300–400 mg in conventional Sinemet® tablets

AMANTADINE HYDROCHLORIDE

Indications: Parkinson's disease (but not drug-induced extrapyramidal symptoms); antiviral, see section 5.3

Cautions: hepatic, or renal impairment (avoid if severe), congestive heart disease (may exacerbate oedema), confused or hallucinatory states, elderly; avoid abrupt discontinuation in Parkinson's disease; **interactions:** Appendix 1 (amantadine)

DRIVING. May affect performance of skilled tasks (e.g. driving)

Contra-indications: epilepsy, history of gastric ulceration, severe renal impairment; pregnancy (toxicity in *animals*), breast-feeding

Side-effects: anorexia, nausea, nervousness, inability to concentrate, insomnia, dizziness, convulsions, hallucinations or feelings of detachment, blurred vision, gastro-intestinal disturbances, livedo reticularis and peripheral oedema; rarely leucopenia, rashes

Dose: 100 mg daily increased after one week to 100 mg twice daily (not later than 4 p.m.), usually in conjunction with other treatment

PoM Symmetrel® (Geigy)

Capsules, red-brown, amantadine hydrochloride 100 mg. Net price 56-cap pack = £10.41. Counselling, driving

Syrup, amantadine hydrochloride 50 mg/5 mL. Net price 150-mL pack = £3.49. Counselling, driving

APOMORPHINE HYDROCHLORIDE

Indications: refractory motor fluctuations in Parkinson's disease ('off' episodes) inadequately controlled by levodopa or other dopaminergics (for capable and motivated patients under specialist supervision)

Cautions: tendency to nausea and vomiting; pulmonary, cardiovascular or endocrine disease, renal impairment; elderly and debilitated, history of postural hypotension (special care on initiation); hepatic, haemopoietic, renal, and cardiovascular monitoring; *on administration with levodopa* test initially and every 6 months for haemolytic anaemia (development calls for specialist haematological care with dose reduction and possible

discontinuation); **interactions:** Appendix 1 (apomorphine)

Contra-indications: respiratory or CNS depression, hypersensitiviy to opioids; neuropsychiatric problems or dementia; not suitable if 'on' response to levodopa marred by severe dyskinesia, hypotonia or psychiatric effects; pregnancy and breast-feeding

Side-effects: dyskinesias during 'on' periods (may require discontinuation); postural instability and falls (impaired speech and balance may not improve), increasing cognitive impairment, personality change and disabling dyskinesias during 'on' phase; nausea and vomiting (see below under Dose); confusion and hallucinations (if continued, specialist observation required with possible gradual dose reduction), sedation, postural hypotension; also euphoria, light-headedness, restlessness, tremors; haemolytic anaemia with levodopa (see Cautions) and rarely eosinophilia; local reactions common (include nodule formation and possible ulceration)—rotate injection sites, dilute with sodium chloride 0.9%, consider ultrasound, ensure no infection

Dose: ADULT over 18 years, *by subcutaneous injection*, usual range (after initiation as below) 3–30 mg daily in divided doses; subcutaneous infusion may be preferable in those requiring division of injections into more than 10 doses daily; max. single dose 10 mg; ADOLESCENT (under 18 years) and CHILD not recommended

By continuous subcutaneous infusion (those requiring division into more than 10 injections daily) initially 1 mg/hour daily increased according to response (not more often than every 4 hours) in max. steps of 500 micrograms/hour to max. 4 mg/hour (15–60 micrograms/kg/hour); change infusion site every 12 hours and give during waking hours only (24-hour infusions not advised unless severe night-time symptoms)—intermittent bolus boosts also usually needed (in those with severe dyskinesias only when absolutely necessary)

Total daily dose by either route (or combined routes) max. 100 mg

REQUIREMENTS FOR INITIATION. *Hospital admission* and at least 3 days of pretreatment with domperidone, *after at least 3 days* withhold existing antiparkinsonian medication overnight to provoke 'off' episode, *determine* threshold dose, *re-establish* other antiparkinsonian drugs, *determine* effective apomorphine regimen, *teach* to administer by subcutaneous injection into lower abdomen or outer thigh at first sign of 'off' episode, *discharge* from hospital, *monitor* frequently and *adjust* dosage regimen as appropriate (domperidone may normally be withdrawn over several weeks or longer)—for full details of initiation requirements see data sheet

PoM Britaject® (Britannia)

Injection, apomorphine hydrochloride 10 mg/mL, net price 2-mL amp = £7.95, 5-mL amp = £15.95

BROMOCRIPTINE

Indications: parkinsonism (but not drug-induced extrapyramidal symptoms); endocrine disorders, see section 6.7.1

Cautions; Side-effects: see section 6.7.1

HYPOTENSIVE REACTIONS. Hypotensive reactions may be disturbing in some patients during the first few days of treatment and particular care should be exercised when driving or operating machinery; tolerance may be reduced by alcohol

Dose: first week 1–1.25 mg at night, second week 2–2.5 mg at night, third week 2.5 mg twice daily, fourth week 2.5 mg 3 times daily then increasing by 2.5 mg every 3–14 days according to response to a usual range of 10–40 mg daily; taken with food

Preparations

See section 6.7.1

LYSURIDE MALEATE

(Lisuride Maleate)

Indications: Parkinson's disease

Cautions: history of pituitary tumour; history of psychotic disturbance; pregnancy; porphyria (see section 9.8.2); **interactions:** Appendix 1 (lysuride)

HYPOTENSIVE REACTIONS. Hypotensive reactions may be disturbing in some patients during the first few days of treatment and particular care should be exercised when driving or operating machinery

Contra-indications: severe disturbances of peripheral circulation; coronary insufficiency

Side-effects: nausea and vomiting; dizziness; headache, lethargy, malaise, drowsiness, psychotic reactions (including hallucinations); occasionally severe hypotension, rashes; rarely abdominal pain and constipation; Raynaud's phenomenon reported

Dose: initially 200 micrograms at bedtime with food increased as necessary at weekly intervals to 200 micrograms twice daily (midday and bedtime) then to 200 micrograms 3 times daily (morning, midday, and bedtime); further increases made by adding 200 micrograms each week first to the bedtime dose, then to the midday dose and finally to the morning dose; max. 5 mg daily in 3 divided doses after food

PoM **Revanil®** (Roche)

Tablets, scored, lysuride maleate 200 micrograms. Net price 100-tab pack = £24.00. Label: 21, counselling, hypotensive reactions

PERGOLIDE

Indications: adjunct to levodopa in Parkinson's disease

Cautions: arrhythmias or underlying cardiac disease, history of confusion or hallucinations, dyskinesia (may cause or exacerbate), pregnancy, breast-feeding; increase dose gradually and avoid abrupt withdrawal; porphyria (see section 9.8.2); **interactions:** Appendix 1 (pergolide)

HYPOTENSIVE REACTIONS. Hypotensive reactions may be disturbing in some patients during the first few days of treatment and particular care should be exercised when driving or operating machinery

Side-effects: hallucinations, confusion, dyskinesia, somnolence, abdominal pain, nausea, dyspepsia, diplopia, rhinitis, dyspnoea, insomnia, constipation or diarrhoea, hypotension, tachycardia and atrial premature contractions reported; neuroleptic malignant syndrome also reported

Dose: 50 micrograms daily for 2 days, increased gradually by 100–150 micrograms every third day over next 12 days, usually given in 3 divided doses; further increases of 250 micrograms every third day; usual maintenance 3 mg daily (above 5 mg daily not evaluated); during pergolide titration levodopa dose may be reduced cautiously

PoM **Celance®** (Lilly)

Tablets, all scored, pergolide (as mesylate) 50 micrograms (ivory), net price 75-tab starter pack = £30.25, 100-tab pack = £40.34; 250 micrograms (green), 100-tab pack = £55.32; 1 mg (pink), 100-tab pack = £199.65. Counselling, hypotensive reactions

SELEGILINE

Indications: Parkinson's disease or symptomatic parkinsonism (but not drug-induced extrapyramidal symptoms), either used alone (in early disease) or as an adjunct to levodopa therapy (but see notes above)

Cautions: side-effects of levodopa may be increased, concurrent levodopa dosage may need to be reduced by 20–50%; **interactions:** Appendix 1 (selegiline)

Side-effects: hypotension, nausea and vomiting, confusion or psychosis, agitation

Dose: 10 mg in the morning, or 5 mg at breakfast and midday; see below

ELDERLY. To avoid initial confusion and agitation, it may be appropriate to start treatment with a dose of 2.5 mg daily, particularly in the elderly

PoM **Selegiline Hydrochloride** (Non-proprietary)

Tablets, selegiline hydrochloride 5 mg, net price 60-tab pack = £26.31; 10 mg, 30-tab pack = £25.84

Available from ASTA Medica (Vivapryl®), Bioglan, Cox, Hillcross, Norton, Opus (Centrapryl®)

PoM **Eldepryl®** (Britannia)

Tablets, both scored, selegiline hydrochloride 5 mg, net price 60-tab pack = £28.08; 10 mg, 30-tab pack = £27.20

Oral liquid, selegiline hydrochloride 10 mg/5 mL, net price 200-mL = £37.44

4.9.2 Antimuscarinic drugs used in parkinsonism

Antimuscarinic drugs (less correctly termed 'anticholinergics') are the other main class of drugs used in Parkinson's disease. They are less effective than levodopa in idiopathic Parkinson's disease although they often usefully supplement its action. Patients with mild symptoms, particularly where tremor predominates, may be treated initially with antimuscarinic drugs (alone or with selegiline, section 4.9.1), levodopa being added or substituted as symptoms progress. They have value in post-encephalitic parkinsonism.

Antimuscarinic drugs exert their antiparkinsonian effect by correcting the relative central cholinergic excess thought to occur in parkinsonism as a result of dopamine deficiency. In most patients their effects are only moderate, reducing tremor and rigidity to some effect but without significant action on bradykinesia. They exert a synergistic effect when used with levodopa and are also useful in reducing sialorrhoea.

The antimuscarinic drugs also reduce the symptoms of drug-induced parkinsonism as seen, for example, with antipsychotic drugs (section 4.2.1) but there is no justification for giving them simultaneously with antipsychotics unless parkinsonian side-effects occur. Tardive dyskinesia is not improved by the antimuscarinic drugs and may be made worse.

No important differences exist between the many synthetic antimuscarinic drugs available but some patients appear to tolerate one better than another. They may be taken before food if dry mouth is troublesome, or after food if gastro-intestinal symptoms predominate. Those most commonly used are **orphenadrine** and **benzhexol; benztropine** and **procyclidine** are also used. Benztropine is similar to benzhexol but is excreted more slowly; changes in dose therefore need to be carried out very gradually. Both procyclidine and benztropine may be given parenterally and are effective emergency treatment for acute drug-induced dystonic reactions which may be severe.

BENZHEXOL HYDROCHLORIDE
(Trihexyphenidyl Hydrochloride)

Indications: parkinsonism; drug-induced extra-pyramidal symptoms (but not tardive dyskinesia, see notes above)

Cautions: cardiovascular disease, hepatic or renal impairment; elderly; avoid abrupt discontinuation of treatment; liable to abuse; **interactions:** Appendix 1 (antimuscarinics)

DRIVING. May affect performance of skilled tasks (e.g. driving)

Contra-indications: untreated urinary retention, closed-angle glaucoma, gastro-intestinal obstruction

Side-effects: dry mouth, gastro-intestinal disturbances, dizziness, blurred vision; less commonly urinary retention, tachycardia, hypersensitivity, nervousness, and with high doses in susceptible patients, mental confusion, excitement, and psychiatric disturbances which may necessitate discontinuation of treatment

Dose: 1 mg daily, gradually increased; usual maintenance dose 5–15 mg daily in 3–4 divided doses; ELDERLY preferably lower end of range

PoM **Artane®** (Lederle)
Tablets, both scored, benzhexol hydrochloride 2 mg, net price 20 = 31p; 5 mg, 20 = 63p. Counselling, before or after food (see notes above), driving

PoM **Broflex®** (Bioglan)
Syrup, pink, benzhexol hydrochloride 5 mg/5 mL. Net price 200-mL pack = £5.78. Counselling, before or after food (see notes above), driving

BENZTROPINE MESYLATE
(Benzatropine Mesilate)

Indications; Cautions; Contra-indications; Side-effects: see under Benzhexol Hydrochloride, but causes sedation rather than stimulation; avoid in children under 3 years

Dose: by mouth, 0.5–1 mg daily usually at bedtime, gradually increased; max. 6 mg daily; usual maintenance dose 1–4 mg daily in single or divided doses; ELDERLY preferably lower end of range

By intramuscular or intravenous injection, 1–2 mg, repeated if symptoms reappear; ELDERLY preferably lower end of range

PoM **Cogentin®** (MSD)
Tablets, scored, benztropine mesylate 2 mg. Net price 20 = 29p. Label: 2
Injection, benztropine mesylate 1 mg/mL. Net price 2-mL amp = 92p

BIPERIDEN

Indications; Cautions; Contra-indications; Side-effects: see under Benzhexol Hydrochloride, but may cause drowsiness; injection may cause hypotension

Dose: by mouth, biperiden hydrochloride 1 mg twice daily, gradually increased to 2 mg 3 times daily; usual maintenance dose 3–12 mg daily in divided doses; ELDERLY preferably lower end of range

By intramuscular or slow intravenous injection, biperiden lactate 2.5–5 mg up to 4 times daily; ELDERLY preferably lower end of range

PoM **Akineton®** (Knoll)
Tablets, scored, biperiden hydrochloride 2 mg. Net price 100-tab pack = £4.60. Label: 2
Injection, biperiden lactate 5 mg/mL. Net price 1-mL amp = 69p

ORPHENADRINE HYDROCHLORIDE

Indications; Cautions; Contra-indications; Side-effects: see under Benzhexol Hydrochloride, but more euphoric; may cause insomnia; porphyria (see section 9.8.2)

Dose: 150 mg daily in divided doses, gradually increased; max. 400 mg daily; ELDERLY preferably lower end of range

PoM **Orphenadrine Hydrochloride** (Non-proprietary)
Oral solution, orphenadrine hydrochloride 50mg/5 mL. Net price 200-mL = £7.00. Counselling, driving
Available from Rosemont (sugar-free)

oM **Biorphen®** (Bioglan)

Elixir, sugar-free, orphenadrine hydrochloride 25 mg/5 mL. Net price 200-mL pack = £6.59. Counselling, driving

oM **Disipal®** (Yamanouchi)

Tablets, yellow, s/c, orphenadrine hydrochloride 50 mg. Net price 20 = 48p. Counselling, driving

Additives: include tartrazine

PROCYCLIDINE HYDROCHLORIDE

Indications; Cautions; Contra-indications; Side-effects: see under Benzhexol Hydrochloride

Dose: by mouth, 2.5 mg 3 times daily, gradually increased if necessary; usual max. 30 mg daily (60 mg daily in exceptional circumstances); ELD ERLY preferably lower end of range

Acute dystonia, *by intramuscular injection,* 5–10 mg repeated if necessary after 20 minutes; max. 20 mg daily; *by intravenous injection,* 5 mg (usually effective within 5 minutes); an occasional patient may need 10 mg or more and may require up to half an hour to obtain relief; ELD ERLY preferably lower end of dose

oM **Procyclidine** (Non-proprietary)

Tablets, procyclidine hydrochloride 5 mg. Net price 20 = £1.15. Counselling, driving

oM **Arpicolin®** (Rosemont)

Syrup, sugar-free, procyclidine hydrochloride 2.5 mg/5 mL, net price 200-mL pack = £4.95; 5 mg/5 mL, 200-mL pack = £8.80. Counselling, driving

oM **Kemadrin®** (Wellcome)

Tablets, scored, procyclidine hydrochloride 5 mg. Net price 20 = £1.17. Counselling, driving

Injection, procyclidine hydrochloride 5 mg/mL. Net price 2-mL amp = £1.49

4.9.3   Drugs used in essential tremor, chorea, tics, and related disorders

Tetrabenazine is mainly used to control movement disorders in Huntington's chorea and related disorders. It may act by depleting nerve endings of dopamine. It has useful action in only a proportion of patients and its use may be limited by the development of depression.

Haloperidol may be useful in improving motor tics and symptoms of Gilles de la Tourette syndrome and related choreas. **Pimozide** (see section 4.2.1 for CSM warning) and more recently **clonidine** (section 4.7.4.2) and **sulpiride** (section 4.2.1), are also used in Gilles de la Tourette syndrome. **Benzhexol** (section 4.9.2) at high dosage may also improve some movement disorders. It sometimes necessary to build the dose up over many weeks, to 20 to 30 mg daily or higher. **Chlorpromazine** and **haloperidol** are used to relieve intractable hiccup (section 4.2.1).

Propranolol or another beta-adrenoceptor blocking drug (see section 2.4) may be useful in treating essential tremor or tremors associated with anxiety or thyrotoxicosis. Propranolol is given in a dosage of 40 mg 2 or 3 times daily, increased if necessary; 80 to 160 mg daily is usually required for maintenance.

Primidone in some cases provides relief from benign essential tremor; the dose is increased slowly to reduce side-effects.

Piracetam has been introduced recently as adjunctive treatment for myoclonus of cortical origin.

Riluzole has been introduced recently to extend life or the time to mechanical ventilation in patients with amyotrophic lateral sclerosis. Treatment should only be initiated by physicians experienced in treating motor neurone disease.

HALOPERIDOL

Indications: motor tics, adjunctive treatment in choreas and Gilles de la Tourette syndrome; other indications, section 4.2.1

Cautions; Contra-indications; Side-effects: see section 4.2.1

Dose: by mouth, 0.5–1.5 mg 3 times daily adjusted according to the response; 10 mg daily or more may occasionally be necessary in Gilles de la Tourette syndrome; CHILD, Gilles de la Tourette syndrome up to 10 mg daily

Preparations

Section 4.2.1

PIRACETAM

Indications: adjunctive treatment of cortical myoclonus

Cautions: avoid abrupt withdrawal; elderly; renal impairment (avoid if severe)

Contra-indications: hepatic and severe renal impairment; pregnancy and breast-feeding

Side-effects: diarrhoea, weight gain; somnolence, insomnia, nervousness, depression; hyperkinesia; rash

Dose: initially 7.2 g daily in 2–3 divided doses, increased according to response by 4.8 g daily every 3–4 days to max. 20 g daily (subsequently, attempts should be made to reduce dose of concurrent therapy); CHILD under 16 years not recommended

ORAL SOLUTION. Follow the oral solution with a glass of water (or soft drink) to reduce bitter taste.

▼ PoM **Nootropil®** (UCB Pharma)

Tablets, f/c, scored, piracetam 800 mg, net price 90-tab pack = £15.80; 1.2 g, 56-tab pack = £14.74. Label: 3

Oral solution, piracetam, 333.3 mg/mL, net price 300-mL pack = £21.93. Label: 3

PRIMIDONE

Indications: essential tremor; epilepsy, see section 4.8.1

Cautions; Contra-indications; Side-effects: see section 4.8.1

Dose: essential tremor, initially 50 mg daily increased gradually over 2–3 weeks according to response; max. 750 mg daily

Preparations

Section 4.8.1

RILUZOLE

Indications: to extend life or the time to mechanical ventilation for patients with amyotrophic lateral sclerosis, initiated by specialist physicians experienced in the management of motor neurone disease

Cautions: history of abnormal hepatic function (see product literature for details); **interactions:** Appendix 1 (riluzole)

BLOOD DISORDERS. Patients or their carers should be told how to recognise signs of neutropenia and advised to seek immediate medical attention if symptoms such as fever occur; white blood cell counts should be determined in febrile illness; neutropenia requires discontinuation of riluzole

DRIVING. Dizziness or vertigo may affect performance of skilled tasks (e.g. driving)

Contra-indications: hepatic and renal impairment; pregnancy and breast-feeding

Side-effects: nausea, vomiting, asthenia, tachycardia, somnolence, headache, dizziness, vertigo, pain, paraesthesia, alterations in liver function tests

Dose: 50 mg twice daily; CHILD not recommended

▼ PoM **Rilutek**® (Rhône-Poulenc Rorer)
Tablets, f/c, riluzole 50 mg. Net price 56-tab pack = £286.00. Counselling, blood disorders, driving

---

TETRABENAZINE

Indications: movement disorders due to Huntington's chorea, senile chorea, and related neurological conditions

Cautions: pregnancy; avoid in breast-feeding; **interactions:** Appendix 1 (tetrabenazine)

DRIVING. May affect performance of skilled tasks (e.g. driving)

Side-effects: drowsiness, gastro-intestinal disturbances, depression, extrapyramidal dysfunction, hypotension

Dose: initially 12.5 mg twice daily (elderly 12.5 mg daily) gradually increased to 12.5–25 mg 3 times daily; max. 200 mg daily

PoM **Tetrabenazine** (Cambridge)
Tablets, pale yellow-buff, scored, tetrabenazine 25 mg. Net price 120-tab pack = £15.26. Label: 2
Note. The brand name Nitoman® was formerly used for tetrabenazine preparations

---

TORSION DYSTONIAS AND OTHER INVOLUNTARY MOVEMENTS

BOTULINUM A TOXIN-HAEMAGGLUTININ COMPLEX

Indications: see under preparations below

Cautions: as a biological product bear in mind potential for anaphylaxis; do not give with (or before) aminoglycoside antibiotics or spectinomycin; other specific cautions, see below; other **interactions:** Appendix 1 (botulinum toxin)

SPECIFIC CAUTIONS WHEN TREATING BLEPHAROSPASM OR HEMIFACIAL SPASM. Avoid deep or misplaced injections—relevant anatomy (and any alterations due to previous surgery) must be understood before injecting; reduced blinking can lead to corneal exposure, persistent

epithelial defect and corneal ulceration (especially in those with VIIth nerve disorders)—careful testing of corneal sensation in previously operated eyes, avoidance of injection in lower lid area and vigorous treatment of epithelial defect needed

SPECIFIC CAUTIONS WHEN TREATING TORTICOLLIS. Only for specialists experienced in diagnosis and management of torticollis and who have received training (provided by Speywood) in administering Dysport®

COUNSELLING. All patients should be alerted to possible side-effects

Contra-indications: generalised disorders of muscle activity (e.g. myasthenia gravis); pregnancy and breast-feeding

Side-effects: increased electrophysiologic jitter in some distant muscles; misplaced injections may paralyse nearby muscle groups and excessive doses may paralyse distant muscles; rash; antibody formation (substantial deterioration in response); transient burning sensation after injection

SPECIFIC SIDE-EFFECTS WHEN TREATING BLEPHAROSPASM OR HEMIFACIAL SPASM. Ptosis, lacrimation and irritation (including dry eye, lagophthalmos and photophobia); also ectropion, keratitis, diplopia and entropion; angle-closure glaucoma reported; bruising, ecchymosis and swelling of soft eyelid tissues minimised by applying gentle pressure at injection site immediately after injection

SPECIFIC SIDE-EFFECTS WHEN TREATING TORTICOLLIS. Dysphagia and pooling of saliva (occurs most frequently after injection into sternomastoid muscle); dry mouth, voice changes, weakness of neck muscles; generalised muscle weakness, diplopia and blurred vision; rarely respiratory difficulties (associated with high doses); CSM has warned of persistent dysphagia and sequelae (including death)—**important**, see also under Cautions

Dose: see under preparations below (**important:** specific to **each individual preparation** and **not interchangeable**)

▼ PoM **Botox**® (Allergan)
Injection, powder for reconstitution, botulinum A toxin-haemagglutinin complex, net price 100-unit vial = £135.00

Dose: Blepharospasm, into medial and lateral orbicularis oculi of upper lid and lateral orbicularis oculi of lower lid (additional sites in brow area, lateral orbicularis and upper facial area may also be injected if spasms interfere with vision), initially 1.25–2.5 units at each site (total of up to 25 units per eye) increased to max. 5 units per site, if response inadequate (e.g. not longer than 2 months); total dose should not exceed 100 units every 12 weeks; CHILD not recommended

Hemifacial spasm or VIIth nerve disorders, as for unilateral blepharospasm (other affected facial muscles being injected with initial doses of 1.25–2.5 units); electromyographic control may be needed to identify affected small circumoral muscles; CHILD not recommended

IMPORTANT. Botox® is licensed **only** for blepharospasm and hemifacial spasm; it is **not** licensed for torticollis

DURATION OF ACTION. Initial effect usually within 3 days with peak after 1–2 weeks. Injections need to be repeated approximately every 12 weeks.

PoM **Dysport**® (Speywood)
Injection, powder for reconstitution, botulinum A toxin-haemagglutinin complex, net price 500-unit vial = £172.50

Dose: Blepharospasm, initially 20 units medially and 40 units laterally into junction between preseptal and orbital parts of both upper and lower orbicularis oculi of each eye (total of 120 units per eye)—see package insert for diagram to aid placement of injections; subsequently, dose may need to be reduced to 20 units medially and 20 units laterally as above (total of 80 units per eye); dose may be further reduced to total of 60 units per eye by omitting medial lower lid injection; CHILD not recommended

Hemifacial spasm, as for unilateral blepharospasm, above; CHILD not recommended

DURATION OF ACTION (BLEPHAROSPAM AND HEMIFACIAL SPASM). Initial effect usually within 2–4 days with peak within 2 weeks. Injections need to be repeated approximately every 8 weeks.

Torticollis, administration by specialist experienced in diagnosis and management (see also Cautions above),

Spasmodic torticollis, initially 500 units divided between 2–3 most active neck muscles

Rotational torticollis, initially 350 units into splenius capitis muscle (ipsilateral to direction of chin/head rotation) and 150 units into sternomastoid muscle (contralateral to rotation)

Laterocollis, initially 350 units into ipsilateral splenius capitis muscle and 150 units into ipsilateral sternomastoid muscle; if associated *with shoulder elevation*, ipsilateral trapezoid or levator scapulae muscles may also require treatment (according to visible hypertrophy of muscle or electromyographic findings); if 3 muscles require treatment, inject 300 units into splenius capitis muscle, 100 units into sternomastoid muscle and 100 units into third muscle

Retrocollis, initially, 250 units into each splenius capitis muscle *then* after 6 weeks may be followed by bilateral trapezius injections (up to 250 units per muscle)—bilateral splenii injections may increase risk of neck muscle weakness

Subsequent injections adjusted according to response and side-effects; max. 1000 units

CHILD not recommended

DURATION OF ACTION (TORTICOLLIS). Initial effect usually within 1 week. Injections need to be repeated every 8–12 weeks or as required

4.10 Drugs used in substance dependence

This section includes drugs used in alcohol dependence, cigarette smoking, and opioid dependence.

The health departments of the UK have produced a report, *Drug Misuse and Dependence* which contains guidelines on clinical management.

Drug Misuse and Dependence, London, HMSO, 1991 can be obtained from:

HMSO Publications Centre
PO Box 276, London SW8 5DT
Telephone orders, 0171-873 9090

or from HMSO bookshops and through good booksellers.

It is **important** to be aware that *people who misuse drugs* may be at risk not only from the intrinsic toxicity of the drug itself but also from the practice of injecting preparations intended for administration by mouth. Excipients used in the production of oral dose forms are usually insoluble and may lead to *abscess formation at the site of injection*, or even to *necrosis and gangrene*; moreover, deposits in the heart or lungs may lead to *severe cardiac or pulmonary toxicity*. Additional hazards include *infection* following the use of a dirty needle or an unsterilised diluent.

ALCOHOL DEPENDENCE

Disulfiram (Antabuse®) is used as an adjunct to the treatment of alcohol dependence. It gives rise to extremely unpleasant systemic reactions after the ingestion of even small amounts of alcohol because it leads to accumulation of acetaldehyde in the body. Reactions include flushing of the face, throbbing headache, palpitations, tachycardia, nausea, vomiting, and, with large doses of alcohol, arrhythmias, hypotension, and collapse. Even the small amounts of alcohol included in many oral medicines may be sufficient to precipitate a reaction (even toiletries containing alcohol should be avoided). It may be advisable for patients to carry a card warning of the danger of administration of alcohol.

Chlormethiazole is used to attenuate withdrawal symptoms but itself has a dependence potential. In order to minimise the risk of dependence, administration of chlormethiazole should be limited to 9 days under inpatient supervision.

Benzodiazepines are also used in the management of withdrawal, but again have dependence potential (see section 4.1).

Acamprosate is a new drug which, in combination with counselling, may be helpful in maintaining abstinence in alcohol-dependent patients. It should be initiated as soon as possible *after* abstinence has been achieved and should be maintained if the patient relapses. Continued alcohol abuse, however, negates the therapeutic benefit of acamprosate.

ACAMPROSATE CALCIUM

Indications: maintenance of abstinence in alcohol dependence

Cautions: continued alcohol abuse (risk of treatment failure); **interactions:** Appendix 1 (acamprosate)

Contra-indications: renal and severe hepatic impairment; pregnancy and breast-feeding

Side-effects: diarrhoea, nausea, vomiting, abdominal pain, pruritus, occasionally maculopapular rash, rarely bullous skin reactions; fluctuation in libido

Dose: ADULT 18–65 years, 60 kg and over, 666 mg (2 tablets) 3 times daily; less than 60 kg, 666 mg (2 tablets) at breakfast, 333 mg (1 tablet) at midday and 333 mg (1 tablet) at night

TREATMENT COURSE. Treatment should be initiated as soon as possible after alcohol withdrawal period and maintained if patient relapses; recommended treatment period 1 year

▼ PoM **Campral EC**® (Lipha)

Tablet, e/c, acamprosate calcium 333 mg. Net price 84-tab pack = £24.95. Label: 5, 21, 25

Electrolytes: Ca²⁺ 0.8 mmol/tablet

BENZODIAZEPINES
Section 4.1.2

CHLORMETHIAZOLE
(Clomethiazole)

Indications: see under Dose; insomnia, restlessness and agitation in the elderly (section 4.1.1); status epilepticus (section 4.8.2); sedation during regional anaesthesia (section 15.1.4.1); eclampsia, see data sheet

Cautions: cardiac and respiratory disease (confusional state may indicate hypoxia); history of drug abuse; marked personality disorder; pregnancy and breast-feeding; elderly (excessive sedation with higher doses); hepatic impairment (especially if severe since sedation can mask hepatic coma); renal impairment; avoid prolonged use (and abrupt withdrawal thereafter); **interactions:** Appendix 1 (anxiolytics and hypnotics)

SPECIAL CAUTIONS FOR INTRAVENOUS INFUSION. Resuscitation facilities must be available; maintain clear airway (risk of mechanical obstruction in deep sedation); *rapid infusion* to be given only under direct medical supervision (risk of apnoea and hypotension—special care in those susceptible to cerebral or cardiac complications, e.g. the elderly); during *continuous infusion* sleep induced may lapse into deep unconsciousness and patient must be kept under close and constant observation; *prolonged infusion* may lead to accumulation and delay recovery, may also cause electrolyte imbalance (infusion contains only Na^+ 32 mmol/litre and no other electrolytes)

DRIVING. Drowsiness may persist the next day and affect performance of skilled tasks (e.g. driving); effects of alcohol enhanced

Contra-indications: acute pulmonary insufficiency; alcohol-dependent patients who continue to drink

Side-effects: nasal congestion and irritation (with sneezing), conjunctival irritation, headache; rarely, paradoxical excitement, confusion, dependence; gastro-intestinal disturbances, rash, urticaria, bullous eruption, anaphylaxis, alterations in liver enzymes also reported; on *intravenous infusion*, localised thrombophlebitis, tachycardia and transient fall in blood pressure (apnoea and hypotension on rapid infusion, see Cautions)

Dose: by mouth, alcohol withdrawal, initially 2–4 capsules, if necessary repeated after some hours; day 1 (first 24 hours), 9–12 capsules in 3–4 divided doses;

day 2, 6–8 capsules in 3–4 divided doses;

day 3, 4–6 capsules in 3–4 divided doses; then gradually reduced over days 4–6; total treatment for not more than 9 days

Note. For an equivalent therapeutic effect 1 capsule ≡ 5 mL syrup

By intravenous infusion, acute alcohol withdrawal, when oral administration not practicable, as a 0.8% solution of chlormethiazole edisylate, initially 3–7.5 mL (24–60 mg)/minute until shallow sleep induced (from which patient can be easily awakened) then reduced to 0.5–1 mL (4–8 mg)/minute to achieve lowest possible rate to maintain shallow sleep and adequate spontaneous respiration; urgent deep sedation (direct medical supervision only) 40–100 mL (320–800 mg) over 3–5 minutes then reduced to maintenance as indicated above

IMPORTANT. See special cautions for intravenous infusion under Cautions (above)

PoM **Heminevrin®** (Astra)

Capsules, grey-brown, chlormethiazole base 192 mg in an oily basis. Net price 60-cap pack = £4.34. Label: 19

Syrup, sugar-free, chlormethiazole edisylate 250 mg/5 mL. Net price 300-mL pack = £3.63. Label: 19

Intravenous infusion 0.8%, chlormethiazole edisylate 8 mg/mL. Net price 500-mL bottle = £5.12

DISULFIRAM

Indications: adjunct in the treatment of chronic alcohol dependence (under specialist supervision)

Cautions: ensure that alcohol not consumed for at least 24 hours before initiating treatment; see also notes above; alcohol challenge **not** recommended on routine basis (if considered essential—specialist units only with resuscitation facilities); hepatic or renal impairment, respiratory disease, diabetes mellitus, epilepsy; **interactions:** Appendix 1 (disulfiram)

ALCOHOL REACTION. Patients should be warned of unpredictable and occasionally severe nature of disulfiram-alcohol interactions. Reactions can occur within 10 minutes and last several hours (may require intensive supportive therapy—oxygen should be available). Patients should not ingest alcohol at all and should be warned of possible presence of alcohol in liquid medicines, remedies, tonics, foods and even in toiletries (alcohol should also be avoided for at least 1 week after stopping)

Contra-indications: cardiac failure, coronary artery disease, history of cerebrovascular accident, hypertension, psychosis, severe personality disorder, suicide risk, pregnancy, breast-feeding

Side-effects: initially drowsiness and fatigue; nausea, vomiting, halitosis, reduced libido; rarely psychotic reactions (depression, paranoia, schizophrenia, mania), allergic dermatitis, peripheral neuritis, hepatic cell damage

Dose: 800 mg as a single dose on first day, reducing over 5 days to 100–200 mg daily; should not be continued for longer than 6 months without review; CHILD not recommended

PoM **Antabuse®** (Dumex)

Tablets, scored, disulfiram 200 mg. Net price 50-tab pack = £17.50. Label: 2, counselling, alcohol reaction

CIGARETTE SMOKING

Nicotine chewing gum, patches or nasal spray may be used as an adjunct to counselling but are not generally available on the NHS.

NICOTINE PRODUCTS

Indications: adjunct to smoking cessation

Cautions: cardiovascular disease (avoid if severe); hyperthyroidism; diabetes mellitus; phaeochromocytoma; renal and hepatic impairment; history of gastritis and peptic ulcers; *patches,* exercise may increase absorption and side-effects, skin disorders (patches should not be placed on broken skin); should not smoke or use nicotine replacement products in combination; **interactions:** Appendix 1 (nicotine and tobacco)

DRIVING. The nasal spray should not be used when driving or operating machinery (sneezing or watering eyes could contribute to accident)

Contra-indications: severe cardiovascular disease (including severe arrhythmias or immediate post-myocardial infarction period); recent cerebrovascular accident (including transient ischaemic attacks); pregnancy and breast-feeding; *patches*, chronic generalised skin disease (patches should not be placed on broken skin); patches not for occasional smokers

Side-effects: nausea, dizziness, headache and cold and influenza-like symptoms, palpitations, dyspepsia, insomnia, vivid dreams, myalgia; other side-effects reported include chest pain, blood pressure changes, anxiety and irritability, somnolence and impaired concentration, dysmenorrhoea; *with patches*, skin reactions (discontinue if severe)—vasculitis also reported; *with spray*, nasal irritation, nose bleeds, watering eyes, ear sensations; *with gum*, increased salivation, aphthous ulceration (sometimes with swelling of tongue); *spray or gum*, throat irritation

Dose: see under preparations, below

NHS Niconil® (Elan)

Patches, self-adhesive, nicotine, *'11 mg'* patch (releasing approx. 11 mg/24 hours), net price 7 = £7.97; *'22 mg'* patch (releasing approx. 22 mg/24 hours), starter pack = £7.97, 7 = £7.97

ADMINISTRATION: apply to dry, non-hairy skin on trunk or upper arm, removing after 24 hours and siting replacement patch on different area (avoid using the same area for several days); initially '22 mg' patch daily usually for 4 weeks; then '11 mg' patch for 2 weeks; review treatment if abstinence not achieved in 3 months; CHILD not recommended

NHS Nicorette® (Pharmacia)

Nicorette chewing gum, sugar-free, nicotine (as resin) 2 mg, net price pack of 30 = £2.98; pack of 105 = £8.05

Nicorette plus chewing gum, sugar-free, nicotine (as resin) 4 mg, net price pack of 30 = £3.98; pack of 105 = £10.80

Note. Also available in mint flavour

Dose: initially one 2-mg piece (**Nicorette®**) chewed slowly for approx. 30 minutes, when urge to smoke occurs; patients needing more than 15 pieces of 2 mg daily may need the 4-mg strength (**Nicorette Plus®**); max. 15 pieces of 4-mg strength daily; withdraw gradually after 3 months; CHILD not recommended

Nicorette patches, self-adhesive, all beige, nicotine, *'5 mg'* patch (releasing approx. 5 mg/16 hours), net price 7 = £7.20; *'10 mg'* patch (releasing approx. 10 mg/16 hours), 7 = £8.36; *'15 mg'* patch (releasing approx. 15 mg/16 hours), 7 = £9.07,

ADMINISTRATION: apply on waking to dry, non-hairy skin on hip, chest or upper arm, removing after approx. 16 hours, usually when retiring; site next patch on different area (avoid using same area for several days); initially '15-mg' patch for 16 hours daily for 8 weeks then '10-mg' patch for 16 hours daily for 2 weeks then '5-mg' patch for 16 hours daily for 2 weeks; review treatment if abstinence not achieved in 3 months; CHILD not recommended

NHS[1] PoM *Nicorette nasal spray*, nicotine 500 micrograms/metered spray. Net price 200-spray unit = £10.99

ADULT. Apply 1 spray into each nostril as required to max. twice an hour for 16 hours daily (max. 64 sprays daily) for 8 weeks, then reduce gradually over next 4 weeks (reduce by half at end of first 2 weeks, stop altogether at end of next 2 weeks); max. treatment length 3 months; CHILD under 16 years not recommended

1. Currently prescribable but prescriptions may be sent to Health Authorities to investigate circumstances under which written.

NHS Nicotinell® (Zyma)

NHS[1] *Chewing gum*, sugar-free, nicotine 2 mg, net price pack of 24 = £2.57; pack of 96 = £7.70

Note. Also available in mint flavour

Dose: initially one 2-mg piece chewed slowly for approx. 30 minutes, when urge to smoke occurs; max. 15 pieces daily; withdraw gradually after 3 months; CHILD not recommended

TTS Patches, self-adhesive, all yellowish-ochre, nicotine, *'10'* patch (releasing approx. 7 mg/24 hours), net price 7 = £8.21; *'20'* patch (releasing approx. 14 mg/24 hours), 7 = £8.64; *'30'* patch (releasing approx. 21 mg/24 hours), 7 = £9.07

ADMINISTRATION: apply to dry, non-hairy skin on trunk or upper arm, removing after 24 hours and siting replacement patch on a different area (avoid using the same area for several days); individuals smoking 20 cigarettes daily or fewer, initially '20' patch daily; individuals smoking more than 20 cigarettes daily, initially '30' patch daily; withdraw gradually, reducing dose every 3–4 weeks; review treatment if abstinence not achieved in 3 months; CHILD under 18 years not recommended

1. Currently prescribable but prescriptions may be sent to Health Authorities to investigate circumstances under which written.

OPIOID DEPENDENCE

Methadone is an opioid *agonist*. It can be substituted for opioids such as diamorphine, preventing the onset of withdrawal symptoms; it is itself addictive and should only be prescribed for those who are physically dependent on opioids. It is administered in a single daily dose usually as methadone mixture 1 mg/mL. The dose is adjusted according to the degree of dependence with the aim of gradual reduction.

Naltrexone is an opioid *antagonist*. It blocks the action of opioids such as diamorphine and precipitates withdrawal symptoms in opioid-dependent subjects. Since the euphoric action of opioid agonists is blocked by naltrexone it is given to former addicts as an aid to relapse prevention.

Lofexidine has been recently introduced for the alleviation of symptoms in patients undergoing opioid withdrawal. Like clonidine it appears to act centrally to produce a reduction in sympathetic tone but reduction in blood pressure is less marked.

LOFEXIDINE HYDROCHLORIDE

Indications: management of symptoms of opioid withdrawal

Cautions: severe coronary insufficiency, recent myocardial infarction, cerebrovascular disease, marked bradycardia (monitor pulse rate frequently); renal impairment; history of depression (on longer treatment); pregnancy and breast-feed-

---

ing; withdraw gradually over 2–4 days (or longer) to minimise risk of rebound hypertension and associated symptoms; **interactions:** Appendix 1 (lofexidine)

Side-effects: drowsiness, dry mucous membranes (particularly dry mouth, throat and nose), hypotension, bradycardia, rebound hypertension on withdrawal (see Cautions); sedation and coma in overdosage

Dose: initially, 200 micrograms twice daily, increased as necessary in steps of 200–400 micrograms daily to max. 2.4 mg daily; recommended duration of treatment 7–10 days if no opioid use (but longer may be required); withdraw gradually over 2–4 days or longer; CHILD not recommended

PoM BritLofex® (Britannia)
Tablets, peach, f/c, lofexidine hydrochloride 200 micrograms. Net price 60-tab pack = £77.95. Label: 2

METHADONE HYDROCHLORIDE
Indications: adjunct in treatment of opioid dependence, see notes above; analgesia, section 4.7.2
Cautions; Contra-indications; Side-effects: section 4.7.2; overdosage: see Emergency Treatment of Poisoning, p. 22

IMPORTANT: Methadone, even in low doses is a **special hazard** for children; non-dependent adults are also at risk; dependent adults are at risk if tolerance is incorrectly assessed during induction

INCOMPATIBILITY. Syrup preserved with hydroxybenzoate esters may be incompatible with methadone hydrochloride.

Dose: initially 10–20 mg daily, increased by 10–20 mg daily until no signs of withdrawal or intoxication; usual dose 40–60 mg daily; CHILD not recommended (see also important note above)

CD Methadone (Non-proprietary)
Mixture 1 mg/mL, methadone hydrochloride 1 mg/mL, net price 30 mL = 46p, 50 mL = 76p, 100 mL = £1.52, 500 mL = £7.59. Label: 2

Available from Hillcross, Link (Methodex®), Martindale, Rosemont, Thornton & Ross—taste and colour of different formulations may vary slightly

IMPORTANT. This preparation is 2½ times the strength of Methadone Linctus and is intended only for drug dependent persons for whom treatment may be ordered on form FP10(HP)(ad) or FP10(MDA), or in Scotland on forms HBP(A) or GP10. The title includes the strength and prescriptions should be written accordingly

Injection and *Tablets,* section 4.7.2

Linctus, see section 3.9.1

CD Methadose® (Rosemont)
Oral concentrate, methadone hydrochloride 10 mg/mL (blue), net price 200 mL = £17.84; 20 mg/mL (brown), 200 mL = £35.68. Label: 2

Note. The final strength of the methadone mixture to be dispensed to the patient must be specified on the prescription

IMPORTANT. This preparation is intended to be diluted as appropriate with Methadose® Diluent (life of diluted solution 3 months) and is for drug dependent persons for whom treatment may be ordered on form FP10(HP)(ad) or FP10(MDA), or in Scotland on forms HBP(A)

NALTREXONE HYDROCHLORIDE
Indications: adjunct to prevent relapse in detoxified formerly opioid-dependent patients (who have remained opioid-free for at least 7–10 days)
Cautions: hepatic and renal impairment; liver function tests needed before and during treatment; test for opioid dependence with naloxone; avoid concomitant use of opioids but increased dose of opioid analgesic may be required for pain (monitor for opioid intoxication); pregnancy, breast-feeding

WARNING FOR PATIENTS. Patients need to be warned that an attempt to overcome the block could result in acute opioid intoxication

Contra-indications: patients currently dependent on opioids; acute hepatitis or liver failure
Side-effects: nausea, vomiting, abdominal pain; anxiety, nervousness, sleeping difficulty, headache, reduced energy; joint and muscle pain; less frequently, loss of appetite, diarrhoea, constipation, increased thirst; chest pain; increased sweating and lachrymation; increased energy, 'feeling down', irritability, dizziness, chills; delayed ejaculation, decreased potency; rash; occasionally, liver function abnormalities; reversible idiopathic thrombocytopenia reported
Dose: (initiate in specialist clinics only) 25 mg initially then 50 mg daily; the total weekly dose may be divided and given on 3 days of the week for improved compliance (e.g. 100 mg on Monday and Wednesday, and 150 mg on Friday); CHILD not recommended

PoM Nalorex® (Du Pont)
Tablets, orange, scored, naltrexone hydrochloride 50 mg. Net price 50-tab pack = £79.49

5: Drugs used in the treatment of
INFECTIONS

In this chapter, drug treatment is discussed under the following headings:

5.1   Antibacterial drugs
5.2   Antifungal drugs
5.3   Antiviral drugs
5.4   Antiprotozoal drugs
5.5   Anthelmintics

5.1   Antibacterial drugs

5.1.1   Penicillins
5.1.2   Cephalosporins, cephamycins and other beta-lactam antibiotics
5.1.3   Tetracyclines
5.1.4   Aminoglycosides
5.1.5   Macrolides
5.1.6   Clindamycin
5.1.7   Some other antibiotics
5.1.8   Sulphonamides and trimethoprim
5.1.9   Antituberculous drugs
5.1.10   Antileprotic drugs
5.1.11   Metronidazole and tinidazole
5.1.12   4-Quinolones
5.1.13   Urinary-tract infections

CHOICE OF A SUITABLE DRUG. Before selecting an antibiotic the clinician must first consider two factors—the patient and the known or likely causative organism. Factors related to the patient which must be considered include history of allergy, renal and hepatic function, resistance to infection (i.e. whether immunocompromised), ability to tolerate drugs by mouth, severity of illness, ethnic origin, age and, if female, whether pregnant, breast-feeding or taking an oral contraceptive.

The known or likely organism and its antibiotic sensitivity, in association with the above factors, will suggest one or more antibiotics, the final choice depending on the microbiological, pharmacological, and toxicological properties.

An example of a rational approach to the selection of an antibiotic is treatment of a urinary-tract infection in a patient complaining of nausea in early pregnancy. The organism is reported as being resistant to ampicillin but sensitive to nitrofurantoin (can cause nausea), gentamicin (can only be given by injection and best avoided in pregnancy), tetracycline (causes dental discoloration) and co-trimoxazole (folate antagonist therefore theoretical teratogenic risk), and cephalexin. The safest antibiotics in pregnancy are the penicillins and cephalosporins; therefore, cephalexin would be indicated for this patient.

The principles involved in selection of an antibiotic must allow for a number of variables including changing renal and hepatic function, increasing bacterial resistance, and new information on side-effects. Duration of therapy, dosage, and route of administration depend on site, type and severity of infection.

ANTIBIOTIC POLICIES. Many hospitals limit the antibiotics that may be used to achieve reasonable economy consistent with adequate cover, and to reduce the development of resistant organisms. An authority may indicate a range of drugs for general use, and permit other drugs only on the advice of the microbiologist or physician responsible for the control of infectious diseases.

BEFORE STARTING THERAPY. The following precepts should be considered before starting:

Viral infections should not be treated with antibiotics.

Samples should be taken for culture and sensitivity testing; **'blind'** prescribing of an antibiotic for a patient ill with unexplained pyrexia usually leads to further difficulty in establishing the diagnosis.

An up-to-date knowledge of **prevalent organisms** and their current sensitivity is of great help in choosing an antibiotic before bacteriological confirmation is available.

The **dose** of an antibiotic will vary according to a number of factors including age, weight, renal function, and severity of infection. The prescribing of the so-called 'standard' dose in serious infections may result in failure of treatment or even death of the patient therefore it is important to prescribe a dose appropriate to the condition. On the other hand, for an antibiotic with a narrow margin between the toxic and therapeutic dose (e.g. an aminoglycoside) it is also important to avoid an excessive dose and plasma concentration monitoring may be required.

The **route** of administration of an antibiotic will often depend on the severity of the infection. Life-threatening infections require intravenous therapy. Whenever possible painful intramuscular injections should be avoided in children.

Duration of therapy depends on the nature of the infection and the response to treatment. Courses should not be unduly prolonged and may be wasteful and may lead to side-effects. However, in certain infections such as tuberculosis or chronic osteomyelitis it is necessary to continue treatment for relatively long periods. Conversely a single dose of an antibiotic may cure uncomplicated urinary-tract infections.

SUPERINFECTION. In general, broad-spectrum antibacterial drugs such as the cephalosporins are more likely to be associated with adverse reactions related to the selection of resistant organisms e.g. *fungal infections* or *antibiotic-associated colitis* (pseudomembranous colitis).

THERAPY. Suggested treatment is shown in table 1. When the pathogen has been isolated treatment may be changed to a more appropriate antibiotic if necessary. If no bacterium is cultured the antibiotic can be continued or stopped on clinical grounds. Infections for which prophylaxis is useful are listed in table 2.

Table 1. Summary of antibacterial therapy

1: Gastro-intestinal system
Gastro-enteritis

Antibiotic not usually indicated
  Frequently nonbacterial aetiology

Campylobacter enteritis

Erythromycin *or* ciprofloxacin

Invasive salmonellosis

Ciprofloxacin *or* trimethoprim
  Includes severe infections which may be invasive

Shigellosis

Ciprofloxacin *or* trimethoprim
  Antibiotic not indicated for mild cases. Ciprofloxacin
  should be used for trimethoprim-resistant strains

Typhoid fever

Chloramphenicol *or* ciprofloxacin
  Infections from Indian subcontinent, Middle-East, and
  South-East Asia may be chloramphenicol-resistant and
  ciprofloxacin may be more appropriate

Antibiotic-associated colitis (pseudomembranous colitis)

Oral vancomycin *or* oral metronidazole

Biliary-tract infection

Gentamicin *or* a cephalosporin

Peritonitis

Gentamicin (*or* a cephalosporin) + metronidazole
(*or* clindamycin)

Peritoneal dialysis-associated peritonitis

Vancomycin[3] + gentamicin added to dialysis fluid
  Discontinue either gentamicin or vancomycin when sensitivity known; treat for 5–10 days

2: Cardiovascular system
Endocarditis caused by Penicillin-sensitive streptococci (e.g. viridans streptococci)

Benzylpenicillin (*or* vancomycin[3] if penicillin-
allergic) + low-dose gentamicin (i.e. 60–80 mg
twice daily)
  Treat for up to 4 weeks; stop gentamicin after 2 weeks if
  organism fully sensitive to penicillin. Oral amoxycillin[1]
  may be substituted for benzylpenicillin after 2 weeks

Endocarditis caused by Streptococci with reduced sensitivity to penicillin e.g. *Streptococcus faecalis*

Benzylpenicillin (*or* vancomycin[3] if penicillin-
allergic) + low-dose gentamicin (i.e. 60–80 mg
twice daily)
  Treat for 4 weeks

Endocarditis caused by Staphylococcus aureus
(and *Staphylococcus epidermidis*)

Flucloxacillin[2] + *either* gentamicin *or* fusidic acid
(*or* vancomycin[3] alone if penicillin-allergic)
  Treat for at least 4 weeks; stop gentamicin after 2 weeks

3: Respiratory system
Haemophilus epiglottitis

Chloramphenicol *or* cefotaxime
  Give intravenously

Exacerbations of chronic bronchitis

Amoxycillin[1] *or* trimethoprim *or* tetracycline
  Note that 20% of pneumococci and 15% of *Haemophilus influenzae* strains tetracycline-resistant; 15% *H.
  influenzae* strains amoxycillin-resistant

Chlamydial infections

Tetracycline *or* erythromycin[4]
  Treat for at least 10–14 days

Pneumonia: Previously healthy chest

Benzylpenicillin *or* amoxycillin[1]
  Add flucloxacillin[2] if Staphylococcus suspected e.g. in
  influenza or measles; add erythromycin[4] if *Mycoplasma
  pneumoniae* or Legionella infection suspected (severe
  Legionella infections may require addition of rifampicin); pneumococci with decreased penicillin sensitivity being isolated but not yet common in UK

Pneumonia: Previously unhealthy chest

Flucloxacillin[2] + amoxycillin[1] *or* erythromycin[4]
alone; *if hospital acquired,* a broad-spectrum
cephalosporin *or* an aminoglycoside
  Substitute erythromycin[4] (*or* rifampicin and
  erythromycin[4], see above) for flucloxacillin if
  Legionella infection suspected; use erythromycin[4] if
  Mycoplasma pneumoniae infection suspected

4: Central nervous system
Meningitis caused by Meningococci

Benzylpenicillin *or* cefotaxime
  Give rifampicin for 2 days before hospital discharge

Meningitis caused by Pneumococci

Cefotaxime
  Substitute benzylpenicillin if organism penicillin-sensitive; if organism highly penicillin- or cephalosporin-
  resistant, add vancomycin

Meningitis caused by Haemophilus influenzae

Chloramphenicol *or* cefotaxime
  For *H. influenzae* type b give rifampicin for 4 days
  before hospital discharge

Meningitis caused by Listeria

Amoxycillin[1] + gentamicin

7: Urinary tract
Acute pyelonephritis or prostatitis

Trimethoprim *or* gentamicin *or* cephalosporin *or* a
4-quinolone
  Treat prostatitis with trimethoprim or a 4-quinolone for
  4 weeks

'Lower' urinary-tract infection

Trimethoprim *or* amoxycillin[1] *or* nitrofurantoin *or*
oral cephalosporin

---

1. Where amoxycillin is suggested ampicillin or an ester of ampicillin (see section 5.1.1.3) may be used.
2. Where flucloxacillin is suggested cloxacillin may be used.
3. Where vancomycin is suggested teicoplanin may be used.
4. Where erythromycin is suggested another macrolide (e.g. azithromycin or clarithromycin) may be used.

Table 1. Summary of antibacterial therapy (*continued*)

7: Genital system

Syphilis

Procaine penicillin (*or* tetracycline *or* erythromycin if penicillin-allergic)

Treat for 10–21 days

Gonorrhoea

Amoxicillin[1] with probenecid (*or* spectinomycin *or* a 4-quinolone if penicillin-allergic)

Single-dose treatment in uncomplicated infection; choice depends on locality where infection acquired; contact-tracing advised; remember chlamydia

Non-gonococcal urethritis

Tetracycline *or* erythromycin[4]

Treat for 7–21 days; contact-tracing advised

Pelvic inflammatory disease

Metronidazole + doxycycline (*or* erythromycin)

Remember gonorrhoea; co-amoxiclav is not active against chlamydia; severely ill patients may require gentamicin (or a 'second-generation' cephalosporin) + a tetracycline

9: Blood

Septicaemia: Initial 'blind' therapy

Aminoglycoside + a broad-spectrum penicillin (*or* aztreonam) *or* a 'third generation' cephalosporin alone *or* imipenem (with cilastatin as *Primaxin*®) alone

In immunocompromised, aminoglycoside + a broad-spectrum penicillin *or* a 'third-generation' cephalosporin alone

Choice depends on local resistance patterns and clinical presentation; add metronidazole if anaerobic infection suspected; add flucloxacillin[2] or vancomycin[3] if Gram-positive infection suspected

10: Musculoskeletal system

Osteomyelitis and septic arthritis

Clindamycin alone *or* flucloxacillin[2] + fusidic acid. If *Haemophilus influenzae* give amoxycillin[1] *or* cefuroxime

Under 5 years of age may be *H. influenzae*. Treat acute disease for at least 6 weeks and chronic infection for at least 12 weeks

11: Eye

Purulent conjunctivitis

Chloramphenicol *or* gentamicin eye-drops

12: Ear, nose, and oropharynx

Dental infections

Phenoxymethylpenicillin (*or* amoxycillin[1]) *or* erythromycin *or* metronidazole

Tetracycline for chronic destructive forms of periodontal disease

Sinusitis

Amoxycillin[1] *or* doxycycline *or* erythromycin[4]

Treat for 2 weeks

Otitis externa

Flucloxacillin[2]

Otitis media

Amoxycillin[1] (*or* erythromycin[4] if penicillin-allergic)

Initial parenteral therapy (in severe infections) with benzylpenicillin, then oral therapy with phenoxymethylpenicillin. Under 5 years of age may be *Haemophilus influenzae*

Throat infections

Phenoxymethylpenicillin (*or* erythromycin[4] if penicillin-allergic) *or* oral cephalosporin

> Avoid amoxycillin if possibility of glandular fever, see section 5.1.1.3

Initial parenteral therapy (in severe infection) with benzylpenicillin, then oral therapy with phenoxymethylpenicillin *or* amoxycillin[1]; treat beta-haemolytic streptococcal infections for at least 10 days. Most infections are caused by viruses

13: Skin

Impetigo

Topical fusidic acid *or* mupirocin; oral flucloxacillin[2] *or* erythromycin if widespread

Topical treatment for 7 days usually adequate; max. duration of topical treatment 10 days

Erysipelas

Phenoxymethylpenicillin

Cellulitis

Phenoxymethylpenicillin + flucloxacillin[2] (*or* erythromycin alone if penicillin-allergic) *or* co-amoxiclav

Severe cellulitis may require parenteral benzylpenicillin + flucloxacillin[2] or co-amoxiclav alone

Animal bites

Co-amoxiclav

Cleanse wound thoroughly and give adsorbed tetanus vaccine; also use tetanus immunoglobulin for serious potentially contaminated wounds

Acne—see section 13.6

---

1. Where amoxycillin is suggested ampicillin or an ester of ampicillin (see section 5.1.1.3) may be used.
2. Where flucloxacillin is suggested cloxacillin may be used.
3. Where vancomycin is suggested teicoplanin may be used.
4. Where erythromycin is suggested another macrolide (e.g. azithromycin or clarithromycin) may be used.

Table 2. Summary of antibacterial prophylaxis

Prevention of recurrence of **rheumatic fever**
Phenoxymethylpenicillin 250 mg twice daily *or* sulphadiazine 1 g daily (500 mg daily for patients under 30 kg)

Prevention of secondary case of **meningococcal meningitis**[1]
Rifampicin 600 mg every 12 hours for 2 days; CHILD 10 mg/kg (under 1 year, 5 mg/kg) every 12 hours for 2 days
or ciprofloxacin 500 mg as a single dose [not licensed for this indication]; CHILD obtain further advice[1]
or i/m ceftriaxone 250 mg as a single dose [not licensed for this indication]; CHILD under 12 years 125 mg

Prevention of secondary case of *Haemophilus influenzae* type b disease[1]
Rifampicin 600 mg once daily for 4 days (optimum regimen for adults); CHILD over 3 months 20 mg/kg once daily for 4 days (max. 600 mg daily)

Prevention of secondary case of **diphtheria** in non-immune patient
Erythromycin 500 mg every 6 hours for 7–10 days; CHILD up to 2 years 125 mg every 6 hours, 2–8 years 250 mg every 6 hours

Prevention of **whooping cough**
ADULT and CHILD erythromycin 50 mg/kg daily (max. 2 g) in 4 divided doses for 7–10 days

Prevention of **pneumococcal infection** following splenectomy or in patients with sickle cell disease
Phenoxymethylpenicillin 500 mg every 12 hours; CHILD under 5 years 125 mg every 12 hours, 6–12 years 250 mg every 12 hours–if cover also needed for *H. influenzae* in CHILD give amoxycillin instead (under 5 years 125 mg every 12 hours, over 5 years 250 mg every 12 hours)

Prevention of **endocarditis**[2] in patients with heart-valve lesion, septal defect, patent ductus, or prosthetic valve

Dental procedures[3] *under local or no anaesthesia*,
patients who have not received more than a single dose of a penicillin in the previous month, including those with a prosthetic valve (but not those who have had endocarditis), oral amoxycillin 3 g 1 hour before procedure; CHILD under 5 years quarter adult dose; 5–10 years half adult dose

patients who are penicillin-allergic or have received more than a single dose of a penicillin in the previous month, oral clindamycin[4] 600 mg 1 hour before procedure; CHILD under 5 years quarter adult dose; 5–10 years half-adult dose

patients who have had endocarditis, amoxycillin + gentamicin, as under general anaesthesia

Dental procedures[3] *under general anaesthesia*,
no special risk (including patients who have not received more than a single dose of a penicillin in the previous month),
either i/m or i/v amoxycillin 1 g at induction, then oral amoxycillin 500 mg 6 hours later; CHILD under 5 years quarter adult dose; 5–10 years half adult dose
or oral amoxycillin 3 g 4 hours before induction then oral amoxycillin 3 g as soon as possible after procedure; CHILD under 5 years quarter adult dose; 5–10 years half adult dose
or oral amoxycillin 3 g + oral probenecid 1 g 4 hours before procedure;

special risk (patients with a prosthetic valve or who have had endocarditis), i/m or i/v amoxycillin 1 g + i/m or i/v gentamicin 120 mg at induction, then oral amoxycillin 500 mg 6 hours later; CHILD under 5 years amoxycillin quarter adult dose, gentamicin 2 mg/kg; 5–10 years amoxycillin half adult dose, gentamicin 2 mg/kg

patients who are penicillin-allergic or who have received more than a single dose of a penicillin in the previous month,
either i/v vancomycin 1 g over at least 100 minutes then i/v gentamicin 120 mg at induction or 15 minutes before procedure; CHILD under 10 years vancomycin 20 mg/kg, gentamicin 2 mg/kg
or i/v teicoplanin 400 mg + gentamicin 120 mg at induction or 15 minutes before procedure; CHILD under 14 years teicoplanin 6 mg/kg, gentamicin 2 mg/kg
or i/v clindamycin[4] 300 mg over at least 10 minutes at induction or 15 minutes before procedure then oral or i/v clindamycin 150 mg 6 hours later; CHILD under 5 years quarter adult dose; 5–10 years half adult dose

---

1. For details of those who should receive chemoprophylaxis contact a consultant in communicable disease control (or a consultant in infectious diseases or the local public health laboratory). Unless there has been mouth to mouth contact, hospital workers do not generally require chemoprophylaxis.
2. Advice on the prevention of endocarditis reflects the recommendations of a Working Party of the British Society for Antimicrobial Chemotherapy, *Lancet*, 1982, **2**, 1323–26; *idem*, 1986, **1**, 1267; *idem*, 1990, **335**, 88–9; *idem*, 1992, **339**, 1292–93; also *J Antimicrob Chemother*, 1993; **31**, 437–8
3. Dental procedures that require antibiotic prophylaxis are, *extractions, scaling,* and *surgery involving gingival tissues.* Antibiotic prophylaxis for dental procedures may be supplemented with *chlorhexidine gluconate gel 1%* or *chlorhexidine gluconate mouthwash 0.2%,* used 5 minutes before procedure
4. If **clindamycin** is used, periodontal or other multistage procedures should not be repeated at intervals of less than 2 weeks

Table 2. Summary of antibacterial prophylaxis (*continued*)

Prevention of **endocarditis**[1] in patients with heart-valve lesion, septal defect, patent ductus, or prosthetic valve (*continued*)

Upper respiratory-tract procedures, as for dental procedures; post-operative dose may be given parenterally if swallowing is painful

Genito-urinary procedures, as for *special risk* patients undergoing dental procedures under general anaesthesia except that clindamycin is not given, see above; if urine infected, prophylaxis should also cover infective organism

Obstetric, gynaecological and gastro-intestinal procedures (prophylaxis required for patients with prosthetic valves or those who have had endocarditis only), as for genito-urinary procedures

Prevention of **gas-gangrene** in high lower-limb amputations or following major trauma
Benzylpenicillin 300–600 mg every 6 hours for 5 days *or* if penicillin-allergic metronidazole 500 mg every 8 hours

Prevention of **tuberculosis** in susceptible close contacts
Isoniazid 300 mg daily for 6 months; CHILD, isoniazid 5–10 mg/kg daily max. 300 mg daily)
or isoniazid 300 mg daily + rifampicin 600 mg daily (450 mg if less than 50 kg) for 3 months; CHILD isoniazid 5–10 mg/kg daily (max. 300 mg daily) + rifampicin 10 mg/kg daily (max. 600 mg daily)

Prevention of infection in **abdominal surgery**
Operations on stomach or oesophagus for carcinoma, or cholecystectomy in patients with possibly infected bile
Single dose of gentamicin *or* a cephalosporin given in 2 hours before operation
Resections of colon and rectum for carcinoma, and resections in inflammatory bowel disease
Single dose of *either* gentamicin + metronidazole *or* cefuroxime + metronidazole given in 2 hours before operation
Hysterectomy
Metronidazole as suppository *or* single i/v dose

1. Advice on the prevention of endocarditis reflects the recommendations of a Working Party of the British Society for Antimicrobial Chemotherapy, *Lancet*, 1982, **2**, 1323–26; *idem*, 1986, **1**, 1267; *idem*, 1990, **335**, 88–9; *idem*, 1992, **339**, 1292–93; also *J Antimicrob Chemother*, 1993; **31**, 437–8

Joint prostheses and dental treatment.

Advice of a Working Party of the British Society for Antimicrobial Chemotherapy is that patients with prosthetic joint implants (including total hip replacements) do not require antibiotic prophylaxis for dental treatment. The Working Party considers that it is unacceptable to expose patients to the adverse effects of antibiotics when there is no evidence that such prophylaxis is of any benefit, but that those who develop any intercurrent infection require prompt treatment with antibiotics to which the infecting organisms are sensitive.

The Working Party has commented that joint infections have rarely been shown to follow dental procedures and are even more rarely caused by oral streptococci.

Immunosuppression and indwelling intraperitoneal catheters

Advice of a Working Party of the British Society for Antimicrobial Chemotherapy is that patients who are immunosuppressed (including transplant patients) and patients with indwelling intraperitoneal catheters do not require antibiotic prophylaxis for dental treatment provided there is no other indication for prophylaxis.

The Working Party has commented that there is little evidence that dental treatment is followed by infection in immunosuppressed and immunodeficient patients nor is there evidence that dental treatment is followed by infection in patients with indwelling intraperitoneal catheters.

5.1.1 Penicillins

5.1.1.1 Benzylpenicillin and phenoxymethylpenicillin
5.1.1.2 Penicillinase-resistant penicillins
5.1.1.3 Broad-spectrum penicillins
5.1.1.4 Antipseudomonal penicillins

The penicillins are bactericidal and act by interfering with bacterial cell wall synthesis. They diffuse well into body tissues and fluids, but penetration into the cerebrospinal fluid is poor except when the meninges are inflamed. They are excreted in the urine in therapeutic concentrations. Probenecid (see section 10.1.4) blocks the renal tubular excretion of the penicillins, producing higher and more prolonged plasma concentrations; it is not recommended in children under 2 years of age.

The most important side-effect of the penicillins is hypersensitivity, which causes rashes and, occasionally, anaphylaxis, which can be fatal. Patients who are allergic to one penicillin will be allergic to all as the hypersensitivity is related to the basic penicillin structure. A rare but serious toxic effect of the penicillins is encephalopathy due to cerebral irritation. This may result from excessively high doses but can also develop with normal doses given to patients with renal failure. The penicillins should **not** be given by intrathecal injection as they can cause encephalopathy which may be fatal.

A second problem relating to high doses of penicillin, or normal doses given to patients with renal failure, is the accumulation of electrolyte since most injectable penicillins contain either sodium or potassium.

Diarrhoea frequently occurs during oral penicillin therapy. It is most common with ampicillin and its derivatives, which can also cause pseudomembranous colitis.

5.1.1.1 BENZYLPENICILLIN AND PHENOXYMETHYLPENICILLIN

Benzylpenicillin (Penicillin G), the first of the penicillins, remains an important and useful antibiotic but is inactivated by bacterial penicillinases (beta-lactamases). It is effective for streptococcal, pneumococcal, gonococcal, and meningococcal infections and also for anthrax, diphtheria, gas-gangrene, leptospirosis, syphilis, tetanus, yaws, and treatment of Lyme disease in children. Pneumococci, meningococci, and gonococci which have decreased sensitivity to penicillin have been isolated; benzylpenicillin is no longer recommended for pneumococcal meningitis. Benzylpenicillin is inactivated by gastric acid and absorption from the gut is low; therefore it is best given by injection. Benzylpenicillin may cause convulsions after high doses by intravenous injection or in renal failure.

Procaine penicillin is a sparingly soluble salt of benzylpenicillin. It is used in intramuscular depot preparations which provide therapeutic tissue concentrations for up to 24 hours. It is the preferred choice for the treatment of syphilis; neurosyphilis requires special consideration.

Phenoxymethylpenicillin (Penicillin V) has a similar antibacterial spectrum to benzylpenicillin, but is less active. It is gastric acid-stable, so is suitable for oral administration. It should not be used for serious infections because absorption can be unpredictable and plasma concentrations variable. It is indicated principally for respiratory-tract infections in children, for streptococcal tonsillitis, and for continuing treatment after one or more injections of benzylpenicillin when clinical response has begun. It should not be used for meningococcal or gonococcal infections. Phenoxymethylpenicillin is used for prophylaxis against streptococcal infections following rheumatic fever and against pneumococcal infections following splenectomy or in sickle cell disease.

BENZYLPENICILLIN
(Penicillin G)

Indications: throat infections, otitis media, streptococcal endocarditis, meningococcal meningitis, pneumonia (see table 1); prophylaxis in limb amputation

Cautions: history of allergy; renal impairment; **interactions:** Appendix 1 (penicillins)

Contra-indications: penicillin hypersensitivity

Side-effects: sensitivity reactions including urticaria, fever, joint pains; angioedema; transient leucopenia and thrombocytopenia; anaphylactic

shock in hypersensitive patients; diarrhoea after administration by mouth

Dose: by intramuscular or by slow intravenous injection or by infusion, 1.2 g daily in 4 divided doses, increased if necessary to 2.4 g daily or more (see also below); PREMATURE INFANT and NEONATE, 50 mg/kg daily in 2 divided doses; INFANT 1–4 weeks, 75 mg/kg daily in 3 divided doses; CHILD 1 month–12 years, 100 mg/kg daily in 4 divided doses (higher doses may be required, see also below)

Bacterial endocarditis, *by slow intravenous injection or by infusion,* 7.2 g daily in 4–6 divided doses

Meningococcal meningitis, *by slow intravenous injection or by infusion,* 2.4 g every 4–6 hours; PREMATURE INFANT and NEONATE, 100 mg/kg daily in 2 divided doses; INFANT 1–4 weeks, 150 mg/kg daily in 3 divided doses; CHILD 1 month–12 years, 180–300 mg/kg daily in 4–6 divided doses

Important. If meningococcal disease is suspected general practitioners are advised to give a single injection of benzylpenicillin by intramuscular or by intravenous injection before transporting the patient urgently to hospital. Suitable doses are: ADULT 1.2 g; INFANT 300 mg; CHILD 1–9 years 600 mg, 10 years and over as for adult

Prophylaxis in limb amputation, section 5.1, table 2

By intrathecal injection, **not** recommended

Note. Benzylpenicillin doses in BNF may differ from those in data sheet

PoM Crystapen® (Britannia)
Injection, powder for reconstitution, benzylpenicillin sodium (unbuffered). Net price 600-mg vial = 44p, 2-vial 'GP pack' = £1.99
Electrolytes: Na+ 1.68 mmol/600-mg vial

PHENOXYMETHYLPENICILLIN
(Penicillin V)

Indications: tonsillitis, otitis media, erysipelas; rheumatic fever and pneumococcal infection prophylaxis (see table 2)

Cautions; Contra-indications; Side-effects: see under Benzylpenicillin; **interactions:** Appendix 1 (penicillins)

Dose: 500 mg every 6 hours increased to 750 mg every 6 hours in severe infections; CHILD, every 6 hours, up to 1 year 62.5 mg, 1–5 years 125 mg, 6–12 years 250 mg

Rheumatic fever and pneumococcal infection prophylaxis, section 5.1, table 2

PoM Phenoxymethylpenicillin (Non-proprietary)
Tablets, phenoxymethylpenicillin (as potassium salt) 250 mg, net price 20 = 30p. Label: 9, 23
Available from APS (Apsin®), Berk, Cox, Evans, Kent (Tenkicin®), Lagap
Oral solution, phenoxymethylpenicillin (as potassium salt) for reconstitution with water, net price 125 mg/5 mL, 100 mL = £1.03; 250 mg/5 mL, 100 mL = £1.25. Label: 9, 23
Available from APS (Apsin®), Cox, Evans, Kent (Tenkicin®)

PROCAINE PENICILLIN

Indications: penicillin-sensitive infections

Cautions; Contra-indications; Side-effects: see under Benzylpenicillin; **not** for intravenous administration

Dose: see below

PoM Bicillin® (Yamanouchi)

Injection, powder for reconstitution, procaine penicillin 1.8 g, benzylpenicillin sodium 360 mg. Net price 6-mL multidose vial = £2.70

Electrolytes: Na+ 1 mmol/vial

Dose: when reconstituted with 4.6 mL water for injections, 1 mL (procaine penicillin 300 mg, benzylpenicillin sodium 60 mg) every 12–24 hours by intramuscular injection

Primary syphilis, by intramuscular injection, 3 mL (4 mL in patients over 80 kg) daily for 10 days (14 days for secondary or latent syphilis)

Note. Reconstitution with 4.6 mL water for injections produces 6 mL

5.1.1.2 PENICILLINASE-RESISTANT PENICILLINS

Most staphylococci are now resistant to benzylpenicillin because they produce penicillinases. **Cloxacillin** and **flucloxacillin**, however, are not inactivated by these enzymes and are thus effective in infections caused by penicillin-resistant staphylococci, which is the sole indication for their use. They are acid-stable and can, therefore, be given by mouth as well as by injection.

Flucloxacillin is better absorbed from the gut than cloxacillin and is, therefore, to be preferred for oral therapy. For CSM warning on cholestatic jaundice see under Flucloxacillin.

Staph. aureus strains resistant to methicillin [now discontinued] (methicillin-resistant *Staphylococcus aureus*, MRSA) and cloxacillin have emerged in some hospitals; some of these organisms are only sensitive to vancomycin (section 5.1.7). Other alternatives include rifampicin and teicoplanin.

Temocillin is a new penicillin with activity against penicillinase-producing Gram-negative bacteria (except *Pseudomonas aeruginosa*); it is not active against Gram-positive bacteria.

CLOXACILLIN

Indications: infections due to penicillinase-producing staphylococci

Cautions; Contra-indications; Side-effects: see under Benzylpenicillin (section 5.1.1.1)

Dose: by mouth, 500 mg every 6 hours, at least 30 minutes before food

By intramuscular injection, 250 mg every 4–6 hours

By slow intravenous injection or by infusion, 500 mg every 4–6 hours

Doses may be doubled in severe infections

CHILD, any route, under 2 years quarter adult dose; 2–10 years half adult dose

Note. Oral liquid preparation no longer marketed

PoM Cloxacillin (Non-proprietary)

Capsules, cloxacillin (as sodium salt) 250 mg, net price 20 = £3.55; 500 mg, 20 = £7.11. Label: 9, 23

Available from Forley (Orbenin®), SmithKline Beecham

Injection, powder for reconstitution, cloxacillin (as sodium salt). Net price 250-mg vial = 91p; 500-mg vial = £1.81

Electrolytes: Na+ 0.59 mmol/250-mg vial, 1.18 mmol/500-mg vial

Available from Forley (Orbenin®), SmithKline Beecham

FLUCLOXACILLIN

Indications: infections due to penicillinase-producing staphylococci including otitis externa; adjunct in pneumonia, impetigo, cellulitis and in staphylococcal endocarditis (section 5.1 table 1)

Cautions; Contra-indications; Side-effects: see under Benzylpenicillin (section 5.1.1.1); hepatitis and cholestatic jaundice reported (see also CSM advice below); caution in porphyria (see section 9.8.2)

CHOLESTATIC JAUNDICE. CSM has advised that cholestatic jaundice may occur up to several weeks after treatment with flucloxacillin has been stopped. Administration for more than 2 weeks and increasing age are risk factors

Dose: by mouth, 250 mg every 6 hours, at least 30 minutes before food

By intramuscular injection, 250 mg every 6 hours

By slow intravenous injection or by infusion, 0.25–1 g every 6 hours

Doses may be doubled in severe infections

CHILD, any route, under 2 years quarter adult dose; 2–10 years half adult dose

PoM Flucloxacillin (Non-proprietary)

Capsules, flucloxacillin (as sodium salt) 250 mg, net price 20 = £1.51; 500 mg, 20 = £2.92. Label: 9, 23

Available from APS, Ashbourne (Fluclomix®), Berk (Ladropen®), Cox, Galen (Galfloxin®), Kent, Lagap, Norton, Yamanouchi (Stafoxil®)

Oral solution (= elixir or syrup), flucloxacillin (as sodium salt) for reconstitution with water, 125 mg/5 mL. Net price 100 mL = £3.33. Label: 9, 23

Available from APS, Berk (Ladropen®), Cox, Kent, Norton

Injection, powder for reconstitution, flucloxacillin (as sodium salt). Net price 250-mg vial = 75p; 500-mg vial = £1.71

Available from Berk (Ladropen®)

PoM Floxapen® (Beecham)

Capsules, both black/caramel, flucloxacillin (as sodium salt) 250 mg, net price 20-cap pack = £5.08, 28-cap pack = £7.11; 500 mg, 28-cap pack = £14.25. Label: 9, 23

Syrup, flucloxacillin (as magnesium salt) for reconstitution with water, 125 mg/5 mL, net price 100 mL = £3.65; 250 mg/5 mL, 100 mL = £7.30. Label: 9, 23

Injection, powder for reconstitution, flucloxacillin (as sodium salt). Net price 250-mg vial = £1.02; 500-mg vial = £2.04; 1-g vial = £4.08

Electrolytes: Na+ 0.57 mmol/250-mg vial, 1.13 mmol/500-mg vial, 2.26 mmol/1-g vial

TEMOCILLIN

Indications: infections due to penicillinase-producing Gram-negative bacteria except pseudomonas

Cautions; Contra-indications; Side-effects: see under Benzylpenicillin (section 5.1.1.1)

Dose: by intramuscular injection or by intravenous injection (over 3–4 minutes) *or by intravenous infusion,* 1–2 g every 12 hours

Acute uncomplicated urinary-tract infections, 1 g daily as a single dose

PoM **Temopen®** (Bencard)

Injection, powder for reconstitution, temocillin (as sodium salt). Net price 1-g vial = £15.00

Electrolytes: Na⁺ 5 mmol/g

5.1.1.3 BROAD-SPECTRUM PENICILLINS

Ampicillin is active against certain Gram-positive and Gram-negative organisms but is inactivated by penicillinases including those produced by *Staphylococcus aureus* and by common Gram-negative bacilli such as *Escherichia coli.* Almost all staphylococci, 50% of *E. coli* strains and 15% of *Haemophilus influenzae* strains are now resistant. The likelihood of resistance should therefore be considered before using ampicillin for the 'blind' treatment of infections; in particular, it should not be used for hospital patients without checking sensitivity.

Ampicillin is well excreted in the bile and urine. It is principally indicated for the treatment of exacerbations of chronic bronchitis and middle ear infections, both of which are usually due to *Streptococcus pneumoniae* and *H. influenzae,* and for urinary-tract infections (section 5.1.13) and gonorrhoea.

Ampicillin can be given by mouth but less than half the dose is absorbed, and absorption is further decreased by the presence of food in the gut. Higher plasma concentrations are obtained with the ampicillin esters **bacampicillin** and **pivampicillin**; their absorption is little affected by the presence of food, and the incidence of diarrhoea is less than with ampicillin.

Maculopapular rashes commonly occur with ampicillin (and amoxycillin) but are not usually related to true penicillin allergy. They almost always occur in patients with glandular fever; broad-spectrum penicillins should not therefore be used for 'blind' treatment of a sore throat. Rashes are also common in patients with chronic lymphatic leukaemia; rashes may also be more common in patients infected with the human immunodeficiency virus (HIV) although initial reports have not been confirmed.

Amoxycillin is a derivative of ampicillin which differs by only one hydroxyl group and has a similar antibacterial spectrum. It is better absorbed than ampicillin when given by mouth, producing higher plasma and tissue concentrations; unlike ampicillin, absorption is not affected by the presence of food in the stomach. Amoxycillin is used for endocarditis prophylaxis (section 5.1, table 2); it may also be used for the treatment of Lyme disease in children.

Co-amoxiclav consists of amoxycillin with the beta-lactamase inhibitor clavulanic acid. Clavulanic acid itself has no significant antibacterial activity but, by inactivating penicillinases, it makes the combination active against penicillinase-producing bacteria that are resistant to amoxycillin. These include most *Staph. aureus,* 50% of *E. coli* strains, and up to 15% of *H. influenzae* strains, as well as many *Bacteroides* and *Klebsiella* spp. Co-amoxiclav may be used for pelvic inflammatory disease and for cellulitis (see section 5.1, table 1). For CSM warning on cholestatic jaundice see under Co-amoxiclav.

Combinations of ampicillin with flucloxacillin (as co-fluampicil) and ampicillin with cloxacillin (Ampiclox®) are available.

AMOXYCILLIN
(Amoxicillin)

Indications: see under Ampicillin; also endocarditis prophylaxis; adjunct in listerial meningitis (section 5.1, table1)

Cautions; Contra-indications; Side-effects: see under Ampicillin

Dose: by mouth, 250 mg every 8 hours, doubled in severe infections; CHILD up to 10 years, 125 mg every 8 hours, doubled in severe infections

Severe or recurrent purulent respiratory infection, 3 g every 12 hours

Endocarditis prophylaxis, section 5.1, table 2

Short-course oral therapy

Dental abscess, 3 g repeated after 8 hours

Urinary-tract infections, 3 g repeated after 10–12 hours

Gonorrhoea, single dose of 2–3 g with probenecid 1 g

Otitis media, CHILD 3–10 years, 750 mg twice daily for 2 days

By intramuscular injection, 500 mg every 8 hours; CHILD, 50–100 mg/kg daily in divided doses

By intravenous injection or infusion, 500 mg every 8 hours increased to 1 g every 6 hours; CHILD, 50–100 mg/kg daily in divided doses

PoM **Amoxycillin** (Non-proprietary)

Capsules, amoxycillin (as trihydrate) 250 mg, net price 20 = 83p; 500 mg, 20 = £1.11. Label: 9

Available from APS, Ashbourne (Amix®), Berk (Almodan®), BHR (Amrit®), Cox, Eastern (Amoram®), Galen (Galenamox®), Kent, Lagap, Norton, Rima (Rimoxallin®)

Oral suspension, amoxycillin (as trihydrate) for reconstitution with water, 125 mg/5 mL, net price 100 mL = £1.09; 250 mg/5 mL, 100 mL = £1.97. Label: 9

Note. Sugar-free versions are available and can be ordered by specifying 'sugar-free' on the prescription

Available from APS, Ashbourne (Amix®), Berk (Almodan®), BHR (Amrit®), Cox, Eastern (Amoram®), Galen (Galenamox®), Kent, Lagap, Norton, Rima (Rimoxallin®)

Sachets, sugar-free, amoxycillin 3 g (as trihydrate)/sachet, net price 2-sachet pack = £4.61, 14-sachet pack = £31.65. Label: 9, 13

Available from Hillcross, Kent, Norton

PoM **Amoxil®** (Bencard)

Capsules, both maroon/gold, amoxycillin (as trihydrate), 250 mg, net price 21-cap pack = £4.04; 500 mg, 21-cap pack = £8.09. Label: 9

Dispersible tablets, sugar-free, amoxycillin 500 mg (as trihydrate). Net price 21-tab pack = £9.33. Label: 9, 13

Fiztab (= chewable tablets), sugar-free, amoxycillin (as trihydrate) 125 mg, net price 20-tab pack = £2.42; 250 mg, 20-tab pack = £4.84; 500 mg, 20-tab pack = £9.68. Label: 9, 10 patient information leaflet

Note. Dose form not suitable for children under 3 years

Syrup SF, both sugar-free, amoxycillin (as trihydrate) for reconstitution with water, 125 mg/5 mL, net price 100 mL = £2.42; 250 mg/5 mL, 100 mL = £4.84. Label: 9

Paediatric suspension, amoxycillin 125 mg (as trihydrate)/1.25 mL when reconstituted with water. Net price 20 mL = £3.63. Label: 9, counselling, use of pipette

Sachets SF, powder, sugar-free, amoxycillin 750 mg (as trihydrate)/sachet, net price 4-sachet pack = £3.15; 3 g/sachet, 2-sachet pack = £5.20. Label: 9, 13

Injection, powder for reconstitution, amoxycillin (as sodium salt). Net price 250-mg vial = 36p; 500-mg vial = 66p; 1-g vial = £1.31

Electrolytes: Na⁺ 3.3 mmol/g

AMPICILLIN

Indications: urinary-tract infections, otitis media, sinusitis, chronic bronchitis, invasive salmonellosis, gonorrhoea

Cautions: history of allergy; renal impairment; erythematous rashes common in glandular fever, chronic lymphatic leukaemia, and possibly HIV infection (see notes above); **interactions:** Appendix 1 (penicillins)

Contra-indications: penicillin hypersensitivity

Side-effects: nausea, diarrhoea; rashes (discontinue treatment); rarely, pseudomembranous colitis; see also under Benzylpenicillin (section 5.1.1.1)

Dose: by mouth, 0.25–1 g every 6 hours, at least 30 minutes before food

Gonorrhoea, 2–3.5 g as a single dose with probenecid 1 g

Urinary-tract infections, 500 mg every 8 hours

By intramuscular injection or intravenous injection or infusion, 500 mg every 4–6 hours; higher doses in meningitis

CHILD under 10 years, any route, half adult dose

PoM **Ampicillin** (Non-proprietary)

Capsules, ampicillin 250 mg, net price 20 = 66p; 500 mg, 20 = £1.27. Label: 9, 23

Available from APS, Berk (Vidopen®), Cox, Kent, Lagap, Norton, Rima (Rimacillin®), Yamanouchi (Amfipen®)

Oral suspension, ampicillin 125 mg/5 mL when reconstituted with water, net price 100 mL = 84p; 250 mg/5 mL, 100 mL = £1.06. Label: 9, 23

Available from APS, Berk, Cox, Kent, Lagap, Norton, Rima (Rimacillin®), Yamanouchi (Amfipen®)

PoM **Penbritin®** (Beecham)

Capsules, both black/red, ampicillin (as trihydrate) 250 mg, net price 28-cap pack = £2.26; 500 mg, 28-cap pack = £4.51. Label: 9, 23

Syrup, ampicillin (as trihydrate) for reconstitution with water, 125 mg/5 mL, net price 100 mL = £1.20; 250 mg/5 mL, 100 mL = £2.39. Label: 9, 23

Paediatric suspension, ampicillin 125 mg (as trihydrate)/1.25 mL. Net price 25 mL = £2.23. Label: 9, 23, counselling, use of pipette

Injection, powder for reconstitution, ampicillin (as sodium salt). Net price 250-mg vial = 37p; 500-mg vial = 74p

Electrolytes: Na⁺ 0.73 mmol/250-mg vial, 1.47 mmol/500-mg vial

With cloxacillin

PoM **Ampiclox®** (Beecham)

Capsules, black/purple, ampicillin 250 mg (as trihydrate), cloxacillin 250 mg (as sodium salt). Net price 20-cap pack = £7.00. Label: 9, 23

Dose: 1–2 capsules every 4–6 hours

Syrup, ampicillin 125 mg (as trihydrate), cloxacillin 125 mg (as sodium salt)/5 mL when reconstituted with water. Net price 100 mL = £5.00. Label: 9, 23

Dose: 10–20 mL every 4–6 hours; CHILD 1 month–2 years, quarter adult dose; 2–12 years, half adult dose

Injection, ampicillin 250 mg (as sodium salt), cloxacillin 250 mg (as sodium salt). Net price per vial = £1.49

Electrolytes: Na⁺ 1.32 mmol/vial

Dose: by intramuscular injection or intravenous injection or infusion, 1–2 vials every 4–6 hours; CHILD up to 2 years quarter adult dose, 2–10 years half adult dose

PoM **Ampiclox Neonatal®** (Beecham)

Suspension, sugar-free, ampicillin 60 mg (as trihydrate), cloxacillin 30 mg (as sodium salt)/0.6 mL when reconstituted with water. Net price 10 mL = £2.27. Label: 9, counselling, use of pipette

Dose: 0.6 mL every 4 hours

Injection, ampicillin 50 mg (as sodium salt), cloxacillin 25 mg (as sodium salt). Net price per vial = 42p.

Electrolytes: Na⁺ <0.5 mmol/vial

Dose: NEONATE and PREMATURE INFANT, by intramuscular injection or by intravenous injection or infusion, 1 vial every 8 hours

With flucloxacillin

See Co-fluampicil

BACAMPICILLIN HYDROCHLORIDE

Indications; Cautions; Contra-indications; Side-effects: see under Ampicillin

Dose: 400 mg 2–3 times daily, doubled in severe infections; CHILD over 5 years, 200 mg 3 times daily

Uncomplicated gonorrhoea, 1.6 g as a single dose with probenecid 1 g

PoM **Ambaxin®** (Upjohn)

Tablets, scored, bacampicillin hydrochloride 400 mg. Net price 20 = £6.34. Label: 9

CO-AMOXICLAV

A mixture of amoxicillin (as the trihydrate or as the sodium salt) and clavulanic acid (as potassium clavulanate); the proportions are expressed in the form *x/y* where *x* and *y* are the strengths in milligrams of amoxicillin and clavulanic acid respectively

Indications; Cautions; Contra-indications; Side-effects: see under Ampicillin and notes above; also caution in hepatic impairment (monitor hepatic function), pregnancy; hepatitis, cholestatic jaundice (see also CSM advice below), erythema multiforme (including Stevens-Johnson syndrome), toxic epidermal necrolysis, exfoliative dermatitis, and interstitial nephritis reported; phlebitis at injection site also reported; treatment not to exceed 14 days without review

CHOLESTATIC JAUNDICE. CSM has advised that cholestatic jaundice may occur up to 6 weeks after treatment with co-amoxiclav has been stopped. Clavulanic acid is likely to be responsible

Dose: *by mouth,* expressed as amoxycillin, 250 mg every 8 hours, dose doubled in severe infections; CHILD see under preparations below (under 6 years Augmentin® '125/31 SF' suspension; 6–12 years Augmentin® '250/62 SF' suspension *or* for short-term treatment with twice daily dosage in CHILD 2–12 years Augmentin-Duo® 400/57 suspension)

Dental infections, expressed as amoxycillin, 250 mg every 8 hours for 5 days

By intravenous injection over 3–4 minutes *or by intravenous infusion,* expressed as amoxycillin, 1 g every 8 hours increased to 1 g every 6 hours in more serious infections; INFANTS up to 3 months 25 mg/kg every 8 hours (every 12 hours in the perinatal period and in premature infants); CHILD 3 months–12 years, 25 mg/kg every 8 hours increased to 25 mg/kg every 6 hours in more serious infections

Surgical prophylaxis, expressed as amoxycillin, 1 g at induction; for high risk procedures (e.g. colorectal surgery) a further 2–3 doses may be given every 8 hours in first 24 hours (longer if significantly increased risk of infection)

PoM Augmentin® (Beecham)

Tablets *375 mg,* f/c, co-amoxiclav 250/125 (amoxycillin 250 mg as trihydrate, clavulanic acid 125 mg as potassium salt). Net price 21-tab pack = £8.09. Label: 9

Tablets *625 mg,* f/c, co-amoxiclav 500/125 (amoxycillin 500 mg as trihydrate, clavulanic acid 125 mg as potassium salt). Net price 21-tab pack = £13.00. Label: 9

Dispersible tablets, sugar-free, co-amoxiclav 250/125 (amoxycillin 250 mg as trihydrate, clavulanic acid 125 mg as potassium salt). Net price 21-tab pack = £9.08. Label: 9, 13

Suspension '125/31 SF', sugar-free, co-amoxiclav 125/31 (amoxycillin 125 mg as trihydrate, clavulanic acid 31 mg as potassium salt)/5 mL when reconstituted with water. Net price 100 mL = £4.15. Label: 9

Note. Suspension contains aspartame 12.5 mg/5 mL (see section 9.4.1)

Dose: CHILD under 1 year 0.8 mL/kg daily in 3 divided doses; 1–6 years (10–18 kg) 5 mL every 8 hours, doubled in severe infections

Suspension '250/62 SF', sugar-free, co-amoxiclav 250/62 (amoxycillin 250 mg as trihydrate, clavulanic acid 62 mg as potassium salt)/5 mL when reconstituted with water. Net price 100 mL = £5.84. Label: 9

Note. Suspension contains aspartame 12.5 mg/5 mL (see section 9.4.1)

Dose: CHILD 6–12 years 5 mL every 8 hours, doubled in severe infections

Injection 600 mg, powder for reconstitution, co-amoxiclav 500/100 (amoxycillin 500 mg as sodium salt, clavulanic acid 100 mg as potassium salt). Net price per vial = £1.35

Electrolytes: Na+ 1.6 mmol, K+ 0.5 mmol/600-mg vial

Injection 1.2 g, powder for reconstitution, co-amoxiclav 1000/200 (amoxycillin 1 g as sodium salt, clavulanic acid 200 mg as potassium salt). Net price per vial = £2.70

Electrolytes: Na+ 3.1 mmol, K+ 1 mmol/1.2-g vial

PoM Augmentin-Duo® (SmithKline Beecham)

Suspension '400/57', sugar-free, co-amoxiclav 400/57 (amoxycillin 400 mg as trihydrate, clavulanic acid 57 mg as potassium salt)/5 mL when reconstituted with water. Net price 35 mL = £4.15, 70 mL = £5.84, 140 mL = £11.45. Label: 9

Note. Suspension contains aspartame 12.5 mg/5 mL (see section 9.4.1)

Dose: CHILD 2–6 years (13–21 kg) 2.5 mL twice daily, 7–12 years (22–40 kg) 5 mL twice daily, doubled in severe infections

CO-FLUAMPICIL

A mixture of equal parts by mass of flucloxacillin and ampicillin

Indications: mixed infections involving penicillinase-producing staphylococci

Cautions; Contra-indications; Side-effects: see under Ampicillin and Flucloxacillin

Dose: *by mouth,* co-fluampicil, 250/250 every 6 hours, dose doubled in severe infections; CHILD under 10 years half adult dose, dose doubled in severe infections

By intramuscular or slow intravenous injection or by intravenous infusion, co-fluampicil 250/250 every 6 hours, dose doubled in severe infections; CHILD under 2 years quarter adult dose, 2–10 years half adult dose, dose doubled in severe infections

PoM Co-fluampicil (Non-proprietary)

Capsules, co-fluampicil 250/250 (flucloxacillin 250 mg as sodium salt, ampicillin 250 mg as trihydrate). Net price 20 = £4.59. Label: 9, 22

Available from Cox, Generics (Flu-Amp®), Kent, Norton

PoM Magnapen® (Beecham)

Capsules, black/turquoise, co-fluampicil 250/250 (flucloxacillin 250 mg as sodium salt, ampicillin 250 mg as trihydrate). Net price 20-cap pack = £6.15. Label: 9, 22

Syrup, co-fluampicil 125/125 (flucloxacillin 125 mg as magnesium salt, ampicillin 125 mg as trihydrate)/5 mL when reconstituted with water. Net price 100 mL = £4.99. Label: 9, 22

Injection 500 mg, powder for reconstitution, co-fluampicil 250/250 (flucloxacillin 250 mg as sodium salt, ampicillin 250 mg as sodium salt). Net price per vial = £1.33

Electrolytes: Na+ 1.3 mmol/vial

PIVAMPICILLIN

Indications: see under Ampicillin

Cautions; Contra-indications; Side-effects: see under Ampicillin; hepatic and renal function tests required in long-term use; avoid in porphyria (see section 9.8.2) and in carnitine deficiency

Dose: 500 mg every 12 hours, doubled in severe infections; CHILD 3 months–1 year 40–60 mg/kg daily in 2–3 divided doses; 1–5 years 350–525 mg daily; 6–10 years 525–700 mg daily; doses can be doubled in severe infections

PoM **Pondocillin**® (Leo)

Tablets, f/c, pivampicillin 500 mg. Net price 20 = £4.12. Label: 5, 9, 21

Suspension, sugar-free, pivampicillin 175 mg/ 5 mL when reconstituted with water. Net price 50 mL = £1.72; 100 mL = £2.77. Label: 5, 9, 21

5.1.1.4 ANTIPSEUDOMONAL PENICILLINS

The carboxypenicillins, **carbenicillin** and **ticarcillin**, are principally indicated for the treatment of serious infections caused by *Pseudomonas aeruginosa* although they also have activity against certain other Gram-negative bacilli including *Proteus* spp. and *Bacteroides fragilis*. Carbenicillin has been replaced by ticarcillin which is more active against these organisms.

Timentin® (ticarcillin with clavulanic ácid, section 5.1.1.3), is active against penicillinase-producing bacteria resistant to ticarcillin.

The ureidopenicillins, **azlocillin** and **piperacillin**, have a broad spectrum and are both more active than ticarcillin against *Ps. aeruginosa*.

Tazocin® (piperacillin with the beta-lactamase inhibitor tazobactam) is active against beta-lactamase producing bacteria resistant to the ureidopenicillins.

For pseudomonas septicaemias (especially in neutropenia or endocarditis) these antipseudomonal penicillins should be given with an aminoglycoside (e.g. gentamicin or netilmicin, section 5.1.4) as there is a synergistic effect. Penicillins and aminoglycosides must not, however, be mixed in the same syringe or infusion.

Owing to the sodium content of many of these antibiotics, high doses may lead to hypernatraemia.

AZLOCILLIN

Indications: infections due to *Pseudomonas aeruginosa*, see notes above

Cautions; Contra-indications; Side-effects: see under Benzylpenicillin (section 5.1.1.1); **interactions:** Appendix 1 (penicillins)

Dose: by intravenous injection, 2 g every 8 hours

Serious infections, *by intravenous infusion,* 5 g every 8 hours; PREMATURE INFANT 50 mg/kg every 12 hours; NEONATE 100 mg/kg every 12 hours; INFANT 7 days–1 year 100 mg/kg every 8 hours; CHILD 1–14 years 75 mg/kg every 8 hours

PoM **Securopen**® (Bayer)

Injection, powder for reconstitution, azlocillin (as sodium salt). Net price 500-mg vial = £1.03; 1-g vial = £2.36; 2-g vial = £2.94

Electrolytes: Na⁺ 1.08 mmol/500-mg vial, 2.17 mmol/1-g vial, 4.33 mmol/2-g vial

Infusion, powder for reconstitution, azlocillin (as sodium salt). Net price 5 g vial = £8.10 (also available with 50 mL water for injections, transfer needle, and infusion bag)

Electrolytes: Na⁺ 10.84 mmol/5-g vial

CARBENICILLIN

Indications: infections due to *Pseudomonas aeruginosa* and *Proteus* spp., see notes above

Cautions; Contra-indications: see under Benzylpenicillin (section 5.1.1.1)

Side-effects: see under Benzylpenicillin (section 5.1.1.1); also hypokalaemia, alteration in platelet function

Dose: Pseudomonal infections and systemic Proteus infections, *by intravenous injection* over 3–4 minutes *or by intravenous infusion,* 5 g every 4–6 hours; CHILD 250–400 mg/kg daily in 3–6 divided doses

Urinary-tract infections and less serious Proteus infections, *by intramuscular injection,* 1–2 g every 6 hours; CHILD 50–100 mg/kg daily in 3–6 divided doses

PoM **Pyopen**® (Link)

Injection, powder for reconstitution, carbenicillin (as sodium salt). Net price 1-g vial = £3.00

Electrolytes: Na⁺ 5.4 mmol/1-g vial

PIPERACILLIN

Indications: infections due to *Pseudomonas aeruginosa,* see notes above

Cautions; Contra-indications; Side-effects: see under Benzylpenicillin (section 5.1.1.1)

Dose: by intramuscular or by slow intravenous injection or by intravenous infusion, 100–150 mg/ kg daily (in divided doses), increased to 200– 300 mg/kg daily in severe infections, and to at least 16 g daily in life-threatening infections; single doses over 2 g intravenous route only

PoM **Pipril**® (Lederle)

Injection, powder for reconstitution, piperacillin (as sodium salt). Net price 1-g vial = £2.79; 2-g vial = £5.53

Infusion, powder for reconstitution, piperacillin 4 g (as sodium salt), with 50-mL bottle water for injections and transfer needle. Net price complete unit = £11.65

Electrolytes: Na⁺ 1.94 mmol/g

With tazobactam

PoM **Tazocin**® (Lederle)

Injection 2.25 g, powder for reconstitution, piperacillin 2 g (as sodium salt), tazobactam 250 mg (as sodium salt). Net price per vial = £7.24

Electrolytes: Na⁺ 4.69 mmol/2.25-g vial

Injection 4.5 g, powder for reconstitution, piperacillin 4 g (as sodium salt), tazobactam 500 mg (as

---

sodium salt). Net price per vial = £13.16; infusion pack (4.5-g infusion bottle, 50-mL bottle water for injections and transfer needle) = £14.48

Electrolytes: Na+ 9.37 mmol/4.5-g vial

Dose: lower respiratory-tract, urinary-tract, intra-abdominal and skin infections, and septicaemia, ADULT and CHILD over 12 years, *by intravenous injection* over 3–5 minutes *or by intravenous infusion,* 2.25–4.5 g every 6–8 hours, usually 4.5 g every 8 hours; CHILD under 12 years, not yet recommended

TICARCILLIN

Indications: infections due to *Pseudomonas* and *Proteus* spp, see notes above

Cautions; Contra-indications; Side-effects: see under Benzylpenicillin (section 5.1.1.1)

Dose: by slow intravenous injection over 3–4 minutes *or by intravenous infusion,* 15–20 g daily in divided doses; CHILD 200–300 mg/kg daily in divided doses

Urinary-tract infections, *by intramuscular or slow intravenous injection,* 3–4 g daily in divided doses; CHILD 50–100 mg/kg daily in divided doses

PoM **Ticar®** (Link)

Injection, powder for reconstitution, ticarcillin (as sodium salt). Net price 1-g vial = £4.20; 5-g vial = £17.09

Electrolytes: Na+ 5.3 mmol/1-g vial, 26.7 mmol/5-g vial

With clavulanic acid

Note. For a CSM warning on cholestatic jaundice possibly associated with clavulanic acid, see under Co-amoxiclav p. 234.

PoM **Timentin®** (Beecham)

Injection 1.6 g, powder for reconstitution, ticarcillin 1.5 g (as sodium salt), clavulanic acid 100 mg (as potassium salt). Net price per vial = £3.04

Injection 3.2 g, powder for reconstitution, ticarcillin 3 g (as sodium salt), clavulanic acid 200 mg (as potassium salt). Net price per vial = £6.08

Electrolytes: Na+ 16 mmol, K+ 1 mmol /3.2-g vial

Dose: by intravenous infusion, 3.2 g every 6–8 hours increased to every 4 hours in more severe infections; CHILD 80 mg/kg every 6–8 hours (every 12 hours in neonates)

5.1.2 Cephalosporins, cephamycins, and other beta-lactam antibiotics

Antibiotics discussed in this section include the **cephalosporins**, such as cefotaxime, ceftazidime, cefuroxime, cephalexin and cephradine, the **cephamycin,** cefoxitin, the **monobactam,** aztreonam, and the **carbapenems** imipenem (a thienamycin derivative) and meropenem.

CEPHALOSPORINS AND CEPHAMYCINS

The cephalosporins are broad-spectrum antibiotics which are used for the treatment of septicaemia, pneumonia, meningitis, biliary-tract infections, peritonitis, and urinary-tract infections. All have a

similar antibacterial spectrum although individual agents have differing activity against certain organisms. The pharmacology of the cephalosporins is similar to that of the penicillins, excretion being principally renal and blocked by probenecid.

The principal side-effect of the cephalosporins is hypersensitivity and about 10% of penicillin-sensitive patients will also be allergic to the cephalosporins. Haemorrhage due to interference with blood clotting factors has been associated with several cephalosporins.

Cephradine and **cephazolin** have generally been replaced by the newer cephalosporins mentioned below.

Cefuroxime and **cephamandole** are 'second generation' cephalosporins and are less susceptible than the earlier cephalosporins to inactivation by penicillinases. They are, therefore, active against certain bacteria which are resistant to the other drugs and have greater activity against *Haemophilus influenzae* and *Neisseria gonorrhoeae.*

Cefotaxime, ceftazidime, ceftizoxime, cefodizime and **ceftriaxone** are 'third generation' cephalosporins with greater activity than the 'second generation' cephalosporins against certain Gram-negative bacteria. However, they are less active than cefuroxime and cephamandole against Gram-positive bacteria, most notably *Staphylococcus aureus.* Their broad antibacterial spectrum may encourage superinfection with resistant bacteria or fungi.

Ceftazidime has good activity against pseudomonas. It is also active against other Gram-negative bacteria.

Ceftriaxone has a longer half-life than other cephalosporins and therefore only needs once daily administration. Indications include serious infections such as septicaemia, pneumonia, and meningitis. The calcium salt of ceftriaxone forms a precipitate in the gall bladder which may rarely cause symptoms but these usually resolve when the antibiotic is stopped.

Cefpirome has been introduced recently for urinary-tract, lower respiratory-tract and skin structure infections, bacteraemia, and infections associated with neutropenia.

Cefoxitin, a cephamycin antibiotic, is active against bowel flora including *Bacteroides fragilis* and because of this it has been recommended for abdominal sepsis such as peritonitis.

ORALLY ACTIVE CEPHALOSPORINS. The orally active 'first generation' cephalosporins, **cephalexin, cephradine,** and **cefadroxil** and the 'second generation' cephalosporin **cefaclor** have a similar antimicrobial spectrum. They are useful for urinary-tract infections which do not respond to other drugs or which occur in pregnancy, respiratory-tract infections, sinusitis, and skin and soft-tissue infections. Cefaclor has good activity against *H. influenzae,* but is associated with protracted skin reactions especially in children. Cefadroxil has a longer duration of action than the other cephalosporins but poor activity against *H. influenzae.* **Cefuroxime axetil,** an ester of the 'second generation' cephalosporin cefuroxime, has the same antibacterial spectrum as the parent compound.

Cefixime has a longer duration of action than the other cephalosporins that are active by mouth. It is presently only licensed for acute infections. **Ceftibuten** is similar to cefixime but is less active against pneumococci.

Cefpodoxime proxetil, is more active than the other oral cephalosporins against respiratory bacterial pathogens and it is licensed for upper and lower respiratory-tract infections.

CEFACLOR

Indications: infections due to sensitive Gram-positive and Gram-negative bacteria, but see notes above

Cautions: penicillin sensitivity; renal impairment (see Appendix 3); pregnancy and breast-feeding (but appropriate to use); false positive urinary glucose (if tested for reducing substances) and false positive Coombs' test; **interactions:** Appendix 1 (cephalosporins)

Contra-indications: cephalosporin hypersensitivity; porphyria (see section 9.8.2)

Side-effects: diarrhoea and rarely pseudomembranous colitis (CSM has warned both more likely with higher doses), nausea and vomiting, abdominal discomfort, headache; allergic reactions including rashes, pruritus, urticaria, serum sickness-like reactions with rashes, fever and arthralgia, and anaphylaxis; erythema multiforme, toxic epidermal necrolysis reported; disturbances in liver enzymes, transient hepatitis and cholestatic jaundice; other side-effects reported include eosinophilia and blood disorders (including thrombocytopenia, leucopenia, agranulocytosis and aplastic anaemia); reversible interstitial nephritis, hyperactivity, nervousness, sleep disturbances, confusion, hypertonia and dizziness

Dose: 250 mg every 8 hours, doubled for severe infections; max. 4 g daily; CHILD over 1 month, 20 mg/kg daily in 3 divided doses, doubled for severe infections, max. 1 g daily; *or* 1 month–1 year, 62.5 mg every 8 hours; 1–5 years, 125 mg; over 5 years, 250 mg; doses doubled for severe infections

PoM Cefaclor (Non-proprietary)
Capsules, cefaclor (as monohydrate) 250 mg, net price 21-cap pack = £9.60; 500 mg 21-cap pack = £22.74. Label: 9
Available from Hillcross, Kent

PoM Distaclor® (Dista)
Capsules, cefaclor (as monohydrate) 500 mg (violet/grey), net price 20 = £21.66. Label: 9
Suspension, both pink, cefaclor (as monohydrate) for reconstitution with water, 125 mg/5 mL, net price 100 mL = £5.16; 250 mg/5 mL, 100 mL = £10.32. Label: 9

PoM Distaclor MR® (Dista)
Tablets, m/r, both blue, cefaclor (as monohydrate) 375 mg, net price 14-tab pack = £6.93; 500 mg, 7-tab pack = £5.95. Label: 9, 21, 25
Dose: 375 mg every 12 hours with food, dose doubled for pneumonia
Lower urinary-tract infections, 375 mg every 12 hours with food *or* 500 mg at night

CEFADROXIL

Indications: see under Cefaclor; see also notes above

Cautions; Contra-indications; Side-effects: see under Cefaclor

Dose: patients over 40 kg, 0.5–1 g twice daily; skin, soft tissue, and simple urinary-tract infections, 1 g daily; CHILD under 1 year, 25 mg/kg daily in divided doses; 1–6 years, 250 mg twice daily; over 6 years, 500 mg twice daily

PoM Baxan® (Bristol-Myers)
Capsules, cefadroxil 500 mg (as monohydrate). Net price 20 = £5.64. Label: 9
Suspension, cefadroxil (as monohydrate) for reconstitution with water, 125 mg/5 mL, net price 60 mL = £1.75; 250 mg/5 mL, 60 mL = £3.48; 500 mg/5 mL, 60 mL = £5.21. Label: 9

CEFIXIME

Indications: see under Cefaclor and notes above

Cautions; Contra-indications; Side-effects: see under Cefaclor

Dose: ADULT and CHILD over 10 years, 200–400 mg daily as a single dose or in 2 divided doses; CHILD over 6 months 8 mg/kg daily as a single dose or in 2 divided doses *or* 6 months–1 year 75 mg daily; 1–4 years 100 mg daily; 5–10 years 200 mg daily

PoM Suprax® (Rhône-Poulenc Rorer)
Tablets, f/c, scored, cefixime 200 mg. Net price 20 = £27.39. Label: 9
Paediatric oral suspension, cefixime 100 mg/5 mL when reconstituted with water. Net price 37.5 mL (with double-ended spoon for measuring 3.75 mL or 5 mL since dilution not recommended) = £6.53; 75 mL = £11.72. Label: 9

CEFODIZIME

Indications: see under Dose

Cautions; Contra-indications; Side-effects: see under Cefaclor

Dose: by intramuscular or intravenous injection or by intravenous infusion, lower respiratory-tract infection (including pneumonia and bronchopneumonia), 1 g every 12 hours
Upper and lower urinary-tract infections (including acute and chronic pyelonephritis and cystitis), 1 g every 12 hours *or* 2 g daily (as a single dose); single doses over 1 g intravenous route only

PoM Timecef® (Roussel)
Injection, powder for reconstitution, cefodizime (as sodium salt), net price 1-g vial = £11.04
Electrolytes: Na+ 3.18 mmol/g

CEFOTAXIME

Indications: see under Cefaclor; surgical prophylaxis; Haemophilus epiglottitis and meningitis (see section 5.1 table 1); see also notes above

Cautions; Contra-indications; Side-effects: see under Cefaclor

Dose: by intramuscular or intravenous injection or by intravenous infusion, moderate to serious infection, 1 g every 8 hours; life-threatening infection, 2 g every 8 hours; exceptionally, for life-threatening infections due to organisms less sensitive to cefotaxime, up to 12 g daily; NEONATE, 50 mg/kg daily in 2–4 divided doses increased to 150–200 mg/kg daily in severe infections; CHILD, 100–150 mg/kg daily in 2–4 divided doses; increased up to 200 mg/kg daily in severe infections

Urinary-tract and mild to moderate infections, 1 g every 12 hours

Gonorrhoea, 1 g as a single dose

PoM Claforan® (Roussel)
Injection, powder for reconstitution, cefotaxime (as sodium salt). Net price 500-mg vial = £2.41; 1-g vial = £4.85; 2-g vial = £9.65
Electrolytes: Na+ 2.09 mmol/g

CEFOXITIN

Indications: see under Cefaclor; surgical prophylaxis; more active against Gram-negative bacteria

Cautions; Contra-indications; Side-effects: see under Cefaclor

Dose: by deep intramuscular or by slow intravenous injection or by infusion, 1–2 g every 6–8 hours, increased up to 12 g daily in divided doses for infections requiring higher doses; CHILD up to 1 week 20–40 mg/kg every 12 hours, 1–4 weeks 20–40 mg/kg every 8 hours, over 1 month 20–40 mg/kg every 6–8 hours, increased up to 200 mg/kg daily in divided doses (max. 12 g daily) in severe infections; intravenous route recommended for children

Uncomplicated urinary-tract infection, *by deep intramuscular injection*, 1 g every 12 hours for 10 days

Uncomplicated gonorrhoea, *by deep intramuscular injection*, 2 g as a single dose with probenecid 1 g by mouth

Surgical prophylaxis, *by deep intramuscular injection or by intravenous injection or infusion*, 2 g 30–60 minutes before surgery, dose repeated every 6 hours for usual max. 24 hours; CHILD 30–40 mg/kg 30–60 minutes before surgery, dose repeated every 6 hours for usual max. 24 hours (second and third doses every 8–12 hours in NEONATES); intravenous route recommended for children

PoM Mefoxin® (MSD)
Injection, powder for reconstitution, cefoxitin (as sodium salt). Net price 1-g vial = £4.92; 2-g vial = £9.84
Electrolytes: Na+ 2.3 mmol/g

CEFPIROME

Indications: see under Cefaclor and notes above

Cautions; Contra-indications; Side-effects: see under Cefaclor; interference with creatinine assays using picrate method; taste disturbance shortly after injection reported

Dose: by intravenous injection or infusion, complicated upper and lower urinary-tract, skin and soft-tissue infections, 1 g every 12 hours increased to 2 g every 12 hours in very severe infections

Lower respiratory-tract infections, 1–2 g every 12 hours

Severe infections including bacteraemia and septicaemia and infections in neutropenic patients, 2 g every 12 hours

CHILD under 12 years not recommended

▼ **PoM Cefrom®** (Roussel)
Injection, powder for reconstitution, cefpirome (as sulphate), net price 1-g vial = £10.75; 2-g vial = £21.50

CEFPODOXIME

Indications: respiratory-tract infections but in pharyngitis and tonsillitis reserved for infections which are recurrent, chronic, or resistant to other antibiotics

Cautions; Contra-indications; Side-effects: see under Cefaclor

Dose: upper respiratory-tract infections, 100 mg twice daily with food (200 mg twice daily in sinusitis)

Lower respiratory-tract infections (including bronchitis and pneumonia), 100–200 mg twice daily with food

CHILD under 15 days not recommended, 15 days–6 months 8 mg/kg daily in 2 divided doses, 6 months–2 years 40 mg twice daily, 3–8 years 80 mg twice daily, over 9 years 100 mg twice daily

PoM Orelox® (Roussel)
Tablets, f/c, cefpodoxime 100 mg (as cefpodoxime proxetil). Net price 10-tab pack = £9.26. Label: 5, 9, 21

Oral suspension, cefpodoxime (as proxetil) for reconstitution with water, 40 mg/5 mL, net price 50 mL = £6.50, 100 mL = £10.89. Label: 5, 9, 21
Note. Suspension contains aspartame (see section 9.4.1)

CEFTAZIDIME

Indications: see under Cefaclor; see also notes above

Cautions; Contra-indications; Side-effects: see under Cefaclor

Dose: by deep intramuscular injection or intravenous injection or infusion, 1 g every 8 hours *or* 2 g every 12 hours; 2 g every 8–12 hours in severe infections; single doses over 1 g intravenous route only; elderly usual max. 3 g daily; CHILD, up to 2 months 25–60 mg/kg daily in 2 divided doses, over 2 months 30–100 mg/kg daily in 2–3 divided doses; up to 150 mg/kg daily (max. 6 g daily) in 3 divided doses if immunocompromised or meningitis; intravenous route recommended for children

Urinary-tract and less serious infections, 0.5–1 g every 12 hours

---

Pseudomonal lung infection in cystic fibrosis, ADULT with normal renal function 100–150 mg/kg daily in 3 divided doses; CHILD up to 150 mg/kg daily (max. 6 g daily) in 3 divided doses; intravenous route recommended for children

Surgical prophylaxis, prostatic surgery, 1 g at induction of anaesthesia repeated if necessary when catheter removed

PoM Fortum® (Glaxo)

Injection, powder for reconstitution, ceftazidime (as pentahydrate), with sodium carbonate, net price 250-mg vial = £2.48, 500-mg vial = £4.95, 1-g vial = £9.90, 2-g vial (for injection and for infusion, both) = £29.00; *infusion kit*, 2-g vial, 50-mL bag sodium chloride intravenous infusion, transfer needle, swab, sealing cap, and label, complete kit = £20.82
Electrolytes: Na⁺ 2.3 mmol/g

PoM Kefadim® (Lilly)

Injection, powder for reconstitution, ceftazidime (as pentahydrate), with sodium carbonate, net price 500-mg vial = £4.95, 1-g vial = £9.90, 2-g vial (for injection and for infusion, both) = £19.80
Electrolytes: Na⁺ 2.3 mmol/g

CEFTIBUTEN

Indications: see under Cefaclor and notes above
Cautions; Contra-indications; Side-effects: see under Cefaclor
Dose: ADULT and CHILD over 10 years (over 45 kg) 400 mg daily as a single dose; CHILD over 6 months, as oral suspension, 9 mg/kg daily as a single dose *or* see under oral suspension below

▼ **PoM Cedax®** (Schering-Plough)

Capsules, ceftibuten (as dihydrate) 400 mg, net price 5-cap pack = £13.03, 7-cap pack = £17.50. Label: 9
Oral suspension, ceftibuten (as dihydrate) for reconstitution with water, 90 mg/5 mL, net price 60 mL = £7.63; 180 mg/5 mL, 60 mL = £15.26. Label: 9
Dose: as oral suspension containing 90 mg/5 mL, CHILD 6 months–1 year 5 mL daily as a single dose, 1–3 years 8 mL daily, 3–6 years 10 mL daily
As oral suspension containing 180 mg/5 mL, CHILD 3–6 years 5 mL daily as a single dose, 6–10 years 8 mL daily, over 10 years 10 mL daily

CEFTIZOXIME

Indications: see under Cefaclor; see also notes above
Cautions; Contra-indications; Side-effects: see under Cefaclor; reduce dose in elderly
Dose: by deep intramuscular or slow intravenous injection or by intravenous infusion, 1–2 g every 8–12 hours increased in severe infections up to 8 g daily (in 3 divided doses); intramuscular doses of 2 g and over divided between more than 1 site; CHILD over 3 months 30–60 mg/kg daily in 2–4 divided doses, increased to 100–150 mg/kg daily for severe infections
Gonorrhoea, *by deep intramuscular injection*, 1 g as a single dose

Urinary-tract infections, *by deep intramuscular or slow intravenous injection or by infusion*, 0.5–1 g every 12 hours

PoM Cefizox® (Wellcome)

Injection, powder for reconstitution, ceftizoxime (as sodium salt). Net price 500-mg vial = £2.76; 1-g vial = £5.50; 2-g vial = £11.00
Electrolytes: Na⁺ 2.6 mmol/g

CEFTRIAXONE

Indications: see under Cefaclor and notes above; surgical prophylaxis
Cautions; Contra-indications; Side-effects: see under Cefaclor; also caution in hepatic impairment if accompanied by renal impairment; may displace plasma bilirubin—contra-indicated in infants under 6 weeks; calcium ceftriaxone may appear as a precipitate in urine or as gallstones
Dose: by deep intramuscular injection, or by intravenous injection over 2–4 minutes, or by intravenous infusion, 1 g daily as a single dose; 2–4 g daily as a single dose in severe infections; intramuscular doses over 1 g divided between more than one site
CHILD over 6 weeks 20–50 mg/kg daily as a single dose; up to 80 mg/kg as a single dose in severe infections; doses over 50 mg/kg by intravenous infusion only
Uncomplicated gonorrhoea, *by deep intramuscular injection*, 250 mg
Surgical prophylaxis, *by deep intramuscular injection or by intravenous injection over 2–4 minutes*, 1 g as a single dose; colorectal surgery, *by intramuscular or by intravenous injection over 2–4 minutes or by intravenous infusion*, 2 g; intramuscular doses over 1 g divided between more than one site
Prophylaxis of meningococcal meningitis, section 5.1 (table 2)

▼ **PoM Rocephin®** (Roche)

Injection, powder for reconstitution, ceftriaxone (as sodium salt), net price 250-mg vial = £2.87; 1-g vial = £11.46; 2-g vial = £22.92
Electrolytes: Na⁺ 3.6 mmol/g

CEFUROXIME

Indications: see under Cefaclor; surgical prophylaxis; more active against *Haemophilus influenzae* and *Neisseria gonorrhoeae*
Cautions; Contra-indications; Side-effects: see under Cefaclor
Dose: by mouth (as cefuroxime axetil), 250 mg twice daily in most infections including mild to moderate lower respiratory-tract infections (e.g. bronchitis); doubled for more severe lower respiratory-tract infections or if pneumonia suspected
Urinary-tract infection, 125 mg twice daily, doubled in pyelonephritis
Gonorrhoea, 1 g as a single dose
CHILD over 3 months, 125 mg twice daily, if necessary doubled in child over 2 years with otitis media

By intramuscular injection or intravenous injection or infusion, 750 mg every 6–8 hours; 1.5 g every 6–8 hours in severe infections; single doses over 750 mg intravenous route only

CHILD usual dose 60 mg/kg daily (range 30–100 mg/kg daily) in 3–4 divided doses (2–3 divided doses in neonates)

Gonorrhoea, 1.5 g as a single dose by intramuscular injection (divided between 2 sites)

Surgical prophylaxis, 1.5 g by intravenous injection at induction; may be supplemented with 750 mg intramuscularly 8 and 16 hours later (abdominal, pelvic, and orthopaedic operations) *or* followed by 750 mg intramuscularly every 8 hours for further 24–48 hours (cardiac, pulmonary, oesophageal, and vascular operations)

Meningitis, 3 g intravenously every 8 hours; CHILD, 200–240 mg/kg daily (in 3–4 divided doses) reduced to 100 mg/kg daily after 3 days or on clinical improvement; NEONATE, 100 mg/kg daily reduced to 50 mg/kg daily

PoM Zinacef® (Glaxo)

Injection, powder for reconstitution, cefuroxime (as sodium salt). Net price 250-mg vial = 88p; 750-mg vial = £2.64; 1.5-g vial (for injection and for infusion) = £5.29; *infusion kit*, 750-mg vial, 50-mL bag sodium chloride intravenous infusion, transfer needle, swab, sealing cap, and label, complete kit = £3.67; *Zinacef/Metronidazole infusion kit*, 750-mg vial, 100-mL bag metronidazole 5 mg/mL, transfer needle, swab, sealing cap and label, complete kit = £3.77
Electrolytes: Na⁺ 1.8 mmol/750-mg vial

PoM Zinnat® (Glaxo)

Tablets, both f/c, cefuroxime 125 mg (as cefuroxime axetil) net price 14-tab pack = £4.73; 250 mg, 14-tab pack = £9.45. Label: 9, 21, 25

Suspension, cefuroxime (as cefuroxime axetil) 125 mg/5 mL when reconstituted with water. Net price 70 mL = £5.40. Label: 9, 21

Sachets, cefuroxime (as cefuroxime axetil) 125 mg/sachet, net price 14-sachet pack = £5.40. Label: 9, 13, 21

CEPHALEXIN
(Cefalexin)

Indications: see under Cefaclor

Cautions; Contra-indications; Side-effects: see under Cefaclor

Dose: 250 mg every 6 hours *or* 500 mg every 8–12 hours increased to 1–1.5 g every 6–8 hours for severe infections; CHILD, 25 mg/kg daily in divided doses, doubled for severe infections, max. 100 mg/kg daily; *or* under 1 year, 125 mg every 12 hours; 1–5 years, 125 mg every 8 hours; 6–12 years, 250 mg every 8 hours

PoM Cephalexin (Non-proprietary)

Capsules, cephalexin 250 mg, net price 20 = £2.13; 500 mg, 20 = £4.19. Label: 9
Available from APS, Berk, Cox, Hillcross, Kent (Tenkorex®)

Tablets, cephalexin 250 mg, net price 20 = £2.29 500 mg, 20 = £4.25. Label: 9
Available from APS, Berk, Cox, Hillcross, Kent (Tenkorex®), Norton

Oral suspension, cephalexin for reconstitution with water, 125 mg/5 mL, net price 100 mL = £1.27; 250 mg/5 mL, 100 mL = £2.55. Label: 9
Available from APS, Berk, Cox, Hillcross, Kent (Tenkorex®)

PoM Ceporex® (Glaxo)

Capsules, both caramel/grey, cephalexin 250 mg net price 28-cap pack = £4.47; 500 mg, 28-cap pack = £8.72. Label: 9

Tablets, all pink, f/c, cephalexin 250 mg, net price 28-tab pack = £4.47; 500 mg, 28-tab pack = £8.72; 1 g (scored), 14-tab pack = £8.72. Label: 9

Syrup, all orange, cephalexin for reconstitution with water, 125 mg/5 mL, net price 100 mL = £1.59; 250 mg/5 mL, 100 mL = £3.19; 500 mg 5 mL, 100 mL = £6.19. Label: 9

PoM Keflex® (Lilly)

Capsules, cephalexin 250 mg (green/white), net price 28-cap pack = £3.57; 500 mg (pale green/dark green), 28-cap pack = £6.97. Label: 9

Tablets, both peach, cephalexin 250 mg, net price 28-tab pack = £3.57; 500 mg (scored), 28-tab pack = £6.97. Label: 9

Suspension, cephalexin for reconstitution with water, 125 mg/5 mL (pink), net price 100 mL = £1.27; 250 mg/5 mL (orange), 100 mL = £2.55 Label: 9

CEPHAMANDOLE
(Cefamandole)

Indications: see under Cefaclor; surgical prophylaxis

Cautions; Contra-indications; Side-effects: see under Cefaclor

Dose: by deep intramuscular injection or by intravenous injection over 3–5 minutes *or* by intravenous infusion, 0.5–2 g every 4–8 hours; CHILD over 1 month, 50–100 mg/kg daily in 3–6 divided doses increased to 150 mg/kg daily for severe infections

Surgical prophylaxis, by intramuscular or intravenous injection, 1–2 g 30–60 minutes before surgery followed by 1–2 g every 6 hours for 24–48 hours (up to 72 hours for implantation of prostheses)

PoM Kefadol® (Dista)

Injection, powder for reconstitution, cephamandole (as nafate) with sodium carbonate. Net price 1-g vial = £3.91
Electrolytes: Na⁺ 3.35 mmol/1-g vial

CEPHAZOLIN
(Cefazolin)

Indications: see under Cefaclor; surgical prophylaxis

Cautions; Contra-indications; Side-effects: see under Cefaclor

Dose: by intramuscular injection or intravenous injection or infusion, 0.5–1 g every 6–12 hours; CHILD, 25–50 mg/kg daily (in divided doses), increased to 100 mg/kg daily in severe infections

PoM **Kefzol**® (Lilly)

Injection, powder for reconstitution, cephazolin (as sodium salt). Net price 500-mg vial = £2.45; 1-g vial = £4.63

Electrolytes: Na⁺ 2.1 mmol/g

CEPHRADINE

(Cefradine)

Indications: see under Cefaclor; surgical prophylaxis

Cautions; Contra-indications; Side-effects: see under Cefaclor

Dose: by mouth, 250–500 mg every 6 hours *or* 0.5–1 g every 12 hours; CHILD, 25–50 mg/kg daily in divided doses

By deep intramuscular injection or by intravenous injection over 3–5 minutes *or by intravenous infusion*, 0.5–1 g every 6 hours, increased to 8 g daily in severe infections; CHILD 50–100 mg/kg daily in 4 divided doses

Surgical prophylaxis, *by deep intramuscular injection or by intravenous injection* over 3–5 minutes, 1–2 g immediately prior to surgery

PoM **Velosef**® (Squibb)

Capsules, cephradine 250 mg (orange/blue), net price 20-cap pack = £3.55; 500 mg (blue), 20-cap pack = £7.00. Label: 9

Syrup, cephradine 250 mg/5 mL when reconstituted with water. Net price 100 mL = £4.22. Label: 9

Injection, powder for reconstitution, cephradine. Net price 500-mg vial = 99p; 1-g vial = £1.95

OTHER BETA-LACTAM ANTIBIOTICS

Aztreonam is a monocyclic beta-lactam ('monobactam') antibiotic with an antibacterial spectrum limited to Gram-negative aerobic bacteria including *Pseudomonas aeruginosa*, *Neisseria meningitidis*, and *Haemophilus influenzae*; it should not be used alone for 'blind' treatment since it is not active against Gram-positive organisms. Aztreonam is also effective against *Neisseria gonorrhoeae* (but not against concurrent chlamydial infection). Side-effects are similar to those of the other beta-lactams although aztreonam may be less likely to cause hypersensitivity in penicillin-sensitive patients.

Imipenem, a carbapenem, has a broad spectrum of activity which includes many aerobic and anaerobic Gram-positive and Gram-negative bacteria. Imipenem is partially inactivated in the kidney by enzymatic activity and is therefore administered in combination with **cilastatin**, a specific enzyme inhibitor, which blocks its renal metabolism. Side-effects are similar to those of other beta-lactam antibiotics; neurotoxicity has been observed at very high dosage or in renal failure. **Meropenem** is similar to imipenem but is stable to the renal enzyme which inactivates imipenem and therefore can be given without cilastatin.

AZTREONAM

Indications: Gram-negative infections including *Pseudomonas aeruginosa*, *Haemophilus influenzae*, and *Neisseria meningitidis*

Cautions: hypersensitivity to beta-lactam antibiotics; hepatic impairment; reduce dose in renal impairment; **interactions:** Appendix 1 (aztreonam)

Contra-indications: aztreonam hypersensitivity; pregnancy and breast-feeding

Side-effects: nausea, vomiting, diarrhoea, abdominal cramps; mouth ulcers, altered taste; jaundice and hepatitis; blood disorders (including thrombocytopenia and neutropenia); urticaria and rashes

Dose: by deep intramuscular injection or by intravenous injection over 3–5 minutes *or by intravenous infusion,* 1 g every 8 hours *or* 2 g every 12 hours; 2 g every 6–8 hours for severe infections (including systemic *Pseudomonas aeruginosa* and lung infections in cystic fibrosis); single doses over 1 g intravenous route only

CHILD over 1 week, *by intravenous injection or infusion*, 30 mg/kg every 6–8 hours increased in severe infections for child of 2 years or older to 50 mg/kg every 6–8 hours; max. 8 g daily

Urinary-tract infections, 0.5–1 g every 8–12 hours

Gonorrhoea/cystitis, *by intramuscular injection*, 1 g as a single dose

PoM **Azactam**® (Squibb)

Injection, powder for reconstitution, aztreonam. Net price 500-mg vial = £4.48; 1-g vial = £8.95; 2-g vial = £17.90

IMIPENEM WITH CILASTATIN

Indications: aerobic and anaerobic Gram-positive and Gram-negative infections; surgical prophylaxis; not indicated for CNS infections

Cautions: hypersensitivity to other beta-lactam antibiotics; renal impairment; CNS disorders (e.g. epilepsy); pregnancy; **interactions:** Appendix 1 (*Primaxin*®)

Contra-indications: hypersensitivity to imipenem or cilastatin; breast-feeding

Side-effects: nausea, vomiting, diarrhoea (pseudomembranous colitis reported), taste disturbances; blood disorders, positive Coombs test; allergic reactions (with rash, pruritus, urticaria, fever, anaphylactic reactions, rarely toxic epidermal necrolysis); myoclonic activity, convulsions, confusion and mental disturbances reported; slight increases in liver enzymes and bilirubin reported; increases in serum creatinine and blood urea; red coloration of urine in children reported; local reactions: erythema, pain and induration, and thrombophlebitis

Dose: by deep intramuscular injection, mild to moderate infections, in terms of imipenem, 500–750 mg every 12 hours; gonococcal urethritis or cervicitis, 500 mg as a single dose

By intravenous infusion, in terms of imipenem, 1–2 g daily (in 3–4 divided doses); less sensitive organisms, up to 50 mg/kg daily (to max. 4 g daily); CHILD 3 months and older, 60 mg/kg (up to max. of 2 g) daily in 4 divided doses

Surgical prophylaxis, *by intravenous infusion*, 1 g at induction of anaesthesia repeated after 3 hours, supplemented in high risk (e.g. colorectal surgery by doses of 500 mg 8 and 16 hours after induction

PoM **Primaxin®** (MSD)
Intramuscular injection, powder for reconstitution, imipenem (as monohydrate) 500 mg with cilastatin (as sodium salt) 500 mg. Net price 15-mL vial = £15.00
Electrolytes: Na⁺ 1.47 mmol/vial
Intravenous infusion, powder for reconstitution, imipenem (as monohydrate) 250 mg with cilastatin (as sodium salt) 250 mg. Net price 60-mL vial = £9.00
Electrolytes: Na⁺ 0.86 mmol/vial
Intravenous infusion, powder for reconstitution, imipenem (as monohydrate) 500 mg with cilastatin (as sodium salt) 500 mg. Net price 120-mL vial = £15.00; *Monovial*, 20-mL vial (with transfer needle) = £15.00
Electrolytes: Na⁺ 1.72 mmol/vial

MEROPENEM
Indications: aerobic and anaerobic Gram-positive and Gram-negative infections
Cautions: hypersensitivity to penicillins, cephalosporins and other beta-lactam antibiotics; hepatic impairment (monitor liver function); renal impairment; pregnancy and breast-feeding
Contra-indications: hypersensitivity to meropenem
Side-effects: nausea, vomiting, diarrhoea (pseudomembranous colitis reported), abdominal pain; disturbances in liver function tests; thrombocytopenia (reduction in partial thromboplastin time reported), positive Coombs' test, eosinophilia, neutropenia; headache, paraesthesia; rash, pruritus, urticaria; convulsions reported, local reactions including pain and thrombophlebitis at injection site
Dose: by intravenous injection over 5 minutes *or by intravenous infusion*, 500 mg every 8 hours, dose doubled in hospital-acquired pneumonia, peritonitis, septicaemia and infections in neutropenic patients; CHILD 3 months–12 years 10–20 mg/kg every 8 hours, over 50 kg body weight adult dose
Meningitis, 2 g every 8 hours; CHILD 3 months–12 years 40 mg/kg every 8 hours, over 50 kg body weight adult dose

▼ PoM **Meronem®** (Zeneca)
Injection, powder for reconstitution, meropenem, net price 250-mg vial = £10.00; 500-mg vial = £15.00; 1-g vial = £30.00
Electrolytes: Na⁺ 3.9 mmol/g

5.1.3   Tetracyclines
The tetracyclines are broad-spectrum antibiotics whose value has decreased owing to increasing bacterial resistance. They remain, however, the treatment of choice for infections caused by chlamydia (trachoma, psittacosis, salpingitis, urethritis, and lymphogranuloma venereum), rickettsia (including Q-fever), mycoplasma (respiratory and genital infections), brucella (doxycycline with rifampicin), and the spirochaete, *Borrelia burgdorferi* (Lyme disease). They are also used in acne, in destructive (refractory) periodontal disease, in exacerbations of chronic bronchitis (because of their activity against *Haemophilus influenzae*), and for leptospirosis in penicillin hypersensitivity (as an alternative to erythromycin).

Microbiologically, there is little to choose between the various tetracyclines, the only exception being **minocycline** which has a broader spectrum; it is active against *Neisseria meningitidis* and has been used for meningococcal prophylaxis but is no longer recommended because of side-effects including dizziness and vertigo (see section 5.1, table 2 for current recommendations).

The tetracyclines are deposited in growing bone and teeth (being bound to calcium) causing staining and occasionally dental hypoplasia, and should **not** be given to children under 12 years or to pregnant or breast-feeding women. With the exception of **doxycycline** and **minocycline** the tetracyclines may exacerbate renal failure and should **not** be given to patients with kidney disease. Absorption of tetracyclines is decreased by milk (except doxycycline and minocycline), antacids, and calcium, iron and magnesium salts.

TETRACYCLINE
Indications: exacerbations of chronic bronchitis; brucellosis (see also notes above), chlamydia, mycoplasma, and rickettsia; pleural effusions due to malignancy or cirrhosis; acne vulgaris (see section 13.6)
Cautions: hepatic impairment (avoid intravenous administration); renal impairment (see Appendix 3); rarely causes photosensitivity; **interactions:** Appendix 1 (tetracyclines)
Contra-indications: renal impairment (see Appendix 3), pregnancy and breast-feeding (see also Appendixes 4 and 5), children under 12 years of age, systemic lupus erythematosus
Side-effects: nausea, vomiting, diarrhoea; erythema (discontinue treatment); headache and visual disturbances may indicate benign intracranial hypertension; hepatotoxicity, pancreatitis and pseudomembranous colitis reported
Dose: by mouth, 250 mg every 6 hours, increased in severe infections to 500 mg every 6–8 hours
Acne, see section 13.6
Primary, secondary, or latent syphilis, 500 mg every 6 hours for 15 days
Non-gonococcal urethritis, 500 mg every 6 hours for 7–14 days (21 days if failure or relapse following the first course)
COUNSELLING. Tablets or capsules should be swallowed whole with plenty of fluid while sitting or standing
By intravenous infusion, 500 mg every 12 hours; max. 2 g daily
Pleural effusions, see under Achromycin® intravenous infusion

---

PoM **Tetracycline** (Non-proprietary)

Tablets, coated, tetracycline hydrochloride 250 mg. Net price 20 = 31p. Label: 7, 9, 23, counselling, posture, see above

Available from Cox, Hillcross, Kent, Norton

PoM **Achromycin**® (Lederle)

Capsules, orange, tetracycline hydrochloride 250 mg. Net price 20 = 96p. Label: 7, 9, 23, counselling, posture, see above

Intravenous infusion, powder for reconstitution, tetracycline hydrochloride. Net price 250-mg vial = £1.48; 500-mg vial = £1.98

Dose: infections, see above

Recurrent pleural effusions, by intrapleural instillation, 500 mg in 30–50 mL sodium chloride intravenous infusion 0.9%

PoM **Sustamycin**® (Boehringer Mannheim)

Capsules, m/r, light blue/dark blue, tetracycline hydrochloride 250 mg. Net price 20 = £2.40. Label: 7, 9, 23, 25

Dose: 2 capsules initially, then 1 every 12 hours

PoM **Tetrachel**® (Berk)

Capsules, orange, tetracycline hydrochloride 250 mg. Net price 20 = 49p. Label: 7, 9, 23, counselling, posture, see above

Tablets, orange, f/c, tetracycline hydrochloride 250 mg. Net price 20 = 34p. Label: 7, 9, 23, counselling, posture, see above

Compound preparations

PoM **Deteclo**® (Lederle)

Tablets, blue, f/c, tetracycline hydrochloride 115.4 mg, chlortetracycline hydrochloride 115.4 mg, demeclocycline hydrochloride 69.2 mg. Net price 20 = £2.48. Label: 7, 9, 11, 23, counselling, posture, see above

Dose: 1 tablet every 12 hours; 3–4 tablets daily in more severe infections

DEMECLOCYCLINE HYDROCHLORIDE

Indications: see under Tetracycline; also inappropriate secretion of antidiuretic hormone, section 6.5.2

Cautions; Contra-indications; Side-effects: see under Tetracycline, but photosensitivity is more common; reversible nephrogenic diabetes insipidus reported

Dose: 150 mg every 6 hours *or* 300 mg every 12 hours

PoM **Ledermycin**® (Lederle)

Capsules, red, demeclocycline hydrochloride 150 mg. Net price 20 = £4.13. Label: 7, 9, 11, 23

DOXYCYCLINE

Indications: see under Tetracycline; brucellosis (with rifampicin); also chronic prostatitis and sinusitis; pelvic inflammatory disease (with metronidazole, section 5.1, table 1)

Cautions; Contra-indications; Side-effects: see under Tetracycline, but may be used in renal impairment; avoid in porphyria (see section 9.8.2)

Dose: 200 mg on first day, then 100 mg daily; severe infections (including chronic urinary-tract infections), 200 mg daily

Acne, 50 mg daily for 6–12 weeks or longer

COUNSELLING. Capsules should be swallowed whole with plenty of fluid during meals while sitting or standing

PoM **Doxycycline** (Non-proprietary)

Capsules, doxycycline (as hydrochloride) 50 mg, net price 28-cap pack = £7.26; 100 mg, 20 = £5.72. Label: 6, 9, 11, 27, counselling, posture, see above

Available from APS, Ashbourne (Demix®), Berk (Cyclodox®), Cox, Hillcross, ISIS (Ramysis®), Kent, Lagap (Doxylar®), Norton

PoM **Nordox**® (Panpharma)

Capsules, green, doxycycline 100 mg (as hydrochloride). Net price 10-cap pack = £4.66. Label: 6, 9, 11, 27, counselling, posture, see above

PoM **Vibramycin**® (Invicta)

Capsules, doxycycline (as hydrochloride) 50 mg (green/ivory), net price 28-cap pack = £7.74; 100 mg (green), 8-cap pack = £4.18. Label: 6, 9, 11, 27, counselling, posture, see above

PoM **Vibramycin-D**® (Invicta)

Dispersible tablets, off-white, doxycycline 100 mg. Net price 8-tab pack = £4.91. Label: 6, 9, 11, 13

LYMECYCLINE

Indications; Cautions; Contra-indications; Side-effects: see under Tetracycline

Dose: 408 mg every 12 hours

PoM **Tetralysal 300**® (Galderma)

Capsules, lymecycline 408 mg (≡ tetracycline 300 mg). Net price 20-cap pack = £2.96. Label: 6, 9

MINOCYCLINE

Indications: see under Tetracycline; also meningococcal carrier state

Cautions; Contra-indications: see under Tetracycline, but may be used in renal impairment

Side-effects: see under Tetracycline; also dizziness and vertigo (more common in women); severe exfoliative rashes, pigmentation (sometimes irreversible), systemic lupus erythematosus and liver damage reported

Dose: 100 mg twice daily

Acne, 50 mg twice daily *or* 100 mg once daily for minimum course of 6 weeks

Gonorrhoea, initially 200 mg then 100 mg every 12 hours for at least 4 days in men; women may require longer treatment

Prophylaxis of asymptomatic meningococcal carrier state (but no longer recommended, see notes above), 100 mg twice daily for 5 days usually followed by rifampicin

PoM Minocycline (Non-proprietary)

Capsules, minocycline (as hydrochloride) 50 mg, net price 56-cap pack = £17.20; 100 mg, 28-cap pack = £14.74. Label: 6, 9, 11
Available from Merck (Aknemin®)

Tablets, minocycline (as hydrochloride) 50 mg, net price 84-tab pack = £19.52; 100 mg, 20 = £9.78. Label: 6, 9, 11
Available from APS, Ashbourne (Blemix®), Berk (Cyclomin®), Cox, Galen (Minogal®), Hillcross, Kent, Lederle (Minocin®), Norton

PoM Minocin MR® (Lederle)

Capsules, m/r, orange/brown (enclosing yellow and orange pellets), minocycline (as hydrochloride) 100 mg. Net price 56-cap pack = £29.12. Label: 6, 11, 25

Dose: acne, 1 capsule daily

OXYTETRACYCLINE

Indications; Cautions; Contra-indications; Side-effects: see under Tetracycline; avoid in porphyria (see section 9.8.2)

Dose: 250–500 mg every 6 hours

PoM Oxytetracycline (Non-proprietary)

Tablets, coated, oxytetracycline dihydrate 250 mg, net price 20 = 27p. Label: 7, 9, 23
Available from APS, Ashbourne (Oxytetramix®), Berk (Berkmycen®, contain tartrazine), Cox, CP, DDSA (Oxymycin®), Kent, Norton

PoM Terramycin® (Pfizer)

Capsules, yellow, oxytetracycline 250 mg (as hydrochloride). Net price 28-cap pack = 96p. Label: 7, 9, 23

Tablets, yellow, s/c, oxytetracycline 250 mg (as dihydrate). Net price 28-tab pack = 96p. Label: 7, 9, 23

5.1.4 Aminoglycosides

These include amikacin, gentamicin, kanamycin, neomycin, netilmicin, streptomycin, and tobramycin. All are bactericidal and active against some Gram-positive and many Gram-negative organisms. Amikacin, gentamicin, and tobramycin are also active against *Pseudomonas aeruginosa*; streptomycin is active against *Mycobacterium tuberculosis* and is now almost entirely reserved for tuberculosis (section 5.1.9).

The aminoglycosides are not absorbed from the gut (although there is a risk of absorption in inflammatory bowel disease and liver failure) and must therefore be given by injection for systemic infections.

Excretion is principally via the kidney and accumulation occurs in renal impairment.

Most side-effects of this group of antibiotics are dose-related therefore care must be taken with dosage and whenever possible treatment should not exceed 7 days. The important side-effects are ototoxicity, and to a lesser degree nephrotoxicity; they occur most commonly in the elderly and in patients with renal failure.

If there is impairment of renal function (or high pre-dose plasma concentrations) the interval between doses must be increased; if the renal impairment is severe the dose itself should be reduced as well.

Aminoglycosides may impair neuromuscular transmission and should not be given to patients with myasthenia gravis; large doses given during surgery have been responsible for a transient myasthenic syndrome in patients with normal neuromuscular function.

Aminoglycosides should not be given with potentially ototoxic diuretics (e.g. frusemide and ethacrynic acid); if concurrent use is unavoidable administration of the aminoglycoside and of the diuretic should be separated by as long a period as practicable.

PLASMA CONCENTRATIONS. Plasma concentration monitoring avoids both excessive and subtherapeutic concentrations thus preventing toxicity and ensuring efficacy. Concentrations should be measured approximately 1 hour after intramuscular or intravenous administration and also just before the next dose.

If possible plasma aminoglycoside concentrations should be measured in all patients and **must** be determined in *infants*, in *elderly*, in *obesity*, and in *cystic fibrosis, or* if *high doses* are being given, *or* if there is *renal impairment, or* if treatment lasts *longer than 7 days.*

ONCE DAILY DOSAGE. Although aminoglycosides are generally given in 2–3 divided doses during the 24 hours, *once daily administration* has been shown to reduce the risk of toxicity (while ensuring adequate plasma concentrations) but **expert advice** about dosage and plasma concentrations should be obtained.

Gentamicin is the most important of the aminoglycosides and is widely used for the treatment of serious infections. It is the aminoglycoside of choice in the UK. It has a broad spectrum but is inactive against anaerobes and has poor activity against haemolytic streptococci and pneumococci. When used for the 'blind' therapy of undiagnosed serious infections it is usually given in conjunction with a penicillin and/or metronidazole.

The daily dose is up to 5 mg/kg given in divided doses every 8 hours (if renal function is normal); whenever possible treatment should not exceed 7 days. Higher doses are occasionally indicated for serious infections, especially in the neonate or the compromised host. A lower dose of 80 mg twice daily (60 mg for lighter or elderly patients) in association with benzylpenicillin is sufficient for endocarditis due to oral streptococci (often termed *Streptococcus viridans*) and gut streptococci.

Amikacin is a derivative of kanamycin and has one important advantage over gentamicin in that it is stable to 8 of the 9 classified aminoglycoside-inactivating enzymes whereas gentamicin is inactivated by 5. It is principally indicated for the treatment of serious infections caused by Gram-negative bacilli resistant to gentamicin.

Kanamycin has been superseded by other aminoglycosides.

Netilmicin has similar activity to gentamicin, but may cause less ototoxicity in those needing treatment for longer than 10 days. Netilmicin is active against a number of gentamicin-resistant Gram-negative bacilli but is less active against *Ps. aeruginosa* than gentamicin or tobramycin.

Tobramycin is similar to gentamicin. It is slightly more active against *Ps. aeruginosa* but shows less activity against certain other Gram-negative bacteria.

Neomycin is too toxic for parenteral administration and can only be used for infections of the skin or mucous membranes or to reduce the bacterial population of the colon prior to bowel surgery or in hepatic failure. Oral administration may lead to malabsorption. Small amounts of neomycin may be absorbed from the gut in patients with hepatic failure and, as these patients may also be uraemic, cumulation may occur with resultant ototoxicity.

PREGNANCY. Where possible, the aminoglycosides should be avoided in pregnancy as they cross the placenta and can cause fetal eighth nerve damage.

GENTAMICIN

Indications: septicaemia and neonatal sepsis; meningitis and other CNS infections; biliary-tract infection, acute pyelonephritis or prostatitis, endocarditis caused by *Strep. viridans* or *Strep. faecalis* (with a penicillin); pneumonia in hospital patients, adjunct in listerial meningitis (section 5.1, table 1)

Cautions: renal impairment, infants and elderly (adjust dose and monitor renal, auditory and vestibular function together with plasma gentamicin concentrations); avoid prolonged use; see also notes above; **interactions:** Appendix 1 (aminoglycosides)

Contra-indications: pregnancy, myasthenia gravis

Side-effects: vestibular and auditory damage, nephrotoxicity; rarely, hypomagnesaemia on prolonged therapy, pseudomembranous colitis; see also notes above

Dose: by intramuscular or by slow intravenous injection over at least 3 minutes *or by intravenous infusion,* 2–5 mg/kg daily in (in divided doses every 8 hours), see also notes above; reduce dose and measure plasma concentrations in renal impairment

CHILD up to 2 weeks, 3 mg/kg every 12 hours; 2 weeks–12 years, 2 mg/kg every 8 hours

By intrathecal injection, 1 mg daily (increased if necessary to 5 mg daily), with 2–4 mg/kg daily *by intramuscular injection* (in divided doses every 8 hours)

Endocarditis prophylaxis, section 5.1, table 2

Note. One-hour ('peak') concentration should not exceed 10 mg/litre; pre-dose ('trough') concentration should be less than 2 mg/litre

PoM **Gentamicin** (Non-proprietary)

Injection, gentamicin (as sulphate), net price 40 mg/mL, 1-mL amp = £1.40, 2-mL amp = £1.86, 2-mL vial = £1.92
Available from David Bull

PoM **Cidomycin®** (Roussel)

Injection, gentamicin 40 mg (as sulphate)/mL. Net price 2-mL amp or vial = £1.55

Paediatric injection, gentamicin 10 mg (as sulphate)/mL. Net price 2-mL vial = 65p

Intrathecal injection, gentamicin 5 mg (as sulphate)/mL. Net price 1-mL amp = 77p

PoM **Genticin®** (Roche)

Injection, gentamicin 40 mg (as sulphate)/mL. Net price 2-mL amp = £1.58

PoM **Isotonic Gentamicin Injection** (Baxter)

Intravenous infusion, gentamicin 800 micrograms (as sulphate)/mL in sodium chloride intravenous infusion 0.9%. Net price 100-mL (80-mg) Viaflex® bag = £1.61
Electrolytes: Na+ 15.4 mmol/100-mL bag

AMIKACIN

Indications: serious Gram-negative infections resistant to gentamicin

Cautions; Contra-indications; Side-effects: see under Gentamicin

Dose: by intramuscular or by slow intravenous injection or by infusion, 15 mg/kg daily in 2 divided doses, see also notes above

Note. One-hour ('peak') concentration should not exceed 30 mg/litre; pre-dose ('trough') concentration should be less than 10 mg/litre

PoM **Amikin®** (Bristol-Myers)

Injection, amikacin 250 mg (as sulphate)/mL. Net price 2-mL vial = £10.14
Electrolytes: Na+ < 0.5 mmol/vial

Paediatric injection, amikacin 50 mg (as sulphate)/mL. Net price 2-mL vial = £2.36
Electrolytes: Na+ < 0.5 mmol/vial

KANAMYCIN

Indications: superseded by other aminoglycosides (see notes above)

Cautions; Contra-indications; Side-effects: see under Gentamicin

Dose: by intramuscular injection, 250 mg every 6 hours *or* 500 mg every 12 hours, see also notes above

By intravenous infusion, 15–30 mg/kg daily in divided doses every 8–12 hours, see also notes above

Note. One-hour ('peak') concentration should not exceed 30 mg/litre; pre-dose ('trough') concentration should be less than 10 mg/litre

PoM **Kannasyn®** (Sanofi Winthrop)

Powder (for preparing injections), kanamycin (as acid sulphate). Net price 1-g vial = £23.77

NEOMYCIN SULPHATE

Indications: bowel sterilisation prior to surgery, see also notes above

Cautions; Contra-indications; Side-effects: see under Gentamicin but too toxic for systemic use, see notes above; avoid in intestinal obstruction and in renal impairment

Dose: by mouth, bowel sterilisation, 1 g every 4 hours

PoM **Mycifradin**® (Upjohn)
Tablets, neomycin sulphate 500 mg. Net price 20 = £3.60

PoM **Nivemycin**® (Knoll)
Tablets, neomycin sulphate 500 mg. Net price 20 = £2.17

NETILMICIN

Indications: serious Gram-negative infections resistant to gentamicin

Cautions; Contra-indications; Side-effects: see under Gentamicin

Dose: by intramuscular injection or by intravenous injection over 3–5 minutes or by intravenous infusion, 4–6 mg/kg daily, as a single daily dose or in divided doses every 8 or 12 hours; in severe infections, up to 7.5 mg/kg daily in divided doses every 8 hours (reduced as soon as clinically indicated, usually within 48 hours) NEONATE up to 1 week, 3 mg/kg every 12 hours; INFANT over 1 week, 2.5–3 mg/kg every 8 hours; CHILD 2–2.5 mg/kg every 8 hours

Urinary-tract infection, 150 mg as a single daily dose for 5 days

Gonorrhoea, 300 mg as a single dose

Note. For divided daily dose regimens, one-hour ('peak') concentration should not exceed 12 mg/litre; pre-dose ('trough') concentration should be less than 2 mg/litre

PoM **Netillin**® (Schering-Plough)
Injection, netilmicin (as sulphate) 10 mg/mL, net price 1.5-mL (15-mg) amp = £1.49; 50 mg/mL, 1-mL (50-mg) amp = £2.21; 100 mg/mL, 1-mL (100-mg) amp = £2.88; 1.5-mL (150-mg) amp = £4.11, 2-mL (200-mg) amp = £5.33

TOBRAMYCIN

Indications: see under Gentamicin and notes above

Cautions; Contra-indications; Side-effects: see under Gentamicin

Dose: by intramuscular injection or by slow intravenous injection or by intravenous infusion, 3 mg/kg daily in divided doses every 8 hours, see also notes above; in severe infections up to 5 mg/kg daily in divided doses every 6–8 hours (reduced to 3 mg/kg as soon as clinically indicated); NEONATE 2 mg/kg every 12 hours; CHILD over 1 week 2–2.5 mg/kg every 8 hours

Urinary-tract infection, *by intramuscular injection,* 2–3 mg/kg daily as a single dose

Note. One-hour ('peak') concentration should not exceed 10 mg/litre; pre-dose ('trough') concentration should be less than 2 mg/litre

PoM **Tobramycin** (Non-proprietary)
Injection, tobramycin (as sulphate) 40 mg/mL, net price 1-mL (40-mg) vial = £1.61, 2-mL (80-mg) vial = £2.89
Available from David Bull

PoM **Nebcin**® (Lilly)
Injection, tobramycin (as sulphate) 10 mg/mL, net price 2-mL (20-mg) vial = £1.19; 40 mg/mL, 1-mL (40-mg) vial = £1.61, 2-mL (80-mg) vial = £2.89

5.1.5 Macrolides

Erythromycin has an antibacterial spectrum that is similar but not identical to that of penicillin; it is thus an alternative in penicillin-allergic patients.

Indications for erythromycin include respiratory infections, whooping cough, legionnaires' disease, and campylobacter enteritis. It has activity against gut anaerobes and has been used with neomycin for prophylaxis before bowel surgery. It is active against many penicillin-resistant staphylococci but some are now also resistant to erythromycin; it has poor activity against *Haemophilus influenzae*. Erythromycin is also active against chlamydia and mycoplasmas.

Erythromycin causes nausea, vomiting, and diarrhoea in some patients; in mild to moderate infections this can be avoided by giving a lower dose (250 mg 4 times daily) but if a more serious infection, such as Legionella pneumonia, is suspected higher doses are needed.

Azithromycin is a macrolide with slightly less activity than erythromycin against Gram-positive bacteria but enhanced activity against some Gram-negative organisms including *H. influenzae*. Plasma concentrations are very low but tissue concentrations are much higher. It has a long tissue half-life and once daily dosage is recommended.

Clarithromycin is an erythromycin derivative with slightly greater activity than the parent compound. Tissue concentrations are higher than with erythromycin. It is given twice daily.

Azithromycin and clarithromycin cause fewer gastro-intestinal side-effects than erythromycin.

Spiramycin is also a macrolide (see section 5.4.7).

ERYTHROMYCIN

Indications: alternative to penicillin in hypersensitive patients; campylobacter enteritis, pneumonia, legionnaires' disease, syphilis, non-gonococcal urethritis, chronic prostatitis, acne vulgaris (see section 13.6); diphtheria and whooping cough prophylaxis

Cautions: hepatic and renal impairment; prolongation of QT interval (ventricular tachycardia reported); porphyria (see section 9.8.2); pregnancy (not known to be harmful) and breast-feeding (only small amounts in milk); **interactions:** Appendix 1 (erythromycin and other macrolides)

ARRHYTHMIAS. Avoid concomitant administration with astemizole or terfenadine, see also pp. 137–8; also avoid with cisapride (see p. 34) [other interactions, Appendix 1]

Contra-indications: estolate contra-indicated in liver disease

Side-effects: nausea, vomiting, abdominal discomfort, diarrhoea (pseudomembranous colitis reported); urticaria, rashes and other allergic reactions; reversible hearing loss reported after large doses; cholestatic jaundice and cardiac effects (including chest pain and arrhythmias) also reported

Dose: by mouth, ADULT and CHILD over 8 years, 250–500 mg every 6 hours *or* 0.5–1 g every 12 hours (see notes above); up to 4 g daily in severe infections; CHILD up to 2 years 125 mg every 6 hours, 2–8 years 250 mg every 6 hours, doses doubled for severe infections

Acne, see section 13.6

Early syphilis, 500 mg 4 times daily for 14 days

By intravenous infusion, ADULT and CHILD severe infections, 50 mg/kg daily by continuous infusion *or* in divided doses every 6 hours; mild infections (oral treatment not possible), 25 mg/kg daily

PoM Erythromycin (Non-proprietary)

Tablets, e/c, erythromycin 250 mg, net price 20 = 81p; 500 mg, 20 = £1.64. Label: 5, 9, 25

Available from Abbott, APS, Ashbourne (Rommix®), Berk (Erycen®), Cox, CP, Kent, Norton

PoM Erythromycin Ethyl Succinate (Non-proprietary)

Oral suspension, erythromycin (as ethyl succinate) for reconstitution with water 125 mg/5 mL, net price 100 mL = £1.18; 250 mg/5 mL, 100 mL = £1.83; 500 mg/5 mL, 100 mL = £3.34. Label: 9

Note. Sugar-free versions are available and can be ordered by specifying 'sugar-free' on the prescription

Available from APS, Ashbourne (Rommix®), Berk, Cox, CP, Hillcross, Kent, Lagap, Norton, Rosemont (Arpimycin®)

PoM Erythromycin Lactobionate (Non-proprietary)

Intravenous infusion, powder for reconstitution, erythromycin (as lactobionate), net price 1-g vial = £9.98

Available from Abbott, David Bull

PoM Erymax® (Elan)

Capsules, opaque orange/clear orange, enclosing orange and white e/c pellets, erythromycin 250 mg. Net price 30-cap pack = £6.08. Label: 5, 9, 25

Dose: 1 every 6 hours *or* 2 every 12 hours; acne, 1 twice daily then 1 daily after 1 month

PoM Erythrocin® (Abbott)

Tablets, both f/c, erythromycin (as stearate), 250 mg, net price 20 = £2.65; 500 mg, 20 = £5.46. Label: 9

PoM Erythroped® (Abbott)

Suspension, erythromycin (as ethyl succinate) for reconstitution with water, 125 mg/5 mL (*Suspension PI*), net price 140 mL = £2.81; 250 mg/5 mL, 140 mL = £5.32; 500 mg/5 mL (*Suspension forte*), 140 mL = £9.43. Label: 9

Suspension SF, sugar-free, erythromycin (as ethyl succinate) for reconstitution with water, 125 mg/5 mL (*Suspension PI SF*), net price 140 mL = £2.89; 250 mg/5 mL, 140 mL = £5.63. Label: 9

Granules, erythromycin (as ethyl succinate), 125 mg/sachet (*Granules PI*), net price 28-sachet pack = £3.94; 250 mg/sachet, 28-sachet pack = £6.64; 500 mg/sachet (*Granules forte*), 28-sachet pack = £10.75. Label: 9, 13

PoM Erythroped A® (Abbott)

Tablets, yellow, f/c, erythromycin 500 mg (as ethyl succinate). Net price 28-tab pack = £9.26. Label: 9

Granules, orange, erythromycin 1 g (as ethyl succinate)/sachet. Net price 14-sachet pack = £10.75. Label: 9, 13

PoM Ilosone® (Dista)

Capsules, ivory/red, erythromycin 250 mg (as estolate). Net price 20 = £6.26. Label: 9

Tablets, pink, erythromycin 500 mg (as estolate). Net price 12-tab pack = £7.48. Label: 9

AZITHROMYCIN

Indications: respiratory-tract infections; otitis media; skin and soft-tissue infections; uncomplicated genital chlamydial infections

Cautions; Side-effects: see under Erythromycin; caution in pregnancy and breast-feeding; mild neutropenia reported; **interactions:** Appendix 1 (erythromycin and other macrolides)

Contra-indications: hepatic impairment

Dose: 500 mg once daily for 3 days; CHILD over 6 months 10 mg/kg once daily for 3 days; *or* body-weight 15–25 kg, 200 mg once daily for 3 days; body-weight 26–35 kg, 300 mg once daily for 3 days; body-weight 36–45 kg, 400 mg once daily for 3 days

Genital chlamydial infections, 1 g as a single dose

PoM Zithromax® (Richborough)

Capsules, azithromycin (as dihydrate) 250 mg. Net price 4-cap pack = £8.95, 6-cap pack = £13.43. Label: 5, 9, 23

Oral suspension, azithromycin (as dihydrate) 200 mg/5 mL when reconstituted with water. Net price 15-mL pack = £5.08, 22.5-mL pack = £7.62, 30-mL pack = £13.80. Label: 5, 9, 23

CLARITHROMYCIN

Indications: respiratory-tract infections, mild to moderate skin and soft tissue infections; adjunct in the treatment of duodenal ulcers by eradication of *Helicobacter pylori*—see section 1.3

Cautions; Side-effects: see under Erythromycin; reduce dose in renal impairment; caution in pregnancy and breast-feeding; also reported, headache, taste disturbances, stomatitis, glossitis, cholestasis, jaundice, hepatitis, and Stevens-Johnson syndrome; on intravenous infusion, local tenderness, phlebitis; **interactions:** Appendix 1 (erythromycin and other macrolides)

ARRHYTHMIAS. Avoid concomitant administration with astemizole or terfenadine, see also pp. 137–8; also avoid with cisapride (see p. 34) [other interactions, Appendix1]

Dose: by mouth, 250 mg every 12 hours for 7 days, increased in severe infections to 500 mg every 12 hours for up to 14 days; CHILD body-weight under 8 kg, 7.5 mg/kg twice daily; 8–11 kg (1–2 years), 62.5 mg twice daily; 12–19 kg (3–6 years), 125 mg twice daily; 20–29 kg (7–9 years), 187.5 mg twice daily; 30–40 kg (10–12 years), 250 mg twice daily
Eradication of *H. pylori,* see section 1.3
By intravenous infusion into larger proximal vein, 500 mg twice daily; CHILD not recommended

PoM Klaricid® (Abbott)
Tablets, both yellow, f/c, clarithromycin 250 mg, net price 14-tab pack = £11.24; 500 mg, 14-tab pack = £22.49. Label: 9
Paediatric suspension, clarithromycin 125 mg/ 5 mL when reconstituted with water. Net price 70 mL = £6.00, 100 mL = £10.32. Label: 9
Intravenous infusion, powder for reconstitution, clarithromycin. Net price 500-mg vial = £12.14
Electrolytes: Na⁺ < 0.5 mmol/500-mg vial

5.1.6   Clindamycin

Clindamycin has only a limited use because of serious side-effects. Its most serious toxic effect is pseudomembranous colitis (see section 1.5) which may be fatal and is most common in middle-aged and elderly women, especially following operation. Although it can occur with most antibiotics it is more frequently seen with clindamycin. Patients should therefore discontinue treatment immediately if diarrhoea develops.

Clindamycin is active against Gram-positive cocci, including penicillin-resistant staphylococci and also against many anaerobes, especially *Bacteroides fragilis.* It is well concentrated in bone and excreted in bile and urine.

Clindamycin is recommended for staphylococcal joint and bone infections such as osteomyelitis, and intra-abdominal sepsis. Clindamycin is also used for endocarditis prophylaxis (section 5.1, table 2).

CLINDAMYCIN

Indications: staphylococcal bone and joint infections, peritonitis; endocarditis prophylaxis, section 5.1, table 2
Cautions: discontinue immediately if diarrhoea or colitis develops; hepatic or renal impairment; monitor liver function and blood counts on prolonged therapy and in neonates and infants; pregnancy; breast-feeding (see Appendix 5); **interactions:** Appendix 1 (clindamycin)
Contra-indications: diarrhoeal states
Side-effects: diarrhoea (discontinue treatment), abdominal discomfort, nausea, vomiting, pseudomembranous colitis; rash; jaundice and altered liver function tests; neutropenia, eosinophilia, agranulocytosis and thrombocytopenia reported; pain, induration, and abscess after intramuscular injection; thrombophlebitis after intravenous injection

Dose: by mouth, 150–300 mg every 6 hours; up to 450 mg every 6 hours in severe infections; CHILD, 3–6 mg/kg every 6 hours
COUNSELLING. Patients should discontinue immediately and contact doctor if diarrhoea develops; capsules should be swallowed with a glass of water.
By deep intramuscular injection or by intravenous infusion, 0.6–2.7 g daily (in 2–4 divided doses); life-threatening infection, up to 4.8 g daily; single doses above 600 mg by intravenous infusion only; single doses by intravenous infusion not to exceed 1.2 g
CHILD over 1 month, 15–40 mg/kg daily in 3–4 divided doses; severe infections, at least 300 mg daily regardless of weight
Endocarditis prophylaxis, section 5.1, Table 2

PoM Dalacin C® (Upjohn)
Capsules, clindamycin (as hydrochloride) 75 mg (lavender), net price 24-cap pack = £6.21; 150 mg, (lavender/maroon), 24-cap pack = £11.43. Label: 9, 27, counselling, see above (diarrhoea)
Paediatric suspension, off-white, clindamycin 75 mg (as palmitate hydrochloride)/5 mL when reconstituted with purified water (freshly boiled and cooled). Net price 100 mL = £6.62. Label: 9, 27, counselling, see above (diarrhoea)
Injection, clindamycin 150 mg (as phosphate)/mL. Net price 2-mL amp = £5.17; 4-mL amp = £10.29

5.1.7   Some other antibiotics

Antibacterials discussed in this section include chloramphenicol, fusidic acid, spectinomycin, glycopeptide antibiotics (vancomycin and teicoplanin), and the polymyxin, colistin.

CHLORAMPHENICOL

Chloramphenicol is a potent, potentially toxic, broad-spectrum antibiotic which should be reserved for the treatment of life-threatening infections, particularly those caused by *Haemophilus influenzae,* and also for typhoid fever.

Its toxicity renders it unsuitable for systemic use except in the circumstances indicated above.

Eye-drops of chloramphenicol (see section 11.3.1) are useful for bacterial conjunctivitis.

CHLORAMPHENICOL

Indications: see notes above
Cautions: avoid repeated courses and prolonged treatment; reduce doses in hepatic or renal impairment; blood counts required before and periodically during treatment; may cause 'grey syndrome' in neonates (monitor plasma concentrations); **interactions:** Appendix 1 (chloramphenicol)
Contra-indications: pregnancy (see also Appendix 4), breast-feeding, porphyria (see section 9.8.2)
Side-effects: blood disorders including reversible and irreversible aplastic anaemia (with reports of resulting leukaemia), peripheral neuritis, optic

neuritis, erythema multiforme, nausea, vomiting, diarrhoea, stomatitis, glossitis; nocturnal haemo-globinuria reported

Dose: by mouth or by intravenous injection or infusion, 50 mg/kg daily in 4 divided doses (exceptionally, can be doubled for severe infections such as septicaemia and meningitis, providing high doses reduced as soon as clinically indicated); CHILD, haemophilus epiglottitis and pyogenic meningitis, 50–100 mg/kg daily in divided doses (high dosages decreased as soon as clinically indicated); INFANTS under 2 weeks 25 mg/kg daily (in 4 divided doses), 2 weeks–1 year 50 mg/kg daily (in 4 divided doses)

Note. Plasma concentration monitoring required in neonates and preferred in those under 4 years of age; recommended peak plasma concentration (measured approx. 1 hour after intravenous injection or infusion) 15–25 mg/litre; pre-dose ('trough') concentration should not exceed 15 mg/litre

PoM Chloramphenicol (Non-proprietary)

Capsules, chloramphenicol 250 mg. Net price 20 = £2.56

Available from Sussex

PoM Chloromycetin® (P-D)

Injection, powder for reconstitution, chloramphenicol (as sodium succinate). Net price 300-mg vial = £5.16; 1.2-g vial = £5.03

Electrolytes: Na+ 0.94 mmol/300-mg vial, 3.75 mmol/1.2-g vial

PoM Kemicetine® (Pharmacia)

Injection, powder for reconstitution, chloramphenicol (as sodium succinate). Net price 1-g vial = £1.21

Electrolytes: Na+ 3.14 mmol/g

FUSIDIC ACID

Fusidic acid and its salts are narrow-spectrum antibiotics. The only indication for their use is in infections caused by penicillin-resistant staphylococci, especially osteomyelitis, as they are well concentrated in bone; they are also used for staphylococcal endocarditis (section 5.1, table 1). A second antistaphylococcal antibiotic is usually required to prevent emergence of resistance.

SODIUM FUSIDATE

Indications: see notes above

Cautions: liver-function tests required

Side-effects: nausea, vomiting, rashes, reversible jaundice, especially after high dosage or rapid infusion (withdraw therapy if persistent)

Dose: see under Preparations, below

PoM Fucidin® (Leo)

Tablets, f/c, sodium fusidate 250 mg. Net price 20 = £13.54. Label: 9

Dose: as sodium fusidate, 500 mg every 8 hours, doubled for severe infections

Suspension, off-white, fusidic acid 250 mg/5 mL. Net price 50 mL = £7.58. Label: 9, 21

Dose: as fusidic acid, ADULT 750 mg every 8 hours; CHILD up to 1 year 50 mg/kg daily (in 3 divided doses),

1–5 years 250 mg every 8 hours, 5–12 years 500 mg every 8 hours

Note. Fusidic acid is incompletely absorbed and doses recommended for suspension are proportionately higher than those for sodium fusidate tablets

Intravenous infusion, powder for reconstitution, sodium fusidate 500 mg (≡ fusidic acid 480 mg), with buffer. Net price per vial (with diluent) = £8.15

Electrolytes: Na+ 3.1 mmol/vial when reconstituted with buffer

Dose: as sodium fusidate, by intravenous infusion, ADULT over 50 kg, 500 mg 3 times daily; ADULT under 50 kg and CHILD, 6–7 mg/kg 3 times daily

SPECTINOMYCIN

Spectinomycin is active against Gram-negative organisms, including *N. gonorrhoeae.* Its only indication is the treatment of gonorrhoea caused by penicillin-resistant organisms or in a penicillin-allergic patient.

SPECTINOMYCIN

Indications: see notes above

Cautions: pregnancy and breast-feeding; **interactions:** Appendix 1 (spectinomycin)

Side-effects: nausea, dizziness, urticaria, fever

Dose: by deep intramuscular injection, 2 g; up to 4 g in difficult-to-treat cases and in geographical areas of resistance; CHILD over 2 years, if no alternative treatment, 40 mg/kg

PoM Trobicin® (Upjohn)

Injection, powder for reconstitution, spectinomycin (as hydrochloride). Net price 2-g vial (with diluent) = £8.16

VANCOMYCIN AND TEICOPLANIN

The glycopeptide antibiotics vancomycin and teicoplanin have bactericidal activity against aerobic and anaerobic Gram-positive bacteria.

Vancomycin has a limited use by the intravenous route in the prophylaxis and treatment of endocarditis and other serious infections caused by Gram-positive cocci including multi-resistant staphylococci. It has a relatively long duration of action and can therefore be given every 12 hours; plasma concentrations should be monitored (especially in patients with renal impairment in whom the dose may need marked reduction). It is ototoxic and nephrotoxic. Vancomycin is **not effective** by mouth for systemic infections.

Vancomycin is effective in the treatment of antibiotic-associated colitis (pseudomembranous colitis, see also section 1.5) for which it is given by mouth; a dose of 125 mg every 6 hours for 7 to 10 days is considered to be adequate. Vancomycin should **not** be given by mouth for systemic infections since it is not significantly absorbed.

Teicoplanin is very similar to vancomycin but has a significantly longer duration of action allowing once daily administration. Unlike vancomycin, teicoplanin can be given by intramuscular as well as by intravenous injection.

VANCOMYCIN

Indications: see notes above

Cautions: avoid rapid infusion (risk of anaphylactoid reactions, see Side-effects); rotate infusion sites; renal impairment; elderly; avoid if history of deafness; blood counts, urinalysis and renal function tests required in all patients; monitor auditory function and plasma-vancomycin concentration in elderly or if renal impairment; pregnancy and breast-feeding; systemic absorption may follow oral administration especially in inflammatory bowel disorders or following multiple doses; **interactions:** Appendix 1 (vancomycin)

Side-effects: after parenteral administration: nephrotoxicity including renal failure and interstitial nephritis; ototoxicity (discontinue if tinnitus occurs); blood disorders including neutropenia (usually after 1 week or cumulative dose of 25 g), rarely agranulocytosis and thrombocytopenia; nausea, chills, fever; eosinophilia, anaphylaxis, rashes (including exfoliative dermatitis, Stevens-Johnson syndrome and vasculitis); phlebitis (irritant to tissue); on rapid infusion, severe hypotension (including shock and cardiac arrest), wheezing, dyspnoea, urticaria, pruritus, flushing of the upper body ('red man' syndrome), pain and muscle spasm of back and chest

Dose: by mouth, antibiotic-associated colitis, 125 mg every 6 hours for 7–10 days, see notes above; CHILD 5 mg/kg every 6 hours, over 5 years, half adult dose

Note. Oral paediatric dose is lower than that on data sheet but is adequate

By intravenous infusion, 500 mg over at least 60 minutes every 6 hours *or* 1 g over at least 100 minutes every 12 hours; NEONATE up to 1 week, 15 mg/kg initially then 10 mg/kg every 12 hours; INFANT 1–4 weeks, 15 mg/kg initially then 10 mg/kg every 8 hours; CHILD over 1 month, 10 mg/kg every 6 hours

Endocarditis prophylaxis, section 5.1, table 2

Note. Plasma concentration monitoring required; peak plasma concentration (measured 2 hours after intravenous infusion) should not exceed 30 mg/litre; pre-dose ('trough') concentration should not exceed 10 mg/litre

PoM **Vancomycin** (Non-proprietary)

Injection, powder for reconstitution, vancomycin (as hydrochloride). 500-mg vial

Note. Can be used to prepare solution for oral administration

Available from Antigen, David Bull

PoM **Vancocin®** (Lilly)

Matrigel capsules, vancomycin (as hydrochloride) 125 mg (blue/peach), net price 20-cap pack = £63.08; 250 mg (blue/grey), 20-cap pack = £126.16

Injection, powder for reconstitution, vancomycin (as hydrochloride). Net price 250-mg vial = £4.76; 500-mg vial = £8.66; 1-g vial = £17.32

Note. Can be used to prepare solution for oral administration

TEICOPLANIN

Indications: potentially serious Gram-positiv infections including endocarditis, dialysis-associ ated peritonitis, and serious infections due to *Sta phylococcus aureus*; prophylaxis in endocarditi and in orthopaedic surgery at risk of infectio with Gram-positive organisms

Cautions: vancomycin sensitivity; blood count and liver and kidney function tests required reduce dose in renal impairment (and monitc renal and auditory function on prolonged admin istration or if other nephrotoxic or neurotoxi drugs given); pregnancy and breast-feeding

Side-effects: nausea, vomiting, diarrhoea; rash fever, bronchospasm, anaphylactic reactions; diz ziness, headache; blood disorders includin eosinophilia, leucopenia, and thrombocytopenia disturbances in liver enzymes, transient increas of serum creatinine; tinnitus, mild hearing los and vestibular disorders also reported; local reac tions include erythema, pain, and thrombophleb itis

Dose: by intravenous injection or infusion, 400 m initially, subsequently 200 mg daily; severe infec tions, 400 mg every 12 hours for 3 doses initiall subsequently 400 mg daily; subsequent doses ca be given *by intramuscular injection;* higher dose may be required in patients of over 85 kg and i severe burns or endocarditis (see data sheet)

CHILD over 2 months *by intravenous injection o infusion,* initially 10 mg/kg every 12 hours for doses, subsequently 6 mg/kg daily (severe infec tions or in neutropenia, 10 mg/kg daily); subse quent doses can be given *by intramuscula injection* (but intravenous administration pre ferred in children); NEONATE *by intravenous infu sion,* initially a single dose of 16 mg/kg subsequently 8 mg/kg daily

Endocarditis prophylaxis, section 5.1, table 2

Orthopaedic surgery prophylaxis, *by intravenou injection,* 400 mg at induction of anaesthesia

PoM **Targocid®** (Merrell)

Injection, powder for reconstitution, teicoplanin net price 200-mg vial (with diluent) = £26.0 400-mg vial (with diluent) = £52.10

Electrolytes: Na⁺ < 0.5 mmol/200- and 400-mg vial

POLYMYXINS

The polymyxin antibiotic, **colistin**, is active agains Gram-negative organisms, including *Pseudomona aeruginosa.* It is **not** absorbed by mouth and thu needs to be given by injection to obtain a systemi effect; however, it is toxic and has few, if any, indi cations for systemic use.

Colistin is used by mouth in bowel sterilisatio regimens in neutropenic patients (usually with nys tatin); it is **not** recommended for gastro-intestina infections. It is also given by inhalation of a neb ulised solution as an adjunct to standard antibioti therapy.

Both colistin and polymyxin B are included i some preparations for topical application.

COLISTIN

Indications: see notes above

Cautions: renal impairment; porphyria (see section 9.8.2); **interactions:** Appendix 1 (colistin)

Contra-indications: myasthenia gravis; pregnancy; breast-feeding

Side-effects: perioral and peripheral paraesthesia, vertigo, muscle weakness, apnoea, nephrotoxicity; rarely vasomotor instability, slurred speech, visual disturbance, confusion and psychosis; neurotoxicity reported with excessive doses; bronchospasm on inhalation

Dose: by mouth, bowel sterilisation, 1.5–3 million units every 8 hours

By intramuscular injection or intravenous injection or infusion, 2 million units every 8 hours (but see notes above)

By inhalation of nebulised solution, patients over 40 kg, 1 million units every 12 hours; patients under 40 kg, 500 000 units every 12 hours

Note. Colistin doses in BNF may differ from those in data sheet

ᵖoM Colomycin® (Pharmax)

Tablets, scored, colistin sulphate 1.5 million units. Net price 50 = £65.11

Syrup, colistin sulphate 250 000 units/5 mL when reconstituted with water. Net price 80 mL = £3.88

Injection, powder for reconstitution, colistin sulphomethate sodium. Net price 500 000-unit vial = £1.27; 1 million-unit vial = £1.88

Electrolytes: (before reconstitution) Na⁺ < 0.5 mmol/500 000- and 1 million-unit vial

5.1.8 Sulphonamides and trimethoprim

The importance of the sulphonamides has decreased as a result of increasing bacterial resistance and their replacement by antibiotics which are generally more active and less toxic.

Sulphamethoxazole and trimethoprim are used in combination (as **co-trimoxazole**) because of their synergistic activity, but see below for important CSM recommendations limiting the use of this combination.

Trimethoprim can be used alone for urinary- and respiratory-tract infections and for prostatitis, shigellosis, and invasive salmonella infections.

Side-effects of the sulphonamides include rashes, Stevens-Johnson syndrome (erythema multiforme), renal failure (especially with the less soluble preparations), and blood dyscrasias, notably marrow depression and agranulocytosis.

The **longer-acting sulphonamide,** sulfametopyrazine which is highly bound to plasma proteins, has the advantage of requiring less frequent administration, but toxic effects due to accumulation are more likely to occur.

For *topical preparations* of sulphonamides used in the treatment of burns see section 13.10.1.1.

Cautionary label wordings, see inside back cover

CSM recommendations. Co-trimoxazole should be limited to the role of drug of choice in Pneumocystis carinii pneumonia; it is also indicated for toxoplasmosis and nocardiasis. It should now only be considered for use in acute exacerbations of chronic bronchitis and infections of the urinary tract when there is good bacteriological evidence of sensitivity to co-trimoxazole and good reason to prefer this combination to a single antibiotic; similarly it should only be used in acute otitis media in children when there is good reason to prefer it. Review of the safety of co-trimoxazole using spontaneous adverse drug reaction data has indicated that the profile of reported adverse reactions with trimethoprim is similar to that with co-trimoxazole; blood and generalised skin disorders are the most serious reactions with both drugs and predominantly have been reported to occur in elderly patients. A recent large post-marketing study has demonstrated that such reactions are very rare with co-trimoxazole; the study did not distinguish between co-trimoxazole and trimethoprim with respect to serious hepatic, renal, blood or skin disorders.

CO-TRIMOXAZOLE

A mixture of trimethoprim and sulphamethoxazole in the proportions of 1 part to 5 parts

Indications: see CSM recommendations above

Cautions: blood counts in prolonged treatment, maintain adequate fluid intake, renal impairment, breast-feeding; photosensitivity; elderly patients (**important:** see CSM recommendations above); G6PD deficiency (see section 9.1.5); **interactions:** Appendix 1 (co-trimoxazole)

BLOOD DISORDERS AND RASHES. A reminder that treatment should be stopped immediately if blood disorders or rashes develop

Contra-indications: pregnancy (see Appendix 4), infants under 6 weeks (risk of kernicterus), renal or hepatic failure, jaundice, blood disorders; porphyria (see section 9.8.2)

Side-effects: nausea, vomiting, diarrhoea, glossitis, rashes, erythema multiforme (includes Stevens-Johnson syndrome); epidermal necrolysis, pancreatitis, eosinophilia, agranulocytosis, granulocytopenia, purpura, leucopenia, thrombocytopenia; megaloblastic anaemia due to trimethoprim; pseudomembranous colitis, jaundice and hepatic necrosis reported

Dose: by mouth, 960 mg every 12 hours, increased to 1.44 g in severe infections; 480 mg every 12 hours if treated for more than 14 days; CHILD, every 12 hours, 6 weeks to 5 months, 120 mg; 6 months to 5 years, 240 mg; 6–12 years, 480 mg

Prophylaxis of recurrent urinary-tract infection, 480 mg at night; CHILD 6–12 mg/kg at night

Gonorrhoea, 1.92 g every 12 hours for 2 days, or 2.4 g followed by a further dose of 2.4 g after 8 hours but see notes above

High-dose therapy for *Pneumocystis carinii* infections, 120 mg/kg daily in divided doses for 14 days

By intravenous infusion, 960 mg every 12 hours increased to 1.44 g every 12 hours in severe infections; CHILD 36 mg/kg daily in 2 divided doses increased to 54 mg/kg daily in severe infections

Note. 480 mg of co-trimoxazole consists of sulphamethoxazole 400 mg and trimethoprim 80 mg

PoM **Co-trimoxazole** (Non-proprietary)

Tablets, co-trimoxazole 480 mg, net price 20 = 61p; 960 mg, 20 = £1.40. Label: 9
Available from APS, Ashbourne (Comixco®), Cox, DDSA (Fectrim®, Fectrim® Forte), Hillcross, Kent, Norton

Dispersible tablets, co-trimoxazole 480 mg. Net price 20 = £1.85. Label: 9, 13
Available from APS, Norton (Comox®)

Paediatric oral suspension, co-trimoxazole 240 mg/5 mL. Net price 100 mL = £1.08. Label: 9
Available from APS, Ashbourne (Comixco®), Lagap (Laratrim®), Norton, Rosemont (Chemotrim®)

Oral suspension, co-trimoxazole 480 mg/5 mL. Net price 100 mL = £3.50. Label: 9
Available from Kent, Lagap (Laratrim®)

Strong sterile solution, co-trimoxazole 96 mg/mL. For dilution and use as an intravenous infusion. Net price 5-mL amp = £1.64, 10-mL amp = £3.06
Available from David Bull

PoM **Bactrim**® (Roche)

Drapsules® (= tablets), orange, f/c, co-trimoxazole 480 mg. Net price 40-tab pack = £4.98. Label: 9

Paediatric syrup, sugar-free, yellow, co-trimoxazole 240 mg/5 mL. Net price 100 mL = £2.09. Label: 9

PoM **Septrin**® (Wellcome)

Tablets, co-trimoxazole 480 mg. Net price 20 = £3.03. Label: 9

Dispersible tablets, orange, sugar-free, co-trimoxazole 480 mg. Net price 20 = £3.55. Label: 9, 13

Forte tablets, scored, co-trimoxazole 960 mg. Net price 20 = £5.05. Label: 9

Adult suspension, co-trimoxazole 480 mg/5 mL. Net price 100 mL = £4.74. Label: 9

Paediatric suspension, sugar-free, co-trimoxazole 240 mg/5 mL. Net price 100 mL = £2.63. Label: 9

Intravenous infusion, co-trimoxazole 96 mg/mL. To be diluted before use. Net price 5-mL amp = £1.59

SULFAMETOPYRAZINE

Indications: urinary-tract infections, chronic bronchitis

Cautions; Contra-indications; Side-effects: see under Co-trimoxazole

Dose: 2 g once weekly

PoM **Kelfizine W**® (Pharmacia)

Tablets, sulfametopyrazine 2 g. Tablets to be taken in water. Net price 5-tab pack = £6.68. Label: 9, 13

SULPHADIAZINE

(Sulfadiazine)

Indications: prevention of rheumatic fever recurrence, toxoplasmosis [unlicensed]—see section 5.4.7

Cautions; Contra-indications; Side-effects: see under Co-trimoxazole; avoid in severe renal impairment

Dose: prevention of rheumatic fever, *by mouth*, 1 g daily (500 mg daily for patients less than 30 kg)

PoM **Sulphadiazine** (Non-proprietary)

Tablets, sulphadiazine 500 mg. Net price 56-ta pack = £14.99. Label: 9, 27
Available from CP

Injection, sulphadiazine (as sodium salt) 250 mg mL. Net price 4-mL amp = £2.00
Available from Rhône-Poulenc Rorer

SULPHADIMIDINE

Indications: urinary-tract infections

Cautions; Contra-indications; Side-effects: se under Co-trimoxazole

Dose: by mouth, 2 g initially, then 0.5–1 g every 6 8 hours

PoM **Sulphadimidine** (Non-proprietary)

Tablets, sulphadimidine 500 mg. Net price 20 £3.00. Label: 9, 27
Available from CP

TRIMETHOPRIM

Indications: urinary-tract infections, acute an chronic bronchitis

Cautions: renal impairment, breast-feeding, pre disposition to folate deficiency, blood coun required on long-term therapy; porphyria (se section 9.8.2); **interactions:** Appendix 1 (tri methoprim)

Contra-indications: severe renal impairmen pregnancy, neonates, blood dyscrasias

Side-effects: gastro-intestinal disturbances inclu ing nausea and vomiting, pruritus, rashes, depres sion of haematopoiesis; rarely erythem multiforme, toxic epidermal necrolysis; asepti meningitis reported

Dose: by mouth, acute infections, 200 mg every 1 hours; CHILD, twice daily, 2–5 months 25 mg, months–5 years 50 mg, 6–12 years 100 mg
Chronic infections and prophylaxis, 100 mg night; CHILD 1–2 mg/kg at night

By slow intravenous injection or infusion, 150 250 mg every 12 hours; CHILD under 12 years, 6 9 mg/kg daily in 2–3 divided doses

PoM **Trimethoprim** (Non-proprietary)

Tablets, trimethoprim 100 mg, net price 20 = 44p 200 mg, 20 = 66p. Label: 9
Available from APS, Ashbourne (Triprimix®), Be (Trimopan®), Cox, Kent, Lagap (Trimogal®), Norton

PoM **Ipral**® (Squibb)

Tablets, trimethoprim 100 mg, net price 20 = 80p 200 mg, 20 = £1.71. Label: 9

PoM **Monotrim**® (Solvay)

Tablets, both scored, trimethoprim 100 mg, ne price 20 = 82p; 200 mg, 20 = £1.44. Label: 9

Suspension, sugar-free, trimethoprim 50 mg/5 m Net price 100 mL = £1.77. Label: 9

Injection, trimethoprim (as lactate) 20 mg/mL. Ne price 5-mL amp = £1.11

PoM **Trimopan**® (Berk)

Suspension, sugar-free, trimethoprim 50 mg/5 m Net price 100 mL = £2.34. Label: 9

5.1.9 Antituberculous drugs

Tuberculosis is treated in two phases—an *initial phase* using at least three drugs and a *continuation phase* using two drugs. Treatment requires specialised knowledge, particularly where the disease involves resistant organisms or non-respiratory organs.

The regimens given below are recommended by the Joint Tuberculosis Committee of the British Thoracic Society for the treatment of tuberculosis in the UK; variations occur in other countries.

INITIAL PHASE. The concurrent use of at least three drugs during the initial phase is designed to reduce the population of viable bacteria as rapidly as possible and to prevent the emergence of drug-resistant bacteria. Treatment of choice for the initial phase is the daily use of isoniazid, rifampicin, and pyrazinamide; ethambutol is added if drug resistance is thought likely. Streptomycin is now rarely used in the UK but it may be added if the organism is resistant to isoniazid. The initial phase drugs should be continued for 2 months.

CONTINUATION PHASE. After the initial phase, treatment is continued for a further 4 months with isoniazid and rifampicin; longer treatment is necessary for bone and joint infections, for meningitis, or for resistant organisms.

Recommended dosage for standard unsupervised 6-month regimen

Isoniazid (for 6 months)	ADULT 300 mg daily; CHILD 10 mg/kg (max. 300 mg) daily
Rifampicin (for 6 months)	ADULT under 50 kg 450 mg daily, 50 kg and over 600 mg daily: CHILD 10 mg/kg daily
Pyrazinamide (for first 2 months only)	ADULT under 50 kg 1.5 g, 50 kg and over 2 g daily; CHILD 35 mg/kg daily

Note. Ethambutol and streptomycin are included in treatment regimens if resistance is suspected; see notes below for doses

PREGNANCY AND BREAST-FEEDING. The standard regimen (above) may be used during pregnancy and breast-feeding; pyridoxine supplements are advisable. Streptomycin should not be given in pregnancy.

CHILDREN. As for adults, children are given isoniazid, rifampicin, and pyrazinamide for the first 2 months followed by isoniazid and rifampicin during the next 4 months. If pyrazinamide is omitted from the initial phase, then treatment with isoniazid and rifampicin should be given for 9 months. Except in exceptional circumstances (e.g. drug resistance) ethambutol should be **avoided** in young children because of the difficulty in testing eyesight and in obtaining reports of visual symptoms (see below).

SUPERVISED TREATMENT. Treatment needs to be fully supervised in patients who cannot be relied upon to comply with the treatment regimen. These patients are given isoniazid, rifampicin, and pyrazinamide 3 times a week under supervision for the first 2 months followed by isoniazid and rifampicin three times a week for a further 4 months.

Recommended dosage for intermittent supervised treatment

Isoniazid (for 6 months)	ADULT and CHILD 15 mg/kg 3 times a week
Rifampicin (for 6 months)	ADULT 600–900 mg 3 times a week; CHILD 15 mg/kg 3 times a week
Pyrazinamide (for first 2 months only)	ADULT under 50 kg 2 g 3 times a week, 50 kg and over 2.5 g; CHILD 50 mg/kg 3 times a week
	or
	ADULT under 50 kg 3 g twice a week, 50 kg and over 3.5 g; CHILD 75 mg/kg twice a week

Note. Ethambutol and streptomycin are included in treatment regimens if resistance is suspected; see notes below for doses

IMMUNOCOMPROMISED PATIENTS. Immunocompromised patients may develop tuberculosis owing to reactivation of previously latent disease or to new infection. Multi-resistant *Mycobacterium tuberculosis* may be present or the infection may be caused by other mycobacteria e.g. *M. avium* complex in which case specialist advice is needed. Culture should always be carried out and the type of organism and its sensitivity confirmed. A minimum duration of treatment of 9 months is currently recommended for *M. tuberculosis* infection.

MONITORING. Since isoniazid, rifampicin and pyrazinamide are associated with liver toxicity (see Appendix 2), *hepatic function* should be checked before and during treatment with these drugs; those dependent on alcohol or who have pre-existing liver disease require special care.

Renal function should be checked before treatment with antituberculous drugs and appropriate dosage adjustments made. Streptomycin or ethambutol should preferably be avoided in patients with renal impairment, but if used require dose reduction and possibly drug concentration monitoring (see Appendix 3).

Visual acuity should be tested before ethambutol is used (see below).

> Major causes of treatment failure are incorrect prescribing by the physician and inadequate compliance by the patient. Avoid both excessive and inadequate dosage. Treatment should be supervised by a specialist physician.

Isoniazid is cheap and highly effective. Like rifampicin it should always be included in any antituberculous regimen unless there is a specific contra-indication. Its only common side-effect is peripheral neuropathy which is more likely to occur where there are pre-existing risk factors such as diabetes and alcoholism and in chronic renal failure and malnutrition. In these circumstances pyridoxine 10 mg daily should be given prophylactically from the start of treatment. Other side-effects such as hepatitis (important: see Monitoring above) and psychosis are rare.

Rifampicin is a key component of any antituberculous regimen. Like isoniazid it should always be included unless there is a specific contra-indication.

During the first two months of rifampicin administration transient disturbance of liver function with elevated serum transaminases is common but generally does not require interruption of treatment. Occasionally more serious liver toxicity requires a change of treatment particularly in those with pre-existing liver disease (important: see Monitoring above).

On intermittent treatment six toxicity syndromes have been recognised—influenzal, abdominal, and respiratory symptoms, shock, renal failure, and thrombocytopenic purpura—and can occur in 20 to 30% of patients.

Rifampicin induces hepatic enzymes which accelerate the metabolism of several drugs including oestrogens, corticosteroids, phenytoin, sulphonylureas, and anticoagulants. **Important:** the effectiveness of oral contraceptives is reduced and alternative family planning advice should be offered (see section 7.3.1).

Rifabutin, a newly introduced rifamycin, is indicated for *prophylaxis* against *M. avium* complex infections in patients with a low CD4 count; it is also licensed for the *treatment* of non-tuberculous mycobacterial disease and pulmonary tuberculosis. As with rifampicin it induces hepatic enzymes and the effectiveness of oral contraceptives is reduced requiring alternative family planning methods.

Pyrazinamide is a bactericidal drug only active against intracellular dividing forms of *Mycobacterium tuberculosis*; it exerts its main effect only in the first two or three months. It is particularly useful in tuberculous meningitis because of good meningeal penetration. It is not active against *M. bovis*. Serious liver toxicity may occasionally occur (important: see Monitoring above).

Ethambutol is included in a treatment regimen if resistance is suspected; it can be omitted if the risk of resistance is low. For unsupervised treatment ethambutol is given in a dose of 25 mg/kg daily in the initial phase followed by 15 mg/kg daily in the continuation phase (*or* 15 mg/kg daily throughout); in fully supervised intermittent treatment ethambutol is given in a dose of 30 mg/kg 3 times a week *or* 45 mg/kg twice a week.

Side-effects of ethambutol are largely confined to visual disturbances in the form of loss of acuity, colour blindness, and restriction of visual fields. These toxic effects are more common where excessive dosage is used or the patient's renal function is impaired, in which case the drug should be **avoided**. The earliest features of ocular toxicity are subjective and patients should be advised to discontinue therapy immediately if they develop deterioration in vision and promptly seek further advice. Early discontinuation of the drug is almost always followed by recovery of eyesight. Patients who cannot understand warnings about visual side-effects should, if possible, be given an alternative drug. In particular, ethambutol should be **avoided** in children until they are at least 6 years old and capable of reporting subjective visual changes accurately.

Ophthalmic examination should be performed before treatment.

Streptomycin is now rarely used in the UK except for resistant organisms. It is given intramuscularly in a standard dose of 1 g daily, reduced to 500–750 mg in patients under 50 kg or those over 40 years of age. For fully supervised intermittent treatment streptomycin is given in a dose of 1 g 3 times a week, reduced to 750 mg 3 times a week in patients under 50 kg. Children are given streptomycin in a dose of 15–20 mg/kg daily or for fully supervised intermittent treatment, 15–20 mg/kg 3 times a week. Plasma drug concentrations should be measured, particularly in patients with impaired renal function in whom streptomycin must be used with great care. Side-effects increase after a cumulative dose of 100 g, which should only be exceeded in exceptional circumstances.

Second-line drugs available for infections caused by resistant organisms, or when first-line drugs cause unacceptable side-effects, include capreomycin, cycloserine, newer macrolides (e.g. azithromycin and clarithromycin), 4-quinolones (e.g. ciprofloxacin and ofloxacin) and prothionamide (no longer on UK market). Advice on the availability of second-line antituberculous drugs can be obtained from Regional Drug Information Services.

CAPREOMYCIN

Indications: in combination with other drugs, tuberculosis resistant to first-line drugs
Cautions: renal, hepatic, or auditory impairment, monitor renal, hepatic, auditory, and vestibular function and electrolytes; pregnancy (teratogenic in *animals*) and breast-feeding; **interactions:** Appendix 1 (capreomycin)
Side-effects: hypersensitivity reactions including urticaria and rashes; leucocytosis or leucopenia, rarely thrombocytopenia; changes in liver function tests; nephrotoxicity, electrolyte disturbances; hearing loss with tinnitus and vertigo, neuromuscular block after large doses, pain and induration at injection site
Dose: by deep intramuscular injection, 1 g daily (not more than 20 mg/kg) for 2–4 months, then 1 g 2–3 times each week

PoM **Capastat**® (Dista)
Injection, powder for reconstitution, capreomycin sulphate 1 million units (≡ capreomycin approx. 1 g). Net price per vial = £17.25

CYCLOSERINE

Indications: in combination with other drugs, tuberculosis resistant to first-line drugs
Cautions: discontinue (or reduce dose) if allergic dermatitis or symptoms of CNS toxicity; reduce dose in renal impairment (avoid if severe); monitor haematological, renal, and hepatic function; pregnancy and breast-feeding; **interactions:** Appendix 1 (cycloserine)

Contra-indications: severe renal impairment, epilepsy, depression, severe anxiety, psychotic states, alcohol dependence, porphyria (see section 9.8.2)

Side-effects: mainly neurological, including headache, dizziness, vertigo, drowsiness, tremor, convulsions; psychosis, depression; rashes; megaloblastic anaemia; changes in liver function tests

Dose: initially 250 mg every 12 hours for 2 weeks increased according to blood concentration and response to max. 500 mg every 12 hours; CHILD initially 10 mg/kg daily adjusted according to blood concentration and response

Note. Blood concentration monitoring required especially in renal impairment or if dose exceeds 500 mg daily or if signs of toxicity; blood concentration should not exceed 30 mg/litre

PoM Cycloserine (Lilly)
Capsules, red/grey cycloserine 250 mg, net price 100-cap pack = £220.69. Label: 2, 8

ETHAMBUTOL HYDROCHLORIDE

Indications: tuberculosis, in combination with other drugs

Cautions: reduce dose in renal impairment; elderly; pregnancy; warn patients to report visual changes—see notes above

Contra-indications: young children (see notes), optic neuritis, poor vision

Side-effects: optic neuritis, red/green colour blindness, peripheral neuritis

Dose: ADULT and CHILD over 6 years, see notes above

PoM Myambutol® (Lederle)
Tablets, ethambutol hydrochloride 100 mg (yellow), net price 100-tab pack = £7.22; 400 mg (grey), 100-tab pack = £25.84. Label: 8

ISONIAZID

Indications: tuberculosis, in combination with other drugs; prophylaxis—section 5.1, Table 2

Cautions: hepatic impairment (monitor hepatic function, see also below); renal impairment; slow acetylator status (increased risk of side-effects); epilepsy; history of psychosis; alcoholism; pregnancy and breast-feeding (see section 9.8.2); **interactions:** Appendix 1 (isoniazid)

HEPATIC DISORDERS. Patients or their carers should be told how to recognise signs of liver disorder, and advised to discontinue treatment and seek immediate medical attention if symptoms such as persistent nausea, vomiting, malaise or jaundice develop

Contra-indications: drug-induced liver disease

Side-effects: nausea, vomiting; peripheral neuritis with high doses (pyridoxine prophylaxis, see notes above), optic neuritis, convulsions, psychotic episodes; hypersensitivity reactions including fever, erythema multiforme, purpura; agranulocytosis; hepatitis (especially over age of 35); systemic lupus erythematosus-like syndrome, pellagra, hyperglycaemia, and gynaecomastia reported

Dose: by mouth or by intramuscular or intravenous injection, see notes above

PoM Isoniazid (Non-proprietary)
Tablets, isoniazid 50 mg, net price 20 = £1.38; 100 mg, 20 = 40p. Label: 8, 22
Available from APS, Norton

Elixir (BPC), isoniazid 50 mg, citric acid monohydrate 12.5 mg, sodium citrate 60 mg, concentrated anise water 0.05 mL, compound tartrazine solution 0.05 mL, glycerol 1 mL, double-strength chloroform water 2 mL, water to 5 mL. Label: 8, 22
'Special order' [unlicensed] product; contact Martindale, Rosemont, or regional hospital manufacturing unit

Injection, isoniazid 25 mg/mL. Net price 2-mL amp = £2.65
Available from Cambridge

PYRAZINAMIDE

Indications: tuberculosis in combination with other drugs

Cautions: hepatic impairment (monitor hepatic function, see also below); renal impairment; diabetes; gout; **interactions:** Appendix 1 (pyrazinamide)

HEPATIC DISORDERS. Patients or their carers should be told how to recognise signs of liver disorder, and advised to discontinue treatment and seek immediate medical attention if symptoms such as persistent nausea, vomiting, malaise or jaundice develop

Contra-indications: liver damage, porphyria (see section 9.8.2)

Side-effects: hepatotoxicity including fever, anorexia, hepatomegaly, jaundice, liver failure; nausea, vomiting, arthralgia, sideroblastic anaemia, urticaria

Dose: see notes above

PoM Zinamide® (MSD)
Tablets, scored, pyrazinamide 500 mg. Net price 20 = £1.44. Label: 8

RIFABUTIN

Indications: see under Dose

Cautions: see under Rifampicin; reduce dose in severe renal impairment

Side-effects: nausea, vomiting; leucopenia, thrombocytopenia, anaemia; raised liver enzymes, jaundice; uveitis following high doses or administration with drugs which raise plasma concentration—see also **interactions:** Appendix 1 (rifamycins); also hypersensitivity reactions including fever, rash, eosinophilia, bronchospasm, shock; urine, saliva and other body secretions coloured orange-red

Dose: prophylaxis of *Mycobacterium avium* complex infections in immunosuppressed patients with low CD4 count (see data sheet), 300 mg daily as a single dose

Treatment of non-tuberculous mycobacterial disease, in combination with other drugs, 450–600 mg daily as a single dose for up to 6 months after cultures negative

Treatment of pulmonary tuberculosis, in combination with other drugs, 150–450 mg daily as a single dose for at least 6 months
CHILD not recommended

▼ PoM **Mycobutin®** (Pharmacia)
Capsules, red-brown, rifabutin 150 mg. Net price 30-cap pack = £82.29. Label: 8, 14, counselling, lenses, see under Rifampicin

RIFAMPICIN

Indications: see under Dose
Cautions: reduce dose in hepatic impairment (see Appendix 2; liver function tests and blood counts in hepatic disorders and on prolonged therapy, see also below); renal impairment (if above 600 mg daily); pregnancy and breast-feeding (see notes above and Appendixes 4 and 5); **important:** advise patients on oral contraceptives to use additional means (see also section 7.3.1); discolours soft contact lenses; see also notes above; **interactions:** Appendix 1 (rifamycins)
Note. If treatment interrupted re-introduce with low dosage and increase gradually; discontinue permanently if serious side-effects develop
HEPATIC DISORDERS. Patients or their carers should be told how to recognise signs of liver disorder, and advised to discontinue treatment and seek immediate medical attention if symptoms such as persistent nausea, vomiting, malaise or jaundice develop
Contra-indications: jaundice, porphyria (see section 9.8.2)
Side-effects: gastro-intestinal symptoms including anorexia, nausea, vomiting, diarrhoea (pseudomembranous colitis reported); those occurring mainly on intermittent therapy include influenzal syndrome (with chills, fever, dizziness, bone pain), respiratory symptoms (including shortness of breath), collapse and shock, haemolytic anaemia, acute renal failure, and thrombocytopenic purpura; alterations of liver function, jaundice; flushing, urticaria, and rashes; other side-effects reported include oedema, muscular weakness and myopathy, leucopenia, eosinophilia, menstrual disturbances; urine, saliva, and other body secretions coloured orange-red; thrombophlebitis reported if infusion used for prolonged period
Dose: brucellosis, legionnaires' disease and serious staphylococcal infections, in combination with other drugs, *by mouth or by intravenous infusion*, 0.6–1.2 g daily (in 2–4 divided doses)
Tuberculosis, in combination with other drugs, see notes above
Leprosy, section 5.1.10
Prophylaxis of meningococcal meningitis and *Haemophilus influenzae* (type b) infection, section 5.1, table 2

PoM **Rifampicin** (Non-proprietary)
Capsules, rifampicin 150 mg, net price 20 = £4.07; 300 mg, 20 = £8.13. Label: 8, 14, 22, counselling, see lenses above
Available from APS, Generics

PoM **Rifadin®** (Merrell)
Capsules, rifampicin 150 mg (blue/red), net price 20 = £3.73; 300 mg (red), 20 = £7.45. Label: 14, 22, counselling, see lenses above
Syrup, red, rifampicin 100 mg/5 mL. Net price 120 mL = £3.62. Label: 8, 14, 22, counselling, se lenses above
Intravenous infusion, powder for reconstitutio rifampicin. Net price 600-mg vial (with solven = £7.80
Electrolytes: Na⁺ < 0.5 mmol/vial

PoM **Rimactane®** (Ciba)
Capsules, rifampicin 150 mg (red), net price 5 tab pack = £11.39; 300 mg (red/brown), 56-ta pack = £22.77. Label: 8, 14, 22, counselling, se lenses above
Syrup, red, rifampicin 100 mg/5 mL. Net pri 100 mL = £3.06. Label: 8, 14, 22, counselling, se lenses above
Intravenous infusion, powder for reconstitutio rifampicin (as sodium salt). Net price 300-mg vi (with diluent) = £8.01
Electrolytes: Na⁺ < 0.5 mmol/vial
Note. Owing to risk of contact sensitisation care must taken to avoid contact during preparation and infusion

Combined preparations
PoM **Rifater®** (Merrell)
Tablets, pink-beige, s/c, rifampicin 120 mg, ison azid 50 mg, pyrazinamide 300 mg. Net price 20 £4.29. Label: 8, 14, 22, counselling, see lense above
Dose: initial treatment of pulmonary tuberculos patients up to 40 kg 3 tablets daily preferably befo breakfast, 40–49 kg 4 tablets daily, 50–64 kg 5 table daily, 65 kg or more, 6 tablets daily; not suitable for u in children

PoM **Rifinah 150®** (Merrell)
Tablets, pink, rifampicin 150 mg, isoniaz 100 mg. Net price 84-tab pack = £16.18. Label: 14, 22, counselling, see lenses above
Dose: ADULT under 50 kg, 3 tablets daily, preferab before breakfast

PoM **Rifinah 300®** (Merrell)
Tablets, orange, rifampicin 300 mg, isoniaz 150 mg. Net price 56-tab pack = £21.38. Label: 14, 22, counselling, see lenses above
Dose: ADULT 50 kg and over, 2 tablets daily, preferab before breakfast

PoM **Rimactazid 150®** (Ciba)
Tablets, pink, s/c, rifampicin 150 mg, isoniaz 100 mg. Net price 84-tab pack = £16.42. Label: 14, 22, counselling, see lenses above
Additives: include gluten
Dose: ADULT under 50 kg, 3 tablets daily, preferab before breakfast

PoM **Rimactazid 300®** (Ciba)
Tablets, orange, s/c, rifampicin 300 mg, isoniaz 150 mg. Net price 56-tab pack = £21.71. Label: 14, 22, counselling, see lenses above
Additives: include gluten
Dose: ADULT 50 kg and over, 2 tablets daily, preferab before breakfast

STREPTOMYCIN

Indications: tuberculosis, in combination wi other drugs

Cautions; Contra-indications; Side-effects: see under Aminoglycosides, section 5.1.4; also hypersensitivity reactions, paraesthesia of mouth
Dose: by deep intramuscular injection, see notes above

PoM **Streptomycin Sulphate** (Evans)
Injection, powder for reconstitution, streptomycin (as sulphate). Net price 1-g vial = £5.62

5.1.10 Antileprotic drugs

Advice from a member of the Panel of Leprosy Opinion is essential for the treatment of leprosy (Hansen's disease). Details of the Panel can be obtained from the Department of Health telephone 0171-972 4480.

The World Health Organization has made recommendations to overcome the problem of dapsone resistance and to prevent the emergence of resistance to other antileprotic drugs. These recommendations are based on the same principles as for the chemotherapy of tuberculosis. Drugs recommended are **dapsone**, **rifampicin**, and **clofazimine**. Other drugs with significant bactericidal activity against *Mycobacterium leprae* include ofloxacin, minocycline and clarithromycin, but none of these are as active as rifampicin; at present they should be reserved as second-line drugs for leprosy.

A three-drug regimen is recommended for *multibacillary leprosy* (lepromatous, borderline-lepromatous, and borderline leprosy) and a two-drug regimen for those suffering from *paucibacillary leprosy* (borderline-tuberculoid, tuberculoid, and indeterminate). These regimens, which are widely applicable throughout the world (with minor local variations), are as follows:

Multibacillary leprosy (3-drug regimen)

Rifampicin	600 mg once-monthly, supervised (450 mg for adults weighing less than 35 kg)
Dapsone	100 mg daily, self-administered (50 mg daily or 1–2 mg/kg daily for adults weighing less than 35 kg)
Clofazimine	300 mg once-monthly, supervised, *and* 50 mg daily (or 100 mg on alternate days), self-administered

Note. When rifampicin cannot be given, a 2-year regimen of clofazimine with two of the following—ofloxacin, minocycline or clarithromycin are used for the first 6 months then clofazimine with either minocycline or ofloxacin for 18 months; when clofazimine cannot be given, ofloxacin or minocycline may be substituted in the standard regimen.

Treatment for multibacillary leprosy should be given for at least 2 years and be continued, wherever possible, up to smear negativity. It should be continued unchanged during both type I (reversal) or type II (erythema nodosum leprosum) reactions. During reversal reactions neuritic pain or weakness can herald the rapid onset of permanent nerve damage. Treatment with prednisolone (initially 40–60 mg daily) should be instituted at once. Mild type II reactions may respond to aspirin or chloroquine. Severe reactions may require corticosteroids;

increased doses of clofazimine 100 mg 3 times daily for the first month with subsequent reductions, are also useful but may take 4–6 weeks to attain full effect.

Paucibacillary leprosy (2-drug regimen)

Rifampicin	600 mg once-monthly, supervised (450 mg for those weighing less than 35 kg)
Dapsone	100 mg daily, self-administered

Treatment for paucibacillary leprosy should be given for 6 months. If treatment is interrupted the regimen should be recommenced where it was left off to complete the full course.

Neither the multibacillary nor the paucibacillary antileprosy regimen is sufficient to treat tuberculosis, therefore patients who also have tuberculosis should be given appropriate antituberculous drugs in addition to the antileprosy regimen.

DAPSONE
Indications: leprosy, dermatitis herpetiformis
Cautions: cardiac or pulmonary disease; anaemia (treat severe anaemia before starting); G6PD-deficiency (including breast-feeding of affected children, see section 9.1.5); pregnancy; avoid in porphyria (see section 9.8.2); **interactions:** Appendix 1 (dapsone)
Side-effects: (dose-related and uncommon at doses used for leprosy), neuropathy, allergic dermatitis (rarely including toxic epidermal necrolysis and Stevens-Johnson syndrome), anorexia, nausea, vomiting, headache, insomnia, anaemia, hepatitis, agranulocytosis; dapsone syndrome (rash with fever and eosinophilia)—discontinue immediately (may progress to exfoliative dermatitis, hepatitis, hypoalbuminaemia, psychosis and death)
Dose: leprosy, 1–2 mg/kg daily, see notes above
Dermatitis herpetiformis, see specialist literature

PoM **Dapsone** (Non-proprietary)
Tablets, dapsone 50 mg, net price 20 = 54p; 100 mg, 20 = 73p. Label: 8
Available from Cox

CLOFAZIMINE
Indications: leprosy
Cautions: hepatic and renal impairment; pregnancy and breast-feeding; may discolour soft contact lenses; avoid if persistent abdominal pain and diarrhoea
Side-effects: nausea, vomiting (hospitalise if persistent), abdominal pain; headache, tiredness; brownish-black discoloration of lesions and skin including areas exposed to light; reversible hair discoloration; dry skin; red discoloration of faeces, urine and other body fluids; also rash, pruritus, photosensitivity, acne-like eruptions, anorexia, eosinophilic enteropathy, bowel obstruction, dry eyes, dimmed vision, macular and subepithelial corneal pigmentation; elevation of blood sugar, weight loss, splenic infarction lymphadenopathy

Dose: leprosy, see notes above
Lepromatous lepra reactions, dosage increased to
300 mg daily for max. of 3 months

PoM **Lamprene®** (Geigy)
Capsules, brown, clofazimine 100 mg. Net price
100-cap pack = £6.66. Label: 8, 14, 21

RIFAMPICIN
Section 5.1.9

5.1.11   Metronidazole and tinidazole

Metronidazole is an antimicrobial drug with high
activity against anaerobic bacteria and protozoa;
indications include trichomonal vaginitis (section
5.4.3), bacterial vaginosis (notably *Gardnerella
vaginalis* infections), and *Entamoeba histolytica*
and *Giardia lamblia* infections (section 5.4.2). It is
also used for surgical and gynaecological sepsis in
which its activity against colonic anaerobes, especially *Bacteroides fragilis*, is important. Metronidazole is also effective in the treatment of antibiotic-
associated colitis (pseudomembranous colitis, see
also section 1.5) in a dose of 400 mg by mouth three
times daily. Topical metronidazole (see section
13.10.1.2) reduces the odour produced by anaerobic
bacteria in fungating tumours; it is also used in the
management of rosacea.

Tinidazole is similar to metronidazole but has a
longer duration of action.

METRONIDAZOLE
Indications: anaerobic infections (including dental), see under Dose below; protozoal infections,
section 5.4.2
Cautions: disulfiram-like reaction with alcohol,
hepatic impairment and hepatic encephalopathy;
pregnancy and breast-feeding (manufacturer
advises avoidance of high-dose regimens); clinical and laboratory monitoring advised if treatment exceeds 10 days; **interactions:** Appendix 1
(metronidazole)
Side-effects: nausea, vomiting, unpleasant taste,
furred tongue, and gastro-intestinal disturbances;
rashes, urticaria and angioedema; rarely drowsiness, headache, dizziness, ataxia, darkening of
urine, and anaphylaxis; on prolonged or intensive
therapy peripheral neuropathy, transient epilepti-
form seizures, and leucopenia
Dose: anaerobic infections (usually treated for 7
days), *by mouth,* 800 mg initially then 400 mg
every 8 hours; *by rectum,* 1 g every 8 hours for 3
days, then 1 g every 12 hours; *by intravenous
infusion,* 500 mg every 8 hours; CHILD, any route,
7.5 mg/kg every 8 hours
Leg ulcers and pressure sores, *by mouth,* 400 mg
every 8 hours for 7 days
Bacterial vaginosis, *by mouth,* 400 mg twice daily
for 7 days *or* 2 g as a single dose
Acute ulcerative gingivitis, *by mouth,* 200 mg
every 8 hours for 3 days; CHILD 1–3 years 50 mg
every 8 hours for 3 days; 3–7 years 100 mg every
12 hours; 7–10 years 100 mg every 8 hours

Acute dental infections, *by mouth,* 200 mg every 8
hours for 3–7 days
Surgical prophylaxis, *by mouth,* 400 mg every 8
hours started 24 hours before surgery, then continued postoperatively *by intravenous infusion* or
by rectum (see below) until oral administration
can be resumed; CHILD 7.5 mg/kg every 8 hours
By rectum, 1 g every 8 hours; CHILD 125–250 mg
every 8 hours
By intravenous infusion, 500 mg shortly before
surgery then every 8 hours until oral administration can be started; CHILD, 7.5 mg/kg every 8
hours

PoM **Metronidazole** (Non-proprietary)
Tablets, metronidazole 200 mg, net price 20 = 39p;
400 mg, 20 = 85p. Label: 4, 9, 21, 25, 27
Available from APS, Cox, DDSA (Vaginyl®), Hillcross,
Kent, Lagap (Metrolyl®), Lederle (Zadstat®), Norton,
Rosemont; 500 mg tablets also available from Dumex
Suspension, metronidazole (as benzoate) 200 mg/
5 mL. Net price 100 mL = £4.19. Label: 4, 9, 23
Available from Hillcross, Rosemont
Intravenous infusion, metronidazole 5 mg/mL. Net
price 20-mL amp = £1.70, 100-mL container =
£3.57
Available from Braun, David Bull, Phoenix
PoM **Anabact®:** see section 13.10.1.2
PoM **Flagyl®** (Rhône-Poulenc Rorer)
Tablets, both f/c, ivory, metronidazole 200 mg, net
price 21-tab pack = £2.14; 400 mg, 14-tab pack =
£3.03. Label: 4, 9, 21, 25, 27
Intravenous infusion, metronidazole 5 mg/mL. Net
price 100-mL Viaflex® bag = £3.41
Electrolytes: Na+ 13.6 mmol/100-mL bag
Suppositories, metronidazole 500 mg, net price 10
= £7.26; 1 g, 10 = £11.02. Label: 4, 9
PoM **Flagyl S®** (Rhône-Poulenc Rorer)
Suspension, metronidazole (as benzoate) 200 mg/
5 mL. Net price 100 mL = £4.85. Label: 4, 9, 23
PoM **Metrogel®:** see section 13.10.1.2
PoM **Metrolyl®** (Lagap)
Intravenous infusion, metronidazole 5 mg/mL. Net
price 100-mL Steriflex® bag = £4.50
Electrolytes: Na+ 14.53 mmol/100-mL bag
Suppositories, metronidazole 500 mg, net price 10
= £4.25; 1 g, 10 = £6.80. Label: 4, 9
PoM **Metrotop®:** see section 13.10.1.2
PoM **Rozex®:** see section 13.10.1.2
PoM **Zadstat®** (Lederle)
Suppositories, metronidazole 500 mg, net price 10
= £4.14; 1 g, 10 = £6.63. Label: 4, 9

With antifungal
PoM **Flagyl Compak®** (Rhône-Poulenc Rorer)
Treatment pack, tablets, off-white, f/c, metronidazole 400 mg, with pessaries, yellow, nystatin
100 000 units. Net price 14 tablets and 14 pessaries (with applicator) = £4.75
Dose: for mixed trichomonal and candidal infections, 1
tablet twice daily for 7 days and 1 pessary inserted twice
daily for 7 days *or* 1 pessary at night for 14 nights

TINIDAZOLE
Indications: anaerobic infections, see under Dose
below; protozoal infections, section 5.4.2

Cautions; Side-effects: see under Metronidazole; pregnancy (manufacturer advises avoidance in first trimester)

Dose: anaerobic infections *by mouth*, 2 g initially, followed by 1 g daily *or* 500 mg twice daily, usually for 5–6 days

Bacterial vaginosis and acute ulcerative gingivitis, a single 2-g dose

Abdominal surgery prophylaxis, a single 2-g dose approximately 12 hours before surgery

PoM **Fasigyn®** (Pfizer)

Tablets, f/c, tinidazole 500 mg. Net price 20-tab pack = £11.50. Label: 4, 9, 21, 25

5.1.12 4-Quinolones

Antibacterials discussed in this section include acrosoxacin, ciprofloxacin, ofloxacin, and the urinary antiseptics cinoxacin, nalidixic acid, and norfloxacin.

Acrosoxacin is used only in the treatment of gonorrhoea in patients allergic to penicillins or who have strains resistant to penicillins and other antibiotics.

Nalidixic acid, **cinoxacin**, and **norfloxacin** are effective in uncomplicated urinary-tract infections.

Ciprofloxacin is active against both Gram-positive and Gram-negative bacteria. It is particularly active against Gram-negative bacteria, including salmonella, shigella, campylobacter, neisseria, and pseudomonas. Ciprofloxacin only has moderate activity against Gram-positive bacteria such as *Streptococcus pneumoniae* and *Strep. faecalis*; it is not the drug of first choice for pneumococcal pneumonia. It is active against chlamydia and some mycobacteria. Most anaerobic organisms are not susceptible. Uses for ciprofloxacin include infections of the respiratory (but not for pneumococcal pneumonia, see above) and urinary tracts, and of the gastro-intestinal system (including typhoid fever), and gonorrhoea and septicaemia caused by sensitive organisms. Although licensed for skin and soft tissue infections there is a high incidence of staphylococcal resistance and it should be avoided in methicillin-resistant *Staphylococcus aureus* (MRSA) infections.

Ofloxacin is used for urinary-tract infections, lower respiratory-tract infections, gonorrhoea, and non-gonococcal urethritis and cervicitis.

CAUTIONS. 4-Quinolones should be used with caution in patients with epilepsy or a history of epilepsy, in hepatic or renal impairment (see Appendixes 2 and 3), in pregnancy, during breast-feeding, and in children or adolescents (arthropathy has developed in weight-bearing joints in young *animals*). The CSM has warned that 4-quinolones may induce **convulsions** in patients with or without a history of convulsions; taking NSAIDs at the same time may also induce them. Other **interactions**: Appendix 1 (4-quinolones)

CSM advice (tendon damage)
At the first sign of pain or inflammation, patients taking 4-quinolones should discontinue the treatment and rest the affected limb until tendon symptoms have resolved.

SIDE-EFFECTS. Common side-effects of the 4-quinolones include nausea, vomiting, abdominal pain, diarrhoea (rarely pseudomembranous colitis), headache, dizziness, sleep disorders, rash, pruritus, fever, anaphylaxis, photosensitivity, increase in blood urea and creatinine, transient disturbances in liver enzymes and bilirubin, arthralgia and myalgia, blood disorders (including eosinophilia, leucopenia, thrombocytopenia, and altered prothrombin concentration). Less frequent side-effects include anorexia, restlessness, depression, hallucinations, confusion, and disturbances in vision, taste, hearing and smell; also isolated reports of intracranial hypertension and tendon damage (especially in the elderly and those taking corticosteroids, see also CSM advice above). Side-effects that have been reported to the CSM also include haemolytic anaemia, renal impairment, hepatic dysfunction, anaphylaxis, and hypoglycaemia. The drug should be **discontinued** if mental, neurological or hypersensitivity reactions occur with the first dose.

CIPROFLOXACIN

Indications: Gram-negative and Gram-positive infections, see notes above; surgical prophylaxis in upper gastro-intestinal procedures

Cautions; Side-effects: see notes above; avoid excessive alkalinity of urine and ensure adequate fluid intake (risk of crystalluria); not recommended in children or growing adolescents; caution in G6PD deficiency (see section 9.1.5); anaphylaxis reported, also reported dyspepsia, flatulence, dysphagia, tremor, convulsions, jaundice and hepatitis with necrosis, renal failure, nephritis, vasculitis, urticaria, erythema nodosum, Stevens-Johnson syndrome, Lyell syndrome, petechiae, haemorrhagic bullae, tenosynovitis and tachycardia; pain and phlebitis at injection site; **interactions:** Appendix 1 (4-quinolones)

DRIVING. May impair performance of skilled tasks (e.g. driving); effects of alcohol enhanced

Dose: by mouth, respiratory-tract infections, 250–750 mg twice daily

Urinary-tract infections, 250–500 mg twice daily (250 mg twice daily for 3 days in acute uncomplicated cystitis)

Gonorrhoea, 250 mg as a single dose; 500 mg may be required in resistant cases

Most other infections, 500–750 mg twice daily

Surgical prophylaxis, 750 mg 60–90 minutes before procedure

Prophylaxis of meningococcal meningitis [not licensed], section 5.1, table 2

By intravenous infusion (over 30–60 minutes), 200–400 mg twice daily

Urinary-tract infections, 100 mg twice daily

Gonorrhoea, 100 mg as a single dose

CHILD not recommended (see above) but where benefit outweighs risk, *by mouth*, 7.5–15 mg/kg daily in 2 divided doses *or by intravenous infusion*, 5–10 mg/kg daily in 2 divided doses

PoM **Ciproxin®** (Baypharm)

Tablets, all f/c, ciprofloxacin (as hydrochloride) 250 mg (scored), net price 10-tab pack = £7.50, 20-tab pack = £15.00; 500 mg (scored), 10-tab pack = £13.75, 20-tab pack = £27.50; 750 mg, 10-tab pack = £20.00. Label: 6, 9, 25, counselling, driving

Intravenous infusion, ciprofloxacin 2 mg (as lactate)/mL, net price 50-mL bottle = £10.18, 100-mL bottle = £19.85, 200-mL bottle = £29.00

Electrolytes: Na⁺ 15.4 mmol/100-mL bottle

ACROSOXACIN

(Rosoxacin)

Indications: gonorrhoea

Cautions; Side-effects: see notes above; avoid frequent repeat doses in patients under 18 years; **interactions:** Appendix 1 (4-quinolones)

DRIVING. May impair performance of skilled tasks (e.g. driving)

Dose: 300 mg as a single dose on an empty stomach

PoM **Eradacin®** (Sanofi Winthrop)

Capsules, red/yellow, acrosoxacin 150 mg. Net price 2 caps = £3.12. Label: 2, 23

CINOXACIN

Indications: urinary-tract infections

Cautions; Side-effects: see notes above; avoid in severe renal impairment; also reported, perineal burning, Stevens-Johnson syndrome; **interactions:** Appendix 1 (4-quinolones)

DRIVING. May impair performance of skilled tasks (e.g. driving)

Dose: 500 mg every 12 hours; prophylaxis, 500 mg at night

PoM **Cinobac®** (Lilly)

Capsules, green/orange, cinoxacin 500 mg. Net price 14-cap pack = £10.41. Label: 9, counselling, driving

NALIDIXIC ACID

Indications: urinary-tract infections

Cautions; Side-effects: see notes above; avoid in porphyria (see section 9.8.2) and if history of convulsive disorders, avoid strong sunlight, false positive urinary glucose (if tested for reducing substances); monitor blood counts, renal and liver function if treatment exceeds 2 weeks; caution in G6PD deficiency (see section 9.1.5); also reported toxic psychosis and convulsions, weakness, increased intracranial pressure, paraesthesia, cranial nerve palsy, cholestasis, metabolic acidosis; **interactions:** Appendix 1 (4-quinolones)

Dose: 1 g every 6 hours for 7 days, reduced in chronic infections to 500 mg every 6 hours; CHILD over 3 months max. 50 mg/kg daily in divided doses; reduced in prolonged therapy to 30 mg/kg daily

PoM **Nalidixic Acid** (Non-proprietary)

Tablets, nalidixic acid 500 mg. Net price 56-tab pack = £12.83. Label: 9, 11

Available from Norton

PoM **Mictral®** (Sanofi Winthrop)

Granules, effervescent, nalidixic acid 660 mg, sodium citrate (as sodium citrate and citric acid) 4.1 g/sachet (Na⁺ 41 mmol/sachet). Net price 9-sachet pack = £5.48. Label: 9, 11, 13

Dose: 1 sachet in water 3 times daily for 3 days

PoM **Negram®** (Sanofi Winthrop)

Tablets, beige, nalidixic acid 500 mg. Net price 56-tab pack = £12.83. Label: 9, 11

Suspension, pink, sugar-free, nalidixic acid 300 mg/5 mL. Net price 150 mL = £12.85. Label: 9, 11

PoM **Uriben®** (Rosemont)

Suspension, pink, nalidixic acid 300 mg/5 mL. Net price 200 mL = £16.95; 500 mL = £38.20. Label: 9, 11

NORFLOXACIN

Indications: see under Dose

Cautions; Side-effects: see notes above; caution in G6PD deficiency (see section 9.1.5); avoid in prepubertal children and growing adolescents; also reported, anorexia, depression, anxiety, tinnitus, toxic epidermal necrolysis, erythema multiforme (Stevens-Johnson syndrome); **interactions:** Appendix 1 (4-quinolones)

DRIVING. May impair performance of skilled tasks (e.g. driving)

Dose: urinary-tract infections, 400 mg twice daily for 7–10 days (for 3 days in uncomplicated lower urinary-tract infections)

Chronic relapsing urinary-tract infections, 400 mg twice daily for up to 12 weeks; may be reduced to 400 mg once daily if adequate suppression within first 4 weeks

PoM **Utinor®** (MSD)

Tablets, scored, norfloxacin 400 mg. Net price 6-tab pack = £2.88, 14-tab pack = £6.72. Label: 6, 9, counselling, driving

OFLOXACIN

Indications: see under Dose

Cautions; Side-effects: see notes above; caution in history of psychiatric illness and in G6PD deficiency; avoid strong sunlight; avoid in epilepsy or history of epilepsy and in children and adolescents; also reported, inflammation and rupture of tendons, erythema mutiforme, vasculitic reactions, angioedema, anxiety, unsteady gait and tremor, paraesthesia, neuropathy, psychotic reactions (discontinue treatment—see notes above); tachycardia, anaemia, agranulocytosis and pancytopenia; on intravenous infusion, hypotension and local reactions (including thrombophlebitis); **interactions:** Appendix 1 (4-quinolones)

DRIVING. May affect performance of skilled tasks (e.g. driving); effects enhanced by alcohol

Dose: by mouth, urinary-tract infections, 200–400 mg daily preferably in the morning, increased if necessary in upper urinary-tract infections to 400 mg twice daily

Lower respiratory-tract infections, 400 mg daily preferably in the morning, increased if necessary to 400 mg twice daily

Skin and soft-tissue infections, 400 mg twice daily

Uncomplicated gonorrhoea, 400 mg as a single dose

Non-gonococcal urethritis and cervicitis, 400 mg daily in single or divided doses

By intravenous infusion (over at least 30 minutes for each 200 mg), complicated urinary-tract infection, 200 mg daily

Lower respiratory-tract infection, 200 mg twice daily

Skin and soft-tissue infections, 400 mg twice daily

Septicaemia, 200 mg twice daily

Severe or complicated infections, dose may be increased to 400 mg twice daily

PoM Tarivid® (Hoechst, Roussel)

Tablets, f/c, scored, ofloxacin 200 mg, net price 10-tab pack = £10.26, 20-tab pack = £20.50; 400 mg (yellow), 5-tab pack = £10.24, 10-tab pack = £20.43. Label: 6, 9, 11, counselling, driving

Intravenous infusion, ofloxacin (as hydrochloride) 2 mg/mL, net price 50-mL bottle = £15.41; 100-mL bottle = £22.01 (both hosp. only)

5.1.13   Urinary-tract infections

Urinary-tract infection is more common in women than in men; when it occurs in men there is frequently an underlying abnormality of the renal tract. Recurrent episodes of infection are an indication for radiological investigation especially in children in whom untreated pyelonephritis may lead to permanent kidney damage.

Escherichia coli is the most common cause of urinary-tract infection. Less common causes include Proteus and Klebsiella spp. *Pseudomonas aeruginosa* infections are almost invariably associated with functional or anatomical abnormalities of the renal tract. *Staphylococcus epidermidis* and *Enterococcus faecalis* infection may complicate catheterisation or instrumentation. Whenever possible a specimen of urine should be collected for culture and sensitivity testing before starting antibiotic therapy.

Uncomplicated lower urinary-tract infections often respond to ampicillin, nalidixic acid, nitrofurantoin, or trimethoprim given for 5–7 days; those caused by fully sensitive bacteria respond to two 3-g doses of amoxycillin (section 5.1.1.3). Bacterial resistance, however, especially to ampicillin (to which approximately 50% of *E. coli* are now resistant), has increased the importance of urine culture prior to therapy. Alternatives for resistant organisms include co-amoxiclav (amoxycillin with clavulanic acid), an oral cephalosporin, ciprofloxacin, and fosfomycin. Hexamine should **not** be used as it is only bacteriostatic, requires acid urine, and frequently causes side-effects.

Long-term low dose therapy may be required in selected patients to prevent *recurrence of infection*; indications include frequent relapses and significant kidney damage. Trimethoprim and nitrofurantoin have been recommended for long-term therapy.

Acute pyelonephritis can be associated with septicaemia and is best treated initially by injection of a broad-spectrum antibiotic such as aztreonam, cefuroxime, ciprofloxacin, or gentamicin especially if the patient is vomiting or severely ill.

Prostatitis can be difficult to cure and requires treatment for several weeks with an antibiotic which penetrates prostatic tissue such as trimethoprim, erythromycin, or ciprofloxacin.

Where infection is localised and associated with an indwelling *catheter* a bladder instillation is often effective (see section 7.4.4).

Patients with *heart-valve lesions* undergoing instrumentation of the urinary tract should be given a parenteral antibiotic to prevent bacteraemia and endocarditis (section 5.1, Table 2).

Urinary-tract infection in *pregnancy* may be asymptomatic and requires prompt treatment to prevent progression to acute pyelonephritis. Penicillins and cephalosporins can be given in pregnancy but trimethoprim, sulphonamides, 4-quinolones, and tetracyclines should be avoided.

In *renal failure* antibiotics normally excreted by the kidney accumulate with resultant toxicity unless the dose is reduced. This applies especially to the aminoglycosides which should be used with great caution; tetracyclines, hexamine, and nitrofurantoin should be avoided altogether.

FOSFOMYCIN

Indications: acute uncomplicated lower urinary-tract infection; prophylaxis in transurethral procedures

Cautions: pregnancy and breast-feeding; not recommended in patients over 75 years or in severe renal impairment (inadequate urinary concentrations); **interactions:** Appendix 1 (fosfomycin)

Side-effects: nausea, diarrhoea, heartburn; rash

Dose: urinary-tract infection, 3 g as a single dose at bedtime after emptying bladder; CHILD not recommended

Prophylaxis in transurethral procedures, 3 g as a single dose 3 hours before procedure followed by 3 g 24 hours after procedure

▼ **PoM Monuril®** (Pharmax)

Granules, fosfomycin (as trometamol) 3 g/sachet, net price 1-sachet pack = £4.45. Label: 13, 23

NITROFURANTOIN

Indications: urinary-tract infections

Cautions: anaemia; diabetes mellitus; electrolyte imbalance; vitamin B and folate deficiency; pulmonary disease; hepatic impairment; monitor lung and liver function on long-term therapy, especially in the elderly; susceptibility to peripheral neuropathy; false positive urinary glucose (if tested for reducing substances); urine may be coloured yellow or brown; **interactions:** Appendix 1 (nitrofurantoin)

Contra-indications: impaired renal function, infants less than 3 months old, G6PD deficiency (including pregnancy at term, and breast-feeding of affected infants, see section 9.1.5 and Appendixes 4 and 5), porphyria (see section 9.8.2)

Side-effects: anorexia, nausea, vomiting, and diarrhoea; acute and chronic pulmonary reactions (may be associated with lupus erythematosus-like syndrome); peripheral neuropathy; also reported, angioedema, urticaria, rash and pruritus; rarely, cholestatic jaundice, hepatitis, exfoliative dermatitis, erythema multiforme, pancreatitis, arthralgia, blood disorders (including agranulocytosis, thrombocytopenia, and aplastic anaemia), benign intracranial hypertension, and transient alopecia

Dose: acute uncomplicated infection, 50 mg every 6 hours with food for 7 days; CHILD over 3 months, 3 mg/kg daily in 4 divided doses
Severe chronic recurrent infection, 100 mg every 6 hours with food for 7 days (dose reduced or discontinued if severe nausea)
Prophylaxis (but see Cautions), 50–100 mg at night; CHILD over 3 months, 1 mg/kg at night

PoM Nitrofurantoin (Non-proprietary)
Tablets, nitrofurantoin 50 mg and 100 mg. Label: 9, 14, 21
Available from Biorex, Cox, Kent

PoM Furadantin® (Procter & Gamble Pharm.)
Tablets, all yellow, scored, nitrofurantoin 50 mg, net price 20 = £1.96; 100 mg, 20 = £3.62. Label: 9, 14, 21
Suspension, yellow, sugar-free, nitrofurantoin 25 mg/5 mL. Net price 300 mL = £4.95. Label: 9, 14, 21

PoM Macrobid® (Procter & Gamble Pharm.)
Capsules, m/r, blue/yellow, nitrofurantoin 100 mg (as nitrofurantoin macrocrystals and nitrofurantoin monohydrate). Net price 14-cap pack = £4.89. Label: 9, 14, 21, 25
Dose: uncomplicated urinary-tract infection, 1 capsule twice daily with food
Genito-urinary surgical prophylaxis, 1 capsule twice daily on day of procedure and for 3 days after

PoM Macrodantin® (Procter & Gamble Pharm.)
Capsules, nitrofurantoin 50 mg (yellow/white), net price 28-cap pack = £3.05; 100 mg (yellow), 20 = £3.84. Label: 9, 14, 21

HEXAMINE HIPPURATE
(Methenamine hippurate)

Indications: prophylaxis and long-term treatment of recurrent urinary-tract infections

Cautions: pregnancy; avoid concurrent administration with sulphonamides (risk of crystalluria) or urinary alkalinising agents; **interactions:** Appendix 1 (hexamine)

Contra-indications: severe renal impairment, dehydration, metabolic acidosis

Side-effects: gastro-intestinal disturbances, bladder irritation, rash

Dose: 1 g every 12 hours (may be increased in patients with catheters to 1 g every 8 hours); CHILD 6–12 years 500 mg every 12 hours

Hiprex® (3M)
Tablets, scored, hexamine hippurate 1 g. Net price 60-tab pack = £7.40. Label: 9

5.2 Antifungal drugs

Fungal infections are frequently associated with a defect in host resistance which should, if possible, be corrected otherwise drug therapy may fail. Similarly, treatment of dermatophyte infection may be unsuccessful until the animal source has been removed or controlled.

For local treatment of fungal infections see also sections 7.2.2 (genital), 7.4.4 (bladder), 11.3.2 (eye), 12.1.1 (ear), 12.3.2 (oropharynx), and 13.10.2 (skin).

POLYENE ANTIFUNGALS. The polyene antifungals include amphotericin and nystatin.

Amphotericin is not absorbed from the gut and is the only polyene antibiotic which can be given parenterally. It is used for the treatment of systemic fungal infections and is active against most fungi and yeasts. It is highly protein bound and penetrates poorly into body fluids and tissues. When given parenterally amphotericin is toxic and side-effects are common.

A formulation of amphotericin encapsulated in liposomes (AmBisome®) is available and is apparently significantly less toxic than the parent compound. Amphotericin is also available as a complex with sodium cholesteryl sulphate (Amphocil®). Another liposomal formulation (Abelcet®) has also recently been introduced. All are recommended for systemic mycoses when amphotericin alone is contra-indicated because of toxicity, especially nephrotoxicity.

Nystatin is not absorbed when given by mouth and is too toxic for parenteral use. It is active against a number of yeasts and fungi but is principally used for *Candida albicans* infections of skin and mucous membranes. It is also used in the treatment of intestinal candidiasis.

IMIDAZOLE ANTIFUNGALS. The imidazole antifungals include clotrimazole, econazole, fenticonazole, isoconazole, ketoconazole, miconazole, sulconazole, and tioconazole; they are active against a wide range of fungi and yeasts. Their main indications are vaginal candidiasis and dermatophyte infections. Clotrimazole, econazole, fenticonazole, isoconazole, sulconazole, and tioconazole are used for local treatment.

Miconazole is used for local treatment and can be given by mouth for oral and intestinal infection.

Ketoconazole is significantly better absorbed after oral administration than the other imidazoles, but has been associated with fatal hepatotoxicity. The CSM has advised that prescribers should weigh the potential benefits of ketoconazole treatment against the liver damage risk and should carefully monitor patients both clinically and biochemically. It should **not** be given for superficial fungal infections.

TRIAZOLE ANTIFUNGALS. The triazole antifungals include fluconazole and itraconazole which are absorbed by mouth.

Fluconazole is an oral triazole antifungal indicated for local and systemic candidiasis and cryptococcal infections.

Itraconazole is indicated for oropharyngeal and vulvovaginal candidiasis, pityriasis versicolor, and tinea corporis and pedis; it is metabolised in the liver and should not be given to patients with a history of liver disease. It is also indicated for systemic fungal infections (including aspergillosis, candidiasis, and cryptococcosis) where other antifungal drugs are inappropriate or ineffective.

OTHER ANTIFUNGALS. **Flucytosine** is a synthetic antifungal drug which is only active against yeasts and has been used for the treatment of systemic candidiasis, cryptococcosis, and torulopsosis. Side-effects are uncommon but bone-marrow depression can occur and weekly blood counts are necessary during prolonged therapy. Synergy has been demonstrated with amphotericin. Resistance to flucytosine is not uncommon and can develop during therapy; sensitivity testing is, therefore, essential before and during treatment.

Griseofulvin is selectively concentrated in keratin and is the drug of choice for widespread or intractable dermatophyte infections. It is well absorbed from the gut but is inactive when applied topically. It is more effective in skin than in nail infections and treatment must be continued for several weeks or even months. Side-effects are uncommon.

Terbinafine, an allylamine antifungal, has recently been introduced for ringworm infections where oral treatment is considered appropriate.

> **Oral versus topical antifungal preparations**. Oral antifungal preparations should preferably be used for those who are resistant to (or intolerant of) topical preparations

AMPHOTERICIN
(Amphotericin B)

Indications: See under Dose

Cautions: when given parenterally, toxicity common (**important:** close supervision necessary and test dose required); hepatic and renal-function tests, blood counts, and plasma electrolyte monitoring required; other nephrotoxic drugs, corticosteroids (avoid except to control reactions), antineoplastics; pregnancy and breast-feeding; frequent change of injection site (irritant); avoid rapid infusion (risk of arrhythmias); **interactions:** Appendix 1 (amphotericin)

Side-effects: when given parenterally, anorexia, nausea and vomiting, diarrhoea, epigastric pain; febrile reactions, headache, muscle and joint pain; anaemia; disturbances in renal function (including hypokalaemia and hypomagnesaemia) and renal toxicity; also cardiovascular toxicity (including arrhythmias), blood disorders, neurological disorders (including hearing loss, diplopia, convulsions, peripheral neuropathy), abnormal liver function (discontinue treatment), rash, anaphylactoid reactions (**important:** test dose required)

Dose: by mouth, intestinal candidiasis, 100–200 mg every 6 hours

Oral and perioral infections, see section 12.3.2

By intravenous infusion, see under preparations, below

PoM **Fungilin®** (Squibb)
Tablets, yellow, scored, amphotericin 100 mg. Net price 56-tab pack = £8.32. Label: 9
Lozenges—see section 12.3.2
Suspension, yellow, sugar-free, amphotericin 100 mg/mL. Net price 12 mL = £2.31. Label: 9, counselling, use of pipette

PoM **Fungizone®** (Squibb)
Intravenous infusion, powder for reconstitution, amphotericin (as sodium deoxycholate complex). Net price 50-mg vial = £3.70
Electrolytes: Na+ < 0.5 mmol/vial
Dose: by intravenous infusion, systemic fungal infections, 250 micrograms/kg daily, gradually increased if tolerated to 1 mg/kg daily; max. (severe infection) 1.5 mg/kg daily or on alternate days; **important:** test dose required
Note. Prolonged treatment usually necessary; if interrupted for longer than 7 days recommence at 250 micrograms/kg daily and increase gradually

Lipid formulations
▼ PoM **Abelcet®** (Liposome Company)
Intravenous infusion, amphotericin 5 mg/mL as lipid complex with L-α-dimyristoylphosphatidylcholine and L-α-dimyristoylphosphatidylglycerol. Net price 20-mL vial = £86.00 (hosp. only)
Dose: severe invasive candidiasis; severe systemic fungal infections in patients not responding to conventional amphotericin or other antifungal drugs or where toxicity or renal impairment precludes conventional amphotericin, including invasive aspergillosis, cryptococcal meningitis and systemic cryptococcosis in AIDS patients, by intravenous infusion, ADULT and CHILD, initial test dose 1 mg over 15 minutes then 5 mg/kg daily for at least 14 days; **important:** test dose required

PoM **AmBisome®** (NeXstar)
Intravenous infusion, powder for reconstitution, amphotericin 50 mg encapsulated in liposomes. Net price 50-mg vial = £145.00
Electrolytes: Na+ < 0.5 mmol/vial
Dose: severe systemic or deep mycoses where toxicity (particularly nephrotoxicity) precludes use of conventional amphotericin, by intravenous infusion, ADULT and CHILD initially 1 mg/kg daily as a single dose increased gradually if necessary to 3 mg/kg daily as a single dose; **important:** test dose required

▼ PoM **Amphocil®** (Zeneca)
Intravenous infusion, powder for reconstitution, amphotericin as a complex with sodium cholesteryl sulphate. Net price 50-mg vial = £109.00, 100-mg vial = £199.00
Electrolytes: Na+ < 0.5 mmol/vial
Dose: severe systemic or deep mycoses where toxicity or renal failure preclude use of conventional amphotericin, by intravenous infusion, ADULT and CHILD initially 1 mg/kg daily as a single dose increased gradually if necessary to 3–4 mg/kg daily as a single dose; **important:** test dose required

---

Cautionary label wordings, see inside back cover   Prices are **net**, see p.1

FLUCONAZOLE

Indications: see under Dose

Cautions: renal impairment; pregnancy (toxicity at high doses in *animal* studies) and breast-feeding; raised liver enzymes (review need for treatment if raised significantly, possible risk of hepatic necrosis); **interactions:** Appendix 1 (antifungals, imidazole and triazole)

CSM **Warning.** Avoid concomitant administration with astemizole or terfenadine, see also pp. 137–8; also avoid with cisapride (see p. 34) [other interactions, Appendix 1]

Side-effects: nausea, abdominal discomfort, diarrhoea, and flatulence; occasionally abnormalities of liver enzymes; rarely rash (discontinue treatment or monitor closely if infection invasive or systemic); angioedema, anaphylaxis, bullous lesions, and Stevens-Johnson syndrome reported; severe cutaneous reactions in AIDS patients also reported

Dose: acute or recurrent vaginal candidiasis, *by mouth*, a single dose of 150 mg

Mucosal candidiasis (except vaginal), *by mouth*, 50 mg daily (100 mg daily in unusually difficult infections) given for 7–14 days in oropharyngeal candidiasis (max. 14 days except in severely immunocompromised patients); for 14 days in atrophic oral candidiasis associated with dentures; for 14–30 days in other mucosal infections (e.g. oesophagitis, candiduria, non-invasive bronchopulmonary infections); CHILD *by mouth or by intravenous infusion*, 3–6 mg/kg on first day then 3 mg/kg daily (every 72 hours in NEONATE up to 2 weeks old, every 48 hours in neonate 2–4 weeks old)

Tinea pedis, corporis, cruris, versicolor, and dermal candidiasis, *by mouth*, 50 mg daily for 2–4 weeks (for up to 6 weeks in tinea pedis); max. duration of treatment 6 weeks

Invasive candidal infections (including candidaemia and disseminated candidiasis) and cryptococcal infections (including meningitis), *by mouth or intravenous infusion*, 400 mg initially then 200 mg daily, increased if necessary to 400 mg daily; treatment continued according to response (at least 6–8 weeks for cryptococcal meningitis); CHILD 6–12 mg/kg daily (every 72 hours in NEONATE up to 2 weeks old, every 48 hours in neonate 2–4 weeks old)

Prevention of relapse of cryptococcal meningitis in AIDS patients after completion of primary therapy, 100–200 mg daily

Prevention of fungal infections in immunocompromised patients following cytotoxic chemotherapy or radiotherapy, 50–400 mg daily adjusted according to risk; 400 mg daily if high risk of systemic infections e.g. following bone-marrow transplantation; commence treatment before anticipated onset of neutropenia and continue for 7 days after neutrophil count in desirable range; CHILD according to extent and duration of neutropenia, 3–12 mg/kg daily (every 72 hours in NEONATE up to 2 weeks old, every 48 hours in neonate 2–4 weeks old)

Diflucan® (Pfizer)

PoM¹ *Capsules,* fluconazole 50 mg (blue/white), net price 7-cap pack = £16.61; 150 mg (blue), single-capsule pack = £7.12; 200 mg (purple/white), 7-cap pack = £66.42. Label: 50 and 200 mg, 9

1. Can be sold to the public for vaginal candidiasis in women aged 16–60 years, in a container or packaging containing not more than 150 mg and labelled to show a max. dose of 150 mg; a proprietary brand (Diflucan® One) containing a single 150-mg capsule is on sale to the public

PoM *Oral suspension,* fluconazole for reconstitution with water, 50 mg/5 mL, net price 35 mL = £16.61; 200 mg/5 mL, 35 mL = £66.42. Label: 9

PoM *Intravenous infusion,* fluconazole 2 mg/mL in sodium chloride intravenous infusion 0.9%, net price 25-mL bottle = £7.32; 100-mL bottle = £29.28

Electrolytes: Na⁺ 15 mmol/100-mL bottle

FLUCYTOSINE

Indications: systemic yeast and fungal infections; adjunct to amphotericin in cryptococcal meningitis, in severe systemic candidiasis and in other severe or long-standing infections

Cautions: hepatic impairment, renal impairment (reduce dose and monitor plasma concentrations), elderly, blood disorders, liver- and kidney-function tests and blood counts required (weekly in renal impairment or blood disorders); pregnancy, breast-feeding

Side-effects: nausea, vomiting, diarrhoea, rashes; less frequently confusion, hallucinations, convulsions, headache, sedation, vertigo, alterations in liver function tests (hepatitis and hepatic necrosis reported); blood disorders including thrombocytopenia, leucopenia, and aplastic anaemia reported

Dose: by intravenous infusion over 20–40 minutes, 200 mg/kg daily in 4 divided doses usually for not more than 7 days; extremely sensitive organisms, 100–150 mg/kg daily may be sufficient; treat for at least 4 months in cryptococcal meningitis

Note. For plasma concentration monitoring blood should be taken shortly before starting the next infusion; plasma concentration for optimum response 25–50 mg/litre (200–400 micromol/litre)—should not be allowed to exceed 80 mg/litre (620 micromol/litre)

PoM **Alcobon®** (Roche)

Intravenous infusion, flucytosine 10 mg/mL. Net price 250-mL infusion bottle = £18.21 (hosp. only)

Electrolytes: Na⁺ 34.44 mmol/250-mL bottle

Note. Flucytosine tablets may be available on a named-patient basis from Bell and Croyden

GRISEOFULVIN

Indications: dermatophyte infections of the skin, scalp, hair and nails, where topical therapy has failed or is inappropriate

Cautions: rarely aggravation or precipitation of systemic lupus erythematosus; breast-feeding; **interactions:** Appendix 1 (griseofulvin)

DRIVING. May impair performance of skilled tasks (e.g. driving); effects of alcohol enhanced

---

Contra-indications: liver failure, lupus erythematosus and related conditions, porphyria (see section 9.8.2); pregnancy (**avoid** pregnancy **during** and for **1 month after** treatment; manufacturer now also states that a man should not father a child within 6 months of treatment)

Side-effects: headache, nausea, vomiting, rashes, photosensitivity; dizziness, fatigue, agranulocytosis and leucopenia reported; lupus erythematosus, erythema multiforme, toxic epidermal necrolysis, peripheral neuropathy, confusion and impaired co-ordination also reported

Dose: 500 mg daily, in divided doses or as a single dose, in severe infection dose may be doubled, reducing when response occurs; CHILD, 10 mg/kg daily in divided doses or as a single dose

PoM Fulcin® (Zeneca)
Tablets, griseofulvin 125 mg (scored), net price 20 = 61p; 500 mg (f/c), 20 = £2.29. Label: 9, 21, counselling, driving
Oral suspension, brown, griseofulvin 125 mg/5 mL. Net price 100 mL = £1.10. Label: 9, 21, counselling, driving

PoM Grisovin® (Glaxo)
Tablets, both f/c, griseofulvin 125 mg, net price 20 = 47p; 500 mg, 20 = £1.75. Label: 9, 21, counselling, driving

ITRACONAZOLE

Indications: oropharyngeal and vulvovaginal candidiasis; pityriasis versicolor and other dermatophyte infections; onychomycosis; histoplasmosis; alternative where other antifungal drugs inappropriate or ineffective in systemic infections (aspergillosis, candidiasis and cryptococcosis including cryptococcal meningitis), and in maintenance treatment of AIDS patients to prevent relapse of underlying fungal infection; prevention of fungal infection in neutropenia when standard therapy inappropriate

Cautions: avoid if history of liver disease; liver function tests required if treatment exceeds 1 month or if anorexia, nausea, vomiting, fatigue, abdominal pain or dark urine (discontinue if test abnormal); renal impairment (bioavailability may be reduced); absorption reduced in AIDS and neutropenia (monitor plasma-itraconazole concentration and increase dose if necessary); discontinue treatment if peripheral neuropathy; breast-feeding; **interactions:** Appendix 1 (antifungals, imidazole and triazole)
CSM Warning. Avoid concomitant administration with astemizole or terfenadine, see also pp. 137–8; also avoid with cisapride (see p. 34) [other interactions, Appendix 1]

Contra-indications: pregnancy (toxicity in *animal* studies)

Side-effects: nausea, abdominal pain, dyspepsia, constipation (diarrhoea with oral liquid), headache, dizziness, raised liver enzymes, menstrual disorders; allergic reactions (including pruritus, rash, urticaria and angioedema), hepatitis and cholestatic jaundice (especially if treatment exceeds 1 month), peripheral neuropathy (discontinue treatment), and Stevens-Johnson syndrome reported; on prolonged use hypokalaemia, oedema and hair loss reported

Dose: oropharyngeal candidiasis, 100 mg daily (200 mg daily in AIDS or neutropenia) for 15 days; see also under *Sporanox®* oral liquid below
Vulvovaginal candidiasis, 200 mg twice daily for 1 day
Pityriasis versicolor, 200 mg daily for 7 days
Tinea corporis and tinea cruris, 100 mg daily for 15 days
Tinea pedis and tinea manuum, 100 mg daily for 30 days
Onychomycosis, *either* 200 mg daily for 3 months *or* course ('pulse') of 200 mg twice daily for 7 days, subsequent courses repeated after 21-day interval; fingernails two courses, toenails three courses
Histoplasmosis, 200 mg 1–2 times daily
Alternative in systemic infections, 200 mg once daily (candidiasis 100–200 mg once daily) increased in invasive or disseminated disease and in cryptococcal meningitis to 200 mg twice daily
Maintenance in AIDS patients and prophylaxis in neutropenia, 200 mg once daily, increased to 200 mg twice daily if low plasma-itraconazole concentration (see Cautions)
CHILD and ELDERLY not recommended

PoM Sporanox® (Janssen)
Capsules, blue/pink, enclosing coated beads, itraconazole 100 mg. Net price 4-cap pack = £5.99; 15-cap pack = £22.46; 28-cap pack (Sporanox-Pulse®) = £41.93; 60-cap pack = £89.84. Label: 5, 9, 21, 25
Oral liquid, itraconazole 10 mg/mL. Net price 150 mL (with 10-mL measuring cup) = £52.28. Label: 9, counselling, administration
Dose: oral or oesophageal candidiasis in HIV-positive or other immunocompromised patients, 20 mL (2 measuring cups) daily in 1–2 divided doses for 1 week (continue for another week if no response)
Fluconazole-resistant oral or oesophageal candidiasis, 20–40 mL (2–4 measuring cups) daily in 1–2 divided doses for 2 weeks (continue for another 2 weeks if no response)
COUNSELLING. Do not take with food; swish around mouth and swallow, do not rinse afterwards

KETOCONAZOLE

Indications: systemic mycoses, serious chronic resistant mucocutaneous candidiasis, serious resistant gastro-intestinal mycoses, chronic resistant vaginal candidiasis, resistant dermatophyte infections of skin or finger nails (not toe nails); prophylaxis of mycoses in immunosuppressed patients

Cautions: **important:** monitor liver function clinically and biochemically—for treatment lasting longer than 14 days perform liver function tests before starting, 14 days after starting, then at monthly intervals (for details see data sheet)—for CSM advice see p. 262; avoid in porphyria (see section 9.8.2); **interactions:** Appendix 1 (antifungals, imidazole and triazole)

CSM Warning. Avoid concomitant administration with astemizole or terfenadine, see also pp. 137–8; also avoid with cisapride (see p. 34) [other interactions, Appendix 1]

Contra-indications: hepatic impairment; pregnancy (teratogenicity in *animal* studies, packs carry a warning to avoid in pregnancy) and breast-feeding

Side-effects: nausea, vomiting, abdominal pain; headache; rashes, urticaria, pruritus; rarely thrombocytopenia, paraesthesia, photophobia, dizziness, alopecia, gynaecomastia and oligospermia; fatal liver damage—see also under Cautions, risk of developing hepatitis greater if given for longer than 14 days

Dose: 200 mg once daily with food, usually for 14 days; if response inadequate after 14 days continue until at least 1 week after symptoms have cleared and cultures become negative; max. 400 mg daily.

CHILD, 3 mg/kg daily

Chronic resistant vaginal candidiasis, 400 mg daily with food for 5 days

PoM **Nizoral®** (Janssen)

Tablets, scored, ketoconazole 200 mg. Net price 30-tab pack = £15.69. Label: 5, 9, 21

Suspension, pink, ketoconazole 100 mg/5 mL. Net price 100 mL with pipette = £7.16. Label: 5, 9, 21, counselling, use of pipette

MICONAZOLE

Indications: see under Dose

Cautions: pregnancy; avoid in porphyria (see section 9.8.2); **interactions:** Appendix 1 (antifungals, imidazole and triazole)

CSM Warning. Avoid concomitant administration with astemizole or terfenadine, see also pp. 137–8; also avoid with cisapride (see p. 34) [other interactions, Appendix 1]

Side-effects: nausea and vomiting, pruritus, rashes

Dose: *by mouth* as tablets, oral and intestinal fungal infections, 250 mg every 6 hours for 10 days or up to 2 days after symptoms clear; as oral gel, see under Daktarin® oral gel

Daktarin® (Janssen)

PoM *Tablets*, scored, miconazole 250 mg. Net price 20-tab pack = £14.89. Label: 9, 21

Note. Can be sucked for oral treatment

PoM[1] *Oral gel*, sugar-free, miconazole 25 mg/mL. Net price 15-g tube = £2.04, 80-g tube = £5.00. Label: 9, counselling advised, hold in mouth, after food

Dose: oral and intestinal fungal infections, 5–10 mL in the mouth after food 4 times daily; retain near lesions before swallowing; CHILD under 2 years, 2.5 mL twice daily, 2–6 years, 5 mL twice daily, over 6 years, 5 mL 4 times daily

Localised lesions, smear on affected area with clean finger

1. 15-g tube can be sold to public

NYSTATIN

Indications: candidiasis

Side-effects: nausea, vomiting, diarrhoea at high doses; oral irritation and sensitisation; rash (including urticaria) and rarely Stevens-Johnson syndrome reported

Dose: *by mouth*, intestinal candidiasis 500 000 units every 6 hours, doubled in severe infections; CHILD 100 000 units 4 times daily

Prophylaxis, 1 million units daily; NEONATE 100 000 units daily as a single dose

For use as a mouthwash in oral candidiasis, see section 12.3.2

PoM **Nystatin** (Non-proprietary)

Oral suspension, nystatin 100 000 units/mL. Net price 30 mL = £2.00. Label: 9, counselling use of pipette

Available from Kent, Lagap, Rosemont (sugar-free, Nystamont®)

PoM **Nystan®** (Squibb)

Tablets, brown, s/c, nystatin 500 000 units. Net price 56-tab pack = £4.70. Label: 9

Pastilles—see section 12.3.2

Pessaries—see section 7.2.2

Suspension, yellow, nystatin 100 000 units/mL. Net price 30 mL with pipette = £2.05. Label: 9, counselling, use of pipette

Suspension, gluten-, lactose-, and sugar-free, nystatin 100 000 units/mL when reconstituted with water. Net price 24 mL with pipette = £1.67. Label: 9, counselling, use of pipette

TERBINAFINE

Indications: dermatophyte infections of the nails, ringworm infections (including tinea pedis, cruris, and corporis) where oral therapy appropriate (due to site, severity or extent)

Cautions: hepatic and renal impairment; pregnancy, breast-feeding; **interactions:** Appendix 1 (terbinafine)

Side-effects: abdominal discomfort, loss of appetite, nausea, diarrhoea; headache; rash and urticaria occasionally with arthralgia or myalgia; serious skin reactions including Stevens-Johnson syndrome and toxic epidermal necrolysis reported (discontinue treatment if progressive skin rash); also reported, taste disturbance, photosensitivity, and rarely liver toxicity including jaundice, cholestasis and hepatitis

Dose: 250 mg daily usually for 2–6 weeks in tinea pedis, 2–4 weeks in tinea cruris, 4 weeks in tinea corporis, 6 weeks–3 months or longer in nail infections; CHILD not recommended

▼ PoM **Lamisil®** (Sandoz)

Tablets, off-white, scored, terbinafine 250 mg (as hydrochloride), net price 14-tab pack = £23.16, 28-tab pack = £44.66. Label: 9

5.3 Antiviral drugs

The specific therapy of virus infections is generally unsatisfactory and treatment is, therefore, primarily symptomatic. Fortunately, the majority of infections resolve spontaneously. For **interferon** preparations used in hepatitis B and C infections, see section 8.2.4.

HERPES SIMPLEX AND VARICELLA–ZOSTER

Aciclovir is active against herpes viruses but does not eradicate them. It is effective only if started at the onset of infection. Uses of aciclovir include the systemic treatment of varicella–zoster (chickenpox–shingles) and the systemic and topical treatment of herpes simplex infections of the skin and mucous membranes (including initial and recurrent genital herpes); it is also used topically in the eye. It can be life-saving in herpes simplex and varicella–zoster infections in the immunocompromised, and is also used in the immunocompromised for prevention of recurrence and prophylaxis. Aciclovir may also be given by mouth to immunocompetent adults and older adolescents with chickenpox; it is not generally indicated for immunocompetent children in whom the disease is milder. See also section 11.3.3 (eye) and section 13.10.3 (skin, including herpes labialis).

Famciclovir, a prodrug of penciclovir, is similar to aciclovir and it is recommended for herpes zoster and genital herpes; unlike aciclovir it only needs to be given 3 times daily (or as a single daily dose in herpes zoster). Penciclovir itself is used as a cream for herpes simplex labialis (see section 13.10.3). **Valaciclovir** is an ester of aciclovir which is licensed for herpes zoster and for herpes simplex infections of the skin and mucous membranes (including initial and recurrent genital herpes).

Idoxuridine is also only effective if started at the onset of infection; it is too toxic for systemic use. It has been used topically in the treatment of herpes simplex lesions of the skin and external genitalia with variable results; it has also been used topically in the treatment of zoster, but evidence of its value is dubious. See also section 13.10.3 (skin, including herpes labialis).

Inosine pranobex has been used by mouth for herpes simplex infections; its effectiveness has not been established.

Amantadine has been used by mouth for herpes zoster but, again, its effectiveness has not been established. Amantadine may be used for prophylaxis during an outbreak of influenza A in:

 unimmunised patients in 'at risk' groups (see under Influenza vaccine, section 14.4), for 2 weeks while the vaccine takes effect

 patients in 'at risk' groups for whom immunisation is contra-indicated, for the duration of the outbreak

 health care workers and other key personnel (to prevent disruption of service), during an epidemic.

ACICLOVIR

(Acyclovir)

Indications: herpes simplex and varicella–zoster (see also under Dose)

Cautions: maintain adequate hydration; renal impairment (see Appendix 3); pregnancy and breast-feeding; **interactions:** Appendix 1 (aciclovir and famciclovir)

Side-effects: rashes; gastro-intestinal disturbances; rises in bilirubin and liver enzymes, increases in blood urea and creatinine, decreases in haematological indices, headache, neurological reactions (including dizziness), fatigue; on intravenous infusion, severe local inflammation (sometimes leading to ulceration), also confusion, hallucinations, agitation, tremors, somnolence, psychosis, convulsions and coma

Dose: by mouth,

Herpes simplex, treatment, 200 mg (400 mg in the immunocompromised or if absorption impaired) 5 times daily, usually for 5 days; CHILD under 2 years, half adult dose, over 2 years, adult dose

Herpes simplex, prevention of recurrence, 200 mg 4 times daily *or* 400 mg twice daily possibly reduced to 200 mg 2 or 3 times daily and interrupted every 6–12 months

Herpes simplex, prophylaxis in the immunocompromised, 200–400 mg 4 times daily; CHILD under 2 years, half adult dose, over 2 years, adult dose

Varicella and herpes zoster, treatment, 800 mg 5 times daily for 7 days; CHILD, varicella, 20 mg/kg (max. 800 mg) 4 times daily for 5 days *or* under 2 years 200 mg 4 times daily, 2–5 years 400 mg 4 times daily, over 6 years 800 mg 4 times daily

By intravenous infusion over 1 hour, herpes simplex or recurrent varicella–zoster 5 mg/kg every 8 hours; doubled in primary and recurrent varicella–zoster in the immunocompromised, and in simplex encephalitis (for which it should be continued for at least 10 days); CHILD up to 3 months 10 mg/kg every 8 hours; 3 months–12 years, 250 mg/m^2 every 8 hours, dose doubled in the immunocompromised and in simplex encephalitis (for which it should be continued for at least 10 days)

By topical application, herpes simplex (*cream* or *eye ointment* as appropriate) every 4 hours (5 times daily), see sections 13.10.3 and 11.3.3

Note. Cream should not be used on mucous membranes

PoM Aciclovir (Non-proprietary)

Tablets, aciclovir 200 mg, net price 25-tab pack = £28.80; 400 mg, 56-tab pack = £105.90; 800 mg, 35-tab pack £107.25. Label:9

Available from CP

Dispersible tablets, aciclovir 200 mg, net price 25-tab pack = £28.89; 400 mg, 56-tab pack = £105.95; 800 mg, 35-tab pack = £107.30. Label: 9

Available from Cox, Hillcross, Norton

PoM Zovirax® (Wellcome)

Tablets, all dispersible, aciclovir 200 mg (blue), net price 25-tab pack = £28.89; 400 mg (pink), 56-tab pack = £105.95; 800 mg (scored, *Shingles Treatment Pack*), 35-tab pack = £107.30. Label: 9

Suspension, both off-white, sugar-free, aciclovir 200 mg/5 mL, net price 125 mL = £28.89; 400 mg/5 mL (*Chickenpox Treatment*) 50 mL = £16.14. Label: 9

Intravenous infusion, powder for reconstitution, aciclovir (as sodium salt). Net price 250-mg vial = £10.91; 500-mg vial = £20.22

Electrolytes: Na⁺ 1.1 mmol/250-mg vial

Cream, see section 13.10.3

Eye ointment, see section 11.3.3

AMANTADINE HYDROCHLORIDE

Indications: see under Dose and notes above; parkinsonism, see section 4.9.1

Cautions; Contra-indications; Side-effects: see section 4.9.1

Dose: herpes zoster, 100 mg twice daily for 14 days, if necessary extended for a further 14 days for post-herpetic neuralgia

Influenza A₂, ADULT and CHILD over 10 years, treatment, 100 mg daily for 4–5 days; prophylaxis, 100 mg daily usually for 6 weeks *or* with influenza vaccination for 2–3 weeks after vaccination

ELDERLY over 65 years, less than 100 mg daily *or* 100 mg at intervals of more than 1 day

Preparations

See section 4.9.1

FAMCICLOVIR

Indications: treatment of herpes zoster and genital herpes simplex

Cautions: renal impairment; pregnancy and breast-feeding; **interactions:** Appendix 1 (aciclovir and famciclovir)

Side-effects: nausea; headache

Dose: herpes zoster, 250 mg 3 times daily for 7 days *or* 750 mg once daily for 7 days

Genital herpes, first episode, 250 mg 3 times daily for 5 days; recurrent infection, 125 mg twice daily for 5 days

CHILD not recommended

▼ PoM **Famvir**® (SmithKline Beecham)

Tablets, both f/c, famciclovir 125 mg, net price 10-tab pack = £25.56; 250 mg, 15-tab pack = £76.68, 21-tab pack = £107.35. Label: 9

IDOXURIDINE

See section 13.10.3 (skin including herpes labialis)

INOSINE PRANOBEX

Indications: see under Dose

Cautions: avoid in renal impairment; history of gout or hyperuricaemia

Side-effects: reversible increases in serum and urinary uric acid

Dose: mucocutaneous herpes simplex, 1 g 4 times daily for 7–14 days

Adjunctive treatment of genital warts, 1 g 3 times daily for 14–28 days

PoM **Imunovir**® (Nycomed)

Tablets, inosine pranobex 500 mg. Net price 100 = £39.50. Label: 9

VALACICLOVIR

Note. Valaciclovir is a pro-drug of aciclovir

Indications: treatment of herpes zoster and of herpes simplex infections of skin and mucous membranes including initial and recurrent genital herpes

Cautions: maintain adequate hydration; renal impairment (see Appendix 3); pregnancy and breast-feeding; **interactions:** Appendix 1 (aciclovir and famciclovir)

Side-effects: as a pro-drug of aciclovir it is anticipated that side-effects will be comparable; nausea and headache reported

Dose: herpes zoster, 1 g 3 times daily for 7 days

Herpes simplex, first episode, 500 mg twice daily for 5 days (up to 10 days if severe); recurrent infection, 500 mg twice daily for 5 days

CHILD not recommended

▼ PoM **Valtrex**® (Wellcome)

Tablets, valaciclovir (as hydrochloride) 500 mg. Net price 10-tab (*HS Treatment*) pack = £23.50, 42-tab (*Shingles Treatment*) pack = £98.50 Label: 9

HUMAN IMMUNODEFICIENCY VIRUS

Zidovudine inhibits the human immunodeficiency virus (HIV) but does not eradicate it from the body; it is not therefore a cure for AIDS but may delay progression of the disease. It is now also being recommended for asymptomatic HIV antibody positive individuals. Zidovudine is toxic and expensive and should only be prescribed by those experienced in its use.

Didanosine is indicated for the treatment of symptomatic HIV infection in adult patients who are intolerant of zidovudine *or* who have shown significant clinical or immunological deterioration during zidovudine therapy *or* when zidovudine is inappropriate. **Zalcitabine** is a recently introduced anti-HIV drug with similar indications.

A combination of zidovudine with either didanosine or zalcitabine is more effective than zidovudine alone and can delay the emergence of HIV strains resistant to zidovudine.

ZIDOVUDINE

(Azidothymidine, AZT)

Note. The abbreviation AZT which has sometimes been used for zidovudine has also been used for another drug

Indications: management of advanced human immunodeficiency virus (HIV) disease such as acquired immunodeficiency syndrome (AIDS) or AIDS-related complex; early symptomatic or asymptomatic HIV infection with markers indicating risk of disease progression; symptomatic or asymptomatic HIV-infected children with markers indicating significant immune suppression; consider for prevention of maternal-fetal HIV transmission (by treating pregnant women and their newborn infants)

Cautions: haematological toxicity (blood tests at least every 2 weeks for first 3 months then at least once a month, early disease with good bone marrow reserves may require less frequent tests e.g. every 1–3 months); vitamin B_{12} deficiency (increased risk of neutropenia); reduce dose or interrupt treatment according to data sheet if anaemia or myelosuppression; renal impairment; hepatic impairment, monitor closely patients at risk of liver disease (especially obese women) including those with hepatomegaly and hepatitis; risk of lactic acidosis, see Side-effects; elderly; pregnancy; breast-feeding not recommended during treatment; **interactions:** Appendix 1 (zidovudine)

Contra-indications: abnormally low neutrophil counts or haemoglobin values (see data sheet); neonates with hyperbilirubinaemia requiring treatment other than phototherapy, or with raised transaminase (see data sheet)

Side-effects: anaemia (may require transfusion), neutropenia, and leucopenia (all more frequent with high dose and advanced disease); also include, nausea and vomiting, anorexia, abdominal pain, dyspepsia, headache, rash, fever, myalgia, paraesthesia, insomnia, malaise, and asthenia; also reported, convulsions (and other cerebral effects), myopathy, pigmentation of nail, skin and oral mucosa, pancytopenia (with bone marrow hypoplasia and rarely thrombocytopenia), liver disorders including fatty change and raised bilirubin and liver enzymes (suspend treatment if progressive hepatomegaly or rapidly elevating plasma aminotransferase), lactic acidosis (with tachypnoea, dyspnoea, and reduced plasma bicarbonate—suspend treatment)

Dose: by mouth, various dosages *including* 500–600 mg daily in 2–5 divided doses *or* 1 g daily in 2 divided doses; CHILD over 3 months 120–180 mg/m² every 6 hours (max. 200 mg every 6 hours)

Prevention of maternal-fetal HIV transmission, women over 14 weeks gestation, *by mouth,* 100 mg 5 times daily until beginning of labour *then* during labour and delivery, *by intravenous infusion* initially 2 mg/kg over 1 hour *then* 1 mg/kg/hour until umbilical cord clamped (for planned caesarean section, start intravenous infusion 4 hours before operation); newborn INFANT starting within 12 hours of birth, *by mouth,* 2 mg/kg every 6 hours continued until 6 weeks old (or if unable to take by mouth, *by intravenous infusion* over 30 minutes, 1.5 mg/kg every 6 hours)

Patients temporarily unable to take zidovudine by mouth, *by intravenous infusion* over 1 hour, 1–2 mg/kg every 4 hours (approximating to 1.5–3 mg/kg every 4 hours by mouth) usually for not more than 2 weeks

PoM **Retrovir**® (Wellcome)

Capsules, zidovudine 100 mg (white/blue band), net price 100 = £124.95; 250 mg (blue/white/dark blue band), 40-cap pack = £124.95

Tablets, zidovudine 300 mg, net price 60 = £224.90

Syrup, zidovudine 50 mg/5 mL. Net price 200-mL pack with 10-mL oral syringe = £24.99

Injection, zidovudine 10 mg/mL. For dilution and use as an intravenous infusion. Net price 20-mL vial = £12.54

DIDANOSINE
(DDI)

Indications: symptomatic HIV infection in patients who are intolerant of zidovudine *or* who have shown significant clinical or immunological deterioration during zidovudine therapy *or* when zidovudine is inappropriate

Cautions: history of pancreatitis (extreme caution, see also below); peripheral neuropathy or hyperuricaemia (see under Side-effects; monitor liver enzymes (suspend if significant elevation)—see also Contra-indications; hepatic and renal impairment (see Appendixes 2 and 3); pregnancy; avoid tetracyclines at same time of day (didanosine tablets contain aluminium and magnesium antacids)

PANCREATITIS. If raised serum amylase suspend treatment (even if asymptomatic) until diagnosis of pancreatitis excluded; on return to normal values re-initiate treatment only if essential (using low dose increased gradually if appropriate). Whenever possible avoid concomitant treatment with other drugs known to cause pancreatic toxicity (e.g. intravenous pentamidine isethionate); monitor closely if concomitant therapy unavoidable. Since significant elevations of triglycerides cause pancreatitis monitor closely if elevated

Contra-indications: hepatic abnormalities due to previous didanosine treatment; breast-feeding

Side-effects: pancreatitis (see also under Cautions); peripheral neuropathy especially in advanced HIV infection—suspend (reduced dose may be tolerated when symptoms resolve); asymptomatic hyperuricaemia (suspend treatment if measures to reduce uric acid concentration fail); diarrhoea (occasionally serious); also reported, nausea, vomiting, confusion, insomnia, chills, fever, headache, pain, rash, pruritus, asthenia, convulsions, pneumonia

Dose: ADULT under 60 kg 125 mg every 12 hours, 60 kg and over 200 mg every 12 hours; CHILD safety and efficacy not established, see data sheet for details

COUNSELLING. Each dose to be taken as 2 tablets (total 4 tablets daily) chewed thoroughly, crushed or dispersed in water; clear apple juice may be added for flavouring

▼ PoM **Videx**® (Bristol-Myers)

Tablets, both with aluminium and magnesium antacids, didanosine 25 mg, net price 60-tab pack = £28.60; 100 mg, 60-tab pack = £88.00. Each tablet contains Al^{3+} 8.4 mmol, Mg^{2+} 7.9 mmol, Na^+ 11.5 mmol. Label: 23, counselling, administration, see above

Additives: include aspartame

ZALCITABINE
(DDC)

Indications: advanced HIV infection in adults intolerant of zidovudine (low haemoglobin concentration, symptomatic anaemia or low neutrophil count) or in whom zidovudine has failed (clinical deterioration, rapidly worsening immunological status)

Cautions: patients at risk of developing peripheral neuropathy (see below); pancreatitis (see also below)—monitor serum amylase in those with history of elevated serum amylase, pancreatitis, alcohol abuse, or receiving parenteral nutrition; cardiomyopathy, history of congestive cardiac failure; hepatotoxicity (see below); monitor full blood count and clinical chemistry periodically; pregnancy (women of childbearing age should use effective contraception during treatment); renal impairment; **interactions:** Appendix 1 (zalcitabine)

PERIPHERAL NEUROPATHY. Discontinue immediately if peripheral neuropathy develops—characterised by numbness and burning dysaesthesia possibly followed by sharp shooting pains or severe continuous burning and potentially irreversible pain; extreme caution and close monitoring required in those at risk of peripheral neuropathy (especially those with low CD4 cell count for whom risk is greater)

PANCREATITIS. Discontinue permanently if clinical pancreatitis develops; suspend if raised serum amylase associated with dysglycaemia, rising triglyceride, decreasing serum calcium or other signs of impending pancreatitis until pancreatitis excluded; suspend if treatment required with another drug known to cause pancreatic toxicity (e.g. intravenous pentamidine isethionate); caution and close monitoring if history of pancreatitis (or of elevated serum amylase) or if risk of pancreatitis

HEPATOTOXICITY. Potentially life-threatening lactic acidosis and severe hepatomegaly with steatosis reported therefore caution in liver disease, liver enzyme abnormalities, or history of alcohol abuse or hepatitis; suspend or discontinue if deterioration in liver function tests, hepatic steatosis, progressive hepatomegaly or unexplained lactic acidosis

Contra-indications: peripheral neuropathy (see also above); breast-feeding

Side-effects: peripheral neuropathy (discontinue immediately, see also above); oral ulcers, nausea, vomiting, dysphagia, anorexia, diarrhoea, abdominal pain, constipation; pharyngitis; headache, dizziness; myalgia, arthralgia; rash, pruritus, sweating, weight loss, fatigue, fever, rigors, chest pain, anaemia, leucopenia, neutropenia, thrombocytopenia, disorders of liver function; less frequently pancreatitis (see also above), oesophageal ulcers (suspend treatment if no response to treatment for specific organisms), jaundice and hepatocellular damage (see also under Cautions); see data sheet for other less frequent side-effects

Dose: 750 micrograms 3 times daily; ELDERLY and CHILD under 13 years safety and efficacy not established

▼ PoM Hivid® (Roche)

Tablets, both f/c, zalcitabine 375 micrograms (beige), net price 100-tab pack = £104.20; 750 micrograms (grey), 100-tab pack = £158.71

CYTOMEGALOVIRUS (CMV)

Ganciclovir is related to aciclovir but is more active against cytomegalovirus; it is also much more toxic than aciclovir. It should therefore only be prescribed when the potential benefit outweighs the risks. It is administered by intravenous infusion. Capsules are available for *maintenance treatment* of CMV retinitis in AIDS patients following intra-

venous therapy if the condition is stable. Ganciclovir causes profound myelosuppression whe given with zidovudine; the two should not normall be given together particularly during initial gancic clovir therapy.

Foscarnet is also active against cytomegaloviru but is recommended only for retinitis in AIDS patients in whom ganciclovir is contra-indicated is inappropriate; it is toxic and can cause ren impairment in up to 50% of patients.

GANCICLOVIR

Indications: life-threatening or sight-threatenin cytomegalovirus infections in immunocompr mised patients only; prevention of cytomegalo virus disease during immunosuppressive therap following organ transplantation

Cautions: close monitoring of blood counts (se data sheet); history of cytopenia; low platele count; concomitant use of myelosuppressants drugs which inhibit rapid cell replication; potenti carcinogen and teratogen; renal impairmen ensure adequate hydration during administratio vesicant—infuse into vein with adequate flo preferably via a plastic cannula; limited experienc in children (possible risk of long-term carcinogen or reproductive toxicity—not for neonatal or co genital cytomegalovirus disease); **interactions** see notes above and Appendix 1 (ganciclovir)

Contra-indications: pregnancy (includes effe tive contraception during treatment and barrie contraception for men during and for 90 day after treatment); breast-feeding (until 72 hour after last dose); hypersensitivity to ganciclovir aciclovir; abnormally low neutrophil or platelet counts (see data sheet)

Side-effects: most frequent, leucopenia and throm bocytopenia; less frequent, anaemia, pancytopeni fever, rash, abnormal liver function tests; als chills, oedema, infections, malaise; nausea, vom ting, mouth ulcers, dyspepsia, dysphagia, diarrhoe anorexia, gastro-intestinal haemorrhage, abdo minal pain; chest pain, arrhythmias, hypertensio hypotension, deep thrombophlebitis, migrain vasodilation; dyspnoea; psychosis, confusio mood disturbances, nervousness, dry mouth, drow siness, dizziness, abnormal gait, ataxia, paraes thesia, tremor, headache, coma; eosinphili decrease in blood glucose; haematuria, raise serum creatinine and blood urea nitrogen; breas pain, urinary frequency, urinary-tract infectio aspermatogenesis; myasthenia, myalgia; distu bances in taste and vision, eye pain, deafness; reti nal detachment in AIDS patients with retiniti alopecia, acne, sweating, rash, pruritus, urticari local inflammation, pain and phlebitis at injectio site

Dose: by intravenous infusion over 1 hour, initia (induction) treatment, 5 mg/kg every 12 hours fo 14–21 days for treatment or for 7–14 days for pre vention; maintenance (for patients at risk relapse of retinitis) 6 mg/kg daily on 5 days pe week *or* 5 mg/kg daily every day; if retiniti progresses initial induction treatment may b repeated

Maintenance treatment in AIDS patients where retinitis stable (following at least 3 weeks of intravenous ganciclovir), *by mouth*, 1 g 3 times daily with food *or* 500 mg 6 times daily with food
In renal impairment, consult data sheet

PoM Cymevene® (Roche)
Capsules, green, ganciclovir 250 mg, net price 84-cap pack = £265.65. Label: 21
Intravenous infusion, powder for reconstitution, ganciclovir (as sodium salt). Net price 500-mg vial = £35.58
Electrolytes: Na⁺ 2 mmol/500-mg vial
CAUTION IN HANDLING. Wear gloves and safety glasses when reconstituting; if solution contacts skin or mucosa immediately wash with soap and water

FOSCARNET SODIUM
Indications: cytomegalovirus retinitis in patients with AIDS in whom ganciclovir is inappropriate
Cautions: renal impairment (avoid if severe), hypocalcaemia, monitor serum creatinine and serum calcium concentrations every second day; ensure adequate hydration
Contra-indications: pregnancy, breast-feeding
Side-effects: nausea, vomiting, headache, fatigue, rash; impairment of renal function including acute renal failure, symptomatic hypocalcaemia; decreased haemoglobin concentration; rarely hypoglycaemia, convulsions; thrombophlebitis if given undiluted by peripheral vein
Dose: by intravenous infusion, 20 mg/kg over 30 minutes then 21–200 mg/kg daily according to renal function for 2–3 weeks

PoM Foscavir® (Astra)
Intravenous infusion, foscarnet sodium hexahydrate 24 mg/mL, net price 250-mL bottle = £31.35, 500-mL bottle = £52.24

RESPIRATORY SYNCYTIAL VIRUS

Tribavirin inhibits a wide range of DNA and RNA viruses. It is given by inhalation for the treatment of severe bronchiolitis caused by the respiratory syncytial virus in infants, especially when they have other serious diseases. It is also effective in Lassa fever.

TRIBAVIRIN
(Ribavirin)
Indications: severe respiratory syncytial virus bronchiolitis in infants and children
Cautions: maintain standard supportive respiratory and fluid management therapy; monitor electrolytes closely; monitor equipment for precipitation
Contra-indications: pregnancy
Side-effects: reticulocytosis; also worsening respiration, bacterial pneumonia, and pneumothorax reported
Dose: by aerosol inhalation or nebulisation (via small particle aerosol generator) of solution containing 20 mg/mL for 12–18 hours for at least 3 days; max. 7 days

PoM Virazid® (ICN)
Inhalation, tribavirin 6 g for reconstitution with 300 mL water for injections. Net price 3 × 6-g vials = £570.38

5.4 Antiprotozoal drugs

5.4.1	Antimalarials
5.4.2	Amoebicides
5.4.3	Trichomonacides
5.4.4	Antigiardial drugs
5.4.5	Leishmaniacides
5.4.6	Trypanocides
5.4.7	Drugs for toxoplasmosis
5.4.8	Drugs for pneumocystis pneumonia

Advice on specific problems available from:

Malaria Reference	
Laboratory	0171-636 8636 (prophylaxis only)
Birmingham	0121-766 6611
Glasgow	0141-946 7120
Liverpool	0151-708 9393
London	0171-387 4411 (treatment)
	0171-388 9600 (travel prophylaxis)
Oxford	(01865) 225217
Recorded advice	
for Travellers	0891 600350
(49p/minute standard rate, 39p/minute cheap rate)	

5.4.1 Antimalarials

Recommendations on the prophylaxis and treatment of malaria reflect guidelines agreed by UK malaria specialists.

The centres listed above should be consulted for advice on special problems.

> WARNING. Settled immigrants (or long-term visitors) to the UK may be unaware that they will have **lost their immunity** and also that the areas where they previously lived **may now be malarious**

TREATMENT OF MALARIA

If the infective species is **not known** or if the infection is **mixed** initial treatment should be with quinine, mefloquine, or halofantrine as for *falciparum malaria*.

FALCIPARUM MALARIA (TREATMENT)

Falciparum malaria (malignant malaria) is caused by *Plasmodium falciparum*. In most parts of the world *P. falciparum* is now resistant to chloroquine which should not therefore be given for treatment[1].

Quinine, **mefloquine**, or **halofantrine** can be given *by mouth* if the patient can swallow tablets and there are no serious manifestations (e.g. impaired consciousness); quinine should be given *by intravenous infusion* (see below) if the patient is seriously ill or unable to take tablets.

Footnote—*see next page*

The adult dosage regimen for **quinine** *by mouth* is:

600 mg (of quinine salt[2]) every 8 hours for 7 days *and* (if quinine resistance known or suspected)

either followed by **Fansidar®** 3 tablets as a single dose

or (if Fansidar®-resistant) *followed by* **tetracycline** 250 mg every 6 hours for 7 days when renal function has returned to normal.

Alternatively **mefloquine** or **halofantrine** (**important:** see warnings on p. 276) may be given instead of quinine but resistance has been reported in several countries. It is not necessary to give Fansidar® or tetracycline after mefloquine or halofantrine treatment.

The adult dosage regimen for **mefloquine** *by mouth* is:

20 mg/kg (of mefloquine base) as a single dose (up to maximum 1.5 g) *or preferably* as 2 divided doses 6–8 hours apart.

The adult dosage regimen for **halofantrine** (**important:** see warnings on p. 276) *by mouth* is:

1.5 g of halofantrine hydrochloride divided into three doses of 500 mg given at intervals of 6 hours (on an empty stomach); this course should be repeated after an interval of 1 week.

If the patient is seriously ill, **quinine** should be given *by intravenous infusion*. The adult dosage regimen for quinine *by infusion* is:

loading dose[3] of 20 mg/kg[4] (up to maximum 1.4 g) of quinine salt[2] infused over 4 hours *then after 8–12 hours* maintenance dose of 10 mg/kg[5] (up to maximum 700 mg) of quinine salt[2] infused over 4 hours every 8–12 hours (until patient can swallow tablets to complete the 7-day course)

---

1. For chloroquine-sensitive strains of falciparum malaria chloroquine is effective *by mouth* in the dosage schedule outlined under benign malarias but it should **not** be used unless there is an **unambiguous exposure history** in one of the few remaining areas of chloroquine sensitivity.
   If the patient with a *chloroquine-sensitive infection* is seriously ill, chloroquine is given *by continuous intravenous infusion*. The dosage (for adults and children) is chloroquine 10 mg/kg (of base) infused over 8 hours, followed by three 8-hour infusions of 5 mg/kg (of base) each. *Oral therapy* is started as soon as possible to complete the course; the total cumulative dose for the course should be 25 mg/kg of base.
2. Valid for quinine hydrochloride, dihydrochloride, and sulphate; not valid for quinine bisulphate which contains a correspondingly smaller amount of quinine.
3. In intensive care units the loading dose can alternatively be given as quinine salt[2] 7 mg/kg infused over 30 minutes followed immediately by 10 mg/kg over 4 hours then (after 8 hours) maintenance dose as described.
4. **Important:** the loading dose of 20 mg/kg should **not** be used if the patient has received quinine (or quinidine) or mefloquine during the previous 24 hours—**for additional warnings** relating to halofantrine, see p. 276
5. Maintenance dose should be reduced to 5–7 mg/kg of salt if parenteral treatment is required for more than 48 hours.
6. Halofantrine and mefloquine are also active in benign malarias but are not required since chloroquine is usually effective; as with chloroquine a radical cure with primaquine is required for *P. vivax* and *P. ovale* infections.

---

either followed by Fansidar® *or* (when renal function has returned to normal) tetracycline as above

CHILDREN.

Oral. Quinine is well tolerated by children although the salts are bitter. The dosage regimen for quinine *by mouth* for children is:

10 mg/kg (of quinine salt[2]) every 8 hours for 7 days *then* (if quinine resistance known or suspected)

Fansidar® as a single dose: up to 4 years ½ tablet, 5–6 years 1 tablet, 7–9 years 1½ tablets, 10–14 years 2 tablets.

Alternatively mefloquine or halofantrine may be given instead of quinine; it is not necessary to give Fansidar® after mefloquine or halofantrine treatment. The dosage regimen for mefloquine *by mouth* for children is calculated on a mg/kg basis as for adults (see above). The dosage regimen for halofantrine *by mouth* (**important:** see warnings on p. 276) for children over 37 kg is the same as for adults (see above); the dosage regimen for halofantrine for smaller children is reduced as follows:

weight under 23 kg, no suitable dose form;

weight 23–31 kg, 3 doses of 250 mg at intervals of 6 hours;

weight 32–37 kg, 3 doses of 375 mg at intervals of 6 hours.

This course of halofantrine should be repeated after an interval of 1 week.

Parenteral. The dosage regimen for quinine *by intravenous infusion* for children is calculated on a mg/kg basis as for adults (see above).

PREGNANCY. Falciparum malaria is particularly dangerous in pregnancy, especially in the last trimester. The adult treatment doses of oral and intravenous quinine given above (including the loading dose) can safely be given to pregnant women. Halofantrine is contra-indicated in pregnancy and tetracycline should be avoided (causes dental discoloration); Fansidar® and mefloquine are also best avoided until more information is available.

BENIGN MALARIAS (TREATMENT)

Benign malaria is usually caused by *Plasmodium vivax* and less commonly by *P. ovale* and *P. malariae*. **Chloroquine**[6] is the drug of choice for the treatment of benign malarias (but chloroquine-resistant *P. vivax* infection has been reported from New Guinea).

The adult dosage regimen for **chloroquine** *by mouth* is:

initial dose of 600 mg (of base) *then*

a single dose of 300 mg after 6 to 8 hours *then*

a single dose of 300 mg daily for 2 days

(approximate total cumulative dose of 25 mg/kg of base)

Chloroquine alone is adequate for *P. malariae* infections but in the case of *P. vivax* and *P. ovale*, a *radical cure* (to destroy parasites in the liver and thus prevent relapses) is required. This is achieved

---

with **primaquine**[7] in an adult dosage of 15 mg daily for 14 to 21 days given after the chloroquine; a 21-day (or even longer) course may be needed for Chesson-type strains of *P. vivax* from south-east Asia and western Pacific.

CHILDREN. The dosage regimen of chloroquine for benign malaria in children is:

initial dose of 10 mg/kg (of base) *then*

a single dose of 5 mg/kg after 6–8 hours *then*

a single dose of 5 mg/kg daily for 2 days

For a *radical cure* children are then given primaquine[7] in a dose of 250 micrograms/kg daily.

PREGNANCY. The adult treatment doses of chloroquine can be given for benign malaria. In the case of *P. vivax* or *P. ovale*, however, the radical cure with primaquine should be **postponed** until the pregnancy is over; instead chloroquine should be continued at a dose of 600 mg each week during the pregnancy.

PROPHYLAXIS AGAINST MALARIA

The recommendations on prophylaxis reflect guidelines agreed by UK malaria specialists; the advice is aimed at residents of the UK who travel to endemic areas for short stays. The choice of drug (see next page) takes account of:

risk of exposure to malaria;

extent of drug resistance;

efficacy of the recommended drugs;

side-effects of the drugs;

patient-related criteria (e.g. age, pregnancy, renal or hepatic impairment).

NETS AND REPELLENTS. The most important point to remember is that **prophylaxis is relative and not absolute**, and that breakthrough can occur with any of the drugs recommended anywhere in the world. Travellers should be warned that **personal protection** against being bitten (e.g. keep well covered, use mosquito nets, repellents etc.) is **very important**.

LENGTH OF PROPHYLAXIS. In order to determine tolerance and to establish habit, prophylaxis should be started one week (preferably two weeks in the case of mefloquine) before travel into an endemic area (or if not possible at earliest opportunity up to 1 or 2 days before travel); it should be continued for **at least 4 weeks after leaving**.

RETURN FROM MALARIAL REGION. It is important to be aware that **any illness** that occurs within 1 year and **especially within 3 months of return might be malaria** even if all recommended precautions against malaria were taken. Travellers should be **warned** of this and told that if they develop any illness **particularly within 3 months** of their return they should go **immediately** to a doctor and specifically mention their exposure to malaria.

7. Before starting primaquine blood should be tested for glucose-6-phosphate dehydrogenase (G6PD) activity since the drug can cause haemolysis in G6PD-deficient patients. In G6PD deficiency primaquine, in a dose for adults of 30 mg once a week (children 500–750 micrograms/kg once a week) for 8 weeks, has been found useful and without undue harmful effects.

CHILDREN. The following prophylactic doses are based on guidelines agreed by UK malaria experts and may differ from advice in data sheets. If in doubt telephone centres listed on p. 271.

Age	Weight (kg)	Fraction of adult dose	
		Chloroquine Proguanil	Maloprim®
0–5 weeks		⅛	—
6 weeks– 11 months		¼	—
1–5 years	10–19	½	¼
6–11 years	20–39	¾	½
12 years	40	adult dose	adult dose

Note. Weight is a better guide than age for children over 6 months old. Specialist advice should be obtained for use of Maloprim® in children under 1 year of age.

For children's doses of mefloquine see p. 277.

Prophylaxis is required in **breast-fed infants**; although antimalarials are excreted in milk, the amounts are too variable to give reliable protection.

EPILEPSY. Both chloroquine and mefloquine are unsuitable for malaria prophylaxis in subjects with a history of epilepsy. In areas *without chloroquine resistance* proguanil 200 mg daily alone is recommended; in areas *with chloroquine resistance* doxycycline may be considered [unlicensed indication, specialist advice needed] but its metabolism may be influenced by antiepileptics (see **interactions**: Appendix 1 (tetracyclines).

RENAL IMPAIRMENT. Avoidance (or dosage reduction) of proguanil or chloroquine is recommended since both are excreted by the kidneys. Although the data sheet remains cautious, the UK malaria experts consider that mefloquine is appropriate to use and does not require dosage reduction. They also consider doxycycline to be appropriate [unlicensed indication, specialist advice needed].

PREGNANCY. Chloroquine and proguanil may be given in usual doses in areas where *P. falciparum* strains are sensitive; in the case of proguanil, folate supplements (folic acid 5 mg daily) should be given. Mefloquine should be avoided in the first trimester (see p. 277). Maloprim® is also contra-indicated in the first trimester; folate supplements should be given if Maloprim® is prescribed in the second and third trimester. The centres listed on p. 271 should be consulted for advice on prophylaxis in resistant areas.

SPECIFIC RECOMMENDATIONS

Where a journey requires two regimens, the highest risk regimen should be used for the whole journey.

North Africa and the Middle East

VERY LOW RISK. Risk *very low* in Abu Dhabi, Algeria, tourist areas of Egypt, Libya, Morocco, Tunisia, most tourist areas of Turkey:

> no prophylaxis recommended but consider malaria if fever presents

LOW RISK. Risk *low* in southern border areas of Azerbaijan, Egypt (El Fayoum only, June–October), rural north Iraq (May–November), north border of Syria (May–October), Turkey (plain around

Adana, Side, south-east Anatolia, March–November), south border areas of Tajikistan:

preferably

chloroquine 300 mg (as base) once weekly

or

(if chloroquine not appropriate)

proguanil hydrochloride 200 mg once daily

RISK. Risk *present* and *chloroquine resistance present* in Afghanistan (below 2000 m, May–November), Iran (March–November), Oman, Saudi Arabia (except Northern, Eastern and Central Provinces, Asir plateau, and western border cities where very little risk), northern rural United Arab Emirates, Yemen:

both
chloroquine 300 mg (as base) once weekly
and
proguanil hydrochloride 200 mg once daily

Sub-Saharan Africa

VERY HIGH RISK. Risk *very high* (or *locally very high*) and *chloroquine resistance very widespread* in Angola, Benin, Burkina Faso, Burundi, Cameroon, Central African Republic, Chad, Comoros, Congo, Djibouti, Equatorial Guinea, Eritrea, Ethiopia, Gabon, Gambia, Ghana, Guinea, Guinea-Bissau, Ivory Coast, Kenya, Liberia, Madagascar, Malawi, Mali, Mozambique, Niger, Nigeria, Principe, Rwanda, São Tomé, Senegal, Sierra Leone, Somalia, Sudan, Swaziland, Tanzania, Togo, Uganda, Zaïre, Zambia, Zimbabwe (Zambezi valley, see also below):

preferably

mefloquine 250 mg once weekly

or

(if mefloquine not appropriate)

both
chloroquine 300 mg (as base) once weekly
and
proguanil hydrochloride 200 mg once daily

RISK. Risk *present* (in *parts of country*) and *some chloroquine resistance* in northern half of Botswana (November–June), Mauritania (all year in southern half; July–October in northern half), northern third of Namibia (November–June), north-east part of South Africa (low altitude areas of north and eastern Transvaal and eastern Natal to 100 kilometres north of Durban), areas below 1200 m in Zimbabwe (November–June; all year in Zambezi valley *where mefloquine preferable*):

preferably

both
chloroquine 300 mg (as base) once weekly
and
proguanil hydrochloride 200 mg once daily

or

(if chloroquine plus proguanil not appropriate)

mefloquine 250 mg once weekly

Note. In Zimbabwe and neighbouring countries, Maloprim® (also known as Deltaprim®) prophylaxis is widely used by local residents (sometimes with chloroquine), but it is not advised by UK malaria experts in order to simplify UK guidelines especially for those travelling to more than one country.

No prophylaxis recommended for Cape Verde and non-rural areas of Mauritius (but consider malaria if fever presents); *chloroquine prophylaxis* appropriate for rural areas of **Mauritius**

South Asia

HIGH RISK. Risk *high* and *chloroquine resistance high* in east Bangladesh (including Chittagong Hill Tracts):

preferably

mefloquine 250 mg once weekly

or

(if mefloquine not appropriate)

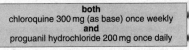

both
chloroquine 300 mg (as base) once weekly
and
proguanil hydrochloride 200 mg once daily

VARIABLE RISK. Risk *variable* and *chloroquine resistance usually moderate* in Bangladesh (except east, see above; no risk in Dhaka city), southern districts of Bhutan, India (no risk in mountain states of north), Nepal (below 1300 m; no risk in Kathmandu), Pakistan (below 2000 m), Sri Lanka (no risk in and just south of Colombo):

both
chloroquine 300 mg (as base) once weekly
and
proguanil hydrochloride 200 mg once daily

South-East Asia

VERY LOW RISK. Risk *very low* in Bali, Brunei (no risk), main tourist areas of China (but *substantial risk* in Yunnan and Hainan, see below; *chloroquine prophylaxis* appropriate for remote areas), Hong Kong, Malaysia (but *substantial risk* in Sabah, see below, and *variable risk* in deep forests, see also below), Sarawak (but *variable risk* in deep forests, see below), Singapore (no risk), Thailand (Bangkok and main tourist centres but *substantial risk* in rural areas, see below, and *great risk* in borders with Cambodia and Myanmar, **important:** see also below):

no prophylaxis recommended but consider malaria if fever presents

VARIABLE RISK. Risk *variable* and *some chloroquine resistance* in Indonesia (no risk in Bali and cities but *substantial risk* in Irian Jaya, see below), rural Philippines below 600 m (no risk in Cebu, Leyte, Bohol, Catanduanes), deep forests of peninsular Malaysia and Sarawak:

both
chloroquine 300 mg (as base) once weekly
and
proguanil hydrochloride 200 mg once daily

Risk may vary in different parts of a country—check under all risk levels

SUBSTANTIAL RISK. Risk *substantial* and *drug resistance common* in Cambodia (no risk in Phnom Penh; **important:** specialist advice needed for western provinces, see below), China (Yunnan and Hainan; *chloroquine prophylaxis* appropriate for other remote areas), Irian Jaya, Laos (no risk in Vientiane), Myanmar (formerly Burma), Sabah, backpacking in rural Thailand (**important:** specialist advice needed for border areas, see below), Vietnam (no risk in cities and delta area):

mefloquine 250 mg once weekly

GREAT RISK. Risk *great* and *mefloquine resistance prevalent* in western provinces of Cambodia, borders of Thailand with Cambodia and Myanmar (but not for routine backpackers):

doxycycline 100 mg once daily
[unlicensed indication—specialist advice needed and not for longer than 3 months]

Oceania

RISK. Risk *high* and *chloroquine resistance high* in Papua New Guinea (below 1800 m), Solomon Islands, Vanuatu:

preferably

mefloquine 250 mg once weekly

or
(if mefloquine not appropriate)

both
Maloprim® 1 tablet once weekly
and
chloroquine 300 mg (as base) once weekly

Latin America

VARIABLE TO LOW RISK. Risk *variable to low* in Argentina (small area in north-west only), rural Belize (except Belize district), rural Costa Rica (below 500 m), Dominican Republic, El Salvador, Guatemala (below 1500 m), Haiti, Honduras, some rural areas of Mexico (not regularly visited by tourists), Nicaragua, Panama (west of Panama Canal but *high risk* east of Panama Canal, see below), rural Paraguay (October–May):

preferably

chloroquine 300 mg (as base) once weekly

or
(if chloroquine not appropriate)

proguanil hydrochloride 200 mg once daily

VARIABLE TO HIGH RISK. Risk *variable to high* and *chloroquine resistance present* in rural areas of Bolivia (below 2500 m), Ecuador (below 1500 m),

rural areas of Peru (below 1500 m), rural areas of Venezuela (except on coast):

preferably

both
chloroquine 300 mg (as base) once weekly
and
proguanil hydrochloride 200 mg once daily

or
(if chloroquine plus proguanil not appropriate)

mefloquine 250 mg once weekly

Note. Maloprim® plus chloroquine prophylaxis is also an alternative

HIGH RISK. Risk *high* and *marked chloroquine resistance* in Bolivia (Amazon basin area), Brazil (throughout 'Legal Amazon' area which includes the Amazon basin region, Mato Grosso and Maranhao only; elsewhere *very low risk*—no prophylaxis), Colombia (most areas below 800 m), French Guiana, all interior regions of Guyana, Panama (east of Panama Canal), Surinam (except Paramaribo and coast), Venezuela (Amazon basin area):

preferably

mefloquine 250 mg once weekly

or
(if mefloquine not appropriate)

both
chloroquine 300 mg (as base) once weekly
and
proguanil hydrochloride 200 mg once daily

STANDBY TREATMENT. Adults travelling for prolonged periods to areas of chloroquine-resistance who are unlikely to have easy access to medical care should carry a standby treatment course. Self-medication should be **avoided** if medical help is accessible; prophylaxis should be continued during and after the attack.

In order to avoid excessive self-medication, the traveller should be provided with **written instructions** that urgent medical attention should be sought if fever (38°C or more) develops 7 days (or more) after arriving in a malarious area and that self treatment is indicated if medical help is not immediately available or the condition is worsening.

In view of the continuing emergence of resistant strains and of the different regimens required for different areas expert advice should be sought on the best treatment course for an individual traveller.

WARNING. Settled immigrants (or long-term visitors) to the UK may be unaware that they will have **lost their immunity** and also that the areas where they previously lived **may now be malarious**

CHLOROQUINE

Chloroquine is used for the *prophylaxis of malaria* in areas of the world where the *risk of chloroquine resistant falciparum malaria is still low*; it is usually given with proguanil (but sometimes alone or with Maloprim®). It is no longer recommended (or is no longer first choice) in areas of the world where *resistance is high* (for details, see specific recommendations by country, pp. 273–5).

Chloroquine it is **no longer recommended** for the *treatment of falciparum malaria* owing to widespread resistance, nor is it recommended if the infective species is *not known* or if the infection is *mixed*; in these cases treatment should be with quinine, mefloquine or halofantrine (for details, see pp. 271–2). It is still recommended for the *treatment of benign malarias* (for details, see p. 272).

CHLOROQUINE

Indications: chemoprophylaxis and treatment of malaria, see notes above; rheumatoid arthritis and lupus erythematosus—see section 10.1.3

Cautions: hepatic impairment, renal impairment (see notes above), pregnancy (but for malaria benefit outweighs risk, see Appendix 4, Antimalarials), may exacerbate psoriasis, neurological disorders (avoid for prophylaxis if history of epilepsy, see notes above), may aggravate myasthenia gravis, severe gastro-intestinal disorders, G6PD deficiency (see section 9.1.5); ophthalmic examination and long-term therapy, see under Chloroquine, section 10.1.3; avoid concurrent therapy with hepatotoxic drugs and with halofantrine (see CSM advice under Halofantrine)—other **interactions**: Appendix 1 (chloroquine)

Side-effects: gastro-intestinal disturbances, headache; also convulsions, visual disturbances, depigmentation or loss of hair, skin reactions (rashes, pruritus); rarely, bone-marrow suppression; other side-effects (not usually associated with malaria prophylaxis or treatment), see under Chloroquine, section 10.1.3; **important:** very toxic in overdosage—immediate advice from poisons centres essential (see also p. 22)

Dose: see notes above

COUNSELLING. Warn travellers about **importance** of avoiding mosquito bites, **importance** of taking prophylaxis regularly, and **importance** of immediate visit to doctor if ill within 1 year and **especially** within 3 months of return. For details, see notes above

PoM ⃰Avloclor® (Zeneca)
Tablets, scored, chloroquine phosphate 250 mg (≡ chloroquine base 155 mg). Net price 20-tab pack = £1.11. Label: 5, counselling, prophylaxis, see above
⃰ Can be sold to the public provided it is licensed and labelled for the prophylaxis of malaria

Nivaquine® (Rhône-Poulenc Rorer)
PoM⃰ *Tablets*, f/c, yellow, chloroquine sulphate 200 mg (≡ chloroquine base 150 mg). Net price 28-tab pack = £1.11. Label: 5, counselling, prophylaxis, see above
PoM⃰ *Syrup*, golden, chloroquine sulphate 68 mg/5 mL (≡ chloroquine base 50 mg/5 mL). Net price 100 mL = £2.33. Label: 5, counselling, prophylaxis, see above
⃰ Can be sold to the public provided it is licensed and labelled for the prophylaxis of malaria
PoM *Injection*, chloroquine sulphate 54.5 mg/mL (≡ chloroquine base 40 mg/mL). Net price 5-mL amp = 63p

HALOFANTRINE

Halofantrine is not suitable for the *prophylaxis of malaria*.

Halofantrine is used for the *treatment of falciparum malaria* (or if the infective species is *not known* or if the infection is *mixed*) (for details, see p. 271–2). It should not be used for the *treatment of benign malarias*, as chloroquine is usually effective. It should not be used where mefloquine has been used for prophylaxis.

HALOFANTRINE HYDROCHLORIDE

Indications: treatment of uncomplicated chloroquine-resistant falciparum malaria or of chloroquine-resistant vivax malaria, see notes above

Cautions: no experience of use in cerebral or complicated malaria; cardiac disease (see below); **interactions:** see below and Appendix 1 (halofantrine)

ARRHYTHMIAS. Halofantrine prolongs QT interval and has a potential for inducing hazardous arrhythmias in susceptible individuals, especially if dose excessive or if taken with food (which enhances absorption). It should **not** be used for standby treatment. Recommendations of the CSM are that halofantrine:
should **not** be taken with meals;
should **not** be taken with other drugs which may induce arrhythmias (e.g. *chloroquine, mefloquine, quinine, tricyclic antidepressants, antipsychotics, certain antiarrhythmics,* and *antihistamines such as astemizole and terfenadine*);
should **not** be taken with drugs causing electrolyte disturbances;
should **not** be administered to those with known prolongation of the QT interval;
should **not** be administered to those with any form of cardiac disease associated with QT interval prolongation or ventricular arrhythmias (e.g. coronary heart disease, cardiomyopathy, and congenital heart disease)

Contra-indications: cardiac disorders including family history of congenital QT interval prolongation (**important:** see also above); other conditions associated with prolonged QT interval (e.g. hypokalaemia, hypomagnesaemia or other electrolyte disorders, thiamine deficiency); unexpected syncopal attacks; pregnancy and breast-feeding (avoid during treatment)

Side-effects: diarrhoea, abdominal pain, nausea, vomiting; transient elevation of serum transaminases; pruritus, rash, intravascular haemolysis, and hypersensitivity reactions also reported; **important:** ventricular arrhythmias (see also above)

Dose: see notes above

▼ PoM **Halfan®** (SK&F)
Tablets, scored, halofantrine hydrochloride 250 mg. Net price 12-tab pack = £13.96. Label: 23

MEFLOQUINE

Mefloquine is used for the *prophylaxis of malaria* in areas of the world where there is a *high risk of chloroquine-resistant falciparum malaria* (for details, see specific recommendations by country, p. 273–5).

Mefloquine is used for the *treatment of falciparum malaria* (or if the infective species is *not known* or if the infection is *mixed*) (for details, see pp. 271–1). It is also effective for the *treatment of benign malarias*, but is not required as chloroquine is usually effective. Mefloquine should not be used for treatment if it has been used for prophylaxis.

MEFLOQUINE

Indications: chemoprophylaxis of malaria, treatment of uncomplicated falciparum malaria and chloroquine-resistant vivax malaria, see notes above

Cautions: exclude pregnancy before starting chemoprophylaxis (see also under Contra-indications); avoid for chemoprophylaxis in severe hepatic impairment; renal impairment (see notes under Prophylaxis against malaria above); cardiac conduction disorders; epilepsy (avoid for prophylaxis); not recommended in young children (under 15 kg); halofantrine must not be given with or after mefloquine (danger of fatal arrhythmias—see also under Halofantrine); other **interactions:** Appendix 1 (mefloquine)

DRIVING. May affect performance of skilled tasks (e.g. driving); effects may persist for up to 3 weeks

Contra-indications: chemoprophylaxis in first trimester of pregnancy (teratogenic in *animals*, **avoid** pregnancy **during** and for **3 months after**), breast-feeding, and history of serious psychiatric disorders or convulsions (or family history of epilepsy); hypersensitivity to quinine

Side-effects: nausea, vomiting, diarrhoea, abdominal pain; dizziness, loss of balance, headache, somnolence, sleep disorders (insomnia, abnormal dreams); also neuropsychiatric reactions (including sensory and motor neuropathies, anxiety, depression, hallucinations, overt psychosis, convulsions), tinnitus and vestibular disorders, visual disturbances, circulatory disorders (hypotension and hypertension), tachycardia, bradycardia, cardiac conduction disorders, muscle weakness, myalgia, arthralgia, rash, urticaria, pruritus, alopecia, disturbances in liver function tests, asthenia, malaise, fatigue, fever, loss of appetite, leucopenia or leucocytosis, thrombocytopenia; rarely Stevens-Johnson syndrome, AV block and encephalopathy

Dose: chemoprophylaxis, 250 mg each week starting 1–2 weeks before departure (see p. 273) and continued for 4 weeks after leaving malarious area; CHILD 15–19 kg (2–5 years) quarter adult dose, 20–30 kg (6–8 years) half adult dose, 31–45 kg (9–11 years) three-quarters adult dose

LONG-TERM CHEMOPROPHYLAXIS. For long-term visitors the UK malaria specialists now recommend that mefloquine prophylaxis can be taken for up to 1 year, although the data sheet still restricts use to 3 months (with the aim of preventing mefloquine resistance)

Treatment, see notes above

COUNSELLING. Warn travellers about **importance** of avoiding mosquito bites, **importance** of taking prophylaxis regularly, and **importance** of immediate visit to doctor if ill within 1 year and **especially** within 3 months of return. For details, see notes above

PoM **Lariam®** (Roche)

Tablets, scored, mefloquine (as hydrochloride) 250 mg. Net price 8-tab pack = £14.53. Label: 21, 25, 27, counselling, driving, prophylaxis, see above

PRIMAQUINE

Primaquine is used to eliminate the liver stages of *P. vivax* or *P. ovale following chloroquine treatment* (for details, see p. 272).

PRIMAQUINE

Indications: adjunct in the treatment of *Plasmodium vivax* and *P. ovale* malaria (eradication of liver stages)

Cautions: G6PD deficiency (see notes above); systemic diseases associated with granulocytopenia (e.g. rheumatoid arthritis, lupus erythematosus); pregnancy and breast-feeding; **interactions:** Appendix 1 (primaquine)

Side-effects: nausea, vomiting, abdominal pain; less commonly methaemoglobinaemia, haemolytic anaemia especially in G6PD deficiency

Dose: see notes above

Primaquine (Non-proprietary)

Tablets, primaquine (as phosphate) 7.5 mg
Available from Durbin [unlicensed—special order]

PROGUANIL

Proguanil is used (usually *with chloroquine*, but occasionally *alone*) for the *prophylaxis of malaria*, (for details, see specific recommendations by country, see pp. 273–5).

Proguanil is not suitable for the *treatment of malaria*.

PROGUANIL HYDROCHLORIDE

Indications: chemoprophylaxis of malaria

Cautions: renal impairment (see notes under Prophylaxis against malaria); pregnancy (folate supplements needed); **interactions:** Appendix 1 (proguanil)

Side-effects: mild gastric intolerance and diarrhoea; occasionally mouth ulcers and stomatitis; skin reaction and hair loss reported

Dose: see notes above

COUNSELLING. Warn travellers about **importance** of avoiding mosquito bites, **importance** of taking prophylaxis regularly, and **importance** of immediate visit to doctor if ill within 1 year and **especially** within 3 months of return. For details, see notes above

Paludrine® (Zeneca)

Tablets, scored, proguanil hydrochloride 100 mg. Net price 98-tab pack = £7.43. Label: 21, counselling, prophylaxis, see above

PYRIMETHAMINE

Pyrimethamine should not be used alone, but is used with sulfadoxine (in *Fansidar®*) and with dapsone (in *Maloprim®*).

Fansidar® is not recommended for the *prophylaxis of malaria*, but it is used in the treatment of *falciparum malaria* and can be used *with (or following) quinine*.

Maloprim® is used with *chloroquine* for the *prophylaxis of malaria* in certain areas where there is a *high risk of chloroquine-resistant falciparum malaria* (for details see specific recommendations by country, see p. 273–5). *Maloprim®* is not suitable for the *treatment of malaria*.

PYRIMETHAMINE

Indications: malaria (but used only in combined preparations incorporating dapsone or sulfadoxine); toxoplasmosis [not licensed]—section 5.4.7

Cautions: hepatic or renal impairment, folate supplements in pregnancy, breast-feeding, blood counts required with prolonged treatment; **interactions:** Appendix 1 (pyrimethamine)

Side-effects: depression of haematopoiesis with high doses, rashes, insomnia

Dose: malaria, no dose stated because not recommended

Toxoplasmosis, section 5.4.7

PoM **Daraprim®** (Wellcome)
Tablets, scored, pyrimethamine 25 mg. Net price 30-tab pack = £2.22

PYRIMETHAMINE WITH SULFADOXINE

Indications: adjunct to quinine in treatment of *Plasmodium falciparum* malaria (see notes above); **not** recommended for prophylaxis

Cautions; Contra-indications; Side-effects: see under Pyrimethamine and under Co-trimoxazole (section 5.1.8); pregnancy and breast-feeding (see Appendixes 4 and 5); severe side-effects on long-term use therefore not recommended for prophylaxis; pulmonary infiltrates (e.g. eosinophilic or allergic alveolitis) reported—discontinue if cough or shortness of breath

Dose: treatment, see notes above
Prophylaxis, not recommended by UK malaria experts

PoM **Fansidar®** (Roche)
Tablets, scored, pyrimethamine 25 mg, sulfadoxine 500 mg. Net price 10-tab pack = £2.77

PYRIMETHAMINE WITH DAPSONE

Indications: prophylaxis of *Plasmodium falciparum* malaria (limited use, see notes above)

Cautions; Contra-indications; Side-effects: see under Pyrimethamine and under Dapsone (section 5.1.10); G6PD deficiency (see section 9.1.5); pregnancy (see notes under Prophylaxis against malaria and Appendix 4) and breast-feeding (see Appendix 5); side-effects including methaemoglobinaemia, thrombocytopenia, mononucleosis-like syndrome, psychosis, jaundice, pneumonia with eosinophilic pulmonary infiltration, and on prolonged treatment hypoalbuminaemia reported

Dose: malaria prophylaxis, see notes above
COUNSELLING. Warn travellers about **importance** of avoiding mosquito bites, **importance** of taking prophylaxis regularly, and **importance** of immediate visit to doctor if ill within 1 year and **especially** within 3 months of return. For details, see notes above

PoM **Maloprim®** (Wellcome)
Tablets, scored, pyrimethamine 12.5 mg, dapsone 100 mg. Net price 30-tab pack = £2.76. Counselling, prophylaxis, see above

QUININE

Quinine is not suitable for the *prophylaxis of malaria*.

Quinine is used for the *treatment of falciparum malaria* (or if the infective species is *not known* or if the infection is *mixed*) (for details see pp. 271–2).

QUININE

Indications: falciparum malaria; nocturnal leg cramps, see section 10.2.2

Cautions: atrial fibrillation, conduction defects, heart block, pregnancy; monitor blood glucose concentration during parenteral treatment; G6PD deficiency (see section 9.1.5); avoid concurrent administration with halofantrine (see CSM advice under Halofantrine), other **interactions:** Appendix 1 (quinine)

Contra-indications: haemoglobinuria, optic neuritis

Side-effects: cinchonism, including tinnitus, headache, hot and flushed skin, nausea, abdominal pain, rashes, visual disturbances (including temporary blindness), confusion; hypersensitivity reactions including angioedema, blood disorders (including thrombocytopenia and intravascular coagulation), and acute renal failure; hypoglycaemia (especially after parenteral administration); cardiovascular effects (see Cautions); **important:** very toxic in overdosage—immediate advice from poisons centres essential (see also p. 22)

Dose: see notes above

Note. Quinine (anhydrous base) 100 mg ≡ quinine bisulphate 169 mg ≡ quinine dihydrochloride 122 mg ≡ quinine hydrochloride 122 mg ≡ quinine sulphate 121 mg. Quinine bisulphate 300-mg tablets are available but provide smaller amounts of quinine than the dihydrochloride, hydrochloride, or sulphate

PoM **Quinine Sulphate** (Non-proprietary)
Tablets, coated, quinine sulphate 200 mg, net price 20 = 76p; 300 mg, 20 = 81p
Available from APS, Cox, CP, Hillcross, Kent

PoM **Quinine Dihydrochloride** (Non-proprietary)
Injection, quinine dihydrochloride 300 mg/mL. For dilution and use as an infusion. 1- and 2-mL amps
Available from Martindale (special order) or from specialist centres (see p. 271)

Note. Intravenous injection of quinine is so hazardous that it has been superseded by infusion

TETRACYCLINES

Doxycycline is used for the *prophylaxis of malaria* [unlicensed indication—specialist advice needed] in areas of *widespread mefloquine and chloroquine resistance* and also as a second-line drug for those who are unable to take chloroquine or mefloquine (for details, see specific recommendations by country, pp. 273–5).

Tetracycline is used as an *adjunct to quinine in the treatment of falciparum malaria* [unlicensed indication] (for details see p. 272).

DOXYCYCLINE
Section 5.1.3

TETRACYCLINE
Section 5.1.3

5.4.2   Amoebicides

Metronidazole is the drug of choice for *acute invasive amoebic dysentery* since it is very effective against vegetative forms of *Entamoeba histolytica* in ulcers; it is given in an adult dose of 800 mg three times daily for 5 days. **Tinidazole** is also effective. Metronidazole and tinidazole are also active against amoebae which may have migrated to the liver. Treatment with metronidazole (or tinidazole) is followed by a 10-day course of diloxanide furoate.

Diloxanide furoate is the drug of choice for asymptomatic patients with *E. histolytica* cysts in the faeces; metronidazole and tinidazole are relatively ineffective. Diloxanide furoate is relatively free from toxic effects and the usual course is of 10 days, given alone for chronic infections or following metronidazole or tinidazole treatment.

For *amoebic abscesses* of the liver **metronidazole** is effective in doses of 400 mg 3 times daily for 5–10 days; tinidazole is an alternative. The course may be repeated after 2 weeks if necessary. Aspiration of the abscess is indicated where it is suspected that it may rupture or where there is no improvement after 72 hours of metronidazole; the aspiration may need to be repeated. Aspiration aids penetration of metronidazole and, for abscesses with more than 100 mL of pus, if carried out in conjunction with drug therapy, may reduce the period of disability.

Rarely, where metronidazole and tinidazole appear to be ineffective, dehydroemetine may be used (but the risk of side-effects is much greater). Diloxanide furoate is not effective against hepatic amoebiasis, but a 10-day course should be given at the completion of metronidazole or tinidazole treatment to destroy any amoebae in the gut.

DILOXANIDE FUROATE
Indications: chronic amoebiasis—see notes
Side-effects: flatulence, vomiting, urticaria, pruritus

Dose: 500 mg every 8 hours for 10 days; CHILD 20 mg/kg daily in 3 divided doses.
See also notes above

PoM Furamide® (Knoll)
Tablets, scored, diloxanide furoate 500 mg. Label: 9

METRONIDAZOLE
Indications: see under Dose below; anaerobic infections, section 5.1.11
Cautions; Side-effects: section 5.1.11
Dose: by mouth, invasive intestinal amoebiasis, 800 mg every 8 hours for 5 days; CHILD 1–3 years 200 mg every 8 hours; 3–7 years 200 mg every 6 hours; 7–10 years 400 mg every 8 hours

Extra-intestinal amoebiasis (including liver abscess) and symptomless amoebic cyst passers, 400–800 mg every 8 hours for 5–10 days; CHILD 1–3 years 100–200 mg every 8 hours; 3–7 years 100–200 mg every 6 hours; 7–10 years 200–400 mg every 8 hours

Urogenital trichomoniasis, 200 mg every 8 hours for 7 days *or* 400 mg every 12 hours for 7 days, *or* 800 mg in the morning and 1.2 g at night for 2 days, *or* 2 g as a single dose; CHILD 1–3 years 50 mg every 8 hours; 3–7 years 100 mg every 12 hours; 7–10 years 100 mg every 8 hours
Giardiasis, 2 g daily for 3 days; CHILD 1–3 years 500 mg daily; 3–7 years 600–800 mg daily; 7–10 years 1 g daily

Preparations
Section 5.1.11

TINIDAZOLE
Indications: see under Dose below; anaerobic infections, section 5.1.11
Cautions; Side-effects: section 5.1.11
Dose: intestinal amoebiasis, 2 g daily for 2–3 days; CHILD 50–60 mg/kg daily for 3 days
Amoebic involvement of liver, 1.5–2 g daily for 3–5 days; CHILD 50–60 mg/kg daily for 5 days
Urogenital trichomoniasis and giardiasis, single 2-g dose (repeated once if necessary); CHILD single dose of 50–75 mg/kg

Preparations
Section 5.1.11

5.4.3   Trichomonacides

Metronidazole (section 5.4.2) is the treatment of choice for *Trichomonas vaginalis* infection.

If metronidazole is ineffective, **tinidazole** may be tried; it is usually given as a single 2-g dose, with food. A further 2-g dose may be given if there is no clinical improvement.

Alcohol should be avoided during treatment with both metronidazole and tinidazole.

5.4.4   Antigiardial drugs

Metronidazole (section 5.4.2) is the treatment of choice for *Giardia lamblia* infections, given by mouth in a dosage of 2 g daily for 3 days or 400 mg every 8 hours for 5 days.

Alternative treatments are **tinidazole** (section 5.4.2) 2 g as a single dose or **mepacrine hydrochloride** 100 mg every 8 hours for 5–7 days.

MEPACRINE HYDROCHLORIDE

Indications: giardiasis

Cautions: hepatic impairment, elderly, history of psychosis; avoid in psoriasis; **interactions:** Appendix 1 (mepacrine)

Side-effects: gastro-intestinal disturbances; dizziness, headache; with large doses nausea, vomiting and occasionally transient acute toxic psychosis and CNS stimulation; on prolonged treatment yellow discoloration of skin and urine, chronic dermatoses (including severe exfoliative dermatitis), hepatitis, aplastic anaemia; also reported blue/black discoloration of palate and nails and corneal deposits with visual disturbances

Dose: 100 mg every 8 hours for 5–7 days; CHILD 2 mg/kg every 8 hours

Mepacrine Hydrochloride

Tablets, mepacrine hydrochloride 100 mg. Label: 4, 9, 14, 21

Available from BCM Specials [unlicensed—special order]

5.4.5   Leishmaniacides

Cutaneous leishmaniasis frequently heals spontaneously but if skin lesions are extensive or unsightly, treatment is indicated, as it is in visceral leishmaniasis (kala-azar).

Sodium stibogluconate, an organic pentavalent antimony compound, is the treatment of choice for visceral leishmaniasis. The dose is 20 mg/kg daily (max. 850 mg) for at least 20 days by intramuscular or intravenous injection; the dosage varies with different geographical regions and expert advice should be obtained. Skin lesions are treated for 10 days.

Pentamidine isethionate (section 5.4.8) has been used in antimony-resistant visceral leishmaniasis, but although the initial response is often good, the relapse rate is high; it is associated with serious side-effects. Other treatments include paromomycin (*Farmitalia Carlo Erba*, not on UK Market) or liposomal amphotericin [section 5.2 but not licensed for leishmaniasis].

SODIUM STIBOGLUCONATE

Indications: leishmaniasis

Cautions: hepatic impairment; pregnancy; intravenous injections must be given slowly over 5 minutes (to reduce risk of local thrombosis) and stopped if coughing or substernal pain; mucocutaneous disease (see below); heart disease (withdraw if conduction disturbances occur); treat intercurrent infection (e.g. pneumonia)

MUCOCUTANEOUS DISEASE. Successful treatment of mucocutaneous leishmaniasis may induce severe inflammation around the lesions (may be life-threatening if pharyngeal or tracheal involvement)—may require corticosteroid

Contra-indications: significant renal impairment; breast-feeding

Side-effects: anorexia, nausea, vomiting, abdominal pain; ECG changes; headache, lethargy, myalgia; raised liver enzymes; coughing and substernal pain (see Cautions); rarely anaphylaxis; also reported, fever, sweating, flushing, vertigo, bleeding from nose or gum, jaundice, rash; pain and thrombosis on intravenous administration, intramuscular injection also painful

Dose: see notes above

PoM **Pentostam®** (Wellcome)

Injection, sodium stibogluconate equivalent to pentavalent antimony 100 mg/mL. Net price 100-mL bottle = £68.01

5.4.6   Trypanocides

The prophylaxis and treatment of trypanosomiasis is difficult and differs according to the strain of organism. Expert advice should therefore be obtained.

5.4.7   Drugs for toxoplasmosis

Most infections caused by *Toxoplasma gondii* are self-limiting, and treatment is not necessary. Exceptions are patients with eye involvement (toxoplasma choroidoretinitis), and those who are immunosuppressed. Toxoplasmic encephalitis is a common complication of AIDS. The treatment of choice is a combination of pyrimethamine and sulphadiazine, given for several weeks (expert advice **essential**). Pyrimethamine is a folate antagonist, and adverse reactions to this combination are relatively common (folinic acid supplements and weekly blood counts needed). Alternative regimens use combinations of pyrimethamine with clindamycin or clarithromycin or azithromycin. Long-term secondary prophylaxis is required after treatment of toxoplasmosis in AIDS.

If toxoplasmosis is acquired in pregnancy, transplacental infection may lead to severe disease in the fetus. Spiramycin (not on UK market) may reduce the risk of transmission of maternal infection to the fetus.

5.4.8   Drugs for Pneumocystis pneumonia

Pneumonia caused by *Pneumocystis carinii* occurs in immunosuppressed or severely debilitated patients. It is the commonest cause of pneumonia in AIDS. **Co-trimoxazole** (section 5.1.8) in high dosage is the drug of choice for the treatment of pneumocystis pneumonia. **Pentamidine isethionate** is an alternative to co-trimoxazole and is particularly indicated for patients with a history of adverse reactions to, or who have not responded to, co-trimoxazole. Pentamidine isethionate is a potentially toxic drug that can cause severe hypotension during or immediately after administration; it should only be administered by those experienced in its use. Pentamidine isethionate is given by intravenous infusion but can also be administered by inhalation which reduces side-effects (although systemic absorption may still occur).

Intermittent *prophylactic inhalation* of pentamidine isethionate may prevent relapse but co-trimoxazole is easier to administer and just as effective (in a dose of 960 mg twice daily) for prophylaxis.

Atovaquone has recently become available for the treatment of mild to moderate Pneumocystis pneumonia in patients who are intolerant of co-trimoxazole.

ATOVAQUONE

Indications: treatment of mild to moderate *Pneumocystis carinii* pneumonia in patients intolerant of co-trimoxazole

Cautions: initial diarrhoea and difficulty in taking with food may reduce absorption (and require alternative therapy); other causes of pulmonary disease should be sought and treated; elderly; hepatic and renal impairment; pregnancy; avoid breast-feeding; **interactions:** Appendix 1 (atovaquone)

Side-effects: diarrhoea, nausea, vomiting; headache, insomnia; rash, fever; elevated liver enzymes and amylase; anaemia; hyponatraemia

Dose: 750 mg 3 times daily with food (particularly high fat) for 21 days; CHILD not recommended

▼ PoM **Wellvone**® (Wellcome)
Tablets, yellow, f/c, atovaquone 250 mg. Net price 189-tab pack = £377.14. Label: 21

CO-TRIMOXAZOLE
Section 5.1.8

PENTAMIDINE ISETHIONATE
(Pentamidine isetionate)

Indications: see under Dose (should only be given by specialists)

Cautions: risk of severe hypotension following administration (establish baseline blood pressure and administer with patient lying down; monitor blood pressure closely during administration, and at regular intervals, until treatment concluded); hepatic and renal impairment; hypertension or hypotension; hyperglycaemia or hypoglycaemia; leucopenia, thrombocytopenia, or anaemia; pregnancy and breast-feeding; carry out laboratory monitoring for all functions according to data sheet

Side-effects: severe reactions, sometimes fatal, due to hypotension, hypoglycaemia, pancreatitis, and arrhythmias; also leucopenia, thrombocytopenia, acute renal failure, hypocalcaemia; also reported: azotaemia, abnormal liver-function

tests, leucopenia, anaemia, hyperkalaemia, nausea and vomiting, dizziness, syncope, flushing, hyperglycaemia, rash, and taste disturbances; Stevens-Johnson syndrome reported; on inhalation, bronchoconstriction (may be prevented by prior use of bronchodilators), cough, shortness of breath, and wheezing; discomfort, pain, induration, abscess formation, and muscle necrosis at injection site

Dose: *Pneumocystis carinii* pneumonia, *by intravenous infusion*, 4 mg/kg daily for at least 14 days (reduced according to data sheet in renal impairment)

By inhalation of nebulised solution (using suitable equipment—see data sheet) 600 mg pentamidine isethionate daily for 3 weeks; secondary prevention, 300 mg every 4 weeks *or* 150 mg every 2 weeks

Visceral leishmaniasis (Kala-azar), *by deep intramuscular injection*, 3–4 mg/kg on alternate days to max. total of 10 injections; course may be repeated if necessary

Cutaneous leishmaniasis, *by deep intramuscular injection*, 3–4 mg/kg once or twice weekly until condition resolves (but see also section 5.4.5)

Trypanosomiasis, *by deep intramuscular injection or intravenous infusion*, 4 mg/kg daily or on alternate days to total of 7–10 injections

Note. Direct bolus intravenous injection should be avoided whenever possible and **never** given rapidly; intramuscular injections should be deep and preferably given into the buttock

PoM **Pentacarinat**® (Rhône-Poulenc Rorer)
Injection, powder for reconstitution, pentamidine isethionate. Net price 300-mg vial = £15.58
Nebuliser solution, pentamidine isethionate. Net price 300-mg bottle = £16.45

5.5 Anthelmintics

5.5.1	Drugs for threadworms
5.5.2	Ascaricides
5.5.3	Drugs for tapeworm infections
5.5.4	Drugs for hookworms
5.5.5	Schistosomicides
5.5.6	Filaricides
5.5.7	Drugs for guinea worms
5.5.8	Drugs for strongyloidiasis

Advice on prophylaxis and treatment of helminth infections is available from:

Birmingham	0121-766 6611
Glasgow	0141-946 7120
Liverpool	0151-708 9393
London	0171-387 4411 (treatment)

5.5.1 Drugs for threadworms
(pinworms, *Enterobius vermicularis*)

Anthelmintics are effective in threadworm infections, but their use needs to be combined with hygienic measures to break the cycle of auto-infection. All members of the family require treatment.

Adult threadworms do not live for longer than 6 weeks and for development of fresh worms, ova must be swallowed and exposed to the action of digestive juices in the upper intestinal tract. Direct multiplication of worms does not take place in the large bowel. Adult female worms lay ova on the peri-anal skin which causes pruritus; scratching the area then leads to ova being transmitted on fingers to the mouth, often via food eaten with unwashed hands. Washing hands and scrubbing nails before each meal and after each visit to the toilet is essential. A bath taken immediately after rising will remove ova laid during the night.

Mebendazole is the drug of choice for patients of all ages over 2 years. It is given as a single dose; as reinfection is very common, a second dose may be given after 2–3 weeks.

Piperazine salts are preferably given daily for 7 days (followed by a second course if necessary 7 days later); single-dose preparations are also available.

MEBENDAZOLE

Indications: threadworm, roundworm, whipworm, and hookworm infections

Cautions: pregnancy (toxicity in *rats*), breast-feeding; **interactions:** Appendix 1 (mebendazole)

Note. The package insert in the Vermox® pack includes the statement that it is not suitable for women known to be pregnant or children under 2 years

Side-effects: rarely abdominal pain, diarrhoea; hypersensitivity reactions (including exanthema, rash, urticaria, and angioedema) reported

Dose: threadworms, ADULT and CHILD over 2 years, 100 mg as a single dose; if reinfection occurs second dose may be needed after 2–3 weeks; CHILD under 2 years, not yet recommended

Whipworms, ADULT and CHILD over 2 years, 100 mg twice daily for 3 days; CHILD under 2 years, not yet recommended

Roundworms—section 5.5.2

Hookworms—section 5.5.4

PoM ¹**Vermox**® (Janssen)

Tablets, orange, scored, chewable, mebendazole 100 mg. Net price 6-tab pack = £1.53

Suspension, mebendazole 100 mg/5 mL. Net price 30 mL = £1.77

1. Can be sold to the public if supplied for oral use in the treatment of enterobiasis in adults and children over 2 years provided its container or package is labelled to show a max. single dose of 100 mg and it is supplied in a container or package containing not more than 400 mg; proprietary brands on sale to the public include *Ovex*® and *Pripsen*® *Mebendazole*.

PIPERAZINE

Indications: threadworm and roundworm infections

Cautions: renal impairment (avoid if severe), liver disease, neurological disease; epilepsy, pregnancy (see also Appendix 4—packs on sale to the general public carry a warning to avoid in epilepsy and pregnancy)

Side-effects: nausea, vomiting, colic, diarrhoea, allergic reactions including urticaria, broncho-spasm, and rare reports of Stevens-Johnson syndrome and angioedema; rarely dizziness, muscular incoordination ('worm wobble'); drowsiness, confusion and clonic contractions in patients with neurological or renal abnormalities

Dose: see under Preparations, below

Piperazine Citrate (Non-proprietary)

Elixir, piperazine hydrate 750 mg/5 mL (as citrate)

Available from Cupal (Expelix®), De Witt (De Witt's Worm Syrup), Seton (Pripsen® Worm Elixir)

Dose: threadworms, 15 mL once daily for 7 days; CHILD under 2 years (on doctor's advice only) 0.3–0.5 mL/kg once daily for 7 days, 2–3 years 5 mL once daily for 7 days, 4–6 years 7.5 mL once daily for 7 days, 7–12 years 10 mL once daily for 7 days; repeat course after 1 week if necessary

Roundworms, 30 mL as a single dose; CHILD under 1 year (on doctor's advice only) 0.8 mL/kg as a single dose, 1–3 years 10 mL as a single dose, 4–5 years 15 mL as a single dose, 6–8 years 20 mL as a single dose, 9–12 years 25 mL as a single dose; repeat dose after 2 weeks

Pripsen® (Seton)

Oral powder, cream, piperazine phosphate 4 g and sennosides 15.3 mg/sachet. Net price two-dose sachet pack = £1.31. Label: 13

Dose: threadworms, stirred into a small glass of milk or water and drunk immediately, ADULT and CHILD over 6, 1 sachet, repeat after 14 days; INFANT 3 months–1 year, one-third sachet (2.5 mL powder), repeat after 14 days; CHILD 1–6 years, two-thirds sachet (5 mL powder), repeat after 14 days

Roundworms, first dose as for threadworms; repeat at monthly intervals for up to 3 months if reinfection risk

5.5.2   Ascaricides
(common roundworm infections)

Levamisole (not on UK market) is very effective against *Ascaris lumbricoides* and is generally considered to be the drug of choice. It is very well tolerated; mild nausea or vomiting has been reported in about 1% of treated patients; it is given as a single dose of 120–150 mg in adults.

Mebendazole (section 5.5.1) is also active against ascaris; the usual dose is 100 mg twice daily for 3 days. **Piperazine** may be given in a single adult dose equivalent to 4–4.5 g of piperazine hydrate see Piperazine, above.

5.5.3   Drugs for tapeworm infections

TAENICIDES

Niclosamide is the most widely used drug for tapeworm infections and side-effects are limited to occasional gastro-intestinal upset, lightheadedness, and pruritus; it is not effective against larval worms. Fears of developing cysticercosis in *Taenia solium* infections have proved unfounded. All the same, it is wise to anticipate this possibility by using an anti-emetic on wakening.

Praziquantel (Biltricide®, not on UK market) is effective as niclosamide and is given as a single ~se of 10–20 mg/kg after a light breakfast (a single ~se of 25 mg/kg for *Hymenolepis nana*).

ICLOSAMIDE

ndications: tapeworm infections—see notes above and under Dose

ide-effects: nausea, retching, abdominal pain; ightheadedness; pruritus

ose: Taenia solium, ADULT and CHILD over 6 years 2 g as a single dose after a light breakfast ollowed by a purgative after 2 hours; CHILD under 2 years 500 mg, 2–6 years 1 g

T. saginata and *Diphyllobothrium latum*, as for *T. solium* but half the dose may be taken after breakfast and the remainder 1 hour later followed by a ourgative 2 hours after last dose

Hymenolepis nana, ADULT and CHILD over 6 years 2 g as a single dose on first day then 1 g daily for 6 days; CHILD under 2 years 500 mg on first day then 250 mg daily for 6 days, 2–6 years 1 g on first day then 500 mg daily for 6 days

COUNSELLING. Tablets should be chewed thoroughly (or crushed) before washing down with water

ɔmesan® (Bayer)
ablets, yellow, chewable, niclosamide 500 mg. Net price 4-tab pack = £1.41. Label: 4, 24, counselling, administration

YDATID DISEASE

ysts caused by *Echinococcus granulosus* grow ɔwly and asymptomatic patients do not always ʒuire treatment. Surgical treatment remains the ʒethod of choice in many situations. **Albendazole** used in conjunction with surgery to reduce the ʒk of recurrence or as primary treatment in inoperǝle cases. Alveolar echinococcosis due to *E. multicularis* is usually fatal if untreated. Surgical ʒoval with albendazole cover is the treatment of ʒoice, but where effective surgery is impossible, ʒeated cycles of albendazole (for a year or more) ʒay help. Careful monitoring of liver function is ʒrticularly important during drug treatment.

LBENDAZOLE

ndications: adjunct to surgery in hydatid cysts caused by *Echinococcus granulosus* or *E. multiǀocularis*, or primary treatment if surgery not possible; strongyloidiasis (section 5.5.8)

autions: blood counts and liver function tests before treatment and twice during each cycle; breast-feeding; exclude pregnancy before starting treatment (non-hormonal contraception during and for 1 month after treatment)

ontra-indications: pregnancy (see also Cautions)
ide-effects: gastro-intestinal disturbances, headache, dizziness, changes in liver enzymes; rarely reversible alopecia; rash, fever, blood disorders including leucopenia and pancytopenia reported; allergic shock if cyst leakage; convulsions and meningism in cerebral disease

Dose: E. granulosus, ADULT over 60 kg, medical treatment, 800 mg daily in divided doses for 28 days followed by 14 tablet-free days; up to 3 cycles of treatment may be given

Adjunct in surgical treatment, *pre-surgery*, 800 mg daily in divided doses for 28 days followed by 14 tablet-free days, repeat cycle once before surgery; *post-surgery* (if viable cysts after pre-surgery treatment, or if no pre-surgery treatment, or if only short pre-surgery course), 800 mg daily in divided doses for 28 days followed by 14 tablet-free days, repeat cycle once

E. multilocularis, ADULT over 60 kg, 800 mg daily in divided doses for 28 days followed by 14 tablet-free days; prolonged treatment may be required, see notes above

PoM **Eskazole®** (SmithKline Beecham)
Tablets, orange, scored, chewable, albendazole 400 mg. Net price 60-tab pack = £72.00. Label: 9

5.5.4 Drugs for hookworms

(ancylostomiasis, necatoriasis)

Hookworms live in the upper small intestine and draw blood from the point of their attachment to their host. An iron-deficiency anaemia may thereby be produced and, if present, effective treatment of the infection requires not only expulsion of the worms but treatment of the anaemia.

Mebendazole (section 5.5.1) has a useful broadspectrum activity, and is effective against hookworms; the usual dose is 100 mg twice daily for 3 days.

5.5.5 Schistosomicides

(bilharziasis)

Adult *Schistosoma haematobium* worms live in the genito-urinary veins and adult *S. mansoni* in those of the colon and mesentery. *S. japonicum* is more widely distributed in veins of the alimentary tract and portal system.

Praziquantel (Biltricide®, not on UK market) is effective against all human schistosomes. The dose is 40 mg/kg in 2 divided doses 4–6 hours apart on one day (60 mg/kg in 3 divided doses on one day for *S. japonicum* infections). No serious toxic effects have been reported. Of all the available schistosomicides, it has the most attractive combination of effectiveness, broad-spectrum activity, and low toxicity.

Metriphonate (Bilarcil®, not on UK market) is effective against *S. haematobium* infections only; it may be used if praziquantel is not available.

Hycanthone, lucanthone, niridazole, oxamniquine, and stibocaptate have now been superseded.

5.5.6 Filaricides

Diethylcarbamazine (Hetrazan®, *Lederle*) is effective against microfilariae and adults of *Loa loa*, *Wuchereria bancrofti*, and *Brugia malayi*. To minimise reactions treatment is commenced with a dose of diethylcarbamazine citrate 1 mg/kg on the first day and increased gradually over 3 days to 6 mg/kg daily in divided doses; this dosage is maintained for 21 days and usually gives a radical cure for these infections. Close medical supervision is necessary particularly in the early phase of treatment.

In heavy infections there may be a febrile reaction, and in heavy *Loa loa* infection there is a small risk of encephalopathy. In such cases treatment must be given under careful in-patient supervision and stopped at the first sign of cerebral involvement (and specialist advice sought).

Ivermectin (Mectizan®, *MSD*, not on UK market) is very effective in *onchocerciasis* and it is now the drug of choice. A single dose of 150 micrograms/kg by mouth produces a prolonged reduction in microfilarial levels. Retreatment at intervals of 6 to 12 months depending on symptoms must be given until the adult worms die out. Reactions are usually slight and most commonly take the form of temporary aggravation of itching and rash. Diethylcarbamazine or suramin should no longer be used for onchocerciasis because of their toxicity.

5.5.7   Drugs for guinea worms
(dracontiasis)

Metronidazole has been reported to be effective against *Dracunculus medinensis* in a dose of 400 mg three times daily for 5 days. In India, **mebendazole** has been reported as effective at a dosage of 200 mg twice daily for 7 days.

5.5.8   Drugs for strongyloidiasis

Adult *Strongyloides stercoralis* live in the gut and produce larvae which penetrate the gut wall and invade the tissues, setting up a cycle of auto-infection. **Thiabendazole** is the drug of choice for adults (but side-effects are much more marked in the elderly); it is given at a dosage of 25 mg/kg (max. 1.5 g) every 12 hours for 3 days. **Albendazole** (section 5.5.3) is an alternative with fewer side-effects; it is given in a dose of 400 mg twice daily for 3 days, repeated after 3 weeks if necessary. **Ivermectin** (not on UK market) in a dose of 200 micrograms/kg daily for 2 days may be the most effective drug for chronic *Strongyloides* infection.

THIABENDAZOLE
(Tiabendazole)

Indications: strongyloidiasis, cutaneous a visceral larva migrans, dracontiasis, symptoms trichinosis; secondary treatment for threadwor when mixed with above infestations; adjunct hookworm, whipworm, or roundworm (but n suitable for mixed infections involving rour worms—risk of migration); not for prophylac use

Cautions: hepatic or renal impairment, elder discontinue if hypersensitivity reactions occ correct anaemia, dehydration or malnutriti preferably before treatment; **interaction** Appendix 1 (thiabendazole)

DRIVING. May impair performance of skilled tasks (e driving)

Contra-indications: pregnancy (teratogenesis *animal* studies) and breast-feeding

Side-effects: include anorexia, nausea, vomitir dizziness, diarrhoea, headache, pruritus, drow ness; hypersensitivity reactions including fev chills, angioedema, rashes, erythema multifor and Stevens-Johnson syndrome; rarely tinnit collapse, parenchymal liver damage (may severe and irreversible), visual disorders

Dose: see notes above

PoM **Mintezol®** (MSD)
Tablets, orange, chewable, thiabendazole 500 m Net price 6-tab pack = 62p. Label: 3, 21, 24

6: Drugs used in the treatment of disorders of the
ENDOCRINE SYSTEM

In this chapter, drug treatment is discussed under the following headings:

6.1   Drugs used in diabetes
6.2   Thyroid and antithyroid drugs
6.3   Corticosteroids
6.4   Sex hormones
6.5   Hypothalamic and pituitary hormones
6.6   Drugs affecting bone metabolism
6.7   Other endocrine drugs

6.1 Drugs used in diabetes

6.1.1   Insulin
6.1.2   Oral antidiabetic drugs
6.1.3   Diabetic ketoacidosis
6.1.4   Treatment of hypoglycaemia
6.1.5   Treatment of diabetic nephropathy and neuropathy
6.1.6   Diagnostic and monitoring agents for diabetes mellitus

6.1.1 Insulin

6.1.1.1   Short-acting insulin
6.1.1.2   Intermediate- and long-acting insulins
6.1.1.3   Hypodermic equipment

Insulin plays a key role in the body's regulation of carbohydrate, fat, and protein metabolism. Diabetes mellitus is due to a deficiency in insulin synthesis and secretion. Patients are generally described as insulin-dependent diabetics (type 1) or non-insulin-dependent diabetics (type 2), although many of the latter need insulin to maintain satisfactory control.

Insulin is a polypeptide hormone of complex structure. It is extracted mainly from pork pancreas and purified by crystallisation; it can also be made biosynthetically by recombinant DNA technology using *Escherichia coli* or semisynthetically by enzymatic modification of porcine material (see under Human Insulins, below). All insulin preparations are to a greater or lesser extent immunogenic in man but immunological resistance to insulin action is uncommon.

Insulin is inactivated by gastro-intestinal enzymes, and must therefore be given by injection; the subcutaneous route is ideal for most circumstances. It is usually injected into the upper arms, thighs, buttocks, or abdomen; there may be increased absorption from a limb site if the limb is used in strenuous exercise. Insulin is most readily administered by injection devices ('pens') (section 6.1.1.3) which hold insulin in cartridge form and meter the required dose. The more conventional syringe and needle is still preferred by many and is also required for insulins not available in cartridge form. Subcutaneous insulin injections generally cause no problems although fat hypertrophy is not rare; to some extent it can be avoided by rotating the injection sites. Local allergic reactions are now scarcely seen.

Insulin can also be given by continuous subcutaneous infusion using soluble insulin in an infusion pump. This technique has a limited place in the treatment of diabetes, and provides for continuous basal insulin infusion with prandial boosts. There are many disadvantages to the technique. Patients using it must be well-motivated, reliable, and able to monitor their own blood glucose, and must have access to expert advice both day and night.

CHOICE OF TREATMENT. About 25% of diabetics require insulin treatment; apart from those presenting in ketoacidosis, insulin is needed by most of those with a rapid onset of symptoms, weight loss, weakness, and sometimes vomiting, often associated with ketonuria. The majority of those who are obese can be managed by restriction of carbohydrate or energy intake alone or with the subsequent administration of oral hypoglycaemic drugs. Most children require insulin from the outset.

MANAGEMENT OF DIABETIC PATIENTS. The aim of treatment is to achieve the best possible control of plasma glucose without making the patient obsessional, and avoiding disabling hypoglycaemia; close co-operation is needed between the patient and the medical team since good control of insulin-dependent patients reduces the incidence of complications. Mixtures of available insulin preparations may be required and these combinations have to be worked out for the individual patient. Insulin requirements may be affected by variations in lifestyle, infection, and corticosteroids. In pregnancy insulin requirements should be assessed frequently by an experienced diabetic physician.

Many patients now monitor their own blood glucose concentrations using blood glucose strips preferably with an electronic meter. Since blood glucose concentrations oscillate substantially throughout the day, 'normoglycaemia' cannot always be achieved throughout a 24-hour period without causing damaging hypoglycaemia. It is therefore best to recommend that patients should maintain blood glucose concentrations of between 4 and 10 mmol/litre for most of the time, while accepting that on occasions, for brief periods, they will be above or below these values. Patients should be advised to look for 'peaks' and 'troughs' of blood glucose, and to adjust their insulin dosage only once or twice weekly. Overall it is ideal to aim for an HbA_{1c} level of less than 7% (normal range 4–6%) or an HbA_1 of less than 8.8% (normal range 5.0–7.5%) although this is not always possible without causing disabling hypoglycaemia. Fructosamine can also be used for assessment of control: this is a simpler and cheaper but less reliable measurement of glycated serum proteins.

The energy and carbohydrate intake must be adequate to allow normal growth and development but obesity must be avoided. The carbohydrate intake must be regulated and should be distributed throughout the day. Fine control of plasma glucose can be achieved by moving portions of carbohydrate from one meal to another without altering the total intake.

Insulin doses are determined on an individual basis, by gradually increasing the dose but avoiding troublesome hypoglycaemic reactions.

There are 3 main types of insulin preparations:

1. those of **short** duration which have a relatively rapid onset of action, namely soluble forms of insulin;
2. those with an **intermediate** action, e.g. Isophane Insulin Injection and Insulin Zinc Suspension; and
3. those whose action is slower in onset and lasts for **long** periods, e.g. Human Ultratard®.

The *duration of action* of different insulin preparations varies considerably from one patient to another, and needs to be assessed for every individual; those indicated below are only approximations. The type of insulin used and its dose and frequency of administration depend on the particular needs of the patient. Most patients are best started on insulins of intermediate action twice daily and a short-acting insulin can later be added to cover any hyperglycaemia which may follow breakfast or evening meal.

EXAMPLES OF RECOMMENDED INSULIN REGIMENS

1. Short-acting insulin *mixed* with Intermediate-acting insulin: twice daily (before meals)

2. Short-acting insulin *mixed* with Intermediate-acting insulin: before breakfast
Short-acting insulin: before evening meal
Intermediate-acting insulin: at bedtime

3. Short-acting insulin: three times daily (before breakfast, midday and evening meal)
Intermediate-acting insulin: at bedtime

4. Intermediate-acting insulin *with or without* Short-acting insulin: once daily either before breakfast or at bedtime suffices for some non-insulin dependent (type2) diabetic patients needing insulin

HUMAN INSULINS. There are differences in the amino-acid sequence in animal insulins, human insulins and the human insulin analogue, insulin lispro. Most available insulins are either porcine in origin or of human sequence prepared by modification of porcine material (emp) or biosynthetically (crb, prb, or pyr). Preparations of human sequence insulin should theoretically be less immunogenic, but in trials no real advantage has been shown.

HYPOGLYCAEMIA. This is a potential hazard for all patients receiving insulin, therefore much of their instruction must be directed towards avoiding it.

The conversion from beef to human sequence insulin should always be undertaken with specialist advice; it is usual to reduce the total dose by about 10%, with careful monitoring for the first few days.

When changing from porcine to human sequence insulin, a dose change is not usually needed, but careful monitoring is advised.

Loss of warning of hypoglycaemia is a common problem among insulin-treated patients and can be a serious hazard, especially for drivers. The cause is not known, but very tight control of diabetes appears to lower the blood glucose concentration needed to trigger hypoglycaemic symptoms. Beta-blockers can also blunt hypoglycaemic awareness (and can delay recovery).

Some patients have reported loss of warning of hypoglycaemia after transfer to human insulin. Patients should be warned of this possibility and if they believe that human insulin is responsible for their loss of warning it is reasonable to transfer them back to porcine insulin. When prescribing insulin great care should be taken to specify whether a human or an animal preparation is required. Indications for changing from animal to human preparations must be very carefully considered in the light of these reported problems. Beef insulin preparations are still available for patients who specifically request them

A very small number of insulin-dependent diabetic patients have been reported to have died in bed without known cause. There is no evidence that human insulin was responsible and the cause is still under investigation.

DRIVING. Car drivers need to be particularly careful to avoid hypoglycaemia (see above) and should be warned of the problems. They should normally check their blood glucose concentration before driving and, on long journeys, at intervals of approximately two hours. If hypoglycaemia occurs a car driver should switch off the ignition until recovery is complete, which may take up to 15 minutes or longer. Driving is not permitted when hypoglycaemic awareness has been lost.

DIABETES AND SURGERY. When an insulin-dependent diabetic patient requires surgery that is likely to require an intravenous infusion for longer than 12 hours the following regimen provides for intravenous administration of insulin (for an indefinite period).

Give an injection of the patient's **usual insulin** *on the night before the operation.*

Start an intravenous infusion of glucose 5% containing potassium chloride 10 mmol per litre *early on the day of the operation* and run at a constant rate appropriate to the patient's fluid requirements (usually 125 mL per hour); make up a solution of **soluble insulin** 1 unit/mL in sodium chloride 0.9% and infuse intravenously using a syringe pump piggybacked to the intravenous infusion.

The rate of the insulin infusion should normally be:

Blood glucose < 4 mmol/litre, *give* 0.5 units/hour
Blood glucose 4–15 mmol/litre, *give* 2 units/hour
Blood glucose 15–20 mmol/litre, *give* 4 units/hour
Blood glucose > 20 mmol/litre, *review*

In resistant cases (such as patients who are shocked or severely ill or those receiving corticosteroids or sympathomimetics) 2–4 times these rates or even more may be needed.

If a syringe pump is not available **soluble insulin** 16 units/litre should be added to the intravenous infusion of glucose 5% containing potassium chloride 10 mmol per litre (provided the patient is not hyperkalaemic) and the infusion run at the rate appropriate to the patient's fluid requirements (usually 125 mL per hour) with the insulin dose adjusted as follows:

Blood glucose < 4 mmol/litre, *give* 8 units/litre
Blood glucose 4–15 mmol/litre, *give* 16 units/litre
Blood glucose 15–20 mmol/litre, *give* 32 units/litre
Blood glucose > 20 mmol/litre, *review*

The rate of intravenous infusion depends on the volume depletion, cardiac function, age, and other factors. Blood glucose concentrations should be measured pre-operatively then every 2 hours until stable then every 6 hours. Intravenous insulin lasts for only a few minutes therefore infusion must not be stopped unless the patient becomes frankly hypoglycaemic (blood glucose < 3 mmol/litre) in which case it should be stopped for up to 30 minutes. The amount of potassium chloride in the infusion needs to be assessed for the individual patient by regular measurement of serum electrolytes (at least once daily). Sodium chloride 0.9% infusion should be substituted for glucose 5% if the blood glucose is persistently above 15 mmol/litre.

After recovery, once the patient starts to eat and drink, give subcutaneous insulin *before breakfast* and stop intravenous insulin 30 minutes later; the dose may need to be 10–20% more than usual if the patient is still in bed or unwell. If the patient was not previously receiving insulin, initially give 30–40 units daily in four divided doses using soluble before meals and intermediate-acting at bedtime and adjust amount from day to day. Patients with hyperglycaemia often relapse after conversion back to subcutaneous insulin calling for one of the following approaches:

additional doses of soluble insulin at any of the four injection times (before meals or bedtime) *or*

temporary addition of intravenous insulin infusion (while continuing the subcutaneous regimen) until blood glucose concentration is satisfactory *or*

complete reversion to the intravenous regimen (especially if the patient is unwell).

UNITS. The word 'unit' should **not** be abbreviated.

6.1.1.1 SHORT-ACTING INSULINS

Soluble Insulin is a short-acting form of insulin. For maintenance regimens it is usual to inject it 15 to 30 minutes before meals.

Soluble insulin is the only appropriate form of insulin for use in diabetic emergencies and at the time of surgical operations. It has the great advantage that it can be given intravenously and intramuscularly, as well as subcutaneously.

When injected subcutaneously, soluble insulin has a rapid onset of action (after 30 to 60 minutes), a peak action between 2 and 4 hours, and a duration of action of up to 8 hours. Human sequence preparations tend to have a more rapid onset and a shorter overall duration.

When injected intravenously, soluble insulin has a very short half-life of only about 5 minutes and its effect disappears within 30 minutes.

The human insulin analogue, **insulin lispro**, has a more rapid onset of action than soluble insulin; it can be given subcutaneously very close to a meal. Insulin lispro has a shorter duration of action than soluble insulin

---

SOLUBLE INSULIN
(Insulin Injection; Neutral Insulin)

A sterile solution of insulin (i.e. bovine or porcine) or of human insulin; pH 6.6–8.0

Indications: diabetes mellitus; diabetic ketoacidosis (section 6.1.3)

Cautions: see notes above; reduce dose in renal impairment; **interactions:** Appendix 1 (antidiabetics)

Side-effects: see notes above; local reactions and fat hypertrophy at injection site; overdose causes hypoglycaemia

Dose: by subcutaneous, intramuscular, or intravenous injection or intravenous infusion, according to patient's requirements

COUNSELLING. Show bottle to patient and confirm that patient is expecting the version dispensed

Highly purified animal

Hypurin Neutral® (CP)

Injection, soluble insulin (bovine, highly purified) 100 units/mL. Net price 10-mL vial = £16.80

*Pork Velosulin® (Novo Nordisk, Wellcome)

Injection, soluble insulin (porcine, highly purified) 100 units/mL. Net price 10-mL vial = £6.58

* formerly Velosulin®

Human sequence

Human Actrapid® (Novo Nordisk)

Injection, soluble insulin (human, pyr) 100 units/mL. Net price 10-mL vial = £9.42; 5 × 1.5-mL Penfill® cartridge (for NHS NovoPen® devices) = £7.50; 5 × 3-mL Actrapid® prefilled disposable injection devices (range 2–78 units, allowing 2-unit dosage adjustments) = £26.33

Human Velosulin® (Novo Nordisk, Wellcome)

Injection, soluble insulin (human, emp) 100 units/mL. Net price 10-mL vial = £9.42

Humulin S® (Lilly)

Injection, soluble insulin (human, prb) 100 units/mL. Net price 10-mL vial = £9.98; 5 × 1.5-mL cartridge (for NHS B-D pen®) = £9.13; 5 × 3-mL Humaject S® prefilled disposable injection devices (range 2–96 units, allowing 2-unit dosage adjustment) = £23.70

Mixed preparations, see Biphasic Insulin and Biphasic Isophane Insulin (section 6.1.1.2)

Cautionary label wordings, see inside back cover

INSULIN LISPRO

(Recombinant human insulin analogue)

Indications: diabetes mellitus

Cautions; Side-effects: see under Soluble Insulin

Dose: by subcutaneous injection, according to patient's response

COUNSELLING. Show bottle to patient and confirm that patient is expecting the version dispensed

▼ **Humalog®** (Lilly)

Injection, insulin lispro (recombinant human insulin analogue) 100 units/mL. Net price 10-mL vial = £15.71; 5 × 1.5-mL cartridge (for NHS B-D Pen® or NHS Diapen®) = £13.39

6.1.1.2 INTERMEDIATE- AND LONG-ACTING INSULINS

When given by subcutaneous injection intermediate- and long-acting insulins have an onset of action of approximately 1–2 hours, a maximal effect at 4–12 hours, and a duration of 16–35 hours. Some are given twice daily in conjunction with short-acting (soluble) insulin, and others are given once daily, particularly in elderly patients. They can be mixed with soluble insulin in the syringe, essentially retaining the properties of the two components, although there may be some blunting of the initial effect of the soluble insulin component (especially on mixing with protamine zinc insulin, see below).

Isophane Insulin is a suspension of insulin with protamine which is of particular value for initiation of twice-daily insulin regimens. Patients usually mix isophane with soluble insulin but ready-mixed preparations may be appropriate (**Biphasic Isophane Insulin**).

Biphasic Insulin is another ready-mixed insulin suitable for twice-daily injection.

Insulin Zinc Suspension (Amorphous) has an intermediate duration of action and **Insulin Zinc Suspension (Crystalline)** a more prolonged duration of action. These preparations may be used independently or in **Insulin Zinc Suspension** (30% amorphous, 70% crystalline).

Protamine Zinc Insulin is usually given once daily in conjunction with short-acting (soluble) insulin. It has the drawback of binding with the soluble insulin when mixed in the same syringe, and is now rarely used.

INSULIN ZINC SUSPENSION

(Insulin Zinc Suspension (Mixed); I. Z. S.)

A sterile neutral suspension of bovine and/or porcine insulin or of human insulin in the form of a complex obtained by the addition of a suitable zinc salt; consists of rhombohedral crystals (10–40 microns) and of particles of no uniform shape (not exceeding 2 microns)

Indications: diabetes mellitus (long acting)

Cautions; Side-effects: see under Soluble Insulin (section 6.1.1.1)

Dose: by subcutaneous injection, according to patient's requirements

COUNSELLING. Show bottle to patient and confirm that patient is expecting the version dispensed

Highly purified animal

Hypurin Lente® (CP)

Injection, insulin zinc suspension (bovine, highly purified) 100 units/mL. Net price 10-mL vial = £16.80

Lentard MC® (Novo Nordisk)

Injection, insulin zinc suspension (bovine and porcine, highly purified) 100 units/mL. Net price 10-mL vial = £5.78

Human sequence

Human Monotard® (Novo Nordisk)

Injection, insulin zinc suspension (human, pyr) 100 units/mL. Net price 10-mL vial = £9.42

Humulin Lente® (Lilly)

Injection, insulin zinc suspension (human, prb) 100 units/mL. Net price 10-mL vial = £10.98

INSULIN ZINC SUSPENSION (AMORPHOUS)

(Amorph. I. Z. S.)

A sterile neutral suspension of bovine or porcine insulin in the form of a complex obtained by the addition of a suitable zinc salt; consists of particles of no uniform shape (not exceeding 2 microns)

Indications: diabetes mellitus (intermediate acting)

Cautions; Side-effects: see under Soluble Insulin (section 6.1.1.1)

Dose: by subcutaneous injection, according to patient's requirements

COUNSELLING. Show bottle to patient and confirm that patient is expecting the version dispensed

Semitard MC® (Novo Nordisk)

Injection, insulin zinc suspension (amorphous) (porcine, highly purified) 100 units/mL. Net price 10-mL vial = £6.28

INSULIN ZINC SUSPENSION (CRYSTALLINE)

(Cryst. I. Z. S.)

A sterile neutral suspension of bovine insulin or of human insulin in the form of a complex obtained by the addition of a suitable zinc salt; consists of rhombohedral crystals (10–40 microns)

Indications: diabetes mellitus (long acting)

Cautions; Side-effects: see under Soluble Insulin (section 6.1.1.1)

Dose: by subcutaneous injection, according to patient's requirements

COUNSELLING. Show bottle to patient and confirm that patient is expecting the version dispensed

Human sequence

Human Ultratard® (Novo Nordisk)

Injection, insulin zinc suspension, crystalline (human, pyr) 100 units/mL. Net price 10-mL vial = £9.42

Humulin Zn® (Lilly)

Injection, insulin zinc suspension, crystalline (human, prb) 100 units/mL. Net price 10-mL vial = £10.98

ISOPHANE INSULIN

(Isophane Insulin Injection; Isophane Protamine Insulin Injection; Isophane Insulin (NPH))

A sterile suspension of bovine or porcine insulin or of human insulin in the form of a complex obtained by the addition of protamine sulphate or another suitable protamine

Indications: diabetes mellitus (intermediate acting)

Cautions; Side-effects: see under Soluble Insulin (section 6.1.1.1); protamine may cause allergic reactions

Dose: by subcutaneous injection, according to patient's requirements

COUNSELLING. Show bottle to patient and confirm that patient is expecting the version dispensed

Highly purified animal
Hypurin Isophane® (CP)

Injection, isophane insulin (bovine, highly purified) 100 units/mL. Net price 10-mL vial = £16.80

* Pork Insulatard® (Novo Nordisk, Wellcome)

Injection, isophane insulin (porcine, highly purified) 100 units/mL. Net price 10-mL vial = £6.58
*formerly Insulatard®—method of manufacture changed, patients should monitor blood glucose regularly during transition

Human sequence
*Human Insulatard® ge (Novo Nordisk)

Injection, isophane insulin (human, pyr) 100 units/mL. Net price 10-mL vial = £9.42; 5 × 1.5-mL Penfill® cartridge (for NHS Novopen® devices) = £7.90; 5 × 3-mL prefilled disposable injection devices (range 2–78 units allowing 2-unit dosage adjustment) = £26.33
*formerly Human Protaphane®

Humulin I® (Lilly)

Injection, isophane insulin (human, prb) 100 units/mL. Net price 10-mL vial = £9.98; 5 × 1.5-mL cartridge (for NHS B-D pen®) = £9.13; 5 × 3-mL Humaject I® prefilled disposable injection devices (range 2–96 units, allowing 2-unit dosage adjustment) = £23.70

Mixed preparations, see Biphasic Isophane Insulin (below)

PROTAMINE ZINC INSULIN

(Protamine Zinc Insulin Injection)

A sterile suspension of insulin in the form of a complex obtained by the addition of a suitable protamine and zinc chloride; this preparation was included in BP 1980 but is not included in BP 1988

Indications: diabetes mellitus (long acting)

Cautions; Side-effects: see under Soluble Insulin (section 6.1.1.1); protamine may cause allergic reactions; see also notes above

Dose: by subcutaneous injection, according to patient's requirements

COUNSELLING. Show bottle to patient and confirm that patient is expecting the version dispensed

Hypurin Protamine Zinc® (CP)

Injection, protamine zinc insulin (bovine, highly purified) 100 units/mL. Net price 10-mL vial = £19.02

BIPHASIC INSULINS

BIPHASIC INSULIN

(Biphasic Insulin Injection)

A sterile suspension of crystals containing bovine insulin in a solution of porcine insulin

Indications: diabetes mellitus (intermediate acting)

Cautions; Side-effects: see under Soluble Insulin (section 6.1.1.1)

Dose: by subcutaneous injection, according to patient's requirements

COUNSELLING. Show bottle to patient and confirm that patient is expecting the version dispensed

Rapitard MC® (Novo Nordisk)

Injection, biphasic insulin (highly purified) 100 units/mL. Net price 10-mL vial = £5.78

BIPHASIC ISOPHANE INSULIN

(Biphasic Isophane Insulin Injection)

A sterile buffered suspension of porcine insulin complexed with protamine sulphate (or another suitable protamine) in a solution of porcine insulin *or* a sterile buffered suspension of human insulin complexed with protamine sulphate (or another suitable protamine) in a solution of human insulin

Indications: diabetes mellitus (intermediate acting)

Cautions; Side-effects: see under Soluble Insulin (section 6.1.1.1); protamine may cause allergic reactions

Dose: by subcutaneous injection, according to the patient's requirements

COUNSELLING. Show bottle to patient and confirm that patient is expecting the version dispensed

Highly purified animal
* Pork Mixtard 30® (Novo Nordisk Wellcome)

Injection, biphasic isophane insulin (porcine, highly purified), 30% soluble, 70% isophane, 100 units/mL. Net price 10-mL vial = £6.58
*formerly Mixtard 30/70®—method of manufacture changed, patients should monitor blood glucose regularly during transition

Human sequence
*Human Mixtard® 30 ge (Novo Nordisk)

Injection, biphasic isophane insulin (human, pyr), 30% soluble, 70% isophane, 100 units/mL. Net price 10-mL vial = £9.42
*formerly Human Actraphane 30/70®

*Human Mixtard® 10 (Novo Nordisk)

Injection, biphasic isophane insulin (human, pyr), 10% soluble, 90% isophane, 100 units/mL. Net price 5 × 1.5-mL Penfill® cartridge (for NHS Novopen® devices) = £7.90; 5 × 3-mL prefilled disposable injection devices (range 2–78 units, allowing 2-unit dosage adjustment) = £26.33
*formerly PenMix 10/90®

*Human Mixtard® 20 (Novo Nordisk)

Injection, biphasic isophane insulin (human, pyr), 20% soluble, 80% isophane, 100 units/mL. Net price 5 × 1.5-mL Penfill® cartridge (for NHS Novopen® devices) = £7.90; 5 × 3-mL prefilled disposable injection devices (range 2–78 units, allowing 2-unit dosage adjustment) = £26.33
*formerly PenMix 20/80®

*Human Mixtard® 30 (Novo Nordisk)

Injection, biphasic isophane insulin (human, pyr), 30% soluble, 70% isophane, 100 units/mL. Net price 5 × 1.5-mL Penfill® cartridge (for NHS Novopen® devices) = £7.90; 5 × 3-mL prefilled disposable injection devices (range 2–78 units, allowing 2-unit dosage adjustment) = £26.33
*formerly PenMix 30/70®

*Human Mixtard® 40 (Novo Nordisk)

Injection, biphasic isophane insulin (human, pyr), 40% soluble, 60% isophane, 100 units/mL. Net price 5 × 1.5-mL Penfill® cartridge (for NHS Novopen® devices) = £7.90; 5 × 3-mL prefilled disposable injection devices (range 2–78 units, allowing 2-unit dosage adjustments) = £26.33
*formerly PenMix 40/60®

*Human Mixtard® 50 (Novo Nordisk)

Injection, biphasic isophane insulin (human, pyr), 50% soluble, 50% isophane, 100 units/mL. Net price 5 × 1.5-mL Penfill® cartridge (for NHS Novopen® devices) = £7.90; 5 × 3-mL prefilled disposable injection devices (range 2–78 units, allowing 2-unit dosage adjustment) = £26.33
*formerly PenMix 50/50®

Humulin M1® (Lilly)

Injection, biphasic isophane insulin (human, prb), 10% soluble, 90% isophane, 100 units/mL. Net price 10-mL vial = £10.98; 5 × 1.5-mL cartridge (for NHS B-D Pen® or NHS Diapen®) = £9.13; 5 × 3-mL cartridge (for NHS B-D Pen® +3,0ml) = £18.26; 5 × 3-mL Humaject M1® prefilled disposable injection devices (range 2–96 units, allowing 2-unit dosage adjustment) = £23.70

Humulin M2® (Lilly)

Injection, biphasic isophane insulin (human, prb), 20% soluble, 80% isophane, 100 units/mL. Net price 10-mL vial = £9.98; 5 × 1.5-mL cartridge (for NHS B-D Pen® or NHS Diapen®) = £9.13; 5 × 3-mL cartridge (for NHS B-D Pen® +3,0ml) = £18.26; 5 × 3-mL Humaject M2® prefilled disposable injection devices (range 2–96 units, allowing 2-unit dosage adjustment) = £23.70

Humulin M3® (Lilly)

Injection, biphasic isophane insulin (human, prb), 30% soluble, 70% isophane, 100 units/mL. Net price 10-mL vial =£9.98; 5 × 1.5-mL cartridge (for NHS B-D Pen® or NHS Diapen®) = £9.13; 5 × 3-mL cartridge (for NHS B-D Pen® +3,0ml) = £18.26; 5 × 3-mL Humaject M3® prefilled disposable injection devices (range 2–96 units, allowing 2-unit dosage adjustment) = £23.70

Humulin M4® (Lilly)

Injection, biphasic isophane insulin (human, prb), 40% soluble, 60% isophane, 100 units/mL. Net price 10-mL vial = £10.98; 5 × 1.5-mL cartridge (for NHS B-D Pen® or NHS Diapen®) = £9.13; 5 × 3-mL cartridge (for NHS B-D Pen® +3,0ml) = £18.26; 5 × 3-mL Humaject M4® prefilled disposable injection devices (range 2–96 units, allowing 2-unit dosage adjustment) = £23.70

Humulin M5® (Lilly)

Injection, biphasic isophane insulin (human, prb), 50% soluble, 50% isophane, 100 units/mL. Net price 10-mL vial = £10.98; 5 × 1.5-mL cartridge (for NHS B-D Pen® or NHS Diapen®) = £9.13; 5 × 3-mL cartridge (for NHS B-D Pen® +3,0ml) = £18.26

6.1.1.3 HYPODERMIC EQUIPMENT

Patients should be advised on the safe disposal of lancets, single-use syringes, and needles. Suitable arrangements for the safe disposal of contaminated waste must be made before these products are prescribed for patients who are carriers of infectious diseases.

Injection devices

NHS Autopen® (Owen Mumford)

Injection device, for use with Lilly and Novo Nordisk 1.5-mL insulin cartridges; allows adjustment of dosage in multiples of one unit, max. 16 units (single unit version); two units, max. 32 units (two unit version). Net price (both) = £13.96

NHS B-D Pen® (Becton Dickinson)

Injection devices, for use with Lilly insulin cartridges; B-D Pen® (for 1.5-mL cartridges) allows adjustment of dosage in multiples of one unit, max. 30 units, net price = £23.86 (also available from clinics); B-D Pen® +3,0m (for 3-mL cartridges) allows adjustment of dosage in multiples of one unit, max. 69 units (available only from clinics)

NHS Diapen® (Lilly)

Injection devices for use with Humulin® 1.5-mL insulin cartridges; allows adjustment of dosage in multiples of one unit, max.18 units (Diapen® 1); two units, max. 36 units (Diapen® 2). Net price (both) = £49.00

NHS NovoPen® (Novo Nordisk)

Injection devices, for use with Penfill® insulin cartridges; allows adjustment of dosage in multiples of two units, max. 36 units (NovoPen® II) *or* one unit, max. 40 units (NovoPen® Classic, NovoPen® Fun). Available only from clinics

NHS Penject® (Hypoguard)

Injection device, for use with B-D U100 1mL syringe; allows adjustment of dosage in multiples of two units. Net price = £21.25

Lancets— sterile, single use

Type A (Drug Tariff). Cylindrical mount fluted longitudinally; compatible with NHS Autoclix® (BM Diagnostics), NHS B-D Lancer® (Becton Dickinson) NHS Glucolet® (Bayer Diagnostics), NHS Monoject® (Sherwood), NHS Penlet® II (Lifescan) and NHS Soft Touch® (BM Diagnostics) finger-pricking devices

Available from Bayer (Baylet®, net price 200-lancet pack = £6.08), Becton Dickinson (B-D Microfine® +, net price 200-lancet pack = £6.13), Gainor Medical (Cleanlet® 25, net price 100-lancet pack = £3.19; 200 lancet pack = £6.08) Owen Mumford (Unilet G® Superlite net price 100-lancet pack = £3.17; 200-lancet pack £6.01; Unilet® Universal ComforTouch, net price 100 lancet pack = £3.17; 200-lancet pack = £6.01), Sherwood (Monolet®, net price 100-lancet pack = £3.28; 200-lancet pack = £6.24; Monolet Extra®, net price 100-lancet pack = £3.28)

Type B (Drug Tariff). Cylindrical mount with concentric ribs; compatible with NHS Autolet® (Owen Mumford) and NHS Glucolet® (Bayer Diagnostics) finger-pricking devices

Available from Bayer Diagnostics (Ames®, net price 100-lancet pack = £3.19; 200-lancet pack = £6.08), Gainor Medical (Cleanlet 25XL, net price 100-lancet pack = £3.19; 200-lancet pack = £6.08), Owen Mumford (Unilet® Superlite, net price 100-lancet pack = £3.17; 200-lancet pack = £6.01; Unilet® Universal Comfer-Touch, net price 100-lancet pack = £3.17; 200-lancet pack = £6.01)

Needles

Hypodermic Needle , Sterile single use (Drug Tariff). For use with re-usable glass syringe, sizes 0.5 mm (25G), 0.45 mm (26G), 0.4 mm (27G). Net price 100-needle pack = £2.20

Available from Becton Dickinson (Microlance®), Sherwood (Monoject®)

Needle Clipping (Chopping) Device (Drug Tariff). Consisting of a clipper to remove needle from its hub and container from which cut-off needles cannot be retrieved; designed to hold 1200 needles, not suitable for use with lancets. Net price = £1.08

Available from Becton Dickinson (B-D Safe-clip®)

Syringes

Clickcount® (Hypoguard). Calibrated glass with Luer taper conical fitting, supplied with dosage chart and strong box for blind patients for whom the Pre-Set syringe is unsuitable. Net price 1 mL = £17.42

Hypodermic Syringe (Drug Tariff). Calibrated glass with Luer taper conical fitting, for use with U100 insulin. Net price 0.5 mL and 1 mL = £13.21

Available from Rand Rocket (Abcare®)

Pre-Set U100 Insulin Syringe (Drug Tariff). Calibrated glass with Luer taper conical fitting, supplied with dosage chart and strong box, for blind patients. Net price 1 mL = £20.11

Available from Rand Rocket

U100 Insulin Syringe with Needle (Drug Tariff). Disposable with fixed or separate needle for single use or single patient-use, colour coded orange, 0.45 mm (26G), 0.4 mm (27G), 0.36 mm (28G), 0.33 mm (29G). Net price 10 (with needle) , 0.3 mL = £1.19; 0.5 mL = £1.15; 1 mL = £1.16

Available from Becton Dickinson (B-D Micro-Fine®+, Plastipak®), Braun (Omnikan®), Rand Rocket (Clinipak®), Sherwood (Monoject® Ultra), Steriseal (Insupak®), Terumo (Myjector®)

Syringe carrying case (Drug Tariff). For use with Clickcount® and Hypodermic insulin syringe. Net price 1 = £1.93; screw cap (to convert for use with Pre-Set U 100 insulin syringe) = 71p

6.1.2   Oral antidiabetic drugs

6.1.2.1 Sulphonylureas
6.1.2.2 Biguanides
6.1.2.3 Other antidiabetics

Oral antidiabetic drugs are used for non-insulin-dependent (type 2) diabetes; they should not be prescribed until patients have been shown not to respond adequately to at least three months' restriction of energy and carbohydrate intake. They should be used to augment the effect of diet, and not to replace it.

6.1.2.1 SULPHONYLUREAS

The sulphonylureas act mainly by augmenting insulin secretion and consequently are effective only when some residual pancreatic beta-cell activity is present; during long-term administration they also have an extrapancreatic action. All may lead to hypoglycaemia 4 hours or more after food but this is usually an indication of overdose, and is relatively uncommon.

There are several sulphonylureas but there is no evidence for any difference in their effectiveness. Only **chlorpropamide** has appreciably more side-effects, mainly because of its very prolonged duration of action and the consequent hazard of hypoglycaemia (but also as a result of the common and unpleasant chlorpropamide-alcohol flush phenomenon). Selection of an individual sulphonylurea depends otherwise on the age of the patient and renal function (see below), or more generally just on personal preference.

Elderly patients are particularly prone to the dangers of hypoglycaemia when long-acting sulphonylureas are used; **chlorpropamide**, and also **glibenclamide**, should be avoided in these patients and replaced by others, such as **gliclazide** or **tolbutamide**.

CAUTIONS AND CONTRA-INDICATIONS. These drugs tend to encourage weight gain and should only be prescribed if poor control and symptoms persist despite adequate attempts at dieting. They should not be used during breast-feeding, and caution is needed in the elderly and those with hepatic and renal insufficiency because of the hazard of hypoglycaemia. The short-acting tolbutamide may be used in renal impairment, as may gliquidone and gliclazide which are principally metabolised and inactivated in the liver. Sulphonylureas should be avoided in porphyria (see section 9.8.2).

Insulin therapy should be instituted temporarily during intercurrent illness (such as myocardial infarction, coma, infection, and trauma) and during surgery since control of diabetes with the sulphonylureas is often inadequate in such circumstances. Insulin therapy is also usually substituted during pregnancy (see also Appendix 4). Sulphonylureas are contra-indicated in the presence of ketoacidosis.

SIDE-EFFECTS. These are generally mild and infrequent and include gastro-intestinal disturbances and headache..

Chlorpropamide may cause facial flushing after drinking alcohol; this effect is not normally witnessed with other sulphonylureas. Chlorpropamide may also enhance antidiuretic hormone and very rarely cause hyponatraemia.

Sensitivity reactions (usually in first 6–8 weeks of therapy) include transient rashes which rarely progress to erythema multiforme and exfoliative dermatitis, fever, and jaundice; photosensitivity has also rarely been reported with chlorpropamide. Blood disorders are rare too but include thrombocytopenia, agranulocytosis, and aplastic anaemia. All these phenomena are very rare.

CHLORPROPAMIDE

Indications: diabetes mellitus (for use in diabetes insipidus, see section 6.5.2)

Cautions; Contra-indications; Side-effects: see notes above; **interactions:** Appendix 1 (antidiabetics)

Dose: initially 250 mg daily (elderly patients 100–125 mg but avoid—see notes above), adjusted according to response; max. 500 mg daily; taken with breakfast

PoM **Chlorpropamide** (Non-proprietary)
Tablets, chlorpropamide 100 mg, net price 20 = 22p; 250 mg, 20 = 32p. Label:4
Available from APS, Cox, CP, Kent

PoM **Diabinese**® (Pfizer)
Tablets, scored, chlorpropamide 100 mg, net price 28-tab pack = 56p; 250 mg, 28-tab pack = £1.23. Label: 4

GLIBENCLAMIDE

Indications: diabetes mellitus

Cautions; Contra-indications; Side-effects: see notes above; **interactions:** Appendix 1 (antidiabetics)

Dose: initially 5 mg daily (elderly patients 2.5 mg (but see also notes above)), adjusted according to response; max. 15 mg daily; taken with breakfast

PoM **Glibenclamide** (Non-proprietary)
Tablets, glibenclamide 2.5 mg, net price 20 = 30p; 5 mg, 20 = 32p
Available from APS (Libanil®), Ashbourne (Diabetamide®), Berk (Calabren®), Cox, CP, Generics, Hillcross, Kent (Gliken®), Lagap (Malix®), Norton

PoM **Daonil**® (Hoechst)
Tablets, scored, glibenclamide 5 mg. Net price 28-tab pack = £2.63

PoM **Semi-Daonil**® (Hoechst)
Tablets, scored, glibenclamide 2.5 mg. Net price 28-tab pack = £1.58

PoM **Euglucon**® (Roussel)
Tablets, glibenclamide 2.5 mg, net price 28-tab pack = £1.58; 5 mg (scored), 28-tab pack = £2.63

GLICLAZIDE

Indications: diabetes mellitus

Cautions; Contra-indications; Side-effects: see notes above; **interactions:** Appendix 1 (antidiabetics)

Dose: initially, 40–80 mg daily, adjusted according to response; up to 160 mg as a single dose, with breakfast; higher doses divided; max. 320 mg daily

PoM **Gliclazide** (Non-proprietary)
Tablets, scored, gliclazide 80 mg. Net price 60-tab pack = £7.00
Available form Norton

PoM **Diamicron**® (Servier)
Tablets, scored, gliclazide 80 mg. Net price 60-tab pack = £7.00

GLIPIZIDE

Indications: diabetes mellitus

Cautions; Contra-indications; Side-effects: see notes above; **interactions:** Appendix 1 (antidiabetics)

Dose: initially 2.5–5 mg daily, adjusted according to response; max. 40 mg daily; up to 15 mg may be given as a single dose before breakfast; higher doses divided

PoM **Glibenese**® (Pfizer)
Tablets, scored, glipizide 5 mg. Net price 56-tab pack = £3.63

PoM **Minodiab**® (Pharmacia)
Tablets, glipizide 2.5 mg, net price 60-tab pack = £3.31; 5 mg (scored), 60-tab pack = £3.54

GLIQUIDONE

Indications: diabetes mellitus

Cautions; Contra-indications; Side-effects: see notes above; **interactions:** Appendix 1 (antidiabetics)

Dose: initially 15 mg daily before breakfast, adjusted to 45–60 mg daily in 2 or 3 divided doses; max. single dose 60 mg, max. daily dose 180 mg

PoM **Glurenorm**® (Sanofi Winthrop)
Tablets, scored, gliquidone 30 mg. Net price 100-tab pack = £17.54

TOLAZAMIDE

Indications: diabetes mellitus

Cautions; Contra-indications; Side-effects: see notes above; **interactions:** Appendix 1 (antidiabetics)

Dose: initially 100–250 mg daily with breakfast adjusted according to response; max. 1 g daily; higher doses divided

PoM **Tolanase**® (Upjohn)
Tablets, both scored, tolazamide 100 mg, net price 100-tab pack = £5.65; 250 mg, 100-tab pack = £12.29

TOLBUTAMIDE

Indications: diabetes mellitus

Cautions; Contra-indications; Side-effects: see notes above; **interactions:** Appendix 1 (antidiabetics)

Dose: 0.5–1.5 g (max. 2 g) daily in divided doses (see notes above)

PoM **Tolbutamide** (Non-proprietary)
Tablets, tolbutamide 500 mg. Net price 20 = 34p
Available from APS, Cox, CP, Hillcross, Norton

PoM **Rastinon**® (Hoechst)
Tablets, scored, tolbutamide 500 mg. Net price 100-tab pack = £3.33

6.1.2.2 BIGUANIDES

Metformin, the only available biguanide, has a different mode of action from the sulphonylureas, and is not interchangeable with them. It exerts its effect mainly by decreasing gluconeogenesis and by increasing peripheral utilisation of glucose; since it only acts in the presence of endogenous insulin it is only effective in diabetics with some residual functioning pancreatic islet cells. Metformin is used in the treatment of non-insulin-dependent diabetics when strict dieting and sulphonylurea treatment have failed to control diabetes, especially in overweight patients, in whom it may be used first. It can be used alone or with a sulphonylurea. An important advantage of metformin is that hypoglycaemia is not usually a problem; other advantages are the lower incidence of weight gain and lower plasma insulin levels. It does not exert a hypoglycaemic action in non-diabetic subjects unless given in overdose. Gastro-intestinal side-effects are initially common, and may persist in some patients, particularly when very high doses such as 3 g daily are given.

Metformin is not free from the hazard of lactic acidosis but this occurs almost exclusively in patients with renal impairment, in whom it should not be used.

METFORMIN HYDROCHLORIDE
Indications: diabetes mellitus (see notes above)
Cautions: see notes above; **interactions:** Appendix 1 (antidiabetics)
Contra-indications: hepatic or renal impairment (withdraw if renal impairment suspected), predisposition to lactic acidosis, heart failure, severe infection or trauma, dehydration, alcohol dependence; pregnancy, breast-feeding
Side-effects: anorexia, nausea, vomiting, diarrhoea (usually transient), lactic acidosis (withdraw treatment), decreased vitamin-B_{12} absorption
Dose: 500 mg every 8 hours *or* 850 mg every 12 hours with or after food; max. 3 g daily in divided doses though most physicians limit this to 2 g daily (see notes above)

PoM **Metformin** (Non-proprietary)
Tablets, coated, metformin hydrochloride 500 mg, net price 20 = 36p; 850 mg, 20 = 60p. Label: 21
Available from APS, Berk, Cox, Hillcross, Lagap (Orabet®), Norton, Opus (Glucamet®)
PoM **Glucophage®** (Lipha)
Tablets, f/c, metformin hydrochloride 500 mg, net price 84-tab pack = £2.00; 850 mg, 56-tab pack = £2.22. Label: 21

6.1.2.3 OTHER ANTIDIABETICS

Acarbose, an inhibitor of intestinal alpha glucosidases, delays the digestion of starch and sucrose and hence the increase in blood glucose levels which follow a carbohydrate-containing meal. It has been recently introduced for the treatment of non-insulin-dependent (type 2) diabetes.

Guar gum, if taken in adequate quantities, results in some reduction of postprandial plasma-glucose concentrations in diabetes mellitus, probably by retarding carbohydrate absorption. It is also used to relieve symptoms of the dumping syndrome.

ACARBOSE
Indications: diabetes mellitus inadequately controlled by diet or by diet with oral hypoglycaemic agents
Cautions: monitor hepatic transaminase levels (higher doses); may enhance hypoglycaemic effects of insulin and sulphonylureas (hypoglycaemic episodes may be treated with oral glucose but not with sucrose); **interactions:** Appendix 1 (antidiabetics)
Contra-indications: pregnancy and breast-feeding; inflammatory bowel disease (e.g. ulcerative colitis, Crohn's disease), partial intestinal obstruction (or predisposition); hepatic impairment, severe renal impairment; hernia, history of abdominal surgery
Side-effects: flatulence, soft stools, diarrhoea (may need to reduce dose or withdraw), abdominal distension and pain
Note. Antacids not recommended for treating side-effects (unlikely to be beneficial)
Dose: 50 mg daily initially (to minimise side-effects) increased to 50 mg 3 times daily, then increased if necessary after 6–8 weeks to 100 mg 3 times daily; max. 200 mg 3 times daily; CHILD under 12 years not recommended
COUNSELLING. The tablets should either be chewed with first mouthful of food or swallowed whole with a little liquid immediately before food. In order to counteract possible hypoglycaemia, patients receiving insulin or a sulphonylurea as well as acarbose need to carry glucose (not sucrose—acarbose interferes with sucrose absorption)

PoM **Glucobay®** (Bayer)
Tablets, acarbose 50 mg, net price 90-tab pack = £14.10; 100 mg (scored). 90-tab pack = £17.70. Counselling, administration

GUAR GUM
Indications: see notes above
Cautions: maintain adequate fluid intake; **interactions:** Appendix 1 (guar gum)
COUNSELLING. Preparations that swell in contact with liquid should always be carefully swallowed with water and should not be taken immediately before going to bed.
Contra-indications: gastro-intestinal obstruction
Side-effects: flatulence, abdominal distension, intestinal obstruction

Guarem® (Rybar)
Granules, ivory, sugar-free, guar gum 5 g/sachet, net price 50 sachets = £8.70; 100 sachets = £15.67. Label: 13, counselling, administration
Dose: 5 g stirred into 200 mL fluid 3 times daily immediately before main meals (or sprinkled on food and eaten accompanied by 200 mL fluid)

6.1.3   Diabetic ketoacidosis

Soluble insulin, the only form of insulin that may be given intravenously, is used in the management of diabetic ketoacidotic and hyperosmolar non-ketotic coma. It is preferable to use the type of soluble insulin that the patient has been using previously. It is necessary to achieve and to maintain an adequate plasma-insulin concentration until the metabolic disturbance is brought under control.

Insulin is best given by *intravenous infusion*, using an infusion pump, and diluted to 1 unit/mL (care in mixing, see Appendix 6). Adequate plasma concentrations can usually be maintained with infusion rates of 6 units/hour for adults and 0.1 units/kg/hour for children. Blood glucose is expected to decrease by about 5 mmol/hour; if the response is inadequate the infusion rate can be doubled or quadrupled. When the plasma glucose has fallen to 10 mmol/litre the infusion rate can be reduced to 3 units/hour for adults (about 0.02 units/kg/hour for children) and continued until the patient is ready to take food by mouth. The insulin infusion should not be stopped before subcutaneous insulin has been started.

No matter how large, a bolus intravenous injection of insulin can only provide an adequate plasma concentration for a short time, therefore if facilities for intravenous infusion are not available the insulin is given by *intramuscular injection*. An initial loading dose of 20 units intramuscularly is followed by 6 units intramuscularly every hour until the plasma glucose concentration has fallen to 10 mmol/litre; intramuscular injections are then given every 2 hours. Although absorption of insulin is usually rapid after intramuscular injection, it may be impaired in the presence of hypotension and poor tissue perfusion; moreover depots of insulin may build up during treatment therefore late hypoglycaemia should be watched for and treated appropriately.

Intravenous replacement of fluid and electrolytes with **sodium chloride** intravenous infusion is an essential part of the management of ketoacidosis; **potassium chloride** is included in the infusion as appropriate to prevent the hypokalaemia induced by the insulin. **Sodium bicarbonate** infusion (1.26% or 2.74%) is only used in cases of extreme acidosis and shock since the acid-base disturbance is normally corrected by the insulin. **Glucose** solution (5%) is infused once the blood glucose has decreased below 10 mmol/litre but insulin infusion must continue. For glucose, see section 9.2.2.

6.1.4   Treatment of hypoglycaemia

Initially, glucose or 3 or 4 lumps of sugar should be taken with a little water. If necessary, this may be repeated in 10 to 15 minutes.

If hypoglycaemia causes unconsciousness, up to 50 mL of **50% glucose intravenous infusion** should be given intravenously (see section 9.2.2).

Glucagon can be given as an alternative to parenteral glucose in hypoglycaemia. It is a polypeptide hormone produced by the alpha cells of the islets of Langerhans. Its action is to increase plasma glucose concentration by mobilising glycogen stored in the liver. It has the advantage that it can be injected by any route (intramuscular, subcutaneous, or intravenous) in a dose of 1 mg (1 unit) in circumstances when an intravenous injection of glucose would be difficult or impossible to administer. It may be issued to close relatives of insulin-treated patients for emergency use in hypoglycaemic attacks. It is often advisable to prescribe on an 'if necessary' basis to hospitalised insulin-treated patients, so that it may be given rapidly by the nurses during a hypoglycaemic emergency. If not effective in 15 minutes intravenous glucose should be given.

GLUCAGON

Indications: see notes above and under Dose

Cautions: see notes above. Ineffective in chronic hypoglycaemia, starvation, and adrenal insufficiency

Contra-indications: insulinoma, phaeochromocytoma, glucagonoma

Side-effects: nausea, vomiting, diarrhoea, hypokalaemia, rarely hypersensitivity reactions

Dose: by subcutaneous, intramuscular, or intravenous injection, adults and children 0.5–1 unit; if no response within 15 minutes intravenous glucose must be given

Diagnostic aid, see data sheet

Beta-blocker poisoning, see p. 22

*Note.*1 unit of glucagon = 1 mg of glucagon or glucagon hydrochloride

PoM Glucagon Injection (Non-proprietary)

Injection powder for reconstitution, glucagon (as hydrochloride, with lactose). Net price 1-unit (1-mg) vial (Lilly) = £7.10;10-mg vial (Novo Nordisk) = £39.98 (both with diluent)

Note. If given in doses higher than 2 units (as in beta-blocker poisoning p. 22) reconstitute with water for injection instead of diluent

▼ **PoM GlucaGen® Kit** (Novo Nordisk)

Injection, powder for reconstitution, glucagon (rys) as hydrochloride with lactose. Net price 1-mg vial (with pre-filled syringe containing water for injection) = £19.95

CHRONIC HYPOGLYCAEMIA

Diazoxide, administered by mouth, is useful in the management of patients with chronic hypoglycaemia from excess endogenous insulin secretion, either from an islet cell tumour or islet cell hyperplasia. It has no place in the management of acute hypoglycaemia.

DIAZOXIDE

Indications: chronic intractable hypoglycaemia (for use in hypertensive crisis see section 2.5.1)

Cautions: ischaemic heart disease, pregnancy, labour, impaired renal function; haematological examinations and blood pressure monitoring required during prolonged treatment; growth, bone, and developmental checks in children; **interactions:** Appendix 1 (diazoxide)

Side-effects: anorexia, nausea, vomiting, hyperuricaemia, hypotension, oedema, tachycardia, arrhythmias, extrapyramidal effects; hypertrichosis on prolonged treatment
Dose: by mouth, adults and children, initially 5 mg/kg daily in 2–3 divided doses

PoM **Eudemine**® (Evans)
Tablets, diazoxide 50 mg. Net price 20 = £7.68

6.1.5 Treatment of diabetic nephropathy and neuropathy

DIABETIC NEPHROPATHY

Regular review of diabetic patients should include a test for urinary protein (using Albustix®). If this test is positive and the proteinuria is considered to be due to diabetic nephropathy then monitoring and treatment of blood pressure is imperative, and renal function should be assessed regularly.

Detection of microalbuminuria (as the earliest sign of nephropathy) is now recommended at least for younger insulin-dependent diabetic patients. If reagent strip tests (NHS Micral-Test®) are used and prove positive, the result should then be confirmed in the laboratory by radio-immunoassay. Test for microalbuminuria should be positive on at least three separate occasions before comments are made or action is taken. Tight control of diabetes is important and antihypertensive therapy is needed when microalbuminuria is established and increasing. The blood pressure must be kept below 140 mmHg systolic and 90 mmHg diastolic.

There is now some evidence that ACE inhibitors (see section 2.5.5.1) may have a specific advantage over other antihypertensive drugs in diabetic nephropathy giving greater protection for the same degree of blood pressure control. ACE inhibitors may potentiate the hypoglycaemic effect of insulin and oral antidiabetic drugs; this effect is more likely during the first weeks of combined treatment and in patients with renal impairment.

Thiazides (see section 2.2.1) have an adverse effect on blood glucose and lipids (although this problem is less marked with the lower doses now given) and should be avoided in diabetes unless the blood pressure cannot be controlled by alternative antihypertensives. Beta-blockers (see section 2.4) can lead to a small deterioration of glucose tolerance and they also interfere with metabolic and autonomic responses to hypoglycaemia; cardioselective beta-blockers (see p. 74) may be preferable but even cardioselective beta-blockers should be avoided in those with frequent episodes of hypoglycaemia).

DIABETIC NEUROPATHY

Note. Several recommendations in this section involve non-licensed indications
Optimal diabetic control is beneficial for the management of *painful neuropathy.* Most patients should be treated with insulin, and relief can probably be accelerated by continuous insulin infusion. **Non-opioid analgesics** such as aspirin and para-

cetamol (see section 4.7.1) are indicated. Relief may also be obtained with the **tricyclic antidepressants,** amitriptyline, imipramine, and nortriptyline (see section 4.3.1) with or without a low dose of a **phenothiazine** (see section 4.2). **Carbamazepine** (see section 4.8.1) or mexiletine may be useful.

In *autonomic neuropathy* diabetic diarrhoea can often be aborted by two or three doses of **tetracycline** 250 mg (see section 5.1.3). Otherwise **codeine phosphate** (see section 1.4.2) is the best drug, but all other antidiarrhoeal preparations can be tried. **Anti-emetics** or **cisapride** may control vomiting in gastroparesis. In the rare cases where they do not, erythromycin (especially when given intravenously) has been shown to be of benefit but further studies are needed.

In *neuropathic postural hypotension* an increased salt intake and the use of the **mineralocorticoid** fludrocortisone 100 to 400 micrograms daily (see section 6.3.1) help by increasing plasma volume but uncomfortable oedema is a common side-effect. Fludrocortisone can also be combined with **flurbiprofen** (see section 10.1.1) and **ephedrine hydrochloride** (see section 3.1.1.2).

Gustatory sweating can be treated with **antimuscarinics** (see section 1.2), poldine methylsulphate is the best but propantheline bromide may also be used; side-effects are common. In some patients with *neuropathic oedema,* **ephedrine hydrochloride** 30 to 60 mg three times daily offers impressive relief.

6.1.6 Diagnostic and monitoring agents for diabetes mellitus

BLOOD GLUCOSE MONITORING

Blood glucose monitoring gives a direct measure of the glucose concentration at the time of the test and can detect hypoglycaemia as well as hyperglycaemia. It is a method of assessing diabetic control, especially where tight control is essential e.g. in pregnancy. Patients should be properly trained in the use of blood glucose monitoring systems and to take appropriate action on the results obtained. Inadequate understanding of the normal fluctuations in blood glucose may lead to confusion and inappropriate action. It is ideal for patients to observe the 'peaks' and 'troughs' of blood glucose over 24 hours and make adjustments of their insulin no more than twice or twice weekly. Daily alterations to the insulin dose are highly undesirable (except during illness).

Blood glucose concentration evaluation is best carried out by means of a meter. Visual colour comparison is often useful but is much less satisfactory. Meters give a more precise reading and are useful for patients with poor eyesight or who are colour blind.

Note. In the U.K. blood glucose concentration is expressed in mmol/litre and the British Diabetic Association advises its members that these units should be used for self blood glucose monitoring. In other European countries units of mg/100 mL (or mg/dL) are commonly used.

It is advisable to check that the meter is pre-set in the correct units.

Test strips

Biocare Glucose VT® (Biocare)

Reagent strips, for blood glucose monitoring, visual range (1.1–44.4 mmol/litre). Net price 50-strip pack = £8.50

BM-Accutest® (BM Diagnostics)

Reagent strips, for blood glucose monitoring, range (1.1–33.3 mmol/litre), for use with NHS Accutrend meter only. Net price 50-strip pack = £13.30

BM-Test 1–44® (BM Diagnostics)

Reagent strips, for blood glucose monitoring, visual range (1–44 mmol/litre) meter range (0.5–27.7 mmol/litre), suitable for use with NHS Reflolux® S. Net price 50-strip pack = £14.01

Dextrostix® (Bayer Diagnostics)

Reagent strips, for blood glucose monitoring, visual range (1.4–14 mmol/litre). Net price 50-strip pack = £13.99

ExacTech® (MediSense)

Biosensor strips, for blood glucose monitoring, range (2.2–25 mmol/litre), for use with NHS ExacTech® meter only. Net price 50-strip pack = £13.45

Glucostix® (Bayer Diagnostics)

Reagent strips, for blood glucose monitoring, visual range (1–44 mmol/litre), meter range (2–22 mmol/litre), suitable for use with NHS Glucometer® GX. Net price 50-strip pack = £13.99

Glucotide® (Bayer Diagnostics)

Reagent strips, for blood glucose monitoring, range (0.6–33.3 mmol/litre), for use with Glucometer® 4 meter only. Net price 50-strip pack = £13.30

Hypoguard® GA (Hypoguard)

Reagent strips, for blood glucose monitoring, visual range (1–22 mmol/litre), meter range (0–22 mmol/litre), suitable for use with NHS Hypocount® GA. Net price 50-strip pack = £12.21

Hypoguard® Supreme (Hypoguard)

Reagent strips, for blood glucose monitoring, visual range 1–22 mmol/litre), meter range (2–22 mmol/litre), suitable for use with NHS Hypocount® Supreme meter. Net price 50-strip pack = £12.73

MediSense G2® (MediSense)

Sensor strips, for blood glucose monitoring, range (1.1–33.3 mmol/litre) for use with NHS MediSense Card® or NHS MediSense Pen® meters only. Net price 50-strip pack = £12.93

Medi-Test® Glycaemie C (BHR)

Reagent strips, for blood glucose monitoring, visual range (1.1–44.4 mmol/litre), meter range (1.1–33.3 mmol/litre), suitable for use with NHS Glycotronic® C meter. Net price 50-strip pack = £12.95

One Touch® (LifeScan)

Reagent strips, for blood glucose monitoring, range (0–33.3 mmol/litre), for use with NHS One Touch® meter only. Net price 50-strip pack = £13.35

Meters

NHS Accutrend® (BM Diagnostics)

Meters for blood glucose monitoring for use with BM-Accutest® test strips. Accutrend = £34.00, Accutrend Alpha = £29.00, Accutrend Mini = £25.00, Accutrend DM = £149.00

NHS ExacTech® (MediSense)

Meters (Sensor) for blood glucose monitoring for use with ExacTech® test strips. ExacTech Card = £24.00, ExacTech Card starter pack = £34.00, ExacTech Pen = £24.00, ExacTech Pen starter pack = £34.00

NHS Glucometer® (Bayer Diagnostics)

Meters for blood glucose monitoring, Glucometer 4 (for use with Glucotide® test strips) = £35.00; Glucometer GX (for use with Glucostix® test strips) = £29.00

NHS Glycotronic® C (BHR)

Meter for blood glucose monitoring (for use with Medi-Test® Glycaemic C test strips) = £31.00

NHS Hypocount® (Hypoguard)

Meters for blood glucose monitoring, Hypocount GA (for use with Hypoguard GA® test strips) = £24.95, Hypocount® Supreme (for use with Hypoguard® Supreme test strips) = £34.95

NHS MediSense® (MediSense)

Meters (Sensor) for blood glucose monitoring for use with MediSense G2® test strips. MediSense Card = £35.00, MediSense Pen = £35.00

NHS One Touch® (LifeScan)

Meters for blood glucose monitoring for use with One Touch® test strips. One Touch Basic system pack = £39.00, One Touch II system pack = £59.00

NHS Reflolux® S (BM Diagnostics)

Meter for blood glucose monitoring (for use with BM-Test 1–44® test strips) = £29.00

URINALYSIS

Urine testing for glucose is useful in patients who find blood glucose monitoring difficult. Tests for glucose range from reagent strips specific to glucose to reagent tablets which detect all reducing sugars. Few patients still use *Clinitest*; *Clinistix* is suitable for screening purposes only. Tests for ketones and proteins are usually performed in clinics and patients are rarely required to do these tests for themselves.

Microalbuminuria can be detected with NHS Micral-Test® but this should be followed by confirmation in the laboratory, since false positive results are common.

Glucose

Clinistix® (Bayer Diagnostics)

Reagent strips, for detection of glucose in urine. Net price 50-strip pack = £2.75

Clinitest® (Bayer Diagnostics)

Reagent tablets, for detection of glucose and other reducing substances in urine. Pocket set (test tube, dropper and 36 tablets), net price = £3.50, 36-tab pack = £1.74, 6-test tube pack = £1.98, 6-dropper pack = £1.98, NHS test tube rack set (6 tubes and 2 droppers) = £5.46

Diabur Test 5000® (BM Diagnostics)

Reagent strips, for detection of glucose in urine. Net price 50-strip pack = £2.28

Diastix® (Bayer Diagnostics)

Reagent strips, for detection of glucose in urine. Net price 50-strip pack = £2.34

Medi-Test® Glucose (BHR)

Reagent strips, for detection of glucose in urine. Net price 50-strip pack = £1.99

Ketones

Acetest® (Bayer Diagnostics)

Reagent tablets, for detection of ketones in urine. Net price 100-tab pack = £3.13

Ketostix® (Bayer Diagnostics)

Reagent strips, for detection of ketones in urine. Net price 50-strip pack = £2.45

Ketur Test® (BM Diagnostics)

Reagent strips, for detection of ketones in urine. Net price 50-strip pack = £2.18

Protein

Albustix® (Bayer Diagnostics)

Reagent strips, for detection of protein in urine. Net price 50-strip pack = £3.37

Albym Test® (BM Diagnostics)

Reagent strips, for detection of protein in urine. Net price 50-strip pack = £2.94

Other reagent strips available for urinalysis include NHS BM-Test-GP® (glucose and protein—BM Diagnostics), NHS Ketodiastix® (glucose and ketones—Bayer Diagnostics), NHS Medi-Test Combi 2® (glucose and protein—BHR), NHS Micral-Test II® (albumin—BM Diagnostics), NHS Microbumintest® (albumin—Bayer Diagnostics), NHS Uristix® (glucose and protein—Bayer Diagnostics)

GLUCOSE TOLERANCE TEST

The **glucose** tolerance test is used in the diagnosis of diabetes mellitus. In the UK this generally involves giving 75 g of glucose BP (= dextrose monohydrate) by mouth to the fasting patient, and measuring plasma concentrations at intervals. At an international level, however, confusion has arisen because in different pharmacopoeias the title 'glucose' can mean the anhydrous form or the monohydrate. Sources at the World Health Organisation have therefore suggested that the form of dextrose should be standardised as anhydrous, and that the standard amount should be 75 g. The equivalent value (and titles) in the UK are:

Anhydrous glucose BP (anhydrous dextrose) 75 g = Glucose BP (dextrose monohydrate) 82.5 g

6.2 Thyroid and antithyroid drugs

6.2.1 Thyroid hormones
6.2.2 Antithyroid drugs

6.2.1 Thyroid hormones

Thyroid hormones are used in hypothyroidism (myxoedema), and also in diffuse non-toxic goitre, Hashimoto's thyroiditis (lymphadenoid goitre), and thyroid carcinoma. Neonatal hypothyroidism requires prompt treatment for normal development.

Thyroxine sodium is the treatment of choice for *maintenance* therapy. The initial dose should not exceed 100 micrograms daily, preferably before breakfast, or 25 to 50 micrograms in elderly patients or those with cardiac disease, increased by 25 to 50 micrograms at intervals of at least 4 weeks. The usual maintenance dose to relieve hypothyroidism is 100 to 200 micrograms daily which can be administered as a single dose.

In infants a daily dose of 10 micrograms/kg up to a maximum of 50 micrograms daily should be given; subsequent therapy should reach 100 micrograms daily by 5 years and 100–200 micrograms by 12 years, guided by clinical response, growth assessment, and measurements of plasma thyroxine and thyroid-stimulating hormone.

Liothyronine sodium has a similar action to thyroxine but is more rapidly metabolised; 20 micrograms is equivalent to 100 micrograms of thyroxine. Its effects develop after a few hours and disappear within 24 to 48 hours of discontinuing treatment. It may be used in *severe hypothyroid states* when a rapid response is desired.

Liothyronine by intravenous injection is the treatment of choice in *hypothyroid coma.* Adjunctive therapy includes intravenous fluids, hydrocortisone, and antibiotics; assisted ventilation is often required.

Dried **thyroid** should **not** be used as its effects are unpredictable.

THYROXINE SODIUM

Indications: hypothyroidism

Cautions: panhypopituitarism or predisposition to adrenal insufficiency from other causes (initiate corticosteroid therapy before starting thyroxine), elderly, cardiovascular disorders (myocardial insufficiency or ECG evidence of myocardial infarction, see Initial Dosage below), diabetes insipidus, diabetes mellitus (dosage increase may be needed for antidiabetic drugs including insulin); pregnancy (monitor serum thyrotrophin levels—dosage adjustment may be necessary) and breast-feeding (see Appendix 5); **interactions:** Appendix 1 (thyroxine)

INITIAL DOSAGE. A pre-therapy ECG is valuable as changes induced by hypothyroidism may be confused with evidence of ischaemia. If too rapid an increase of metabolism is produced (causing diarrhoea, nervousness, rapid pulse, insomnia, tremors and sometimes anginal pain where there is latent myocardial ischaemia), reduce dosage or withhold for 1–2 days and start again at a lower dose

Contra-indications: thyrotoxicosis

Side-effects: usually at excessive dosage (see Initial Dosage under Cautions) include anginal pain, cardiac arrhythmias, palpitation, skeletal muscle cramps, tachycardia, diarrhoea, vomiting, tremors, restlessness, excitability, insomnia, headache, flushing, sweating, excessive loss of weight and muscular weakness

Dose: ADULT, initially 50–100 micrograms (50 micrograms for those over 50 years) daily, preferably before breakfast, adjusted in steps of 50 micrograms every 3–4 weeks until normal metabolism maintained (usually 100–200 micrograms daily); where there is cardiac disease, initially 25 micrograms daily *or* 50 micrograms on alternate days, adjusted in steps of 25 micrograms every 4 weeks; CHILD (see also notes above), congenital hypothyroidism, 25 micrograms daily adjusted in steps of 25 micrograms every 2–4 weeks until mild toxic symptoms appear then reduce dose slightly; juvenile myxoedema (child over 1 year), initially 2.5–5 micrograms/kg daily

PoM **Thyroxine** (Non-proprietary)

Tablets, thyroxine sodium 25 micrograms, net price 20 = 30p; 50 micrograms, 20 = 3p; 100 micrograms, 20 = 5p

Various strengths available from APS, Cox, CP, Goldshield (including Eltroxin®), Kent, Norton

LIOTHYRONINE SODIUM

(L-Tri-iodothyronine sodium)

Indications: see notes above

Cautions; Contra-indications; Side-effects: see under Thyroxine Sodium; has a more rapid effect

Dose: by mouth, initially 20 micrograms daily gradually increased to 60 micrograms daily in 2–3 divided doses; elderly patients should receive smaller initial doses, gradually increased; CHILD, adult dose reduced in proportion to body-weight

By slow intravenous injection, hypothyroid coma, 5–20 micrograms repeated every 12 hours or more frequently (every 4 hours if necessary); alternatively 50 micrograms initially then 25 micrograms every 8 hours reducing to 25 micrograms twice daily

PoM **Tertroxin®** (Link)

Tablets, scored, liothyronine sodium 20 micrograms. Net price 100-tab pack = £14.92

PoM **Triiodothyronine** (Link)

Injection, powder for reconstitution, liothyronine sodium (with dextran). Net price 20-microgram amp = £31.63

6.2.2   Antithyroid drugs

Antithyroid drugs are used to prepare patients for thyroidectomy. They are also used for prolonged periods in the hope of inducing life-long remission. In the UK carbimazole is the most commonly used drug. Propylthiouracil may be used in patients who suffer sensitivity reactions to carbimazole as sensitivity is not necessarily displayed to both drugs. Both drugs act primarily by interfering with the synthesis of thyroid hormones.

CSM warning

(neutropenia and agranulocytosis)

Doctors are reminded of the importance of recognising bone marrow suppression induced by carbimazole and the need to stop treatment promptly.

1. Patient should be asked to report symptoms and signs suggestive of infection, especially sore throat.

2. A white blood cell count should be performed if there is any clinical evidence of infection.

3. Carbimazole should be stopped promptly if there is clinical or laboratory evidence of neutropenia.

Carbimazole is given in a daily dose of 20 to 60 mg and maintained at this dose until the patient becomes euthyroid, usually after 4 to 8 weeks; the dose may then be progressively reduced to a maintenance of between 5 and 15 mg daily; therapy is usually given for 18 months. Children may be given an initial dose of 15 mg daily, adjusted according to response. Rashes are common, and propylthiouracil may then be substituted. Pruritus and rashes can also be treated with antihistamines without discontinuing therapy, however patients should be advised to report any sore throat immediately because of the rare complication of agranulocytosis (see CSM warning, above).

Propylthiouracil is given in a daily dose of 300 to 600 mg and maintained on this dose until the patient becomes euthyroid; the dose may then be progressively reduced to a maintenance of between 50 and 150 mg daily.

Although antithyroid drugs have a short half-life they need only be given once daily because of their prolonged effect on the thyroid. Over-treatment with the rapid development of hypothyroidism is not uncommon and should be avoided particularly during pregnancy since it can cause fetal goitre.

A combination of carbimazole, 20 to 60 mg daily with thyroxine, 50 to 150 micrograms daily, may be used in a *blocking-replacement regimen*; therapy is again usually given for 18 months. The blocking-replacement regimen is **not** suitable during pregnancy.

Unless operation or use of radioactive iodine is planned, treatment should be for at least a year.

Before partial thyroidectomy **iodine** may be given for 10 to 14 days in addition to carbimazole or propylthiouracil to assist control and reduce vascularity of the thyroid. Iodine should not be used for long-term treatment since its antithyroid action tends to diminish.

Radioactive sodium iodide (^{131}I) solution is used increasingly for the treatment of thyrotoxicosis at all ages, particularly where medical therapy or compliance is a problem, in patients with cardiac disease, and in patients who relapse after thyroidectomy.

Propranolol is useful for rapid relief of thyrotoxic symptoms and may be used in conjunction with antithyroid drugs or as an adjunct to radioactive iodine. Beta-blockers are also useful in neonatal thyrotoxicosis and in supraventricular arrhythmias due to hyperthyroidism. Propranolol may be used in conjunction with iodine to prepare mildly thyrotoxic patients for surgery but it is still preferable to make the patient euthyroid with carbimazole before surgery. Laboratory tests of thyroid function are not altered by beta-blockers. Most experience in treating thyrotoxicosis has been gained with propranolol but **nadolol** is also used. For doses and preparations of beta-blockers see section 2.4.

Thyrotoxic crisis ('thyroid storm') requires emergency treatment with intravenous administration of fluids, propranolol (5 mg) and hydrocortisone (100 mg every 6 hours, as sodium succinate), as well as oral iodine solution and carbimazole or propylthiouracil which may need to be administered by nasogastric tube.

PREGNANCY AND BREAST-FEEDING. Radioactive iodine therapy is contra-indicated during pregnancy. Propylthiouracil and carbimazole can be given but the blocking-replacement regimen (see above) is **not** suitable. Both drugs cross the placenta and in high doses may cause fetal goitre and hypothyroidism—the lowest dose that will control the hyperthyroid state should be used (requirements in Graves' disease tend to fall during pregnancy). Rarely, carbimazole has been associated with aplasia cutis of the neonate.

Carbimazole and propylthiouracil transfer to breast milk but this does not preclude breast-feeding as long as neonatal development is closely monitored and the lowest effective dose is used.

CARBIMAZOLE

Indications: hyperthyroidism

Cautions: large goitre; liver disorders, pregnancy, breast-feeding (see notes)

Side-effects: nausea, headache, rashes and pruritus, arthralgia; rarely alopecia, agranulocytosis (**see CSM warning above**), jaundice

Dose: see notes above

COUNSELLING. Warn patient to tell doctor immediately if sore throat, mouth ulcers, bruising, fever, malaise, or non-specific illness develops

PoM **Neo-Mercazole®** (Roche)
Tablets, both pink, carbimazole 5 mg, net price 100-tab pack = £2.74; 20 mg, 100-tab pack = £10.14. Counselling, blood disorder symptoms

IODINE AND IODIDE

Indications: thyrotoxicosis (pre-operative)
Cautions: pregnancy, children; not for long-term treatment
Contra-indications: breast-feeding
Side-effects: hypersensitivity reactions including coryza-like symptoms, headache, lachrymation, conjunctivitis, pain in salivary glands, laryngitis, bronchitis, rashes; on prolonged treatment depression, insomnia, impotence; goitre in infants of mothers taking iodides

Aqueous Iodine Oral Solution (Lugol's Solution), iodine 5%, potassium iodide 10% in purified water, freshly boiled and cooled, total iodine 130 mg/mL. Net price 100 mL = £1.20. Label: 27
Dose: 0.1–0.3 mL 3 times daily well diluted with milk or water

PROPYLTHIOURACIL

Indications: hyperthyroidism
Cautions; Side-effects: see under Carbimazole; also rarely tendency to haemorrhage; reduce dose in renal impairment; systemic lupus erythematosus reported
Dose: see notes above

PoM **Propylthiouracil** (Non-proprietary)
Tablets, propylthiouracil 50 mg. Net price 20 = £8.95
Available from CP, Hillcross, Norton

6.3   Corticosteroids

6.3.1   Replacement therapy
6.3.2   Glucocorticoid therapy

6.3.1   Replacement therapy

The adrenal cortex normally secretes hydrocortisone (cortisol) which has glucocorticoid activity and weak mineralocorticoid activity. It also secretes the mineralocorticoid aldosterone.

In deficiency states, physiological replacement is best achieved with a combination of **hydrocortisone**[1] and the mineralocorticoid **fludrocortisone**; hydrocortisone alone does not usually provide sufficient mineralocorticoid activity for complete replacement.

In *Addison's disease* or following adrenalectomy, **hydrocortisone** 20 to 30 mg daily by mouth is usually required. This is given in 2 doses, the larger in the morning and the smaller in the evening, mimicking the normal diurnal rhythm of cortisol secretion. The optimum daily dose is determined on the basis of clinical response. Glucocorticoid therapy is supplemented by fludrocortisone 50 to 300 micrograms daily.

In *acute adrenocortical insufficiency*, **hydrocortisone** is given intravenously (preferably as sodium succinate) in doses of 100 mg every 6 to 8 hours in sodium chloride intravenous infusion 0.9%.

In *hypopituitarism* glucocorticoids should be given as in adrenocortical insufficiency, but since the production of aldosterone is also regulated by the renin-angiotensin system a mineralocorticoid is not usually required. Additional replacement therapy with thyroxine (section 6.2.1) and sex hormones (section 6.4) should be given as indicated by the pattern of hormone deficiency.

Corticosteroid cover for *adrenalectomy*, for *hypophysectomy* or for operations on patients on long-term treatment with corticosteroids is determined logically from the knowledge that in a normal person major stress will not lead to the secretion of more than 300 mg of cortisol in 24 hours; once the stress is over, cortisol production rapidly returns to its usual level of approximately 20 mg per 24 hours. A simple way of mimicking this is to administer hydrocortisone. On the day of operation hydrocortisone 100 mg (usually as the sodium succinate) is given by intramuscular or intravenous injection with the premedication, and repeated every 8 hours. In the absence of complications, the dose can be halved every 24 hours until a normal maintenance dose of 20 to 30 mg per 24 hours is reached on the 5th postoperative day.

CORTISONE ACETATE
Section 6.3.2

FLUDROCORTISONE ACETATE

Indications: mineralocorticoid replacement in adrenocortical insufficiency
Cautions; Contra-indications; Side-effects: section 6.3.2
Dose: adrenocortical insufficiency, 50–300 micrograms daily; CHILD 5 micrograms/kg daily

PoM **Florinef®** (Squibb)
Tablets, pink, scored, fludrocortisone acetate 100 micrograms. Net price 56-tab pack = £2.69. Label: 10 steroid card

HYDROCORTISONE
Section 6.3.2

---

1. Cortisone has been superseded by hydrocortisone.

Cautionary label wordings, see inside back cover

6.3.2   Glucocorticoid therapy

In comparing the relative potencies of corticosteroids in terms of their anti-inflammatory (glucocorticoid) effects it should be borne in mind that high anti-inflammatory (glucocorticoid) activity in itself is of no advantage unless it occurs in conjunction with relatively low mineralocorticoid activity so that the mineralocorticoid effect on water and electrolytes is not also increased. The mineralocorticoid activity of **fludrocortisone** (section 6.3.1) is so high that its anti-inflammatory activity is of no clinical relevance.. The table below shows equivalent anti-inflammatory doses.

Equivalent Anti-inflammatory Doses of Corticosteroids

This table takes no account of mineralocorticoid effects, nor does it take account of variations in duration of action

Prednisolone 5 mg
≡ Betamethasone 750 micrograms
≡ Cortisone acetate 25 mg
≡ Dexamethasone 750 micrograms
≡ Hydrocortisone 20 mg
≡ Methylprednisolone 4 mg
≡ Prednisone 5 mg
≡ Triamcinolone 4 mg

The mineralocorticoid effects of **cortisone** and **hydrocortisone** are too high for them to be used on a long-term basis for disease suppression since fluid retention would be too great, but they are suitable for adrenal replacement therapy (section 6.3.1); hydrocortisone is preferred because cortisone is only active after conversion in the liver to hydrocortisone. Hydrocortisone is used on a short-term basis by intravenous injection for the emergency management of some conditions. The relatively moderate anti-inflammatory potency of hydrocortisone also makes it a first-choice topical corticosteroid for the management of inflammatory skin conditions because side-effects (both topical and those associated with absorption) are less marked (see section 13.4); cortisone is not active topically.

Prednisolone has predominantly glucocorticoid activity and is the corticosteroid most commonly used by mouth for long-term disease suppression. **Prednisone** has a similar level of glucocorticoid activity but is only active after conversion in the liver to prednisolone; it is therefore not recommended.

Betamethasone and **dexamethasone** have very high glucocorticoid activity in conjunction with insignificant mineralocorticoid activity. This makes them particularly suitable for high-dose therapy in conditions where water retention would be a disadvantage (e.g. *cerebral oedema*).

They also have a long duration of action and this, coupled with their lack of mineralocorticoid action makes them particularly suitable for conditions which require suppression of corticotrophin secretion (e.g. *congenital adrenal hyperplasia*). Some esters of betamethasone and of **beclomethasone** exert a considerably more marked topical effect (e.g. on the skin or the lungs) than when given by mouth; use is made of this to obtain topical effects without corresponding systemic activity (e.g. for skin applications and asthma inhalations).

DISADVANTAGES OF CORTICOSTEROIDS

Overdosage or prolonged use may exaggerate some of the normal physiological actions of corticosteroids leading to mineralocorticoid and glucocorticoid side-effects.

Mineralocorticoid side-effects include *hypertension, sodium and water retention and potassium loss*. They are most marked with fludrocortisone, but are significant with cortisone, hydrocortisone, corticotrophin, and tetracosactrin. Mineralocorticoid actions are negligible with the high potency glucocorticoids, betamethasone and dexamethasone, and occur only slightly with methylprednisolone, prednisolone, prednisone, and triamcinolone.

Glucocorticoid side-effects include *diabetes* and *osteoporosis*, which is a danger, particularly in the elderly, as it may result in osteoporotic fractures for example of the hip or vertebrae; in addition administration of high doses is associated with *avascular necrosis* of the femoral head. *Mental disturbances* may occur; a serious paranoid state or depression with risk of suicide may be induced, particularly in patients with a history of mental disorder. *Euphoria* is frequently observed. *Muscle wasting* (proximal myopathy) may also occur. Corticosteroid therapy is also weakly linked with *peptic ulceration* (the use of soluble or enteric-coated preparations to reduce the risk is speculative only).

High doses of corticosteroids may cause *Cushing's syndrome*, with moon face, striae, and acne; it is usually reversible on withdrawal of treatment, but this must always be gradually tapered to avoid symptoms of acute adrenal insufficiency (**important**: see also Adrenal Suppression p. 302).

In children, administration of corticosteroids may result in *suppression of growth*. Corticosteroids given in high dosage during *pregnancy* may affect adrenal development in the child (but see also Appendix 4).

Modification of tissue reactions may result in spread of *infection*; suppression of clinical signs may allow diseases such as septicaemia and tuberculosis to reach an advanced stage before being recognised—**important:** see also Infections p. 302.

Adrenal atrophy can persist for years after stopping prolonged corticosteroid therapy, therefore any illness or surgical emergency may require temporary reintroduction of corticosteroid therapy to compensate for lack of sufficient adrenocortical response. Anaesthetists **must** therefore know whether a patient is taking or has been taking corticosteroids to avoid a precipitous fall in blood pressure during anaesthesia or in the immediate postoperative period. Patients should therefore carry cards giving details of their dosage and possible complications.

Steroid cards can be obtained from the local Health
Authority in England and Wales. In Scotland steroid
cards are available from Health Boards. In Northern Ireland they may be obtained from Central Services
Agency, 27 Adelaide St, Belfast BT2 8FH.

Community pharmacists may also obtain steroid cards
from the Royal Pharmaceutical Society of Great Britain.

For other references to the adverse effects of corticosteroids see section 11.4 (eye) and section 13.4
(skin).

CLINICAL MANAGEMENT

Corticosteroids should not be used unless the benefits justify the hazards; the lowest dose that will
produce an acceptable response should be used (see
also under Administration, below). Dosage varies
widely in different diseases and in different
patients.

If the use of a corticosteroid can save or prolong
life, as in *exfoliative dermatitis*, *pemphigus*, *acute
leukaemia* or *acute transplant rejection*, high doses
may need to be given, as the complications of therapy are likely to be less serious than the effects of
the disease itself.

When long-term corticosteroid therapy is used in
relatively benign chronic diseases such as *rheumatoid arthritis* the danger of treatment may become
greater than the disabilities produced by the disease. To minimise side-effects the maintenance
dose should be kept as low as possible (see also section 10.1.2.1).

When potentially less harmful measures are ineffective corticosteroids are used topically for the
treatment of *inflammatory conditions of the skin*
(see section 13.4). Corticosteroids should be
avoided or used only under specialist supervision in
psoriasis (see section 13.5).

Corticosteroids are used both topically (by rectum) and systemically (by mouth or intravenously)
in the management of *ulcerative colitis* and *Crohn's
disease* (see sections 1.5 and 1.7.2).

Use can be made of the mineralocorticoid activity
of fludrocortisone to treat *postural hypotension* in
autonomic neuropathy (see section 6.1.5).

Very high doses of corticosteroids have been
given by intravenous injection in *septic shock*.
However a recent study (using methylprednisolone
sodium succinate) did not demonstrate efficacy and,
moreover, suggested a higher mortality in some
subsets of patients given the high-dose corticosteroid therapy.

Dexamethasone and betamethasone have little if
any mineralocorticoid action and their long duration of action makes them particularly suitable for
suppressing corticotrophin secretion in *congenital
adrenal hyperplasia* where the dose should be tailored to the individual on clinical grounds and by
measurement of adrenal androgens and 17-
hydroxyprogesterone. In common with all glucocorticoids their suppressive action on the hypo-
thalamic-pituitary-adrenal axis is greatest and most
prolonged when they are given at night. In most

normal subjects a single dose of 1 mg of
dexamethasone at night, depending on weight, is
sufficient to inhibit corticotrophin secretion for 24
hours. This is the basis of the 'overnight
dexamethasone suppression test' for diagnosing
Cushing's syndrome.

Betamethasone and dexamethasone are also
appropriate for conditions where water retention
would be a disadvantage, as for example in treating
traumatic *cerebral oedema* with doses of 12 to
20 mg daily.

In acute hypersensitivity reactions such as *angioedema* of the upper respiratory tract and *anaphylactic shock*, corticosteroids are indicated as an adjunct
to emergency treatment with adrenaline (see section
3.4.3). In such cases hydrocortisone (as sodium
succinate) by intravenous injection in a dose of 100
to 300 mg may be required.

Corticosteroids are preferably used by inhalation
in the management of *asthma* (see section 3.2) but
systemic therapy in association with bronchodilators is required for the emergency treatment of
severe acute asthma (see section 3.1.1).

Corticosteroids may also be useful in conditions
such as *rheumatic fever*, *chronic active hepatitis*,
and *sarcoidosis*; they may also lead to remissions of
acquired *haemolytic anaemia*, and some cases of
the *nephrotic syndrome* (particularly in children)
and *thrombocytopenic purpura*.

Corticosteroids can improve the prognosis of serious conditions such as *systemic lupus erythematosus*, *temporal arteritis*, and *polyarteritis nodosa*;
the effects of the disease process may be suppressed
and symptoms relieved, but the underlying condition is not cured, although it may ultimately burn
itself out. It is usual to begin therapy in these conditions at fairly high dose, such as 40 to 60 mg prednisolone daily, and then to reduce the dose to the
lowest commensurate with disease control.

For other references to the use of corticosteroids
see section 11.4 (eye), 12.1.1 (otitis externa), 12.2.1
(allergic rhinitis), and 12.3.1 (aphthous ulcers).

ADMINISTRATION

Whenever possible *local treatment* with creams,
intra-articular injections, inhalations, eye-drops, or
enemas should be used in preference to *systemic
treatment*. The suppressive action of a corticosteroid on cortisol secretion is least when it is given
in the morning, therefore in an attempt to reduce
pituitary-adrenal suppression a corticosteroid (usually prednisolone) should normally be taken as a
single dose in the morning. In an attempt to reduce
pituitary-adrenal suppression further, the total dose
for two days can sometimes be taken as a single
dose on alternate days; alternate-day administration has not been very successful in the management
of asthma (see section 3.2) but it can be suitable for
rheumatoid arthritis (see section 10.1.2). Pituitary-
adrenal suppression can also be reduced by means
of intermittent therapy with short courses. In some
conditions it may be possible to reduce the dose of
corticosteroid by adding a small dose of an immunosuppressive drug (see section 8.2.1).

PREDNISOLONE

Indications: suppression of inflammatory and allergic disorders; see also notes above; inflammatory bowel disease, section 1.5; asthma, section 3.2; immunosuppression, section 8.2.2; rheumatic disease, section 10.1.2

Cautions: adrenal suppression (see below), infection (see below), children and adolescents (growth retardation which may be irreversible—prolonged or continuous treatment rarely justified), elderly (side-effects more serious—close supervision required particularly on long-term treatment); frequent monitoring required in those with history of tuberculosis (or X-ray changes), hypertension, recent myocardial infarction (rupture reported), congestive heart failure, liver failure, renal impairment, diabetes mellitus including family history, osteoporosis (post-menopausal women at special risk), glaucoma (including family history), severe affective disorders (particularly those with previous history of steroid-induced psychosis), epilepsy, peptic ulceration, hypothyroidism, history of steroid myopathy; pregnancy and breast-feeding (see Appendixes 4 and 5); **interactions:** Appendix 1 (corticosteroids)

ADRENAL SUPPRESSION. During prolonged therapy *adrenal atrophy* may develop and persist for years after stopping. Too rapid a reduction of dosage, following a prolonged course (7 days or longer), can lead to acute adrenal insufficiency, hypotension and death. Therefore withdrawal must always be gradual, tapered off over weeks or months depending on dosage and duration of therapy. Withdrawal may also be associated with fever, myalgia, arthralgia, rhinitis, conjunctivitis, painful itchy skin nodules and loss of weight.

Any intercurrent illness, trauma, or surgical procedure requires a temporary increase in dosage, or if already stopped, a temporary re-introduction of corticosteroid. Patients should carry a steroid treatment card giving clear guidance on precautions to be taken to minimise risk and providing details of prescriber, drug, dosage and duration of treatment.

INFECTIONS. Susceptibility and severity of infections may be increased and clinical presentation may be atypical. Serious infections such as *septicaemia* and *tuberculosis* may reach an advanced stage before being recognised. *Amoebiasis* or *strongyloidiasis* may be activated or exacerbated (exclude before initiating corticosteroid in those at risk or with suggestive symptoms). *Ocular infections* (fungal or viral) may also be exacerbated (see also section 11.4.1). Infections such as *chickenpox* and *measles* are also of particular concern (for details see below).

Chickenpox: unless they have had chickenpox, all patients receiving oral or parenteral corticosteroids for purposes other than replacement should be regarded as being *at risk of severe chickenpox.* Manifestations of fulminant illness include pneumonia, hepatitis and disseminated intravascular coagulation; rash is not necessarily a prominent feature. Patients (or parents of children) at risk should be advised to take reasonable steps *to avoid close personal contact* with chickenpox or herpes zoster and *to seek urgent medical attention* if exposed to chickenpox. Passive immunisation with varicella-zoster immunoglobulin (see section 14.5) is needed by exposed non-immune patients receiving systemic corticosteroids or who have used them within the previous 3 months (preferably given within 3 days of exposure—not later than 10 days). If a diagnosis of chickenpox is confirmed, the illness warrants specialist care and urgent treatment. Corticosteroids should not be stopped (dosage may need to be increased). Currently there is no good evidence that topical, inhaled or rectal corticosteroids are associated with an increased risk of severe chickenpox.

Measles: Patients should be advised to take particular care to avoid exposure to measles and to seek medical advice without delay if exposure occurs; prophylaxis with intramuscular normal immunoglobulin (see section 14.5) may be needed.

Contra-indications: systemic infection (unless specific antimicrobial therapy given); avoid live virus vaccines in those receiving immunosuppressive doses (serum antibodies may not be obtained)

Side-effects: minimised by using lowest effective dose for minimum period possible; *gastro-intestinal effects* include dyspepsia, peptic ulceration (with perforation and haemorrhage), abdominal distension, acute pancreatitis, oesophageal ulceration and candidiasis; *musculoskeletal effects* include proximal myopathy, osteoporosis, vertebral and long bone fractures avascular osteonecrosis, tendon rupture; *endocrine effects* include adrenal suppression (see under Cautions above), menstrual irregularities and amenorrhoea, Cushings syndrome (on using high doses, usually reversible on withdrawal), hirsutism, weight gain, negative nitrogen and calcium balance, increased appetite; increased susceptibility to and severity of infection (see under Cautions above); *neuropsychiatric effects* include euphoria, psychological dependence, depression, insomnia, increased intracranial pressure with papilloedema in children (usually after withdrawal), psychosis and aggravation of schizophrenia, aggravation of epilepsy; *ophthalmic effects* include increased intra-ocular pressure, glaucoma, papilloedema, posterior subcapsular cataracts, corneal or scleral thinning and exacerbation of ophthalmic viral or fungal disease; *other side-effects* include impaired healing, skin atrophy, bruising, striae, telangiectasia, acne, myocardial rupture following recent myocardial infarction, fluid and electrolyte disturbance, leucocytosis, hypersensitivity reactions (including anaphylaxis), thromboembolism, nausea, malaise, hiccups

Dose: *by mouth,* initially, up to 10–20 mg daily (severe disease, up to 60 mg daily), preferably taken in the morning after breakfast; can often be reduced within a few days but may need to be continued for several weeks or months

Maintenance, usual range, 2.5–15 mg daily, but higher doses may be needed; cushingoid side-effects increasingly likely with doses above 7.5 mg daily

By intramuscular injection, prednisolone acetate, 25–100 mg once or twice weekly (for preparation see section 10.1.2.2)

PoM **Prednisolone** (Non-proprietary)

Tablets, prednisolone 1 mg, net price 20 = 7p; 5 mg, 20 = 18p. Label: 10 steroid card, 21

Available from APS, Cox, CP, Hillcross, Norton, Roussel (Precortisyl®)

Tablets, both e/c, prednisolone 2.5 mg (brown), net price 30-tab pack = 26p; 5 mg (red), 30-tab pack = 43p. Label: 5, 10 steroid card, 25

Available from APS, Biorex, Cox, Lagap, Norton (2.5 mg), Pfizer (Deltacortril Enteric®)

Injection, see section 10.1.2.2

PoM Precortisyl Forte® (Roussel)

Tablets, scored, prednisolone 25 mg. Net price 56-tab pack = £4.26. Label: 10 steroid card, 21

PoM Prednesol® (Glaxo)

Tablets, pink, scored, soluble, prednisolone 5 mg (as sodium phosphate). Net price 100-tab pack = £5.76. Label: 10 steroid card, 13, 21

BETAMETHASONE

Indications: suppression of inflammatory and allergic disorders; congenital adrenal hyperplasia; cerebral oedema; see also notes above; ear, section 12.1.1; eye, section 11.4.1; nose, section 12.2.1

Cautions; Contra-indications; Side-effects: see notes above and under Prednisolone

Dose: by mouth, usual range 0.5–5 mg daily. See also Administration (above)

By intramuscular injection or slow intravenous injection or infusion, 4–20 mg, repeated up to 4 times in 24 hours; CHILD, *by slow intravenous injection*, up to 1 year 1 mg, 1–5 years 2 mg, 6–12 years 4 mg

PoM Betnelan® (Evans)

Tablets, scored, betamethasone 500 micrograms. Net price 100-tab pack = £3.63. Label: 10 steroid card, 21

PoM Betnesol® (Evans)

Tablets, pink, scored, soluble, betamethasone 500 micrograms (as sodium phosphate). Net price 100-tab pack = £3.20. Label: 10 steroid card, 13, 21

Injection, betamethasone 4 mg (as sodium phosphate)/mL. Net price 1-mL amp = 65p. Label: 10 steroid card

CORTISONE ACETATE

Indications: section 6.3.1

Cautions; Contra-indications; Side-effects: see notes above and under Prednisolone

Dose: by mouth, for replacement therapy, 25–37.5 mg daily in divided doses

PoM Cortisyl® (Roussel)

Tablets, scored, cortisone acetate 25 mg. Net price 56-tab pack = £3.24. Label: 10 steroid card, 21

DEXAMETHASONE

Indications: suppression of inflammatory and allergic disorders; shock; diagnosis of Cushing's disease, congenital adrenal hyperplasia; cerebral oedema; see also notes above; rheumatic disease, section 10.1.2; eye, section 11.4.1

Cautions; Contra-indications; Side-effects: see notes above and under Prednisolone; perineal irritation may follow intravenous administration of the phosphate ester

Dose: by mouth, usual range 0.5–10 mg daily. See also Administration (above)

Chemotherapy emesis, see section 8.1

By intramuscular injection or slow intravenous injection or infusion (as dexamethasone phosphate), initially 0.5–20 mg; CHILD 200–500 micrograms/kg daily

Cerebral oedema (as dexamethasone phosphate), *by intravenous injection*, 10 mg initially, then 4 mg *by intramuscular injection* every 6 hours as required for 2–10 days

PoM Dexamethasone (Organon)

Tablets, dexamethasone 500 micrograms, net price 20 = 64p; 2 mg, 20 = £1.73. Label: 10 steroid card, 21

Injection, dexamethasone sodium phosphate 5 mg/mL (≡ dexamethasone 4 mg/mL ≡ dexamethasone phosphate 4.8 mg/mL). Net price 1-mL amp = 83p; 2-mL vial = £1.27. Label: 10 steroid card

PoM Decadron® (MSD)

Tablets, scored, dexamethasone 500 micrograms. Net price 30-tab pack = 96p. Label: 10 steroid card, 21

Injection, dexamethasone phosphate 4 mg/mL (≡ dexamethasone 3.33 mg/mL ≡ dexamethasone sodium phosphate 4.17 mg/mL). Net price 2-mL vial = £1.76. Label: 10 steroid card

Note. Injection containing dexamethasone phosphate 4 mg/mL (as sodium phosphate) is also available from David Bull

PoM Decadron Shock-Pak® (MSD)

Injection, dexamethasone 20 mg/mL (≡ dexamethasone sodium phosphate 25 mg/mL). Net price 5-mL vial = £15.13. Label: 10 steroid card

Note. Injection containing dexamethasone 20 mg/mL is also available from David Bull

Dose: shock, *by intravenous injection or infusion*, 2–6 mg/kg, repeated if necessary after 2–6 hours (but see section 6.3.2)

FLUDROCORTISONE
See section 6.3.1

HYDROCORTISONE

Indications: adrenocortical insufficiency (section 6.3.1); shock; see also notes above; hypersensitivity reactions (such as anaphylactic shock and angioedema), section 3.4.5; inflammatory bowel disease, section 1.5; haemorrhoids, section 1.7.2; rheumatic disease, section 10.1.2; eye, 11.4.1; skin, section 13.4

Cautions; Contra-indications; Side-effects: see notes above and under Prednisolone; perineal irritation may follow intravenous administration of the phosphate ester

Dose: by mouth, replacement therapy, 20–30 mg daily in divided doses—see section 6.3.1; CHILD 10–30 mg

By intramuscular injection or slow intravenous injection or infusion, 100–500 mg, 3–4 times in 24 hours or as required; CHILD *by slow intravenous injection* up to 1 year 25 mg, 1–5 years 50 mg, 6–12 years 100 mg

Oral preparations
PoM Hydrocortone® (MSD)

Tablets, scored, hydrocortisone 10 mg, net price 30-tab pack = 70p; 20 mg, 30-tab pack = £1.07. Label: 10 steroid card, 21

Parenteral preparations
PoM Efcortesol® (Glaxo)

Injection, hydrocortisone 100 mg (as sodium phosphate)/mL. Net price 1-mL amp = 75p; 5-mL amp = £3.40. Label: 10 steroid card

Note. Perineal irritation may follow intravenous injection of the phosphate ester

PoM Solu-Cortef® (Upjohn)

Injection, powder for reconstitution, hydrocortisone (as sodium succinate). Net price 100-mg vial (with 2-mL amp water for injections) = £1.02; without water for injections = 96p. Label: 10 steroid card

METHYLPREDNISOLONE

Indications: suppression of inflammatory and allergic disorders; cerebral oedema; see also notes above; rheumatic disease, section 10.1.2; skin, section 13.4

Cautions; Contra-indications; Side-effects: see notes above and under Prednisolone; rapid intravenous administration of large doses has been associated with cardiovascular collapse

Dose: by mouth, usual range 2–40 mg daily. See also Administration (above)

By intramuscular injection or slow intravenous injection or infusion, initially 10–500 mg; graft rejection, up to 1 g daily *by intravenous infusion* for up to 3 days

Oral preparations
PoM Medrone® (Upjohn)

Tablets, scored, methylprednisolone 2 mg (pink), net price 30-tab pack = £2.69; 4 mg, 30-tab pack = £5.16; 16 mg, 30-tab pack = £14.31; 100 mg (blue), 20-tab pack = £40.27. Label: 10 steroid card, 21

Parenteral preparations
PoM Methylprednisolone (Non-proprietary)

Injection, powder for reconstitution, methylprednisolone (as sodium succinate). Net price 500-mg vial = £7.42; 1-g vial = £11.68
Available from David Bull

PoM Solu-Medrone® (Upjohn)

Injection, powder for reconstitution, methylprednisolone (as sodium succinate) (all with solvent). Net price 40-mg vial = £1.32; 125-mg vial = £3.96; 500-mg vial = £8.00; 1-g vial = £14.42; 2-g vial = £27.38. Label: 10 steroid card

Intramuscular depot
PoM Depo-Medrone® (Upjohn)

Injection (aqueous suspension), methylprednisolone acetate 40 mg/mL. Net price 1-mL vial = £2.70; 2-mL vial = £4.87; 3-mL vial = £7.05. Label: 10 steroid card

Dose: by deep intramuscular injection into gluteal muscle, 40–120 mg, a second injection may be given after 2–3 weeks if required

PREDNISONE

Indications: suppression of inflammatory and allergic disorders; see also notes above

Cautions; Contra-indications; Side-effects: see notes above and under Prednisolone; avoid in liver disease

Dose: see Prednisolone

PoM Prednisone (Non-proprietary)

Tablets, prednisone 5 mg, net price 20 = 15p. Label: 10 steroid card, 21

TRIAMCINOLONE

Indications: suppression of inflammatory and allergic disorders; see also notes above; rheumatic disease, section 10.1.2; mouth, section 12.3.1; skin, section 13.4

Cautions; Contra-indications; Side-effects: see notes above and under Prednisolone; triamcinolone in high dosage has a greater tendency to cause proximal myopathy and should be avoided in chronic therapy

Dose: by mouth, 2–24 mg daily. See also Administration (above)

By deep intramuscular injection, into gluteal muscle, 40 mg of acetonide for depot effect, repeated at intervals according to the patient's response; max. single dose 100 mg

PoM Kenalog® (Squibb)

Injection (aqueous suspension), triamcinolone acetonide 40 mg/mL. Net price 1-mL vial (intramuscular/intra-articular) = £1.70; 1-mL syringe (intramuscular only) = £2.11; 2-mL syringe (intramuscular only) = £3.66. Label: 10 steroid card

PoM Ledercort® (Lederle)

Tablets, triamcinolone 2 mg (blue), net price 60-tab pack = £5.69; 4 mg, 60-tab pack = £11.33. Label: 10 steroid card, 21

6.4   Sex hormones

Sex hormones are described under the following section headings:

6.4.1   Female sex hormones
6.4.2   Male sex hormones and antagonists
6.4.3   Anabolic steroids

6.4.1   Female sex hormones

6.4.1.1   Oestrogens and HRT
6.4.1.2   Progestogens

6.4.1.1 OESTROGENS AND HRT

Oestrogens are necessary for the development of female secondary sexual characteristics; they also stimulate myometrial hypertrophy with endometrial hyperplasia.

In terms of oestrogenic activity *natural oestrogens* (oestradiol, oestrone, and oestriol) have a more appropriate profile for hormone replacement therapy (HRT) than *synthetic oestrogens* (ethinyloestradiol, mestranol, and stilboestrol); the profile of *conjugated oestrogens* resembles that of natural oestrogens.

Oestrogen therapy is given cyclically or continuously for a number of gynaecological conditions. If long-term therapy is required a progestogen should be added to prevent cystic hyperplasia of the endometrium and possible transformation to cancer. This addition of a progestogen is not necessary if the patient has had a hysterectomy or in the case of tibolone.

Oestrogens are no longer used to *suppress lactation* because of their association with thromboembolism.

HORMONE REPLACEMENT THERAPY (HRT). Menopausal *vasomotor symptoms* and menopausal *vaginitis* are alleviated by administration of small doses of oestrogen. There is also good evidence that small doses of oestrogen given for several years starting in the perimenopausal period will diminish postmenopausal *osteoporosis* and reduce the incidence of *stroke and myocardial infarction*. There is an increased risk of *endometrial cancer* (countered by a progestogen, see below) and, after some years of use, possibly a slightly increased risk of *breast cancer*.

Hormone replacement therapy (HRT) is indicated for menopausal women whose lives are inconvenienced by *vaginal atrophy* or *vasomotor instability*. Vaginal atrophy may respond to a short course of oestrogen cream given for a few weeks and repeated if necessary. Oral therapy is needed for vasomotor symptoms and should be given for at least a year; in a woman with a uterus a progestogen should be added to reduce the risk of endometrial cancer (see above). Hormone replacement therapy is also indicated for women with *early natural or surgical menopause (before age 45)*, since they are at high risk of osteoporosis; in a woman with a uterus a progestogen should again be added to reduce the risk of endometrial cancer (see above); hormone replacement therapy should be given to the age of at least 50 and possibly for a further 10 years.

Long-term hormone replacement therapy in general is almost certainly favourable in risk-benefit terms for menopausal women *without a uterus* because they do not require progestogen therapy; it should probably be continued for about 10 years. The picture is less clear for menopausal women *with a uterus* because the need for administration of progestogen may blunt the protective effect of low-dose oestrogen against myocardial infarction and stroke; any effect of the progestogen (favourable or otherwise) on breast cancer is not yet known. Nevertheless, risk factors for osteoporosis should be borne in mind and, if there are several, consideration given to hormone replacement therapy. Risk factors include *recent corticosteroid therapy or any disease predisposing to osteoporosis, family history,* *thinness, lack of exercise, alcoholism or smoking, and fracture of a hip or forearm before the age of 65; women of Afro-Caribbean origin appear to be less susceptible than those who are white or Asian.*

Choice. The choice of oestrogen for hormone replacement therapy is not straightforward and depends on an overall balance of indication, risk, and convenience. Vaginitis in a woman with a uterus can be treated for only a few weeks with an oestrogen, without addition of cyclical progestogen; this constraint includes topical cream (see section 7.2.1) since a significant amount is absorbed through the vaginal mucosa. Oestrogen therapy alone is suitable for long-term continuous therapy in a woman without a uterus. A woman with a uterus requires a regimen of oestrogen with cyclical progestogen for the last 10 to 13 days of the cycle (or administration of a preparation which combines both oestrogenic and progestogenic activity). All oral preparations of oestrogen are subject to first-pass metabolism in the intestine and liver, therefore subcutaneous or transdermal administration reflects more closely endogenous hormone activity. In the case of subcutaneous implants, problems have been encountered with the recurrence of vasomotor symptoms at supraphysiological plasma concentrations; moreover, there is evidence of prolonged endometrial stimulation after discontinuation (calling for continued cyclical progestogen).

Providing calcium intake is adequate calcium supplements do not confer additional benefit on hormone replacement therapy (see section 9.5.1).

Surgery. For hormone replacement therapy the evidence of an increased thrombotic risk is questionable, which suggests that it need not normally be stopped before major elective surgery (particularly as heparin prophylaxis is usual in this age group). For reference to supraphysiological concentrations of oestradiol implants see notes above.

OESTROGENS FOR HRT
Note. Relates only to small amounts of oestrogens given for hormone replacement therapy
 Indications: see notes above and under preparations
 Cautions: prolonged exposure to unopposed oestrogens may increase risk of development of endometrial cancer (see notes above); migraine (or migraine-like headaches); history of breast nodules or fibrocystic disease—closely monitor breast status (breast cancer, see notes above); pre-existing uterine fibroids may increase in size, symptoms of endometriosis may be exacerbated; increased risk of gall bladder disease reported; porphyria (see section 9.8.2); **interactions:** Appendix 1 (oestrogens)
 OTHER CONDITIONS. The data sheets and patient information leaflets also advise caution in a number of other conditions including hypertension, cardiac or renal disease, diabetes, asthma, epilepsy, melanoma, otosclerosis, multiple sclerosis, systemic lupus erythematosus. Evidence for the need for caution in these conditions is unsatisfactory and many women with these conditions may stand to benefit from HRT.

Contra-indications: pregnancy; oestrogen-dependent cancer, active thrombophlebitis or thromboembolic disorders, liver disease (where liver function tests have failed to return to normal), Dubin-Johnson and Rotor syndromes (or monitor closely), undiagnosed vaginal bleeding, breast-feeding

Side-effects: nausea and vomiting, weight changes, breast enlargement and tenderness, premenstrual-like syndrome, fluid retention, changes in liver function, cholestatic jaundice, rashes and chloasma, depression, headache, contact lenses may irritate; transdermal delivery systems may cause contact sensitisation (possible severe hypersensitivity reaction on continued exposure), and headache has been reported on vigorous exercise

WITHDRAWAL BLEEDING. Cyclical HRT (where a progestogen is taken for 10–14 days of each 28-day oestrogen treatment cycle) usually results in a *regular withdrawal bleed* towards the end of the progestogen. The aim of continuous combined HRT (where a combination of oestrogen and progestogen is taken, usually in a single tablet, throughout each 28-day treatment cycle) is to avoid bleeding, but *irregular bleeding* may occur during the early treatment stages (if it continues endometrial abnormality should be excluded and consideration given to cyclical HRT instead)

Dose: see under preparations

COUNSELLING ON PATCHES. Patch should be removed after 3–4 days (or once a week in case of 7-day patch) and replaced with fresh patch on slightly different site; recommended sites: clean, dry, unbroken areas of skin on trunk below waistline; not to be applied on or near breasts or under waistband. If patch falls off in bath allow skin to cool before applying new patch

---

Women with Uterus

The following preparations contain a **progestogen** as well as an **oestrogen** and are therefore suitable for a woman with an **intact uterus**; they are **not** suitable for use as (or with) hormonal contraceptives

Conjugated oestrogens with progestogen
PoM Premique® (Wyeth)

Premique® tablets, s/c, blue, conjugated oestrogen 625 micrograms, medroxyprogesterone acetate 5 mg. Net price 3 × 28-tab pack = £20.55

Dose: menopausal symptoms (including osteoporosis prophylaxis), if uterus intact, 1 tablet daily on a continuous basis, starting on 1st day of menstruation (or any time if cycles have ceased or are infrequent)

Note. Unsuitable for use in women under 54 years or within 12 months of last menstrual period; may cause irregular bleeding in early stages of treatment—if bleeding continues exclude endometrial abnormality and consider changing to cycle therapy, see below

Premique® Cycle Calendar pack, 28 maroon (s/c) tablets, conjugated oestrogens 625 micrograms; 14 white tablets, medroxyprogesterone acetate 10 mg. Net price 3 × 42-tab pack = £20.55

Dose: menopausal symptoms (including osteoporosis prophylaxis), if uterus intact, 1 maroon tablet daily on a continuous basis starting on 1st day of menstruation (or at any time if cycles have ceased or are infrequent) and 1 white tablet daily on days 15–28 of each 28-day treatment cycle; subsequent courses are repeated without interval

PoM Prempak-C® (Wyeth)

Prempak C® 0.625 Calendar pack, all s/c, 28 maroon tablets, conjugated oestrogens 625 micrograms; 12 light brown tablets, norgestrel 150 micrograms (≡ levonorgestrel 75 micrograms). Net price 3 × 40-tab pack = £12.15

Dose: menopause symptoms (including osteoporosis prophylaxis), if uterus intact, 1 maroon tablet daily on continuous basis, starting on 1st day of menstruation (or at any time if cycles have ceased or are infrequent), and 1 brown tablet daily on days 17–28 of each 28-day treatment cycle; subsequent courses are repeated without interval

Prempak C® 1.25 Calendar pack, all s/c, 28 yellow tablets, conjugated oestrogens 1.25 mg; 12 light brown tablets, norgestrel 150 micrograms (≡ levonorgestrel 75 micrograms). Net price 3 × 40-tab pack = £12.15

Dose: see under 0.625 Calendar pack, but taking 1 yellow tablet daily on continuous basis (instead of 1 maroon tablet) if symptoms not fully controlled with lower strength

Mestranol with progestogen
PoM Menophase® (Searle)

Tablets, 5 pink, mestranol 12.5 micrograms; 8 orange, mestranol 25 micrograms; 2 yellow, mestranol 50 micrograms; 3 green, mestranol 25 micrograms and norethisterone 1 mg; 6 blue, mestranol 30 micrograms and norethisterone 1.5 mg; 4 lavender, mestranol 20 micrograms and norethisterone 750 micrograms. Net price per pack = £3.25

Dose: menopausal symptoms (including osteoporosis prophylaxis), if uterus intact 1 tablet daily, starting with a pink tablet on Sunday, then in sequence (without interruption)

Oestradiol with progestogen
PoM Climagest® (Sandoz)

Climagest® 1-mg tablets, 16 grey-blue, oestradiol valerate 1 mg; 12 white, oestradiol valerate 1 mg and norethisterone 1 mg. Net price 28-tab pack = £4.38; 3 × 28-tab pack = £12.75

Dose: menopausal symptoms (but not osteoporosis prophylaxis), 1 grey-blue tablet daily for 16 days, starting on 1st day of menstruation (or at any time if cycles have ceased or are infrequent) then 1 white tablet for 12 days; subsequent courses are repeated without interval

Climagest® 2-mg tablets, 16 blue, oestradiol valerate 2 mg; 12 yellow, oestradiol valerate 2 mg and norethisterone 1 mg. Net price 28-tab pack = £4.38; 3 × 28-tab pack = £12.75

Dose: see Climagest® 1-mg, but starting with 1 blue tablet daily (instead of 1 grey-blue tablet) if symptoms not controlled with lower strength

PoM Climesse® (Sandoz)

Tablets, pink, oestradiol valerate 2 mg, norethisterone 700 micrograms. Net price 1 × 28-tab pack = £7.90; 3 × 28-tab pack = £23.70

Dose: menopausal symptoms (including osteoporosis prophylaxis), if uterus intact, 1 tablet daily on a continuous basis

Note. Unsuitable for use in the perimenopause or within 12 months of the last menstrual period; may cause irregular bleeding in early stages of treatment—if bleeding continues exclude endometrial abnormality and consider changing to cyclical HRT

PoM Cyclo-Progynova® (Schering Health)

Cyclo-Progynova® 1-mg Tablets, all s/c, 11 beige, oestradiol valerate 1 mg; 10 brown, oestradiol valerate 1 mg and levonorgestrel 250 micrograms. Net price per pack = £3.50

Dose: menopausal symptoms (including osteoporosis prophylaxis), if uterus intact, 1 beige tablet daily for 11 days, starting on 5th day of menstruation (or at any time if cycles have ceased or are infrequent), then 1 brown tablet daily for 10 days, followed by a 7-day interval

Cyclo-Progynova® 2-mg Tablets, all s/c, 11 white, oestradiol valerate 2 mg; 10 brown, oestradiol valerate 2 mg and norgestrel 500 micrograms (≡ levonorgestrel 250 micrograms). Net price per pack = £3.50

Dose: see Cyclo-Progynova® 1-mg, but starting with 1 white tablet daily (instead of 1 beige tablet) if symptoms not fully controlled with lower strength

PoM Elleste-Duet® (Searle)

Tablets, 16 orange, oestradiol 2 mg; 12 grey, oestradiol 2 mg, norethisterone acetate 1 mg. Net price 3 × 28-tab pack = £9.72

Dose: menopausal symptoms (including osteoporosis prophylaxis) 1 orange tablet daily for 16 days, starting on 2nd day of menstruation (or at any time if cycles have ceased or are infrequent) then 1 grey tablet daily for 12 days; subsequent courses are repeated without interval

PoM Estracombi® (Ciba)

Combination pack of 4 self-adhesive patches of *Estraderm TTS® 50* (releasing oestradiol approx. 50 micrograms/24 hours) and 4 patches of *Estragest TTS®* (releasing oestradiol approx. 50 micrograms/24 hours and norethisterone acetate 250 micrograms/24 hours). Net price per pack = £11.14. Label: 10 patient information leaflet, counselling, administration

Dose: menopausal symptoms (including osteoporosis prophylaxis) if uterus intact, starting within 5 days of onset of menstruation (or any time if cycles have ceased or are infrequent), 1 *Estraderm TTS® 50* patch to be applied twice weekly for 2 weeks followed by 1 *Estragest TTS®* patch twice weekly for 2 weeks; subsequent courses are repeated without interval

PoM Estrapak 50® (Ciba)

Calendar pack, 8 self-adhesive patches, releasing oestradiol approx. 50 micrograms/24 hours, and 12 tablets, red, norethisterone acetate 1 mg. Net price per pack = £9.48. Label: 10 patient information leaflet, counselling, administration

Dose: menopausal symptoms (including osteoporosis prophylaxis) if uterus intact, starting within 5 days of onset of menstruation (or at any time if cycles have ceased or are infrequent), apply 1 patch twice weekly on continuous basis, and take 1 tablet daily on days 15–26 of each 28-day treatment cycle

PoM Evorel® Pak (Cilag)

Calendar pack, 8 self-adhesive patches (releasing oestradiol approx. 50 micrograms/24 hours) and 12 tablets, norethisterone 1 mg. Net price per pack = £8.45. Label:10 patient information leaflet, counselling, administration

Dose: menopausal symptoms (but not osteoporosis prophylaxis), if uterus intact, apply 1 patch twice weekly on a continuous basis (increased if necessary to 2 patches twice weekly after first month) and take 1 tablet daily on days 15–26 of each 28-day treatment cycle

PoM Femapak® 80 (Solvay)

Combination pack of 8 self-adhesive patches of *Fematrix® 80* (releasing oestradiol approx. 80 micrograms/24 hours) and 14 tablets of *Duphaston®* (dydrogesterone 10 mg). Net per pack = £8.95. Label: 10 patient information leaflet, counselling, administration

Dose: menopausal symptoms (but not osteoporosis prophylaxis), if uterus intact, starting within 5 days of onset of menstruation (or any time if cycles have ceased or are infrequent), apply 1 patch twice weekly on a continuous basis and take 1 tablet daily on days 15–28 of each 28-day treatment cycle

PoM Femoston® (Solvay)

Femoston® 1/10 tablets, both f/c, 14 white, oestradiol 1 mg; 14 grey, oestradiol 1 mg, dydrogesterone 10 mg. Net price 28-tab pack = £4.99; 3 × 28-tab pack = £14.97

Dose: menopausal symptoms (but not osteoporosis prophylaxis) if uterus intact, 1 white tablet daily for 14 days, starting within 5 days of onset of menstruation (or any time if cycles have ceased or are infrequent) then 1 grey tablet for 14 days; subsequent courses are repeated without interval

Femoston® 2/10 tablets, both f/c, 14 orange, oestradiol 2 mg; 14 yellow, oestradiol 2 mg, dydrogesterone 10 mg. Net price 28-tab pack = £4.99; 3 × 28-tab pack = £14.97

Dose: menopausal symptoms (including osteoporosis prophylaxis) if uterus intact, 1 orange tablet daily for 14 days, starting within 5 days of onset of menstruation (or any time if cycles have ceased or are infrequent) then 1 yellow tablet daily for 14 days; subsequent courses are repeated without interval; where therapy is required for control of menopausal symptoms alone, *Femoston® 1/10* is given initially and *Femoston® 2/10* substituted if symptom control is not achieved

Femoston® 2/20 tablets, both f/c, 14 orange, oestradiol 2 mg; 14 blue, oestradiol 2 mg, dydrogesterone 20 mg. Net price 28-tab pack = £7.48; 3 × 28-tab pack = £22.44

Dose: see Femoston® 2/10, but taking 1 blue tablet (instead of 1 yellow tablet) if withdrawal bleed is early or endometrial biopsy shows inadequate progestational response

PoM Kliofem® (Novo Nordisk)

Tablets, yellow, oestradiol 2 mg, norethisterone acetate 1 mg. Net price 3 × 28-tab pack = £25.95

Dose: menopausal symptoms (including osteoporosis prophylaxis), if uterus intact, 1 tablet daily on a continuous basis; start at end of scheduled bleed if changing from sequential HRT

Note. Unsuitable for use in the perimenopause or within 12 months of the last menstrual period; may cause irregular bleeding in first 6 cycles—if bleeding continues, discontinue or change to sequential HRT

PoM Nuvelle® (Schering Health)

Tablets, all s/c, 16 white, oestradiol valerate 2 mg; 12 pink, oestradiol valerate 2 mg and levonorgestrel 75 micrograms. Net price 3 × 28-tab pack = £13.77

Dose: menopausal symptoms (including osteoporosis prophylaxis), 1 white tablet daily for 16 days, starting on 5th day of menstruation (or any time if cycles have ceased or are infrequent) then 1 pink tablet daily for 12 days; subsequent courses are repeated without interval

PoM Tridestra® (Sanofi Winthrop)

Tablets, 70 white, oestradiol valerate 2 mg; 14 blue, oestradiol valerate 2 mg and medroxyprogesterone acetate 20 mg; 7 yellow, placebo. Net price 91-tab pack = £24.90

Dose: menopausal symptoms (including osteoporosis prophylaxis), if uterus intact, 1 white tablet daily for 70 days, starting on 5th day of menstruation (or at anytime if cycles have ceased or are infrequent), then 1 blue tablet daily for 14 days, then 1 yellow tablet daily for 7 days; subsequent courses are repeated without interval

Oestradiol and oestriol with progestogen

PoM Trisequens® (Novo Nordisk)

Trisequens® tablets, 12 blue, oestradiol 2 mg, oestriol 1 mg; 10 white, oestradiol 2 mg, oestriol 1 mg, norethisterone acetate 1 mg; 6 red, oestradiol 1 mg, oestriol 500 micrograms. Net price 3 × 28-tab pack = £20.55

Dose: menopausal symptoms (including osteoporosis prophylaxis), if uterus intact, 1 blue tablet daily, starting on 5th day of menstruation (or at any time if cycles have ceased or are infrequent), then 1 tablet daily in sequence (without interruption)

Trisequens Forte® tablets, 12 yellow, oestradiol 4 mg, oestriol 2 mg; 10 white, oestradiol 4 mg, oestriol 2 mg, norethisterone acetate 1 mg; 6 red, oestradiol 1 mg, oestriol 500 micrograms. Net price 3 × 28-tab pack = £20.55

Dose: menopausal symptoms (but not osteoporosis prophylaxis), see under Trisequens®, starting with 1 yellow tablet daily (instead of 1 blue tablet) if symptoms not fully controlled with lower strength

Piperazine oestrone sulphate with progestogen

PoM Improvera® (Upjohn)

Tablets, both scored, 28 peach, piperazine oestrone sulphate 1.5 mg; 12 white, medroxyprogesterone acetate 10 mg. Net price per pack = £11.85

Dose: menopausal symptoms (including osteoporosis prophylaxis), if uterus intact, 1 peach tablet daily on a continuous basis starting on 5th day of menstruation (or at any time if cycles have ceased or are infrequent) and 1 white tablet on days 17–28 of each 28-day treatment cycle; subsequent courses are repeated without interval

---

Women without Uterus

The following preparations do **not** contain a **progestogen**; if the uterus is intact they need to be given with a progestogen in which case packs incorporating a suitable progestogen tablet are preferred (see above)

Conjugated oestrogens only

PoM Premarin® (Wyeth)

Tablets, all s/c, conjugated oestrogens 625 micrograms (maroon), net price 3 × 28-tab pack = £6.69; 1.25 mg (yellow), 3 × 28-tab pack = £9.08

Dose: menopausal symptoms (including osteoporosis prophylaxis, (with progestogen for 12–14 days per cycle if uterus intact), 0.625–1.25 mg daily

Note. Premarin® tablets 2.5 mg (purple, net price 20 = £2.30) are still available, but no longer have a product licence for palliative care in breast cancer (and provide a higher dose than that having a product licence for osteoporosis prophylaxis)

Oestradiol only

PoM Oestradiol Implants (Organon)

Implant, oestradiol 25 mg, net price each = £9.59; 50 mg, each = £19.16; 100 mg, each = £33.40

Dose: by implantation, oestrogen replacement, including osteoporosis prophylaxis (with cyclical progestogen on 10–13 days of each cycle if uterus intact, see notes above), 25–100 mg as required (usually every 4–8 months) according to oestrogen levels—check before each implant

PoM Climaval® (Sandoz)

Tablets, oestradiol valerate 1 mg (grey-blue), net price 1 × 28-tab pack = £2.34; 3 × 28-tab pack = £7.02;

2 mg (blue), 1 × 28-tab pack = £2.34, 3 × 28-tab pack = £7.02

Dose: menopausal symptoms (if patient has had a hysterectomy), 1–2 mg daily

PoM Elleste-Solo® (Searle)

Elleste-Solo® 1-mg tablets, oestradiol 1 mg. Net price 3 × 28-tab pack = £5.34

Dose: menopausal symptoms (but not osteoporosis prophylaxis), with progestogen for 12–14 days per cycle if uterus intact, 1 mg daily

Note. Elleste-Solo® tablets can be given continuously or cyclically (21 days out of 28)

Elleste-Solo® 2-mg tablets, oestradiol 2 mg. Net price 3 × 28-tab pack = £5.34

Dose: menopausal symptoms not controlled with lower strength (or osteoporosis prophylaxis), with progestogen for 12–14 days per cycle if uterus intact, 2 mg daily

Note. Elleste-Solo® tablets can be given continuously or cyclically (21 days out of 28)

PoM Estraderm MX® (Ciba)

Patches, self-adhesive, oestradiol *MX 25 patch* (releasing approx. 25 micrograms/24 hours), net price 8-patch pack = £6.75, 24-patch pack = £20.25; *MX 50 patch* (releasing approx. 50 micrograms/24 hours), 8-patch pack = £7.45, 24-patch pack = £22.35, 20-patch pack (hosp. only) = £16.76; *MX 100 patch* (releasing approx. 100 micrograms/24 hours), 8-patch pack = £8.20, 24-patch pack = £24.60. Label: 10 patient information leaflet, counselling, administration

Dose: menopausal symptoms (including osteoporosis prophylaxis in case of Estraderm MX® 50 **only**) 1 patch to be applied twice weekly on a continuous basis; give progestogen for 12 days a month (unless patient has had hysterectomy); therapy should be initiated with MX 50 for first month, subsequently adjusted to lowest effective dose

PoM Estraderm TTS® (Ciba)

Patches, self-adhesive, oestradiol, *TTS 25 patch* (releasing approx. 25 micrograms/24 hours), net price, 8-patch pack = £6.75, 24-patch pack = £20.25; *TTS 50 patch* (releasing approx. 50 micrograms/24 hours), 8-patch pack = £7.45, 24-patch pack = £22.35; *TTS 100 patch* (releasing approx. 100 micrograms/24 hours), 8-patch pack = £8.20, 24-patch pack = £24.60, 20-patch pack (hosp. only) = £16.76 . Label: 10 patient information leaflet, counselling, administration

Dose: menopausal symptoms (including osteoporosis prophylaxis in case of Estraderm TTS® 50 **only**), 1 patch to be applied twice weekly on continuous basis; give progestogen for 12 days a month (unless patient has had hysterectomy); therapy should be initiated with TTS 50 for first month, subsequently adjusted to lowest effective dose

PoM Evorel® (Cilag)

Patches, self-adhesive, oestradiol *'25' patch* (releasing approx. 25-micrograms/24 hours), net price 8-patch pack = £6.75; *'50' patch* (releasing approx. 50 micrograms/24 hours), 8-patch pack = £7.45; *'75' patch* (releasing approx. 75-micrograms/24 hours), 8-patch pack = £7.90; *'100' patch* (releasing approx. 100 micrograms/24 hours), 8-patch pack = £8.20. Label: 10 patient information leaflet, counselling, administration

Dose: menopausal symptoms (but not osteoporosis prophylaxis), 1 patch to be applied twice weekly on a continuous basis; give progestogen for 12 days a month (unless patient has had hysterectomy); therapy should be initiated with *'50' patch* for first month, subsequently adjusted to lowest effective dose

---

PoM **Fematrix**® (Solvay)

Patches, self-adhesive, oestradiol '40' patch (releasing approx. 40 micrograms/24 hours), net price 8-patch pack = £6.45; '80' patch (releasing approx. 80 micrograms/24 hours), 8-patch pack = £6.95. Label:10 patient information leaflet, counselling, administration

Dose: menopausal symptoms (but not osteoporosis prophylaxis) 1 patch to be applied twice weekly on a continuous basis starting within 5 days of onset of menstruation (or at any time if cycles have ceased or are infrequent); give progestogen for 12–14 days of each cycle (unless patient has had hysterectomy); therapy should be initiated with '40' patch in those with menopausal symptoms, prolonged oestrogen deficiency or anticipated intolerence to higher strength—may be increased to '80' patch if required (then subsequently adjusted to lowest effective dose)

PoM **FemSeven**® (Merck)

Patches, self-adhesive, releasing oestradiol approx. 50 micrograms/24 hours. Net price 4-patch pack = £6.44. Label:10 patient information leaflet, counselling, administration

Dose: menopausal symptoms (including osteoporosis prophylaxis), 1 patch to be applied once a week on a continuous basis, increased if necessary after first month to max. 2 patches/week; give progestogen for 12 days a month (unless patient has had hysterectomy)

PoM **Menorest**® (Rhône-Poulenc Rorer)

Patches, self-adhesive, oestradiol '37.5' patch (releasing approx. 37.5 micrograms/24 hours), net price 8-patch pack = £6.34; '50' patch (releasing approx. 50 micrograms/24 hours), 8-patch pack = £6.44; '75' patch (releasing approx. 75 micrograms/24 hours), 8-patch pack = £7.50. Label: 10 patient information leaflet, counselling administration

Dose: menopausal symptoms (but not osteoporosis prophylaxis) 1 patch to be applied every 3–4 days on a continuous basis; give progestogen on 12 days a month (unless patient has had hysterectomy); therapy should be initiated with '50' patch for first month, subsequently adjusted to lowest effective dose

PoM **Oestrogel**® (Hoechst, Roussel)

Gel, oestradiol 0.06%. Net price 64-measure pack = £7.95. Label: 10 patient information leaflet, counselling, administration

Dose: menopausal symptoms (but not osteoporosis prophylaxis), 2 measures once daily to be applied over an area twice that of the template provided; may be increased after one month to max. 4 measures

COUNSELLING. Apply gel to clean, dry, intact areas of skin such as arms, shoulders or inner thighs and allow to dry for 5 minutes before covering skin with clothing. Not to be applied on or near breasts or on vulval region. Avoid skin contact with another person (particularly male) and other skin products or washing the area for at least 1 hour after application

PoM **Progynova**® (Schering Health)

Tablets, both s/c, oestradiol valerate 1 mg (beige), net price 28-tab pack = £2.34; 2 mg (blue), 28-tab pack = £2.34

Dose: menopausal symptoms (if patient has had hysterectomy), 1–2 mg daily

PoM **Progynova**® TS (Schering Health)

Patches, self-adhesive, *Progynova*® TS (releasing oestradiol approx. 50 micrograms/24 hours), net price 12-patch pack = £19.32; *Progynova*® TS *forte* (releasing oestradiol approx. 100 micrograms/24 hours), 12-patch pack = £25.00. Label: 10 patient information leaflet, counselling, administration

Dose: menopausal symptoms (but not osteoporosis prophylaxis) 1 patch to be applied once a week on a continuous or cyclical basis (1 patch per week for three weeks followed by a 7-day patch-free interval); give progestogen for 12 days a month (unless patient has had hysterectomy)

PoM **Zumenon**® (Solvay)

Tablets, blue, f/c, oestradiol 2 mg, net price 28-tab pack = £2.55

Dose: menopausal symptoms (but not osteoporosis prophylaxis), with progestogen for 10–14 days per cycle if uterus intact, starting on the 5th day of menstruation (or any time if cycles have ceased or are infrequent) 1–2 tablets daily

Oestradiol, oestriol and oestrone only

PoM **Hormonin**® (Shire)

Tablets, pink, oestradiol 600 micrograms, oestriol 270 micrograms, oestrone 1.4 mg. Net price 90-tab pack = £6.44

Dose: menopausal symptoms (including osteoporosis prophylaxis), with progestogen for 12–13 days per cycle if uterus intact, 1–2 tablets daily

Note. Hormonin® tablets can be given continuously or cyclically (21 days out of 28)

Oestriol only

PoM **Ovestin**® (Organon)

Tablets, scored, oestriol 1 mg. Net price 30-tab pack = £4.40. Label: 25

Dose: genito-urinary symptoms associated with oestrogen-deficiency states, 0.5–3 mg daily, as single dose, for up to 1 month, then 0.5–1 mg daily until restoration of epithelial integrity (short-term use)

Piperazine oestrone sulphate only

PoM **Harmogen**® (Upjohn)

Tablets, peach, scored, piperazine oestrone sulphate 1.5 mg. Net price 28-tab pack = £3.14

Dose: menopausal symptoms (including osteoporosis prophylaxis), 1.5 mg daily on continuous basis (with progestogen for 10–13 days per 28-day cycle if uterus intact); up to 3 mg daily (in single or divided doses) for vasomotor symptoms and menopausal vaginitis

TIBOLONE

Tibolone combines oestrogenic and progestogenic activity with weak androgenic activity. It has recently been introduced for the treatment of vasomotor symptoms of the menopause. It is given continuously, without cyclical progestogen.

TIBOLONE

Indications: see under Dose

Cautions: renal impairment, epilepsy, migraine, diabetes mellitus, hypercholesterolaemia; withdraw if signs of thrombo-embolic disease, abnormal liver function tests or cholestatic jaundice; see also Note below; **interactions:** Appendix 1 (tibolone)

Contra-indications: hormone-dependent tumours, history of cardiovascular or cerebrovascular disease (e.g. thrombophlebitis, thrombo-embolism), uninvestigated vaginal bleeding, severe liver disease, pregnancy, breast-feeding

Side-effects: weight changes, ankle oedema, dizziness, seborrhoeic dermatitis, vaginal bleeding, headache, gastro-intestinal disturbances, increased facial hair; migraine, visual disturbances, liver-function changes, rash and pruritus also reported

Dose: vasomotor symptoms following natural or surgical menopause, 2.5 mg daily

Note. Unsuitable for use in the premenopause and as or with an oral contraceptive; also unsuitable for use within 12 months of the last menstrual period (may cause irregular bleeding); induce withdrawal bleeding with a progestogen if transferring from another form of HRT

PoM **Livial®** (Organon)

Tablets, tibolone 2.5 mg. Net price 28-tab pack = £13.66; 3 × 28-tab pack = £40.98

ETHINYLOESTRADIOL

Ethinyloestradiol has been used as hormone replacement for menopausal symptoms in a dose of 10–20 micrograms daily. This has now been largely replaced by more appropriate forms of oestrogen.

Ethinyloestradiol is occasionally used, under **specialist supervision**, for the management of *hereditary haemorrhagic telangiectasia* (but evidence of any beneficial effect is uncertain). Side-effects include nausea, fluid retention, and thrombosis. Impotence and gynaecomastia occur in men.

For use in breast cancer, see section 8.3.1

ETHINYLOESTRADIOL

Indications: see notes above

Cautions; Contra-indications; Side-effects: cardiovascular disease (sodium retention with oedema, thromboembolism), hepatic impairment (jaundice), feminising effects in men; see also under Combined Oral Contraceptives (section 7.3.1), and under Oestrogen for HRT (above)

Dose: see notes above

PoM **Ethinyloestradiol** (Non-proprietary)

Tablets, ethinyloestradiol 10 micrograms, net price 20 = £2.08; 50 micrograms, 20 = £3.04; 1 mg, 20 = £6.24

Available from Norton

STILBOESTROL

See section 8.3.1

6.4.1.2 PROGESTOGENS

There are two main groups of progestogen, *progesterone and its analogues* (dydrogesterone, hydroxyprogesterone, and medroxyprogesterone) and *testosterone analogues* (norethisterone and norgestrel). The newer progestogens (desogestrel, norgestimate, and gestodene) are all derivatives of norgestrel; levonorgestrel is the active isomer of norgestrel and has twice its potency. Progesterone and its analogues are less androgenic than the testosterone derivatives and neither progesterone nor dydrogesterone causes virilisation. Other synthetic derivatives are variably metabolised into testosterone and oestrogen; thus side-effects vary with the preparation and the dose.

Where *endometriosis* requires drug treatment, it may respond to a progestogen, e.g. norethisterone, administered on a continuous basis. Danazol, gestrinone, and gonadorelin analogues are also available (see section 6.7.2).

Although oral progestogens have been used widely for *menorrhagia* they are relatively ineffective compared with tranexamic acid (see section 2.11) or, particularly where dysmenorrhoea is also a factor, mefenamic acid (see section 10.1.1); the levonorgestrel-releasing intra-uterine device (see section 7.3.2.3) may be particularly useful for women also requiring contraception [currently licensed only as a contraceptive]. Oral progestogens have also been used for *severe dysmenorrhoea*, but where contraception is also required in younger women the best choice is a combined oral contraceptive (see section 4.7.1)

Progestogens have also been advocated for the alleviation of *premenstrual symptoms*, but no convincing physiological basis for such treatment has been shown.

Progestogens have been used in *habitual abortion* but there is no evidence of benefit. If they are used for this purpose they should be of the true progesterone-derivative type, e.g. **hydroxyprogesterone hexanoate** to avoid any masculinisation of a female fetus.

HORMONE REPLACEMENT THERAPY. In post-menopausal women receiving *long-term oestrogen therapy for hormone replacement*, a progestogen needs to be added to prevent cystic hyperplasia of the endometrium and possible transformation to cancer; it can be added on a cyclical or a continuous basis. Combined packs incorporating suitable progestogen tablets are available, see p. 306.

ORAL CONTRACEPTION. Desogestrel, ethynodiol, levonorgestrel, and norethisterone are used in *combined oral contraceptives* and in *progestogen-only contraceptives* (see sections 7.3.1 and 7.3.2).

CANCER. Progestogens also have a role in *neoplastic disease* (see section 8.3.2).

DESOGESTREL

Ingredient of combined oral contraceptives (section 7.3.1)

DYDROGESTERONE

Indications: see under Dose and notes above

Cautions; Contra-indications; Side-effects: see under Medroxyprogesterone Acetate and notes above; breakthrough bleeding may occur (increase dose)

Dose: endometriosis, 10 mg 2–3 times daily from 5th to 25th day of cycle or continuously

Infertility, irregular cycles, 10 mg twice daily from 11th to 25th day for at least 6 cycles (but not recommended)

Habitual abortion, 10 mg twice daily from day 11 to day 25 of cycle until conception, then continuously until 20th week of pregnancy and gradually reduced (but see notes above)

Dysfunctional uterine bleeding, 10 mg twice daily (together with an oestrogen) for 5–7 days to arrest bleeding; 10 mg twice daily (together with an oestrogen) from 11th to 25th day of cycle to prevent bleeding

Dysmenorrhoea, 10 mg twice daily from 5th to 25th day of cycle

Amenorrhoea, 10 mg twice daily from 11th to 25th day of cycle with oestrogen therapy from 1st to 25th day of cycle

Premenstrual syndrome, 10 mg twice daily from 12th to 26th day of cycle increased if necessary (but not recommended, see notes above)

Hormone replacement therapy, with continuous oestrogen therapy, see under *Duphaston*® HRT below

PoM Duphaston® (Solvay)
Tablets, yellow, scored, dydrogesterone 10 mg. Net price 60-tab pack = £11.87

PoM Duphaston® HRT (Solvay)
Tablets, yellow, scored, dydrogesterone 10 mg. Net price 42-tab pack = £8.31
Dose: 10 mg daily on days 15–28 of each 28-day oestrogen HRT cycle, increased to 10 mg twice daily if withdrawal bleed is early or endometrial biopsy shows inadequate progestational response

ETHYNODIOL DIACETATE
Ingredient of combined and progestogen-only oral contraceptives (sections 7.3.1 and 7.3.2).

GESTODENE
Ingredient of combined oral contraceptives (section 7.3.1)

GESTRONOL HEXANOATE
See section 8.3.2

HYDROXYPROGESTERONE HEXANOATE
(Hydroxyprogesterone Caproate)
Indications: habitual abortion but see notes above
Cautions; Contra-indications; Side-effects: see under Medroxyprogesterone acetate and notes above
Dose: by slow intramuscular injection, 250–500 mg weekly during first half of pregnancy

PoM Proluton* Depot® (Schering Health)
Injection (oily), hydroxyprogesterone hexanoate 250 mg/mL. Net price 1-mL amp = £2.35; 2-mL amp = £3.69
*formerly Primolut Depot®

LEVONORGESTREL
Ingredient of combined and progestogen-only contraceptives (sections 7.3.1 and 7.3.2)

MEDROXYPROGESTERONE ACETATE
Indications: see under Dose; contraception, see section 7.3.2.2; malignant disease, see section 8.3.2
Cautions: diabetes, hypertension, cardiac or renal disease; **interactions:** Appendix 1 (progestogens)
Contra-indications: pregnancy, undiagnosed vaginal bleeding, hepatic impairment or active liver disease, severe arterial disease, breast or genital tract carcinoma; porphyria (see section 9.8.2)
Side-effects: acne, urticaria, fluid retention, weight changes, gastro-intestinal disturbances, changes in libido, breast discomfort, premenstrual symptoms, irregular menstrual cycles; also depression, insomnia, somnolence, alopecia, hirsutism, anaphylactoid-like reaction; rarely jaundice
Dose: by mouth, 2.5–10 mg daily for 5–10 days beginning on 16th–21st day of cycle, repeated for 2 cycles in dysfunctional uterine bleeding and 3 cycles in secondary amenorrhoea
Mild to moderate endometriosis, 10 mg 3 times daily for 90 consecutive days, beginning on 1st day of cycle

PoM Provera® (Upjohn)
Tablets, all scored, medroxyprogesterone acetate 2.5 mg (orange), net price 30-tab pack = £1.93; 5 mg (blue), 10-tab pack = £1.29; 10 mg (white), 10-tab pack = £2.59, 90-tab pack = £23.20

Combined preparations
See section 6.4.1.1

MEGESTROL ACETATE
See section 8.3.2

NORETHISTERONE
Indications: see under Dose; HRT, see section 6.4.1.1; contraception, see sections 7.3.1 and 7.3.2; malignant disease, see section 8.3.2
Cautions; Contra-indications; Side-effects: see under Medroxyprogesterone Acetate but more virilising and greater incidence of liver disturbances and jaundice; avoid in pregnancy; exacerbation of epilepsy and migraine

Cautionary label wordings, see inside back cover

Prices are **net**, see p.1

Dose: endometriosis 10 mg daily starting on 5th day of cycle (increased if spotting occurs to 20–25 mg daily, reduced once bleeding has stopped)

Menorrhagia, 5 mg 3 times daily for 10 days to arrest bleeding; to prevent bleeding 5 mg twice daily from 19th to 26th day

Dysmenorrhoea, 5 mg 3 times daily from 5th to 24th day for 3–4 cycles

Premenstrual syndrome, 5 mg 2–3 times daily from 19th to 26th day for several cycles (but not recommended, see notes above)

Postponement of menstruation, 5 mg 3 times daily starting 3 days before anticipated onset (menstruation occurs 2–3 days after stopping)

Progestogenic opposition of menopausal oestrogen HRT, see under *Micronor® HRT*, below

Tablets of 5 mg
Note. **Not** licensed for HRT purposes
PoM **Menzol®** (Schwarz)
Tablets, scored, norethisterone 5 mg. Net price 3 × 24-tab (8-day) 'Planapak' = £7.70; 3 × 60-tab (20-day) 'Planapak' = £19.35
PoM **Primolut N®** (Schering Health)
Tablets, norethisterone 5 mg. Net price 30-tab pack = £2.16
PoM **Utovlan®** (Searle)
Tablets, scored, norethisterone 5 mg. Net price 100 = £6.54
Note. Norethisterone 5 mg tablets are also available from Cox

Tablets of 1 mg for HRT purposes
PoM **Micronor® HRT** (Cilag)
Tablets, norethisterone 1 mg. Net price 3 × 12-tab pack = £3.75
Dose: 1 tablet daily on days 15–26 of each 28-day oestrogen HRT cycle

Combined preparations
See section 6.4.1.1

NORETHISTERONE ACETATE
Ingredient of combined oral contraceptives (section 7.3.1) and combined preparations for HRT (section 6.4.1.1)

NORGESTIMATE
Ingredient of combined oral contraceptive (section 7.3.1)

NORGESTREL
Ingredient of progestogen-only oral contraceptives (section 7.3.2) and combined preparations for HRT (section 6.4.1.1)

PROGESTERONE
Indications: see under preparations
Cautions: diabetes, breast-feeding, hypertension; hepatic, cardiac, or renal disease; **interactions:** Appendix 1 (progestogens)

Contra-indications: undiagnosed vaginal bleeding, missed or incomplete abortion, severe arterial disease, mammary carcinoma; porphyria (see section 9.8.2)

Side-effects: acne, urticaria, fluid retention, weight changes, gastro-intestinal disturbances, changes in libido, breast discomfort, premenstrual symptoms, irregular menstrual cycles; also chloasma, depression, pyrexia, insomnia, somnolence, alopecia, hirsutism; rarely jaundice. Injection may be painful

PoM **Cyclogest®** (Hoechst)
Pessaries, progesterone 200 mg, net price 15 = £5.27; 400 mg, 15 = £7.63
Dose: by vagina or rectum, premenstrual syndrome, 200 mg daily to 400 mg twice daily starting at day 12–14 and continued until onset of menstruation (but not recommended, see notes above); rectally if barrier methods of contraception are used, or if vaginal infection
PoM **Gestone®** (Ferring)
Injection, progesterone 25 mg/mL, net price 1-mL amp = 34p; 50 mg/mL, 1-mL amp = 44p, 2-mL amp = 58p
Dose: by deep intramuscular injection into buttock, embryo transfer, consult data sheet

6.4.2　Male sex hormones and antagonists

Androgens cause masculinisation; they may be used as replacement therapy in castrated adults and in those who are hypogonadal due to either pituitary or testicular disease. In the normal male they inhibit pituitary gonadotrophin secretion and depress spermatogenesis. Androgens also have an anabolic action which led to the development of anabolic steroids (section 6.4.3).

Androgens are useless as a treatment of impotence and impaired spermatogenesis unless there is associated hypogonadism; they should not be given until the hypogonadism has been properly investigated. Treatment should be under expert supervision.

When given to patients with hypopituitarism they can lead to normal sexual development and potency but not to fertility. If fertility is desired, the usual treatment is with gonadotrophins or pulsatile gonadotrophin-releasing hormone (section 6.5.1) which will stimulate spermatogenesis as well as androgen production.

Caution should be used when androgens or chorionic gonadotrophin are used in treating boys with delayed puberty since the fusion of epiphyses is hastened and may result in short stature.

Androgens are still quite useful in occasional women with disseminated cancer of the breast despite their masculinising effects.

Intramuscular depot preparations of **testosterone esters** are preferred for replacement therapy. Testosterone enanthate or propionate or alternatively Sustanon®, which consists of a mixture of testosterone esters and has a longer duration of action, may be used. Satisfactory replacement therapy can sometimes be obtained with 1 mL of Sustanon 250®, given by intramuscular injection once a month, although more frequent dose intervals are often necessary. Implants of testosterone have been superseded for hypogonadism but are still occasionally used. Menopausal women are also sometimes given implants of testosterone (in a dose of 50–100 mg every 4–8 months) as an adjunct to hormone replacement therapy.

Of the orally available preparations, **testosterone undecanoate** and **mesterolone** are available. Methyltestosterone and other 17α-alkyl derivatives of testosterone are no longer on the UK market because they sometimes cause dose-related cholestatic jaundice.

TESTOSTERONE AND ESTERS

Indications: see under preparations

Cautions: cardiac, renal, or hepatic impairment (see Appendix 2), elderly, ischaemic heart disease, hypertension, epilepsy, migraine, skeletal metastases (risk of hypercalcaemia), pre-pubital boys (see notes above)

Contra-indications: breast cancer in men, prostatic cancer, hypercalcaemia, pregnancy, breast-feeding, nephrosis

Side-effects: sodium retention with oedema, hypercalcaemia, increased bone growth, priapism, precocious sexual development and premature closure of epiphyses in pre-pubertal males, virilism in women, and suppression of spermatogenesis in men

Oral

PoM **Restandol®** (Organon)

Capsules, red-brown, testosterone undecanoate 40 mg in oily solution. Net price 28-cap pack = £8.69; 56-cap pack = £17.38. Label: 21, 25

Dose: androgen deficiency, 120–160 mg daily for 2–3 weeks; maintenance 40–120 mg daily

Intramuscular

PoM **Primoteston Depot®** (Schering Health)

Injection (oily), testosterone enanthate 250 mg/mL. Net price 1-mL amp = £4.13

Dose: by slow intramuscular injection, hypogonadism, initially 250 mg every 2–3 weeks; maintenance 250 mg every 3–6 weeks

Breast cancer, 250 mg every 2–3 weeks

PoM **Sustanon 100®** (Organon)

Injection (oily), testosterone propionate 20 mg, testosterone phenylpropionate 40 mg, and testosterone isocaproate 40 mg/mL. Net price 1-mL amp = £1.22

Note. Contains arachis (peanut) oil

Dose: by deep intramuscular injection, androgen deficiency, 1 mL every 2 weeks

PoM **Sustanon 250®** (Organon)

Injection (oily), testosterone propionate 30 mg, testosterone phenylpropionate 60 mg, testosterone isocaproate 60 mg, and testosterone decanoate 100 mg/mL. Net price 1-mL amp = £2.87

Note. Contains arachis (peanut) oil

Dose: by deep intramuscular injection, androgen deficiency, 1 mL usually every 3 weeks

PoM **Virormone®** (Ferring)

Injection, testosterone propionate 50 mg/mL. Net price 2-mL amp = 46p

Dose: by intramuscular injection, androgen deficiency, 50 mg 2–3 times weekly

Delayed puberty, 50 mg weekly

Breast cancer, 100 mg 2–3 times weekly

Implant

PoM **Testosterone** (Organon)

Implant, testosterone 100 mg, net price = £7.40; 200 mg = £13.79

Dose: by implantation, male hypogonadism, 100–600 mg; 600 mg usually maintains plasma testosterone levels within the normal range for 4–5 months

Menopausal women, see notes above

MESTEROLONE

Indications: see under Dose

Cautions; Contra-indications; Side-effects: see under Testosterone Esters; spermatogenesis unimpaired

Dose: androgen deficiency, 25 mg 3–4 times daily for several months, reduced to 50–75 mg daily in divided doses for maintenance

PoM **Pro-Viron®** (Schering Health)

Tablets, scored, mesterolone 25 mg. Net price 30-tab pack = £4.75

ANTI-ANDROGENS

Cyproterone acetate is an anti-androgen used in the treatment of severe hypersexuality and sexual deviation in the male. It inhibits spermatogenesis and produces reversible infertility (but is not a male contraceptive); abnormal sperm forms are produced. Fully informed consent is recommended and an initial spermatogram. As hepatic tumours have been produced in *animal* studies, careful consideration should be given to the risk/benefit ratio before treatment. Cyproterone acetate is also used as an adjunct in prostatic cancer (see section 8.3.4) and in the treatment of acne and hirsutism in women (see section 13.6.2).

Finasteride is a specific inhibitor of the enzyme 5α-reductase which metabolises testosterone into the more potent androgen, dihydrotestosterone. This inhibition of testosterone metabolism leads to reduction in prostate size, with improvement in urinary flow rate and obstructive symptoms. It is an effective alternative to alpha-blockers (see section 7.4.1) in treatment of benign prostatic hyperplasia.

CYPROTERONE ACETATE

Indications: see notes above; prostate cancer, see section 8.3.4.2

Cautions: ineffective for male hypersexuality in chronic alcoholism (relevance to prostate cancer not known); blood counts initially and throughout treatment; monitor hepatic function regularly (liver function tests should be performed before treatment, see also under Side-effects below); monitor adrenocortical function regularly; diabetes mellitus (see also Contra-indications)

DRIVING. May impair performance of skilled tasks (e.g. driving)

Contra-indications: (do not apply in prostate cancer) hepatic disease, severe diabetes (with vascular changes); sickle-cell anaemia, malignant or wasting disease, severe depression, history of thrombo-embolic disorders; youths under 18 years (may arrest bone maturation and testicular development)

Side-effects: fatigue and lassitude, breathlessness, weight changes, reduced sebum production (may clear acne), changes in hair pattern, gynaecomastia (rarely leading to galactorrhoea and benign breast nodules); rarely osteoporosis; inhibition of spermatogenesis (see notes above); hepatotoxicity reported (including jaundice, hepatitis and hepatic failure usually in men given 200–300 mg daily for prostatic cancer, see section 8.3.4.2 for details and warnings)

Dose: male hypersexuality, 50 mg twice daily after food

PoM **Androcur**® (Schering Health)

Tablets, scored, cyproterone acetate 50 mg. Net price 56-tab pack = £32.23. Label: 3, 21

Note. Tablets containing cyproterone acetate 50 mg are also available from Cox, Generics, Hillcross, Lagap

FINASTERIDE

Indications: benign prostatic hyperplasia

Cautions: obstructive uropathy, prostate cancer (may decrease markers such as prostate specific antigen); use of condoms recommended if sexual partner is pregnant or is likely to become pregnant (finasteride excreted in semen); women of child-bearing potential should avoid handling crushed or broken tablets

Side-effects: impotence, decreased libido and ejaculate volume, breast tenderness and enlargement, hypersensitivity reactions (including lip swelling and rash)

Dose: 5 mg daily, review treatment after 6 months (may require several months treatment before benefit is obtained)

PoM **Proscar**® (MSD)

Tablets, blue, f/c, finasteride 5 mg. Net price 28-tab pack = £24.90

6.4.3   Anabolic steroids

All the anabolic steroids have some androgenic activity but they cause less virilisation than androgens in women. Their protein-building property led to the hope that they might be widely useful in medicine but this hope has not been realised. Their use as body builders or tonics is quite unjustified; they are abused by some athletes.

Anabolic steroids have also been given for osteoporosis in women but are no longer advocated for this purpose.

Anabolic steroids are used in the treatment of some *aplastic anaemias* (see section 9.1.3) and to reduce the itching of *chronic biliary obstruction* (see Prescribing in Palliative Care p. 13).

NANDROLONE

Indications: osteoporosis in postmenopausal women (but not recommended, see notes above); aplastic anaemia see section 9.1.3

Cautions: cardiac and renal impairment, hepatic impairment (see Appendix 2), hypertension, diabetes mellitus epilepsy, migraine; monitor skeletal maturation in young patients; skeletal metastases (risk of hypercalcaemia) **interactions:** Appendix 1 (anabolic steroids)

Contra-indications: severe hepatic impairment, prostate cancer, male breast cancer, pregnancy and breast-feeding, porphyria (see section 9.8.2)

Side-effects: acne, sodium retention with oedema, virilisation with high doses including voice changes (sometimes irreversible), amenorrhoea, inhibition of spermatogenesis, premature epiphyseal closure; abnormal liver-function tests reported with high doses; liver tumours reported occasionally on prolonged treatment with anabolic steroids

Dose: see below

PoM **Deca-Durabolin**® (Organon)

Injection (oily), nandrolone decanoate 25 mg/mL, net price 1-mL amp = £1.92; 50 mg/mL, 1-mL amp = £3.71

Note. Contains arachis (peanut) oil

Dose: by deep intramuscular injection, 50 mg every 3 weeks

PoM **Deca-Durabolin 100**® see section 9.1.3

STANOZOLOL

Indications: see under Dose

Cautions: cardiac or renal impairment; premature closure of epiphyses in children; peliosis hepatis and hepatic tumours reported on long-term treatment breast cancer (possibility of hypercalcaemia); monitor liver function, haematocrit and haemoglobin; diabetes mellitus (possible dosage adjustments for oral hypoglycaemic drugs and avoid in insulin-dependent diabetes); **interactions:** Appendix 1 (anabolic steroids)

Contra-indications: pregnancy, breast-feeding, established liver disease (if history of jaundice—liver function tests before starting treatment); prostate cancer, insulin-dependent diabetes mellitus; not indicated for treatment of loss of appetite, unexplained weight loss, or failure to thrive in children; porphyria (see section 9.8.2)

Side-effects: androgenic effects (generally mild and reversible on stopping treatment) include acne hirsutism, amenorrhoea, sodium retention with oedema; voice change—usually at higher dosage (discontinue); menstrual irregularity, headache muscle cramp, dyspepsia, rash, hair loss, euphoria depression, increased haematocrit and haemoglobin cholestatic jaundice and rarely peliosis hepatis and hepatic tumours also reported; changes in liver enzymes, in lipoproteins, and in thyroid hormones also premature epiphyseal closure (on prolonged treatment)

Dose: by mouth, vascular manifestations of Behcet's disease, 10 mg daily

Hereditary angioedema, 2.5–10 mg daily to control attacks, reduced for maintenance (2.5 mg 3 times weekly may be sufficient); CHILD 1–6 years initially 2.5 mg daily, 6–12 years initially 2.5–5 mg daily reduced for maintenance

Note. In hereditary angioedema restricted to well-established cases who have experienced serious attacks (and not for premenopausal women except in life-threatening situations)

PoM **Stromba**® (Sanofi Winthrop)
Tablets, scored, stanozolol 5 mg. Net price 56-tab pack = £26.26

6.5 Hypothalamic and pituitary hormones and anti-oestrogens

Hypothalamic and pituitary hormones are described under the following section headings:

6.5.1 Hypothalamic and anterior pituitary hormones and anti-oestrogens

6.5.2 Posterior pituitary hormones and antagonists

Use of preparations in these sections requires detailed prior investigation of the patient and *should be reserved for specialist centres.*

6.5.1 Hypothalamic and anterior pituitary hormones and anti-oestrogens

ANTI-OESTROGENS

The anti-oestrogens **clomiphene** and **tamoxifen** are used in the treatment of female infertility due to oligomenorrhoea or secondary amenorrhoea (e.g. associated with polycystic ovarian disease). They induce gonadotrophin release by occupying oestrogen receptors in the hypothalamus, thereby interfering with feedback mechanisms; chorionic gonadotrophin is sometimes used as an adjunct. Patients should be warned that there is a risk of multiple pregnancy (*rarely* more than twins).

CLOMIPHENE CITRATE

Indications: anovulatory infertility—see notes above

Cautions: see notes above; polycystic ovary syndrome (cysts may enlarge during treatment), ovarian hyperstimulation syndrome (OHSS), uterine fibroids, ectopic pregnancy, incidence of multiple births increased (consider ultrasound monitoring), visual symptoms (discontinue and initiate ophthalmological examination)

CSM Advice. The CSM has recommended that clomiphene should not normally be used for longer than 6 cycles (possible increased risk of ovarian cancer in patients treated for longer than recommended).

Contra-indications: hepatic disease, ovarian cysts, hormone dependent tumours or abnormal uterine bleeding of undetermined cause, pregnancy

Side-effects: visual disturbances (withdraw), ovarian hyperstimulation (withdraw), hot flushes, abdominal discomfort, occasionally nausea, vomiting, depression, insomnia, breast tenderness, headache, intermenstrual spotting, menorrhagia, endometriosis, convulsions, weight gain, rashes, dizziness, hair loss

Dose: 50 mg daily for 5 days, starting within about 5 days of onset of menstruation (preferably on 2nd day) or at any time (normally preceded by a progestogen-induced withdrawal bleed) if cycles have ceased; second course of 100 mg daily for 5 days may be given in absence of ovulation; most patients who are going to respond will do so to first course; 3 courses should constitute adequate therapeutic trial; long-term cyclical therapy not recommended—see CSM advice, above

PoM **Clomid**® (Merrell)
Tablets, yellow, scored, clomiphene citrate 50 mg. Net price 30-tab pack = £11.27; 100-tab pack = £32.80

PoM **Serophene**® (Serono)
Tablets, scored, clomiphene citrate 50 mg. Net price 10-tab pack = £4.12; 30-tab pack = £11.56; 100-tab pack = £33.64

TAMOXIFEN
See section 8.3.4

ANTERIOR PITUITARY HORMONES

CORTICOTROPHINS

Tetracosactrin an analogue of corticotrophin (ACTH) is used to test adrenocortical function; corticotrophin itself is no longer commercially available in the UK. Failure of the plasma cortisol concentration to rise after intramuscular administration indicates adrenocortical insufficiency.

Both corticotrophin and tetracosactrin were formerly used as alternatives to corticosteroids in conditions such as Crohn's disease or rheumatoid arthritis; their value was limited by the variable and unpredictable therapeutic response and by the waning of their effect with time.

TETRACOSACTRIN
(Tetracosactide)

Indications: see notes above

Cautions; Contra-indications; Side-effects: see section 6.3.2; important risk of anaphylaxis (medical supervision; see data sheet)

PoM **Synacthen**® (Ciba)
Injection, tetracosactrin 250 micrograms (as acetate)/mL. Net price 1-mL amp = £1.03p
Dose: diagnostic (30-minute test), *by intramuscular or intravenous injection*, 250 micrograms as a single dose

PoM **Synacthen Depot**® (Ciba)
Injection (aqueous suspension), tetracosactrin 1 mg (as acetate)/mL, with zinc phosphate complex; also contains benzyl alcohol. Net price 1-mL amp = £2.09
Dose: diagnostic (5-hour test), *by intramuscular injection*, 1 mg as a single dose
Note. Formerly used therapeutically by intramuscular injection, in an initial dose of 1 mg daily (or every 12 hours in acute cases); reduced to 1 mg every 2–3 days, then 1 mg weekly (or 500 micrograms every 2–3 days) but value was limited (see notes above)

GONADOTROPHINS

Follicle-stimulating hormone (FSH) and luteinising hormone (LH) together (as in **human menopausal gonadotrophin**) or follicle-stimulating hormone alone (as in **urofollitrophin** or **follitropin alpha**), are used in the treatment of infertile women with proven hypopituitarism or who have not responded to clomiphene, or in superovulation treatment for assisted conception (such as *in vitro* fertilisation).

The gonadotrophins are also occasionally used in the treatment of oligospermia associated with hypopituitarism. There is no justification for their use in primary gonadal failure.

Chorionic gonadotrophin has also been used in delayed puberty in the male to stimulate endogenous testosterone production, but has little advantage over testosterone (section 6.4.2).

CHORIONIC GONADOTROPHIN

(Human Chorionic Gonadotrophin; HCG)

A preparation of a glycoprotein fraction secreted by the placenta and obtained from the urine of pregnant women having the action of the pituitary luteinising hormone

Indications: see notes above

Cautions: see notes above; cardiac or renal impairment, asthma, epilepsy, migraine

Side-effects: oedema (particularly in males—reduce dose), headache, tiredness, mood changes, gynaecomastia, local reactions; sexual precocity with high doses; may aggravate ovarian hyperstimulation

Dose: by subcutaneous or intramuscular injection, according to patient's response

PoM **Gonadotraphon LH®** (Paines & Byrne)

Injection, powder for reconstitution, chorionic gonadotrophin. Net price 500-unit amp = 98p; 1000-unit amp = £1.25; 5000-unit amp = £3.47 (all with solvent). For intramuscular injection

PoM **Pregnyl®** (Organon)

Injection, powder for reconstitution, chorionic gonadotrophin. Net price 1500-unit amp = £2.48; 5000-unit amp = £3.69 (both with solvent). For intramuscular injection

PoM **Profasi®** (Serono)

Injection, powder for reconstitution, chorionic gonadotrophin. Net price 500-unit amp = 83p; 1000-unit amp = £1.14; 2000-unit amp = £2.10; 5000-unit amp = £3.56; 10 000-unit amp = £7.39 (all with solvent). For subcutaneous or intramuscular injection

FOLLITROPIN ALPHA

(Recombinant human follicle stimulating hormone)

Indications: see notes above

Cautions; Side-effects: see under Human Menopausal Gonadotrophins

Dose: by subcutaneous injection, according to patient's response

▼ PoM **Gonal-F®** (Serono)

Injection, powder for reconstitution, follitropin alpha 75 units, 1 amp = £29.00; 150 units, 1 amp = £58.34 (both with diluent)

HUMAN MENOPAUSAL GONADOTROPHINS

Purified extract of human post-menopausal urine containing follicle-stimulating hormone (FSH) and luteinising hormone (LH); the relative *in vivo* activity is designated a ratio; the 1:1 ratio is also known as menotrophin

Indications: see notes above

Cautions: ovarian cysts, adrenal or thyroid disorders, hyperprolactinoma or pituitary tumour

Side-effects: ovarian hyperstimulation, multiple pregnancy; local reactions

Dose: by deep intramuscular injection, according to patient's response

PoM **Humegon®** (Organon)

Injection, powder for reconstitution, menotrophin as follicle-stimulating hormone 75 units, luteinising hormone 75 units net price per amp = £8.60; follicle-stimulating hormone 150 units, luteinising hormone 150 units, 1 amp = £16.00 (both with solvent)

PoM **Normegon®** (Organon)

Injection, powder for reconstitution. human menopausal gonadotrophins as follicle-stimulating hormone 75 units, luteinising hormone 25 units net price per amp = £10.21; follicle-stimulating hormone 150 units, luteinising hormone 50 units, 1 amp = £20.41 (both with solvent)

PoM **Pergonal®** (Serono)

Injection, powder for reconstitution, menotrophin as follicle-stimulating hormone 75 units, luteinising hormone 75 units. Net price per amp (with solvent) = £9.91

UROFOLLITROPHIN

Extract of the urine of postmenopausal women containing follicle-stimulating hormone

Indications: see notes above

Cautions; Side-effects: see under Human Menopausal Gonadotrophins

Dose: by subcutaneous or intramuscular injection, according to patient's response

PoM **Metrodin High Purity®** (Serono)

Injection, powder for reconstitution, urofollitrophin as follicle-stimulating hormone, net price 75-unit amp = £18.62; 150-unit amp = £37.23 (both with solvent). For subcutaneous or intramuscular injection

PoM **Orgafol®** (Organon)

Injection, powder for reconstitution, urofollitrophin as follicle-stimulating hormone, net price 75-unit amp (with solvent) = £9.50. For intramuscular injection

GROWTH HORMONE

Growth hormone is used in the treatment of growth hormone deficiency (including short stature in Turner syndrome); only the human type is effective as growth hormone is species specific. Growth hormone of human origin (HGH; somatrophin) has been replaced by a growth hormone of human sequence, **somatropin**, produced using recombinant DNA technology.

SOMATROPIN
(Synthetic Human Growth Hormone)

Indications: see under Dose

Cautions: diabetes mellitus (adjustment of antidiabetic therapy may be necessary), papilloedema (see under Side-effects), relative deficiencies of other pituitary hormones (notably hypothyroidism—periodic thyroid function tests recommended), history of malignant disease, slipped epiphysis of the hip (monitor for limping), resolved intracranial hypertension (monitor closely), avoid in pregnancy (interrupt treatment if pregnancy occurs)

Contra-indications: evidence of tumour activity (complete antitumour therapy and ensure intracranial lesions inactive before starting); not to be used after renal transplantation or for growth promotion in children with closed epiphyses

Side-effects: funduscopy for papilloedema recommended if severe or recurrent headache, visual problems, nausea and vomiting occur—if papilloedema confirmed consider benign intracranial hypertension (rare cases reported); fluid retention (peripheral oedema, arthralgia, myalgia), anti-body formation, hypothyroidism, transient reactions at injection site; leukaemia in children with growth hormone deficiency also reported

Dose: by subcutaneous injection, weekly dosage tailored for each individual and given in 3, 6 or 7 divided doses (rotate injection sites to prevent lipoatrophy); alternatively *by intramuscular injection,* weekly dosage given in 3 divided doses (but more painful)

Gonadal dysgenesis (Turner syndrome), 0.6–1 unit/kg weekly (18–28 units/m² body-surface area weekly) in divided doses given by subcutaneous injection

Insufficient secretion of growth hormone in children, 0.5–0.7 units/kg weekly (14–20 units/m² body-surface area weekly) in divided doses given by subcutaneous or intramuscular injection

Chronic renal insufficiency in children (renal function decreased to less than 50%), approx. 1 unit/kg weekly (30 units/m² body-surface area weekly) divided into daily subcutaneous injections, higher doses may be needed; adjustment may be required after 6 months

Adult growth hormone deficiency, initially 0.125 units/kg weekly (divided into daily subcutaneous injections) gradually increased if required to max. 0.25 units/kg weekly; use minimum effective dose (requirements may decrease with age)

PoM Genotropin® (Pharmacia)
Injection, powder for reconstitution, somatropin (rbe), net price 4-unit vial (with diluent) = £30.50. For subcutaneous injection

Injection, two-compartment cartridge containing powder for reconstitution, somatropin (rbe) and diluent. Net price 16-unit cartridge = £122.00, 36-unit cartridge = £274.50. For use with NHS Genotropin® Pen device (available free from clinics). For subcutaneous injection

KabiQuick injection, two-compartment single-dose syringe containing powder for reconstitution, somatropin (rbe) and diluent. Net price 2-unit syringe = £16.00, 3-unit syringe = £24.00, 4-unit syringe = £32.00. For subcutaneous injection

KabiVial injection, two-compartment cartridge containing powder for reconstitution, somatropin (rbe) and diluent. Net price 4-unit vial = £30.50, 16-unit vial = £122.00. For subcutaneous injection

PoM Humatrope® (Lilly)
Injection, powder for reconstitution, somatropin (rbe), net price 4-unit vial = £30.50; 16-unit vial = £122.00 (both with diluent). For subcutaneous or intramuscular injection

PoM Norditropin® (Novo Nordisk)
Injection, powder for reconstitution, somatropin (epr), net price 12-unit vial (with diluent) = £89.21. For subcutaneous injection

PenSet 12 injection, powder for reconstitution, somatropin (epr), net price 12-unit vial (with diluent in cartridge and needle) = £93.68. For use with NHS Nordiject®12 device (available free from clinics). For subcutaneous injection

PenSet 24 injection, powder for reconstitution, somatropin (epr), net price 24-unit vial (with diluent in cartridge and needle) = £187.35. For use with NHS Nordiject® 24 device (available free from clinics). For subcutaneous injection

PoM Saizen® (Serono)
Injection, powder for reconstitution, somatropin (rmc), net price 4-unit vial (with diluent) = £30.50; 10-unit vial (with diluent) = £76.25. For subcutaneous or intramuscular injection

PoM Zomacton® (Ferring)
Injection, powder for reconstitution, somatropin (rbe), net price 12-unit vial (with diluent) = £83.28. For subcutaneous injection

HYPOTHALAMIC HORMONES

Gonadorelin when injected intravenously in normal subjects leads to a rapid rise in plasma concentrations of both luteinising hormone (LH) and follicle-stimulating hormone (FSH). It has not proved to be very helpful, however, in distinguishing hypothalamic from pituitary lesions. Gonadorelin is also used for treatment of infertility, particularly in the female. **Gonadorelin analogues** are indicated in endometriosis and infertility (see section 6.7.2) and in breast and prostate cancer (see section 8.3.4).

Protirelin may be of value in difficult cases of hyperthyroidism but has been superseded largely by immunoassays. Failure of plasma thyrotrophin (TSH) concentration to rise after intravenous injection indicates excess circulating thyroid hormones. Impaired or absent responses also occur in some euthyroid patients with single adenoma, multinodular goitre, or endocrine exophthalmos; patients with hypopituitarism show a reduced or delayed rise.

Sermorelin, an analogue of growth hormone releasing hormone (somatorelin, GHRH), has recently been introduced as a diagnostic test for secretion of growth hormone.

GONADORELIN

(Gonadotrophin-releasing hormone; GnRH; LH–RH)

Indications: see preparations below

Side-effects: rarely, nausea, headache, abdominal pain, increased menstrual bleeding; rarely, hypersensitivity reaction on repeated administration of large doses; irritation at injection site

Dose: see under preparations

PoM **Fertiral**® (Hoechst)

Injection, gonadorelin 500 micrograms/mL. Net price 2-mL amp = £33.44

> For amenorrhoea and infertility due to abnormal release of LH–RH (endogenous gonadorelin), *by pulsatile subcutaneous infusion*, initially 10–20 micrograms over 1 minute, repeated every 90 minutes until conception occurs or for max. of 6 months; *pulsatile intravenous infusion* (in association with heparin) may be required

PoM **HRF**® (Monmouth)

Injection, powder for reconstitution, gonadorelin. Net price 100-microgram vial = £13.45; 500-microgram vial = £29.39 (both with diluent) (hosp. only)

> For assessment of pituitary function (adults), *by subcutaneous or intravenous injection*, 100 micrograms

PoM **Relefact LH–RH**® (Hoechst)

Injection, gonadorelin 100 micrograms/mL. Net price 1-mL amp = £9.44

> For assessment of pituitary function, *by intravenous injection*, 100 micrograms

PoM **Relefact LH-RH/TRH**® (Hoechst)

Injection, gonadorelin 100 micrograms, protirelin 200 micrograms/mL. Net price 1-mL amp = £10.90

> For assessment of anterior pituitary reserve, *by intravenous injection*, 1 mL

PROTIRELIN

(Thyrotrophin-releasing hormone; TRH)

Indications: assessment of thyroid function and thyroid stimulating hormone reserve

Cautions: severe hypopituitarism, myocardial ischaemia, bronchial asthma and obstructive airways disease, pregnancy

Side-effects: after rapid intravenous administration desire to micturate, flushing, dizziness, nausea, strange taste; transient increase in pulse rate and blood pressure; rarely bronchospasm

Dose: by intravenous injection, 200 micrograms; CHILD 1 microgram/kg

PoM **TRH-Cambridge**® (Cambridge)

Injection, protirelin 100 micrograms/mL. Net price 2-mL amp = £6.60 (hosp. only)

SERMORELIN

Indications: see notes above

Cautions: epilepsy; discontinue growth hormone therapy 1–2 weeks before test; untreated hypothyroidism, antithyroid drugs; obesity, hyperglycaemia, elevated plasma fatty acids; avoid preparations which affect release of growth hormone (includes those affecting release of somatostatin, insulin or glucocorticoids and cyclooxygenase inhibitors such as aspirin and indomethacin)

Contra-indications: pregnancy and breast-feeding

Side-effects: occasional facial flushing and pain at injection site

Dose: by intravenous injection, 1 microgram/kg in the morning after an overnight fast

▼ PoM **Geref 50**® (Serono)

Injection, powder for reconstitution, sermorelin 50 micrograms (as acetate). Net price per amp (with solvent) = £55.00

6.5.2   Posterior pituitary hormones and antagonists

POSTERIOR PITUITARY HORMONES

DIABETES INSIPIDUS. **Vasopressin** (antidiuretic hormone, ADH) is used in the treatment of *pituitary* ('cranial') *diabetes insipidus* as its analogues **lypressin** or **desmopressin**. Dosage is tailored to produce a slight diuresis every 24 hours to avoid water intoxication. Treatment may be required for a limited period only in diabetes insipidus following trauma or pituitary surgery.

Desmopressin has a longer duration of action than vasopressin or lypressin; unlike vasopressin and lypressin it has no vasoconstrictor effect. It is given by mouth or intranasally for maintenance therapy and by injection in the postoperative period or in unconscious patients. Desmopressin is also used in the differential diagnosis of diabetes insipidus. Following a dose of 2 micrograms intramuscularly or 20 micrograms intranasally, restoration of the ability to concentrate urine after water deprivation confirms a diagnosis of cranial diabetes insipidus. Failure to respond occurs in nephrogenic diabetes insipidus.

In *nephrogenic* and *partial pituitary diabetes insipidus* benefit may be gained from the paradoxical antidiuretic effect of thiazides (see section 2.2.1) e.g. chlorthalidone 100 mg twice daily reduced to maintenance dose of 50 mg daily.

Chlorpropamide (section 6.1.2.1) is also useful in partial pituitary diabetes insipidus, and probably acts by sensitising the renal tubules to the action of remaining endogenous vasopressin; it is given in doses of up to 350 mg daily in adults and 200 mg daily in children, care being taken to avoid hypoglycaemia. Carbamazepine (see section 4.8.1) is also sometimes useful (in a dose of 200 mg once or twice daily) [unlicensed]; its mode of action may be similar to that of chlorpropamide.

OTHER USES. Desmopressin injection is also used to boost factor VIII concentrations in mild to moderate haemophilia. For a comment on use of desmopressin in nocturnal enuresis see section 7.4.2.

Vasopressin infusion is used to control variceal bleeding in portal hypertension, prior to more definitive treatment and with variable results. Terlipressin, a derivative of vasopressin, is used similarly.

Oxytocin, another posterior pituitary hormone, is indicated in obstetrics (see section 7.1.1).

VASOPRESSIN

Indications: pituitary diabetes insipidus; bleeding from oesophageal varices

Cautions: heart failure, asthma, epilepsy, migraine or other conditions which might be aggravated by water retention; renal impairment (see also contra-indications); pregnancy; avoid fluid overload

Contra-indications: vascular disease (especially disease of coronary arteries) unless extreme caution, chronic nephritis (until reasonable blood nitrogen concentrations attained)

Side-effects: pallor, nausea, belching, abdominal cramps, desire to defaecate, hypersensitivity reactions, constriction of coronary arteries (may cause anginal attacks and myocardial ischaemia)

Dose: by subcutaneous or intramuscular injection, diabetes insipidus, 5–20 units every four hours

By intravenous infusion, initial control of variceal bleeding, 20 units over 15 minutes

Synthetic vasopressin

PoM Pitressin® (P-D)

Injection, argipressin (synthetic vasopressin) 20 units/mL. Net price 1-mL amp = £10.00 (hosp. only)

DESMOPRESSIN

Indications: see under Dose

Cautions: see under Vasopressin; less pressor activity, but still considerable caution in renal impairment, in cardiovascular disease and in hypertension (not indicated for nocturnal enuresis or nocturia in these circumstances); also considerable caution in cystic fibrosis; avoid fluid overload—in nocturia periodic blood pressure and weight checks needed to monitor for fluid overload; **interactions:** Appendix 1 (desmopressin)

HYPONATRAEMIC CONVULSIONS. The CSM has advised that patients being treated for primary nocturnal enuresis should be warned to avoid fluid overload (including during swimming) and to stop taking desmopressin during an episode of vomiting or diarrhoea (until fluid balance normal). The risk of hyponatraemic convulsions can also be minimised by keeping to the recommended starting doses and by avoiding concomitant use of drugs which increase secretion of vasopressin (e.g. tricyclic antidepressants)

Side-effects: fluid retention, and hyponatraemia (in more serious cases with convulsions) on administration without restricting fluid intake; headache, nausea, vomiting, and epistaxis also reported

Dose: by mouth

Diabetes insipidus, treatment, ADULT and CHILD, initially 300 micrograms daily (in three divided doses); maintenance, 300–600 micrograms daily; range 0.2–1.2 mg daily

Primary nocturnal enuresis (with normal urine concentrating ability), ADULT and CHILD over 5 years (preferably over 7 years), 200 micrograms at bedtime, only increased to 400 micrograms if lower dose not effective (**important:** see also Cautions; withdraw for at least one week for reassessment after 3 months

Postoperative polyuria/polydipsia, adjust dose according to urine osmolality

Intranasally

Diabetes insipidus, diagnosis, ADULT and CHILD, 20 micrograms

Diabetes insipidus, treatment, ADULT, 10–40 micrograms daily (in one or two divided doses); CHILD, 5–20 micrograms; infants may require lower doses

Primary nocturnal enuresis (with normal urine concentrating ability), ADULT and CHILD over 5 years (preferably over 7 years), initially 20 micrograms at bedtime, only increased to 40 micrograms if lower dose not effective (**important:** see also Cautions); withdraw for at least one week for reassessment after 3 months

Nocturia associated with multiple sclerosis (when other treatments have failed), ADULT (under 65 years), 10–20 micrograms at bedtime (**important:** see also cautions)

Renal function testing (empty bladder at time of testing), ADULT, 40 micrograms; CHILD (1–15 years), 20 micrograms; CHILD (under 1 year), 10 micrograms (restrict fluid intake to 50% at next two feeds to avoid fluid overload)

By injection

Diabetes insipidus, diagnosis (*subcutaneous or intramuscular*), ADULT and CHILD, 2 micrograms

Diabetes insipidus, treatment (*subcutaneous, intramuscular or intravenous*), ADULT, 1–4 micrograms daily; CHILD 400 nanograms

Renal function testing (*subcutaneous or intramuscular*), ADULT and CHILD, 2 micrograms

Mild to moderate haemophilia and von Willebrands disease, post lumbar puncture headache, fibrinolytic response testing, consult data sheet

PoM DDAVP® (Ferring)

Tablets, both scored, desmopressin acetate 100 micrograms, net price 90-tab pack = £45.95; 200 micrograms, 90-tab pack = £91.90. Counselling, fluid intake, see above

Intranasal solution, desmopressin 100 micrograms/mL. Net price 2.5-mL dropper bottle and catheter = £9.50. Counselling, fluid intake, see above

Injection, desmopressin 4 micrograms/mL. Net price 1-mL amp = £1.07

PoM Desmotabs® (Ferring)

Tablets, scored, desmopressin acetate 200 micrograms, net price 28-tab pack = £29.00. Counselling, fluid intake, see above

PoM Desmospray® (Ferring)

Nasal spray, desmopressin 10 micrograms/metered spray. Net price 5-mL unit = £22.90. Counselling, fluid intake, see above

Note. Children requiring dose of less than 10 micrograms should be given DDAVP® intranasal solution

LYPRESSIN

Indications: pituitary diabetes insipidus

Cautions; Contra-indications; Side-effects: see under Vasopressin; less hypersensitivity; also nasal congestion with ulceration of mucosa

Dose: intranasally, 5–10 units 3–4 times daily

PoM **Syntopressin**® (Sandoz)

Nasal spray, lypressin 50 units/mL, 5 units/squeeze. Net price 5-mL bottle = £3.40

TERLIPRESSIN

Indications: bleeding from oesophageal varices

Cautions; Contra-indications; Side-effects: see under Vasopressin, but effects are milder

Dose: by intravenous injection, 2 mg followed by 1 or 2 mg every 4 to 6 hours until bleeding is controlled, for up to 72 hours

PoM **Glypressin**® (Ferring)

Injection, terlipressin, powder for reconstitution. Net price 1-mg vial with 5 mL diluent = £19.00 (hosp. only)

ANTIDIURETIC HORMONE ANTAGONISTS

Demeclocycline (see section 5.1.3) may be used in the treatment of hyponatraemia resulting from inappropriate secretion of antidiuretic hormone. It is thought to act by directly blocking the renal tubular effect of antidiuretic hormone. Initially 0.9 to 1.2 g is given daily in divided doses, reduced to 600–900 mg daily for maintenance.

6.6 Drugs affecting bone metabolism

6.6.1   Calcitonin
6.6.2   Bisphosphonates

See also calcium (section 9.5.1.1), phosphorus (section 9.5.2), vitamin D (section 9.6.4), and oestrogens in postmenopausal osteoporosis (section 6.4.1.1).

6.6.1   Calcitonin

Calcitonin is involved with parathyroid hormone in the regulation of bone turnover and hence in the maintenance of calcium balance and homoeostasis. It is used to lower the plasma-calcium concentration in some patients with hypercalcaemia (notably when associated with malignant disease). In the treatment of severe Paget's disease of bone it is used mainly for relief of pain but it is also effective in relieving some of the neurological complications, for example deafness. The prolonged use of porcine calcitonin can lead to the production of neutralising antibodies. **Salcatonin** (synthetic salmon calcitonin) is less immunogenic and thus more suitable for long-term therapy. When changing treatment in Paget's disease, calcitonin (pork) 80 units is equivalent to salcatonin 50 units.

CALCITONIN (PORK)

Indications: Paget's disease of bone; hypercalcaemia

Cautions: see notes above; may contain trace of thyroid; skin test if history of allergy; pregnancy and breast-feeding (avoid—inhibits lactation in *animals*)

Side-effects: nausea, vomiting, flushing, tingling of hands, unpleasant taste, inflammatory reactions at injection site

Dose: hypercalcaemia, *by subcutaneous or intramuscular injection*, initially 4 units/kg daily adjusted according to clinical and biochemical response (higher doses more conveniently given as salcatonin, see below)

Paget's disease of bone, *by subcutaneous or intramuscular injection*, dose range 80 units 3 times weekly to 160 units daily in single or divided doses; in patients with bone pain or nerve compression syndromes, 80–160 units daily for 3–6 months

PoM **Calcitare**® (Rhône-Poulenc Rorer)

Injection, powder for reconstitution, porcine calcitonin. Net price 160-unit vial (with gelatin diluent) = £12.18

SALCATONIN
(Calcitonin (salmon))

Indications: see under Dose (all short term)

Cautions; Side-effects: see under Calcitonin (pork) and notes above

Dose: hypercalcaemia, *by subcutaneous or intramuscular injection*, range from 5–10 units/kg daily *to* 400 units every 6–8 hours adjusted according to clinical and biochemical response (no additional benefit with over 8 units/kg every 6 hours); *by slow intravenous infusion* (Miacalcic® only), 5–10 units/kg over at least 6 hours

Paget's disease of bone, *by subcutaneous or intramuscular injection*, dose range 50 units 3 times weekly to 100 units daily, in single or divided doses; in patients with bone pain or nerve compression syndromes, 50–100 units daily for 3–6 months

Bone pain in neoplastic disease, *by subcutaneous or intramuscular injection*, 200 units every 6 hours *or* 400 units every 12 hours for 48 hours may be repeated at discretion of physician

Postmenopausal osteoporosis, *by subcutaneous or intramuscular injection*, 100 units daily with dietary calcium and vitamin D supplements (see sections 9.5.1.1 and 9.6.4)

PoM **Calsynar**® (Rhône-Poulenc Rorer)

Injection, salcatonin 100 units/mL in saline/acetate, net price 1-mL amp = £7.92; 200 units/mL in saline/acetate, 2-mL vial = £28.47
For subcutaneous or intramuscular injection only

PoM **Miacalcic**® (Sandoz)

Injection, salcatonin 50 units/mL, net price 1-mL amp = £3.56; 100 units/mL, 1-mL amp = £7.13; 200 units/mL, 2-mL vial = £25.62
For subcutaneous or intramuscular injection and for dilution and use as an intravenous infusion

---

6.6.2 Bisphosphonates

Bisphosphonates are used mainly in the treatment of *Paget's disease* of bone. They are adsorbed onto hydroxyapatite crystals, so slowing both their rate of growth and dissolution, and reduce the increased rate of bone turnover associated with the disease. They are also used in the treatment of *hypercalcaemia of malignancy* (see section 9.5.1.2). Bisphosphonates may also have an important role in treating *osteoporosis in postmenopausal women*.

ALENDRONIC ACID
Indications: postmenopausal osteoporosis
Cautions: upper gastro-intestinal disorders (dysphagia, symptomatic oesophageal disease, gastritis, duodenitis, or ulcers—see also under Contra-indications and Side-effects); correct disturbances of calcium and mineral metabolism (e.g. vitamin D deficiency, hypocalcaemia) before starting; exclude other causes of osteoporosis; avoid concomitant use with aspirin or NSAIDs; **interactions:** Appendix 1 (bisphosphonates)
Contra-indications: abnormalities of oesophagus and other factors which delay emptying (e.g. stricture or achalasia), hypocalcaemia (ensure adequate calcium intake), renal impairment, pregnancy and breast-feeding; inability to stand or sit upright for 30 minutes (see Counselling below)
Side-effects: oesophageal reactions (see below), abdominal pain and distension, diarrhoea or constipation, flatulence, musculoskeletal pain, headache; rash, erythema and transient decreases in serum calcium and phosphate also reported
OESOPHAGEAL REACTIONS. Severe oesophageal reactions (oesophagitis, oesophageal ulcers and oesophageal erosions) have been reported; patients should be advised to stop taking the tablets and to seek medical attention if they develop symptoms of oesophageal irritation such as dysphagia, new or worsening heartburn, pain on swallowing or retrosternal pain
Dose: 10 mg daily at least 30 minutes before breakfast
COUNSELLING. Swallow the tablets whole with a full glass of water on an empty stomach at least 30 minutes before breakfast (and any other oral medication); stand or sit upright for at least 30 minutes and do not lie down until after eating breakfast. Do not take the tablets at bedtime or before rising.

▼ PoM **Fosamax**® (MSD)
Tablets, alendronic acid 10 mg (as alendronate sodium). Net price 28-tab pack = £25.69. Counselling, administration

DISODIUM ETIDRONATE
Indications: see under Dose
Cautions: reduce dose in mild renal impairment (avoid if moderate to severe); **interactions:** Appendix 1 (bisphosphonates)
Contra-indications: moderate to severe renal impairment; pregnancy and breast-feeding; not indicated for osteoporosis in presence of hypercalcaemia or hypercalciuria or for osteomalacia

Side-effects: nausea, diarrhoea; asymptomatic hypocalcaemia; increased bone pain in Paget's disease, also increased risk of fractures with high doses in Paget's disease (discontinue if fractures occur); rarely skin reactions (including angio-edema urticaria and pruritus), transient hyperphosphataemia, abdominal pain, constipation, headache, paraesthesia, peripheral neuropathy reported; blood disorders (including leucopenia, agranulocytosis and pancytopenia) also reported
Dose: Paget's disease of bone, *by mouth*, 5 mg/kg as a single daily dose for up to 6 months; doses above 10 mg/kg daily for up to 3 months may be used with caution but doses above 20 mg/kg daily are not recommended; after interval of not less than 3 months may be repeated where evidence of reactivation—including biochemical indices (avoid premature retreatment)
MONITORING. Serum phosphate, serum alkaline phosphatase and (if possible) urinary hydroxyproline should be measured before starting and at intervals of 3 months—see data sheet for further details
Established vertebral osteoporosis, see under *Didronel PMO*®

COUNSELLING. Avoid food for at least 2 hours before and after oral treatment, particularly calcium-containing products e.g. milk; also avoid iron and mineral supplements and antacids

PoM **Didronel**® (Procter & Gamble Pharm.)
Tablets, disodium etidronate 200 mg. Net price 60-tab pack = £43.88. Counselling, food and calcium (see above)

With calcium carbonate
For cautions and side-effects of calcium carbonate see section 9.5.1.1
PoM **Didronel PMO**® (Procter & Gamble Pharm.)
Tablets, 14 white, disodium etidronate 400 mg; 76 pink, effervescent, calcium carbonate 1.25 g (Cacit®). Net price per pack = £40.20. Label: 10 patient information leaflet, counselling, food and calcium (see above)
Dose: established vertebral osteoporosis (90-day cycles) 1 etidronate daily for 14 days, then 1 calcium daily for 76 days

DISODIUM PAMIDRONATE
Disodium pamidronate was formerly called aminohydroxypropylidenediphosphonate disodium (APD)
Indications: see under Dose
Cautions: renal impairment—monitor renal function in those with pre-existing renal disease or predisposition to renal impairment (e.g. in multiple myeloma or tumour-induced hypercalcaemia); cardiac disease (especially in elderly); previous thyroid surgery (risk of hypocalcaemia); monitor serum electrolytes, calcium and phosphate—possibility of convulsions due to electrolyte changes; avoid concurrent use with other bisphosphonates; **interactions:** Appendix 1 (bisphosphonates)
DRIVING. Patients should be warned against driving or operating machinery immediately after treatment (somnolence or dizziness may occur)

Contra-indications: pregnancy and breast-feeding

Side-effects: asymptomatic hypocalcaemia, hypophosphataemia, transient rise in body temperature, fever and influenza-like symptoms (sometimes accompanied by malaise, rigors, fatigue and flushes), oliguria; occasionally transient bone pain, arthralgia, myalgia, nausea, vomiting, headache lymphocytopenia, hypomagnesaemia; rarely muscle cramps, anorexia, abdominal pain, diarrhoea, constipation, dyspepsia, agitation, confusion, dizziness, insomnia, somnolence, lethargy, anaemia, leucopenia, hypotension or hypertension, rash, pruritus, hyperkalaemia or hypokalaemia, hypernatraemia, symptomatic hypocalcaemia (with paraesthesia, tetany); isolated cases of seizures, hallucinations, thrombocytopenia, haematuria, acute renal failure, deterioration of pre-existing renal disease, conjunctivitis and other ocular symptoms, abnormal liver function tests, reactivation of herpes simplex and zoster also reported; also local reactions at injection site

Dose: by slow intravenous infusion (via cannula in a relatively large vein), see also Appendix 6

Hypercalcaemia of malignancy, according to serum calcium concentration 15–60 mg in single infusion or in divided doses over 2–4 days; max. 90 mg per treatment course

Osteolytic lesions and bone pain in bone metastases associated with breast cancer or multiple myeloma, 90 mg every 4 weeks (or every 3 weeks to coincide with chemotherapy in breast cancer)

Paget's disease of bone, 30 mg once a week for 6 weeks (total dose 180 mg) *or* 30 mg in first week then 60 mg every other week (total dose 210 mg); max. total 360 mg (in divided doses of 60 mg) per treatment course; may be repeated every 6 months

CALCIUM AND VITAMIN D SUPPLEMENTS. Oral supplements are advised for those with Paget's disease at risk of calcium or vitamin D deficiency (e.g. through malabsorption or lack of exposure to sunlight) to minimise potential risk of hypocalcaemia

PoM **Aredia Dry Powder®** (Ciba)

Injection, powder for reconstitution, disodium pamidronate, for use as an infusion. Net price 15-mg vial = £27.27; 30-mg vial = £54.53; 90-mg vial = £155.80 (all with diluent). Counselling, driving, see above

SODIUM CLODRONATE

Indications: see under Dose

Cautions: monitor renal and hepatic function and white cell count; also monitor serum calcium and phosphate periodically; renal dysfunction reported in patients receiving concomitant NSAIDs; maintain adequate fluid intake during treatment; **interactions:** Appendix 1 (bisphosphonates)

Contra-indications: moderate to severe renal impairment; pregnancy and breast-feeding

Side-effects: nausea, diarrhoea; asymptomatic hypocalcaemia; skin reactions

Dose: osteolytic lesions, hypercalcaemia and bone pain associated with skeletal metastases in patients with breast cancer or multiple myeloma, *by mouth,* 1.6 g daily in single or 2 divided dose increased if necessary to a max. of 3.2 g daily

COUNSELLING. Avoid food for 1 hour before and after treatment, particularly calcium-containing products e.g. milk; also avoid iron and mineral supplements and antacids; maintain adequate fluid intake

Hypercalcaemia of malignancy, *by slow intravenous infusion,* 300 mg daily for max. 7–10 day *or* by single-dose infusion of 1.5 g

PoM **Bonefos®** (Boehringer Ingelheim)

Capsules, yellow, sodium clodronate 400 mg. Net price 30-cap pack = £45.59; 112-cap pack = £170.23, 120-cap pack = £182.39. Counselling, food and calcium

Tablets, f/c, scored, sodium clodronate 800 mg. Net price 10-tab pack = £30.40; 60-tab pack = £182.39. Counselling, food and calcium

Concentrate (= intravenous solution), sodium clodronate 60 mg/mL, for dilution and use as infusion. Net price 5-mL amp = £14.43

PoM **Loron®** (Boehringer Mannheim)

Loron® capsules, sodium clodronate 400 mg. Net price 120-cap pack = £202.65. Label: 10 patient information leaflet, counselling, food and calcium

Loron 520® tablets, f/c, scored, sodium clodronate 520 mg. Net price 10-tab pack = £30.40; 60-tab pack = £182.39. Label: 10 patient information leaflet, counselling, food and calcium

Dose: 2 tablets daily in single or two divided doses; may be increased to max. 4 tablets daily

Note. Due to greater bioavailability one *Loron 520®* tablet (520 mg) is equivalent to two *Loron®* capsules (2 × 400 mg)

PoM **Loron® for infusion** (Boehringer Mannheim)

Intravenous solution, sodium clodronate 30 mg/mL, for dilution and use as infusion. Net price 10-mL amp = £14.43

TILUDRONIC ACID

Indications: Paget's disease of bone

Cautions: renal impairment (monitor renal function regularly, see under Contra-indications); correct disturbances of calcium metabolism disorders (e.g. vitamin D deficiency, hypocalcaemia) before starting; avoid concomitant use of indomethacin; **interactions:** Appendix 1 (bisphosphonates)

Contra-indications: severe renal impairment, juvenile Paget's disease, pregnancy and breast-feeding

Side-effects: stomach pain, nausea, diarrhoea; rarely asthenia, dizziness, headache and skin reactions

Dose: 400 mg daily as a single dose for 12 weeks; may be repeated if necessary after 6 months

COUNSELLING. Avoid food for 2 hours before and after treatment, particularly calcium-containing products e.g. milk; also avoid antacids

▼ PoM **Skelid**® (Sanofi Winthrop)

Tablets, tiludronic acid (as tiludronate disodium) 200 mg. Net price 28-tab pack = £99.00. Counselling, food and calcium

6.7 Other endocrine drugs

This section includes:

6.7.1 Bromocriptine and other dopamine-receptor stimulants

6.7.2 Danazol, gestrinone, and gonadorelin analogues

6.7.3 Metyrapone and trilostane

6.7.1 Bromocriptine and other dopamine-receptor stimulants

Bromocriptine is a stimulant of dopamine receptors in the brain; it also inhibits release of prolactin by the pituitary. Bromocriptine is used for the treatment of galactorrhoea and cyclical benign breast disease, and for the treatment of prolactinomas (when it reduces both plasma prolactin concentration and tumour size). Bromocriptine also inhibits the release of growth hormone and is sometimes used in the treatment of acromegaly, the success rate is much lower than with prolactinomas.

Cabergoline has actions and uses similar to those of bromocriptine, but its duration of action is longer. Its profile of side-effects appears to differ from that of bromocriptine, which means that patients intolerant of bromocriptine may be able to tolerate cabergoline (and *vice versa*).

Quinagolide has been introduced recently; its actions and uses are similar to those of bromocriptine, but its profile of side-effects differs slightly.

SUPPRESSION OF LACTATION. Although bromocriptine and cabergoline are licensed to suppress lactation, they are **not** recommended for routine suppression (or for the relief of symptoms of post-partum pain and engorgement) that can be adequately treated with simple analgesics and breast support. Quinagolide is not licensed for the suppression of lactation.

BROMOCRIPTINE

Indications: see notes above and under Dose; parkinsonism, see section 4.9.1

Cautions: specialist evaluation—monitor for pituitary enlargement, particularly during pregnancy, annual gynaecological assessment (post-menopausal, every 6 months), monitor for peptic ulceration in acromegalic patients; contraceptive advice if appropriate (oral contraceptives may increase prolactin concentrations); caution in patients with history of serious mental disorders (especially psychotic disorders) or with cardiovascular disease or Raynaud's syndrome and monitor for retroperitoneal fibrosis; hepatic and renal impairment (see appendixes 2 and 3); por-

phyria (see section 9.8.2); **interactions:** Appendix 1 (bromocriptine and cabergoline)

HYPOTENSIVE REACTIONS. Hypotensive reactions may be disturbing in some patients during the first few days of treatment and particular care should be exercised when driving or operating machinery; tolerance may be reduced by alcohol

Contra-indications: hypersensitivity to bromocriptine or other ergot alkaloids; toxaemia of pregnancy and hypertension in postpartum women or in puerperium (see also below); advise women not to breast-feed if lactation prevention fails

POSTPARTUM OR PUERPERIUM. Should not be used postpartum or in puerperium in women with high blood pressure, coronary artery disease or symptoms (or history) of serious mental disorder; monitor blood pressure carefully (especially during first few days) in postpartum women. Very rarely hypertension, myocardial infarction, seizures or stroke (both sometimes preceded by severe headache) and mental disorders have been reported in postpartum women given bromocriptine for lactation suppression—caution with antihypertensive therapy and avoid other ergot alkaloids. Discontinue immediately if hypertension, unremitting headache or signs of CNS toxicity develop

Side-effects: nausea, vomiting, constipation, headache, dizziness, postural hypotension, drowsiness, vasospasm of fingers and toes particularly in patients with Raynaud's syndrome; *high doses,* confusion, psychomotor excitation, hallucinations, dyskinesia, dry mouth, leg cramps, pleural effusions (may necessitate withdrawal of treatment), retroperitoneal fibrosis reported (monitoring required)

Dose: prevention/suppression of lactation (but see notes above and under Contra-indications), 2.5 mg on 1st day (prevention) or daily for 2–3 days (suppression); then 2.5 mg twice daily for 14 days

Hypogonadism/galactorrhoea, infertility, initially 1–1.25 mg at bedtime, increased gradually; usual dose 7.5 mg daily in divided doses, increased if necessary to a max. of 30 mg daily. Usual dose in infertility without hyperprolactinaemia, 2.5 mg twice daily

Cyclical benign breast disease and cyclical menstrual disorders (particularly breast pain), 1–1.25 mg at bedtime, increased gradually; usual dose 2.5 mg twice daily

Acromegaly, initially 1–1.25 mg at bedtime, increase gradually to 5 mg every 6 hours

Prolactinoma, initially 1–1.25 mg at bedtime; increased gradually to 5 mg every 6 hours (occasional patients may require up to 30 mg daily)

CHILD under 15, not recommended

PoM **Bromocriptine** (Non-proprietary)

Tablets, bromocriptine (as mesylate), 2.5 mg, net price 30-tab pack = £5.28. Label: 21, counselling, hypotensive reactions

Available from APS, Berk, Cox, Kent, Norton

PoM **Parlodel**® (Sandoz)

Tablets, both scored, bromocriptine (as mesylate) 1 mg, net price 100-tab pack = £9.05; 2.5 mg, 30-tab pack = £5.28. Label: 21, counselling, hypotensive reactions

---

Capsules, bromocriptine (as mesylate) 5 mg (blue/white), net price 100-cap pack = £34.34; 10 mg (white), 100-cap pack = £63.53. Label: 21, counselling, hypotensive reactions

CABERGOLINE
Indications: see notes above and under Dose
Cautions; Contra-indications; Side-effects: see under Bromocriptine (but profile of side-effects may differ, see notes above); palpitations, epigastric and abdominal pain, epistaxis and hemianopia, syncope, asthenia, hot flushes also reported; exclude pregnancy before starting and avoid until at least 1 month after successful treatment (ovulatory cycles persist for 6 months)—monthly pregnancy tests during the amenorrhoeic period; advise non-hormonal contraception if pregnancy not desired; discontinue if pregnancy occurs during treatment (specialist advice needed); **interactions:** Appendix 1 (bromocriptine and cabergoline)
HYPOTENSIVE REACTIONS. Hypotensive reactions may be disturbing in some patients during the first few days of treatment and particular care should be exercised when driving or operating machinary; tolerance may be reduced by alcohol
Dose: prevention of lactation (but see notes above), during first day postpartum, 1 mg as a single dose; suppression of established lactation (but see notes above) 250 micrograms every 12 hours for 2 days
Hyperprolactinaemic disorders, 500 micrograms weekly (as a single dose *or* as 2 divided doses on separate days) increased at monthly intervals in steps of 500 micrograms until optimal therapeutic response (usually 1 mg weekly, range 0.25–2 mg weekly) with monthly monitoring of serum prolactin levels; reduce initial dose and increase more gradually if patient intolerant; over 1 mg weekly give as divided doses; up to 4.5 mg weekly has been used in hyperprolactinaemic patients
CHILD under 16, not recommended

▼ PoM **Dostinex®** (Pharmacia)
Tablets, scored, cabergoline 500 micrograms. Net price 8-tab pack = £31.46. Label: 21, counselling, hypotensive reactions

QUINAGOLIDE
Indications: see notes above and under Dose
Cautions; Contra-indications; Side-effects: see under Bromocriptine (but profile of side-effects may differ, see notes above); hypersensitivity to quinagolide (but not ergot alkaloids); syncope, anorexia, abdominal pain, diarrhoea, insomnia, oedema, flushing and nasal congestion also reported; advise non-hormonal contraception if pregnancy not desired; discontinue if pregnancy occurs during treatment (specialist advice needed); **interactions:** Appendix 1 (quinagolide)
HYPOTENSIVE REACTIONS. Hypotensive reactions may be disturbing in some patients during the first few days of treatment—monitor blood pressure for a few days after starting treatment and following dosage increases; particular care should be exercised when driving or operating machinery; tolerance may be reduced by alcohol

Dose: hyperprolactinaemia, 25 micrograms at bedtime for 3 days; increased at intervals of 3 days in steps of 25 micrograms to usual maintenance dose of 75–150 micrograms daily; for doses higher than 300 micrograms daily increase in steps of 75–150 micrograms at intervals of not less than 4 weeks
CHILD not recommended

▼ PoM **Norprolac®** (Sandoz)
Tablets, quinagolide, net price 75 micrograms (white), 30-tab pack = £57.00; 150 micrograms (white), 30-tab pack = £100.00; starter pack of 3 × 25-microgram tabs (pink) with 3 × 50-microgram tabs (blue) = £5.00. Label: 21, counselling, hypotensive reactions

6.7.2   Danazol, gestrinone and gonadorelin analogues

Danazol inhibits pituitary gonadotrophins; it combines androgenic activity with antioestrogenic and antiprogestogenic activity. It is used in the treatment of *endometriosis* and has also been used for *mammary dysplasia*, and *gynaecomastia* where other measures proved unsatisfactory; it has been used for *menorrhagia* and other *menstrual disorders* but in view of its side-effects, treatment with other drugs may be preferable (see section 6.4.1.2) It may also be effective in the long-term management of *hereditary angioedema* [unlicensed indication].

Gestrinone has general actions similar to those of danazol and is indicated for the treatment of endometriosis.

DANAZOL
Indications: see notes above and under Dose
Cautions: cardiac, hepatic, or renal impairment (avoid if severe), elderly, polycythaemia, epilepsy, diabetes mellitus, hypertension, migraine lipoprotein disorder, history of thrombosis; withdraw if virilisation (may be irreversible on continued use); non-hormonal contraceptive methods should be used, if appropriate; **interactions** Appendix 1 (danazol)
Contra-indications: pregnancy, ensure that patients with amenorrhoea are not pregnant breast-feeding; severe hepatic, renal or cardiac impairment; thrombo-embolic disease; uninvestigated vaginal bleeding; androgen-dependent tumours; porphyria (see section 9.8.2)
Side-effects: nausea, dizziness, rashes, backache nervousness, headache, weight gain; menstrual disturbances, flushing and reduction in breast size; skeletal muscle spasm, hair loss; androgenic effects including acne, oily skin, oedema, hirsutism, voice changes and rarely clitoral hypertrophy (see also Cautions); insulin resistance leucopenia and thrombocytopenia reported benign intracranial hypertension and visual disturbances also reported; rarely cholestatic jaundice

Dose: usual range 200–800 mg daily in up to 4 divided doses; in women all doses should start during menstruation, preferably on the first day

Endometriosis, initially 400 mg daily in up to 4 divided doses, adjusted according to response, usually for 6 months

Menorrhagia (but see notes above), 200 mg daily, usually for 3 months

Severe cyclical mastalgia, 200–300 mg daily usually for 3–6 months

Benign breast cysts, 300 mg daily usually for 3–6 months

Gynaecomastia, 400 mg daily in divided doses for 6 months (adolescents 200 mg daily, increased to 400 mg daily if no response after 2 months)

For pre-operative thinning of endometrium, 400–800 mg daily for 3–6 weeks

PoM Danazol (Non-proprietary)
Capsules, danazol 100 mg, net price 20 = £5.46; 200 mg, 20 = £10.87
Available from APS, Cox, Generics, Hillcross, Kent, Norton

PoM Danol® (Sanofi Winthrop)
Capsules, danazol 100 mg (grey/white), net price 100-cap pack = £29.74; 200 mg (pink/white), 56-cap pack = £32.98

GESTRINONE

Indications: endometriosis

Cautions; Contra-indications; Side-effects: see under Danazol; **interactions:** Appendix 1 (gestrinone)

Dose: 2.5 mg twice weekly starting on first day of cycle with second dose 3 days later, repeated on same two days preferably at same time each week; duration of treatment usually 6 months

MISSED DOSES. One missed dose — 2.5 mg as soon as possible and maintain original sequence; two or more missed doses — discontinue, re-start on first day of new cycle (following negative pregnancy test)

PoM Dimetriose® (Roussel)
Capsules, gestrinone 2.5 mg, net price 8-cap pack = £73.12

GONADORELIN ANALOGUES

Gonadorelin analogues, after an initial stimulation phase, down-regulate pituitary gonadotrophin secretion, leading to inhibition of ovarian steroid secretion and are thus effective in the treatment of endometriosis.

BUSERELIN

Indications: see under Dose; prostate cancer, see section 8.3.4.2

Contra-indications: pregnancy (use non-hormonal method of contraception), breast-feeding; undiagnosed vaginal bleeding

Side-effects: initially menstrual-like and subsequently breakthrough bleeding, menopause-like symptoms including hot flushes, palpitations, increased sweating, vaginal dryness and change in libido; headache or migraine, nausea, mood changes including depression, changes in breast size, breast tenderness, abdominal pain, fatigue, weight changes, nervousness, dizziness, drowsiness, acne, dry skin, back pain; muscle pain; ovarian cysts (may require withdrawal); decrease in trabecular bone density (repeat courses not recommended); urticaria, rash and pruritus, constipation, vomiting, sleep disorders, leucorrhoea, paraesthesia or sensitivity of extremities, blurred vision, and changes in body hair also reported; irritation of nasal mucosa (spray formulations only)

Dose: endometriosis, 300 micrograms (one 150-microgram spray in each nostril) 3 times daily (starting on 1st or 2nd day of menstruation); max. duration of treatment 6 months (do not repeat)

Pituitary densensitisation before induction of ovulation by gonadotrophins for *in vitro* fertilisation (under specialist supervision), 150 micrograms (one spray in one nostril) 4 times daily starting in early follicular phase (day 1) *or,* after exclusion of pregnancy, in midluteal phase (day 21) and continued until down-regulation achieved (usually about 2–3 weeks) then maintained for few more days during gonadotrophin administration (stopping on administration of chorionic gonadotrophin at follicular maturity)

COUNSELLING. Avoid use of nasal decongestants before and for at least 30 minutes after treatment.

PoM Suprecur® (Hoechst)
Nasal spray, buserelin 150 micrograms (as acetate)/metered spray. Net price 2 × 100-dose pack (with metered dose pumps) = £78.98. Counselling, see above

---

GOSERELIN

Indications: endometriosis and for endometrial thinning before ablation or resection; prostate cancer and advanced breast cancer, see section 8.3.4

Cautions; Contra-indications; Side-effects: see under Buserelin; also bruising at injection site

Dose: by subcutaneous injection into anterior abdominal wall, endometriosis, 3.6 mg every 28 days; max. duration of treatment 6 months (do not repeat); endometrial thinning, 3.6 mg (may be repeated after 28 days if uterus is large or to allow flexible surgical timing)

PoM Zoladex® (Zeneca)
Implant, goserelin 3.6 mg (as acetate) in syringe applicator. Net price each = £122.27

LEUPRORELIN ACETATE

Indications: endometriosis; prostate cancer, see section 8.3.4.2

Cautions; Contra-indications; Side-effects: see under Buserelin; also irritation at injection site, rotate injection site periodically

---

Dose: by subcutaneous or by intramuscular injection, 3.75 mg every 4 weeks, starting during the first 5 days of menstrual cycle; max. duration of treatment 6 months (do not repeat)

Preparations

See section 8.3.4.2

NAFARELIN

Indications: see under Dose

Cautions; Contra-indications; Side-effects: see under Buserelin

Dose: women over 18 years, endometriosis, 200 micrograms twice daily as one spray in one nostril in the morning and one spray in the other nostril in the evening (starting on 2nd, 3rd or 4th day of menstruation), max. duration of treatment 6 months (do not repeat)

Pituitary desensitisation before induction of ovulation by gonadotrophins for *in vitro* fertilisation (under specialist supervision), 400 micrograms (one spray in each nostril) twice daily starting in early follicular phase (day 2) or, after exclusion of pregnancy, in midluteal phase (day 21) and continued until down-regulation achieved (usually within 4 weeks) then maintained for few more days during gonadotrophin administration (stopping on administration of chorionic gonadotrophin at follicular maturity); discontinue if down-regulation not achieved within 12 weeks

COUNSELLING. Avoid use of nasal decongestants before and for at least 30 minutes after treatment; repeat dose if sneezing occurs during or immediately after administration

PoM Synarel® (Searle)

Nasal spray, nafarelin 200 micrograms (as acetate)/metered spray. Net price 30-dose unit = £30.74; 60-dose unit = £53.01. Label: 10 patient information leaflet, counselling, see above

---

BREAST PAIN (MASTALGIA)

Once any serious underlying cause has been ruled out, most women will respond to reassurance and reduction in dietary fat; withdrawal of an oral contraceptive or of hormone replacement therapy may help resolve the pain.

Women whose symptoms persist for longer than 6 months may require drug treatment. Danazol is the most effective but may be unacceptable owing to its unpleasant side-effects (which occur in about one-third of patients). Bromocriptine (section 6.7.1) like danazol is associated with unpleasant side-effects. Gamolenic acid (section 13.5) can be useful and, with its lack of antioestrogenic side-effects, may be preferred particularly in younger women who wish to continue taking an oral contraceptive; whereas bromocriptine and danazol act within 2 months, gamolenic acid may require 8–12 weeks to take effect.

Symptoms recur in about 50% of women within 2 years of withdrawal of therapy but may be less severe.

6.7.3   Metyrapone and trilostane

Metyrapone is a competitive inhibitor of 11β-hydroxylation in the adrenal cortex; the resulting inhibition of cortisol (and to a lesser extent aldosterone) production leads to an increase in ACTH production which, in turn, leads to increased synthesis and release of cortisol precursors. It may be used as a test of anterior pituitary function.

Although most types of *Cushing's syndrome* are treated surgically, that which occasionally accompanies carcinoma of the bronchus is not usually amenable to surgery. Metyrapone has been found helpful in controlling the symptoms of the disease; it is also used in other forms of Cushing's syndrome to prepare the patient for surgery. The dosages used are either low, and tailored to cortisol production, or high, in which case corticosteroid replacement therapy is also needed.

Trilostane reversibly inhibits 3β-hydroxysteroid dehydrogenase/delta 5-4 isomerase in the adrenal cortex; the resulting inhibition of the synthesis of mineralocorticoids and glucocorticoids may be useful in *Cushing's syndrome* and *primary hyperaldosteronism*. Trilostane appears to be less effective than metyrapone for Cushing's syndrome (where it is tailored to corticosteroid production). It also has a minor role in post-menopausal breast cancer that has relapsed following initial oestrogen antagonist therapy (corticosteroid replacement therapy is also required).

See also aminoglutethimide (section 8.3.4)

METYRAPONE

Indications: see notes above and under Dose (specialist supervision in hospital)

Cautions: gross hypopituitarism (risk of precipitating acute adrenal failure); hypertension on long-term administration; hypothyroidism or hepatic impairment (delayed response); many drugs interfere with diagnostic estimation of steroids

DRIVING. Drowsiness may affect the performance of skilled tasks (e.g. driving)

Contra-indications: adrenocortical insufficiency (see Cautions); pregnancy, breast-feeding

Side-effects: occasional nausea, vomiting, dizziness, headache, hypotension, sedation; rarely abdominal pain, allergic skin reactions, hypoadrenalism, hirsutism

Dose: differential diagnosis of ACTH-dependent Cushing's syndrome, 750 mg every 4 hours for 6 doses; CHILD 15 mg/kg (minimum 250 mg) every 4 hours for 6 doses

Management of Cushing's syndrome, range 0.25–6 g daily, tailored to cortisol production; see notes above

Resistant oedema due to increased aldosterone secretion in cirrhosis, nephrosis, and congestive heart failure (with glucocorticoid replacement therapy) 3 g daily in divided doses

PoM Metopirone® (Ciba)

Capsules, metyrapone 250 mg. Net price 100-tab pack = £20.92. Label: 21, counselling, driving

---

TRILOSTANE

Indications: see notes above and under Dose (specialist supervision)

Cautions: breast cancer (concurrent corticosteroid replacement therapy needed, see under Dose), adrenal cortical hyperfunction (tailored to cortisol and electrolytes, concurrent corticosteroid therapy may be needed, see under Dose); hepatic and renal impairment; **interactions:** Appendix 1 (trilostane)

Contra-indications: pregnancy (use non-hormonal method of contraception) and breast-feeding; children

Side-effects: flushing, tingling and swelling of mouth, rhinorrhoea, nausea, vomiting, diarrhoea, and rashes reported; rarely granulocytopenia

Dose: adrenal cortical hyperfunction, 240 mg daily in divided doses for at least 3 days then tailored according to response with regular monitoring of plasma electrolytes and circulating corticosteroids (both mineralocorticoid and glucocorticoid replacement therapy may be needed); usual dose: 120–480 mg daily (may be increased to 960 mg)

Postmenopausal breast cancer (with glucocorticoid replacement therapy) following relapse to initial oestrogen receptor antagonist therapy, initially 240 mg daily increased every 3 days in steps of 240 mg to a maintenance dose of 960 mg daily (720 mg daily if not tolerated)

PoM Modrenal® (Wanskerne)

Capsules, trilostane 60 mg (pink/black), net price 100-cap pack = £39.60; 120 mg (pink/yellow), 100-cap pack = £79.20. Label: 21

7: Drugs used in

OBSTETRICS, GYNAECOLOGY, and URINARY-TRACT DISORDERS

In this chapter, drugs are discussed under the following headings:

7.1 Drugs used in obstetrics
7.2 Treatment of vaginal and vulval conditions
7.3 Contraceptives
7.4 Drugs for genito-urinary disorders
7.5 Appliances for urinary disorders

For hormonal therapy of gynaecological disorders see sections 6.4.1, 6.5.1 and 6.7.2.

7.1 Drugs used in obstetrics

7.1.1 Prostaglandins and oxytocics
7.1.2 Mifepristone
7.1.3 Myometrial relaxants

Note. Because of the complexity of dosage regimens in obstetrics, in all cases **detailed specialist literature** should be consulted.

7.1.1 Prostaglandins and oxytocics

Prostaglandins and oxytocics are used to induce abortion or induce or augment labour and to minimise blood loss from the placental site. They include oxytocin, ergometrine, and the prostaglandins. All induce uterine contractions with varying degrees of pain according to the strength of contractions induced.

INDUCTION OF ABORTION. **Gemeprost**, administered vaginally, and **dinoprostone**, given by the extra-amniotic route, are the preferred prostaglandins for the *medical induction of late therapeutic abortion*. Gemeprost is a prostaglandin available in the form of pessaries to ripen and soften the cervix *before surgical abortion*, particularly in primigravida. Extra-amniotic **dinoprostone** is also of value as an adjunct in 'priming' the cervix prior to *suction termination* but is rarely used nowadays.

INDUCTION AND AUGMENTATION OF LABOUR. **Oxytocin** (*Syntocinon®*) is administered by slow intravenous infusion, using an infusion pump, to *induce or augment labour*, usually in conjunction with amniotomy. Uterine activity must be monitored carefully and hyperstimulation avoided. Large doses of oxytocin may result in excessive fluid retention.

Dinoprostone is available as vaginal tablets, pessaries and vaginal gels for the *induction of labour*. The intravenous and oral routes are rarely used.

PREVENTION AND TREATMENT OF HAEMORRHAGE. Bleeding due to *incomplete abortion* can be controlled with **ergometrine** and **oxytocin** (*Syntometrine®*) given intramuscularly, the dose being adjusted according to the patient's condition and blood loss. This is commonly used prior to surgical evacuation of the uterus, particularly when surgery is delayed. Oxytocin and ergometrine combined are more effective in early pregnancy than either drug alone.

For the routine management of the *third stage of labour* ergometrine 500 micrograms with oxytocin 5 units (*Syntometrine®* 1 mL) is given by intramuscular injection with or after delivery of the shoulders. For the prevention of postpartum haemorrhage in *high-risk cases*, intravenous injection of *either* ergometrine 125–250 micrograms alone *or* oxytocin 5–10 units is recommended, after delivery of the shoulders (repeated if necessary); alternatively intravenous infusion of oxytocin 10–20 units/500 mL can be given after delivery of the shoulders, particularly when the uterus is *atonic*. The use of **carboprost** now has an important role for severe events.

Provided causes such as infection or retained products of conception have been excluded, small secondary postpartum haemorrhage may be treated in domiciliary practice with **ergometrine** by mouth in a dose of 500 micrograms three times daily for 3 days.

CARBOPROST

Indications: postpartum haemorrhage due to uterine atony in patients unresponsive to ergometrine and oxytocin

Cautions: history of glaucoma or raised intra-ocular pressure, asthma, hypertension, hypotension, anaemia, jaundice, diabetes, epilepsy; uterine scars; excessive dosage may cause uterine rupture

Contra-indications: acute pelvic inflammatory disease; cardiac, renal, pulmonary, or hepatic disease

Side-effects: nausea, vomiting and diarrhoea, hyperthermia and flushing, bronchospasm; less frequent effects include raised blood pressure, dyspnoea, and pulmonary oedema; chills, headache, diaphoresis, dizziness; cardiovascular collapse also reported; erythema and pain at injection site reported

Dose: by deep intramuscular injection, 250 micrograms repeated if necessary at intervals of 1½ hours (in severe cases the interval may be reduced but should not be less than 15 minutes); total dose should not exceed 2 mg (8 doses)

PoM **Hemabate®** (Upjohn)

Injection, carboprost as trometamol salt (trometh-amine salt) 250 micrograms/mL, net price 1-mL amp = £16.50 (hosp. only)

DINOPROSTONE

Indications: see notes above

Cautions: history of asthma, glaucoma and raised intra-ocular pressure; cardiac, hepatic or renal impairment; hypertension; history of epilepsy; monitor uterine activity and fetal status (particular care if history of uterine hypertony); uterine rupture; see also notes above; effect of oxytocin enhanced (care needed in monitoring uterine activity when used in sequence)—see also under *Propess-RS®* and Appendix 1 (oxytocin)

Contra-indications: hypersensitivity to prosta-glandins; active cardiac, pulmonary, renal or hepatic disease; placenta praevia or unexplained vaginal bleeding during pregnancy, ruptured membranes, major cephalopelvic disproportion or fetal malpresentation, history of caesarean section or major uterine surgery, untreated pelvic infection, fetal distress, grand multiparas and multiple pregnancy, history of difficult or traumatic delivery; avoid extra-amniotic route in cervicitis or vaginitis

Side-effects: nausea, vomiting, diarrhoea; other side-effects include uterine hypertonus, severe uterine contractions, pulmonary or amniotic fluid embolism, abruptio placenta, fetal distress, maternal hypertension, bronchospasm, rapid cervical dilation, fever, backache; uterine hypercontractility with or without fetal bradycardia, low Apgar scores; cardiac arrest, uterine rupture, stillbirth or neonatal death also reported; vaginal symptoms (warmth, irritation, pain); after intravenous administration—flushing, shivering, headache, dizziness, temporary pyrexia and raised white blood cell count; also local tissue reaction and erythema after intravenous administration and possibility of infection after extra-amniotic administration

Dose: see under Preparations, below

IMPORTANT. Do not confuse dose of **Prostin E2®** vaginal **gel** with that of **Prostin E2®** vaginal **tablets**—not bioequivalent. In addition, do not confuse **Prostin E2®** vaginal gel with **Prepidil®** cervical gel—different site of administration and different indication—see under Preparations, below

PoM **Prepidil®** (Upjohn)

Cervical gel, dinoprostone 200 micrograms/mL in disposable syringe. Net price 2.5-mL syringe (500 micrograms) = £14.12

Dose: by cervix, pre-induction cervical softening and dilation, inserted into cervical canal (just below level of internal cervical os), 500 micrograms [single dose gel]

▼ PoM **Propess®-RS** (Ferring)

Pessaries (within retrieval system), releasing dino-prostone approx. 5 mg over 12 hours. Net price 4-pessary pack = £173.75

Dose: by vagina, cervical ripening and induction of labour at term, 1 pessary inserted high into posterior fornix; if cervical ripening insufficient, remove pessary 8–12 hours later and replace with a second pessary (which should also be removed not more than 12 hours later); max. 2 consecutive pessaries

IMPORTANT. Effect of oxytocin enhanced—particular care needed to monitor uterine activity when oxytocin used in sequence (remove pessary beforehand)

PoM **Prostin E2®** (Upjohn)

Tablets, dinoprostone 500 micrograms. Net price 10-tab pack = £14.93 (hosp. only)

Dose: by mouth, induction of labour, 500 micrograms, followed by 0.5–1 mg (max. 1.5 mg) at hourly intervals

Intravenous solution, for dilution and use as an infusion, dinoprostone 1 mg/mL, net price 0.75-mL amp = £7.43; 10 mg/mL, 0.5-mL amp = £16.05 (both hosp. only; rarely used, see data sheet for dose and indications)

Extra-amniotic solution, dinoprostone 10 mg/mL. Net price 0.5-mL amp (with diluent) = £16.05 (hosp. only; less commonly used nowadays, see data sheet for dose and indications)

Vaginal gel, dinoprostone 400 micrograms/mL, net price 2.5 mL (1 mg) = £14.52; 800 micrograms/mL, 2.5 mL (2 mg) = £16.00

Dose: by vagina, induction of labour, inserted high into posterior fornix (avoid administration into cervical canal), 1 mg (unfavourable primigravida 2 mg), followed after 6 hours by 1–2 mg if required; max. [gel] 3 mg (unfavourable primigravida 4 mg)

Vaginal tablets, dinoprostone 3 mg. Net price 8-vaginal tab pack = £65.04

Dose: by vagina, induction of labour, inserted high into posterior fornix, 3 mg, followed after 6–8 hours by 3 mg if labour is not established; max. 6 mg [vaginal tablets]

Note. Prostin E2 Vaginal Gel and Vaginal Tablets are **not** bioequivalent

DINOPROST

Indications: see under preparation, below

Cautions; Contra-indications; Side-effects: see under Dinoprostone

PoM **Prostin F2 alpha®** (Upjohn)

Intra-amniotic injection, dinoprost 5 mg (as trometamol salt)/mL. Net price 4-mL amp = £19.71 (hosp. only; rarely used, see data sheet for dose and indications)

ERGOMETRINE MALEATE

Indications: see notes above

Cautions: cardiac disease, hypertension, hepatic, and renal impairment, multiple pregnancy; porphyria (see section 9.8.2)

Contra-indications: induction of labour, 1st and 2nd stages of labour, vascular disease, severe cardiac disease, impaired pulmonary function, severe hepatic and renal impairment, sepsis, severe hypertension, eclampsia

Side-effects: nausea, vomiting, headache, dizziness, tinnitus, abdominal pain, chest pain, palpitation, dyspnoea, bradycardia, transient hypertension, vasoconstriction; stroke, myocardial infarction and pulmonary oedema also reported

Dose: see notes above

PoM **Ergometrine Tablets,** ergometrine maleate 500 micrograms. Net price 20 = £5.90

Available from Norton

PoM **Ergometrine Injection,** ergometrine maleate 500 micrograms/mL. Net price 1-mL amp = 30p

Available from Antigen, Phoenix

With oxytocin

PoM **Syntometrine**® (Sandoz)

Injection, ergometrine maleate 500 micrograms, oxytocin 5 units/mL. Net price 1-mL amp = 18p

Dose: by intramuscular injection, 1 mL; by intravenous injection, no longer recommended

GEMEPROST

Indications: see under Dose

Cautions: obstructive airways disease, cardiovascular insufficiency, raised intra-ocular pressure, cervicitis or vaginitis

IMPORTANT. For warnings relating to use of gemeprost in a patient undergoing termination with mifepristone, see under Mifepristone

Contra-indications: hypersensitivity to gemeprost or other prostaglandins

Side-effects: vaginal bleeding and uterine pain; nausea, vomiting, or diarrhoea; headache, muscle weakness, dizziness, flushing, chills, backache, dyspnoea, chest pain, palpitations and mild pyrexia; uterine rupture reported (most commonly in multiparas or if history of uterine surgery or if given with intravenous oxytocics)

Dose: by vagina in pessaries, softening and dilation of the cervix to facilitate transcervical operative procedures in first trimester, inserted into posterior fornix, 1 mg 3 hours before surgery

Second trimester abortion, inserted into posterior fornix, 1 mg every 3 hours for max. of 5 administrations; second course may begin 24 hours after start of treatment (if treatment fails pregnancy should be terminated by another method)

Second trimester intra-uterine death, inserted into posterior fornix, 1 mg every 3 hours for max. of 5 administrations only; monitor for coagulopathy

PoM **Gemeprost** (Farillon)

Pessaries, gemeprost 1 mg. Net price 5-pessary pack = £121.12

OXYTOCIN

Indications: see under Dose and notes above

Cautions: particular caution needed when given for *induction or enhancement of labour* in presence of borderline cephalopelvic disproportion (avoid if significant), mild or moderate pregnancy-induced hypertension or cardiac disease, women over 35 years or with history of lower-uterine segment caesarean section (see also under contra-indications below); if fetal death in utero or meconium-stained amniotic fluid avoid tumultuous labour (may cause amniotic fluid embolism); water intoxication and hyponatraemia—avoid large infusion volumes and restrict fluid intake by mouth (see also Appendix 6); effects enhanced by concomitant prostaglandins (very careful monitoring), caudal block anaesthesia (may enhance hypertensive effects of sympathomimetic vasopressors), see also **interactions:** Appendix 1 (oxytocin)

Contra-indications: hypertonic uterine contractions, mechanical obstruction to delivery, fetal distress; any condition where spontaneous labour or vaginal delivery inadvisable (e.g. significant cephalopelvic disproportion, malpresentation, placenta praevia, vasa praevia, placental abruption, cord presentation or prolapse, predisposition to uterine rupture as in multiple pregnancy, polyhydramnios, grand multiparity and presence of uterine scar from major surgery—including caesarean section); avoid prolonged administration in oxytocin-resistant uterine inertia, severe pre-eclamptic toxaemia or severe cardiovascular disease

Side-effects: uterine spasm (may occur at low doses); uterine hyperstimulation (usually with excessive doses—may cause fetal distress, asphyxia and death, or may lead to hypertonicity, tetanic contractions, soft tissue damage or uterine rupture); water intoxication and hyponatraemia associated with high doses with large infusion volumes of electrolyte-free fluid (see also under Dose below); also nausea, vomiting, arrhythmias; rashes and anaphylactoid reactions (with dyspnoea, hypotension or shock) also reported; placental abruption and amniotic fluid embolism also reported on overdose

Dose: induction of labour for medical reasons or stimulation of labour in hypotonic uterine inertia, *by intravenous infusion* 1–4 milliunits/minute increased at intervals of not less than 20 minutes until labour pattern established similar to normal (usually less than 10 milliunits/minute for pregnancy at term); max. recommended rate 20 milliunits/minute (use solution containing 10 units/500 mL if higher rate required); do not use total of more than 5 units in any one day (may be repeated the following day starting again at 1–4 milliunits/minute)

IMPORTANT. Careful monitoring of fetal heart rate and uterine motility essential so that dosage can be adjusted to individual response (never give intravenous injection); discontinue immediately in event of uterine hyperactivity or fetal distress

Caesarean section, *by slow intravenous injection* immediately after delivery, 5 units

Postpartum haemorrhage, *prevention of postpartum haemorrhage* 5 units *by slow intravenous injection* after delivery of placenta; if infusion used for induction or enhancement of labour, continue at increased rate during third stage of labour and for next few hours; *treatment of postpartum haemorrhage* 5 units *by slow intravenous injection* followed, in severe cases, *by intravenous infusion* of 5–20 units in 500 mL of non-hydrating diluent (e.g. glucose 5% solution) at a rate sufficient to control uterine atony

IMPORTANT. Avoid rapid intravenous injection (may cause acute short-lasting drop in blood pressure); prolonged administration, see warning below

Incomplete, inevitable or missed abortion, 5 units *by slow intravenous injection* followed if necessary *by intravenous infusion* at rate of 20–40 milliunits/minute or higher

IMPORTANT. Prolonged intravenous administration at high doses with large volume of fluid (as possible in inevitable or missed abortion or postpartum haemorrhage) may cause water intoxication with hyponatraemia. To avoid: use electrolyte-containing diluent (i.e. not glucose), increase oxytocin concentration to reduce fluid, restrict fluid intake by mouth; monitor fluid and electrolytes

PoM **Syntocinon**® (Sandoz)

Injection, oxytocin, net price 5 units/mL, 1-mL amp = 20p; 10 units/mL, 1-mL amp = 22p

With ergometrine, see Syntometrine®, above

7.1.1.1 DUCTUS ARTERIOSUS

MAINTENANCE OF PATENCY

Alprostadil (prostaglandin E₁) is used to maintain patency of the ductus arteriosus in neonates with congenital heart defects, prior to corrective surgery in centres where intensive care is immediately available.

ALPROSTADIL

Indications: congenital heart defects in neonates prior to corrective surgery; erectile dysfunction, see section 7.4.5

Cautions: see notes above; history of haemorrhage, avoid in hyaline membrane disease, monitor arterial pressure

Side-effects: apnoea (particularly in infants under 2 kg), flushing, bradycardia, hypotension, tachycardia, cardiac arrest, oedema, diarrhoea, fever, convulsions, disseminated intravascular coagulation, hypokalaemia; cortical proliferation of long bones, weakening of the wall of the ductus arteriosus and pulmonary artery may follow prolonged use; gastric-outlet obstruction reported

Dose: by *intravenous infusion*, initially 50–100 nanograms/kg/minute, then decreased to lowest effective dose

PoM **Prostin VR**® (Upjohn)
Intravenous solution, alprostadil 500 micrograms/mL in alcohol. For dilution and use as an infusion. Net price 1-mL amp = £62.66 (hosp. only)

CLOSURE OF DUCTUS ARTERIOSUS
Prostaglandin E₁ has the role of dilating the ductus arteriosus; **indomethacin** is believed to close it by inhibiting prostaglandin synthesis.

INDOMETHACIN
(Indometacin)

Indications: patent ductus arteriosus in premature infants (under specialist supervision in neonatal intensive care unit); rheumatoid disease, see section 10.1.1

Cautions: may mask symptoms of infection; may reduce urine output by 50% or more (monitor carefully—see also under Anuria or Oliguria, below) and precipitate renal insufficiency especially in infants with depletion of extracellur volume (from any cause), heart failure, sepsis, or hepatic impairment, or who are receiving nephrotoxic drugs; may induce hyponatraemia; monitor renal function and electrolytes; inhibition of platelet aggregation (monitor for signs of bleeding); avoid extravasation; **interactions:** Appendix 1 (NSAIDs)

ANURIA OR OLIGURIA. If anuria or marked oliguria (urinary output of 0.6 mL/kg/hour) is evident at time of scheduled 2nd or 3rd dose, delay until renal function returns to normal

Contra-indications: untreated infection, bleeding (especially with active intracranial haemorrhage or gastro-intestinal bleeding), congenital heart disease where patency of ductus arteriosus necessary for satisfactory pulmonary or systemic blood flow; thrombocytopenia, coagulation defects, necrotising enterocolitis, renal impairment

Side-effects: include haemorrhagic, renal, gastro-intestinal, metabolic, and coagulation disorders; pulmonary hypertension, intracranial bleeding, fluid retention, and exacerbation of infection

Dose: by *intravenous injection*, over 5–10 seconds, 3 doses at intervals of 12–24 hours (provided urine output remains adequate), age less than 48 hours, 200 micrograms/kg then 100 micrograms/kg then 100 micrograms/kg; age 2–7 days, 200 micrograms/kg then 200 micrograms/kg then 200 micrograms/kg; age over 7 days, 200 micrograms/kg then 250 micrograms/kg then 250 micrograms/kg; solution prepared with 1–2 mL sodium chloride 0.9% or water for injections (not glucose and no preservatives)

If ductus arteriosus reopens a second course of 3 injections may be given

PoM **Indocid PDA**® (Morson)
Injection, powder for reconstitution, indomethacin (as sodium trihydrate). Net price 3 × 1-mg vials = £22.50 (hosp. only)

7.1.2 Mifepristone

MIFEPRISTONE

Indications: medical alternative to surgical termination of intra-uterine pregnancy of up to 63 days gestation (based on first day of last menstrual period and/or ultrasound scan)

Cautions: asthma, chronic obstructive airways disease; cardiovascular disease or risk factors; prosthetic heart valves or history of infective endocarditis (prophylaxis recommended, see section 5.1 table 2); not recommended in hepatic or renal impairment; avoid aspirin and NSAIDs for at least 8–12 days after mifepristone administration

Contra-indications: pregnancy of 64 days gestation and over, suspected ectopic pregnancy; chronic adrenal failure, long-term corticosteroid therapy, haemorrhagic disorders and anticoagulant therapy; smokers over 35 years of age (smoking and alcohol must be avoided when taking and for at least 2 days after the gemeprost pessary); porphyria (see section 9.8.2)

Side-effects: vaginal bleeding (may be severe), malaise, faintness, nausea, vomiting, rashes; uterine pain after gemeprost (may be severe and require parenteral opioids); uterine and urinary-tract infections reported

Dose: by *mouth*, 600 mg in a single dose in presence of doctor and observed for at least 2 hours after administration; followed 36–48 hours later (unless abortion already complete) by gemeprost 1 mg *by vagina* as pessaries, observed for at least 6 hours after insertion with follow-up visit 8–12 days later (if treatment fails essential that pregnancy be terminated by another method)

Note. Careful monitoring essential for 6 hours after administration of gemeprost pessary (risk of profound hypotension)

▼ PoM **Mifegyne**® (Roussel)
Tablets, yellow, mifepristone 200 mg. Net price 3-tab pack = £41.83 (supplied to NHS hospitals and premises approved under Abortion Act 1967). Label: 10 patient information leaflet

7.1.3 Myometrial relaxants

Beta₂-adrenoceptor stimulants (beta₂-sympathomimetics) relax uterine muscle and are used in selected cases in an attempt to inhibit *premature delivery.*

Their main purpose is to permit a delay in delivery of at least 48 hours; no statistically significant effect on perinatal mortality has as yet been observed. The greatest benefit is gained by using the delay to administer corticosteroid therapy or to implement other measures known to improve peri-natal health. They are indicated for the inhibition of *uncomplicated* premature labour *between 24 and 33 weeks* of gestation. After successful parenteral ther-apy oral therapy may be used for maintenance (but **not** initially).

RITODRINE HYDROCHLORIDE

Indications: uncomplicated premature labour (see notes above)

Cautions: suspected cardiac disease (physician experi-enced in cardiology to assess), hypertension, hyper-thyroidism, hypokalaemia (special risk with potassium-depleting diuretics), diabetes mellitus (closely monitor blood glucose during intravenous treatment), mild to moderate pre-eclampsia (avoid if severe—see Contra-indications), monitor blood pressure and pulse rate (should not exceed 135–140 beats per minute) and avoid over hydration (see Appendix 6); **important:** pulm-onary oedema—closely monitor state of hydration (dis-continue immediately and institute diuretic therapy if pulmonary oedema occurs); beta-blockers (effect antag-onised—may be used to reverse increased tendency to uterine bleeding following Caesarean section); drugs likely to enhance sympathomimetic side-effects or induce arrhythmias, see also **interactions**, Appendix 1 (sympathomimetics *and* sympathomimetics, beta$_2$)

Contra-indications: cardiac disease, eclampsia and severe pre-eclampsia, intra-uterine infection, intra-uterine fetal death, antepartum haemorrhage (requires immediate delivery), placenta praevia, cord compres-sion; not for use in first or second trimesters

Side-effects: nausea, vomiting, flushing, sweating, tremor; hypokalaemia, tachycardia, palpitations, and hypotension (left lateral position throughout infusion to minimise risk), increased tendency to uterine bleeding (see Cautions); pulmonary oedema (see below and under Cautions); chest pain or tightness (with or without ECG changes) and arrhythmias reported; salivary gland enlargement also reported; on prolonged administration (several weeks) leucopenia and agranulocytosis reported; liver function abnormalities (including increased transaminase levels and hepatitis) reported

Dose: by intravenous infusion (**important:** minimum fluid volume, see below), premature labour, initially 50 micrograms/minute, gradually increased to 150–350 micrograms/minute and continued for 12–48 hours after contractions have ceased (max. rate of 350 micrograms/minute should not be exceeded); or *by intramuscular injection*, 10 mg every 3–8 hours continued for 12–48 hours after contractions have ceased; then *by mouth*, 10 mg 30 minutes before termination of intra-venous infusion, repeated every 2 hours for 24 hours, followed by 10–20 mg every 4–6 hours, max. oral dose 120 mg daily

IMPORTANT. The company has issued a reminder that although *fatal pulmonary oedema* associated with ritodrine infusion is almost certainly multifactorial in origin the balance of evidence suggests that **fluid over-load** is the most important single factor. The volume of infusion fluid administered should therefore be kept to a minimum (normally using dextrose 5% as the diluent), for further guidance see Appendix 6. For specific guid-ance on infusion rates to achieve the required dose, see data sheet

PoM Yutopar® (Solvay)
Tablets, yellow, scored, ritodrine hydrochloride 10 mg. Net price 90-tab pack = £19.80
Injection, ritodrine hydrochloride 10 mg/mL. Net price 5-mL amp = £2.15

SALBUTAMOL

Indications: uncomplicated premature labour (see notes above); asthma, see section 3.1.1

Cautions; Contra-indications; Side-effects: see under Ritodrine Hydrochloride

Dose: by intravenous infusion, 10 micrograms/minute gradually increased to max. of 45 micrograms/minute until contractions have ceased, then gradually reduced; or *by intravenous or intramuscular injection,* 100–250 micrograms repeated according to patient's response; subsequently *by mouth* 4 mg every 6–8 hours

Preparations
See section 3.1.1.1

TERBUTALINE SULPHATE

Indications: uncomplicated premature labour (see notes above); asthma, see section 3.1.1

Cautions; Contra-indications; Side-effects: see under Ritodrine Hydrochloride

Dose: by intravenous infusion, 5 micrograms/minute for 20 minutes, increased every 20 minutes in steps of 2.5 micrograms/minute until contractions have ceased (more than 10 micrograms/minute should **seldom** be given—20 micrograms/minute should **not** be exceeded), continue for 1 hour at level at which contractions have ceased then decrease every 20 minutes in steps of 2.5 micrograms/minute to lowest dose that maintains suppression, continue at this level for 12 hours then *by mouth* 5 mg every 8 hours for as long as physician con-siders it desirable to prolong pregnancy (or alternatively follow the *intravenous infusion* by *subcutaneous injec-tion* 250 micrograms every 6 hours for a few days then *by mouth* as above)

Preparations
See section 3.1.1.1

7.2   Treatment of vaginal and vulval conditions

7.2.1   Preparations for vaginal atrophy
7.2.2   Anti-infective drugs

Symptoms are primarily referable to the vulva, but infections almost invariably involve the vagina which should also be treated. Applications to the vulva alone are likely to give only symptomatic relief without cure.

Aqueous medicated douches may disturb normal vaginal acidity and bacterial flora.

Topical anaesthetic agents give only symptomatic relief and may cause sensitivity reactions. They are indicated only in cases of pruritus where specific local causes have been excluded.

Systemic drugs are required in the treatment of infections such as gonorrhoea and syphilis (see sec-tion 5.1).

7.2.1   Preparations for vaginal atrophy

TOPICAL HRT

Application of *cream* containing an oestrogen may be used on a short-term basis to improve the quality of the vaginal epithelium in *menopausal atrophic*

...aginitis. It is **important** to bear in mind that topical oestrogens should be used in the **minimum effective amount** to minimise absorption of the oestrogen; if they are used on a long-term basis, some require **oral progestogen** for 10–14 days of each month to combat endometrial hyperplasia (for details see under preparations below). *Modified-release vaginal tablets* and an *impregnated vaginal ring* are now also available.

Topical oestrogens are also used *prior to vaginal surgery* in postmenopausal women for prolapse when there is epithelial atrophy.

For a general comment on HRT, including the role of topical oestrogens, see section 6.4.1.1.

OESTROGENS, TOPICAL

Indications: see notes above

Cautions; Contra-indications; Side-effects: see Oestrogen for HRT (section 6.4.1.1); contra-indicated in pregnancy and lactation; discontinue treatment and examine patients periodically to assess need for further treatment

PoM Ortho® Dienoestrol (Cilag)
Cream, dienoestrol 0.01%. Net price 78 g with applicator = £2.61
Condoms: damages latex condoms and diaphragms
Insert 1–2 applicatorfuls daily for 1–2 weeks, then gradually reduced to 1 applicatorful 1–3 times weekly if necessary; attempts to reduce or discontinue should be made at 3–6 month intervals with re-examination

PoM Ortho-Gynest® (Cilag)
Intravaginal cream, oestriol 0.01%. Net price 80 g with applicator = £2.72
Condoms: damages latex condoms and diaphragms
Insert 1 applicatorful daily, preferably in evening; reduced to 1 applicatorful twice a week; attempts to reduce or discontinue should be made at 3–6 month intervals with re-examination
Pessaries, oestriol 500 micrograms. Net price 15 pessaries = £5.29
Condoms: damages latex condoms and diaphragms
Insert 1 pessary daily, preferably in the evening, until improvement occurs; maintenance 1 pessary twice a week; attempts to reduce or discontinue should be made at 3–6 month intervals with re-examination

PoM Ovestin® (Organon)
Intravaginal cream, oestriol 0.1%. Net price 15 g with applicator = £5.21
Condoms: effect on latex condoms and diaphragms not yet known
Insert 1 applicator-dose daily for 2–3 weeks, then reduce to twice a week (discontinue every 2–3 months for 4 weeks to assess need for further treatment); postmenopausal surgery, 1 applicator-dose daily for 2 weeks, resuming 2 weeks after surgery

PoM Premarin® (Wyeth)
Vaginal cream, conjugated oestrogens 625 micrograms/g. Net price 42.5 g with calibrated applicator = £2.19
Condoms: effect on latex condoms and diaphragms not yet known
Insert 1–2 g daily, starting on 5th day of cycle, for 3 weeks, followed by 1-week interval; if therapy long term, oral progestogen for 10–14 days at end of each cycle essential

PoM Tampovagan® (Norgine)
Pessaries, stilboestrol 500 micrograms, lactic acid 5%. Net price 10 pessaries = £5.00
Condoms: no evidence of damage to latex condoms and diaphragms
Insert 2 pessaries at night for 2–3 weeks (short-term only, see notes above)

PoM Vagifem® (Novo Nordisk)
Vaginal tablets, f/c, m/r, oestradiol 25 micrograms in disposable applicators. Net price 15-applicator pack = £14.62
Condoms: no evidence of damage to latex condoms and diaphragms
Insert 1 tablet daily for 2 weeks then reduce to 1 tablet twice weekly; discontinue after 3 months to assess need for further treatment

Vaginal ring
Note. For the treatment of urogenital complaints in postmenopausal women—not suitable for vasomotor symptoms or osteoporosis prophylaxis

PoM Estring® (Pharmacia-Leiras)
Vaginal ring, releasing oestradiol approx. 7.5 micrograms/24 hours. Net price 1-ring pack = £32.90. Label: 10 patient information leaflet
To be inserted into upper third of vagina and worn continuously; replace after 3 months; max. duration of continuous treatment 2 years

NON-HORMONAL PREPARATIONS

Non-hormonal preparations include **NHS** Replens® and **NHS** Senselle® which have a high moisture content and remain *in situ* for up to 24 hours or longer.

See section 7.2.2 for the pH-modifying preparation Aci-jel®.

7.2.2 Anti-infective drugs

Effective specific treatments are available for the common vaginal infections.

FUNGAL INFECTIONS

Candidal vulvitis can be treated locally with cream but is almost invariably associated with vaginal infection which should be treated as well. *Vaginal candidiasis* is treated primarily with antifungal pessaries or cream inserted high into the vagina (including the time of menstruation).

Nystatin is a well established treatment (but stains clothing yellow). One or two pessaries are inserted for 14 to 28 nights; they may be supplemented with cream for vulvitis and to treat other superficial sites of infection.

Imidazole drugs (clotrimazole, econazole, isoconazole, and miconazole) appear to be equally effective in shorter courses of 3 to 14 days according to the preparation used; single dose preparations are also available, which is an advantage when compliance is a problem. Vaginal applications may be supplemented with cream for vulvitis and to treat other superficial sites of infection.

Recurrence is common if the full course of treatment is not completed and is also particularly likely if there are predisposing factors such as antibiotic therapy, oral contraceptive use, pregnancy, or diabetes mellitus. Possible reservoirs of infection may also lead to recontamination and should be treated. These include other skin sites such as the digits, nail beds, and umbilicus as well as the gut and the bladder. The partner may also be the source of re-infection and should be treated with cream at the same time.

Oral treatment with fluconazole or itraconazole should be reserved for resistant or recurrent infection (see section 5.2); oral ketoconazole has been associated with fatal hepatotoxicity (see section 5.2 for CSM warning).

PREPARATIONS FOR VAGINAL AND VULVAL CANDIDIASIS
Side-effects: occasional local irritation

Canesten® (Baypharm)
Cream (topical), clotrimazole 1%. Net price 20 g = £1.77; 50 g = £4.15
  Condoms: effect on latex condoms and diaphragms not yet known
  Apply to anogenital area 2–3 times daily
Vaginal cream, clotrimazole 2%. Net price 35 g (with 5-g applicators) = £5.09
  Condoms: effect on latex condoms and diaphragms not yet known
  Insert 5 g twice daily for 3 days or once nightly for 6 nights
Vaginal cream (10% VC®), clotrimazole 10%. Net price 5-g applicator pack = £3.34
  Condoms: effect on latex condoms and diaphragms not yet known
  Insert 5 g at night as a single dose
Pessaries, clotrimazole 100 mg, net price 6 pessaries with applicator = £3.29; 200 mg, 3 pessaries with applicator = £3.29
  Insert 200 mg for 3 nights *or* 100 mg for 6 nights
Pessary (Canesten 1®), clotrimazole 500 mg. Net price 1 with applicator = £3.29
  Insert 1 at night as a single dose
Combi, clotrimazole 500-mg pessary and cream (topical) 1%. Net price 1 pessary and 20 g cream = £4.25
  Condoms: effect on latex condoms and diaphragms not yet known
Duopak, clotrimazole 100-mg pessary and cream (topical) 1%. Net price 6 pessaries and 20 g cream = £4.24
  Condoms: effect on latex condoms and diaphragms not yet known

Ecostatin® (Squibb)
Cream (topical), econazole nitrate 1%. Net price 15 g = £1.49; 30 g = £2.75
  Condoms: damages latex condoms and diaphragms
  Apply to anogenital area twice daily
PoM[1] *Pessaries,* econazole nitrate 150 mg. Net price 3 with applicator = £3.35
  Condoms: damages latex condoms and diaphragms
  Insert 1 pessary for 3 nights
PoM[1] *Pessary (Ecostatin 1®),* econazole nitrate 150 mg, formulated for single-dose therapy. Net price 1 pessary with applicator = £3.35
  Condoms: damages latex condoms and diaphragms
  Insert 1 pessary at night as a single dose

PoM[1] *Twinpack,* econazole nitrate 150-mg pessaries and cream 1%. Net price 3 pessaries and 15 cream = £4.35
  Condoms: damages latex condoms and diaphragms

Femeron® (Janssen)
Cream, miconazole nitrate 2%. Net price 15g £1.91
  Condoms: damages latex condoms and diaphragms
  Apply to anogenital area twice daily
Soft pessary, miconazole nitrate 1.2 g. Net price = £3.41
  Condoms: damages latex condoms and diaphragms
  Insert 1 pessary at night as a single dose
PoM **Flagyl Compak®** see section 5.1.11

PoM [1] Gyno-Daktarin® (Janssen)
Intravaginal cream, miconazole nitrate 2%. N price 78 g with applicators = £4.95
  Condoms: damages latex condoms and diaphragms
  Insert 5-g applicatorful twice daily for 7 days; *topica* apply to anogenital area twice daily
Pessaries, miconazole nitrate 100 mg. Net price **1** = £3.35
  Condoms: damages latex condoms and diaphragms
  Insert 1 pessary twice daily for 7 days
Combipack, miconazole nitrate 100-mg pessari and cream (topical) 2%. Net price 14 pessari and 15 g cream = £4.35
  Condoms: damages latex condoms and diaphragms
Ovule (= vaginal capsule) *(Gyno-Daktarin 1®* miconazole nitrate 1.2 g in a fatty basis. Net pri 1 ovule (with finger stall) = £3.35
  Condoms: damages latex condoms and diaphragms
  Insert 1 ovule at night as a single dose

Gyno-Pevaryl® (Cilag)
Cream, econazole nitrate 1%. Net price 15 g £1.50; 30 g = £3.45
  Condoms: no evidence of damage to latex condoms and diaph gms
  Insert 5-g applicatorful intravaginally and apply to vul at night for 14 nights; males, apply to penis and und foreskin daily for 14 days
PoM[1] *Pessaries,* econazole nitrate 150 mg. N price 3 pessaries = £3.17
  Condoms: damages latex condoms and diaphragms
  Insert 1 pessary for 3 nights
PoM[1] *Pessary (Gyno-Pevaryl 1®),* econazo nitrate 150 mg, formulated for single-dose th apy. Net price 1 pessary with applicator = £3.37
  Condoms: damages latex condoms and diaphragms
  Insert 1 pessary at night as a single dose
PoM[1] *Combipack,* econazole nitrate 150-mg pess ries, econazole nitrate 1% cream. Net price 3 pe saries and 15 g cream = £4.35
  Condoms: damages latex condoms and diaphragms
PoM[1] *CP pack (Gyno-Pevaryl 1®),* econazo nitrate 150-mg pessary, econazole nitrate 1 cream. Net price 1 pessary and 15 g cream £4.35
  Condoms: damages latex condoms and diaphragms

1. Can be sold to the public for the treatment of *vagin* candidiasis. Until packs labelled 'P' are available, tho labelled 'PoM' can be sold providing the pharmac *deletes* PoM from the pack and *substitutes* a capital P a provides *each purchaser* with a copy of the **patient info** **mation leaflet** supplied by the Royal Pharmaceutical Soc ety of Great Britain.

▼ PoM **Lomexin**® (Upjohn)

Pessaries, fenticonazole nitrate 200 mg, net price 3 pessaries = £3.29; 600 mg, 1 pessary = £3.29

Condoms: damages latex condoms and diaphragms

Insert 600 mg for 1 night *or* 200 mg for 3 nights

Masnoderm® (Dominion)

Cream, clotrimazole 1%. Net price 20 g = £1.54

Condoms: damages latex condoms and diaphragms

Apply to anogenital area 2–3 times daily

PoM **Nizoral**® (Janssen)

Cream (topical), ketoconazole 2%. Net price 30 g = £3.81

Apply to anogenital area once or twice daily

PoM **Nystan**® (Squibb)

Cream and *Ointment*, see section 13.10.2

Gel (topical), nystatin 100 000 units/g. Net price 30 g = £2.66

Condoms: no evidence of damage to latex condoms and diaphragms

Apply to anogenital area 2–4 times daily

Vaginal cream, nystatin 100 000 units/4-g application. Net price 60 g with applicator = £2.77

Condoms: damages latex condoms and diaphragms

Insert 1–2 applicatorfuls at night for at least 14 nights

Pessaries, yellow, nystatin 100 000 units. Net price 28-pessary pack = £1.96

Condoms: no evidence of damage to latex condoms and diaphragms

Insert 1–2 pessaries at night for at least 14 nights

Tablets, see section 5.2

Pevaryl® (Cilag)

Cream, econazole nitrate 1%. Net price 30 g = £2.65

Condoms: effect on latex condoms and diaphragms not yet known

Apply to anogenital area 2–3 times daily

Lotion and *Dusting powder*, see section 13.10.2

PoM †**Travogyn**® (Schering Health)

Vaginal tablets (= pessaries), isoconazole nitrate 300 mg. Net price 2 = £3.37

Condoms: effect on latex condoms and diaphragms not yet known

Insert 2 pessaries as a single dose preferably at night

OTHER INFECTIONS

Vaginal preparations intended to restore normal acidity (Aci-Jel®) may prevent recurrence of vaginal infections and permit the re-establishment of the normal vaginal flora.

 Trichomonal infections commonly involve the lower urinary tract as well as the genital system and need systemic treatment with metronidazole or tinidazole (see section 5.4.2).

 Bacterial infections with Gram-negative organisms are particularly common in association with gynaecological operations and trauma. Metronidazole is effective against certain Gram-negative organisms, especially *Bacteroides* spp. and may be used prophylactically in gynaecological surgery.

 Antibacterial creams such as Sultrin® are used in the treatment of mixed bacterial infections but are of unproven value; they are ineffective against *Candida* spp. and *Trichomonas vaginalis*. A cream containing clindamycin is now also available.

1. See footnote 1 on p. 334

The antiviral drugs aciclovir, famciclovir and valaciclovir (see section 5.3) may be used in the treatment of genital infection due to *herpes simplex virus*, the HSV type 2 being a major cause of genital ulceration. It has a beneficial effect on virus shedding and healing, generally giving relief from pain and other symptoms. See section 5.3 for systemic preparations, and section 13.10.3 for cream.

PREPARATIONS FOR OTHER VAGINAL INFECTIONS

Aci-Jel® (Cilag)

Vaginal jelly, acetic acid 0.92% in a buffered (pH 4) basis. Net price 85 g with applicator = £3.37

Condoms: no evidence of damage to latex condoms and diaphragms

Non-specific infections, insert 1 applicatorful twice daily to restore vaginal acidity

Betadine® (Seton)

Cautions: avoid in pregnancy (also if planned) and in breast-feeding; renal impairment (see Appendix 3); avoid regular use in thyroid disorders

Side-effects: rarely sensitivity; may interfere with thyroid function

Vaginal Cleansing Kit, solution, povidone-iodine 10%. Net price 250 mL with measuring bottle and applicator = £2.92

Condoms: effect on latex condoms and diaphragms not yet known

To be diluted and used once daily, preferably in the morning; may be used with Betadine® pessaries or vaginal gel

Pessaries, brown, povidone-iodine 200 mg. Net price 28 pessaries with applicator = £6.34

Condoms: effect on latex condoms and diaphragms not yet known

Vaginal gel, brown, povidone-iodine 10%. Net price 80 g with applicator = £2.92

Condoms: effect on latex condoms and diaphragms not yet known

Vaginal infections or pre-operatively, insert 1 moistened pessary night and morning for up to 14 days *or* use morning pessary with 5-g gel at night *or* morning douche with pessary (or 5-g gel) at night

PoM **Dalacin**® (Upjohn)

Cream, clindamycin 2% (as phosphate). Net price 40-g pack with 7 applicators = £9.05

Condoms: damages latex condoms and diaphragms

Bacterial vaginosis, insert 5-g applicatorful intravaginally at night for 7 nights

PoM **Sultrin**® (Cilag)

Contra-indications: pregnancy

Side-effects: sensitivity

Cream, sulphathiazole 3.42%, sulphacetamide 2.86%, sulphabenzamide 3.7%. Net price 78 g with applicator = £3.48

Condoms: damages latex condoms and diaphragms

Bacterial vaginosis, insert 1 applicatorful of cream twice daily for 10 days, then once daily if necessary (but see also notes above)

Cautionary label wordings, see inside back cover

7.3   Contraceptives

7.3.1   Combined oral contraceptives
7.3.2   Progestogen-only contraceptives
7.3.3   Spermicidal contraceptives
7.3.4   Contraceptive devices

The criteria by which contraceptive methods should be judged are effectiveness, acceptability, and freedom from side-effects.

Hormonal contraception is the most effective method of fertility control, short of sterilisation, but has unwanted major and minor side-effects, especially for certain groups of women.

Intra-uterine devices have a high use-effectiveness but may produce undesirable side-effects, especially menorrhagia, or be otherwise unsuitable in a significant proportion of women; their use is generally inadvisable in nulliparous women because of the increased risk of pelvic sepsis and infertility.

Barrier methods alone (condoms, diaphragms, and caps) are less effective but can be very reliable for well-motivated couples if used in conjunction with a **spermicide**. Occasionally sensitivity reactions occur. The female condom (Femidom®) is now also available; it is prelubricated but does not contain a spermicide.

7.3.1   Combined oral contraceptives

Oral contraceptives containing an oestrogen and a progestogen are the most effective preparations for general use. Their advantages include:

reliability;
avoidance of dysmenorrhoea;
less iron-deficiency anaemia;
avoidance of pre-menstrual tension;
less benign breast disease;
protection against endometrial and ovarian cancer;
protection against pelvic inflammatory disease.

CHOICE. The oestrogen content ranges from 20 to 50 micrograms and generally a preparation with the lowest oestrogen and progestogen content (but within the guidelines of the CSM advice below) which gives good cycle control and minimal side-effects in the individual woman is chosen.

Low strength preparations (containing ethinyl-oestradiol 20 micrograms) are particularly appropriate for obese or older women provided a combined oral contraceptive is otherwise suitable (but see also CSM advice below).

Standard strength preparations (containing ethinyl-oestradiol 30 or 35 micrograms or in 30/40 microgram *phased* preparations) are appropriate for standard use in the case of those also containing *ethynodiol, levonorgestrel* or *norethisterone*—but in the case of those also containing *desogestrel* or *gestodene*, see CSM advice below. Phased preparations are more complex to take, but provide better cycle control than the equivalent 'monophasic' levonorgestrel or norethisterone formulations.

High strength preparations (containing either ethinyloestradiol 50 micrograms or mestranol

50 micrograms) provide greater contraceptive security but with an increase in the possibility of side-effects. These are used mainly in circumstances of reduced bioavailability (e.g. during long-term use of enzyme-inducing antiepileptics, see FPA advice under Interactions on p. 337).

The progestogens desogestrel, gestodene and norgestimate in combination with ethinyloestradiol have been reported to have less adverse effects on lipids than ethynodiol, levonorgestrel and norethisterone in combination with ethinyloestradiol. However, desogestrel and gestodene have also been associated with an increased risk of *venous thromboembolism* (see CSM advice below)

CSM advice. The CSM has advised that results of studies on the safety of oral contraceptives in relation to venous thromboembolism have provided reassurance about thromboembolic risks associated with oral contraceptives containing *levonorgestrel, norethisterone or ethynodiol* (excess risk around 5 to 10 cases per 100 000 women per annum). The studies indicated, however, that combined oral contraceptives containing *desogestrel* and *gestodene* are associated with around a two-fold increase in the risk, compared with those containing other progestogens. There is insufficient information to know whether there is any increased risk of thromboembolism associated with combined oral contraceptives containing *norgestimate*.

The CSM has therefore advised that combined oral contraceptives containing *gestodene or desogestrel* should **not** be used by women with risk factors for *venous thromboembolism*, including obesity (body mass index 30 kg/m²), varicose veins, or a previous history of thrombosis from any cause [it should *also* be noted that *any personal history* of venous or arterial thrombosis is already a contra-indication to *any* combined oral contraceptive].

Combined oral contraceptives containing *desogestrel or gestodene* should **only** be used by women who are intolerant of other combined oral contraceptives, and are prepared to accept an increased risk of thromboembolism.

This advice **only** affects combined oral preparations containing *desogestrel* (Marvelon®, Mercilon®), or *gestodene* (Femodene® ED, Femodene®, Minulet® Triadene®, Tri-Minulet®).

MISSED PILL. It is important to bear in mind that the critical time for loss of protection is when a pill is omitted at the *beginning* or *end* of a cycle (which lengthens the pill-free interval). The following advice is now recommended by family planning organisations:

'If you forget a pill, take it as soon as you remember, and the next one at your normal time. If you are 12 or more hours late with any pill (especially the first in the packet) the pill may not work. As soon as you remember, continue normal pill taking. However, you will not be protected for the next seven days and must either not have sex or use another method such as the sheath. If these seven days run beyond the end of your packet, start the next packet at once when you have finished the present one, i.e. do not have a gap between packets. This will mean you may not have a period until the end of two packets but this does you no harm. Nor does it matter if you see some bleeding on tablet-taking days. If you are using everyday (ED) pills—miss out the seven inactive pills. If you are not sure which these are, ask your doctor.'

DIARRHOEA AND VOMITING. Vomiting and severe diarrhoea can interfere with absorption and limit effectiveness. Additional precautions should therefore be used during and for 7 days after recovery. If the vomiting and diarrhoea occurs during the last 7 tablets, the next pill-free interval should be omitted (in the case of ED tablets the inactive ones should be omitted).

INTERACTIONS. The effectiveness of both *combined* and *progestogen-only* oral contraceptives may be considerably reduced by interaction with drugs that induce hepatic enzyme activity [e.g. **carbamazepine, griseofulvin, phenytoin, phenobarbitone, primidone, topiramate**, and, above all, **the rifamycins (rifabutin and rifampicin)**].

Family Planning Association (FPA) advice relating to a *short-term course of an enzyme-inducing drug* (important: rifampicin, see also below) is that additional contraceptive precautions should be taken whilst taking the enzyme-inducing drug and for at least 7 days after stopping it; if these 7 days run beyond the end of a packet the new packet should be started immediately without a break (in the case of ED tablets the inactive ones should be omitted). **Important**: it should be noted that **rifampicin** is such a potent enzyme-inducing drug that even if a course lasts for less than 7 days the additional contraceptive precautions should be continued for at least 4 weeks after stopping it.

FPA advice relating to a *long-term course of an enzyme-inducing drug* (important: rifampicin, see also below) in a woman unable to use an alternative method of contraception is to take an oral contraceptive containing ethinyloestradiol 50 micrograms or more; 'tricycling' with standard ('monophasic') tablets (i.e. taking 3 packets without a break followed by a short tablet-free interval of 4 days) is recommended. **Important**: it should be noted that **rifampicin** is such a potent enzyme-inducing drug that an alternative method of contraception (such as an IUD) is **always** recommended. Since the excretory function of the liver does not return to normal for several weeks after stopping an enzyme-inducing drug, FPA advice relating to *withdrawal* is that appropriate contraceptive measures are required for 4 to 8 weeks after stopping.

In the case of *combined* oral contraceptives some **broad-spectrum antibiotics** (e.g. ampicillin) may reduce their efficacy by impairing the bacterial flora responsible for recycling of ethinyloestradiol from the large bowel. FPA advice is that additional contraceptive precautions should be taken whilst taking a *short course of a broad-spectrum antibiotic* and for 7 days after stopping. If these 7 days run beyond the end of a packet the next packet should be started immediately without a break (in the case of ED tablets the inactive ones should be omitted). If the course *exceeds 2 weeks*, resistance to this interference develops, and additional precautions become unnecessary.

SURGERY. Oestrogen-containing oral contraceptives should be discontinued (and adequate alternative contraceptive arrangements made) 4 weeks before major elective surgery and all surgery to the legs; they should normally be recommenced at the first menses occurring at least 2 weeks after full mobilisation. When discontinuation is not possible, e.g. after trauma or if, by oversight, a patient admitted for an elective procedure is still on an oestrogen-containing oral contraceptive, some consideration should be given to subcutaneous heparin prophylaxis. These recommendations do not apply to minor surgery with short duration of anaesthesia, e.g. laparoscopic sterilisation or tooth extraction, or

to women taking oestrogen-free hormonal contraceptives (whether by mouth or by injection).

REASON TO STOP IMMEDIATELY. Combined oral contraceptives should be stopped (pending investigation and treatment), if any of the following symptoms occur:

Sudden severe pain in chest (whether or not radiating to the left arm);

Sudden breathlessness (or cough with blood-stained sputum);

Severe pain in calf of one leg;

Severe pain in stomach;

Unusual severe, prolonged headache—especially if first time or getting progressively worse, or associated with: sudden partial or complete loss of vision; diplopia; dysphasia; vertigo; bad fainting attack or collapse (with or without focal epilepsy); weakness or very marked numbness suddenly affecting one side or one part of body; motor disturbances.

COMBINED ORAL CONTRACEPTIVES
('COC')

Indications: contraception; menstrual symptoms, see section 6.4.1.2

Cautions: risk factor for arterial disease (avoid if two or more risk factors present) including cigarette smoking (avoid in those over 35 years), hypertension, obesity (if 50% above ideal weight for height)—see also CSM advice in notes above, diabetes mellitus (avoid if either retinopathy or nephropathy present), family history of arterial disease (ischaemic heart disease, ischaemic cerebrovascular accident) especially in a first-degree relative under 45 years; varicose veins (avoid if associated with venous thrombosis)—see also CSM advice in notes above; severe depression, long-term immobilisation, sickle-cell disease, inflammatory bowel disease including Crohn's disease; **interactions:** see above and Appendix 1 (contraceptives, oral)

Contra-indications: pregnancy; severe or multiple risk factors for arterial disease (see Cautions), history of arterial or venous thrombosis—see also CSM advice in notes above; valvular heart disease associated with pulmonary hypertension or risk of mural thrombi, ischaemic heart disease, severe hypertension, varicose veins (during sclerosing treatment or where history of thrombosis)—see also CSM advice in notes above; conditions where risk of intravascular thrombosis is higher such as an atherogenic lipid profile (e.g. familial hyperlipidaemia together with cholesterol above 6.5 mmol/litre), or any known prothrombotic coagulation abnormality; focal migraine, severe migraine, crescendo migraine, transient cerebral ischaemic attacks without headaches; liver disease including disorders of hepatic excretion (e.g. Dubin-Johnson or Rotor syndromes), infective hepatitis (until liver function returns to normal), porphyria (see section 9.8.2), and liver adenoma; gall-stones; after evacuation of hydatidiform mole (until return to normal of urine and plasma gonadotrophin values); history of haemolytic uraemic syndrome or during pregnancy of pruritus, chorea, pemphigoid gestationis, cholestatic jaundice, or deterioration of otosclerosis; breast or genital tract carcinoma; undiagnosed vaginal bleeding; breast-feeding (until weaning or for 6 months after birth)

Side-effects: nausea, vomiting, headache, breast tenderness, changes in body weight, thrombosis (more common in blood groups A, B, and AB than O), changes in libido, depression, chloasma, hypertension, contact lenses may irritate, impairment of liver function, hepatic tumours, reduced menstrual loss, 'spotting' in early cycles, absence of withdrawal bleeding; rarely photosensitivity

BREAST CANCER. There is a small increase in the risk of breast cancer during use and for 10 years after stopping the combined oral contraceptive pill; this relative risk does not appear to be related to duration of use. The CSM has advised that a small increase in the risk of breast cancer is more than counterbalanced by the protective effect against cancers of the ovary and endometrium

Dose: each tablet should be taken at approximately same time each day; if delayed by longer than 12 hours contraceptive protection may be lost

21-day combined (monophasic) preparations, 1 tablet daily for 21 days; subsequent courses repeated after a 7-day interval (during which withdrawal bleeding occurs); first course usually started on 1st day of cycle—if starting on 4th day of cycle or later additional precautions (barrier methods) necessary during first 7 days

Every day (ED) combined (monophasic) preparations, 1 tablet daily starting with an *active* tablet usually on 1st day of cycle—if starting on 4th day of cycle or later additional precautions (barrier methods) necessary during first 14 days (14 rather than 7 in case course accidentally started with *inactive* tablets); withdrawal bleeding occurs when *inactive* tablets are being taken; subsequent courses repeated without interval

Biphasic and triphasic preparations, see under individual preparations below

CHANGING TO COMBINED PREPARATION CONTAINING DIFFERENT PROGESTOGEN. *21-day combined preparations:* continue current pack until last tablet and start first tablet of new brand the next day. If a 7-day break is taken before starting new brand, additional precautions (barrier methods) should be used during first 7 days of taking the new brand.

Every Day (ED) combined preparations: start the new brand (first tablet a of *21-day preparation* or the first *active* tablet of an *ED preparation*) the day after taking the last *active* tablet of previous brand (omitting the *inactive* tablets). If not possible to avoid taking the *inactive* tablets of an *ED preparation,* additional precautions (barrier methods) necessary during first 14 days of taking the new brand

CHANGING FROM PROGESTOGEN-ONLY TABLET: start on 1st day of menstruation or any day if amenorrhoea present and pregnancy has been excluded

SECONDARY AMENORRHOEA (exclude pregnancy): start any day, additional precautions (barrier methods) necessary during first 7 days

AFTER CHILDBIRTH (*not* breast-feeding): start 3 weeks postpartum (increased risk of thrombosis if

started earlier); later than 3 weeks postpartum additional precautions (barrier methods) necessary for first 7 days

Not recommended if woman breast-feeding—oral progestogen-only contraceptive preferred

AFTER ABORTION OR MISCARRIAGE: start same day

Low Strength

Ethinyloestradiol with Norethisterone
PoM **Loestrin 20**® (P-D)

Tablets, norethisterone acetate 1 mg, ethinyloestradiol 20 micrograms. Net price 3 × 21-tab pack = £2.58

Dose: 1 tablet daily for 21 days; subsequent courses repeated after 7-day interval (during which withdrawal bleeding occurs); for 'starting routines' see under 'Dose' in monograph above

Ethinyloestradiol with Desogestrel
See **CSM advice** in notes above before prescribing
PoM **Mercilon**® (Organon)

Tablets, desogestrel 150 micrograms, ethinyloestradiol 20 micrograms. Net price 3 × 21-tab pack = £8.97

Dose: 1 tablet daily for 21 days; subsequent courses repeated after 7-day interval (during which withdrawal bleeding occurs); for 'starting routines' see under 'Dose' in monograph above

---

Standard Strength

Ethinyloestradiol with Levonorgestrel
PoM **Eugynon 30**® (Schering Health)

Tablets, levonorgestrel 250 micrograms, ethinyloestradiol 30 micrograms. Net price 21-tab pack = 69p

Dose: 1 tablet daily for 21 days; subsequent courses repeated after 7-day interval (during which withdrawal bleeding occurs); for 'starting routines' see under 'Dose' in monograph above

PoM **Logynon**® (Schering Health)

6 *light brown tablets,* ethinyloestradiol 30 micrograms, levonorgestrel 50 micrograms;
5 *white tablets,* ethinyloestradiol 40 micrograms, levonorgestrel 75 micrograms;
10 *ochre tablets,* ethinyloestradiol 30 micrograms, levonorgestrel 125 micrograms.
Net price 21-tab pack = £1.09

Dose: 1 tablet daily for 21 days, starting with light brown tablet marked 1 on 1st day of cycle; repeat after 7-day interval

PoM **Logynon ED**® (Schering Health)

As for Logynon® with additional 7 white placebo tablets. Net price 28-tab pack = £1.09

Dose: 1 tablet daily starting in red sector on 1st day of cycle; continue in sequence without interruption

PoM **Microgynon 30**® (Schering Health)

Tablets, levonorgestrel 150 micrograms, ethinyloestradiol 30 micrograms. Net price 21-tab pack = 62p

Dose: 1 tablet daily for 21 days; subsequent courses repeated after 7-day interval (during which withdrawal bleeding occurs); for 'starting routines' see under 'Dose' in monograph above

PoM **Ovran 30**® (Wyeth)

Tablets, levonorgestrel 250 micrograms, ethinyloestradiol 30 micrograms. Net price 21-tab pack = 57p

Dose: 1 tablet daily for 21 days; subsequent courses repeated after 7-day interval (during which withdrawal bleeding occurs); for 'starting routines' see under 'Dose' in monograph above

---

PoM **Ovranette**® (Wyeth)

Tablets, levonorgestrel 150 micrograms, ethinyloestradiol 30 micrograms. Net price 3 ×21-tab pack = £1.86

Dose: 1 tablet daily for 21 days; subsequent courses repeated after 7-day interval (during which withdrawal bleeding occurs); for 'starting routines' see under 'Dose' in monograph above

PoM **Trinordiol**® (Wyeth)

6 light brown tablets, ethinyloestradiol 30 micrograms, levonorgestrel 50 micrograms;

5 white tablets, ethinyloestradiol 40 micrograms, levonorgestrel 75 micrograms;

10 ochre tablets, ethinyloestradiol 30 micrograms, levonorgestrel 125 micrograms.

Net price 3 × 21-tab pack = £3.28

Dose: 1 tablet daily for 21 days, starting with light brown tablet marked 1 on 1st day of cycle; repeat after 7 day interval

Ethinyloestradiol with Norethisterone

PoM **BiNovum**® (Ortho)

7 white tablets, ethinyloestradiol 35 micrograms, norethisterone 500 micrograms;

14 peach tablets, ethinyloestradiol 35 micrograms, norethisterone 1mg.

Net price 3 × 21-tab pack = £2.24

Dose: 1 tablet daily for 21 days, starting with white tablet on 1st day of cycle; repeat after 7 day interval

PoM **Brevinor**® (Searle)

Tablets, norethisterone 500 micrograms, ethinyloestradiol 35 micrograms. Net price 3 × 21-tab pack = £1.67

Dose: 1 tablet daily for 21 days; subsequent courses repeated after 7-day interval (during which withdrawal bleeding occurs); for 'starting routines' see under 'Dose' in monograph above

PoM **Loestrin 30**® (P-D)

Tablets, norethisterone acetate 1.5 mg, ethinyloestradiol 30 micrograms. Net price 3 × 21-tab pack = £3.78

Dose: 1 tablet daily for 21 days; subsequent courses repeated after 7-day interval (during which withdrawal bleeding occurs); for 'starting routines' see under 'Dose' in monograph above

PoM **Norimin**® (Searle)

Tablets, norethisterone 1 mg, ethinyloestradiol 35 micrograms. Net price 3 × 21-tab pack = £1.90

Dose: 1 tablet daily for 21 days; subsequent courses repeated after 7-day interval (during which withdrawal bleeding occurs); for 'starting routines' see under 'Dose' in monograph above

PoM **Ovysmen**® (Ortho)

Tablets, norethisterone 500 micrograms, ethinyloestradiol 35 micrograms. Net price 3 × 21-tab pack = £1.70

Dose: 1 tablet daily for 21 days; subsequent courses repeated after 7-day interval (during which withdrawal bleeding occurs); for 'starting routines' see under 'Dose' in monograph above

PoM **Synphase**® (Searle)

7 white tablets, ethinyloestradiol 35 micrograms, norethisterone 500 micrograms;

9 yellow tablets, ethinyloestradiol 35 micrograms, norethisterone 1 mg;

5 white tablets, ethinyloestradiol 35 micrograms, norethisterone 500 micrograms.

Net price 21-tab pack = £1.08

Dose: 1 tablet daily for 21 days, starting with white tablet marked 1 on 1st day of cycle; repeat after 7 day interval

PoM **TriNovum**® (Ortho)

7 white tablets, ethinyloestradiol 35 micrograms, norethisterone 500 micrograms;

7 light peach tablets, ethinyloestradiol 35 micrograms, norethisterone 750 micrograms;

7 peach tablets, ethinyloestradiol 35 micrograms, norethisterone 1 mg.

Net price 3 × 21-tab pack = £2.83

Dose: 1 tablet daily for 21 days, starting with white tablet on 1st day of cycle; repeat after 7-day interval

Ethinyloestradiol with Norgestimate

PoM **Cilest**® (Cilag)

Tablets, norgestimate 250 micrograms, ethinyloestradiol 35 micrograms. Net price 3 × 21-tab pack = £5.84

Dose: 1 tablet daily for 21 days; subsequent courses repeated after 7-day interval (during which withdrawal bleeding occurs); for 'starting routines' see under 'Dose' in monograph above

Ethinyloestradiol with Desogestrel

See **CSM advice** in notes above before prescribing

PoM **Marvelon**® (Organon)

Tablets, desogestrel 150 micrograms, ethinyloestradiol 30 micrograms. Net price 3 × 21-tab pack = £5.85

Dose: 1 tablet daily for 21 days; subsequent courses repeated after 7-day interval (during which withdrawal bleeding occurs); for 'starting routines' see under 'Dose' in monograph above

Ethinyloestradiol with Gestodene

See **CSM advice** in notes above before prescribing

PoM **Femodene**® (Schering Health)

Tablets, gestodene 75 micrograms, ethinyloestradiol 30 micrograms. Net price 3 × 21-tab pack = £5.70

Dose: 1 tablet daily for 21 days; subsequent courses repeated after 7-day interval (during which withdrawal bleeding occurs); for 'starting routines' see under 'Dose' in monograph above

PoM **Femodene ED**® (Schering Health)

Tablets, gestodene 75 micrograms, ethinyloestradiol 30 micrograms. Net price 3 × 28-tab (7 are inactive) pack = £5.70

Dose: 1 tablet daily for 28 days (withdrawal bleeding occurs when inactive tablets are being taken); subsequent courses repeated without interval; for 'starting routines' see under 'Dose' in monograph above

PoM **Minulet**® (Wyeth)

Tablets, gestodene 75 micrograms, ethinyloestradiol 30 micrograms. Net price 3 × 21-tab pack = £5.70

Dose: 1 tablet daily for 21 days; subsequent courses repeated after 7-day interval (during which withdrawal bleeding occurs); for 'starting routines' see under 'Dose' in monograph above

PoM **Triadene**® (Schering Health)

6 beige tablets, ethinyloestradiol 30 micrograms, gestodene 50 micrograms;

5 dark brown tablets, ethinyloestradiol 40 micrograms, gestodene 70 micrograms;

10 white tablets, ethinyloestradiol 30 micrograms, gestodene 100 micrograms.

Net price 3 × 21-tab pack = £7.95

Dose: 1 tablet daily for 21 days, starting with beige tablet marked 'start' on 1st day of cycle; repeat after 7-day interval

---

Cautionary label wordings, see inside back cover

Prices are **net**, see p.1

PoM **Tri-Minulet®** (Wyeth)

6 beige tablets, ethinyloestradiol 30 micrograms, gestodene 50 micrograms;
5 dark brown tablets, ethinyloestradiol 40 micrograms, gestodene 70 micrograms;
10 white tablets, ethinyloestradiol 30 micrograms, gestodene 100 micrograms.
Net price 3 × 21-tab pack = £7.95
Dose: 1 tablet daily for 21 days, starting with beige tablet marked 1 on the 1st day of the cycle; repeat after 7 day interval

High Strength

Ethinyloestradiol with Levonorgestrel

PoM **Ovran®** (Wyeth)

Tablets, levonorgestrel 250 micrograms, ethinyloestradiol 50 micrograms. Net price 21-tab pack = 37p
Dose: 1 tablet daily for 21 days; subsequent courses repeated after 7-day interval (during which withdrawal bleeding occurs); for 'starting routines' see under 'Dose' in monograph above

Mestranol with Norethisterone

PoM **Norinyl-1®** (Searle)

Tablets, norethisterone 1 mg, mestranol 50 micrograms. Net price 3 × 21-tab pack = £1.83
Dose: 1 tablet daily for 21 days; subsequent courses repeated after 7-day interval (during which withdrawal bleeding occurs); for 'starting routines' see under 'Dose' in monograph above

PoM **Ortho-Novin 1/50®** (Ortho)

Tablets, norethisterone 1 mg, mestranol 50 micrograms. Net price 3 × 21-tab pack = £2.35
Dose: 1 tablet daily for 21 days; subsequent courses repeated after 7-day interval (during which withdrawal bleeding occurs); for 'starting routines' see under 'Dose' in monograph above

EMERGENCY CONTRACEPTION

HORMONAL METHOD. The hormonal (Yuzpe) method of emergency contraception is suitable for occasional use. It involves taking two tablets, each containing ethinyloestradiol 50 micrograms and levonorgestrel 250 micrograms, followed 12 hours later by a further two tablets. The method has only been established as effective if the first dose is taken within 72 hours (3 days) of the unprotected intercourse; it is less effective than insertion of an intra-uterine device. Providing any delay does not extend beyond 72 hours, the timing of the first dose should be such that the second dose can conveniently be taken at the correct interval *exactly 12 hours later.* It is not suitable for women with a history of thrombosis or for those with focal migraine at the time of presentation. Side-effects include nausea, vomiting, headache, dizziness, breast discomfort, and menstrual irregularities. If vomiting occurs within 2–3 hours of taking the tablets, two replacement tablets can be given with an anti-emetic (preferably not metoclopramide which is liable to cause extrapyramidal effects in young women); alternatively insertion of an intra-uterine device (see below) may be needed.

The doctor should explain to the patient:
that her next period may be *early or late*;
that she needs to use a *barrier method of contraception* until her next period;

that she should return promptly if she has any *lower abdominal pain or heavy bleeding* (and also in 3 to 4 weeks if her subsequent period is abnormally light, heavy or brief, or is absent, or she is otherwise concerned)

Pregnancy despite treatment: see Appendix 4 (contraceptives, oral)—doctor information leaflet also available

PoM **Schering PC4®** (Schering Health)

Tablets, s/c, levonorgestrel 250 micrograms, ethinyloestradiol 50 micrograms. Net price 4-tab pack = £1.60

For post-coital contraception as an occasional emergency measure; should not be administered if menstrual bleeding overdue or if unprotected intercourse occurred more than 72 hours previously
Dose: 2 tablets as soon as possible after coitus (up to 72 hours) then 2 further tablets 12 hours later
Note. **Ovran®** also contains levonorgestrel 250 micrograms and ethinyloestradiol 50 micrograms but is not licensed or packed for post-coital contraception

IUD. An intra-uterine contraceptive device (see section 7.3.4) can be inserted up to 120 hours (5 days) after unprotected intercourse, care being taken to exclude any sexually transmitted diseases. If exposure has occurred more than 5 days previously, the device can still be inserted up to 5 days after the earliest likely calculated ovulation (i.e. within the minimum period before implantation). Insertion of an intra-uterine device is more effective than the hormonal method.

7.3.2 Progestogen-only contraceptives

7.3.2.1 Oral progestogen-only contraceptives
7.3.2.2 Parenteral progestogen-only contraceptives
7.3.2.3 Intra-uterine progestogen-only contraceptive

7.3.2.1 ORAL PROGESTOGEN-ONLY CONTRACEPTIVES

Oral progestogen-only preparations may offer a suitable alternative when oestrogens are contra-indicated, but have a higher failure rate than combined preparations. They are suitable for older women, for heavy smokers, and for those with hypertension, valvular heart disease, diabetes mellitus, and migraine. Menstrual irregularities (oligomenorrhoea, menorrhagia) are more common but tend to resolve on long-term treatment.

INTERACTIONS. Effectiveness of oral progestogen-only preparations is not affected by broad-spectrum antibiotics but is reduced by enzyme-inducing drugs—see p. 337 and Appendix 1 (progestogens).

SURGERY. All progestogen-only contraceptives (including those given by injection) are suitable for use as an alternative to combined oral contraceptives before major elective surgery.

STARTING ROUTINE. 1 tablet daily, on a continuous basis, starting on 1st day of cycle and taken at the same time each day (if delayed by longer than 3 hours contraceptive protection may be lost). Additional contraceptive precautions are not necessary when initiating treatment.

Changing from a combined oral contraceptive: start on the day following completion of the combined oral contraceptive course without a break (or in the case of ED tablets omitting the inactive ones).

After childbirth: start any time after 3 weeks postpartum (increased risk of breakthrough bleeding if started earlier)—lactation is not affected.

MISSED PILL. The following advice is now recommended by family planning organisations:

'If you forget a pill, take it as soon as you remember and carry on with the next pill at the right time. If the pill was more than three hours overdue you are not protected. Continue normal pill-taking but you must also use another method, such as the sheath, for the next 7 days'.

DIARRHOEA AND VOMITING. Vomiting and severe diarrhoea can interfere with absorption and limit effectiveness. Additional precautions should be used during and for 7 days after recovery.

ORAL PROGESTOGEN-ONLY CONTRACEPTIVES

(Progestogen-only pill, 'POP')

Indications: contraception

Cautions: heart disease, past ectopic pregnancy, malabsorption syndromes, functional ovarian cysts, active liver disease, recurrent cholestatic jaundice, history of jaundice in pregnancy; **interactions:** p. 337 and Appendix 1 (progestogens)

HYPERTENSION. Monitor blood pressure regularly in women receiving progestogen-only contraceptives—but suitable for women with history of hypertension associated with combined pill (and those with other forms of hypertension providing controlled).

Contra-indications: pregnancy, undiagnosed vaginal bleeding; severe arterial disease; liver adenoma, porphyria (see section 9.8.2); after evacuation of hydatidiform mole (until return to normal of urine and plasma gonadotrophin values); breast and genital tract carcinoma

Side-effects: menstrual irregularities (see also notes above); nausea, vomiting, headache, breast discomfort, depression, skin disorders, weight changes

Dose: 1 tablet daily at same time each day, starting on 1st day of cycle then continuously; if tablet delayed for 3 hours or more it should be regarded as a 'missed pill', see notes above

PoM **Femulen®** (Searle)
Tablets, ethynodiol diacetate 500 micrograms. Net price 28-tab pack = 92p

PoM **Micronor®** (Ortho)
Tablets, norethisterone 350 micrograms. Net price 3 × 28-tab pack = £1.89

PoM **Microval®** (Wyeth)
Tablets, levonorgestrel 30 micrograms. Net price 35-tab pack = 82p

PoM **Neogest®** (Schering Health)
Tablets, brown, s/c, norgestrel 75 micrograms (≡ levonorgestrel 37.5 micrograms). Net price 35-tab pack = 82p

PoM **Norgeston®** (Schering Health)
Tablets, s/c, levonorgestrel 30 micrograms. Net price 35-tab pack = 82p

PoM **Noriday®** (Searle)
Tablets, norethisterone 350 micrograms. Net price 3 × 28-tab pack = £1.75

7.3.2.2 PARENTERAL PROGESTOGEN-ONLY CONTRACEPTIVES

Medroxyprogesterone acetate (Depo-Provera®) is a long-acting progestogen given by intramuscular injection; it is as effective as the combined oral preparations but because of its prolonged action should never be given without *full counselling backed by the manufacturer's approved leaflet.* It may be used as a short-term or long-term contraceptive for women who have been appropriately counselled concerning the likelihood of menstrual disturbance and the potential for a delay in return to full fertility. Delayed return of fertility and irregular cycles may occur after discontinuation of treatment but there is no evidence of permanent infertility. Heavy bleeding has been reported in patients given medroxyprogesterone acetate in the immediate puerperium (the first dose is best delayed until 5 to 6 weeks postpartum). If the woman is not breast-feeding, the first injection may be given within 5 days postpartum (she should be warned that the risk of heavy or prolonged bleeding may be increased). Reduction in bone mineral density has also been reported. **Norethisterone enanthate** (Noristerat®) is a long-acting progestogen given as an oily injection which provides contraception for 8 weeks to provide short-term interim contraception e.g. before vasectomy becomes effective. The **cautions** and **contra-indications** of progestogen-only contraceptives given by injection are as for the oral preparations except that as the injection also reliably inhibits ovulation, it protects against ectopic pregnancy and functional ovarian cysts.

A **levonorgestrel-releasing implant system** (Norplant®) is now also available; it has comparable efficacy to injectable medroxyprogesterone acetate but lasts for 5 years. The **cautions** and **contra-indications** are again as for oral preparations, but irregular and prolonged bleeding and amenorrhoea are common; unlike the injectable preparations the method is almost immediately reversible on removal of the implants. The risk of ectopic pregnancy is believed to be reduced overall but may be relatively higher in the later years after an insertion; since functional ovarian cysts may also be more common they need to be distinguished from ectopic pregnancy. *The doctor administering the system should be fully trained in the technique and should provide full counselling backed by the manufacturer's approved leaflet.*

INTERACTIONS. Effectiveness of parenteral progestogen-only contraceptives is not affected by broad-spectrum antibiotics but may be reduced by enzyme-inducing drugs—see p. 337 and Appendix 1 (progestogens)

PARENTERAL PROGESTOGEN-ONLY CONTRACEPTIVES

Indications: contraception, see also notes above and under preparations (roles vary according to preparation)

Cautions; Contra-indications; Side-effects: see notes above and under preparations; **interactions:** see notes above, p. 337 and Appendix 1 (progestogens)

COUNSELLING. Full counselling backed by *manufacturer's approved leaflet* required before administration

Dose: see under preparations

Injectable preparations

PoM Depo-Provera® (Upjohn)

Injection (aqueous suspension), medroxyprogesterone acetate 150 mg/mL, net price 1-mL vial = £4.55; 1-mL prefilled syringe = £4.55. Counselling, see patient information leaflet

Dose: by deep intramuscular injection, 150 mg within first 5 days of cycle or within first 5 days after parturition (delay until 6 weeks after parturition if breast-feeding); for long-term contraception, repeated every 12 weeks (if interval greater than 12 weeks, exclude pregnancy before next injection and advise patient to use additional contraceptive measures (e.g. barrier) for 14 days after the injection)

Note. The 150 mg/mL strength of Depo-Provera® is also available in a 3.3mL vial for use in cancer (see section 8.3.2)

PoM Noristerat® (Schering Health)

Injection (oily), norethisterone enanthate 200 mg/mL. Net price 1-mL amp = £3.00. Counselling, see patient information leaflet

Dose: by deep intramuscular injection into gluteal muscle, short-term contraception, 200 mg within first 5 days of cycle or immediately after parturition (duration 8 weeks); may be repeated once after 8 weeks (withhold breast-feeding for neonates with severe or persistent jaundice requiring medical treatment)

Implants

▼ PoM Norplant® (Roussel)

Implant capsules, containing levonorgestrel 38 mg/implant capsule. Net price 6-implant capsule pack = £179.00. Counselling, see patient information leaflet

Dose: by subdermal implantation, set of 6 implant capsules inserted within first 5 days of cycle (preferably on 1st day—after 1st day additional precautions necessary for following 7 days) *or* on 21st day after parturition (after this day additional precautions necessary for following 7 days); remove within 5 years of insertion

7.3.2.3 INTRA-UTERINE PROGESTOGEN-ONLY CONTRACEPTIVE

Levonorgestrel is released directly in to the uterine cavity from an intra-uterine system (Mirena®). Effects are therefore mainly local and hormonal including prevention of proliferation of the endometrium, thickening of cervical mucus, and suppression of ovulation in some women (in some cycles); the physical presence of the system in the uterus may also make a minor contribution to the overall contraceptive effect. Return of fertility after removal is rapid and appears to be complete. Advantages over copper intra-uterine devices are that there may be an improvement in any dysmenorrhoea and a reduction in blood loss; there is also evidence that the frequency of pelvic inflammatory disease may be reduced (particularly in the youngest age groups who are most at risk). Generally the **cautions** and **contra-indications** are as for standard intra-uterine devices (see section 7.3.4) but the risk of ectopic pregnancy is considerably reduced and pre-existing heavy menses may be alleviated. Moreover, since the progestogen is released close to the site of the main contraceptive action (on cervical mucus and endometrium) progestogenic side-effects and **interactions** are less likely to be a problem—in particular, enzyme-inducing drugs are unlikely to have much influence on the contraceptive effect. Initially changes in the pattern and duration of menstrual bleeding (spotting or prolonged bleeding) are common and full counselling (backed by patient information leaflet) should be undertaken before insertion. Improvement usually occurs a few months after insertion and bleeding may often become scanty or absent, this may therefore be a method of choice for women who have excessively heavy menses. Functional ovarian cysts (usually asymptomatic) may occur and may resolve spontaneously (ultrasound monitoring and other measures are recommended).

INTRA-UTERINE PROGESTOGEN-ONLY CONTRACEPTIVE

Indications: contraception

Cautions; Contra-indications; Side-effects: see notes above; in case of pregnancy—remove system (teratogenicity cannot be excluded); not suitable for emergency contraception; **interactions:** see notes above and Appendix 1 (progestogens)

▼ PoM Mirena® (Pharmacia-Leiras)

Intra-uterine system, T-shaped plastic frame (impregnated with barium sulphate and with threads attached to base) with polydimethylsiloxane reservoir releasing levonorgestrel 20 micrograms/24 hours. Net price = £99.25. Counselling, see patient information leaflet

Insert into uterine cavity within 7 days of onset of menstruation (anytime if replacement) or immediately after first-trimester termination by curettage; postpartum insertions should be delayed until 6 weeks after delivery; effective for 3 years

7.3.3   Spermicidal contraceptives

Spermicidal contraceptives are useful additional safeguards but do **not** give adequate protection if used alone; they are suitable for use with barrier methods. They have two components: a spermicide and a vehicle which itself may have some inhibiting effect on sperm activity.

Condoms: no evidence of harm to latex condoms and diaphragms with the products listed below

Delfen® (Ortho)
Foam, nonoxinol '9' 12.5%, pressurised aerosol unit in a water-miscible basis. Net price 20 g (with applicator) = £4.65
Double Check® (FP)
Pessaries, nonoxinol '9' 6% in a water-soluble basis. Net price 10 pessaries = £1.08
Duracreme® (LRC)
Cream, nonoxinol '9' 2% in a water-soluble basis. Net price 100-g tube = £2.60; applicator = 75p
Duragel® (LRC)
Gel, nonoxinol '9' 2% in a water-soluble basis. Net price 100-g tube = £2.60; applicator = 75p
Gynol II® (Ortho)
Jelly, nonoxinol '9' 2% in a water-soluble basis. Net price 81 g = £2.61; applicator = 75p
Ortho-Creme® (Ortho)
Cream, nonoxinol '9' 2% in a water-miscible basis. Net price 70 g = £2.44; applicator = 75p
Orthoforms® (Ortho)
Pessaries, nonoxinol '9' 5% in a water-soluble basis. Net price 15 pessaries = £2.40

7.3.4 Contraceptive devices

INTRA-UTERINE DEVICES

The intra-uterine device (IUD) is suitable for older parous women but should be a last-resort contraceptive for young nulliparous women because of the increased risk of pelvic inflammatory disease and infertility. Inert intra-uterine devices are no longer on the UK market but may still be worn by some women.

Smaller devices have now been introduced in order to minimise side-effects; these consist of a plastic carrier wound with copper wire or fitted with copper bands; some also have a central core of silver with the aim of preventing fragmentation of the copper. Family planning organisations now recommend that the replacement time for these devices should be 5 years (8 years for Gyne-T® 380 Slimline which also has a copper collar); any copper intrauterine device licensed currently in the UK, which is fitted in a woman over the age of 40, may remain in the uterus until menopause.

The timing and technique of fitting an intra-uterine device play a critical part in its subsequent performance and call for proper training and experience. Devices should not be fitted during the heavy days of the period; they are best fitted after the end of menstruation and before the calculated time of implantation. The main excess risk of infection occurs in the first 20 days after insertion and is believed to be related to pre-existing carriage of a sexually transmitted disease, therefore pre-screening (at least for chlamydia) should ideally be performed. The woman should be advised to attend *as an emergency* if she experiences sustained pain during the next 20 days.

An intra-uterine device should not be removed in mid-cycle unless an additional contraceptive was used for the previous 7 days. If removal is essential (e.g. to treat severe pelvic infection) post-coital contraception should be considered.

If an intra-uterine device fails and the woman wishes to continue to full-term the device should be removed in the first trimester if possible.

INTRA-UTERINE CONTRACEPTIVE DEVICES

Indications: see notes above
Cautions: anaemia, heavy menses, history of pelvic inflammatory disease, diabetes, valvular heart disease (antibiotic cover needed)—avoid if prosthetic valve or past attack of infective endocarditis; epilepsy, increased risk of expulsion if inserted before uterine involution; gynaecological examination before insertion, 6 weeks after (or sooner if there is a problem), then after 6 months, then yearly; remove if pregnancy occurs; anticoagulant therapy (avoid if possible); if pregnancy occurs, increased likelihood that it may be tubal
Contra-indications: pregnancy, severe anaemia, known HIV infection, very heavy menses, history of ectopic pregnancy or tubal surgery, distorted or small uterine cavity, genital malignancy, pelvic inflammatory disease, immunosuppressive therapy, *copper devices:* copper allergy, Wilson's disease, medical diathermy
Side-effects: uterine or cervical perforation, displacement, pelvic infection may be exacerbated, heavy menses, dysmenorrhoea, allergy; *on insertion:* some pain (helped by giving an NSAID, such as ibuprofen half-an-hour before insertion) and bleeding, occasionally, epileptic seizure, vasovagal attack

PoM **Multiload®** Cu250 (Organon)
Intra-uterine device, copper wire, surface area approx. 250 mm² wound on vertical stem of plastic carrier, 3.6 cm length, with 2 down-curving flexible arms, monofilament thread attached to base of vertical stem; preloaded in inserter. Net price = £7.42
For uterine length over 7 cm; replacement every 3 years (but see notes above)
PoM **Multiload® Cu250 Short** (Organon)
Intra-uterine device, as above, with vertical stem length 2.5 cm. Net price = £7.42
For uterine length 5–7 cm; replacement every 3 years (but see notes above)
PoM **Multiload®Cu375** (Organon)
Intra-uterine device, as above, with copper surface area approx. 375 mm². Net price = £9.62
For uterine length over 7 cm; replacement every 5 years (see notes above)

PoM **Novagard**® (Pharmacia)

Intra-uterine device, copper wire with silver core, surface area approx. 200 mm² wound on vertical stem of T-shaped plastic carrier, impregnated with barium sulphate for radio-opacity, monofilament thread attached to base of vertical stem; partially preloaded in inserter. Dimensions: transverse arms, vertical stem, both 3.2 cm. Net price = £9.90

For uterine length over 5.5 cm; replacement every 5 years (see notes above)

PoM **Nova-T**® (Schering Health)

Intra-uterine device, copper wire with silver core, surface area approx. 200 mm² wound on vertical stem of T-shaped plastic carrier, impregnated with barium sulphate for radio-opacity, threads attached to base of vertical stem. Net price = £9.90

For uterine length over 6.5 cm; replacement every 5 years (see notes above)

PoM **Ortho Gyne-T**® **380 Slimline** (Ortho)

Intra-uterine device, copper wire surface area 320 mm² wound on vertical stem of T-shaped plastic carrier (impregnated with radiopaque substance), plastic thread attached to base of vertical stem, and copper collar surface 30 mm² on distal portion of each arm. Net price = £9.40

For uterine length over 6.5 cm; replacement every 8 years (see notes above)

OTHER CONTRACEPTIVE DEVICES

Contraceptive caps

Type A contraceptive pessary. Opaque rubber, sizes 1 to 5 (55–75 mm rising in steps of 5 mm), net price = £6.40

Available from Lamberts (Dumas Vault Cap®)

Type B contraceptive pessary Opaque rubber, sizes 22 to 31 mm (rising in steps of 3 mm), net price = £7.45

Available from Lamberts (Prentif Cavity Rim Cervical Cap®)

Type C contraceptive pessary Opaque rubber, sizes 1 to 3 (42, 48 and 54 mm), net price = £6.40

Available from Lamberts (Vimule Cap®)

Contraceptive diaphragms

Type A Diaphragm with flat metal spring. Transparent rubber with flat metal spring, sizes 55–95 mm (rising in steps of 5 mm), net price = £5.49

Available from Cilag (Ortho-White®), Lamberts (Reflexions®)

Type B Diaphragm with coiled metal rim. Opaque rubber with coiled metal rim, sizes 55–95 mm (rising in steps of 5 mm), net price = £5.53

Available from Cilag (Ortho®)

Type C Arcing Spring Diaphragm. Opaque rubber with arcing spring, sizes 55–95 mm (rising in steps of 5 mm), net price = £6.29

Available from Cilag (All-Flex®), LRC (Durex Arcing Spring®)

Fertility thermometer

Fertility (Ovulation) Thermometer (Zeal)

Mercury in glass thermometer, range 35 to 39°C (graduated in 0.1°C). Net price = £1.59

For monitoring ovulation for the fertility awareness method of contraception

---

7.4   Drugs for genito-urinary disorders

7.4.1	Drugs for urinary retention
7.4.2	Drugs for urinary frequency, enuresis, and incontinence
7.4.3	Drugs used in urological pain
7.4.4	Bladder instillations and urological surgery
7.4.5	Drugs for impotence

For drugs used in the treatment of urinary-tract infections see section 5.1.13.

7.4.1   Drugs for urinary retention

Acute retention is painful and is treated by catheterisation.

Chronic retention is painless and often long-standing. Catheterisation is unnecessary unless there is deterioration of renal function. After the cause has initially been established and treated, drugs may be required to increase detrusor muscle tone.

ALPHA-BLOCKERS

The selective alpha-blockers **alfuzosin, doxazosin, indoramin, prazosin , tamsulosin** and **terazosin** relax smooth muscle in benign prostatic hyperplasia producing an increase in urinary flow-rate and an improvement in obstructive symptoms. Side-effects of selective alpha-blockers include *sedation, dizziness* and *hypotension (notably postural hypotension, particularly after the first dose); other side-effects* associated with this group of drugs include *drowsiness, weakness* and *lack of energy, depression, headache, dry mouth, nausea, urinary frequency and incontinence*, and *tachycardia and palpitations*. They should be avoided in patients with *a history of orthostatic hypotension* and special care (and reduced dosage) is needed when initiating them in the *elderly*, and in *renal* and possibly *hepatic impairment*. Since selective alpha-blockers are also antihypertensive, patients receiving *antihypertensive treatment* require reduced dosage and specialist supervision (as do those with *cardiac disorders*). **Interactions:** see Appendix 1 (alpha-blockers).

DRIVING. Selective alpha-blockers may cause drowsiness and so affect ability to drive or operate machinery.

ALFUZOSIN HYDROCHLORIDE

Indications; Cautions; Contra-indications; Side-effects: see notes above

Dose: 2.5 mg 3 times daily, max. 10 mg daily; ELDERLY 2.5 mg twice daily initially

FIRST DOSE EFFECT. First dose may cause collapse due to hypotensive effect (therefore should be taken on retiring to bed). Patient should be warned to lie down if symptoms such as dizziness, fatigue or sweating develop, and to remain lying down until they abate completely

---

▼ PoM **Xatral**® (Lorex)

Tablets, f/c, alfuzosin hydrochloride 2.5 mg. Net price 60-tab pack = £19.00; 90-tab pack = £25.00. Label: 3, counselling, see dose above

Modified release

▼ PoM **Xatral**® **SR** (Lorex)

Tablets, m/r, yellow, f/c, alfuzosin hydrochloride 5 mg. Net price 60-tab pack = £23.80. Label: 3, 25, counselling, see above

Dose: 5 mg twice daily (elderly, dose form not appropriate for initial dose titration)

DOXAZOSIN

Indications; Cautions; Contra-indications; Side-effects: see notes above and section 2.5.4

Dose: initially 1 mg daily; increased if necessary at intervals of 1–2 weeks to max. 8 mg daily; usual maintenance 2–4 mg daily

PoM **Cardura**® (Invicta)

Tablets, doxazosin (as mesylate) 1 mg, net price 28-tab pack = £10.56; 2 mg, 28-tab pack = £14.08; 4 mg, 28-tab pack = £17.60

INDORAMIN

Indications; Cautions; Contra-indications; Side-effects: see notes above and section 2.5.4

Dose: 20 mg twice daily; increased if necessary by 20 mg every 2 weeks to max. 100 mg daily in divided doses; ELDERLY, 20 mg at night maybe adequate

PoM **Doralese**® (Bencard)

Tablets, yellow, f/c, indoramin 20 mg. net price 60-tab pack = £11.18. Label: 2

PRAZOSIN HYDROCHLORIDE

Indications; Cautions; Contra-indications; Side-effects: see notes above and section 2.5.4

Dose: initially 500 micrograms twice daily for 3–7 days, subsequently adjusted according to response; usual maintenance (and max.) 2 mg twice daily; ELDERLY initiate with lowest possible dose

FIRST DOSE EFFECT. First dose may cause collapse due to hypotensive effect (therefore should be taken on retiring to bed). Patient should be warned to lie down if symptoms such as dizziness, fatigue or sweating develop, and to remain lying down until they abate completely

PoM **Hypovase**® **Benign Prostatic Hypertrophy** (Invicta)

Tablets, prazosin hydrochloride 500 micrograms, net price 56-tab pack = £2.09; 1 mg (orange, scored), 56-tab pack = £2.69; 2 mg (scored), 56-tab pack = £3.66; starter pack of 8 × 500-microgram tabs with 32 × 1-mg tabs = £2.52. Label: 3, counselling, see dose above

TAMSULOSIN HYDROCHLORIDE

Indications; Cautions; Contra-indications; Side-effects: see notes above; avoid in severe liver impairment

Dose: 400 micrograms daily after breakfast

FIRST DOSE EFFECT. First dose may cause collapse due to hypotensive effect (therefore should be taken on retiring to bed). Patient should be warned to lie down if symptoms such as dizziness, fatigue or sweating develop, and to remain lying down until they abate completely

▼ PoM **Flomax**® **MR** (Yamanouchi)

Capsules, m/r, tamsulosin hydrochloride 400 micrograms. Net price 30-cap pack = £23.90. Label: 3, 25, counselling, see dose above

TERAZOSIN

Indications; Cautions; Contra-indications; Side-effects: see notes above and section 2.5.4

Dose: initially 1 mg at bedtime; dose may be doubled at weekly intervals according to response, to max. 10 mg once daily; usual maintenance 5–10 mg daily

FIRST DOSE EFFECT. First dose may cause collapse due to hypotensive effect (therefore should be taken on retiring to bed). Patient should be warned to lie down if symptoms such as dizziness, fatigue or sweating develop, and to remain lying down until they abate completely

PoM **Hytrin BPH**® (Abbott)

Tablets, terazosin (as hydrochloride) 2 mg (yellow), net price 28-tab pack = £12.55; 5 mg (tan), 28-tab pack = £18.89; 10 mg (blue), 28-tab pack = £26.59; starter pack of 7 × 1-mg tab with 7 × 2-mg tab = £6.34. Label: 3, counselling, see dose above

ANTI-ANDROGENS

FINASTERIDE

See section 6.4.2

PARASYMPATHOMIMETICS

Parasympathomimetics produce the effects of parasympathetic nerve stimulation; they possess the muscarinic rather than the nicotinic effects of acetylcholine and improve voiding efficiency by increasing detrusor muscle contraction. In the absence of obstruction to the bladder outlet they have a limited role in the relief of urinary retention. Generalised parasympathomimetic side-effects such as sweating, bradycardia, and intestinal colic may occur, particularly in the elderly.

Carbachol and **bethanechol** are choline esters that have been used in postoperative urinary retention. Bethanechol has a more selective action on the bladder than carbachol but the use of both has now been superseded by catheterisation.

Distigmine inhibits the breakdown of acetylcholine. It may help patients with an upper motor neurone neurogenic bladder.

BETHANECHOL CHLORIDE

Indications: urinary retention (but see notes above)

Contra-indications: intestinal or urinary obstruction or where increased muscular activity of urinary or gastro-intestinal tract harmful; asthma, bradycardia, hyperthyroidism, recent myocardial infarction, epilepsy, hypotension, parkinsonism, vagotonia, peptic ulceration, pregnancy; **interactions**: Appendix 1 (parasympathomimetics)

Side-effects: parasympathomimetic effects such as nausea, vomiting, sweating, blurred vision, bradycardia, and intestinal colic

Dose: 10–25 mg 3–4 times daily half an hour before food

PoM **Myotonine**® (Glenwood)

Tablets, both scored, bethanechol chloride 10 mg, net price 20 = 90p; 25 mg, 20 = £1.15. Label: 22

CARBACHOL

Indications: urinary retention, but see notes above

Contra-indications; Side-effects: see under Bethanechol Chloride but side-effects more acute

Dose: by mouth, 2 mg 3 times daily half an hour before food

By subcutaneous injection (acute symptoms, postoperative urinary retention) 250 micrograms, repeated twice if necessary at 30-minute intervals

Note. Inadvertent intravenous administration of carbachol is **extremely hazardous** and calls for emergency treatment with atropine

PoM **Carbachol** (Non-proprietary)

Tablets, carbachol 2 mg. Net price 20 = £2.57. Label: 22

Note. Supplies may be difficult to obtain

Injection, carbachol 250 micrograms/mL

DISTIGMINE BROMIDE

Indications: urinary retention (see notes above) ; myasthenia gravis, see section 10.2.1

Cautions: asthma, bradycardia, hyperthyroidism, recent myocardial infarction, epilepsy, hypotension, parkinsonism, vagotonia, peptic ulceration, pregnancy; **interactions:** Appendix 1 (parasympathomimetics)

Contra-indications: intestinal or urinary obstruction or where increased muscular activity of urinary or gastro-intestinal tract harmful

Side-effects: see under Bethanechol Chloride, but action slower therefore side-effects less acute; see also Neostigmine (section 10.2.1)

Dose: by mouth, 5 mg daily or on alternate days, half an hour before breakfast

By intramuscular injection, 500 micrograms 12 hours after surgery to prevent urinary retention; may be repeated every 24 hours

PoM **Ubretid**® (Rhône-Poulenc Rorer)

Tablets, scored, distigmine bromide 5 mg. Net price 30-tab pack = £21.86. Label: 22

Injection, distigmine bromide 500 micrograms/mL. Net price 1-mL amp = £1.00

7.4.2 Drugs for urinary frequency, enuresis, and incontinence

URINARY INCONTINENCE

Antimuscarinic drugs such as **oxybutynin** and **flavoxate** are used to treat *urinary frequency*; they increase bladder capacity by diminishing unstable detrusor contractions. All these drugs may cause dry mouth and blurred vision and may precipitate glaucoma. Oxybutynin has a high level of side-effects which limits its use; the dosage needs to be carefully assessed, particularly in the elderly. Flavoxate has less marked side-effects but is also less effective. **Propantheline** was formerly widely used in urinary incontinence but had a low response rate with a high incidence of side-effects; it is now primarily indicated in adult enuresis. The **tricyclic antidepressants** imipramine, amitriptyline, and nortriptyline (see section 4.3.1) are sometimes effective in the management of the unstable bladder because of their antimuscarinic properties.

Purified bovine collagen implant (Contigen®, Bard) is indicated for use in the treatment of *urinary incontinence* caused by intrinsic sphincter deficiency (poor or non-functioning bladder outlet mechanism). The implant is injected (with the aid of a cystoscope) in the tissues around the neck of the bladder creating increased tissue bulk so that resistance to urine outflow is achieved. It should only be used by surgeons or physicians familiar with the use of a cystoscope and trained in the technique for injection of the implant.

FLAVOXATE HYDROCHLORIDE

Indications: urinary frequency and incontinence, dysuria, urgency; bladder spasms due to catheterisation

Cautions; Contra-indications: see under Oxybutynin Hydrochloride (antimuscarinic effect considerably less marked)

Side-effects: antimuscarinic side-effects (see Atropine Sulphate, section 1.2); see also notes above

Dose: 200 mg 3 times daily; CHILD under 12 years not recommended

PoM **Urispas**® (Roche)

Tablets, s/c, flavoxate hydrochloride 200 mg, net price 20 = £2.40

OXYBUTYNIN HYDROCHLORIDE

Indications: urinary frequency and incontinence, neurogenic bladder instability and nocturnal enuresis

Cautions: frail elderly; hepatic or renal impairment; hyperthyroidism; cardiac disease where increase in rate undesirable; prostatic hypertrophy; hiatus hernia with reflux oesophagitis; pregnancy and breast-feeding; porphyria (see section 9.8.2); **interactions:** Appendix 1 (antimuscarinics)

Contra-indications: intestinal obstruction or atony, severe ulcerative colitis or toxic megacolon; significant bladder outflow obstruction; glaucoma

Side-effects: include dry mouth, constipation, blurred vision, nausea, abdominal discomfort, facial flushing (more marked in children), difficulty in micturition (less commonly urinary retention); also headache, dizziness, drowsiness, dry skin, diarrhoea, arrhythmia; see also notes above

Dose: 5 mg 2–3 times daily increased if necessary to max. 5 mg 4 times daily

ELDERLY 2.5–3 mg twice daily initially, increased to 5 mg twice daily according to response and tolerance

CHILD over 5 years, neurogenic bladder instability, 2.5–3 mg twice daily increased to 5 mg twice daily (max. 5 mg 3 times daily); nocturnal enuresis (preferably over 7 years, see notes below), 2.5–3 mg twice daily increased to 5 mg 2–3 times daily (last dose before bedtime)

PoM **Cystrin**® (Pharmacia)

Tablets, oxybutynin hydrochloride 3 mg, net price 100-tab pack = £16.34; 5 mg (scored), 100-tab pack = £27.24. Label: 3

The 5 mg strength is also available from Pharmacia as a non-proprietary

PoM **Ditropan**® (S&N Hlth.)

Tablets, both blue, scored, oxybutynin hydrochloride 2.5 mg, net price 84-tab pack = £11.74; 5 mg, 84-tab pack = £22.88. Label: 3

Elixir, oxybutynin hydrochloride 2.5 mg/5 mL. Net price 150-mL pack = £4.78. Label: 3.

PROPANTHELINE BROMIDE

Indications: adult enuresis, see notes above

Cautions; Contra-indications: see under Oxybutynin Hydrochloride

Side-effects: antimuscarinic side-effects (see Atropine Sulphate, section 1.2); see also notes above

Dose: 15–30 mg 2–3 times daily one hour before meals

Preparations

See section 1.2

NOCTURNAL ENURESIS

Nocturnal enuresis is a normal occurrence in young children but persists in as many as 5% by 10 years of age. In the absence of urinary-tract infection simple measures such as *bladder training* or the use of an *alarm system* may be successful. Drug therapy is not appropriate for children under 7 years of age and should be reserved for when alternative measures have failed preferably on a short-term basis to cover periods away from home. The possible side-effects and the **toxicity** of these drugs if taken in **overdose** should be borne in mind when they are prescribed.

Desmopressin (see section 6.5.2), an analogue of vasopressin, is used for nocturnal enuresis; particular care is needed to avoid fluid overload and treatment should not be continued for longer than 3 months without stopping for a week for full re-assessment.

Tricyclics (see section 4.3.1) such as **amitriptyline**, **imipramine**, and less often **nortriptyline** are also used but behaviour disturbances may occur and relapse is common after withdrawal. Treatment should not normally exceed 3 months unless a full physical examination (including ECG) is given and the child is fully re-assessed.

7.4.3   Drugs used in urological pain

The acute pain of *ureteric colic* may be relieved with **pethidine** (section 4.7.2); **diclofenac** (section 10.1.1) is also effective and compares favourably with pethidine.

Lignocaine gel is a useful topical application in *urethral pain* or to relieve the discomfort of catheterisation (see section 15.2).

ALKALINISATION OF URINE

Alkalinisation of urine may be undertaken with **sodium bicarbonate**, or alternatively with potassium citrate. The alkalinising action may relieve the discomfort of *cystitis* caused by lower urinary tract infections. Sodium bicarbonate, in particular, is also used as a urinary alkalinising agent in some metabolic and renal disorders (see section 9.2.1.3).

POTASSIUM CITRATE

Indications: relief of discomfort in mild urinary-tract infections; alkalinisation of urine

Cautions: renal impairment, cardiac disease; elderly; **interactions:** Appendix 1 (potassium salts)

Side-effects: hyperkalaemia on prolonged high dosage, mild diuresis

Potassium Citrate Mixture (BP)

(Potassium Citrate Oral Solution)

Oral solution, potassium citrate 30%, citric acid monohydrate 5% in a suitable vehicle with a lemon flavour. Extemporaneous preparations should be recently prepared according to the following formula: potassium citrate 3 g, citric acid monohydrate 500 mg, syrup 2.5 mL, quillaia tincture 0.1 mL, lemon spirit 0.05 mL, double-strength chloroform water 3 mL, water to 10 mL. Contains about 28 mmol K^+/10 mL. Label: 27

Dose: 10 mL 3 times daily well diluted with water

Note. Concentrates for preparation of Potassium Citrate Mixture BP are available from Hillcross

Proprietary brands of potassium citrate on sale to the public for the relief of discomfort in mild urinary-tract infections include Cystopurin® (Roche Consumer Health) and Effercitrate® (Typharm)

SODIUM BICARBONATE

Indications: relief of discomfort in mild urinary-tract infections; alkalinisation of urine

Cautions; Side-effects: see section 1.1.2; also caution in elderly

Dose: 3 g in water every 2 hours until urinary pH exceeds 7; maintenance of alkaline urine 5–10 g daily

Sodium Bicarbonate Powder. Label: 13

SODIUM CITRATE

Indications: relief of discomfort in mild urinary-tract infections

Cautions: renal impairment, cardiac disease, pregnancy, patients on a sodium-restricted diet; elderly

Side-effects: mild diuresis

Note. Proprietary brands of Sodium Citrate on sale to the public for the relief of discomfort in mild urinary-tract infections include Cymalon® (Sterling Health), Cystemme® (Abbott), and Cystoleve® (Cupal)

ACIDIFICATION OF URINE

Acidification of urine has been undertaken with **ascorbic acid** but it is not always reliable. Large doses may cause gastro-intestinal disturbances including diarrhoea; renal stones have also been reported in patients with hyperoxaluria.

For pH-modifying solutions for the maintenance of indwelling urinary catheters, see section 7.4.4.

ASCORBIC ACID

Indications: acidification of urine but see notes above

Dose: by mouth, 4 g daily in divided doses

Preparations

See section 9.6.3

OTHER PREPARATIONS FOR URINARY DISORDERS

A terpene mixture (Rowatinex®) is claimed to be of benefit in *urolithiasis* for the expulsion of calculi.

Rowatinex® (Monmouth)

Capsules, yellow, e/c, anethol 4 mg, borneol 10 mg, camphene 15 mg, cineole 3 mg, fenchone 4 mg, pinene 31 mg. Net price 50 = £7.35. Label: 25

Dose: 1–2 capsules 3–4 times daily before food; CHILD not recommended

7.4.4   Bladder instillations and urological surgery

INFECTED BLADDERS. Various solutions are available as irrigations or washouts.

Aqueous **chlorhexidine** (see section 13.11.2) may be used in the management of common infections of the bladder but it is ineffective against most *Pseudomonas* spp. Solutions containing 1 in 5000 (0.02%) are used but they may irritate the mucosa and cause burning and haematuria (in which case they should be discontinued); sterile **sodium chloride solution 0.9%** (physiological saline) is usually adequate and is preferred as a mechanical irrigant.

Bladder irrigations of **amphotericin** 100 micrograms/mL (see section 5.2) may be of value in mycotic infections.

DISSOLUTION OF BLOOD CLOTS. Clot retention is usually treated by irrigation with sterile **sodium chloride solution 0.9%** but sterile **sodium citrate solution for bladder irrigation 3%** may also be helpful. **Streptokinase-streptodornase** (Varidase Topical®, see section 13.11.7) is an alternative.

LOCALLY ACTING CYTOTOXIC DRUGS. **Doxorubicin** (see section 8.1.2) is used for recurrent superficial bladder tumours, and some papillary tumours. A solution (50 mg in 50 mL of sterile sodium chloride solution 0.9%) is instilled monthly. Although systemic side-effects are few, it may cause frequency, urgency, dysuria, and occasionally reduction in bladder capacity.

Epirubicin (see section 8.1.2) is used for papillary tumours. A solution (50 mg in 50 mL of sterile water or sodium chloride solution 0.9%) is instilled weekly for 8 weeks (for prophylaxis, weekly for 4 weeks then monthly for 11 months).

Mitomycin (see section 8.1.2) is used for recurrent superficial bladder tumours. A solution (10 to 40 mg in 20 to 40 mL of sterile water) is instilled weekly or three times weekly for a total of 20 doses.

Thiotepa (see section 8.1.1) is used for recurrent superficial bladder tumours. A solution (15 to 60 mg in 60 mL of sterile water) is instilled weekly for 4 weeks then after a break of 2 weeks, at intervals of 1 to 2 weeks for a further 4 doses. The concentration should be reduced if there is evidence of bone-marrow suppression.

INTERSTITIAL CYSTITIS. **Dimethyl sulphoxide** may be used for symptomatic relief in patients with interstitial cystitis (Hunner's ulcer). 50 mL of a 50% solution (Rimso-50®) is instilled into the bladder, retained for 15 minutes, and voided by the patient. Treatment is repeated at intervals of 2 weeks. Bladder spasm and hypersensitivity reactions may occur and long-term use requires ophthalmic, renal, and hepatic assessment at intervals of 6 months.

CHLORHEXIDINE

Indications: bladder washouts, see notes above and section 13.11.2

DIMETHYL SULPHOXIDE

Indications: bladder washouts, see notes above

PoM **Rimso-50®** (Britannia)

Bladder instillation, sterile, dimethyl sulphoxide 50%, in aqueous solution. Net price 50 mL = £19.31

SODIUM CHLORIDE

Indications: bladder washouts, see notes above

Available from Baxter, Kendall

SODIUM CITRATE

Indications: bladder washouts, see notes above

Sterile Sodium Citrate Solution for Bladder Irrigation, sodium citrate 3%, dilute hydrochloric acid 0.2%, in purified water, freshly boiled and cooled, and sterilised

UROLOGICAL SURGERY

Endoscopic surgery within the urinary tract requires an isotonic irrigant as there is a high risk of fluid absorption; if this occurs in excess, hypervolaemia, haemolysis, and renal failure may result. **Glycine irrigation solution 1.5%** is the irrigant of choice for transurethral resection of the prostate gland and bladder tumours; **sterile sodium chloride solution 0.9%** (physiological saline) is used for percutaneous renal surgery.

GLYCINE

Indications: bladder irrigation during urological surgery; see notes above
Cautions; Side-effects: see notes above

Glycine Irrigation Solution (Non-proprietary)
Irrigation solution, glycine 1.5% in water for injections
Available from Baxter, Kendall

MAINTENANCE OF INDWELLING URINARY CATHETERS

The deposition which occurs in catheterised patients is usually chiefly composed of phosphate and to minimise this the catheter (if latex) should be changed at least as often as every 6 weeks. If the catheter is to be left for longer periods a silicone catheter should be used together with the appropriate use of catheter maintenance solutions. Repeated blockage usually indicates that the catheter needs to be changed.

CATHETER PATENCY SOLUTIONS

Chlorhexidine 0.02%. Available from CliniFlex (Uro-Tainer Chlorhexidine®, 100-mL sachet = £2.41), Galen (Uriflex C®, 100-mL sachet = £2.03)
Mandelic acid 1% Available from CliniFlex (Uro-Tainer Mandelic Acid®, 100-mL sachet = £2.41)
Sodium chloride 0.9%. Available from CliniFlex (Uro-Tainer Sodium Chloride®, 100-mL sachet = £2.29, Uro-Tainer M®, with integral drug additive port, 50- and 100-mL sachets = £2.71), Galen (Uriflex S®, 100-mL sachet = £1.91, Uriflex SP® with integral drug additive port, 100-mL sachet = £1.96)
Solution G, citric acid 3.23%, magnesium oxide 0.38%, sodium bicarbonate 0.7%, disodium edetate 0.01%. Available from CliniFlex (Uro-Tainer Suby G®, 100-mL sachet = £2.41), Galen (Uriflex G®, 100-mL sachet = £2.03)
Solution R, citric acid 6%, gluconolactone 0.6%, magnesium carbonate 2.8%, disodium edetate 0.01%. Available from CliniFlex (Uro-Tainer Solution R®, 100-mL sachet = £2.41), Galen (Uriflex R®, 100-mL sachet = £2.03)

7.4.5 Drugs for impotence

Reasons for failure to produce a satisfactory erection include *psychogenic, vascular, neurogenic,* and *endocrine abnormalities; many drugs* are also liable to induce impotence. Intracavernosal injection of vasoactive drugs under careful medical supervision is used for both diagnostic and therapeutic purposes.

ALPROSTADIL

Alprostadil (prostaglandin E_1) is given by intracavernosal injection for the management of erectile dysfunction (after exclusion of treatable medical causes); it is also used as a diagnostic test.

ALPROSTADIL

Indications: erectile dysfunction (including aid to diagnosis); neonatal congenital heart defects, see section 7.1.1.1
Cautions: prolonged erection (priapism)—patients should be instructed to report any erection lasting 4 hours or longer; treatment of prolonged erection should not be delayed more than 6 hours—for recommendations, see below; anatomical deformations of penis (painful erection more likely)—follow up regularly to detect signs of penile fibrosis (discontinue if angulation, cavernosal fibrosis or Peyronie's disease develop)
Contra-indications: predisposition to prolonged erection (as in sickle cell anaemia, multiple myeloma or leukaemia), anatomical deformity (angulation, cavernosal fibrosis or Peyronie's disease); not for use with other agents for erectile dysfunction or when sexual activity medically inadvisable
Side-effects: penile pain, prolonged erection (see below and under Cautions); reactions at injection site include haematoma; ecchymosis, penile rash, penile oedema, penile fibrosis, haemorrhage, inflammation, itching, swelling; other local reactions include balanitis, urethral bleeding, penile warmth, numbness, yeast infection, irritation, sensitivity, phimosis, pruritus, erythema, venous leak, painful erection and abnormal ejaculation; systemic effects reported include testicular pain, testicular swelling, scrotal erythema, pain or tightness, changes in micturition, hypotension or hypertension, vasodilatation, supraventricular extrasystole, peripheral vascular disorder, dizziness, buttock weakness, localised pain (buttocks, legs, genital, abdominal), headache, pelvic pain, back pain, influenza-like syndrome
PRIAPISM. If priapism should occur treatment should not be delayed more than 6 hours and is as follows:
Initial therapy by penile aspiration—using aseptic technique a 19–21 gauge butterfly needle inserted into the corpus cavernosum and 20–50 mL of blood aspirated; if necessary the procedure may be repeated on the opposite side.
If aspiration unsuccessful, *cautious* intracavernosal injection of a sympathomimetic with action on alpha-adrenergic receptors, continuously monitoring blood pressure and pulse (*extreme caution:* coronary heart disease, hypertension, cerebral ischaemia or if taking antidepressant) as follows:

—intracavernosal injections of phenylephrine 100–200 micrograms (0.5–1 mL of a 200 microgram/mL solution) every 5–10 minutes; max. total dose 1 mg [unlicensed indication][*important:* if suitable strength of phenylephrine injection not available may be specially prepared by diluting 0.1 mL of the phenylephrine 1% (10 mg/mL) injection to 5 mL with sodium chloride 0.9%];
alternatively
—intracavernosal injections of adrenaline 10–20 micrograms (0.5–1mL of a 20 microgram/mL solution) every 5–10 minutes; max. total dose 100 micrograms [*important:* if suitable strength of adrenaline not available may be specially prepared by diluting 0.1 mL of the adrenaline 1 in 1000 (1mg/mL) injection to 5 mL with sodium chloride 0.9%];
alternatively
—intracavernosal injection of metaraminol (*caution: has been associated with fatal hypertensive crises*) [see notes below for a suggested dilution and dose];
If necessary the sympathomimetic injections can be followed by further aspiration of blood through the same butterfly needle.
If sympathomimetics unsuccessful, urgent surgical referral for management (possibly including shunt procedure).

Dose: *by direct intracavernosal injection,* erectile dysfunction, first dose 2.5 micrograms, second dose 5 micrograms (if some response to first dose) *or* 7.5 micrograms (if no response to first dose), increasing in steps of 5–10 micrograms to obtain dose suitable for producing erection not lasting more than 1 hour (neurological dysfunction, first dose 1.25 micrograms, second dose 2.5 micrograms, third dose 5 micrograms, increasing in steps of 5 micrograms to obtain suitable dose); usual range 10–20 micrograms; max. 60 micrograms (max. frequency of injection not more than once in any 1 day and not more than 3 times in any 1 week)
Note. The first dose must be given by medically trained personnel; self administration may only be undertaken after proper training
Aid to diagnosis, 20 micrograms as a single dose (where evidence of neurological dysfunction, initially 5 micrograms and max. 10 micrograms)—consult data sheet for details

▼ PoM **Caverject®** (Upjohn)
Injection, powder for reconstitution, alprostadil. Net price 10-microgram vial = £7.70; 20-microgram vial (with diluent-filled syringe) = £9.95

PAPAVERINE and PHENTOLAMINE

Although not licensed the smooth muscle relaxant **papaverine** is also given by intracavernosal injection for impotence. The usual dose of papaverine by intracavernosal injection is 7.5 mg initially increased according to response to a range of 30–60 mg. Patients with neurological or psychogenic impotence are more sensitive to the effect of papaverine than those with vascular abnormalities. **Phentolamine** (0.25–1.25 mg) is added if the response is inadequate [unlicensed indication].

Persistence of the erection for longer than 4 hours is an emergency requiring aspiration of the corpora; if aspiration fails, 1 mg of metaraminol [0.1 mL of 10 mg/mL metaraminol injection] can be diluted to 5 mL with sodium choride injection 0.9% and given by careful slow injection into the corpora [unlicensed indication] [*caution:* has been associated with fatal hypertensive crisis—consider also advice under Alprostadil, above].

Other side-effects include vasovagal attacks and syncope; caution is needed in patients with cardiovascular disease and ischaemic attacks; predisposition to prolonged erection is a contra-indication.

Local side-effects include haematoma and burning pain at the site of injection and fibrotic changes in the corpora cavernosa (which may lead to Peyronie-like erectile distortion).

PAPAVERINE
Indications; Cautions; Side-effects: see notes above
Note. Papaverine is available as a 'special order' [unlicensed] product, contact BCM Specials, Martindale, or regional hospital manufacturing unit

PHENTOLAMINE
Indications; Cautions; Side-effects: see notes above; phaeochromocytoma, see section 2.5.4
Note. Phentolamine is not licensed for use in erectile dysfunction

7.5   Appliances for urinary disorders

For details of **appliances for urinary disorders**, see Appendix 8.

8: Drugs used in the treatment of
MALIGNANT DISEASE and for IMMUNOSUPPRESSION

In this chapter, drug treatment is discussed under the following headings:

8.1 Cytotoxic drugs
8.2 Drugs affecting the immune response
8.3 Sex hormones and hormone antagonists in malignant disease

Malignant disease may be treated by surgery, radiotherapy, and chemotherapy. Certain tumours are highly sensitive to chemotherapy but many are not, and inappropriate drug administration in these circumstances can only increase morbidity or mortality.

8.1 Cytotoxic drugs

8.1.1 Alkylating drugs
8.1.2 Cytotoxic antibiotics
8.1.3 Antimetabolites
8.1.4 Vinca alkaloids and etoposide
8.1.5 Other antineoplastic drugs

The chemotherapy of cancer is complex and should be confined to specialists in oncology. Cytotoxic drugs have both anti-cancer activity and the potential for damage to normal tissue. Chemotherapy may be given with a curative intent or it may aim to prolong life or to palliate symptoms. In an increasing number of cases chemotherapy may be combined with radiotherapy or surgery or both as either neoadjuvant treatment (initial chemotherapy aimed at shrinking the primary tumour, thereby rendering local therapy less destructive or more effective) or as adjuvant treatment (which follows definitive treatment of the primary disease, when the risk of sub-clinical metastatic disease is known to be high). All chemotherapy drugs cause side-effects and a balance has to be struck between likely benefit and acceptable toxicity.

CRM guidelines on cytotoxic drug handling:

1. Trained personnel should reconstitute cytotoxics;

2. Reconstitution should be carried out in designated areas;

3. Protective clothing (including gloves) should be worn;

4. The eyes should be protected and means of first aid should be specified;

5. Pregnant staff should not handle cytotoxics;

6. Adequate care should be taken in the disposal of waste material, including syringes, containers, and absorbent material.

Cytotoxic drugs may be used either singly, or in combination. In the latter case, the initial letters of the approved or proprietary names of the drugs, identify the regimen used. Drug combinations are frequently more toxic than single drugs but may have the advantage in certain tumours of enhanced response and increased survival. However for some tumours, single-agent chemotherapy remains the treatment of choice.

> Most cytotoxic drugs are teratogenic, and all may cause life-threatening toxicity; administration should, where possible, be confined to those experienced in their use.
>
> Because of the complexity of dosage regimens in the treatment of malignant disease, dose statements have been omitted from some of the drug entries in this chapter. *In all cases detailed specialist literature should be consulted.*
>
> Prescriptions should **not** be repeated except on the instructions of a specialist.

Cytotoxic drugs fall naturally into a number of classes, each with characteristic antitumour activity, sites of action, and toxicity. A knowledge of sites of metabolism and excretion is important because impaired drug handling as a result of disease is not uncommon and may result in enhanced toxic effects. A number of side-effects are characteristic of particular agents or groups of drugs, e.g. neurotoxicity of vinca alkaloids, and details will be provided in the appropriate sections. Most toxic effects are, however, common to many of these drugs and will be briefly outlined here.

EXTRAVASATION OF INTRAVENOUS DRUGS. A number of drugs will cause severe local tissue necrosis if leakage into the extravascular compartment occurs. Recommended modes of administration must be adhered to. Infusion of vesicant drugs should be stopped immediately if local pain is experienced. Where doubt exists as to whether significant leakage has occurred, the infusion should be discontinued and the cannula resited in another vein. There are no proven antidotes for extravasation, but general recommendations include elevation of the limb and application of ice packs three or four times daily until pain and swelling settle; if ulceration occurs plastic surgery may be required.

HYPERURICAEMIA. Hyperuricaemia, which can result in uric acid crystal formation in the urinary tract with associated renal dysfunction is a complication of the treatment of non-Hodgkin's lymphoma and leukaemia. Allopurinol (see section 10.1.4) should be started 24 hours before treating such tumours, and should be continued for 7 to 10 days (it is not required again unless further therapy is given for tumour relapse); patients should be adequately hydrated. The dose of mercaptopurine or azathioprine should be reduced if allopurinol needs to be given concomitantly (see Appendix 1).

NAUSEA AND VOMITING. Nausea and vomiting are a source of considerable distress to many patients receiving chemotherapy. It should be anticipated and, where possible, prevented with anti-emetic treatment tailored to the chemotherapy regimen and the response of the patient.

If first-line anti-emetics are ineffective treatment should be escalated as below. Hospital admission may be necessary.

Group 1: severe emesis unlikely
Drugs in this group include alkylating drugs by mouth, intravenous fluorouracil, vinca alkaloids, and methotrexate given as single therapy; they cause little emesis.

Phenothiazines (e.g. prochlorperazine) or domperidone, given by mouth, when necessary, will often suffice. Premedication with these drugs is often useful before intravenous chemotherapy, treatment being continued for up to 24 hours afterwards. Both prochlorperazine and domperidone are also available as suppositories which is useful for patients who develop vomiting despite oral therapy.

Group 2: moderate emesis
Drugs in this group include intravenous cyclophosphamide and doxorubicin; premedication is essential for all drugs in this group. Most patients can be treated on an out-patient basis therefore, if possible, the anti-emetics should be given by mouth.

Anti-emetics in group 1 are given when necessary but it is usually preferable to also give dexamethasone 6–10 mg by mouth before chemotherapy. Additional treatment with a specific ($5HT_3$) serotonin antagonist (e.g. ondansetron 8 mg by mouth or intravenously) is often necessary. If emesis remains a problem, lorazepam 1–2 mg by mouth may be helpful; it has the advantage of causing drowsiness and amnesia, but patients cannot drive after it. Nabilone is little used and may cause dysphoria.

Patients in group 1 with an unsatisfactory response can be transferred to drugs in this group.

Group 3: severe emesis
Drugs in this group include mustine, dacarbazine, and cisplatin. They commonly cause severe emesis, particularly if used in combination.

The specific ($5HT_3$) serotonin antagonists (i.e. granisetron, ondansetron, tropisetron) are perhaps the most effective drugs for controlling early emesis associated with drugs in this group, but are relatively ineffective at controlling late (after 24 hours) emesis. Intravenous administration of a single dose, usually with dexamethasone, is widely used for patients in this group together with other anti-emetics (e.g. lorazepam, domperidone) as required.

Intravenous high-dose metoclopramide (see section 4.6) has now been largely replaced by the $5HT_3$ antagonists.

Patients in group 2 with an unsatisfactory response can be transferred to drugs in this group.

BONE-MARROW SUPPRESSION. All cytotoxic drugs except vincristine and bleomycin cause marrow depression. This commonly occurs 7 to 10 days after administration, but is delayed for certain drugs, such as carmustine, lomustine, and melphalan. Peripheral blood counts must be checked prior to each treatment, and doses should be reduced or therapy delayed if marrow recovery has not occurred. Fever occurring in a neutropenic patient (neutrophil count less than 0.8×10^9/litre) is an indication for immediate parenteral broad-spectrum antibiotic therapy (see section 5.1, table 1), once appropriate bacteriological investigations have taken place.

It is now possible, in selected patients, to lessen both the duration and the depth of neutropenia by the use of parenterally administered bone marrow growth factors known as colony stimulating factors (see section 9.1.6) or (in patients with ovarian carcinoma receiving cisplatin and cyclophosphamide) by the use of amifostine (section 9.1.6); these tend to be used on an individual basis.

IMPAIRED IMMUNE RESPONSIVENESS. Modification of tissue reactions caused by corticosteroids and other immunosuppressive drugs may result in the rapid *spread of infection*. Suppression of clinical signs may allow diseases such as septicaemia or tuberculosis to reach an advanced stage before being recognised—**important:** for advice relating to measles and chickenpox (varicella) exposure, see p. 515 (measles) and p. 516 (varicella).

ALOPECIA. Reversible hair loss is a common complication, although it varies in degree between drugs and individual patients. No pharmacological methods of preventing this are available.

REPRODUCTIVE FUNCTION. Most cytotoxic drugs are teratogenic and should not be administered during pregnancy, especially during the first trimester (but for transplant therapy, see below).

Contraceptive advice should be offered where appropriate before cytotoxic therapy begins (and should cover the duration of contraception required after therapy has ended). Regimens that do not contain an alkylating drug may have less effect on fertility, but those with an alkylating drug carry the risk of causing permanent male sterility (there is no effect on potency). Pre-treatment counselling and consideration of sperm storage may be appropriate. Females are less severely affected, though the span of reproductive life may be shortened by the onset of a premature menopause. No increase in fetal abnormalities or abortion-rate has been recorded in patients who remain fertile after cytotoxic chemotherapy.

Transplant therapy. Female transplanted patients immunosuppressed with azathioprine should not discontinue it on becoming pregnant; there is no evidence that azathioprine used properly is teratogenic. There is less experience of cyclosporin in pregnancy but it does not appear to be any more harmful than azathioprine. Any risk to the offspring of azathioprine-treated men is small. Tacrolimus and mycophenolate mofetil have been introduced recently and are contra-indicated by the manufacturers in pregnancy.

8.1.1 Alkylating drugs

Extensive experience is available with these drugs, which are among the most widely used in cancer chemotherapy. They act by damaging DNA, thus interfering with cell replication. In addition to the side-effects common to many cytotoxic drugs (section 8.1), there are two problems associated with prolonged usage. Firstly, gametogenesis is often severely affected (see above). Secondly, prolonged use of these drugs, particularly when combined with extensive irradiation, is associated with a marked increase in the incidence of acute non-lymphocytic leukaemia.

Cyclophosphamide is widely used in the treatment of chronic lymphocytic leukaemia, the lymphomas, and solid tumours. It is given *by mouth* or *intravenously* and is inactive until metabolised by the liver. A urinary metabolite of cyclophosphamide, acrolein, may cause haemorrhagic cystitis; this is a rare but very serious complication; if it occurs cyclophosphamide is not normally used again. An increased fluid intake, for 24–48 hours after intravenous injection, will help avoid this complication. When high-dose therapy (e.g. more than 2 g intravenously) is used or when the patient is considered to be at high risk of cystitis (e.g. previous pelvic irradiation) mesna (given initially intravenously then by mouth) will also help prevent this.

Ifosfamide is related to cyclophosphamide and is given *intravenously*; it is *routinely* given with mesna to reduce urothelial toxicity.

Chlorambucil is commonly used to treat chronic lymphocytic leukaemia, the indolent non-Hodgkin's lymphomas, Hodgkin's disease, and ovarian cancer. It is given *by mouth*. Side-effects, apart from marrow suppression, are uncommon. However occasional patients develop severe widespread rashes which can progress to Stevens-Johnson syndrome or to toxic epidermal necrolysis. If a rash occurs further chlorambucil is contra-indicated and cyclophosphamide is substituted.

Melphalan is used to treat myeloma and occasionally solid tumours and lymphomas. It is usually given *by mouth*, but may also be given *intravenously*. Marrow toxicity is delayed and it is usually given at intervals of 4–6 weeks.

Busulphan is used almost exclusively to treat chronic myeloid leukaemia and is given *by mouth*. Frequent blood counts are necessary as excessive myelosuppression may result in irreversible bone-marrow aplasia. Hyperpigmentation of the skin is a common side-effect and, rarely, progressive pulmonary fibrosis may occur.

Lomustine is a lipid-soluble nitrosourea and is given *by mouth*. It is mainly used to treat Hodgkin's disease and certain solid tumours. Marrow toxicity is delayed, and the drug is therefore given at intervals of 4 to 6 weeks. Permanent marrow damage

may occur with prolonged use. Nausea and vomiting are common and moderately severe.

Carmustine is given *intravenously*. It has similar activity and toxicities to lomustine and is most commonly given to patients with myeloma, lymphoma, and brain tumours. Cumulative renal damage and delayed pulmonary fibrosis may occur.

Mustine is now much less commonly used. It is a very toxic drug which causes severe vomiting. The freshly prepared injection must be given into a fast-running *intravenous infusion*. Local extravasation causes severe tissue necrosis.

Estramustine is a combination of an oestrogen and mustine used predominantly in prostate cancer. It is given *by mouth* and has both an antimitotic effect and (by reducing testosterone concentrations) a hormonal effect.

Treosulfan is given *by mouth* or *intravenously* and is used to treat ovarian cancer.

Thiotepa is usually used as an *intracavitary* drug for the treatment of malignant effusions or bladder cancer (see section 7.4.4). It is also occasionally used to treat breast cancer, but requires parenteral administration.

Mitobronitol is occasionally used to treat chronic myeloid leukaemia; it is available on a named-patient basis only (as *Myelobromol®*, Sinclair).

BUSULPHAN

Indications: chronic myeloid leukaemia

Cautions; Side-effects: see section 8.1 and notes above; avoid in porphyria (see section 9.8.2)

Dose: induction of remission, 60 micrograms/kg to max. 4 mg daily; maintenance, 0.5–2 mg daily

PoM Myleran® (Wellcome)

Tablets, busulphan 500 micrograms, net price 25 = £3.53; 2 mg, 25 = £5.32

CARMUSTINE

Indications: see notes above

Cautions; Side-effects: see section 8.1 and notes above; irritant to tissues

PoM BiCNU® (Bristol-Myers)

Injection, powder for reconstitution, carmustine. Net price 100-mg vial (with diluent) = £12.50

CHLORAMBUCIL

Indications: see notes above (for use as an immunosuppressant see section 8.2.1)

Cautions; Side-effects: see section 8.1 and notes above; caution in renal impairment; avoid in porphyria (see section 9.8.2)

Dose: used alone, usually 100–200 micrograms/kg daily for 4–8 weeks

PoM Leukeran® (Wellcome)

Tablets, both yellow, chlorambucil 2 mg, net price 25 = £8.55; 5 mg, 25 = £13.04

CYCLOPHOSPHAMIDE

Indications: see notes above
Cautions; Side-effects: see section 8.1 and notes above; reduce dose in renal impairment; avoid in porphyria (see section 9.8.2); **interactions:** Appendix 1 (cyclophosphamide)

PoM **Cyclophosphamide** (Pharmacia)
Tablets, pink, s/c, cyclophosphamide (anhydrous) 50 mg. Net price 20 = £2.12. Label: 27
Injection, powder for reconstitution, cyclophosphamide. Net price 100-mg vial = £1.06; 200-mg vial = £1.50; 500-mg vial = £2.62; 1-g vial = £4.58
PoM **Endoxana**® (ASTA Medica)
Tablets, s/c, cyclophosphamide 50 mg, net price 100-tab pack = £10.50 Label: 27
Injection, powder for reconstitution, cyclophosphamide. Net price 100-mg vial = £1.04; 200-mg vial = £1.49; 500-mg vial = £2.61; 1-g vial = £4.54

ESTRAMUSTINE PHOSPHATE

Indications: prostate cancer
Cautions: see section 8.1
Contra-indications: peptic ulceration, severe liver or cardiac disease
Side-effects: see section 8.1; also gynaecomastia, altered liver function, cardiovascular disorders (angina and rare reports of myocardial infarction)
Dose: 0.14–1.4 g daily in divided doses (usual initial dose 560 mg daily)
COUNSELLING. Each dose should be taken not less than 1 hour before or 2 hours after meals and should not be taken with dairy products

PoM **Estracyt**® (Pharmacia)
Capsules, estramustine phosphate 140 mg (as disodium salt). Net price 100-cap pack = £149.46. Label: 23 counselling, see above

IFOSFAMIDE

Indications: see notes above
Cautions; Side-effects: see section 8.1 and notes under Cyclophosphamide; reduce dose in renal impairment; **interactions:** Appendix 1 (cyclophosphamide and ifosfamide)

PoM **Mitoxana**® (ASTA Medica)
Injection, powder for reconstitution, ifosfamide. Net price 1-g vial = £19.15; 2-g vial = £35.38 (hosp. only)

LOMUSTINE

Indications: see notes above
Cautions; Side-effects: see section 8.1 and notes above
Dose: used alone, 120–130 mg/m² body-surface every 6–8 weeks

PoM **CCNU**® (Lundbeck)
Capsules, lomustine 10 mg (blue/white), net price 20 = £9.42; 40 mg (blue), 20 = £23.69

MELPHALAN

Indications: myelomatosis; see also notes above
Cautions; Side-effects: see section 8.1 and notes above; reduce dose in renal impairment; **interactions:** Appendix 1 (melphalan)
*Dose: by mouth,*150–300 micrograms/kg daily for 4–6 days, repeated after 4–8 weeks

PoM **Alkeran**® (Wellcome)
Tablets, melphalan 2 mg, net price 25 = £11.73; 5 mg, 25 = £20.75
Injection, powder for reconstitution, melphalan 50 mg (as hydrochloride). Net price 50-mg vial (with solvent-diluent) = £28.26

MUSTINE HYDROCHLORIDE

(Chlormethine Hydrochloride)
Indications: Hodgkin's disease—see notes above
Cautions; Side-effects: see section 8.1 and notes above; irritant to tissues (also caution in handling—vesicant and a nasal irritant)

PoM **Mustine Hydrochloride** (Knoll)
Injection, powder for reconstitution, mustine hydrochloride. Net price 10-mg vial = £15.00

THIOTEPA

Indications: see notes above and section 7.4.4
Cautions; Side-effects: see section 8.1; **interactions:** Appendix 1 (thiotepa)

PoM **Thiotepa** (Lederle)
Injection, powder for reconstitution, thiotepa, net price 15-mg vial = £4.73

TREOSULFAN

Indications: see notes above
Cautions; Side-effects: see section 8.1
Dose: by mouth, courses of 1–2 g daily in 4 divided doses to provide total dose of 21–28 g over initial 8 weeks

PoM **Treosulfan** (Medac)
Capsules, treosulfan 250 mg. Net price 20 = £25.40. Label: 25
Also Available from Farillon
Injection, powder for reconstitution, treosulfan. Net price 1 g = £15.20; 5 g = £59.60 (both in infusion bottle with transfer needle)
Also available from Farillon

UROTHELIAL TOXICITY

Urothelial toxicity, commonly manifest by haemorrhagic cystitis, is a problem peculiar to the use of cyclophosphamide or ifosfamide and is caused by a metabolite (acrolein). **Mesna** reacts specifically with this metabolite in the urinary tract, preventing toxicity. Mesna is used routinely (preferably by mouth) in patients receiving ifosfamide, and in patients receiving cyclophosphamide by the intravenous route at a high dose (e.g. more than 2 g) or in patients with previous urothelial toxicity from cyclophosphamide.

MESNA

Indications: see notes above

Contra-indications: hypersensitivity to thiol-containing compounds

Side-effects: above max. therapeutic doses, nausea, vomiting (use intravenous route), colic, diarrhoea, fatigue, headache, limb and joint pains, depression, irritability, lack of energy, rash, hypotension and tachycardia; rarely hypersensitivity reactions (more common in patients with autoimmune disorders)

Dose: calculated according to oxazaphosphorine (cyclophosphamide or ifosfamide) treatment—for details see data sheet; when given *by mouth*, dose is given 2 hours *before* oxazaphosphorine treatment and repeated 2 and 6 hours *after* treatment; when given *by intravenous injection*, dose is given *with* oxazaphosphorine treatment and repeated 4 and 8 hours *after* treatment

PoM Uromitexan® (ASTA Medica)

Tablets, f/c, mesna 400 mg, net price 10-tab pack = £18.25; 600 mg, 10-tab pack = £23.70

Injection, mesna 100 mg/mL. Net price 4-mL amp = £1.69; 10-mL amp = £3.79

Note. For oral administration contents of ampoule are taken in a flavoured drink such as orange juice or cola which may be stored in a refrigerator for up to 24 hours in a sealed container

8.1.2   Cytotoxic antibiotics

Drugs within this group are widely used. Many cytotoxic antibiotics act as radiomimetics and simultaneous use of radiotherapy should be **avoided** as it may result in markedly enhanced normal tissue toxicity.

Doxorubicin is one of the most successful and widely used antitumour drugs, and is used to treat the acute leukaemias, lymphomas, and a variety of solid tumours. It is given by fast running *infusion*, commonly at 21-day intervals. Local extravasation will cause severe tissue necrosis. Common toxic effects include nausea and vomiting, myelosuppression, alopecia, and mucositis. This drug is largely excreted by the biliary tract, and an elevated bilirubin concentration is an indication for reducing the dose. Supraventricular tachycardia related to drug administration is an uncommon complication. Higher cumulative doses are associated with development of a cardiomyopathy. It is customary to limit total cumulative doses to 450 mg/m² body-surface area as symptomatic and potentially fatal heart failure is increasingly common above this level. Patients with pre-existing cardiac disease, the elderly, and those who have received myocardial irradiation should be treated cautiously. Cardiac monitoring, for example by sequential radionuclide ejection fraction measurement, may assist in safely limiting total dosage. Evidence is available to suggest that weekly low dose administration may be associated with less cardiac damage. Doxorubicin is also given by *bladder instillation* (see section 7.4.4).

Epirubicin is structurally related to doxorubicin and clinical trials suggest that it is as effective in the treatment of breast cancer. A maximum cumulative dose of 0.9–1 g/m² is recommended to help avoid cardiotoxicity. Like doxorubicin it is given *intravenously* and by *bladder instillation* (see section 7.4.4).

Aclarubicin and **idarubicin** are newly introduced anthracyclines with general properties similar to those of doxorubicin. They are both given *intravenously*. Idarubicin may also be given *by mouth*.

Daunorubicin also has general properties similar to those of doxorubicin; a liposomal formulation for *intravenous* use has recently been licensed for advanced HIV-related Kaposi's sarcoma.

Mitozantrone is structurally related to doxorubicin and preliminary work suggests that it has equal activity in breast cancer. It is given *intravenously* and is well tolerated apart from myelosuppression and dose-related cardiotoxicity; cardiac examinations are recommended after a cumulative dose of 160 mg/m² if this complication is to be avoided.

Bleomycin is given *intravenously* or *intramuscularly* to treat the lymphomas, certain solid tumours and, by the *intracavitary route*, malignant effusions. It is unusual in that it causes little marrow suppression. Dermatological toxicity is common; increased pigmentation particularly affecting the flexures and subcutaneous sclerotic plaques may occur. Mucositis is also relatively common and an association with Raynaud's phenomenon is reported. Hypersensitivity reactions manifest by chills and fevers commonly occur a few hours after drug administration and may be prevented by simultaneous administration of a corticosteroid, for example hydrocortisone intravenously. The principal problem associated with the use of bleomycin is progressive pulmonary fibrosis. This is dose related, occurring more commonly at cumulative doses greater than 300 units and in the elderly. Basal lung crepitations or suspicious chest X-ray changes are an indication to stop therapy with this drug. Patients who have received extensive treatment with bleomycin (e.g. cumulative dose more than 100 units) may be at risk of developing respiratory failure if a general anaesthetic is given with high inspired oxygen concentrations. Anaesthetists should be warned of this.

Dactinomycin is principally used to treat paediatric cancers; it is given *intravenously*. Its side-effects are similar to those of doxorubicin, except that cardiac toxicity is not a problem.

Mitomycin is given *intravenously* to treat upper gastro-intestinal and breast cancers. It causes delayed marrow toxicity and is usually administered at 6-weekly intervals. Prolonged use may result in permanent marrow damage. It is a relatively toxic drug and may cause lung fibrosis and renal damage. It is also given by *bladder instillation* (see section 7.4.4).

ACLARUBICIN

Indications: acute non-lymphocytic leukaemia in patients who have relapsed or are resistant or refractory to first-line chemotherapy

---

Cautions; Side-effects: see section 8.1 and notes above; caution in hepatic and renal impairment; irritant to tissues

PoM **Aclacin®** (Lundbeck)
Injection, powder for reconstitution, aclarubicin 20 mg (as hydrochloride). Net price 20-mg vial = £29.20

BLEOMYCIN

Indications: squamous cell carcinoma; see also notes above
Cautions; Side-effects: see section 8.1 and notes above; reduce dose in renal impairment; also caution in handling—irritant to skin

PoM **Bleomycin** (Lundbeck)
Injection, powder for reconstitution, bleomycin (as sulphate). Net price 15-unit amp = £16.29
Note. Ampoules previously labelled as containing '15 mg' of bleomycin contained 15 units. The ampoules are now labelled only as units.

DACTINOMYCIN
(Actinomycin D)
Indications: see notes above
Cautions; Side-effects: see section 8.1 and notes above; irritant to tissues

PoM **Cosmegen Lyovac®** (MSD)
Injection, powder for reconstitution, dactinomycin, net price 500-microgram vial = £1.50

DAUNORUBICIN

Indications: advanced HIV-related Kaposi's sarcoma
Cautions; Side-effects: see section 8.1 and notes above

▼ PoM **DaunoXome®** (NeXstar)
Injection, daunorubicin encapsulated in liposomes. For dilution and use as an infusion. Net price 50-mg vial = £155.00

DOXORUBICIN HYDROCHLORIDE

Indications: see notes above and section 7.4.4
Cautions; Side-effects: see section 8.1 and notes above; reduce dose in hepatic impairment; also caution in handling—irritant to skin and tissues; **interactions:** see Appendix 1 (doxorubicin)

PoM **Doxorubicin Rapid Dissolution**
(Pharmacia)
Injection, powder for reconstitution, doxorubicin hydrochloride, net price 10-mg vial = £18.72; 50-mg vial = £93.60
*Note.*This preparation has replaced Adriamycin®
PoM **Doxorubicin Solution for Injection**
(Pharmacia)
Injection, doxorubicin hydrochloride 2 mg/mL, net price 5-mL vial = £20.60; 25-mL vial = £103.00
Various strengths and sizes also available from David Bull

EPIRUBICIN HYDROCHLORIDE

Indications: see notes above and section 7.4.4
Cautions; Side-effects: see section 8.1 and notes above; reduce dose in hepatic impairment; irritant to tissues

PoM **Pharmorubicin® Rapid Dissolution**
(Pharmacia)
Injection, powder for reconstitution, epirubicin hydrochloride. Net price 10-mg vial = £16.85; 20-mg vial = £33.70; 50-mg vial = £84.24
PoM **Pharmorubicin® Solution for Injection**
(Pharmacia)
Injection, epirubicin hydrochloride 2 mg/mL, net price 5-mL vial = £18.54; 25-mL vial = £92.70

IDARUBICIN HYDROCHLORIDE

Indications: advanced breast cancer after failure of frontline chemotherapy (not including anthracyclines); acute leukaemias—see notes above
Cautions; Side-effects: see section 8.1 and notes above; caution in hepatic and renal impairment; also caution in handling—irritant to skin and tissues

PoM **Zavedos®** (Pharmacia)
Capsules, idarubicin hydrochloride, 5 mg (orange), net price 1-cap pack = £28.80; 10 mg (red/white), 1-cap pack = £57.60; 25 mg (orange/white), 1-cap pack = £144.00. Label: 25
Injection, powder for reconstitution, idarubicin hydrochloride, net price 5-mg vial = £72.80; 10-mg vial = £145.60

MITOMYCIN

Indications: see notes above and section 7.4.4
Cautions; Side-effects: see section 8.1 and notes above; irritant to tissues

PoM **Mitomycin C Kyowa®** (Kyowa Hakko)
Injection, powder for reconstitution, mitomycin. Net price 2-mg vial = £6.16; 10-mg vial = £20.28; 20-mg vial = £38.68 (hosp. only)

MITOZANTRONE
(Mitoxantrone)
Indications: see notes above
Cautions; Side-effects: see section 8.1 and notes above; intrathecal administration not recommended

PoM **Novantrone®** (Lederle)
Intravenous infusion, mitozantrone 2 mg (as hydrochloride)/mL, net price 10-mL vial = £150.43; 12.5-mL vial = £188.05; 15-mL vial = £225.60

8.1.3   Antimetabolites

Antimetabolites are incorporated into new nuclear material or combine irreversibly with vital cellular enzymes, preventing normal cellular division.

Methotrexate inhibits the enzyme dihydrofolate reductase, essential for the synthesis of purines and pyrimidines. It is given *by mouth, intravenously, intramuscularly,* or *intrathecally.* High-dose methotrexate cannot generally be recommended except in clinical trials.

Methotrexate is used as maintenance therapy for childhood acute lymphoblastic leukaemia. Other uses include choriocarcinoma, non-Hodgkin lymphomas, and a number of solid tumours. Intrathecal methotrexate is used in the CNS prophylaxis of childhood acute lymphoblastic leukaemia, and as a therapy for established meningeal cancer or lymphoma.

Methotrexate causes myelosuppression, mucositis, and rarely pneumonitis. It is **contra-indicated** if significant renal impairment is present, as the kidney is its route of excretion. It should also be **avoided** if a significant pleural effusion or ascites is present as it tends to accumulate at these sites, and its subsequent return to the circulation will be associated with myelosuppression. For similar reasons blood counts should be carefully monitored when intrathecal methotrexate is given.

Oral or parenteral folinic acid (see below) will help prevent, and speed recovery from, methotrexate mucositis or myelosuppression.

Cytarabine acts by interfering with pyrimidine synthesis. It is given *subcutaneously, intravenously,* or *intrathecally.* Its predominant use is in the induction of remission of acute myeloblastic leukaemia. It is a potent myelosuppressant and requires careful haematological monitoring.

Fludarabine is recommended for patients with B-cell chronic lymphocytic leukaemia (CLL) after initial treatment with an alkylating agent has failed; it is given *intravenously* daily for 5 days every 28 days. Fludarabine is generally well tolerated but does, however, cause myelosuppression (which may be cumulative), and immunosuppression (with an increased risk of opportunistic infection). Idiosyncratic CNS and pulmonary toxicity have been reported rarely. Dose reduction is recommended in renal impairment.

Cladribine is an effective but potentially toxic drug given by continuous *intravenous infusion* over 7 days for the treatment of hairy cell leukaemia. Myelosuppression may be severe and use is confined to experienced specialists.

Gemcitabine is given *intravenously* for palliative treatment in patients with locally advanced or metastatic non-small cell lung cancer. It is generally well tolerated but may cause mild gastro-intestinal side-effects and rashes; renal impairment and influenza-like symptoms have also been reported. Gemcitabine should not be used concurrently with radical radiotherapy.

Fluorouracil may be given *by mouth* but is usually given *intravenously.* It is used to treat a number of solid tumours, including colon and breast cancer. It may also be used topically for certain malignant skin lesions. Toxicity is unusual, but may include myelosuppression, mucositis, and rarely a cerebellar syndrome. It is also used *topically* as a cream.

Raltitrexed, a thymidylate synthase inhibitor, is given *intravenously* for palliation of metastatic colon cancer. It is probably of similar efficacy to fluorouracil. Raltitrexed is generally well tolerated, but may cause gastro-intestinal side-effects. Caution is advised in hepatic and renal impairment.

Mercaptopurine is used almost exclusively as maintenance therapy for the acute leukaemias. The dose should be reduced if the patient is receiving concurrent allopurinol as this drug interferes with the metabolism of mercaptopurine.

Thioguanine is given *by mouth* to induce remission in acute myeloid leukaemia.

Azathioprine, a derivative of the antimetabolite mercaptopurine is given *by mouth*; as with mercaptopurine the dose needs to be reduced if the patient is receiving concurrent allopurinol. It is commonly used as an immunosuppressant (section 8.2.1).

CLADRIBINE

Indications: see notes above

Cautions; Side-effects: see section 8.1 and notes above

▼ **PoM Leustat**® (Janssen-Cilag)

Injection, cladribine 1 mg/mL. For dilution and use as an infusion. Net price 10-mL vial = £364.57

CYTARABINE

Indications: acute leukaemias

Cautions; Side-effects: see section 8.1 and notes above

PoM Cytarabine (Non-proprietary)

Injection, cytarabine 20 mg/mL. Net price 5-mL vial = £3.84

Injection, cytarabine 100 mg/mL. Net price 1-mL vial = £3.84; 5-mL vial = £19.00; 10-mL vial = £37.83; 20-mL vial = £71.88

All available from David Bull

PoM Alexan® (Pfizer)

Injection, cytarabine 20 mg/mL. Net price 2-mL amp = £1.16; 5-mL amp = £2.91

PoM Alexan® **100** (Pfizer)

Injection, cytarabine 100 mg/mL. Net price 10-mL amp = £26.46. For intravenous infusion only

PoM Cytosar® (Upjohn)

Injection, powder for reconstitution, cytarabine. Net price 100-mg vial = £3.01, 100-mg vial (with diluent) = £3.17; 500-mg vial = £14.95, 500-mg vial (with diluent) = £15.45. For intravenous injection or infusion and subcutaneous injection only

---

FLUDARABINE PHOSPHATE

Indications: see notes above

Cautions; Side-effects: see section 8.1 and notes above; **interactions:** Appendix 1 (Fludarabine)

▼ PoM **Fludara**® (Schering Health)

Injection, powder for reconstitution, fludarabine phosphate. Net price 50-mg vial = £130.00

FLUOROURACIL

Indications: see notes above

Cautions; Side-effects: see section 8.1; also caution in handling—irritant; **interactions:** Appendix 1 (fluorouracil)

Dose: by mouth, maintenance 15 mg/kg weekly; max. in one day 1 g

PoM **Fluorouracil** (Non-proprietary)

Capsules, fluorouracil 250 mg.

Available from Cambridge on a named patient basis

Injection, fluorouracil 25 mg/mL (as sodium salt). Net price 10-mL vial = £2.06; 20-mL vial = £3.97; 100-mL vial = £19.23

Available from David Bull

PoM **Efudix**® (Roche)

Cream, fluorouracil 5%. Net price 20 g = £4.13

GEMCITABINE

Indications: see notes above

Cautions; Side-effects: see section 8.1 and notes above

▼ PoM **Gemzar**® (Lilly)

Injection, powder for reconstitution, gemcitabine (as hydrochloride), net price 200-mg vial = £18.75;1-g vial = £93.75 (both hosp. only)

MERCAPTOPURINE

Indications: acute leukaemias

Cautions; Side-effects: see section 8.1 and notes above; reduce dose in renal impairment; avoid in porphyria (see section 9.8.2); **interactions:** Appendix 1 (mercaptopurine)

Dose: initially 2.5 mg/kg daily

PoM **Puri-Nethol**® (Wellcome)

Tablets, fawn, scored, mercaptopurine 50 mg. Net price 25 = £19.22

METHOTREXATE

Indications: see notes above and under Dose; rheumatoid arthritis, see section 10.1.3; psoriasis, see section 13.5.2

Cautions; Side-effects: see section 8.1, notes above and p. 471; reduce dose in renal impairment; dose-related toxicity in hepatic impairment; porphyria (see section 9.8.2); **interactions:** Appendix 1 (methotrexate)

Dose: by mouth, leukaemia in children (maintenance), 15 mg/m^2 weekly in combination with other drugs

PoM **Methotrexate** (Non-proprietary)

Tablets, yellow, methotrexate 2.5 mg. Net price 100 (David Bull) = £13.78; (Lederle) = £10.59; (Pharmacia, Maxtrex®) = £10.43. Counselling, NSAIDs, see p. 472

Tablets, yellow, methotrexate 10 mg. Net price 100 (David Bull) = £53.47; (Pharmacia, Maxtrex®) = £47.29. Counselling, NSAIDs, see p. 472

Injection, methotrexate 2.5 mg (as sodium salt)/mL. Net price 2-mL vial (David Bull) = £1.63

Injection, methotrexate 25 mg (as sodium salt)/mL. Net price 2-mL vial (David Bull) = £4.45, (Lederle) = £2.62; 8-mL vial (Lederle) = £10.02; 20-mL vial (David Bull) = £37.95, (Lederle) = £25.07; 40-mL vial (Lederle) = £44.57; 200-mL vial (Lederle) = £200.57

Injection, methotrexate 100 mg/mL (not for intrathecal use). Net price 10-mL vial (David Bull) = £76.05; 50-mL vial (David Bull) = £380.07

RALTITREXED

Indications: see notes above

Cautions; Side-effects: see section 8.1 and notes above

▼ PoM **Tomudex**® (Zeneca)

Injection, powder for reconstitution, raltitrexed. Net price 2-mg vial = £116.00

THIOGUANINE

Indications: acute leukaemias

Cautions; Side-effects: see section 8.1 and notes above; reduce dose in renal impairment

Dose: initially 2–2.5 mg/kg daily

PoM **Lanvis**® (Wellcome)

Tablets, yellow, scored, thioguanine 40 mg. Net price 25-tab pack = £46.48

FOLINIC ACID RESCUE

Folinic acid (given as calcium folinate) is used to counteract the folate-antagonist action of methotrexate and thus speed recovery from methotrexate-induced mucositis or myelosuppression. It is generally given 24 hours after the methotrexate, in a dose of 15 mg by mouth every 6 hours, for 2–8 doses (depending on the dose of methotrexate). It does not counteract the antibacterial activity of folate antagonists such as trimethoprim.

Folinic acid also interacts with fluorouracil; when the two are used together in metastatic colonic cancer a favourable effect has been demonstrated on response-rate.

CALCIUM FOLINATE

(Calcium leucovorin)

Indications: see notes above

Cautions: avoid simultaneous administration of methotrexate; as for Folic Acid (section 9.1.2) **not** indicated for pernicious anaemia or other megaloblastic anaemias where vitamin B$_{12}$ deficient

Side-effects: rarely, pyrexia after parenteral administration

Dose: expressed in terms of folinic acid

As an antidote to methotrexate (started 8–24 hours after the beginning of methotrexate infusion), in general up to 120 mg in divided doses over 12–24 hours *by intramuscular or intravenous injection or infusion*, followed by 12–15 mg *intramuscularly or* 15 mg *by mouth* every 6 hours for the next 48–72 hours

Suspected methotrexate overdosage, immediate administration of an equal or higher dose of folinic acid

PoM **Calcium Folinate** (Non-proprietary)

Tablets, scored, folinic acid (as calcium salt) 15 mg. Net price 10-tab pack (David Bull) = £36.75, (Hillcross) = £27.32, (Lagap) = £39.84, (Lederle) = £41.22; 30-tab pack (Pharmacia, Refolinon®) = £94.50

Injection, folinic acid 3 mg (as calcium salt)/ml. Net price 1-mL amp (David Bull) = £2.21, (Lederle) = £1.06; 10-mL amp (Pharmacia, Refolinon®) = £5.70

Injection, folinic acid 7.5 mg (as calcium salt)/mL. Net price 2-mL amp (David Bull) = £7.57

Injection, folinic acid 10 mg (as calcium salt)/mL. Net price 5-mL vial (David Bull) = £18.84; 10-mL vial (David Bull) = £35.09; 30-mL vial (David Bull) = £91.93; 35-mL vial (Lederle, Lederfolin®) = £90.98

Injection, powder for reconstitution, folinic acid (as calcium salt). Net price 15-mg vial (Lederle) = £4.46; 30-mg vial (Lederle) = £8.36

8.1.4   Vinca alkaloids and etoposide

The vinca alkaloids (vinblastine, vincristine, and vindesine) are used to treat the acute leukaemias, lymphomas, and some solid tumours (e.g. breast and lung cancer). They commonly cause peripheral and autonomic neuropathy. This side-effect is most obvious with vincristine, and is manifest by peripheral paraesthesia, loss of deep tendon reflexes, and abdominal bloating and constipation. If these symptoms are severe, doses should be reduced. Significant new motor weakness is a **contra-indication** to further use of these drugs. Recovery of the nervous system is generally slow but complete. Intrathecal administration of **all** vinca alkaloids is **contra-indicated** (usually fatal).

Vincristine causes virtually no myelosuppression. Its use may be associated with alopecia; hyponatraemia, as a result of inappropriate ADH secretion, has been described. It is given *intravenously.*

Vinblastine is a more myelosuppressive drug than vincristine, but causes less neurotoxicity. It is given *intravenously.*

Vindesine is the most recent addition to the vinca alkaloid group. It has a similar range of clinical activity, and side-effects intermediate between those of the above two drugs. It is given *intravenously.*

Etoposide may be given *by mouth* or *intravenously*, the dose when used orally being double that when given intravenously. There is evidence to suggest that administration in divided doses over 3–5 days may be beneficial; courses may not be repeated more frequently than at intervals of 21 days. It has useful activity in small cell carcinoma of the bronchus, the lymphomas, and testicular teratoma. Toxic effects include alopecia, myelosuppression, nausea, and vomiting.

ETOPOSIDE

Indications: see notes above

Cautions; Contra-indications; Side-effects: see section 8.1 and notes above; irritant to tissues

PoM **Etoposide** (Du Pont)

Injection concentrate, etoposide 20 mg/mL. To be diluted. Net price 5-mL vial = £13.50

PoM **Vepesid®** (Bristol-Myers)

Capsules, etoposide 50 mg, net price 20 = £113.95; 100 mg, 10-cap pack = £99.57

Injection, etoposide 20 mg/mL. To be diluted. Net price 5-mL vial = £14.58

VINBLASTINE SULPHATE

Indications: see notes above

Cautions; Contra-indications; Side-effects: see section 8.1 and notes above; caution in handling—avoid contact with eyes; irritant to tissues

IMPORTANT. Intrathecal injection **contra-indicated**

PoM **Vinblastine** (Non-proprietary)

Injection, vinblastine sulphate 1 mg/mL. Net price 10-mL vial = £12.71

Available from David Bull

PoM **Velbe®** (Lilly)

Injection, powder for reconstitution, vinblastine sulphate. Net price 10-mg amp (with diluent) = £14.15

VINCRISTINE SULPHATE

Indications: see notes above

Cautions; Contra-indications; Side-effects: see section 8.1 and notes above; caution in handling—avoid contact with eyes; irritant to tissues

IMPORTANT. Intrathecal injection **contra-indicated**

PoM **Vincristine** (Non-proprietary)

Injection, vincristine sulphate 1 mg/mL. Net price 1-mL vial = £10.92; 2-mL vial = £21.17; 5-mL vial = £44.16; 1-mL syringe = £11.34; 2-mL syringe = £20.55

Available from David Bull

PoM **Oncovin®** (Lilly)

Injection, vincristine sulphate 1 mg/mL, net price 1-mL vial = £14.18; 2-mL vial = £28.05

VINDESINE SULPHATE

Indications: see notes above

Cautions; Contra-indications; Side-effects: see section 8.1 and notes above; caution in handling—avoid contact with eyes; irritant to tissues IMPORTANT. Intrathecal injection **contra-indicated**

PoM Eldisine® (Lilly)

Injection, powder for reconstitution, vindesine sulphate, net price 5-mg vial (with diluent) = £78.30 (hosp. only)

8.1.5   Other antineoplastic drugs

AMSACRINE

Amsacrine has an action and toxic effects similar to those of doxorubicin (section 8.1.2) and is given *intravenously*. It is used in acute myeloid leukaemia. Side-effects include myelosuppression and mucositis; electrolytes should be monitored as fatal arrhythmias have occurred in association with hypokalaemia.

AMSACRINE

Indications: see notes above

Cautions; Side-effects: see section 8.1 and notes above; reduce dose in renal or hepatic impairment; also caution in handling—irritant to skin and tissues

PoM Amsidine® (P-D)

Concentrate for intravenous infusion, amsacrine 5 mg/mL, when reconstituted by mixing two solutions. Net price 1.5-mL amp with 13.5-mL vial = £30.90. (hosp. only)

Note. Use glass apparatus for reconstitution

CARBOPLATIN

Carboplatin, a derivative of cisplatin which has probably equivalent activity in ovarian cancer, is given *intravenously*. It is also active in small cell lung cancer and is under trial in a variety of other malignancies. Carboplatin is better tolerated than cisplatin; nausea and vomiting are reduced in severity and nephrotoxicity, neurotoxicity, and ototoxicity are much less of a problem than with cisplatin. It is, however, more myelosuppressive than cisplatin.

CARBOPLATIN

Indications: see notes above

Cautions; Side-effects: see section 8.1 and notes above; reduce dose in renal impairment

PoM Carboplatin (Non-proprietary)

Injection, carboplatin 10 mg/mL. Net price 15-mL vial = £65.83; 45-mL vial = £197.48

Available from David Bull

PoM Paraplatin® (Bristol-Myers)

Injection, carboplatin 10 mg/mL. Net price 5-mL vial = £22.86; 15-mL vial = £65.83; 45-mL vial = £197.48

CISPLATIN

Cisplatin has an alkylating action and is given *intravenously*. It has useful antitumour activity in certain solid tumours including ovarian cancer and testicular teratoma. It is, however, a toxic drug. Common problems include severe nausea and vomiting, nephrotoxicity (pretreatment hydration mandatory and renal function should be closely monitored), myelotoxicity, ototoxicity (high tone hearing loss and tinnitus), peripheral neuropathy, and hypomagnesaemia. These toxic effects commonly necessitate dose reduction or drug withdrawal. It is preferable that treatment with this drug be supervised by specialists familiar with its use.

CISPLATIN

Indications: see notes above

Cautions; Side-effects: see section 8.1 and notes above; reduce dose in renal impairment; **interactions:** Appendix 1 (cisplatin)

PoM Cisplatin (Non-proprietary)

Injection, cisplatin 1 mg/mL. Net price 10-mL vial = £5.85; 50-mL vial = £28.11; 100-mL vial = £55.64

Available from David Bull

Injection, powder for reconstitution, cisplatin. Net price 50-mg vial = £17.00

Available from Pharmacia

CRISANTASPASE

Crisantaspase is the enzyme asparaginase produced by *Erwinia chrysanthemi*. It is given *intramuscularly* or *subcutaneously* almost exclusively in acute lymphoblastic leukaemia. Facilities for the management of anaphylaxis should be available. Side-effects also include nausea, vomiting, CNS depression, and liver function and blood lipid changes; careful monitoring is therefore necessary and the urine is tested for glucose to exclude hyperglycaemia.

CRISANTASPASE

Indications; Cautions; Side-effects: see notes above

PoM Erwinase® (Speywood)

Injection, powder for reconstitution, crisantaspase. Net price 20 × 10 000-unit vial = £858.00

DACARBAZINE

Dacarbazine is not commonly used on account of its toxicity. It has been used to treat melanoma and, in combination therapy, the soft tissue sarcomas. It is also a component of a commonly used combination for Hodgkin's disease (ABVD—doxorubicin [Adriamycin®], bleomycin, vinblastine, and dacarbazine). It is given *intravenously*. The predominant side-effects are myelosuppression and intense nausea and vomiting.

DACARBAZINE

Indications: see notes above

Cautions; Side-effects: see section 8.1; also caution in handling—irritant to skin and tissues

PoM DTIC-Dome® (Bayer)

Injection, powder for reconstitution, dacarbazine. Net price 100-mg vial = £4.83; 200-mg vial = £7.40

HYDROXYUREA

Hydroxyurea is an orally active drug used mainly in the treatment of chronic myeloid leukaemia. It is occasionally used for polycythaemia (the usual treatment is venesection). Myelosuppression, nausea, and skin reactions are the most common toxic effects.

HYDROXYUREA

(Hydroxycarbamide)

Indications: see notes above

Cautions; Side-effects: see section 8.1 and notes above

Dose: 20–30 mg/kg daily *or* 80 mg/kg every third day

PoM Hydrea® (Squibb)

Capsules, pink/green, hydroxyurea 500 mg. Net price 20 = £2.39

PENTOSTATIN

Pentostatin is highly active in hairy cell leukaemia. It is given *intravenously* on alternate weeks and is capable of inducing prolonged complete remission. It is potentially toxic, causing myelosuppression, immunosuppression and a number of other side-effects which may be severe. Its use is probably best confined to specialist centres.

PENTOSTATIN

Indications: see notes above

Cautions; Contra-indications; Side-effects: see section 8.1 and notes above; **interactions:** Appendix 1 (pentostatin)

▼ **PoM Nipent®** (Lederle)

Injection, powder for reconstitution, pentostatin. Net price 10-mg vial = £774.00

PROCARBAZINE

Procarbazine is most often used in Hodgkin's disease, for example in MOPP (mustine, vincristine [Oncovin®], procarbazine, and prednisolone) chemotherapy. It is given *by mouth*. Toxic effects include nausea, myelosuppression, and a hypersensitivity rash preventing further use of this drug. It is a mild monoamine-oxidase inhibitor but dietary restriction is not considered necessary. Alcohol ingestion may cause a disulfiram-like reaction.

PROCARBAZINE

Indications: see notes above

Cautions; Side-effects: see section 8.1 and notes above; reduce dose in renal impairment; **interactions:** Appendix 1 (procarbazine)

Dose: initially 50 mg daily, increased by 50 mg daily to 250–300 mg daily in divided doses; maintenance (on remission) 50–150 mg daily to cumulative total of at least 6 g

PoM Natulan® (Cambridge)

Capsules, ivory, procarbazine 50 mg (as hydrochloride). Net price 50-cap pack = £13.50. Label: 4

RAZOXANE

Razoxane has limited activity in the leukaemias, and is little used.

RAZOXANE

Indications: see notes above

Cautions; Side-effects: see section 8.1

Dose: acute leukaemias, 150–500 mg/m^2 daily for 3–5 days

PoM Razoxin® (Cambridge)

Tablets, scored, razoxane 125 mg. Net price 30-tab pack = £26.87

TAXANES

Paclitaxel is the first of a new group of drugs termed the taxanes. It is given by *intravenous infusion*. It is licensed for patients with ovarian cancer in whom standard platinum-containing therapy has failed (generally taken to indicate patients with an initially poor response or whose disease progresses within six months of treatment). It is also licensed for patients with metastatic breast cancer where treatment with an anthracycline has failed or is regarded as inappropriate. Paclitaxel is relatively toxic and it is recommended that its use be confined to experienced specialists. Routine premedication with a corticosteroid, an antihistamine and a histamine H$_2$-receptor antagonist is recommended to prevent severe hypersensitivity reactions; despite premedication these reactions may still rarely occur, more commonly only bradycardia or asymptomatic hypotension occur.

In addition to hypersensitivity, side-effects of paclitaxel include myelosuppression, peripheral neuropathy, and cardiac conduction defects with arrhythmias (which are nearly always asymptomatic). It also causes alopecia and muscle pain; nausea and vomiting is mild to moderate.

Only a minority of patients respond to paclitaxel, but the responses are sometimes prolonged.

Docetaxel is licensed for use in anthracycline-resistant breast cancer. The side-effects are similar to those for paclitaxel but persistent fluid retention (commonly seen as leg oedema which worsens during treatment) can be resistant to treatment; hypersensitivity reactions also occur. Dexamethasone by mouth for five days, starting on the day before each

---

course of docetaxel, is recommended for reducing these problems. Caution is advised in hepatic impairment.

DOCETAXEL

Indications: advanced breast cancer where adjuvant cytotoxic chemotherapy (including anthracycline) has failed

Cautions; Contra-indications; Side-effects: see section 8.1 and notes above; **interactions:** Appendix 1 (docetaxel)

▼ PoM **Taxotere®** (Rhône-Poulenc Rorer)
Concentrate for intravenous infusion, docetaxel 40 mg/mL. Net price 0.5-mL vial = £175.00, 2-mL vial = £575.00 (both with diluent). Hosp. only

PACLITAXEL

Indications: metastatic ovarian cancer where standard platinum-containing therapy has failed; metastatic breast carcinoma where standard anthracycline-containing therapy has failed or is inappropriate

Cautions; Contra-indications; Side-effects: see section 8.1 and notes above; **interactions:** Appendix 1 (paclitaxel)

▼ PoM **Taxol®** (Bristol-Myers, Squibb)
Concentrate for intravenous infusion, paclitaxel 6 mg/mL. Net price 5-mL vial = £124.79 (hosp. only)
Note. Contains polyethoxylated castor oil which has been associated with anaphylaxis

8.2 Drugs affecting the immune response

8.2.1	Cytotoxic immunosuppressants
8.2.2	Corticosteroids and other immunosuppressants
8.2.3	Immunostimulants
8.2.4	Interferons
8.2.5	Aldesleukin

8.2.1 Cytotoxic immunosuppressants

These drugs are used to suppress rejection in organ transplant recipients and are also used to treat a variety of auto-immune and collagen diseases (see section 10.1.3). They are non-specific in their action and careful monitoring of peripheral blood counts is required, with dose adjustments for marrow toxicity. Patients receiving these drugs will be prone to atypical infections.

Azathioprine is widely used for transplant recipients and is also used to treat a number of auto-immune conditions, usually when corticosteroid therapy alone has provided inadequate control. This drug is metabolised to mercaptopurine, and doses should be reduced when concurrent therapy with allopurinol is given. The predominant toxic effect is

myelosuppression, although hepatic toxicity is also well recognised.

Mycophenolate mofetil is metabolised to mycophenolic acid which has a more selective mode of action than that of azathioprine. It is licensed for the prophylaxis of acute renal transplant rejection when used in combination with cyclosporin and corticosteroids. There is evidence that compared with similar regimens incorporating azathioprine, mycophenolate mofetil reduces the risk of acute rejection episodes; the risk of opportunistic infections (particularly due to tissue-invasive cytomegalovirus) and the occurrence of blood disorders such as leucopenia may be higher.

Cyclophosphamide and chlorambucil (section 8.1.1) are less commonly prescribed as immunosuppressants.

IMPAIRED IMMUNE RESPONSIVENESS. For general comments and warnings relating to immunosuppression see p. 352 (Impaired Immune Responsiveness)

AZATHIOPRINE

Indications: see notes above

Cautions: should not be prescribed unless adequate monitoring available throughout duration of treatment; monitoring required includes full blood counts carried out at least weekly for the first 8 weeks (more frequently with higher doses or if hepatic or renal impairment) then at least every 3 months thereafter; reduce dose in severe hepatic and renal impairment and in elderly; **interactions:** Appendix 1 (azathioprine)
BONE MARROW SUPPRESSION. Patients should be warned to report immediately any evidence of infection, unexpected bruising or bleeding, or other manifestations of bone marrow suppression

Contra-indications: hypersensitivity to azathioprine or mercaptopurine (see also under Side-effects); decision to maintain or discontinue in pregnancy depends on condition being treated (see also p. 352) but as general rule should not be initiated during pregnancy

Side-effects: hypersensitivity reactions–including malaise, dizziness, vomiting, fever, rigors, muscular pains, arthralgia, disturbed liver function, cholestatic jaundice, arrhythmias and hypotension (calling for immediate and permanent withdrawal); dose-related bone marrow suppression (see also Cautions); hair loss and increased susceptibility to infections in transplant recipients also receiving corticosteroids; nausea; rarely pancreatitis and pneumonitis

Dose: by mouth or *intravenously*, initially, rarely more than 3 mg/kg daily, reduced according to response; maintenance 1–3 mg/kg daily; consider withdrawal if no improvement in 3 months

Suppression of transplant rejection, loading dose, *by mouth* or *intravenously* up to 5 mg/kg; maintenance 1–4 mg/kg daily

Note. Intravenous injection is alkaline and very irritant, intravenous route should therefore be used **only** if oral route not feasible, see also Appendix 6

PoM **Azathioprine** (Non-proprietary)

Tablets, azathioprine 50 mg. Net price 20 = £4.28. Label: 21

Available from APS, Ashbourne (Immunoprin®), Berk (Berkaprine®), Cox, Hillcross, Lagap, Lennon (Oprisine®), Norton, Penn (Azamune®)

PoM **Imuran**® (Wellcome)

Tablets, both f/c, azathioprine 25 mg (orange), net price 100-tab pack = £39.35; 50 mg (yellow), 100-tab pack = £65.61. Label: 21

Injection, powder for reconstitution, azathioprine (as sodium salt). Net price 50-mg vial = £16.54

MYCOPHENOLATE MOFETIL

Indications: prophylaxis of acute renal transplant rejection (in combination with cyclosporin and corticosteroids) under specialist supervision

Cautions: full blood counts every week for 4 weeks then twice a month for 2 months then every month in the first year (possibly interrupt treatment if neutropenia develops); elderly (increased risk of infection, gastro-intestinal haemorrhage and pulmonary oedema); acute serious gastro-intestinal disease (risk of haemorrhage, ulceration and perforation); **interactions:** Appendix 1 (mycophenolate mofetil)

Contra-indications: pregnancy (exclude before starting and avoid for 6 weeks after discontinuation); breast-feeding

Side-effects: diarrhoea, vomiting, constipation, nausea, abdominal pain; hypertension, oedema, chest pain; dyspnoea, cough; dizziness, insomnia, headache, tremor; infection (including cytomegalovirus viraemia, herpes simplex, candidiasis, aspergillosis, urinary-tract infection and pneumonia); leucopenia (see also Cautions), anaemia, thrombocytopenia, leucocytosis; electrolyte disturbances, hyperglycaemia, hypercholesterolaemia; asthenia; renal damage, haematuria; acne; lymphoproliferative disease; less frequently, abnormal liver-function tests, hepatitis, gingivitis, mouth ulceration, haemorrhage, influenza-like syndrome, hypotension, tachycardia, hypoglycaemia, weight gain; allergic reactions reported

Dose: 1 g twice daily starting within 72 hours of transplantation

COUNSELLING. Capsules to be swallowed whole with water on an empty stomach

▼ PoM **CellCept**® (Roche)

Capsules, blue/brown, mycophenolate mofetil 250 mg, net price 300-cap pack = £356.25. Counselling, administration

8.2.2   Corticosteroids and other immunosuppressants

Prednisolone is widely used in oncology. It has a marked antitumour effect in acute lymphoblastic leukaemia, Hodgkin's disease, and the non-Hodgkin lymphomas. It is also active in hormone-sensitive breast cancer and may cause useful disease regression. Finally, it has a role in the palliation of symptomatic end-stage malignant disease when it may produce a sense of well-being.

The corticosteroids are also powerful immunosuppressants. They are used to prevent organ transplant rejection, and in high dose to treat rejection episodes.

Cyclosporin is a fungal metabolite and potent immunosuppressant which is virtually non-myelotoxic but markedly nephrotoxic. It has found particular use in the field of organ and tissue transplantation, for prevention of graft rejection following bone marrow, kidney, liver, pancreas, heart, and heart-lung transplantation, and for prophylaxis of graft-versus-host disease.

Tacrolimus is a macrolide immunosuppressant that has been recently introduced. Although not chemically related to cyclosporin it has a similar mode of action and side-effects, but the incidence of neurotoxicity and nephrotoxicity appears to be greater; cardiomyopathy has also been reported. Disturbance of glucose metabolism also appears to be significant; hypertrichosis appears to be less of a problem than with cyclosporin.

IMPAIRED IMMUNE RESPONSIVENESS. For general comments and warnings relating to corticosteroids and immunosuppressants see section 6.3.2 (under Prednisolone) and p. 352 (Impaired Immune Responsiveness).

CYCLOSPORIN
(Ciclosporin)

Indications: see notes above, and under Dose; atopic dermatitis and psoriasis, see section 13.5.2; rheumatoid arthritis, see section 10.1.3

Cautions: monitor kidney function—dose dependent increase in serum creatinine and urea during first few weeks may necessitate dose reduction in transplant patients (exclude rejection if kidney transplant) or discontinuation in non-transplant patients; monitor liver function (dosage adjustment based on bilirubin and liver enzymes may be needed); monitor blood pressure—discontinue if hypertension develops that cannot be controlled by antihypertensives; hyperuricaemia; monitor serum potassium especially in marked renal dysfunction (and avoid high dietary potassium); measure blood lipids before treatment and thereafter as appropriate; pregnancy (see p. 352) and breast-feeding (see Appendix 5); porphyria (see section 9.8.2); apart from specialist use in transplant patients preferably avoid other immunosuppressants with the exception of corticosteroids (over-suppression may increase susceptibility to infection and lymphoma); **interactions:** Appendix 1 (cyclosporin)

ADDITIONAL CAUTIONS. Atopic Dermatitis and Psoriasis, see section 13.5.2; Rheumatoid Arthritis, see section 10.1.3

Side-effects: commonly dose-dependent increase in serum creatinine and urea during first few weeks (see also under Cautions), and less commonly renal structural changes on long-term administration; also hypertrichosis, tremor, hypertension (especially in heart transplant patients) hepatic dysfunction, fatigue, gingival hypertrophy, gastro-intestinal disturbances, and burning sensation in hands and feet (usually during first week); *occasionally* headache, rash (possibly allergic), mild anaemia, hyperkalaemia, hyperuricaemia, gout, hypomagnesaemia, hypercholesterolaemia, weight increase, oedema, pancreatitis, neuropathy, confusion, paraesthesia, convulsions, dysmenorrhoea or amenorrhoea; muscle weakness, cramps, myopathy, gynaecomastia (in patients receiving concomitant spironolactone), colitis also reported; thrombocytopenia (sometimes with haemolytic uraemic syndrome) also reported; incidence of malignancies and lymphoproliferative disorders similar to that with conventional immunosuppressive therapy

Dose: organ transplantation, used alone, 10–15 mg/kg *by mouth* 4–12 hours before transplantation followed by 10–15 mg/kg daily for 1–2 weeks post-operatively then reduced to 2–6 mg/kg daily for maintenance (dose should be adjusted by monitoring blood concentrations and renal function); dose lower if given concomitantly with other immunosuppressant therapy (e.g. corticosteroids); if necessary one-third oral dose can be given *by intravenous infusion* over 2–6 hours

Bone-marrow transplantation, prevention and treatment of graft-versus-host disease, 3–5 mg/kg daily *by intravenous infusion* over 2–6 hours from day before transplantation to 2 weeks post-operatively (or 12.5–15 mg/kg daily *by mouth*) then 12.5 mg/kg daily *by mouth* for 3–6 months then tailed off (may take up to a year after transplantation)

CONVERSION (from oral *Sandimmun®* to *Neoral®*). Measure trough blood-cyclosporin concentration, serum creatinine and blood pressure then give same dose (mg for mg) of *Neoral®* as previous oral *Sandimmun®*; repeat measurements 4–7 days after conversion (further measurements may be needed in first 2 months, e.g. week 2 and week 4) and adjust dose accordingly. Unlike oral *Sandimmun®* which may be taken either as a single daily dose (transplant recipients) or in 2 divided doses, the daily dose of *Neoral®* is always taken in 2 divided doses.

Because of differences in bioavailability, the brand to be dispensed should be specified by the prescriber

PoM **Neoral®** (Sandoz)

Capsules, cyclosporin 25 mg (blue/grey), net price 30-cap pack = £20.54; 50 mg (yellow/white), 30-cap pack = £40.22; 100 mg (blue/grey), 30-cap pack = £76.33. Counselling, administration

Oral solution, yellow, sugar-free, cyclosporin 100 mg/mL. Net price 50 mL = £114.38. Counselling, administration

COUNSELLING. Total daily dose should be taken in 2 divided doses. Avoid grapefruit or grapefruit juice for 1 hour before dose.

Mix solution with orange juice (or squash) or apple juice (to improve taste) or with water immediately before taking (and rinse with more to ensure total dose). Do not mix with grapefruit juice. Keep medicine measure away from other liquids (including water)

PoM **Sandimmun®** (Sandoz)

Capsules, cyclosporin 25 mg (pale pink), net price 30-cap pack = £20.54; 50 mg (yellow), 30-cap pack = £40.22; 100 mg (dusky pink), 30-cap pack = £76.33. Counselling, administration

Oral solution, oily, yellow, sugar-free, cyclosporin 100 mg/mL. Net price 50 mL = £114.38. Counselling, administration

COUNSELLING. Total daily dose may be taken as a single dose (transplant recipients) or in 2 divided doses. Avoid grapefruit or grapefruit juice for 1 hour before dose

To mask taste, mix solution with cold milk, cold chocolate drink, cola, or orange juice immediately before taking (and rinse with more to ensure total dose). Do not mix with grapefruit juice. Do not use plastic cup. Keep medicine measure away from other liquids (including water)

Concentrate for intravenous infusion (oily), cyclosporin 50 mg/mL. To be diluted before use. Net price 1-mL amp = £1.77; 5-mL amp = £8.38

Note. Contains polyethoxylated castor oil which has been associated with anaphylaxis—observe for at least 30 minutes after starting infusion and at frequent intervals thereafter

PREDNISOLONE
See section 6.3.2

TACROLIMUS

Indications: primary immunosuppression in liver and kidney allograft recipients and allograft rejection resistant to conventional immunosuppressive regimens; see also notes above

Cautions: see under Cyclosporin; also monitor ECG (**important:** also echocardiography, see CSM warning below), visual status, blood glucose, haematological and neurological parameters; **interactions:** Appendix 1 (tacrolimus)

DRIVING. May affect performance of skilled tasks (e.g. driving)

Contra-indications: hypersensitivity to macrolides; pregnancy (exclude before starting—if contraception needed non-hormonal methods should be used), breast-feeding; avoid concurrent administration with cyclosporin (care if patient has previously received cyclosporin)

Side-effects: see notes above and under Cyclosporin; other side-effects reported include CNS and sensory disorders (including agitation, anxiety, depression, euphoria, dream and thinking abnormalities, somnolence, dizziness, decreased reflexes, migraine, amblyopia, cataract, photophobia, deafness and tinnitus); cardiovascular disorders (including ECG changes, tachycardia and cardiomyopathy—**important:** see CSM warning below); respiratory disorders (including asthma, dyspnoea and pleural effusion); hyperglycaemia, diabetes mellitus, hyperkalaemia, hypokalaemia

CSM Warning. Hypertrophic cardiomyopathy has been reported in children given tacrolimus after transplantation. Patients using the drug should be monitored carefully by echocardiography for hypertrophic changes; dose reduction or discontinuation should be considered if these occur

---

Dose: liver allograft, ADULT initially *by intravenous infusion* 10–50 micrograms/kg over 24 hours starting 6 hours after surgery; max. 100 micrograms/kg over 24 hours; then *by mouth* 100–200 micrograms/kg daily in 2 divided doses; max. 300 micrograms/kg daily; CHILD 1.5–2 times initial adult dose

Kidney allograft, ADULT *by mouth* 150–400 micrograms/kg daily in 2 divided doses or *by intravenous infusion* 50–100 micrograms/kg over 24 hours starting within 24 hours after surgery; CHILD 1.5–2 times initial adult dose

▼ PoM **Prograf**® (Fujisawa)

Capsules, tacrolimus 1 mg (white), net price 50-cap pack = £89.45; 5 mg (greyish-red), 50-cap pack = £447.20. Label: 23, counselling, driving

Concentrate for intravenous infusion, tacrolimus 5 mg/mL. To be diluted before use. Net price 1-mL amp = £67.67

Note. Contains polyethoxylated castor oil which has been associated with anaphylaxis

8.2.3   Immunostimulants

A suspension of inactivated *Corynebacterium parvum* organisms (Coparvax®) was formerly used by the intracavitary route to treat malignant effusions. It has now been discontinued.

8.2.4   Interferons

Interferons are naturally occurring proteins with complex effects on immunity and cell function.

INTERFERON ALFA

Interferon alfa (formerly called leucocyte interferon or lymphoblastoid interferon) has shown some antitumour effect in certain lymphomas and solid tumours. The precise role of interferons in cancer treatment is controversial and often ill-defined. They are toxic and their use is often best confined to trials designed to evaluate their antitumour efficacy. Side-effects are dose-related, but commonly include nausea, influenza-like symptoms, lethargy, ocular side-effects and depression (suicidal behaviour reported). Myelosuppression may also occur, particularly affecting granulocyte counts. Cardiovascular problems (hypotension, hypertension, and arrhythmias), and hepatotoxicity have been reported. Other side-effects include hypersensitivity reactions, thyroid abnormalities, psoriasiform rash, confusion, and coma and seizures (usually with high doses in the elderly).

INTERFERON ALFA

Indications: see under preparations

Cautions; Contra-indications; Side-effects: see notes above—but for full details (including monitoring and dosage details) consult data sheets; pregnancy (Appendix 4); **interactions:** Appendix 1 (interferons)

PoM **Intron A**® (Schering-Plough)

Injection, interferon alfa-2b (rbe) 5-million units/mL, net price 2-mL vial = £56.52; 5-mL vial = £141.30 (all with injection equipment). For subcutaneous and intramuscular injection

Injection, powder for reconstitution, interferon alfa-2b (rbe). Net price 3-million unit vial = £16.96; 5-million unit vial = £28.26; 10-million unit vial = £56.52 (all with injection equipment and water for injection). For subcutaneous and intramuscular injection

Both for use in AIDS-related Kaposi's sarcoma, hairy cell leukaemia, non-Hodgkins lymphoma, chronic myelogenous leukaemia, condylomata acuminata (intralesional injection), chronic active hepatitis B, chronic hepatitis C and maintenance of remission in multiple myeloma

PoM **Roferon-A**® (Roche)

Injection, interferon alfa-2a (rbe). Net price 3-million units/mL, 1-mL vial = £16.96; 4.5-million units/mL, 1-mL vial = £25.44; 6-million units/mL, 1-mL vial = £33.92, 3-mL vial = £101.77; 9-million units/mL, 1-mL vial = £50.88. For subcutaneous and intramuscular injection

Injection, powder for reconstitution, interferon alfa-2a (rbe). Net price 18 million-unit vial (with syringe, needle, and water for injection) = £101.77. For subcutaneous and intramuscular injection

Both for use in AIDS-related Kaposi's sarcoma, hairy cell leukaemia, chronic myelogenous leukaemia, recurrent or metastatic renal cell carcinoma, progressive cutaneous T-cell lymphoma, chronic active hepatitis B and chronic hepatitis C; follicular non-Hodgkins lymphoma (solution for injection only)

PoM **Viraferon**® (Schering-Plough)

Injection, interferon alfa-2b (rbe) 5-million units/mL, net price 2-mL vial = £56.52; 5-mL vial = £141.30. For subcutaneous injection

For use in chronic active hepatitis B and chronic hepatitis C

PoM **Wellferon**® (Wellcome)

Injection, interferon alfa-N1 (lns) 3 million units/mL, net price 1-mL vial = £16.96; 10 million units/mL, net price 1-mL vial = £56.52. For subcutaneous and intramuscular injection

For use in hairy cell leukaemia and chronic active hepatitis B

INTERFERON BETA

Interferon beta (formerly called fibroblast interferon) has been recently licensed for use in patients with relapsing, remitting *multiple sclerosis* (characterised by at least two attacks of neurological dysfunction over the previous two-year period, followed by complete or incomplete recovery) who are able to walk unaided. It is indicated for the reduction of frequency and degree of severity of clinical relapses. There is no evidence of an effect on the progression of the disease, on duration of exacerbations (or on symptoms between exacerbations), or on disability. Not all patients respond and a deterioration in the bouts has been observed in some.

Interferon beta should not be used in those with a history of severe depressive illness (or of suicidal ideation), epilepsy inadequately controlled by treatment, or decompensated hepatic impairment. Caution is advised in those with a history of the above conditions or with cardiac disorders or myelosuppression. Most frequently reported side-effects include irritation at injection site (including inflammation, pain, hypersensitivity, necrosis) and flu-like symptoms (fever, chills, myalgia, malaise or sweating) but these decrease over time. Other side-effects include hypersensitivity reactions (including bronchospasm, anaphylaxis and urticaria), menstrual disorders, depression, anxiety, emotional lability, depersonalisation, convulsions, suicide attempts and confusion.

INTERFERON BETA
Indications: see notes above
> *Note.* The Standing Medical Advisory Committee on the use of Interferon Beta-1b in Relapsing-Remitting Multiple Sclerosis in Adults has recommended that patients who apparently fulfil the indications for treatment should be referred to a neurologist for a decision on whether treatment in indicated

Cautions; Contra-indications; Side-effects: see notes above—but for full details (including monitoring and dosage details consult data sheet; pregnancy (Appendix 4—advise contraceptive measures if appropriate), breast-feeding (Appendix 5); **interactions:** Appendix 1 (interferons)

▼ PoM **Betaferon®** (Schering Health)
Injection, powder for reconstitution, interferon beta-1b. Net price 300-micrograms (9.6 million units) vial (with diluent), 15 = £806.20. For subcutaneous injection

INTERFERON GAMMA
See section 14.5

8.2.5   Aldesleukin

Aldesleukin (recombinant interleukin-2) is licensed for use by intravenous infusion in metastatic renal cell carcinoma. This is a very toxic drug which, although responsible for tumour shrinkage in a small proportion of patients, has not been shown to increase survival. Toxicity is universal and often severe. A common acute problem is the development of a capillary leak syndrome causing pulmonary oedema and hypotension. Bone marrow, hepatic, renal, thyroid, and CNS toxicity is also common. It is for use in **specialist units only**. **Interactions:** Appendix 1 (aldesleukin)

PoM **Proleukin®** (Chiron)
Injection, powder for reconstitution, aldesleukin. Net price 18-million unit vial = £140.00
> For metastatic renal cell carcinoma, **excluding** patients in whom all three of the following prognostic factors are present; performance status of Eastern Co-operative Oncology Group of 1 or greater, more than one organ with metastatic disease sites, and a period of less than 24 months between initial diagnosis of primary tumour and date of evaluation of treatment.

8.3   Sex hormones and hormone antagonists in malignant disease

8.3.1   Oestrogens
8.3.2   Progestogens
8.3.3   Androgens
8.3.4   Hormone antagonists

Hormonal manipulation has an important role in the treatment of metastatic breast, prostate, and endometrial cancer, and a more marginal role in the treatment of hypernephroma. These treatments are not curative, but may provide excellent palliation of symptoms in selected patients, sometimes for a period of years. Tumour response, and treatment toxicity should be carefully monitored and treatment changed if progression occurs or side-effects exceed benefit.

8.3.1   Oestrogens

Stilboestrol is now rarely used to treat prostate cancer because of its side-effects. It is also occasionally used in postmenopausal women with breast cancer. Toxicity is common and dose-related side-effects include nausea, fluid retention, and venous and arterial thrombosis. Impotence and gynaecomastia always occur in men, and withdrawal bleeding may be a problem in women. Hypercalcaemia and bone pain may also occur in breast cancer.

Fosfestrol is also used for prostate cancer; it is activated by the enzyme acid phosphatase to produce stilboestrol. Side-effects are as for stilboestrol; in addition, perineal pain may complicate intravenous use.

Ethinyloestradiol is the most potent oestrogen available; unlike other oestrogens it is only slowly metabolised in the liver. It is used in breast cancer.

Polyestradiol is a long-acting oestrogen.

STILBOESTROL
(Diethylstilbestrol)
Indications: see notes above
Cautions; Side-effects: cardiovascular disease (sodium retention with oedema, thromboembolism), hepatic impairment (jaundice), feminising effects in men; see also notes above
Dose: breast cancer, 10–20 mg daily
Prostate cancer, 1–3 mg daily

PoM **Stilboestrol** (Non-proprietary)
Tablets, stilboestrol 1 mg, net price 56 = £8.33; 5 mg, 28 = £7.08
Available from APS (Apstil®)

ETHINYLOESTRADIOL
Indications: see notes above; other indications, see section 6.4.1.1
Cautions; Side-effects: see under Stilboestrol and notes above
Dose: breast cancer, 1–3 mg daily

Preparations
See section 6.4.1.1

FOSFESTROL TETRASODIUM

Indications: prostate cancer

Cautions; Contra-indications; Side-effects: see under Stilboestrol and notes above; nausea and vomiting; after intravenous injection, perineal irritation and pain in bony metastases

Dose: by slow intravenous injection, 600–1200 mg daily for at least 5 days; maintenance 300 mg 1–4 times weekly

By mouth, maintenance, initially up to 240 mg 3 times daily for 7 days then reducing over 14 days to 120–360 mg daily in divided doses

PoM **Honvan**® (ASTA Medica)

Tablets, f/c, fosfestrol tetrasodium 120 mg. Net price 100-tab pack = £15.51

Note. Fosfestrol tetrasodium 100 mg tablets have now been replaced by 120 mg tablets

Injection, fosfestrol tetrasodium 60 mg/mL. Net price 5-mL amp = £1.50

POLYESTRADIOL PHOSPHATE

Indications: prostate cancer

Cautions; Side-effects: see under Stilboestrol and notes above

Dose: by deep intramuscular injection, 80–160 mg every 4 weeks; maintenance 40–80 mg

PoM **Estradurin**® (Pharmacia)

Injection, powder for reconstitution, polyestradiol phosphate (with mepivacaine and nicotinamide). Net price 80-mg vial (with diluent) = £3.86

8.3.2 Progestogens

Progestogens are used largely as second- or third-line therapy in breast cancer. They are also used to treat endometrial cancer and hypernephroma, but are little used for prostate cancer. **Medroxyprogesterone** or **megestrol** are usually chosen and can be given orally; high-dose or parenteral treatment cannot be recommended. Side-effects are mild but may include nausea, fluid retention, and weight gain.

GESTRONOL HEXANOATE

(Gestronone Caproate)

Indications: see notes above; benign prostatic hypertrophy

Cautions; Contra-indications; Side-effects: see under Medroxyprogesterone acetate (section 6.4.1.2) and notes above

Dose: endometrial cancer, *by intramuscular injection,* 200–400 mg every 5–7 days

Benign prostatic hypertrophy, *by intramuscular injection,* 200 mg every week, increased to 300–400 mg every week if necessary

PoM **Depostat**® (Schering Health)

Injection (oily), gestronol hexanoate 100 mg/mL. Net price 2-mL amp = £4.28

MEDROXYPROGESTERONE ACETATE

Indications: see notes above; other indications, see section 6.4.1.2

Cautions; Contra-indications; Side-effects: see section 6.4.1.2 and notes above; glucocorticoid effects at high dose may lead to a cushingoid syndrome; **interactions:** see Appendix 1 (progestogens)

Dose: by mouth, endometrial, prostate, and renal cancer, 100–500 mg daily; breast cancer, various doses in range 0.4–1.5 g daily

By deep intramuscular injection into the gluteal muscle, various doses in range 1 g daily down to 250 mg weekly

PoM **Depo-Provera**® (Upjohn)

Injection, medroxyprogesterone acetate 150 mg/mL. Net price 3.3-mL (500-mg) vial = £12.49

PoM **Farlutal**® (Pharmacia)

Tablets, both scored, medroxyprogesterone acetate 100 mg, net price 20 = £8.12; 250 mg, 50 = £50.73

Tablets, scored, medroxyprogesterone acetate 500 mg. Net price 56 = £113.63. Label: 27

Injection, medroxyprogesterone acetate 200 mg/mL. Net price 2.5-mL vial = £13.88; 5-mL vial = £23.14

PoM **Provera**® (Upjohn)

Tablets, medroxyprogesterone acetate 100 mg (scored), net price 60-tab pack = £24.98; 200 mg (scored), 30-tab pack = £24.71; 400 mg, 30-tab pack = £48.89

Tablets, medroxyprogesterone acetate 2.5 mg, 5 mg and 10 mg, see section 6.4.1.2

MEGESTROL ACETATE

Indications: see notes above

Cautions; Contra-indications; Side-effects: see under Medroxyprogesterone acetate (section 6.4.1.2) and notes above

Dose: breast cancer, 160 mg daily in single or divided doses; endometrial cancer, 40–320 mg daily in divided doses

PoM **Megace**® (Bristol-Myers)

Tablets, both scored, megestrol acetate 40 mg, net price 20 = £5.08; 160 mg (off-white), 30-tab pack = £29.30

NORETHISTERONE

Indications: see notes above; other indications, see section 6.4.1.2

Cautions; Contra-indications; Side-effects: see section 6.4.1.2 and notes above; **interactions:** see Appendix 1 (progestogens)

Dose: breast cancer, 40 mg daily, increased to 60 mg daily if required

Preparations

See section 6.4.1.2

8.3.3   Androgens

The androgens are given parenterally and are occasionally still used as second- or third-line therapy for metastatic breast cancer.

TESTOSTERONE ESTERS

Indications: see notes above; other indications, see section 6.4.2

Cautions; Contra-indications; Side-effects: see under Testosterone and Esters (section 6.4.2)

Dose: see under Preparations

PoM **Primoteston Depot**® (Schering Health)
See section 6.4.2

PoM **Virormone**® (Paines & Byrne)
See section 6.4.2

8.3.4   Hormone antagonists

8.3.4.1 BREAST CANCER

Tamoxifen is an oestrogen receptor antagonist and at a dose of 20 mg daily is the hormonal treatment of choice for breast cancer in postmenopausal women with metastatic disease; it is also increasingly commonly used as a first-line treatment for premenopausal women. Overall, approximately 30% of patients with metastatic breast cancer respond to hormonal manipulation. This figure is increased to 60% in patients with oestrogen receptor positive tumours; receptor negative tumours respond in less than 10%.

Adjuvant hormonal treatment with tamoxifen 20 mg daily is also the treatment of choice in postmenopausal patients with high-risk breast cancer after treatment of the primary. Such treatment has consistently prolonged the period between diagnosis and the development of metastates and has also clearly increased survival. Tamoxifen is also increasingly commonly used as adjuvant treatment for premenopausal women with early breast cancer.

Side-effects are unusual with tamoxifen but patients with bony metastases may experience an exacerbation of pain, sometimes associated with hypercalcaemia. This reaction commonly precedes tumour response. Amenorrhoea commonly develops in premenopausal women. For details of endometrial changes see under Cautions (below) and for CSM advice see under Dose (below)

Patients with non-threatening metastases unresponsive to tamoxifen may still respond to a secondary hormonal treatment. Certainly patients who initially respond to tamoxifen should receive second-line hormone treatment. No clear guidelines are available; for premenopausal patients oophorectomy or a progestogen (section 8.3.2) may be used; for postmenopausal patients a progestogen or aminoglutethimide (see below) may be used. Patients who respond can be given further hormones on relapse; refractory patients are better treated with chemotherapy or palliative therapy.

Toremifene, also an oestrogen receptor antagonist, is licensed for hormone-dependent metastatic breast cancer in postmenopausal women.

Aminoglutethimide has largely replaced adrenalectomy in postmenopausal women with breast cancer; it acts predominantly by inhibiting the conversion of androgens to oestrogens in the peripheral tissues. Corticosteroid replacement therapy is necessary (see section 6.3.1). Early toxicity is common and may include drowsiness, drug fever, and a morbilliform eruption; these side-effects generally settle spontaneously. The dose of aminoglutethimide is usually increased to 500 mg daily over 2 to 4 weeks. Hepatic enzyme induction occurs, and may require modification of the doses of other drugs (e.g. oral anticoagulants).

Trilostane (section 6.7.3) is also indicated for postmenopausal breast cancer. It is quite well tolerated but diarrhoea and abdominal discomfort may be a problem. Like aminoglutethimide, trilostane is an adrenal antagonist therefore corticosteroid replacement therapy is needed.

Formestane, an inhibitor of the enzyme aromatase (which metabolises androgens to oestrogens) is indicated for breast cancer in women with natural or artificial postmenopausal status.

Anastrozole is a selective non-steroidal aromatase inhibitor used to treat advanced postmenopausal breast cancer; steroid replacement therapy is not necessary.

Goserelin, a gonadorelin analogue is now also indicated for management of advanced breast cancer in premenopausal women.

TAMOXIFEN

Indications: see under Dose and notes above

Cautions: occasional cystic ovarian swellings in premenopausal women, occasional hypercalcaemia if bony metastases; increased risk of thromboembolic events when used with cytotoxics; porphyria (see section 9.8.2); **interactions:** Appendix 1 (tamoxifen)

ENDOMETRIAL CHANGES. An increased incidence of endometrial changes, including hyperplasia, polyps and cancer, has been reported in association with tamoxifen. Abnormal vaginal bleeding including menstrual irregularities, vaginal discharge and symptoms such as pelvic pain or pressure in those receiving (or who have previously received) tamoxifen should be promptly investigated.

Contra-indications: pregnancy (exclude before commencing and advise non-hormonal contraception if appropriate) and breast-feeding

Side-effects: hot flushes, vaginal bleeding (**important:** see also Cautions) or suppression of menstruation in some pre-menopausal women, vaginal discharge (**important:** see also Cautions) pruritus vulvae, gastro-intestinal disturbances, light-headedness, tumour flare, falls in platelet counts; occasionally fluid retention, alopecia, rashes, uterine fibroids; also visual disturbances (including corneal changes, cataracts, retinopathy—usually with very high doses); leucopenia (sometimes with anaemia and thrombocytopenia), rarely neutropenia; liver enzyme changes (rarely fatty liver, cholestasis, hepatitis); see also notes above

Dose: breast cancer, 20 mg daily

CSM ADVICE. The CSM has advised that tamoxifen in a dose of 20 mg daily substantially increases survival in early breast cancer, and that no further benefit has been demonstrated with higher doses. Patients should be told of the small risk of endometrial cancer (see under Cautions above) and encouraged to report relevant symptoms early. They can, however, be reassured that the benefits of treatment far outweigh the risks

Anovulatory infertility, 20 mg daily on second, third, fourth and fifth days of cycle; if necessary the daily dose may be increased to 40 mg then 80 mg for subsequent courses; if cycles irregular, start initial course on any day, with subsequent course starting 45 days later *or* on second day of cycle if menstruation occurs

oM **Tamoxifen** (Non-proprietary)

Tablets, tamoxifen (as citrate) 10 mg, net price 30-tab pack = £2.95; 20 mg, 30-tab pack = £3.70; 40 mg, 30-tab pack = £15.07
Various strengths available from APS, Ashbourne (Oestrifen®), Berk (Emblon®), Cox, CP, Kent, Lagap, Lederle (Noltam®), Norton, Opus (Fentamox®), Pharmacia (Tamofen®)

oM **Nolvadex®** (Zeneca)

Tablets, tamoxifen (as citrate) 10 mg, net price 30-tab pack = £6.05; 20 mg (Nolvadex-D®), 30-tab pack = £9.12; 40 mg (scored, Nolvadex-Forte®), 30-tab pack = £21.45

AMINOGLUTETHIMIDE

Indications: see notes above and under Dose

Cautions: see notes above; adrenal hypofunction (see below); monitor blood pressure, plasma electrolytes, blood counts, and thyroid function; **interactions:** Appendix 1 (aminoglutethimide)

ADRENAL HYPOFUNCTION. May cause adrenal hypofunction especially under conditions of stress (such as surgery, trauma, or acute illness), therefore corticosteroid replacement therapy is necessary (see section 6.3.1). If a synthetic glucocorticoid such as dexamethasone is used instead of hydrocortisone a relatively high dose may be needed (metabolism of synthetic corticosteroids accelerated)

Contra-indications: pregnancy (advise non-hormonal contraceptive methods if appropriate) and breast-feeding; porphyria (see section 9.8.2)

Side-effects: see notes above; drowsiness, lethargy, rash (sometimes with fever—usually in first 2 weeks and resolves despite continued administration); occasionally dizziness, nausea; other side-effects reported include ataxia, headache, depression, insomnia, pruritus, urticaria, diarrhoea, vomiting, constipation, anorexia, sweating, hypotension, adrenal insufficiency, hyponatraemia, hypoglycaemia, agranulocytosis, leucopenia, thrombocytopenia, hyperkalaemia, exfoliaive dermatitis, Stevens-Johnson syndrome, hypothyroidism, inappropriate ADH-secretion, masculinisation and hirsuitism in females, renal impairment, pancytopenia, anaemia, allergy, anaphylactic reactions, allergic alveolitis (withdraw immediately if suspected), cholestatic hepatitis, confusion

Dose: advanced breast or prostate cancer, 250 mg daily, increased once a week to max. 250 mg 4 times daily (in breast cancer 250 mg twice daily has proved sufficient in some patients; in prostate cancer up to 750 mg daily is usually satisfactory); given with a glucocorticoid (and sometimes with a mineralocorticoid as well)

Cushing's syndrome due to malignant disease, 250 mg daily, increased gradually to 1 g daily in divided doses (occasionally 1.5–2 g daily); glucocorticoid given only if necessary

PoM Orimeten® (Ciba)

Tablets, scored, aminoglutethimide 250 mg. Net price 56-tab pack = £20.22. Label: 2
Note. Tablets containing aminoglutethimide 250 mg are also available from Pharmacia

ANASTROZOLE

Indications: advanced breast cancer in postmenopausal women

Cautions: laboratory test for menopause if doubt

Contra-indications: pregnancy and breast-feeding; moderate or severe hepatic disease, severe renal impairment; not for premenopausal women

Side-effects: hot flushes, vaginal dryness, hair thinning, anorexia, nausea, vomiting, diarrhoea, headache, rash; asthenia and somnolence—may initially affect ability to drive or operate machinery; slight increases in total cholesterol levels reported

Dose: 1 mg daily

▼ **PoM Arimidex®** (Zeneca)

Tablets, f/c, anastrozole 1 mg. Net price 28-tab pack = £83.16 (also 84-tab pack, hosp. only)

FORMESTANE

Indications: advanced breast cancer in women with natural or artificial postmenopausal status

Cautions: no studies performed in diabetes mellitus (monitor blood glucose)

DRIVING. Drowsiness may affect performance of skilled tasks (e.g. driving)

Contra-indications: not indicated for premenopausal women; pregnancy and breast-feeding

Side-effects: occasionally rash, pruritus, exanthema, hot flushes; facial hypertrichosis, alopecia, lethargy, drowsiness, emotional lability, headache, dizziness, oedema of lower leg, thrombophlebitis, vaginal bleeding, pelvic cramps, nausea, vomiting, constipation, arthralgia, muscle cramps, sore throat, and anaphylactoid reaction also reported; pain and irritation common at injection site (with occasional sterile abscess and haematoma)

Dose: by deep intramuscular injection in the gluteal muscle, 250 mg every 2 weeks (alternate sites)

▼ **PoM Lentaron®** (Ciba)

Injection, powder for reconstitution, formestane 250 mg. Net price 250-mg vial (with diluent) = £72.73. Counselling, driving

---

GOSERELIN

See section 8.3.4.2

TOREMIFENE

Indications: hormone-dependent metastatic breast cancer in postmenopausal women

Cautions: hypercalcaemia may occur (especially if bone metastases and usually at beginning of treatment); **interactions:** Appendix 1 (toremifene)

ENDOMETRIAL CHANGES. There is a risk of increased endometrial changes including hyperplasia, polyps and cancer. Abnormal vaginal bleeding including menstrual irregularities, vaginal discharge and symptoms such as pelvic pain or pressure should be promptly investigated

Contra-indications: endometrial hyperplasia, severe hepatic impairment, history of severe thromboembolic disease; pregnancy and breast-feeding

Side-effects: hot flushes, vaginal bleeding or discharge (**important:** see also Cautions), dizziness, oedema, sweating, nausea, vomiting, chest or back pain, fatigue, headache, skin discoloration, weight increase, insomnia, constipation, dyspnoea, paresis, tremor, vertigo, pruritus, anorexia, corneal opacity (reversible), asthenia; thromboembolic events reported; rarely dermatitis, alopecia, emotional lability, depression, jaundice, stiffness

Dose: 60 mg daily

▼ PoM **Fareston®** (Orion)

Tablets, toremifene (as citrate) 60 mg. Net price 30-tab pack = £31.80

TRILOSTANE

See section 6.7.3

8.3.4.2 PROSTATE CANCER

Metastatic cancer of the prostate is commonly responsive to hormonal treatment designed to deprive the cancer of androgen. Treatment is probably best reserved for symptomatic metastatic disease. The standard treatment is bilateral subcapsular orchidectomy, which commonly results in responses lasting 12–18 months. Alternatively, a gonadorelin analogue such as **buserelin**, **goserelin**, **leuprorelin**, or **triptorelin** may be given. These are as effective as orchidectomy or **stilboestrol** (section 8.3.1) but are expensive and require parenteral administration, at least initially. They cause initial stimulation of luteinising hormone release by the pituitary, which in turn causes testosterone secretion by the testis; this is followed by inhibition of luteinising hormone release with achievement of an anorchic state. During the first 1 to 2 weeks of treatment a number of patients develop a tumour 'flare' which may cause spinal cord compression or increased bone pain. When such problems are anticipated, alternative treatments (e.g. orchidectomy) or the additional use of an anti-androgen such as cyproterone acetate or flutamide (see below) are recommended; anti-androgen treatment should be started 3 days before the gonadorelin analogue and continued for 3 weeks. Other side-effects of gonadorelin analogues are similar to those of orchidectomy.

Cyproterone acetate, flutamide and **bicalutamide** are anti-androgens which can be used to cover the tumour 'flare' which may occur after commencing gonadorelin analogue administration.

Alternative therapies if disease progression occurs despite orchidectomy or administration of gonadorelin analogue, include the use of radiotherapy, strontium, aminoglutethimide or prednisolone. Such second-line treatment may palliate symptoms well, but rarely results in appreciable disease regression.

AMINOGLUTETHIMIDE

See section 8.3.4.1

BICALUTAMIDE

Indications: advanced prostate cancer, see notes above

Cautions: hepatic impairment (monitor hepatic function); **interactions:** Appendix 1 (bicalutamide)

Side-effects: hot flushes, pruritus, breast tenderness, gynaecomastia, asthenia, somnolence; transient elevation of transaminase levels, cholestasis and jaundice (rarely hepatic failure); rarely thrombocytopenia, cardiovascular disorders (including angina, heart failure, conduction defects, arrhythmias and ECG changes); other effects (more common in elderly) include anorexia, dry mouth, dyspepsia, constipation, flatulence, dizziness, insomnia, decreased libido, impotence, dyspnoea, nocturia, alopecia, rashes, sweating, hyperglycaemia, peripheral oedema, weight changes, chest and abdominal pain

Dose: 50 mg daily (see also notes above)

▼ PoM **Casodex®** (Zeneca)

Tablets, f/c, bicalutamide 50 mg. Net price 28-tab pack = £128.00

BUSERELIN

Indications: advanced prostate cancer; other indications, see section 6.7.2

Cautions: during first month monitor patients at risk of ureteric obstruction or spinal cord compression; see notes above

Side-effects: initial increase in bone pain (due to transient increases in plasma testosterone); hot flushes, decreased libido, depression, headache, dizziness, nausea, vomiting, and diarrhoea, infrequent gynaecomastia, urticaria; irritation of nasal mucosa (spray formulation only)

Dose: by *subcutaneous injection*, 500 micrograms every 8 hours for 7 days, then *intranasally*, 1 spray into each nostril 6 times daily (see also notes above)

COUNSELLING. Avoid use of nasal decongestants before and for at least 30 minutes after treatment.

PoM Suprefact® (Hoechst)

Injection, buserelin 1 mg (as acetate)/mL. Net price 2 × 5.5-mL vial = £29.61

Nasal spray, buserelin 100 micrograms (as acetate)/metered spray. Net price treatment pack of 4 × 10-g bottle with spray pump = £97.42. Counselling, see above

CYPROTERONE ACETATE

Indications: prostate cancer, see notes above and for CSM advice see below; other indications, see section 6.4.2

RESTRICTION ON USE. The CSM has advised that in view of the hepatotoxicity associated with long-term doses of 300 mg daily the use of cyproterone acetate in prostate cancer should be restricted to short courses to cover testosterone flare associated with gonadorelin analogues, treatment of hot flushes after orchidectomy or gonadorelin analogues and for patients who have not responded to (or are intolerant of) other treatments

Cautions: in prostate cancer, blood counts initially and throughout treatment, monitor hepatic function (liver function tests should be performed before treatment, see also under Side-effects below); monitor adrenocortical function regularly; risk of recurrence of thromboembolic disease; diabetes mellitus, sickle-cell anaemia, severe depression (in other indications some of these are contra-indicated, see section 6.4.2)

Contra-indications: none in prostate cancer; for contra-indications relating to other indications see section 6.4.2

Side-effects: see section 6.4.2

HEPATOTOXICITY. Direct hepatic toxicity including jaundice, hepatitis and hepatic failure have been reported (usually after several months) in patients treated with cyproterone acetate 200–300 mg daily. Liver function tests should be performed before treatment and whenever symptoms suggestive of hepatotoxicity occur—if confirmed cyproterone should normally be withdrawn unless the hepatotoxicity can be explained by another cause such as metastatic disease (in which case cyproterone should be continued only if the perceived benefit exceeds the risk)

Dose: flare with initial gonadorelin therapy, 300 mg daily in 2–3 divided doses, reduced to 200 mg daily if necessary

Long-term palliative therapy where gonadorelin analogues or orchidectomy contra-indicated, not tolerated, or where oral therapy preferred, 200–300 mg daily

Hot flushes with gonadorelin therapy or after orchidectomy, 50 mg daily; usual range 50–150 mg daily in 1–3 divided doses

PoM Cyprostat® (Schering Health)

Tablets, scored, cyproterone acetate 50 mg net price 168-tab pack = £96.70; 100 mg, 84-tab pack = £96.70. Label: 3, 21

Note. Tablets containing cyproterone acetate 50 mg are also available from Cox, Generics, Hillcross, Lagap

FLUTAMIDE

Indications: advanced prostate cancer, see notes above

Cautions: cardiac disease (sodium retention with oedema); monitor hepatic function (hepatotoxic); **interactions:** Appendix 1 (flutamide)

Side-effects: gynaecomastia (sometimes with galactorrhoea); nausea, vomiting, diarrhoea, increased appetite, insomnia, tiredness; other side-effects reported include decreased libido, inhibition of spermatogenesis, gastric and chest pain, headache, dizziness, oedema, blurred vision, thirst, rashes, pruritus, haemolytic anaemia, systemic lupus erythematosus-like syndrome, and lymphoedema; hepatic injury (with transaminase abnormalities, cholestatic jaundice, hepatic necrosis, encephalopathy and occasional fatality) reported

Dose: 250 mg 3 times daily (see also notes above)

PoM Drogenil® (Schering-Plough)

Tablets, yellow, scored, flutamide 250 mg, net price 84-tab pack = £110.00

Note. Tablets containing flutamide 250 mg are also available from Cox

GOSERELIN

Indications: prostate cancer; advanced breast cancer; endometriosis and endometrial thinning, see section 6.7.2

Cautions; Side-effects: see under Buserelin; also rashes (reversible without stopping therapy); bruising at injection site; rarely hypercalcaemia in breast cancer patients

Dose: see under individual preparations

PoM Zoladex® (Zeneca)

Implant, goserelin 3.6 mg (as acetate) in syringe applicator. Net price each = £122.27

Dose: advanced breast cancer and prostate cancer by *subcutaneous injection* into anterior abdominal wall, 3.6 mg every 28 days (see also notes above)

PoM Zoladex® LA (Zeneca)

Implant, goserelin 10.8 mg (as acetate) in syringe applicator. Net price each = £366.81

Dose: prostate cancer, by *subcutaneous injection* into anterior abdominal wall, 10.8 mg every 12 weeks (see also notes above); not indicated for female patients

LEUPRORELIN ACETATE

Indications: advanced prostate cancer; endometriosis, see section 6.7.2

Cautions; Side-effects: see under Buserelin; also, infrequently, peripheral oedema, fatigue, nausea, irritation at injection site; rotate injection site periodically

Dose: by *subcutaneous or by intramuscular injection,* 3.75 mg every 4 weeks (see also notes above)

PoM Prostap SR® (Lederle)

Injection (microcapsule powder for aqueous suspension), leuprorelin acetate, net price 3.75-mg vial with 2-mL vehicle-filled syringe = £125.40

TRIPTORELIN

Indications: advanced prostate cancer

Cautions; Side-effects: see under Buserelin; also phlebitis, transient hypertension; rarely gastric pain, dry mouth, recurrence af asthma, dysuria, fever, pruritus, sweating, paraesthesia, insomnia, excessive salivation, vertigo, slight hair loss; pain, erythema and induration at injection site also reported

Dose: by intramuscular injection, 3 mg every 4 weeks (see also notes above)

▼ PoM **De-capeptyl**® **sr** (Speywood)
Injection (copolymer microsphere powder for aqueous suspension), triptorelin. Net price 4.2-mg vial (with diluent) = £110.00

8.3.4.3 GASTRO-ENTEROPANCREATIC TUMOURS

Octreotide is a long-acting analogue of the hypothalamic release-inhibiting hormone somatostatin; it is indicated for the relief of symptoms associated with gastro-enteropancreatic endocrine tumours and acromegaly.

OCTREOTIDE

Indications: see under Dose

Cautions: occasional sudden escape from symptomatic control with rapid recurrence of severe symptoms; in insulinoma may increase depth and duration of hypoglycaemia (close observation initially and with dose changes; marked fluctuations may be reduced by increasing administration frequency); in diabetes mellitus may reduce insulin or oral antidiabetic requirements; monitor thyroid function on long-term therapy; inhibits gallbladder motility, bile secretion and flow—ultrasonic examination of gall bladder before and at intervals of 6–12 months during treatment; avoid abrupt withdrawal (see side-effects below); **interactions:** Appendix 1 (octreotide)

Contra-indications: pregnancy (unless compelling reasons) and breast-feeding

Side-effects: gastro-intestinal disturbances including anorexia, nausea, vomiting, abdominal pa and bloating, flatulence, diarrhoea, and steato rhoea; symptoms may be reduced by injectin between meals or at bedtime; impairment of pos prandial glucose tolerance (rarely persiste hyperglycaemia on chronic administration hepatic disturbance reported; gall stone formatic reported after long-term treatment (abrupt wit drawal may result in biliary hypercontractili with associated biliary colic and pancreatitis pain and irritation at injection site (rotate sites)

Dose: symptoms associated with carcino tumours with features of carcinoid syndrom VIPomas, glucagonomas, *by subcutaneous inje tion*, initially 50 micrograms once or twice dail gradually increased according to response 200 micrograms 3 times daily (higher dos required exceptionally); maintenance doses vari ble; in carcinoid tumours discontinue after 1 wee if no effect; if rapid response required, initial do *by intravenous injection* (with ECG monitorin and after dilution to a concentration of 10–50 with sodium chloride 0.9% injection)

Acromegaly, short-term treatment before pituita surgery *or* long-term treatment in those inad quately controlled by other treatment *or* un radiotherapy becomes fully effective *by subcut neous injection*, 100–200 micrograms 3 time daily; discontinue if no improvement within months

PoM **Sandostatin**® (Sandoz)
Injection, octreotide (as acetate)
    50 micrograms/mL, 1-mL amp = £2.90;
    100 micrograms/mL, 1-mL amp = £5.46;
    200 micrograms/mL 5-mL vial = £54.39;
    500 micrograms/mL, 1-mL amp = £26.45

9: Drugs affecting
NUTRITION and BLOOD

In this chapter drugs and preparations are discussed under the following headings:

9.1   Anaemias and some other blood disorders
9.2   Fluids and electrolytes
9.3   Intravenous nutrition
9.4   Oral nutrition
9.5   Minerals
9.6   Vitamins
9.7   Bitters and tonics
9.8   Metabolic disorders

9.1   Anaemias and some other blood disorders

9.1.1   Iron-deficiency anaemias
9.1.2   Megaloblastic anaemias
9.1.3   Hypoplastic and haemolytic anaemias
9.1.4   Autoimmune thrombocytopenic purpura
9.1.5   G6PD deficiency
9.1.6   Drugs used in neutropenia

Before initiating treatment for anaemia it is essential to determine which type is present. Iron salts may be harmful and result in iron overload if given alone to patients with anaemias other than those due to iron deficiency.

9.1.1 Iron-deficiency anaemias

9.1.1.1 Oral iron
9.1.1.2 Parenteral iron

Treatment is only justified in the presence of a demonstrable iron-deficiency state.
Prophylaxis is justifiable in pregnancy for women who have additional risk factors for iron deficiency (e.g. poor diet), menorrhagia, after subtotal or total gastrectomy, and in the management of low birth-weight infants such as premature babies, twins, and in infants delivered by caesarean section.

9.1.1.1 ORAL IRON

Iron salts should be given by mouth unless there are good reasons for using another route.

Ferrous salts show only marginal differences between one another in efficiency of absorption of iron, but ferric salts are much less well absorbed. Haemoglobin regeneration rate is little affected by the type of salt used provided sufficient iron is given, and in most patients the time factor is not critical. Choice of preparation is thus usually decided by incidence of side-effects and cost.

The oral dose of elemental iron for deficiency should be 100 to 200 mg daily. It is customary to give this as dried **ferrous sulphate**, 200 mg (≡ 65 mg elemental iron) three times daily; a dose of ferrous sulphate 200 mg once or twice daily may be effective for prophylaxis or for mild iron defi-ciency. If side-effects arise, dosage can be reduced or a change made to an alternative iron salt. It should be remembered, however, that an apparent improvement in tolerance on changing to another salt may be due to its lower content of elemental iron. The incidence of side-effects due to ferrous sulphate is no greater than with other iron salts when compared on the basis of equivalent amounts of elemental iron.

Iron content of different iron salts

Iron salt	Amount	Content of ferrous iron
Ferrous fumarate	200 mg	65 mg
Ferrous gluconate	300 mg	35 mg
Ferrous succinate	100 mg	35 mg
Ferrous sulphate	300 mg	60 mg
Ferrous sulphate, dried	200 mg	65 mg

THERAPEUTIC RESPONSE. The haemoglobin concentration should rise by about 100–200 mg per 100 mL (1–2 g per litre) per day *or* 2 g/100 mL (20 g/litre) over 3–4 weeks. After the haemoglobin has risen to normal, treatment should be continued for a further three months in an attempt to replenish the iron stores. Epithelial tissue changes such as atrophic glossitis and koilonychia are usually improved although the response is often slow.

COMPOUND PREPARATIONS. Some oral preparations contain ascorbic acid to aid absorption, or the iron is in the form of a chelate, which can be shown experimentally to produce a modest increase in absorption of iron. However, the therapeutic advantage is minimal and cost may be increased.

There is neither theoretical nor clinical justification for the inclusion of other therapeutically active ingredients, such as the B group of vitamins (except folic acid for pregnant women, see Iron and Folic Acid below and p. 377).

MODIFIED-RELEASE CAPSULES AND TABLETS. These are designed to release iron gradually as the capsule or tablet passes along the gut so that a smaller amount of iron is present in the lumen at any one time. It is claimed that each dose unit contains enough iron for 24 hours, thus permitting once daily dosage.

These preparations are likely to carry the iron past the first part of the duodenum into an area of the gut where conditions for iron absorption are poor. The low incidence of side-effects may well be because of the small amounts of iron available under these conditions and so the preparations have no therapeutic advantage and should not be used.

SIDE-EFFECTS. Because iron salts are astringent, gastro-intestinal irritation may occur. Nausea and

---

Cautionary label wordings, see inside back cover   Prices are **net**, see p. 1

epigastric pain are dose-related but the relationship between dose and altered bowel habit (constipation or diarrhoea) is less clear. Oral iron, particularly modified-release preparations, may exacerbate diarrhoea in patients with inflammatory bowel disease; care is also needed in patients with intestinal strictures and diverticulae.

Iron preparations taken orally may have a constipating effect particularly in older patients, occasionally leading to faecal impaction.

FERROUS SULPHATE

Indications: iron-deficiency anaemia

Cautions: pregnancy; **interactions:** Appendix 1 (iron)

Side-effects: see notes above

Dose: see under preparations below

COUNSELLING. Although iron preparations are best absorbed on an empty stomach they may be taken after food to reduce gastro-intestinal side-effects; they may discolour stools

Ferrous Sulphate (Non-proprietary)

Tablets, coated, dried ferrous sulphate 200 mg (65 mg iron), net price 20 = 11p

Dose: prophylactic, 1 tablet daily; therapeutic, 1 tablet 2–3 times daily

Ferrous Sulphate Oral Solution, Paediatric, BP
(Paediatric Ferrous Sulphate Mixture)

Mixture, ferrous sulphate 1.2% and a suitable antioxidant in a suitable vehicle with an orange flavour. Extemporaneous preparations should be recently prepared according to the following formula: ferrous sulphate 60 mg, ascorbic acid 10 mg, orange syrup 0.5 mL, double-strength chloroform water 2.5 mL, water to 5 mL

Dose: therapeutic, CHILD up to 1 year, 5 mL 3 times daily; 1–5 years, 10 mL 3 times daily; 6–12 years, 15 mL 3 times daily *or* 25 mL twice daily. To be taken well diluted with water

Modified-release preparations

NHS **Feospan®** (Evans)

Spansule® (= capsules m/r), clear/red, enclosing green and brown pellets, dried ferrous sulphate 150 mg (47 mg iron). Net price 30-cap pack = 90p. Label: 25

Dose: 1–2 capsules daily; CHILD over 1 year 1 capsule daily; can be opened and sprinkled on food

Ferrograd® (Abbott)

Filmtabs® (= tablets f/c), m/r, red, dried ferrous sulphate 325 mg (105 mg iron). Net price 30-tab pack = 54p. Label: 25

Dose: 1 tablet daily before food

Slow-Fe® (Ciba)

Tablets, m/r, dried ferrous sulphate 160 mg (50 mg iron). Net price 28-tab pack = 25p. Label: 25

Dose: prophylactic, 1 tablet daily; therapeutic, 2 tablets daily; CHILD over 6 years, 1 tablet daily

FERROUS FUMARATE

Indications; Cautions; Side-effects: see under Ferrous Sulphate

Dose: see under preparations below

Fersaday® (Goldshield)

Tablets, orange, f/c, ferrous fumarate 322 mg (100 mg iron). Net price 28-tab pack = 50p

Dose: prophylactic, 1 tablet daily; therapeutic, 1 tablet twice daily

Fersamal® (Forley)

Tablets, brown, ferrous fumarate 200 mg (65 mg iron). Net price 20 = 23p

Dose: 1–2 tablets 3 times daily

Syrup, brown, ferrous fumarate 140 mg (45 mg iron)/5 mL. Net price 200 mL = £2.35

Dose: 10–20 mL twice daily; PREMATURE INFANT 0.6–2.4 mL/kg daily; CHILD up to 6 years 2.5–5 mL twice daily

Galfer® (Galen)

Capsules, red/green, ferrous fumarate 305 mg (100 mg iron). Net price 20 = 36p

Dose: 1 capsule 1–2 times daily before food

Syrup, brown, sugar-free ferrous fumarate 140 mg (45 mg iron)/5 mL. Net price 300 mL = £4.86

Dose: 10 mL 1–2 times daily before food; CHILD (full-term infant and young child) 2.5–5 mL 1–2 times daily

FERROUS GLUCONATE

Indications; Cautions; Side-effects: see under Ferrous Sulphate

Dose: see under preparations below

Ferrous Gluconate (Non-proprietary)

Tablets, red, coated, ferrous gluconate 300 mg (35 mg iron). Net price 20 = 11p

Dose: prophylactic, 2 tablets daily before food; therapeutic, 4–6 tablets daily in divided doses before food; CHILD 6–12 years, prophylactic and therapeutic, 1–3 tablets daily

FERROUS GLYCINE SULPHATE

Indications; Cautions; Side-effects: see under Ferrous Sulphate

Dose: see under preparations below

Plesmet® (Link)

Syrup, ferrous glycine sulphate equivalent to 25 mg iron/5 mL. Net price 100 mL = 65p

Dose: 5–10 mL 3 times daily; CHILD 2.5–5 mL 1–3 times daily, according to age

Modified-release preparations

Ferrocontin Continus® (ASTA Medica)

Tablets, m/r, red, f/c, ferrous glycine sulphate equivalent to 100 mg iron. Net price 30-tab pack = 94p. Label: 25

Dose: 1 tablet daily

POLYSACCHARIDE-IRON COMPLEX

Indications; Cautions; Side-effects: see under Ferrous Sulphate

Dose: see under preparations below

Niferex® (Tillomed)

Elixir, brown, sugar-free, polysaccharide-iron complex equivalent to 100 mg of iron/5 mL. Net price 240-mL pack = £6.06; NHS* 30-mL dropper bottle for paediatric use = £2.16. Counselling, use of dropper

Dose: prophylactic, 2.5 mL daily; therapeutic, 5 mL daily; INFANT, 1 drop (from dropper bottle) per pound (450 g) body-weight 3 times daily; CHILD 2–6 years, 2.5 mL daily, 6–12 years 5 mL daily

* except 30 mL paediatric dropper bottle for prophylaxis and treatment of iron deficiency in infants born prematurely and endorsed 'SLS' ('S2B' in Scotland)

Niferex-150® (Tillomed)

Capsules, brown/orange, polysaccharide-iron complex equivalent to 150 mg of iron. Net price 20 = £2.28

Dose: 1–2 capsules daily

SODIUM IRONEDETATE

(Sodium feredetate)

Indications; Cautions; Side-effects: see under Ferrous Sulphate

Dose: see under preparations below

Sytron® (Link)

Elixir, sugar-free, sodium ironedetate 190 mg equivalent to 27.5 mg of iron/5 mL. Net price 100 mL = 99p

Dose: 5 mL increasing gradually to 10 mL 3 times daily; INFANT and PREMATURE INFANT 2.5 mL twice daily (smaller doses should be used initially); CHILD 1–5 years 2.5 mL 3 times daily, 6–12 years 5 mL 3 times daily

IRON AND FOLIC ACID

These preparations are used for the prevention of iron and folic acid deficiences in pregnancy; they should be distinguished from those used for the prevention of neural tube defects in women planning a pregnancy (see p. 377).

It is important to note that the small doses of folic acid contained in these preparations are inadequate for the treatment of megaloblastic anaemias.

NHS Fefol® (Evans)

Spansule® (=capsules m/r), clear/green, enclosing brown, yellow, and white pellets, dried ferrous sulphate 150 mg (47 mg iron), folic acid 500 micrograms. Net price 30-cap pack = £1.00. Label: 25

Dose: 1 capsule daily

Ferrocontin Folic Continus® (ASTA Medica)

Tablets, orange, f/c, ferrous glycine sulphate equivalent to 100 mg iron for sustained release, folic acid 500 micrograms. Net price 30-tab pack = £1.10. Label: 25

Dose: 1 tablet daily

Ferrograd Folic® (Abbott)

Filmtabs® (= tablets f/c), red/yellow, dried ferrous sulphate 325 mg (105 mg iron) for sustained release, folic acid 350 micrograms. Net price 30-tab pack = 60p. Label: 25

Dose: 1 tablet daily before food

Folex-350® (Rybar)

Tablets, pink, s/c, ferrous fumarate 308 mg (100 mg iron), folic acid 350 micrograms. Net price 30-tab pack = £2.00

Dose: 1 tablet daily

Fortespan® (SmithKline Beecham)

Spansule® (= capsules m/r), clear/green, enclosing red, yellow, and white pellets, dried ferrous sulphate 150 mg (47 mg iron), folic acid 500 micrograms. Net price 30-cap pack = £2.64. Label: 25

Dose: 1 capsule daily

Galfer FA® (Galen)

Capsules, red/yellow, ferrous fumarate 305 mg (100 mg iron), folic acid 350 micrograms. Net price 20 = 40p

Dose: 1 capsule daily before food

PoM **Lexpec with Iron-M®** (Rosemont)

Syrup, brown, sugar-free, ferric ammonium citrate equivalent to 80 mg iron, folic acid 500 micrograms/5 mL. Net price 125 mL = £3.60

Dose: 5–10 mL daily before food

Note. Lexpec with Iron-M® contains five times less folic acid than Lexpec with Iron®

Meterfolic® (Sinclair)

Tablets, grey, f/c, ferrous fumarate equivalent to 100 mg iron, folic acid 400 micrograms. Net price 30-tab pack = 60p

Dose: 1 tablet 1–2 times daily

Prevention of neural tube defects, 1 tablet daily started before conception and continued for at least first trimester

Pregaday® (Evans)

Tablets, brown, f/c, ferrous fumarate equivalent to 100 mg iron, folic acid 350 micrograms. Net price 28-tab pack = 51p

Dose: 1 tablet daily

PoM **Slow-Fe Folic®** (Ciba)

Tablets, m/r, ivory, f/c, dried ferrous sulphate 160 mg (50 mg iron), folic acid 400 micrograms. Net price 28-tab pack = 28p. Label: 25

Dose: 1–2 tablets daily

Higher folic acid content

Appropriate in context of prevention of *recurrence of neural tube defects*, see recommendations on p. 377 *Cautions:* have the theoretical disadvantage of masking anaemia due to vitamin-B_{12} deficiency (which could allow vitamin-B_{12} neuropathy to develop).

PoM **Ferfolic SV®** (Sinclair)

Tablets, pink, ferrous gluconate 250 mg (30 mg iron), folic acid 4 mg, ascorbic acid 10 mg. Net price 20 = 40p

Dose: anaemia, 1–3 tablets daily after food

Prophylaxis of neural tube defects in women known to be at risk, 1 tablet daily started before conception and continued for at least first trimester; see also recommendations on p. 377

PoM **Lexpec with Iron®** (Rosemont)

Syrup, brown, sugar-free, ferric ammonium citrate equivalent to 80 mg iron, folic acid 2.5 mg/5 mL. Net price 125 mL = £3.60

Dose: 5–10 mL daily before food

Note. Lexpec with Iron® contains five times as much folic acid as Lexpec with Iron-M®

COMPOUND IRON PREPARATIONS

There is no justification for prescribing compound iron preparations, except for preparations of iron and folic acid for prophylactic use in pregnancy (see above).

Ferrous Sulphate Tablets, Compound, green, s/c, dried ferrous sulphate equivalent to 170 mg of $FeSO_4$, copper sulphate 2.5 mg, manganese sulphate 2.5 mg. Net price 20 tabs = 43p

Dose: 1–2 tablets daily

Dencyl® (SmithKline Beecham)

Spansule® (= capsules m/r), blue/clear, enclosing red, yellow, and white pellets, dried ferrous sulphate 150 mg (47 mg iron), folic acid 500 micrograms, zinc sulphate monohydrate 61.8 mg (22.5 mg zinc). Net price 30-cap pack = £4.74. Label: 25

Dose: 1 capsule daily during pregnancy

Ditemic® (SmithKline Beecham)

Spansule® (= capsules m/r), orange/clear, enclosing red, orange, and white pellets, dried ferrous sulphate 150 mg (47 mg iron), zinc sulphate monohydrate 61.8 mg (22.5 mg zinc) with vitamins B group and C. Net price 30-cap pack = £7.40. Label: 25

Dose: 1–2 capsules daily; CHILD over 1 year 1 capsule daily

NHS **Fefol Z®** (Evans)

Spansule® (= capsules m/r), blue/clear, enclosing brown, yellow, and white pellets, dried ferrous sulphate 150 mg (47 mg iron), folic acid 500 micrograms, zinc sulphate monohydrate 61.8 mg (22.5 mg zinc). Net price 30-cap pack = £1.79. Label: 25

Dose: 1 capsule daily during pregnancy

NHS **Ferrograd C®** (Abbott)

Filmtabs® (= tablets f/c), red, dried ferrous sulphate 325 mg (105 mg iron) for sustained release, ascorbic acid 500 mg (as sodium salt). Net price 30-tab pack = £1.56. Label: 25

Dose: 1 tablet daily before food

NHS **Fesovit Z®** (Evans)

Spansule® (= capsules m/r), orange/clear, enclosing brown, orange, and white pellets, dried ferrous sulphate 150 mg (47 mg iron), zinc sulphate monohydrate 61.8 mg (22.5 mg zinc) with vitamins B group and C. Net price 30-cap pack = £2.80. Label: 25

Dose: 1–2 capsules daily; CHILD over 1 year 1 capsule daily

NHS **Givitol®** (Galen)

Capsules, red/maroon, ferrous fumarate 305 mg (100 mg iron) with vitamins B group and C. Net price 20 = 82p

Dose: 1 capsule daily before food

9.1.1.2 PARENTERAL IRON

The only valid reason for administering iron **parenterally** is failure of oral therapy due to lack of patient cooperation, severe gastro-intestinal side-effects, continuing severe blood loss or malabsorption. Provided that the oral iron preparation is taken reliably and is absorbed, then the haemoglobin response is not significantly faster with the parenteral route. The need for a more rapid cure of the anaemia is therefore not met by parenteral administration of iron.

A suitable parenteral preparation contains a complex of iron, sorbitol and citric acid as **iron sorbitol injection** (Jectofer®). It is **not** suitable for intravenous injection and, although the low mean molecular weight allows rapid absorption from the injection site, excretion in the saliva and substantial urinary losses also occur.

It is usual to give a course of *deep intramuscular* injections. The manufacturer's dosage schedules should be consulted; these usually include a supplement for reconstitution of iron stores.

To prevent leakage along the needle track with subsequent staining of the skin, intramuscular injections should be deep with suitable technique.

IRON SORBITOL INJECTION

Contains 5% (50 mg/mL) of iron

Indications: iron-deficiency anaemia

Cautions: oral iron should be stopped at least 24 hours before; other injectable iron preparations should be stopped a week before; urine may darken on standing

Contra-indications: liver disease, kidney disease (particularly pyelonephritis), untreated urinary tract infections; early pregnancy; preferably avoid in patients with pre-existing cardiac abnormalities (e.g. angina or arrhythmias)

Side-effects: nausea, vomiting, taste disturbances, dizziness, flushing, occasionally severe arrhythmias

Dose: by deep intramuscular injection, calculated according to weight and iron deficit, see notes above and manufacturer's literature

PoM **Jectofer®** (Astra)

Injection, iron sorbitol injection. Net price 2-mL amp = 45p

9.1.2   Drugs used in megaloblastic anaemias

Most megaloblastic anaemias are due to lack of either vitamin B_{12} or folate and it is essential to establish in every case which deficiency is present and the underlying cause. In emergencies, where delay might be dangerous, it is sometimes necessary to administer both substances after the bone marrow test while plasma assay results are awaited. Normally, however, appropriate treatment should be instituted only when the results of tests are available.

The most common cause of megaloblastic anaemia in the UK is *pernicious anaemia* in which lack of gastric intrinsic factor due to an auto-immune gastritis causes malabsorption of vitamin B_{12}.

Vitamin B_{12} is also needed in the treatment of megaloblastosis due to *prolonged nitrous oxide anaesthesia,* which inactivates the vitamin, and in the rare syndrome of *congenital transcobalamin II deficiency.*

Vitamin B_{12} should be given prophylactically after *total gastrectomy* or *total ileal resection* (or after *partial gastrectomy* if a vitamin B_{12} absorption test shows vitamin B_{12} malabsorption).

Apart from dietary deficiency, all other causes of vitamin-B_{12} deficiency are attributable to *malabsorption* so there is little place for the use of vitamin B_{12} orally and none for vitamin B_{12} intrinsic factor complexes given by mouth.

Hydroxocobalamin has completely replaced cyanocobalamin as the form of vitamin B_{12} of choice for therapy; it is retained in the body longer than cyanocobalamin and thus for maintenance therapy need only be given at intervals of 3 months. Although a haematological response in vitamin-B_{12} deficiency may be obtained by small doses, it is customary to start treatment with 1 mg by intramuscular injection repeated 5 times at intervals of 2 to 3 days to replenish the depleted body stores. Thereafter, maintenance treatment, which is usually for life, can be instituted. There is no evidence that larger doses provide any additional benefit in vitamin-B_{12} neuropathy.

Folic acid has few indications for long-term therapy since most causes of folate deficiency are self-limiting or will yield to a short course of treatment. It should not be used in undiagnosed megaloblastic anaemia unless vitamin B_{12} is administered concur-

---

rently otherwise neuropathy may be precipitated (see above).

In *folate-deficient megaloblastic anaemia* (e.g. due to poor nutrition, pregnancy, or antiepileptics), standard treatment to bring about a haematological remission and replenish body stores, is oral administration of folic acid 5 mg daily for 4 months; up to 15 mg daily may be necessary in malabsorption states.

For *prophylaxis in chronic haemolytic states or in renal dialysis*, it is sufficient to give folic acid 5 mg daily or even weekly, depending on the diet and the rate of haemolysis.

For *prophylaxis in pregnancy* the dose of folic acid is 200–500 micrograms daily (see Iron and Folic Acid, section 9.1.1.1). See also below.

PREVENTION OF NEURAL TUBE DEFECTS. Recommendations of an expert advisory group of the Department of Health include the advice that:

To prevent *recurrence of neural tube defect* women who wish to become pregnant (or who are at risk of becoming pregnant) should be advised to take folic acid supplements at a dose of 5 mg daily (reduced to 4 mg daily if a suitable preparation becomes available); supplementation should continue until the twelfth week of pregnancy. Women receiving antiepileptic therapy need individual counselling by their doctor before starting folic acid.

To prevent *first occurrence of neural tube defect* women who are planning a pregnancy should be advised to take folic acid as a medicinal or food supplement at a dose of 400 micrograms daily before conception and during the first 12 weeks of pregnancy. Women who have not been supplementing and who suspect they are pregnant should start at once and continue until the twelfth week of pregnancy.

There is **no** justification for prescribing multiple-ingredient vitamin preparations containing vitamin B_{12} or folic acid.

HYDROXOCOBALAMIN

Indications: Pernicious anaemia, other causes of vitamin-B_{12} deficiency, subacute combined degeneration of the spinal cord
Cautions: should not be given before diagnosis fully established but see also notes above
Dose: by intramuscular injection, initially 1 mg repeated 5 times at intervals of 2–3 days; maintenance dose 1 mg every 3 months; CHILD, dosage as for adult

PoM **Hydroxocobalamin Injection,** hydroxocobalamin 1 mg/mL. Net price 1-mL amp = £2.27
Note. The BP directs that when vitamin B_{12} injection is prescribed or demanded hydroxocobalamin injection shall be dispensed or supplied
The brand names NHS Cobalin-H® (Link) and NHS Neo-Cytamen® (Evans) are used for hydroxocobalamin injection

CYANOCOBALAMIN

Indications: see notes above
Dose: by mouth, vitamin-B_{12} deficiency of dietary origin, 50–150 micrograms or more daily taken between meals; CHILD 35–50 micrograms twice daily
By intramuscular injection, initially 1 mg repeated 10 times at intervals of 2–3 days, maintenance 1 mg every month, but see notes above

Cyanocobalamin (Non-proprietary)
NHS *Tablets*, cyanocobalamin 50 micrograms. Net price 50-tab pack = £2.36
* except to treat or prevent vitamin-B_{12} deficiency in a patient who is a vegan or who has a proven vitamin-B_{12} deficiency of dietary origin and endorsed 'SLS' ('S2B' in Scotland)
Note. The brand name NHS Cytacon® (Goldshield) is used for cyanocobalamin tablets
NHS *Liquid*, cyanocobalamin 35 micrograms/5 mL. Net price 200 mL = £2.36
Note. The brand name NHS Cytacon® (Goldshield) is used for cyanocobalamin liquid
PoM *Injection*, cyanocobalamin 1 mg/mL. Net price 1-mL amp = £1.67
Note. The BP directs that when vitamin B_{12} injection is prescribed or demanded hydroxocobalamin injection shall be dispensed or supplied
The brand name NHS Cytamen® (Evans) is used for cyanocobalamin injection

FOLIC ACID

Indications: see notes above
Cautions: should never be given alone in the treatment of Addisonian pernicious anaemia and other vitamin B_{12}-deficiency states because it may precipitate the onset of subacute combined degeneration of the spinal cord. Do not use in malignant disease unless megaloblastic anaemia due to folate deficiency is an important complication (some malignant tumours are folate-dependent); **interactions:** Appendix 1 (vitamins)
Dose: initially, 5 mg daily for 4 months (see notes above); maintenance, 5 mg every 1–7 days depending on underlying disease; CHILD up to 1 year, 500 micrograms/kg daily; over 1 year, as adult
Prevention of neural tube defects, see notes above

PoM [1] **Folic Acid** (Non-proprietary)
Tablets, folic acid 400 micrograms, net price = 90-tab pack = £2.08; 5 mg, 20 = 6p
Note. 400-microgram tablets available from Lane (Preconceive®), 5-mg tablets available from various suppliers
1. Can be sold to the public provided daily doses do not exceed 500 micrograms
Syrup, folic acid 2.5 mg/5 mL. Net price 125 mL = £6.75
Available from Hillcross, Rosemont (Lexpec®, sugar-free)

CALCIUM FOLINATE
See section 8.1.3

9.1.3   Drugs used in hypoplastic, haemolytic, and renal anaemias
Anabolic steroids, pyridoxine, antilymphocyte immunoglobulin, and various corticosteroids are used in hypoplastic and haemolytic anaemias.

The place of **anabolic steroids** in the therapy of *aplastic anaemia* remains somewhat controversial and their effectiveness is unclear. There is a wide variation in the reported successful responses. Occasional patients, however, do seem to derive benefit. Since nandrolone decanoate requires intramuscular injection it is unsuitable in aplastic anaemia or cytotoxic aplasia because of the low platelet count. Controlled trials have shown that antilymphocyte globulin produces a response in 50% of acquired cases; higher response rates have been reported when cyclosporin is given as well.

It is unlikely that dietary deprivation of **pyridoxine** (section 9.6.2) produces haematological effects in man. However, certain forms of *sideroblastic anaemia* respond to pharmacological doses, possibly reflecting its role as a co-enzyme during haemoglobin synthesis. Pyridoxine is indicated in both *idiopathic acquired* and *hereditary sideroblastic anaemias*. Although complete cures have not been reported, some increase in haemoglobin may occur; the dose required is usually high, up to 400 mg daily. *Reversible sideroblastic anaemias* respond to treatment of the underlying cause but in pregnancy, haemolytic anaemias, and alcohol dependence, or during isoniazid treatment, pyridoxine is also indicated.

Corticosteroids (see section 6.3) have an important place in the management of a wide variety of haematological disorders. They include conditions with an immune basis such as *auto-immune haemolytic anaemia*, *immune thrombocytopenias* and *neutropenias*, and *major transfusion reactions*. They are also used in chemotherapy schedules for many types of *lymphoma*, *lymphoid leukaemias*, and *paraproteinaemias*, including *myelomatosis*. Corticosteroids are used in *aplastic anaemias*, where their value is more debatable.

NANDROLONE

Indications: aplastic anaemia but see notes above; postmenopausal osteoporosis, see section 6.4.3

Cautions; Contra-indications; Side-effects: see section 6.4.3

Dose: by deep intramuscular injection, aplastic anaemia (but not recommended, see notes above), nandrolone decanoate 50–100 mg weekly

PoM **Deca-Durabolin 100**® (Organon)
Injection (oily), nandrolone decanoate 100 mg/mL. Net price 1-mL amp = £7.34

Note. Contains arachis (peanut) oil

ERYTHROPOIETIN

Epoetin (recombinant human erythropoietin) is used for the anaemia associated with erythropoietin deficiency in chronic renal failure where there is a failure of erythropoietin production. It is indicated for patients both on and off either haemodialysis or peritoneal dialysis. The clinical efficacy of epoetin alfa and epoetin beta is similar. Epoietin alfa is also used to increase the haemoglobin in normal individuals to increase the yield of autologous blood pre-surgery and in patients receiving platinum-containing chemotherapy to shorten the period of anaemia.

Other factors which contribute to the anaemia of chronic renal failure such as iron or folate deficiency should be corrected; aluminium toxicity, concurrent infection or other inflammatory disease may also impair the response to epoetin.

EPOETIN ALFA and BETA
(Recombinant human erythropoietins)

Indications: see under preparations, below

Cautions: inadequately treated or poorly controlled blood pressure (monitor closely blood pressure, haemoglobin, and electrolytes), interrupt treatment if blood pressure uncontrolled; exclude other causes of anaemia (e.g. folic acid or vitamin B_{12} deficiency) and give iron supplements if necessary (see also notes above); ischaemic vascular disease; thrombocytosis (monitor platelet count for first 8 weeks); history of convulsions; malignant disease; chronic liver failure; sudden stabbing migraine-like pain is warning of hypertensive crisis; increase in heparin dose may be needed; pregnancy and breast-feeding; **interactions:** Appendix 1 (epoetin)

Contra-indications: uncontrolled hypertension

Side-effects: dose-dependent increase in blood pressure or aggravation of hypertension; in isolated patients with normal or low blood pressure, hypertensive crisis with encephalopathy-like symptoms and generalised tonic-clonic seizures requiring immediate medical attention; dose-dependent increase in platelet count (but thrombocytosis rare) regressing during treatment; influenza-like symptoms (may be reduced if intravenous injection given over 5 minutes); shunt thrombosis especially if tendency to hypotension or arteriovenous shunt complications; isolated reports of hyperkalaemia, increase in plasma creatinine, urea and phosphate, convulsions, skin reactions, palpebral oedema, anaphylaxis

Dose: aimed at increasing haemoglobin concentration at rate not exceeding 2 g/100 mL/month to stable level of 10–12 g/100 mL (9.5–11 g/100 mL in children); see under preparations, below

Note. Although epoetin alfa and beta are clinically indistinguishable the prescriber must specify which is required

Epoetin alfa
PoM **Eprex**® (Cilag)
Injection, epoetin alfa 2000 units/mL, net price 0.5-mL (1000-unit) vial = £8.78, 0.5-mL (1000-unit) pre-filled syringe = £9.23, 1-mL (2000-unit) vial = £17.55; 4000 units/mL, 0.5-mL (2000-unit) pre-filled syringe = £18.00, 1-mL (4000-unit) vial = £35.10; 10 000 units/mL, 0.3-mL (3000-unit) pre-filled syringe = £26.78, 0.4-mL (4000-unit) pre-filled syringe = £35.55, 1-mL (10 000-unit) vial = £87.75, 1-mL (10 000-unit) pre-filled syringe = £88.20

Dose: anaemia associated with chronic renal failure in patients on haemodialysis, *by subcutaneous injection* (max. 1 mL per injection site) or *by intravenous injection* over 2 minutes, initially 50 units/kg 3 times weekly increased according to response in steps of 25 units/kg at intervals of 4 weeks; omit one of the weekly doses if haemoglobin rise exceeds 2 g/100 mL per month with the initial dose; max. 600 units/kg weekly in 3 divided doses; maintenance dose (when haemoglobin concentration of 10–12 g/100 mL achieved), usually 100–300 units/kg weekly in 2–3 divided doses; CHILD (intravenous route only) initially as for adults; maintenance

---

dose (when haemoglobin concentration of 9.5–11 g/ 100 mL achieved), under 10 kg usually 75–150 units/kg 3 times weekly, 10–30 kg usually 60–150 units/kg 3 times weekly, over 30 kg usually 30–100 units/kg 3 times weekly

Anaemia associated with chronic renal failure in adults on peritoneal dialysis, *by subcutaneous injection* (max. 1 mL per injection site) or *by intravenous injection* over 2 minutes, initially 50 units/kg twice weekly increased according to response in steps of 25 units/kg at intervals of 4 weeks; maintenance dose (when haemoglobin concentration of 10–12 g/100 mL achieved), 50–100 units/ kg weekly in 2 equally divided doses

Severe symptomatic anaemia of renal origin in adults with renal insufficiency not yet on dialysis, preferably *by subcutaneous injection* (max. 1 mL per injection site), initially 50 units/kg 3 times weekly increased according to response in steps of 25 units/kg at intervals of 4 weeks; max. 600 units/kg weekly in 3 divided doses; maintenance dose (when haemoglobin concentration of 10–12 g/100 mL achieved), 50–100 units/kg weekly in 3 divided doses

Anaemia in adults receiving platinum-containing chemotherapy, *by subcutaneous injection* (max. 1 mL per injection site), initially 150 units/kg 3 times weekly, increased if appropriate rise in haemoglobin (or reticulocyte count) not achieved after 4 weeks to 300 units/kg 3 times weekly; discontinue if inadequate response after 4 weeks at higher dose; reduce dose by 25–50% if haemoglobin rise exceeds 2 g/100 mL per month; suspend if haemoglobin exceeds 14 g/100 mL until it falls below 12 g/100 mL and reinstate with dose at 25% below previous dose; continue epoetin for 1 month after end of chemotherapy

To increase yield of autologous blood (to avoid homologous blood) in predonation programme in moderate anaemia *either* when large volume of blood required for elective major surgery *or* if insufficient period to obtain required volume of blood, *by intravenous injection* over 2 minutes, 600 units/kg twice weekly for 3 weeks before surgery; see data sheet for details and advice on ensuring high iron stores

Note. Subcutaneous dose generally about 20–30% lower than intravenous; when changing route give same dose then adjust according to weekly haemoglobin measurements

poetin beta
oM **Recormon**® (Boehringer Mannheim)
njection, powder for reconstitution, epoetin beta. Net price 1000-unit vial = £8.78; 2000-unit vial = £17.55; 5000-unit vial = £43.88; 10 000-unit vial = £87.75 (all with water for injections)
Note. Avoid contact of reconstituted injection with glass; use only plastic materials

Recormon® S injection (for subcutaneous use), powder for reconstitution, epoetin beta. Net price 1000-unit vial = £8.78; 2000-unit vial = £17.55; 5000-unit vial = £43.88; 10 000-unit vial = £87.75 (all with syringe and water for injections)
Dose: anaemia associated with chronic renal failure in dialysis patients, symptomatic anaemia of renal origin in patients not yet on dialysis, ADULT and CHILD over 2 years,

By subcutaneous injection, initially 20 units/kg 3 times weekly for 4 weeks, increased according to response at monthly intervals in steps of 20 units/kg; maintenance dose (when haemoglobin concentration of 10–12 g/ 100 mL achieved), initially reduce dose by half then adjust according to response at intervals of 1–2 weeks

By intravenous injection over 2 minutes (or *by short-term intravenous infusion*), initially 40 units/kg 3 times weekly for 4 weeks, increased if initial haemoglobin rise less than 1 g/100 mL per month to 80 units/kg 3 times weekly with further increases if needed at monthly intervals in steps of 20 units/kg; maintenance dose (when haemoglobin concentration of 10–12 g/100 mL achieved), initially reduce dose by half then adjust according to response at intervals of 1–2 weeks

Max. by either route 720 units/kg weekly

IRON OVERLOAD

Severe tissue iron overload may occur in aplastic and other refractory anaemias, mainly as the result of repeated blood transfusions. It is a particular problem in refractory anaemias with hyperplastic bone marrow, especially *thalassaemia major*, where excessive iron absorption from the gut and inappropriate iron therapy may add to the tissue siderosis.

Venesection therapy is contra-indicated, but the long-term administration of the iron chelating compound **desferrioxamine mesylate** is useful. Subcutaneous infusions of desferrioxamine (20–40 mg/kg over 8–12 hours) are given on 3 to 7 nights each week. Desferrioxamine (up to 2 g per unit of blood) may also be given through the infusion line at the time of blood transfusion.

Iron excretion induced by desferrioxamine is enhanced by administration of vitamin C (section 9.6.3) in a dose of 200 mg daily (100 mg in infants); it should be given separately from food since it also enhances iron absorption. Vitamin C should be avoided for 1–2 weeks after starting desferrioxamine treatment.

Infusion of desferrioxamine may be used to treat *aluminium overload* in dialysis patients; theoretically 100 mg of desferrioxamine binds with 4.1 mg of aluminium.

Orally active iron chelators are under clinical study but are not available for general use.

DESFERRIOXAMINE MESYLATE

Indications: see notes above; iron poisoning, see Emergency Treatment of Poisoning

Cautions: renal impairment; eye and ear examinations before treatment and at 3-month intervals during treatment; aluminium-related encephalopathy (may exacerbate neurological dysfunction); pregnancy, breast-feeding; **interactions:** Appendix 1 (desferrioxamine)

Side-effects: gastro-intestinal disturbances; hepatic and renal impairment; arrhythmias, hypotension (especially when given too rapidly by intravenous injection); anaphylaxis; dizziness; convulsions; Yersinia infection more frequent; disturbances of hearing and vision (including lens opacity and retinopathy); skin reactions; pain on intramuscular injection; local irritation on subcutaneous infusion (usually if infusion concentration or dose too high)

Dose: see notes above; iron poisoning, see Emergency Treatment of Poisoning, p. 23
Note. For full details and warnings relating to administration, consult data sheet

Preparations
See under Emergency Treatment of Poisoning

9.1.4 Drugs used in autoimmune thrombocytopenic purpura

It is usual to commence the treatment of autoimmune (idiopathic) thrombocytopenic purpura with corticosteroids, e.g. prednisolone of the order of 1 mg/kg daily, gradually reducing the dosage over the subsequent weeks. In patients who fail to achieve a satisfactory platelet count or relapse when corticosteroid dosage is reduced or withdrawn, splenectomy is considered.

Other therapy that has been tried in refractory cases includes azathioprine (see section 8.2.1), cyclophosphamide (see section 8.1.1), vincristine or vinblastine (see section 8.1.4) (or vinblastine-loaded platelets), cyclosporin (see section 8.2.2), and danazol (section 6.7.3). Intravenous immunoglobulins (see section 14.5), have also been used in refractory cases or where a temporary rapid rise in platelets is needed, as in pregnancy or pre-operatively. For patients with chronic severe thrombocytopenia refractory to other therapy, tranexamic acid (see section 2.11) may be given to reduce the severity of haemorrhage.

9.1.5 G6PD deficiency

Glucose 6-phosphate dehydrogenase (G6PD) deficiency is highly prevalent in populations originating from most parts of Africa, from most parts of Asia, from Oceania, and from Southern Europe; it can also be encountered, rarely, in any other population.

Subjects with G6PD deficiency are susceptible to developing acute haemolytic anaemia on taking a number of common drugs. They are also susceptible to developing acute haemolytic anaemia upon ingestion of fava beans (*Vicia faba*); this is termed *favism* and tends to be more severe in children or when the fresh fava beans are eaten raw.

When prescribing drugs for patients who are G6PD deficient, the following three points should be kept in mind:

1. G6PD deficiency is genetically heterogeneous; different genetic variants entail different susceptibility to the haemolytic risk from drugs; thus, a drug found to be safe in some G6PD-deficient subjects may not be equally safe in others;
2. no test specifically designed to identify potential risk in G6PD-deficient subjects is currently carried out by manufacturers;
3. the risk and severity of haemolysis is almost always dose-related.

The table below should be read with these points in mind. Whenever possible, a test for G6PD deficiency should be done before prescribing a drug in the list, especially if the patient belongs to a population group in which G6PD deficiency is common.

A very small group of G6PD-deficient individuals, with chronic non-spherocytic haemolytic anaemia, have haemolysis even in the absence of an exogenous trigger. These patients must be regarded as being at high risk of severe exacerbation of haemolysis following administration of any of the drugs listed below.

Drugs with definite risk of haemolysis in most G6PD-deficient subjects

Dapsone and other sulphones (higher doses for dermatit herpetiformis more likely to cause problems)
Methylene blue
Niridazole [not on UK market]
Nitrofurantoin
Pamaquin [not on UK market]
Primaquine (30 mg weekly for 8 weeks has been found be without undue harmful effects in Afro and Asian pe ple, see section 5.4.1)
4-Quinolones (including ciprofloxacin, nalidixic aci norfloxacin, and ofloxacin)
Sulphonamides (including co-trimoxazole; son sulphonamides, e.g. sulphadiazine, have been tested an found not to be haemolytic in many G6PD-deficie subjects)

Drugs with possible risk of haemolysis in some G6PD-deficient subjects

Aspirin (acceptable in a dose of at least 1 g daily in mo G6PD-deficient subjects)
Chloroquine (acceptable in acute malaria)
Menadione, water-soluble derivatives (e.g. menadiol so ium phosphate)
Probenecid
Quinidine (acceptable in acute malaria)
Quinine (acceptable in acute malaria)

Note. Mothballs may contain naphthalene which als causes haemolysis in subjects with G6PD-deficiency.

9.1.6 Drugs used in neutropenia

Recombinant human granulocyte-colony stimulating factor (rhG-CSF) stimulates the production of neutrophils and may reduce the duration of chemo therapy-induced neutropenia and thereby reduce th incidence of associated sepsis; there is as yet no evidence that it improves overall survival. **Filgrastim** (unglycosylated rhG-CSF) and **lenograstim** (glycosylated rhG-CSF) have similar effects; both have been used in a variety of clinical settings but they do not have any clear-cut routine indication In congenital neutropenia filgrastim usually ele vates the neutrophil count with appropriate clinic response. Prolonged use may be associated with a increased risk of myeloid malignancy.

Molgramostim (recombinant human granulocyt macrophage-colony stimulating factor) stimulate the production of all granulocytes and monocyte It has more side-effects than granulocyte-color stimulating factor and is ineffective in congenit neutropenia.

Treatment with recombinant human growth fac tors should only be administered by those experi enced in their use.

FILGRASTIM

(Recombinant human granulocyte-colony stimulatir factor, G-CSF)

Indications: (specialist use only) reduction in dur tion of neutropenia and incidence of febrile neutrop nia in cytotoxic chemotherapy of non-myelo malignancy; reduction in duration of neutropen (and associated sequelae) in myeloablative therap

    Prices are **net**, see p.

followed by bone-marrow transplantation; mobilisation of peripheral blood progenitor cells for harvesting and subsequent autologous infusion; severe congenital neutropenia, cyclic neutropenia, or idiopathic neutropenia and history of severe or recurrent infections (distinguish carefully from other haematological disorders, see data sheet); reversal of neutropenia in advanced HIV infection to allow scheduled myelosuppressive or antiviral therapy

Cautions: tumours with myeloid characteristics (risk of tumour growth), pre-malignant myeloid conditions; reduced myeloid precursors; monitor leucocyte count (discontinue treatment if leucocytosis, see data sheet); monitor platelet count and haemoglobin; regular morphological and cytogenetic bone marrow examinations recommended in severe congenital neutropenia (possible risk of myelodysplastic syndromes or leukaemia); monitor spleen size; osteoporotic bone disease (monitor bone density if given for more than 6 months); does not prevent other toxic effects of high-dose chemotherapy; pregnancy, breast-feeding

Contra-indications: severe congenital neutropenia (Kostman's syndrome) with abnormal cytogenetics

Side-effects: musculoskeletal pain, transient hypotension, disturbances in liver enzymes and serum uric acid; thrombocytopenia; urinary abnormalities including dysuria; allergic reactions (more common after intravenous infusion), proteinuria, haematuria , and transient decrease in blood glucose reported; on long-term use cutaneous vasculitis also reported, also splenic enlargement, hepatomegaly, headache, diarrhoea, anaemia, epistaxis, alopecia, osteoporosis, and rash

Dose: cytotoxic-induced neutropenia, *by subcutaneous injection or by intravenous infusion* (over 30 minutes), 500 000 units/kg started not less than 24 hours after cytotoxic chemotherapy, continued until neutrophil count in normal range, usually for up to 14 days

Myeloablative therapy followed by bone-marrow transplantation, *by intravenous infusion* over 30 minutes *or over 24 hours or by subcutaneous infusion* over 24 hours, 1 million units/kg daily, started not less than 24 hours following cytotoxic chemotherapy (and within 24 hours of bone-marrow infusion), then adjusted according to absolute neutrophil count (see data sheet)

Mobilisation of peripheral blood progenitor cells, used alone, *by subcutaneous injection or by subcutaneous infusion* over 24 hours, 1 million units/kg daily for 6 days; used following adjunctive myelosuppressive chemotherapy (to improve yield), *by subcutaneous injection*, 500 000 units/kg daily, started the day after completion of chemotherapy and continued until neutrophil count in normal range; for timing of leukapheresis see data sheet

Severe chronic neutropenia, *by subcutaneous injection*, ADULT and CHILD, in severe congenital neutropenia, initially 1.2 million units/kg daily in single or divided doses (initially 500 000 units/kg daily in idiopathic or cyclic neutropenia), adjusted according to response (see data sheet)

Reversal of neutropenia in advanced HIV infection, *by subcutaneous injection*, initially 10 000 units/kg daily adjusted according to response up to a max. of 400 000 units/kg daily until neutrophil count in normal range; maintenance of normal neutrophil count, initially 30 million units three times a week then adjusted according to absolute neutrophil count (see data sheet); reduce dose and then stop filgrastim if myelosuppressive therapy discontinued and there is no recurrence of neutropenia

▼ PoM **Neupogen®** (Amgen, Roche)
Injection, filgrastim 30 million units (300 micrograms)/mL; net price 1-mL vial = £77.03, 1.6-mL (48 million-unit) vial = £122.85

LENOGRASTIM
(Recombinant human granulocyte-colony stimulating factor, rHuG-CSF)

Indications: (specialist use only) reduction in the duration of neutropenia and associated complications following bone-marrow transplantation for non-myeloid malignancy or following treatment with cytotoxic chemotherapy associated with a significant incidence of febrile neutropenia

Cautions; Side-effects: see under Filgrastim

Dose: following bone-marrow transplantation, *by intravenous infusion*, ADULT and CHILD over 2 years 19.2 million units/m² daily started the day after transplantation, continued until neutrophil count stable in acceptable range (max. 28 days)

Cytotoxic-induced neutropenia, *by subcutaneous injection*, ADULT and CHILD over 2 years 19.2 million units/m² daily started the day after completion of chemotherapy, continued until neutrophil count stable in acceptable range (max. 28 days)

▼ PoM **Granocyte®** (Chugai)
Injection, powder for reconstitution, lenograstim, net price 33.6 million-unit (263-microgram) vial (with 1-mL amp water for injections) = £77.03

MOLGRAMOSTIM
(Recombinant human granulocyte macrophage-colony stimulating factor, GM-CSF)

Indications: (specialist use only) reduction of severity of neutropenia (and risk of infection) in cytotoxic chemotherapy; acceleration of myeloid recovery following bone-marrow transplantation; neutropenia in patients treated with ganciclovir in AIDS-related cytomegalovirus retinitis

Cautions: monitor serum albumin concentration and full blood count including differential white cell, platelet and haemoglobin; monitor closely patients with pulmonary disease; history of or predisposition to autoimmune disease; pregnancy and breast-feeding; not recommended for patients under 18 years

Contra-indications: myeloid malignancies

Side-effects: nausea, diarrhoea, vomiting, anorexia; dyspnoea; asthenia, fatigue; rash, fever, rigors, flushing, musculoskeletal pain; local reaction following subcutaneous injection; also reported, non-specific chest pain, stomatitis, headache, increased sweating, abdominal pain, pruritus, peripheral oedema, dizziness, paraesthesia, and myalgia; serious reactions reported include anaphylaxis, cardiac failure, capillary leak syndrome, cerebrovascular disorders, confusion, convulsions, hypotension, cardiac rhythm abnormalities, intracranial hypertension, pericardial effusion, pericarditis, pleural effusion, pulmonary oedema, syncope

Dose: (first dose under medical supervision)
Cytotoxic chemotherapy, *by subcutaneous injection*, 60 000–110 000 units/kg daily, starting 24 hours after last dose of chemotherapy, continued for 7–10 days

Bone-marrow transplantation, *by intravenous infusion*, 110 000 units/kg daily, starting day after transplantation, continued until absolute neutrophil count in desirable range (see data sheet); max. duration of treatment 30 days

Adjunct in ganciclovir treatment, *by subcutaneous injection*, 60 000 units/kg daily for 5 days then adjusted to maintain desirable absolute neutrophil count and white blood cell count

▼ PoM **Leucomax®** (Sandoz, Schering-Plough)
Injection, powder for reconstitution, molgramostim, net price 1.67 million-unit (150-microgram) vial = £38.51; 3.33 million-unit (300-microgram) vial = £77.02; 4.44 million-unit (400 microgram) vial = £102.69

CYTOTOXIC-INDUCED NEUTROPENIC INFECTION

Amifostine is specifically licensed for the reduction of risk of infection related to neutropenia in patients undergoing treatment with cisplatin and cyclophosphamide for advanced ovarian carcinoma; it should be given within 30 minutes before chemotherapy.

Other drugs for the reduction of risk of infection associated with neutropenia include granulocyte-colony stimulating factor and granulocyte macrophage-colony stimulating factor.

AMIFOSTINE

Indications: (specialist use only) reduction of neutropenia-related risk of infection due to cyclophosphamide and cisplatin treatment in patients with advanced ovarian carcinoma

Cautions: ensure adequate hydration before treatment; infuse with patient supine and monitor arterial blood pressure (interrupt infusion if blood pressure decreases significantly, see data sheet); interrupt antihypertensive therapy 24 hours beforehand and monitor patients closely; infuse over 15 minutes (longer infusion associated with higher incidence of side-effects); administer antiemetic drugs with amifostine and before highly emetogenic chemotherapy; monitor serum calcium in patients at risk of hypocalcaemia; not recommended in renal and hepatic impairment; pregnancy and breast-feeding; **interactions:** Appendix 1 (amifostine)

Side-effects: hypotension (reversed by infusion of physiological saline and postural management), nausea, vomiting, flushing, chills, dizziness, somnolence, hiccups, sneezing; rarely clinical hypocalcaemia; allergic reactions

Dose: by intravenous infusion over 15 minutes, 910 mg/m² once daily started within 30 minutes before chemotherapy (reduced to 740 mg/m² for subsequent cycles if full dose could not be given first time due to hypotension lasting more than 5 minutes after interruption, see data sheet); CHILD and ELDERLY (over 70 years) not recommended

▼ PoM **Ethyol®** (Schering-Plough)
Intravenous infusion, powder for reconstitution, amifostine. Net price 500-mg vial = £160.00

9.2 Fluids and electrolytes

9.2.1 Oral administration
9.2.2 Intravenous administration
9.2.3 Plasma and plasma substitutes

The following tables give a selection of useful electrolyte values:

Electrolyte concentrations—intravenous fluids

Intravenous infusion	Millimoles per litre				
	Na⁺	K⁺	HCO₃⁻	Cl⁻	Ca²⁺
Normal Plasma Values	142	4.5	26	103	2.5
Sodium Chloride 0.9%	150	—	—	150	—
Compound Sodium Lactate (Hartmann's)	131	5	29	111	2
Sodium Chloride 0.18% and Glucose 4%	30	—	—	30	—
Potassium Chloride 0.3% and Glucose 5%	—	40	—	40	—
Potassium Chloride 0.3% and Sodium Chloride 0.9%	150	40	—	190	—
To correct metabolic acidosis					
Sodium Bicarbonate 1.26%	150	—	150	—	—
Sodium Bicarbonate 8.4% for cardiac arrest	1000	—	1000	—	—
Sodium Lactate (M/6)	167	—	167	—	—

Electrolyte content—gastro-intestinal secretions

Type of fluid	Millimoles per litre				
	H⁺	Na⁺	K⁺	HCO₃⁻	Cl⁻
Gastric	40–60	20–80	5–20	—	100–150
Biliary	—	120–140	5–15	30–50	80–120
Pancreatic	—	120–140	5–15	70–110	40–80
Small bowel	—	120–140	5–15	20–40	90–130

Faeces, vomit, or aspiration should be saved and analysed where possible if abnormal losses are suspected; where this is impracticable the approximations above may be helpful in planning replacement therapy

9.2.1 Oral administration

9.2.1.1 Oral potassium
9.2.1.2 Oral sodium and water
9.2.1.3 Oral bicarbonate

Sodium and potassium salts, which may be given by mouth to prevent deficiencies or to treat established deficiencies of mild or moderate degree, are discussed in this section. Oral preparations for removing excess potassium and preparations for oral rehydration therapy are also included here. Oral bicarbonate, for metabolic acidosis, is also described in this section.

For reference to calcium, magnesium, and phosphate, see section 9.5.

9.2.1.1 ORAL POTASSIUM

Compensation for potassium loss is especially necessary:
1. in those taking digoxin or anti-arrhythmic drugs, where potassium depletion may induce arrhythmias;
2. in patients in whom secondary hyperaldosteronism occurs, e.g. renal artery stenosis, cirrhosis of the liver, the nephrotic syndrome, and severe heart failure;
3. in patients with excessive losses of potassium in the faeces, e.g. chronic diarrhoea associated with intestinal malabsorption or laxative abuse.

Measures to compensate for potassium loss may also be required in the elderly since they frequently take inadequate amounts of potassium in the diet (but see below for **warning** on **renal insufficiency**). Measures may also be required during long-term administration of drugs known to induce potassium loss (e.g. corticosteroids). Potassium supplements are **seldom required** with the small doses of diuretics given to treat hypertension; **potassium-sparing diuretics** (rather than potassium supplements) are recommended for prevention of hypokalaemia due to diuretics such as frusemide or the thiazides when these are given to eliminate oedema.

DOSAGE. If potassium salts are used for the *prevention of hypokalaemia*, then doses of potassium chloride 2 to 4 g (approx. 25 to 50 mmol) daily by mouth are suitable in patients taking a normal diet. *Smaller doses must be used if there is renal insufficiency (common in the elderly)* otherwise there is **danger of hyperkalaemia**. Potassium salts cause nausea and vomiting therefore poor compliance is a major limitation to their effectiveness; where appropriate, potassium-sparing diuretics are preferable (see also above). When there is *established potassium depletion* larger doses may be necessary, the quantity depending on the severity of any continuing potassium loss (monitoring of plasma-potassium concentration and specialist advice would be required). Potassium depletion is frequently associated with chloride depletion and with metabolic alkalosis, and these disorders require correction.

ADMINISTRATION. Potassium salts are preferably given as a liquid (or effervescent) preparation, rather than modified-release tablets; they should be given as the chloride (the use of effervescent potassium tablets BPC 1968 should be restricted to *hyperchloraemic states*, section 9.2.1.3).
Salt substitutes. A number of salt substitutes which contain significant amounts of potassium chloride are readily available as health food products (e.g. Losalt® and Ruthmol®). These should not be used by patients with renal failure as potassium intoxication may result.

POTASSIUM BICARBONATE
Section 9.2.1.3

POTASSIUM CHLORIDE
Indications: potassium depletion (see notes above)
Cautions: elderly, mild to moderate renal impairment (close monitoring required), intestinal stricture, history of peptic ulcer, hiatus hernia (for sustained-release preparations); **important:** special hazard if given with drugs liable to raise plasma potassium concentration such as potassium-sparing diuretics, ACE inhibitors, or cyclosporin, for other **interactions:** Appendix 1 (potassium salts)
Contra-indications: severe renal impairment, plasma potassium concentrations above 5 mmol/litre

Side-effects: nausea and vomiting (severe symptoms may indicate obstruction), oesophageal or small bowel ulceration
Dose: see notes above
Note. Do not confuse Effervescent Potassium Tablets BPC 1968 (section 9.2.1.3) with effervescent potassium chloride tablets. Effervescent Potassium Tablets BPC 1968 do not contain chloride ions and their use should be restricted to hyperchloraemic states (section 9.2.1.3). Effervescent Potassium Chloride Tablets BP are usually available in two strengths, one containing 6.7 mmol each of K+ and Cl- (corresponding to Kloref®), the other containing 12 mmol K+ and 8 mmol Cl- (corresponding to Sando-K®). Generic prescriptions must specify the strength required.

Kay-Cee-L® (Geistlich)
Syrup, red, sugar-free, potassium chloride 7.5% (1 mmol/mL each of K+ and Cl-). Net price 500 mL = £3.00. Label: 21

Kloref® (Cox)
Tablets, effervescent, betaine hydrochloride, potassium benzoate, bicarbonate, and chloride, equivalent to potassium chloride 500 mg (6.7 mmol each of K+ and Cl-). Net price 50 = £1.66. Label: 13, 21

Kloref-S® (Cox)
Granules, effervescent, sugar-free, betaine hydrochloride, potassium bicarbonate and chloride equivalent to potassium chloride 1.5 g (20 mmol each of K+ and Cl-)/sachet. Net price 30 sachets = £3.30. Label: 13, 21

Sando-K® (Sandoz)
Tablets, effervescent, potassium bicarbonate and chloride equivalent to potassium 470 mg (12 mmol of K+) and chloride 285 mg (8 mmol of Cl-). Net price 20 = 34p. Label: 13, 21

Modified-release preparations
Avoid unless effervescent tablets or liquid preparations inappropriate
Slow-K® (Ciba)
Tablets, m/r, orange, s/c, potassium chloride 600 mg (8 mmol each of K+ and Cl-). Net price 20 = 10p. Label: 25, 27, counselling, swallow whole with fluid during meals while sitting or standing

POTASSIUM CITRATE
See section 7.4.3

POTASSIUM REMOVAL

Ion-exchange resins may be used to remove excess potassium in *mild hyperkalaemia* or in *moderate hyperkalaemia* when there are not ECG changes; intravenous therapy is required in emergencies (section 9.2.2).

POLYSTYRENE SULPHONATE RESINS
Indications: hyperkalaemia associated with anuria or severe oliguria, and in dialysis patients
Cautions: children (impaction of resin with excessive dosage or inadequate dilution)

Contra-indications: avoid calcium-containing resin in hyperparathyroidism, multiple myeloma, sarcoidosis, or metastatic carcinoma; avoid sodium-containing resin in congestive heart failure and severe renal impairment

Side-effects: rectal ulceration following rectal administration

Dose: *by mouth*, 15 g 3–4 times daily in water (not fruit juice which has a high K$^+$ content)

By rectum, as an enema, 30 g in methylcellulose solution, retained for 9 hours

CHILD, either route, 0.5–1 g/kg daily

Calcium Resonium® (Sanofi Winthrop)
Powder, buff, calcium polystyrene sulphonate. Net price 300 g = £43.23. Label: 13

Resonium A® (Sanofi Winthrop)
Powder, buff, sodium polystyrene sulphonate. Net price 454 g = £58.53. Label: 13

9.2.1.2 ORAL SODIUM AND WATER

Sodium chloride is indicated in states of sodium depletion and usually needs to be given intravenously (section 9.2.2). In chronic conditions associated with mild or moderate degrees of sodium depletion, e.g. in salt-losing bowel or renal disease, oral supplements of sodium chloride or bicarbonate (section 9.2.1.3), according to the acid-base status of the patient, may be sufficient.

SODIUM BICARBONATE
Section 9.2.1.3

SODIUM CHLORIDE
Indications: sodium depletion; see also section 9.2.2.

Slow Sodium® (Ciba)
Tablets, m/r, sodium chloride 600 mg (approx. 10 mmol each of Na$^+$ and Cl$^-$). Net price 100-tab pack = 55p. Label: 25
Dose: prophylaxis of sodium chloride deficiency 4–8 tablets daily with water (in severe depletion up to max. 20 tablets daily)
Chronic renal salt wasting, up to 20 tablets daily with appropriate fluid intake
CHILD, according to requirements

ORAL REHYDRATION THERAPY (ORT)

As a worldwide problem *diarrhoea* is by far the most important indication for fluid and electrolyte replacement. Intestinal absorption of sodium and water is enhanced by glucose (and other carbohydrates). Replacement of fluid and electrolytes lost through diarrhoea can therefore be achieved by giving solutions containing sodium, potassium, and glucose.

Oral rehydration solutions should:
enhance the absorption of water and electrolytes;
replace the electrolyte deficit adequately and safely;
contain an alkalising agent to counter acidosis;
be slightly hypo-osmolar (about 250 mmol/litre);
be simple to use in hospital and at home;
be palatable and acceptable, especially to children;
be readily available.

It is the policy of the World Health Organization (WHO) to promote a single oral rehydration solution but use it flexibly (e.g. by giving extra water between drinks of oral rehydration solution to moderately dehydrated infants).

Oral rehydration solutions used in the UK are lower in sodium (35–60 mmol/litre) and higher in glucose (up to 200 mmol/litre) than the WHO formulation. They are of benefit for *mild to moderate diarrhoea*, when the body's homoeostatic mechanisms are still working and will not be harmful, but they may be suboptimal in correction of fluid loss and electrolyte imbalance. In the *more severe diarrhoeas* the WHO formulation is marginally more effective in correcting dehydration; it carries no danger of hypernatraemia if used correctly. In acute diarrhoea normal feeding can continue as soon as the fluid deficit has been corrected; breast-feeding in particular should be offered between oral rehydration drinks.

For intravenous rehydration see section 9.2.2.

ORAL REHYDRATION SALTS (ORS)
Indications: fluid and electrolyte loss in diarrhoea, see notes above

Dose: according to fluid loss, usually 200–400 mL solution after every loose motion; INFANT 1–1½ times usual feed volume; CHILD 200 mL after every loose motion

UK formulations
Note. After reconstitution any unused solution should be discarded no later than 1 hour after preparation unless stored in a refrigerator when it may be kept for up to 24 hours.

Diocalm Junior® (SmithKline Beecham Healthcare)
Oral powder, sodium chloride 350 mg, potassium chloride 300 mg, sodium citrate 590 mg, anhydrous glucose 4 g/sachet. Net price 5-sachet pack (orange-flavoured) = £1.29

Reconstitute one sachet with 200 mL of water (freshly boiled and cooled for infants)

Note. Five sachets reconstituted with 1 litre of water provide Na$^+$ 60 mmol, K$^+$ 20 mmol, Cl$^-$ 50 mmol, citrate 10 mmol, and glucose 111 mmol

Dioralyte® (Rhône-Poulenc Rorer)
Effervescent tablets, sodium chloride 117 mg, sodium bicarbonate 336 mg, potassium chloride 186 mg, citric acid anhydrous 384 mg, anhydrous glucose 1.62 g. Net price 10-tab pack (blackcurrant- or citrus-flavoured) = £1.23

Reconstitute 2 tablets with 200 mL of water (only for adults and for children over 1 year)

Note. Ten tablets when reconstituted with 1 litre of water provide Na$^+$ 60 mmol, K$^+$ 25 mmol, Cl$^-$ 45 mmol, citrate 20 mmol, and glucose 90 mmol

Oral powder, sodium chloride 470 mg, potassium chloride 300 mg, disodium hydrogen citrate 530 mg, glucose 3.56 g/sachet. Net price 20 sachet-pack (blackcurrant- or citrus-flavoured or plain) = £4.47

Reconstitute one sachet with 200 mL of water (freshly boiled and cooled for infants)

Note. Five sachets reconstituted with 1 litre of water provide Na$^+$ 60 mmol, K$^+$ 20 mmol, Cl$^-$ 60 mmol, citrate 10 mmol, and glucose 90 mmol

Electrolade® (Eastern)

Oral powder, sodium chloride 236 mg, potassium chloride 300 mg, sodium bicarbonate 500 mg, anhydrous glucose 4 g/sachet (banana-, blackcurrent-, melon-, or orange-flavoured). Net price 6-sachet (multiflavoured) pack = £1.33, 20-sachet (single- or multiflavoured) pack = £4.25

Reconstitute one sachet with 200 mL of water (freshly boiled and cooled for infants)

Note. Five sachets when reconstituted with 1 litre of water provide Na$^+$ 50 mmol, K$^+$ 20 mmol, Cl$^-$ 40 mmol, HCO$_3^-$ 30 mmol, and glucose 111 mmol

Gluco-lyte® (Cupal)

Oral powder, sodium chloride 200 mg, potassium chloride 300 mg, sodium bicarbonate 300 mg, glucose 8 g/sachet. Net price 6 sachets = £1.42

Reconstitute one sachet with 200 mL of water (freshly boiled and cooled for infants)

Note. Five sachets when reconstituted with 1 litre of water provide Na$^+$ 35 mmol, K$^+$ 20 mmol, Cl$^-$ 37 mmol, HCO$_3^-$ 18 mmol, and glucose 200 mmol (corresponds to Oral Rehydration Salts—Formula A, BP)

Rehidrat® (Searle)

Oral powder, sodium chloride 440 mg, potassium chloride 380 mg, sodium bicarbonate 420 mg, citric acid 440 mg, glucose 4.09 g, sucrose 8.07 g, fructose 70 mg/sachet. Net price 24-sachet pack (orange, blackcurrant or lemon and lime flavour) = £6.44; 16-sachet pack (mixed flavours) = £4.29

Note. Lemon and lime version stains vomit green; blackcurrant version contains greater amounts of glucose (4.13 g) and sucrose (8.17 g), and less fructose (10 mg)

Reconstitute one sachet with 250 mL of water (freshly boiled and cooled for infants)

Note. Four sachets when reconstituted with 1 litre of water provide Na$^+$ 50 mmol, K$^+$ 20 mmol, Cl$^-$ 50 mmol, HCO$_3^-$ 20 mmol, citrate 9 mmol, glucose approx. 91 mmol, sucrose approx. 94 mmol, and fructose approx. 1–2 mmol

WHO formulations
WHO Oral Rehydration Salts

Oral powder, sodium chloride 3.5 g, potassium chloride 1.5 g, sodium citrate 2.9 g, anhydrous glucose 20 g. To be dissolved in sufficient water to produce 1 litre (providing Na$^+$ 90 mmol, K$^+$ 20 mmol, Cl$^-$ 80 mmol, citrate 10 mmol, glucose 111 mmol/litre).

Note. Recommended by the WHO and the United Nations Childrens Fund but not commonly used in the UK. Corresponds to Oral Rehydration Salts—Citrate (Formula C) BP; the alternative WHO formulation corresponds to Oral Rehydration Salts—Bicarbonate (Formula B) BP and is less stable

9.2.1.3 ORAL BICARBONATE

Sodium bicarbonate is given by mouth for *chronic acidotic states* such as uraemic acidosis or renal tubular acidosis. The dose for correction of metabolic acidosis is not predictable and the response must be assessed; 4.8 g daily (57 mmol each of Na$^+$ and HCO$_3^-$) or more may be required. For severe metabolic acidosis, sodium bicarbonate can be given intravenously (section 9.2.2).

Sodium bicarbonate may also be used to make the pH of the urine alkaline (see section 7.4.3); for use in dyspepsia see section 1.1.2.

Sodium supplements may increase blood pressure or cause fluid retention and pulmonary oedema in those at risk; hypokalaemia may be exacerbated.

Where *hyperchloraemic acidosis* is associated with potassium deficiency, as in some renal tubular and gastro-intestinal disorders it may be appropriate to give oral **potassium bicarbonate**, although acute or severe deficiency should be managed by intravenous therapy.

SODIUM BICARBONATE

Indications: see notes above

Cautions: see notes above; avoid in respiratory acidosis; **interactions:** Appendix 1 (antacids and adsorbents)

Dose: see notes above

Sodium Bicarbonate (Non-proprietary)

Capsules, sodium bicarbonate 500 mg (approx. 6 mmol each of Na$^+$ and HCO$_3^-$). Net price 20 = 42p

Available from Norton

Tablets, sodium bicarbonate 600 mg, net price 20 tabs = 48p

POTASSIUM BICARBONATE

Indications: see notes above

Cautions: cardiac disease, renal impairment; **interactions:** Appendix 1 (potassium salts)

Contra-indications: hypochloraemia; plasma potassium concentration above 5 mmol/litre

Side-effects: nausea and vomiting

Dose: see notes above

Potassium Tablets, Effervescent, potassium bicarbonate 500 mg, potassium acid tartrate 300 mg, each tablet providing 6.5 mmol of K$^+$. To be dissolved in water before administration. Net price 100 = £3.58. Label: 13, 21

Available from APS, Cox, Evans, Hillcross

Note. These tablets do not contain chloride; for effervescent tablets containing potassium and chloride, see under Potassium Chloride, section 9.2.1.1

WATER

The term water used without qualification means either potable water freshly drawn direct from the public supply and suitable for drinking or freshly boiled and cooled purified water. The latter should be used if the public supply is from a local storage tank or if the potable water is unsuitable for a particular preparation. (Water for injections, section 9.2.2.)

9.2.2   Intravenous administration

Solutions of electrolytes are given intravenously, to meet normal fluid and electrolyte requirements or to replenish substantial deficits or continuing losses, when the patient is nauseated or vomiting and is unable to take adequate amounts by mouth. When intravenous administration is not possible large volumes of fluid can also be given subcutaneously by hypodermoclysis.

In an individual patient the nature and severity of the electrolyte imbalance must be assessed from the history and clinical and biochemical examination. Sodium, potassium, chloride, magnesium, phosphate, and water depletion can occur singly and in combination with or without disturbances of acid-base balance; for reference to the use of magnesium and phosphates, see section 9.5.

Isotonic solutions may be infused safely into a peripheral vein. Solutions more concentrated than plasma, for example 20% glucose are best given through an indwelling catheter positioned in a large vein.

INTRAVENOUS SODIUM

Sodium chloride in isotonic solution provides the most important extracellular ions in near physiological concentration and is indicated in *sodium depletion* which may arise from such conditions as gastro-enteritis, diabetic ketoacidosis, ileus, and ascites. In a severe deficit of from 4 to 8 litres, 2 to 3 litres of isotonic sodium chloride may be given over 2 to 3 hours; thereafter infusion can usually be at a slower rate.

Excessive administration should be avoided; the jugular venous pressure should be assessed, the bases of the lungs should be examined for crepitations, and in elderly or seriously ill patients it is often helpful to monitor the right atrial (central) venous pressure.

Compound sodium lactate (Hartmann's solution) can be used instead of isotonic sodium chloride solution during surgery or in the initial management of the injured or wounded.

Sodium chloride and glucose solutions are indicated when there is combined *water and sodium depletion*. A 1:1 mixture of isotonic sodium chloride and 5% glucose allows some of the water (free of sodium) to enter body cells which suffer most from dehydration while the sodium salt with a volume of water determined by the normal plasma Na$^+$ remains extracellular. Combined sodium, potassium, chloride, and water depletion may occur, for example, with severe diarrhoea or persistent vomiting; replacement is carried out with sodium chloride intravenous infusion 0.9% and glucose intravenous infusion 5% with potassium as appropriate

SODIUM CHLORIDE

Indications: electrolyte imbalance, also section 9.2.1.2

Cautions: restrict intake in impaired renal function, cardiac failure, hypertension, peripheral and pulmonary oedema, toxaemia of pregnancy

Side-effects: administration of large doses may give rise to sodium accumulation and oedema

Dose: see notes above

PoM **Sodium Chloride Intravenous Infusion,** usual strength sodium chloride 0.9% (9 g, 150 mmol each of Na$^+$ and Cl$^-$/litre), this strength being supplied when normal saline for injection is requested. Net price 2-mL amp = 26p; 5-mL amp = 31p; 10-mL amp = 35p; 20-mL amp = 89p; 50-mL amp = £2.25

In hospitals, 500- and 1000-mL packs, and sometimes other sizes, are available

Note. The term 'normal saline' should **not** be used to describe sodium chloride intravenous infusion 0.9%; the term 'physiological saline' is acceptable but it is preferable to give the composition (i.e. sodium chloride intravenous infusion 0.9%).

With other ingredients

PoM **Sodium Chloride and Glucose Intravenous Infusion,** usual strength sodium chloride 0.18% (1.8 g, 30 mmol each of Na$^+$ and Cl$^-$/litre) and 4% of anhydrous glucose

In hospitals, 500- and 1000-mL packs, and sometimes other sizes are available

PoM **Ringer's Solution for Injection,** calcium chloride (dihydrate) 322 micrograms, potassium chloride 300 micrograms, sodium chloride 8.6 mg/mL, providing the following ions (in mmol/litre), Ca^{2+} 2.2, K$^+$ 4, Na$^+$ 147, Cl$^-$ 156

In hospitals, 500- and 1000-mL packs, and sometimes other sizes, are available

PoM **Sodium Lactate Intravenous Infusion, Compound** (Hartmann's Solution for Injection; Ringer-Lactate Solution for Injection), sodium chloride 0.6%, sodium lactate 0.25%, potassium chloride 0.04%, calcium chloride 0.027% (containing Na$^+$ 131 mmol, K$^+$ 5 mmol, Ca^{2+} 2 mmol, HCO$_3^-$ (as lactate) 29 mmol, Cl$^-$ 111 mmol/litre)

In hospitals, 500- and 1000-mL packs, and sometimes other sizes, are available

INTRAVENOUS GLUCOSE

Glucose solutions (5%) are mainly used to replace water deficits and should be given alone when there is no significant loss of electrolytes. Average water requirements in a healthy adult are 1.5 to 2.5 litres daily and this is needed to balance unavoidable losses of water through the skin and lungs and to provide sufficient for urinary excretion. Water depletion (dehydration) tends to occur when these losses are not matched by a comparable intake, as for example may occur in coma or dysphagia or in the aged or apathetic who may not drink water in sufficient amount on their own initiative.

Excessive loss of water without loss of electrolytes is uncommon, occurring in fevers, hyperthyroidism, and in uncommon water-losing renal states such as diabetes insipidus or hypercalcaemia.

Abbreviations and symbols, see inside front cover

Prices are **net**, see p. 1

The volume of glucose solution needed to replace deficits varies with the severity of the disorder, but usually lies within the range of 2 to 6 litres.

Glucose solutions are also given in regimens with calcium, bicarbonate, and insulin for the emergency management of *hyperkalaemia*. They are also given, after correction of hyperglycaemia, during treatment of diabetic ketoacidosis, when they must be accompanied by continuing insulin infusion.

GLUCOSE
(Dextrose Monohydrate)

Note. Glucose BP is the monohydrate but Glucose Intravenous Infusion BP is a sterile solution of anhydrous glucose or glucose monohydrate, potency being expressed in terms of anhydrous glucose

Indications: fluid replacement (see notes above), provision of energy (section 9.3)

Side-effects: glucose injections especially if hypertonic may have a low pH and may cause venous irritation and thrombophlebitis

Dose: water replacement, see notes above; energy source, 1–3 litres daily of 20–50% solution

PoM **Glucose Intravenous Infusion,** glucose or anhydrous glucose (potency expressed in terms of anhydrous glucose), usual strength 5% (50 mg/mL). 25% solution, net price 25-mL amp = £2.21; 50% solution, 25-mL amp = £3.11, 50-mL amp = £1.76
In hospitals, 500- and 1000-mL packs, and sometimes other sizes, are available; also available from IMS (Min-I-Jet® Glucose, 50% in 50-ml disposable syringe).

INTRAVENOUS POTASSIUM

Potassium chloride and sodium chloride intravenous infusion and **potassium chloride and glucose** intravenous infusion are used to correct severe *hypokalaemia* and depletion and when sufficient potassium cannot be taken by mouth. Potassium chloride, as ampoules containing 1.5 g (20 mmol K^+) in 10 mL[1], may be added to 500 mL of sodium chloride or glucose intravenous infusion and given slowly over 2 to 3 hours with specialist advice and ECG monitoring in difficult cases[2]. Repeated measurements of plasma potassium are necessary to determine whether further infusions are required and to avoid the development of hyperkalaemia; this is *especially liable to occur* in renal impairment.

1. **Important**: mix infusion solution **thoroughly** after adding potassium chloride; use ready-prepared solutions when possible
2. Higher concentrations may be given in severe cases but require infusion pump control

POTASSIUM CHLORIDE

Indications: electrolyte imbalance; see also oral potassium supplements, section 9.2.1.1
Cautions: for intravenous infusion the concentration of solution should not usually exceed 3.2 g (43 mmol)/litre; specialist advice and ECG monitoring (see notes above)
Side-effects: rapid infusion toxic to heart

Dose: by slow intravenous infusion, depending on the deficit or the daily maintenance requirements, see also notes above

PoM **Potassium Chloride and Glucose Intravenous Infusion,** usual strength potassium chloride 0.3% (3 g, 40 mmol each of K^+ and Cl^-/litre) with 5% of anhydrous glucose
In hospitals, 500- and 1000-mL packs, and sometimes other sizes, are available

PoM **Potassium Chloride and Sodium Chloride Intravenous Infusion,** usual strength potassium chloride 0.3% (3 g/litre) and sodium chloride 0.9% (9 g/litre), containing 40 mmol of K^+, 150 mmol of Na^+, and 190 mmol of Cl^-/litre
In hospitals, 500- and 1000-mL packs, and sometimes other sizes, are available

PoM **Potassium Chloride, Sodium Chloride, and Glucose Intravenous Infusion,** sodium chloride 0.18% (1.8 g, 30 mmol of Na^+/litre) with 4% of anhydrous glucose and usually sufficient potassium chloride to provide 10–40 mmol of K^+/litre (to be specified by the prescriber)
In hospitals, 500- and 1000-mL packs, and sometimes other sizes, are available

PoM **Potassium Chloride Solution, Strong,** (sterile), potassium chloride 15% (150 mg, approximately 2 mmol each of K^+ and Cl^-/mL). Net price 10-mL amp = 45p
IMPORTANT. Must be diluted with **not less** than 50 times its volume of sodium chloride intravenous infusion 0.9% or other suitable diluent and **mixed well**
Solutions containing 10 and 20% of potassium chloride are also available in both 5- and 10-mL ampoules

BICARBONATE AND LACTATE

Sodium bicarbonate is used to control severe *metabolic acidosis* (as in renal failure). Since this condition is usually attended by sodium depletion, it is reasonable to correct this first by the administration of isotonic sodium chloride intravenous infusion, provided the kidneys are not primarily affected and the degree of acidosis is not so severe as to impair renal function. In these circumstances, isotonic sodium chloride alone is usually effective as it restores the ability of the kidneys to generate bicarbonate. In renal acidosis or in severe metabolic acidosis of any origin (for example blood pH < 7.1) sodium bicarbonate (1.26%) may be infused with isotonic sodium chloride when the acidosis remains unresponsive to correction of anoxia or fluid depletion; a total volume of up to 6 litres (4 litres of sodium chloride and 2 litres of sodium bicarbonate) may be necessary in the adult. In severe shock due for example to cardiac arrest (see section 2.7), metabolic acidosis may develop without sodium depletion; in these circumstances sodium bicarbonate is best given in a small volume of hypertonic solution, such as 50 mL of 8.4% solution intravenously; plasma pH should be monitored.

Sodium bicarbonate infusion is also used in the emergency management of *hyperkalaemia* (see also under Glucose).

Sodium lactate intravenous infusion is obsolete in metabolic acidosis, and carries the risk of producing lactic acidosis, particularly in seriously ill patients with poor tissue perfusion or impaired hepatic function.

SODIUM BICARBONATE

Indications: metabolic acidosis

Dose: by slow intravenous injection, a strong solution (up to 8.4%), or *by continuous intravenous infusion,* a weaker solution (usually 1.26%), an amount appropriate to the body base deficit (see notes above)

PoM **Sodium Bicarbonate Intravenous Infusion,** usual strength sodium bicarbonate 1.26% (12.6 g, 150 mmol each of Na+ and HCO₃⁻/litre); various other strengths available

In hospitals, 500- and 1000-mL packs, and sometimes other sizes, are available

PoM **Min-I-Jet® Sodium Bicarbonate** (IMS)

Intravenous injection, sodium bicarbonate in disposable syringe, net price 4.2%, 10 mL = £4.81; 8.4%, 10 mL = £5.19, 50 mL = £7.75

SODIUM LACTATE

Indications: see notes above

PoM **Sodium Lactate Intravenous Infusion,** sodium lactate M/6, contains the following ions (in mmol/litre), Na+ 167, HCO₃⁻ (as lactate) 167

WATER

PoM **Water for Injections.** Net price 1-mL amp = 16p; 2-mL amp = 15p; 5-mL amp = 22p; 10-mL amp = 26p; 20-mL amp = 57p; 50-mL amp = £1.52

9.2.3   Plasma and plasma substitutes

Plasma and albumin solutions, prepared from whole blood, contain soluble proteins and electrolytes but no clotting factors, blood group antibodies, or pseudocholinesterases; they may be given without regard to the recipient's blood group.

Plasma and albumin solutions are used for the treatment of severe hypoproteinaemia, particularly when associated with a low plasma volume. The use of these solutions in acute plasma or blood loss may be wasteful; plasma substitutes are more appropriate. Concentrated albumin solutions may also be used to obtain a diuresis in hypoalbuminaemic patients (e.g. in hepatic cirrhosis).

ALBUMIN SOLUTION

(Human Albumin Solution)

A solution containing protein derived from plasma, serum, or normal placentas; at least 95% of the protein is albumin. The solution may be isotonic (containing 4–5% protein) or concentrated (containing 15–25% protein).

Indications: see under preparations, below

Cautions: history of cardiac or circulatory disease (administer slowly to avoid rapid rise in blood pressure and cardiac failure, and monitor cardiovascular and respiratory function); correct dehydration when administering concentrated solution

Contra-indications: cardiac failure; severe anaemia

Side-effects: allergic reactions with nausea, vomiting, increased salivation, fever, and chills reported

Isotonic solutions

Indications: acute or sub-acute loss of plasma volume e.g. in burns, pancreatitis, trauma, and complications of surgery; plasma exchange

Available as: *Human Albumin Solution 4.5%* (50-, 100-, 250-, and 400-mL bottles—Immuno); *Albuminar-5®* (500-mL vials—Armour); *Albutein®* 5% (250- and 500-mL vials—Alpha); *Buminate®* 5.0% (250- and 500-mL bottles—Baxter); *Zenalb®* 4.5 (50-, 100-, 250-, and 500-mL bottles—BPL)

Concentrated solutions (20–25%)

Indications: severe hypoalbuminaemia associated with low plasma volume and generalised oedema where salt and water restriction with plasma volume expansion are required; adjunct in the treatment of hyperbilirubinaemia by exchange transfusion in the newborn

Available as: *Albumin Solution 20%* (100-mL vials—SNBTS); *Human Albumin Solution 20%* (10-, 50-, and 100-mL vials—Immuno); *Albutein®* 20% (50- and 100-mL vials—Alpha); *Albutein®* 25% (20-, 50-, and 100-mL vials—Alpha); *Buminate®* 20% (50- and 100-mL vials—Baxter); *Zenalb®* 20 (5-, 50-, and 100-mL bottles—BPL)

PLASMA PROTEIN SOLUTION

(Plasma Protein Fraction, PPF)

An isotonic solution containing 4–5% protein derived from plasma or serum; at least 85% of the protein is albumin.

Indications: see notes above

Cautions; Contra-indications; Side-effects: see under Albumin Solution

Preparations

Available as: *Plasma Protein Solution 4.5%* (100- and 500-mL bottles—SNBTS); *Plasmatein®* 5% (250- and 500-mL vials—Alpha)

PLASMA SUBSTITUTES

Dextrans, gelatin, and the etherified starches, **hetastarch** and **pentastarch** are macromolecular substances which are slowly metabolised; they may be used at the outset to expand and maintain blood volume in shock arising from conditions such as burns or septicaemia. They are rarely needed when shock is due to sodium and water depletion as, in these circumstances, the shock responds to water and electrolyte repletion. They should not be used to maintain plasma volume in conditions such as burns or peritonitis where there is loss of plasma protein, water and electrolytes over periods of several days or weeks. In these situations, plasma or plasma protein fractions containing large amounts of albumin should be given. Plasma substitutes may be used as an immediate short-term measure to treat haemorrhage until blood is available.

Dextrans may interfere with blood group cross-matching or biochemical measurements and these should be carried out before infusion is begun. Dextran 70 by intravenous infusion is used predominantly for volume expansion. Dextran 40 intravenous infusion is used in an attempt to improve peripheral blood flow in ischaemic disease of the limbs. Dextrans 40 and 70 have also been used in the prophylaxis of thromboembolism but are now rarely used for this purpose.

Dosage. Because of the complex requirements relating to blood volume expansion and the primary significance of blood, plasma protein, and electrolyte replacement, detailed dose statements have been omitted. *In all cases data sheets and specialist literature should be consulted.*

DEXTRAN 40 INTRAVENOUS INFUSION

Dextrans of weight average molecular weight about '40 000' 10% in glucose intravenous infusion 5% or in sodium chloride intravenous infusion 0.9%

Indications: conditions associated with peripheral local slowing of the blood flow; prophylaxis of post-surgical thrombo-embolic disease (but see notes above)

Cautions; Contra-indications; Side-effects: see under Dextran 70 Intravenous Infusion; correct dehydration before infusion and give adequate fluids during therapy; very special care in those at risk of vascular overloading

Dose: by intravenous infusion, initially 500–1000 mL; further doses are given according to the patient's condition (see notes above)

PoM **Gentran 40**® (Baxter)
Intravenous infusion, dextran 40 intravenous infusion in glucose intravenous infusion 5% or in sodium chloride intravenous infusion 0.9%. Net price 500-mL bottle (both) = £4.78
PoM [1] **Rheomacrodex**® (Pharmacia)
Intravenous infusion, dextran 40 intravenous infusion in glucose intravenous infusion 5% or in sodium chloride intravenous infusion 0.9%. Net price 500-mL bottle (both) = £6.35
1. May no longer be available from Pharmacia—contact Cambridge

DEXTRAN 70 INTRAVENOUS INFUSION

Dextrans of weight average molecular weight about '70 000' 6% in glucose intravenous infusion 5% or in sodium chloride intravenous infusion 0.9%

Indications: short-term blood volume expansion; prophylaxis of post-surgical thrombo-embolic disease (but see notes above)

Cautions: congestive heart failure, renal impairment; blood samples for cross-matching should ideally be taken before infusion

Contra-indications: severe congestive heart failure; renal failure; bleeding disorders such as thrombocytopenia and hypofibrinogenaemia

Side-effects: urticarial and other hypersensitivity reactions—rarely severe anaphylactoid reactions

Dose: by intravenous infusion, after moderate to severe haemorrhage or in the shock phase of burn injury (initial 48 hours), 500–1000 mL rapidly initially followed by 500 mL later if necessary (see also notes above); total dosage should not exceed 20 mL/kg during initial 24 hours; CHILD total dosage should not exceed 20 mL/kg

PoM **Gentran 70**® (Baxter)
Intravenous infusion, dextran 70 intravenous infusion in glucose intravenous infusion 5% or in sodium chloride intravenous infusion 0.9%. Net price 500-mL bottle (both) = £4.90
PoM [1] **Macrodex**® (Pharmacia)
Intravenous infusion, dextran 70 intravenous infusion in glucose intravenous infusion 5% or in sodium chloride intravenous infusion 0.9%. Net price 500-mL bottle (both) = £4.01
1. May no longer be available from Pharmacia—contact Cambridge

GELATIN

Note. The gelatin is partially degraded
Indications: low blood volume
Cautions; Contra-indications; Side-effects: see under Dextran 70 Intravenous Infusion; increased risk of hypersensitivity reactions
Dose: by intravenous infusion, initially 500–1000 mL of a 3.5–4% solution (see notes above)

PoM **Gelofusine**® (Braun)
Intravenous infusion, succinylated gelatin (modified fluid gelatin, average molecular weight 30 000) 4%, sodium chloride 0.9%. Net price 500-mL bottle = £4.50
PoM **Haemaccel**® (Hoechst)
Intravenous infusion, polygeline (degraded and modified gelatin, average molecular weight 30 000) 35 g, Na^+ 145 mmol, K^+ 5.1 mmol, Ca^{2+} 6.25 mmol, Cl^- 145 mmol/litre. Net price 500-mL bottle = £3.71

ETHERIFIED STARCH

A starch composed of more than 90% of amylopectin that has been etherified with hydroxyethyl groups; hetastarch has a higher degree of etherification than pentastarch
Indications: low blood volume
Cautions; Contra-indications; Side-effects: see under Dextran 70 Intravenous Infusion; pruritus reported
Dose: see under preparations below

Hetastarch
PoM **Hespan**® (Geistlich)
Intravenous infusion, hetastarch (weight average molecular weight 450 000) 6% in sodium chloride intravenous infusion 0.9%. Net price 500-mL Steri-flex® bag = £16.30
Dose: by intravenous infusion, 500–1000 mL; usual daily max. 1500 mL (see notes above)

Hexastarch
PoM **eloHAES**® (Fresenius)
Intravenous infusion, hexastarch (weight average molecular weight 200 000) 6% in sodium chloride intravenous infusion 0.9%. Net price 500-mL Mono-flac® bag = £12.50
Dose: by intravenous infusion, 500–1000 mL; usual daily max. 1500 mL (see notes above)

Pentastarch
PoM HAES-steril® (Fresenius)

Intravenous infusion, pentastarch (weight average molecular weight 200 000), net price (both in sodium chloride intravenous infusion 0.9%) 6%, 500 mL = £10.50; 10%, 500 mL = £16.50

Dose: by intravenous infusion, usual range 500–1000 mL (see notes above)

PoM Pentaspan® (Geistlich)

Intravenous infusion, pentastarch (weight average molecular weight 250 000) 10% in sodium chloride intravenous infusion 0.9%. Net price 500-mL Intraflex bag = £11.25

Dose: by intravenous infusion, 500–2000 mL; usual daily max. 2000 mL (see notes above)

9.3   Intravenous nutrition

When adequate feeding via the alimentary tract is not possible, nutrients may be given by intravenous infusion. This may be in addition to ordinary oral or tube feeding—**supplemental parenteral nutrition**, or may be the sole source of nutrition—**total parenteral nutrition** (TPN). Indications for this method include preparation of undernourished patients for surgery, chemotherapy, or radiation therapy; severe or prolonged disorders of the gastro-intestinal tract; major surgery, trauma, or burns; prolonged coma or refusal to eat; and some patients with renal or hepatic failure. The composition of proprietary preparations available is in the table below.

Total parenteral nutrition requires the use of a solution containing amino acids, glucose, fat, electrolytes, trace elements, and vitamins. This is now commonly provided by the pharmacy in the form of the 3-litre bag. Loading doses of vitamin B_{12} and folic acid are advised and other vitamins are given parenterally twice weekly.

The nutrition solution is infused through a central venous catheter inserted under full surgical precautions. Alternatively infusion through a peripheral vein is used for supplementary as well as total parenteral nutrition for periods of up to a month, depending on the availability of peripheral veins; factors prolonging cannula life and preventing thrombophlebitis include the use of soft polyurethane paediatric cannulae and use of feeds of low osmolality and normal pH. Only nutritional fluids should be given by the intravenous line.

Before starting, the patient should be well oxygenated with a near normal circulating blood volume and attention should be given to renal function and acid-base status. Appropriate biochemical tests should have been carried out beforehand and serious deficits corrected. Nutritional and electrolyte status must be monitored throughout treatment.

Protein is given as mixtures of essential and non-essential synthetic L-amino acids. Ideally, all essential amino acids should be included with a wide variety of non-essential ones to provide sufficient nitrogen together with electrolytes (see also section 9.2.2). Available solutions vary in their composition of amino acids; they often contain an energy source (usually glucose) and electrolytes.

Energy is provided in a ratio of 0.6 to 1.1 megajoules (150–250 kcals) per gram of protein nitrogen. Energy requirements must be met if amino acids are to be utilised for tissue maintenance. A mixture of carbohydrate and fat energy sources (usually 30–50% as fat) gives better utilisation of amino acids than glucose alone.

Glucose is the preferred source of carbohydrate, but if more than 180 g is given per day frequent monitoring of blood glucose is required, and insulin may be necessary. Glucose in various strengths from 10 to 50% must be infused through a central venous catheter to avoid thrombosis.

Fructose and sorbitol have been used in an attempt to avoid the problem of hyperosmolar hyperglycaemic non-ketotic acidosis but other metabolic problems may occur, as with xylitol and ethanol which are now rarely used.

Fat emulsions have the advantages of a high energy to fluid volume ratio, neutral pH, and iso-osmolarity with plasma, and provide essential fatty acids. Available preparations are soya bean oil emulsions. Several days of adaptation may be required to attain maximal utilisation. Reactions include occasional febrile episodes (usually only with 20% emulsions) and rare anaphylactic responses. Interference with biochemical measurements such as those for blood gases and calcium may occur if samples are taken before fat has been cleared. Daily checks are necessary to ensure complete clearance from the plasma in conditions where fat metabolism may be disturbed. **Additives may only be mixed with fat emulsions where compatibility is known.**

SUPPLEMENTARY PREPARATIONS

Administration. Because of the complex requirements relating to parenteral nutrition full details relating to administration have been omitted. In all cases *data sheets and specialist literature should be consulted.*

PoM Addiphos® (Pharmacia)

Solution, sterile, phosphate 40 mmol, K^+ 30 mmol, Na^+ 30 mmol/20 mL. For addition to Vamin® solutions and glucose intravenous infusions. Net price 20-mL vial = £1.15

PoM Additrace® (Pharmacia)

Solution, trace elements for addition to Vamin® solutions, traces of Fe^{3+}, Zn^{2+}, Mn^{2+}, Cu^{2+}, Cr^{3+}, Se^{4+}, Mo^{6+}, F^-, I^-. For adult use. Net price 10-mL amp = £1.75

PoM Cernevit® (Clintec)

Solution, *dl*-alpha tocopherol 11.2 units, ascorbic acid 125 mg, biotin 69 micrograms, cholecalciferol 220 units, cyanocobalamin 6 micrograms, folic acid 414 micrograms, glycine 250 mg, nicotinamide 46 mg, pantothenic acid (as dexpanthenol) 17.25 mg, pyridoxine hydrochloride 5.5 mg, retinol (as palmitate) 3500 units, riboflavine (as dihydrated sodium phosphate) 4.14 mg, thiamine (as cocarboxylase tetrahydrate) 3.51 mg. Dissolve in 5 mL water for injections. Net price per vial = £2.90

oprietary Infusion Fluids for Parenteral Feeding

Preparation	Nitrogen g/litre	[1]Energy kJ/litre	K+	Mg2+	Na+	Acet-	Cl-	Other components/litre
ninoplasmal L5 (Braun) Net price 500 mL = £8.40	8.03		25	2.5	48	59	31	acid phosphate 9 mmol, malate 7.5 mmol
ninoplasmal L10 (Braun) Net price 500 mL = £15.89	16.06		25	2.5	48	59	62	acid phosphate 9 mmol, malate 7.5 mmol
ninoplex 12 (Geistlich) Net price 500 mL = £11.31; 1000 mL = £19.07	12.44		30	2.5	35	5	67	malic acid 4.6 g
ninoplex 24 (Geistlich) Net price 250 mL = £9.79; 500 mL = £17.28	24.9		30	2.5	35	5	67	malic acid 4.5 g
inimix N9G20E (Clintec) Net price (dual compartment bag of amino acids with electrolytes 1000 mL and glucose 20% with calcium 1000 mL) = £29.00	4.55	1680	30	2.5	35	50	40	Ca2+ 2.25 mmol, phosphate 15 mmol, anhydrous glucose 100 g
inimix N14G30E (Clintec) Net price (dual compartment bag of amino acids with electrolytes 1000 mL and glucose 30% with calcium 1000 mL) = £33.00	7	2520	30	2.5	35	70	40	Ca2+ 2.25 mmol, phosphate 15 mmol, anhydrous glucose 150 g
eAmine III 8.5% (Fresenius) Net price 500 mL = £11.99; 1000 mL = £21.06	13.0				10	72	<3	phosphate 10 mmol
eAmine III 10% (Fresenius) Net price 500 mL = £13.60; 1000 mL = £23.50	15.3				10	88	<2	phosphate 20 mmol
eAmine HBC 6.9% (Fresenius) Net price 750 mL = £14.43	9.73				10	57	<3	
ucoplex 1000 (Geistlich) Net price 500 mL = £3.30; 1000 mL = £4.71		4200	30	2.5	50		67	acid phosphate 18 mmol, Zn2+ 0.046 mmol, anhydrous glucose 240 g
ucoplex 1600 (Geistlich) Net price 500 mL = £3.64; 1000 mL = £4.88		6700	30	2.5	50		67	acid phosphate 18 mmol, Zn2+ 0.046 mmol, anhydrous glucose 400 g
epanutrin (Geistlich) Net price 500 mL = £15.74	15.6							
eplexAmine 8% (Fresenius) Net price 500 mL = £16.28	12				10	61	<3	phosphate 10 mmol
yperamine 30 (Braun) Net price 500 mL = £22.04	30				5			
rafusin 22 (Pharmacia) Net price 500 mL = £14.38	22.8							
tralipid 10% (Pharmacia) Net price 100 mL = £3.90; 500 mL = £8.58		4600						fractionated soya oil 100 g, glycerol 22.5 g, phosphate 15 mmol
tralipid 20% (Pharmacia) Net price 100 mL = £5.85; 250 mL = £9.65; 00 mL = £12.87		8400						fractionated soya oil 200 g, glycerol 22.5 g, phosphate 15 mmol
tralipid 30% (Pharmacia) Net price 333 mL = £14.40		12600						fractionated soya oil 300 g, glycerol 16.7 g, phosphate 15 mmol
elip 10% (Clintec) Net price 100 mL = £4.78; 500 mL = £9.51		4600						soya oil 100 g, glycerol 25 g
elip 20% (Clintec) Net price 100 mL = £6.58; 500 mL = £14.53; 000 mL = £25.84		8400						soya oil 200 g, glycerol 25 g
abiMix 9 (Pharmacia) Net price 2580 mL = £64.00	3.49	2596	23	1.9	31		31	Ca2+ 1.9 mmol, anhydrous glucose 58.14 g, phosphate 10.9 mmol, fractionated soya oil 38.76 g, glycerol 4.26 g
abiMix 14 (Pharmacia) Net price 2580 mL = £70.00	5.23	3570	23	1.9	31		31	Ca2+ 1.9 mmol, anhydrous glucose 116.28 g, phosphate 10.9 mmol, fractionated soya oil 38.76 g, glycerol 4.26 g
pofundin MCT/LCT 10% (Braun) Net price 100 mL = £7.17; 500 mL = £12.01		4430						soya oil 50 g, medium chain triglycerides 50 g
pofundin MCT/LCT 20% (Braun) Net price 100 mL = £8.18; 250 mL = £10.52; 00 mL = £17.86		8000						soya oil 100 g, medium chain triglycerides 100 g
pofundin S 10% (Braun) Net price 100 mL = £6.70; 500 mL = £10.95		4470						soya oil 100 g
pofundin S 20% (Braun) Net price 100 mL = £7.81; 500 mL = £17.11		8520						soya oil 200 g
ephramine 5.4% (Fresenius) Net price 250 mL = £14.72	6.4				5	44	<3	essential amino acids only

[1]Excludes protein- or amino acid-derived energy

Note. 1000 kcal = 4200 kJ; 1000 kJ = 238.8 kcal. All entries are PoM

Proprietary Infusion Fluids for Parenteral Feeding (*continued*)

Preparation	Nitrogen g/litre	[1]Energy kJ/litre	K+	Mg2+	Na+	Acet−	Cl−	Other components/litre
Lipovenous 10% (Fresenius) Net price 500 mL = £9.50		4600						fractionated soya oil 100 g, egg lecithin 12 g, glycerol 25 g
Lipovenous 20% (Fresenius) Net price 100 mL = £4.90; 250 mL = £5.60; 500 mL = £14.50		8400						fractionated soya oil 100 g, egg lecithin 12 g, glycerol 25 g
Nutracel 400 (Clintec) Net price 500 mL = £2.54		3400		18		0.16	66	Ca2+ 15 mmol, Mn2+ 0.01 mmol, Zn2+ 0.08 mmol, anhydrous glucose 200 g
Nutracel 800 (Clintec) Net price 1000 mL = £4.39		3400		9		0.08	33	Ca2+ 7.5 mmol, Mn2+ 0.005 mmol, Zn2+ 0.04 mmol, anhydrous glucose 200 g
Nutriflex Basal (Braun) Net price (dual compartment bag of 800 mL and 1200 mL) = £27.50	4.6	2095	30	5.7	49.9	35	50	Ca2+ 3.6 mmol, phosphate 12.8 mmol, anhydrous glucose 125 g
Nutriflex Peri 40/80 (Braun) Net price (dual compartment bag of 800 mL and 1200 mL) = £34.00	5.7	1340	15	4	27	19.5	31.6	Ca2+ 2.5 mmol, phosphate 5.7 mmol, anhydrous glucose 80 g
Nutriflex Plus (Braun) Net price (dual compartment bag of 800 mL and 1200 mL) = £39.00	6.8	2510	25	5.7	37.2	22.9	35.5	Ca2+ 3.6 mmol, phosphate 20 mmol, anhydrous glucose 150 g
Nutriflex Special (Braun) Net price (dual compartment bag of 750 mL and 750 mL) = £43.00	10	4020	25.7	5	40.5	22	49.5	Ca2+ 4.1 mmol, phosphate 15 mmol, anhydrous glucose 240 g
Plasma-Lyte 148 (water) (Baxter) Net price 1000 mL = £1.63			5	1.5	140	27	98	gluconate 23 mmol
Plasma-Lyte 148 (dextrose 5%) (Baxter) Net price 1000 mL = £1.63		840	5	1.5	140	27	98	gluconate 23 mmol, anhydrous glucose 50 g
Plasma-Lyte M (dextrose 5%) (Baxter) Net price 1000 mL = £1.36		840	16	1.5	40	12	40	Ca2+ 2.5 mmol, lactate 12 mmol, anhydrous glucose 50 g
[2]Primene 10% (Clintec) Net price 100 mL = £6.05; 250 mL = £8.29	15					15.6		
Soyacal 10% (Alpha) Net price 50 mL = £2.75; 100 mL = £4.25; 250 mL = £7.25; 500 mL = £9.50		4600						purified soya oil 100 g, glycerol 22.1 g
Soyacal 20% (Alpha) Net price 50 mL = £4.25; 100 mL = £6.50; 250 mL = £10.75; 500 mL = £14.00		8400						purified soya oil 200 g, glycerol 22.1 g
Synthamin 9 (Clintec) Net price 500 mL = £6.97; 1000 mL = £12.92	9.1		60	5	70	100	70	acid phosphate 30 mmol
Synthamin 14 (Clintec) Net price 500 mL = £10.09; 1000 mL = £17.94; 3000 mL = £51.29	14.0		60	5	70	140	70	acid phosphate 30 mmol
Synthamin 14 without electrolytes (Clintec) Net price 500 mL = £10.34; 1000 mL = £18.33	14.0					68	34	
Synthamin 17 (Clintec) Net price 500 mL = £13.26; 1000 mL = £24.08	16.5		60	5	70	150	70	acid phosphate 30 mmol
Synthamin 17 without electrolytes (Clintec) Net price 500 mL = £13.26	16.5					82	40	
Vamin 9 (Pharmacia) Net price 500 mL = £5.85; 1000 mL = £10.04	9.4		20	1.5	50		50	Ca2+ 2.5 mmol
Vamin 9 Glucose (Pharmacia) Net price 100 mL = £3.02; 500 mL = £6.14; 1000 mL = £11.02	9.4	1700	20	1.5	50		50	Ca2+ 2.5 mmol, anhydrous glucose 100 g
Vamin 14 (Pharmacia) Net price 500 mL = £8.63; 1000 mL = £14.67	13.5		50	8	100	135	100	Ca2+ 5 mmol, SO4 2− 8 mmol
Vamin 14 (Electrolyte-Free) (Pharmacia) Net price 500 mL = £8.29; 1000 mL = £14.67	13.5							
Vamin 18 (Electrolyte-Free) (Pharmacia) Net price 500 mL = £10.97; 1000 mL = £19.74	18							
Vaminolact (Pharmacia) Net price 100 mL = £3.36; 500 mL = £7.75	9.3							
Vitrimix KV (Pharmacia) Net price (combined pack of Intralipid 20% 250 mL and Vamin 9 glucose 750 mL) = £19.40	7.0	3340	15	1.1	38		38	Ca2+ 1.9 mmol, anhydrous glucose 75 g

1. Excludes protein- or amino acid-derived energy
2. For use in neonates and children only

Note. 1000 kcal = 4200 kJ; 1000 kJ = 238.8 kcal. All entries are **PoM**

PoM Multibionta® (Merck)

Solution, ascorbic acid 500 mg, dexpanthenol 25 mg, nicotinamide 100 mg, pyridoxine hydrochloride 15 mg, riboflavine sodium phosphate 10 mg, thiamine hydrochloride 50 mg, tocopheryl acetate 5 mg, vitamin A 10 000 units. For addition to infusion solutions. Net price 10-mL amp = £1.61

Contra-indications: not for use in neonates owing to presence of benzyl alcohol as additive

PoM Peditrace® (Pharmacia)

Solution, trace elements for addition to Vaminolact®, Vamin® 14 Electrolyte-Free solutions and glucose intravenous infusions, traces of Zn^{2+}, Cu^{2+}, Mn^{2+}, Se^{4+}, F^-, I^-. For use in infants (when kidney function established, usually second day of life) and children. Net price 10-mL vial = £2.71

Cautions: reduced biliary excretion especially in cholestatic liver disease or in markedly reduced urinary excretion (careful biochemical monitoring required); total parenteral nutrition exceeding 1 month (measure serum manganese concentration and check liver function before commencing treatment and regularly during treatment)—discontinue if manganese concentration raised or if cholestasis develops

PoM Solivito N® (Pharmacia)

Solution, powder for reconstitution, biotin 60 micrograms, cyanocobalamin 5 micrograms, folic acid 400 micrograms, glycine 300 mg, nicotinamide 40 mg, pyridoxine hydrochloride 4.9 mg, riboflavine sodium phosphate 4.9 mg, sodium ascorbate 113 mg, sodium pantothenate 16.5 mg, thiamine mononitrate 3.1 mg. Dissolve in water for injections or glucose intravenous infusion for adding to glucose intravenous infusion or Intralipid®; dissolve in Vitlipid N® or Intralipid® for adding to Intralipid® only. Net price per vial = £1.75

PoM Vitlipid N® (Pharmacia)

Emulsion, adult, vitamin A 330 units, ergocalciferol 20 units, *dl*-alpha tocopherol 1 unit, phytomenadione 15 micrograms/mL. For addition to Intralipid®. Net price 10-mL amp = £1.71

Emulsion, infant, vitamin A 230 units, ergocalciferol 40 units, *dl*-alpha tocopherol 0.7 unit, phytomenadione 20 micrograms/mL. For addition to Intralipid®. Net price 10-mL amp = £1.71

9.4 Oral nutrition

9.4.1   Foods for special diets
9.4.2   Enteral nutrition

9.4.1   Foods for special diets

These are preparations that have been modified to eliminate a particular constituent from a food or are nutrient mixtures formulated as substitutes for the food. They are for patients who either cannot tolerate or cannot metabolise certain common constituents of food.

PHENYLKETONURIA. Phenylketonuria (phenylalaninaemia), which results from the inability to metabolise phenylalanine, is managed by restricting its dietary intake to a small amount sufficient for tissue building and repair. Aspartame (as a sweetener in some foods and medicines) contributes to the phenylalanine intake and may affect control of phenylketonuria. Where the presence of aspartame is specified on a data sheet this is indicated in the BNF against the preparation.

COELIAC DISEASE. Coeliac disease, which results from an intolerance to gluten, is managed by completely eliminating gluten from the diet.

> **ACBS.** In certain clinical conditions some foods may have the characteristics of drugs and the Advisory Committee on Borderline Substances advises as to the circumstances in which such foods may be regarded as drugs and so can be prescribed in the NHS. Prescriptions for these foods issued in accordance with the advice of this committee and endorsed 'ACBS' will normally not be investigated. See Appendix 7 for details of these foods and a listing by clinical condition (consult Drug Tariff for late amendments).

Preparations
See Appendix 7

9.4.2   Enteral nutrition

The body's reserves of protein rapidly become exhausted in severely ill patients, especially during chronic illness or in those with severe burns, extensive trauma, pancreatitis, or intestinal fistula. Much can be achieved by frequent meals and by persuading the patient to take supplementary snacks of ordinary food between the meals.

However, extra calories, protein, other nutrients, and vitamins are often best given by supplementing ordinary meals with sip or tube feeds of one of the nutritionally complete foods.

When patients cannot feed normally at all, for example patients with severe facial injury, oesophageal obstruction, or coma, a diet composed solely of nutritionally complete foods must be given. This is planned by a dietitian who will take into account the protein and total energy requirement of the patient and decide on the form and relative contribution of carbohydrate and fat to the energy requirements.

There are a number of nutritionally complete foods available and their use reduces an otherwise heavy workload in hospital or in the home. Most contain protein derived from milk or soya. Some contain protein hydrolysates or free amino acids and are only appropriate for patients who have diminished ability to break down protein, as may be the case in inflammatory bowel disease or pancreatic insufficiency.

Even when nutritionally complete feeds are being given it may be important to monitor water and electrolyte balance. Extra minerals (e.g. magnesium and zinc) may be needed in patients where gastrointestinal secretions are being lost. Additional vitamins may also be needed. Regular haematological and biochemical tests may be needed particularly in the unstable patient.

Some feeds are supplemented with vitamin K; for drug interactions of vitamin K see Appendix 1/ (vitamins).

CHILDREN. Infants and young children have special requirements and in most situations liquid feeds prepared for adults are totally unsuitable and should not be given. Expert advice should be sought.

Preparations
See Appendix 7

9.5   Minerals

9.5.1	Calcium and magnesium
9.5.2	Phosphorus
9.5.3	Fluoride
9.5.4	Zinc

See section 9.1.1 for iron salts.

9.5.1   Calcium and magnesium

9.5.1.1	Calcium supplements
9.5.1.2	Hypercalcaemia
9.5.1.3	Magnesium

9.5.1.1 CALCIUM SUPPLEMENTS

Calcium supplements are usually only required where dietary calcium intake is deficient. This dietary requirement varies with age and is relatively greater in childhood, pregnancy, and lactation, due to an increased demand, and in old age, due to impaired absorption. In osteoporosis a daily supplement of 800 mg (20 mmol) calcium (as a suitable salt) may reduce the rate of bone loss, but larger doses have not been shown to be more effective.

In hypocalcaemic tetany an initial intravenous injection of 10 mL (2.25 mmol) of calcium gluconate injection 10% may be followed by the continuous infusion of about 40 mL (9 mmol) daily, but plasma calcium should be monitored. This regimen can also be used, immediately but temporarily, to reduce the toxic effects of hyperkalaemia.

Calcium may also be used in cardiac resuscitation (see section 2.7.3).

CALCIUM SALTS

Indications: see notes above; calcium deficiency
Cautions: renal impairment; sarcoidosis; **interactions:** Appendix 1 (calcium salts)
Contra-indications: conditions associated with hypercalcaemia and hypercalciuria (eg. some forms of malignant disease)
Side-effects: mild gastro-intestinal disturbances; bradycardia, arrhythmias, and irritation after intravenous injection
Dose: by mouth, daily in divided doses, see notes above
By slow intravenous injection, acute hypocalcaemia, calcium gluconate 1–2 g (2.25–4.5 mmol of Ca^{2+})
CHILD obtain paediatric advice

Oral preparations
Calcium Gluconate (Non-proprietary)
Tablets, calcium gluconate 600 mg (53.4 mg calcium or 1.35 mmol Ca^{2+}). Net price 20 = 51p. Label: 24
Effervescent tablets, calcium gluconate 1 g (89 mg calcium or 2.25 mmol Ca^{2+}). Net price 100 = £7.68. Label: 13
Note. Each tablet usually contains 4.46 mmol Na^+

Calcium Lactate (Non-proprietary)
Tablets, calcium lactate 300 mg (39 mg calcium or 1 mmol Ca^{2+}). Net price 20 = 22p

Cacit® (Procter & Gamble Pharm.)
Tablets, effervescent, pink, calcium carbonate 1.25 g, providing calcium citrate when dispersed in water (500 mg calcium or 12.6 mmol Ca^{2+}). Net price 76-tab pack = £16.72. Label: 13

Calcichew® (Shire)
Tablets (both chewable), calcium carbonate 1.25 g (500 mg calcium or 12.6 mmol Ca^{2+}), net price 100-tab pack = £10.97; 2.5 g (*Calcichew Forte*®, 1 g calcium or 25 mmol Ca^{2+}), 100-tab pack = £21.94. Label: 24
Additives: include aspartame

Calcidrink® (Shire)
Granules, effervescent, calcium carbonate 2.52 g (1 g calcium or 25 mmol Ca^{2+}). Net price 30-sachet pack = £8.48. Label: 13

Calcium-500 (Martindale)
Tablets, pink, f/c, calcium carbonate 1.25 g (500 mg calcium or 12.5 mmol Ca^{2+}). Net price 100-tab pack = £9.97. Label: 25

Calcium-Sandoz® (Sandoz)
Syrup, calcium glubionate 1.09 g, calcium lactobionate 723 mg (108.3 mg calcium or 2.7 mmol Ca^{2+})/ 5 mL. Net price 500 mL = £2.41

Citrical® (Shire)
Granules, calcium carbonate 1.26 g (500 mg calcium or 12.6 mmol Ca^{2+})/sachet. Net price 90-sachet pack = £23.40. Label: 13

Ossopan® (Sanofi Winthrop)
Tablets, buff, f/c, hydroxyapatite 830 mg (calcium 178 mg or 4.4 mmol Ca^{2+}). Net price 50 = £10.09
Granules, brown, hydroxyapatite 3.32 g (calcium 712 mg or 17.8 mmol Ca^{2+})/sachet. Net price 28-sachet pack = £18.04

Ostram® (Merck)
Powder, calcium phosphate 3.3 g (1.2 g calcium or 29.9 mmol Ca^{2+})/sachet. Net price 30-sachet pack = £5.95. Label: 13

Sandocal® (Sandoz)
Sandocal-400 tablets, effervescent, calcium lactate gluconate 930 mg, calcium carbonate 700 mg, anhydrous citric acid 1.189 g, providing calcium 400 mg (10 mmol Ca^{2+}). Net price 5 × 20-tab pack = £7.20. Label: 13
Sandocal-1000 tablets, effervescent, calcium lactate gluconate 2.327 g, calcium carbonate 1.75 g, anhydrous citric acid 2.973 g providing 1 g calcium (25 mmol Ca^{2+}). Net price 3 × 10-tab pack = £6.45. Label: 13

Titralac®, section 9.5.2.2

Parenteral preparations
PoM **Calcium Gluconate** (Non-proprietary)
Injection, calcium gluconate 10% (8.9 mg calcium or 220 micromol Ca^{2+}/mL). Net price 10-mL amp = 47p

Available from Antigen, Phoenix

PoM Min-I-Jet® Calcium Chloride 10% (IMS)
Injection, calcium chloride 100 mg/mL (27.3 mg calcium or 680 micromol Ca^{2+}/mL). Net price 10-mL disposable syringe = £4.02

9.5.1.2 HYPERCALCAEMIA

Severe hypercalcaemia calls for urgent treatment before detailed investigation of the cause. After rehydration (if necessary with intravenous infusion of **sodium chloride 0.9%**) a **loop diuretic** may be given to deal with heart failure, but is not effective for reducing severe hypercalcaemia and care needs to be taken to avoid dehydration. Drugs (such as thiazides and vitamin D compounds) which promote hypercalcaemia, should be discontinued and dietary calcium should be restricted.

If *severe hypercalcaemia persists* drugs which inhibit mobilisation of calcium from the skeleton may be required. The **bisphosphonates** are useful and disodium pamidronate (see section 6.6.2) is probably the most effective.

Corticosteroids (see section 6.3) are widely given, but may only be useful where hypercalcaemia is due to sarcoidosis or vitamin D intoxication; they often take several days to achieve the desired effect.

Calcitonin (see section 6.6.1) is relatively non-toxic but is expensive and its effect can wear off after a few days despite continued use; it is rarely effective where bisphosphonates have failed to reduce serum calcium adequately.

Intravenous chelating drugs such as **trisodium edetate** are rarely used; they usually cause pain in the limb receiving the infusion and may cause renal damage.

After treatment of severe hypercalcaemia the underlying cause must be established. *Further treatment* is governed by the same principles as for initial therapy. Salt and water depletion and drugs promoting hypercalcaemia should be avoided; oral administration of a bisphosphonate may be useful. **Sodium cellulose phosphate**, which binds calcium in the gut, is rarely helpful, and any associated increase in serum phosphate may be harmful. Similarly, oral and intravenous phosphate may only achieve a reduction in serum calcium by precipitating calcium phosphate in the tissues, resulting in nephrocalcinosis and impairment of renal function. Parathyroidectomy may be indicated for hyperparathyroidism.

BISPHOSPHONATES
See section 6.6.2

CALCITONIN
See section 6.6.1

CORTICOSTEROIDS
See section 6.3.2

SODIUM CELLULOSE PHOSPHATE
Indications: reduction of calcium absorption from food in conditions such as hypercalciuria and hypercalcaemia (but see also notes above)
Cautions: renal impairment (avoid if severe); pregnancy and breast-feeding; growing children
Contra-indications: congestive heart failure and other conditions in which low sodium intake essential, severe renal impairment
Side-effects: occasional diarrhoea; magnesium deficiency reported
Dose: 5 g 3 times daily with meals; CHILD 10 g daily in 3 divided doses with meals

Calcisorb® (3M)
Sachets, sodium cellulose phosphate 5 g. Net price 90-sachet pack = £18.72. Label: 13, 21, counselling, may be sprinkled on food

TRISODIUM EDETATE
Indications: hypercalcaemia (but see notes above); lime burns in the eye (see under Preparations)
Cautions: repeated plasma-calcium determinations important; caution in tuberculosis; avoid rapid infusion, see under Dose
Contra-indications: impaired renal function
Side-effects: nausea, diarrhoea, cramp; in overdosage renal damage
Dose: hypercalcaemia, *by intravenous infusion* over 2–3 hours, up to 70 mg/kg daily; CHILD up to 60 mg/kg daily
IMPORTANT. Ensure rate of infusion and concentration correct (see Appendix 6); too rapid a rate or too high a concentration is extremely hazardous and repeated measurements of plasma calcium concentrations are important for control and maintenance of near normal ionised calcium concentrations. Decrease infusion rate on signs of increased muscle reactivity; discontinue if tetany occurs and restart cautiously only after plasma ionised and total calcium concentrations indicate need for further treatment (and tetany has stopped)

PoM Limclair® (Sinclair)
Injection, trisodium edetate 200 mg/mL. For dilution and use as an intravenous infusion. Net price 5-mL amp = £4.76
Note. For topical use in the eye, dilute 1 mL to 50 mL with sterile purified water

9.5.1.3 MAGNESIUM

Magnesium is an essential constituent of many enzyme systems, particularly those involved in energy generation; the largest stores are in the skeleton.

Magnesium salts are not well absorbed from the gastro-intestinal tract which explains the use of magnesium sulphate (section 1.6.4) as an osmotic laxative.

Magnesium is mainly excreted by the kidneys and is therefore retained in renal failure although significant *hypermagnesaemia* (causing muscle weakness and arrhythmias) is rare.

HYPOMAGNESAEMIA. Since magnesium is secreted in large amounts in the gastro-intestinal fluid, excessive losses in diarrhoea, stoma or fistula are the most common of the causes of *hypomagnesaemia*; deficiency may also occur in alcoholism or diuretic therapy and it has been reported after prolonged treatment with aminoglycosides. Hypomagnesaemia often causes secondary hypocalcaemia (with which it may be confused) and also hypokalaemia and hyponatraemia.

Symptomatic *hypomagnesaemia* is associated with a deficit of 0.5–1 mmol/kg; up to 160 mmol Mg^{2+} over up to 5 days may be required to replace the deficit (allowing for urinary losses). Magnesium is given initially by intravenous infusion or by intramuscular injection of **magnesium sulphate**; the intramuscular injection is painful. Plasma magnesium concentrations should be measured to determine the rate and duration of infusion and the dose should be reduced in renal impairment. To prevent *recurrence of the deficit*, magnesium may be given by mouth in a dose of 24 mmol Mg^{2+} daily in divided doses; a suitable preparation is magnesium glycerophosphate tablets [not licensed]. For maintenance (e.g. in intravenous nutrition), parenteral doses of magnesium are of the order of 10–20 mmol Mg^{2+} daily (often about 12 mmol Mg^{2+} daily).

ARRHYTHMIAS. Magnesium sulphate has also been recommended for the emergency treatment of *serious arrhythmias*, especially in the presence of hypokalaemia (when hypomagnesaemia may also be present) and when salvos of rapid ventricular tachycardia show the characteristic twisting wave front known as *torsades de pointes*. The usual dose of magnesium sulphate is intravenous injection of 8 mmol Mg^{2+} over 10–15 minutes (repeated once if necessary).

MYOCARDIAL INFARCTION. Evidence suggesting a sustained reduction in mortality in patients with *suspected myocardial infarction* given an initial intravenous injection of magnesium sulphate 8 mmol Mg^{2+} over 20 minutes followed by an intravenous infusion of 65–72 mmol Mg^{2+} over the following 24 hours, has not been borne out by a larger study. Some workers, however, continue to hold the view that magnesium is beneficial if given immediately (and for as long as there is a likelihood of reperfusion taking place).

ECLAMPSIA. Magnesium sulphate has been shown to have a major role in *eclampsia* for the prevention of recurrent seizures. Regimens in the UK may vary between hospitals but typically involve initial intravenous administration of magnesium sulphate 4 g (approx. 16 mmol Mg^{2+}) over up to 20 minutes followed by intravenous infusion at a rate of 1 g (approx. 4 mmol Mg^{2+}) every hour; recurrence of seizures may require an additional intravenous bolus of 2–4 g (approx. 8–16 mmol Mg^{2+}). ECG monitoring is carried out as is monitoring of blood pressure and of clinical signs of overdosage (loss of patellar reflexes, weakness, nausea, sensation of warmth, flushing, drowsiness, double vision, and slurred speech—calcium gluconate injection is used for the management of magnesium toxicity); plasma-magnesium concentration is monitored where it is considered necessary. It is also essential to monitor the fetal heart rate continuously.

MAGNESIUM SULPHATE

Indications: see notes above; constipation, section 1.6.4; paste for boils, section 13.10.5

Cautions: hepatic impairment (see Appendix 2) renal impairment (risk of accumulation); monitor magnesium and other electrolytes closely; in severe hypomagnesaemia administer initially via controlled infusion device (preferably syringe pump); **interactions:** Appendix 1 (magnesium salts)

Side-effects: generally associated with hypermagnesaemia, nausea, vomiting, thirst, flushing of skin, hypotension, arrhythmias, coma, respiratory depression, drowsiness, confusion, loss of tendon reflexes, muscle weakness; colic and diarrhoea following oral administration

Dose: see notes above

PoM Magnesium Sulphate (Non-proprietary)
Injection, magnesium sulphate 50% (approx 2 mmol Mg^{2+}/mL). Net price 2-mL (1-g) amp = £4.18
Available from Evans

9.5.2   Phosphorus

9.5.2.1   Phosphate supplements
9.5.2.2   Phosphate-binding agents

9.5.2.1 PHOSPHATE SUPPLEMENTS

Oral phosphate supplements may be required in addition to vitamin D in a small minority of patient with hypophosphataemic vitamin D-resistant rickets. Diarrhoea is a common side-effect and should prompt a reduction in dosage.

Phosphate infusion is occasionally needed in alcohol dependence or in phosphate deficiency arising from use of parenteral nutrition deficient in phosphate supplements; phosphate depletion also occurs in severe diabetic ketoacidosis. For *established hypophosphataemia*, monobasic potassium phosphate may be infused at a maximum rate of 9 mmol every 12 hours. Excessive doses of phosphates may cause hypocalcaemia and metastatic calcification; it is *essential* to monitor closely plasma concentrations of calcium, phosphate potassium, and other electrolytes.

In *total parenteral nutrition* regimens, it is necessary to provide adequate phosphate in order to allow phosphorylation of the glucose; between 20 and 30 mmol of phosphate is required daily.

Phosphate-Sandoz® (Sandoz)
Tablets, effervescent, anhydrous sodium acid phosphate 1.936 g, sodium bicarbonate 350 mg potassium bicarbonate 315 mg, equivalent to phosphorus 500 mg (16.1 mmol phosphate), sodium 468.8 mg (20.4 mmol Na^+), potassium 123 mg (3.1 mmol K^+). Net price 20 = 73p. Label 13
Dose: hypercalcaemia, up to 6 tablets daily adjusted according to response; CHILD under 5 years up to 3 tablets daily
Vitamin D-resistant hypophosphataemic osteomalacia 4–6 tablets daily; CHILD under 5 years 2–3 tablets daily

5.2.2 PHOSPHATE-BINDING AGENTS

Aluminium-containing and calcium-containing antacids are used as phosphate-binding agents in the management of hyperphosphataemia complicating renal failure. Calcium-containing phosphate-binding agents are contra-indicated in hypercalcaemia or hypercalciuria. Phosphate-binding agents which contain aluminium may increase plasma aluminium in dialysis patients.

ALUMINIUM HYDROXIDE

Indications: hyperphosphataemia

Cautions: hyperaluminaemia; porphyria (see section 9.8.2); see also notes above; **interactions:** Appendix 1 (antacids and adsorbents)

Aluminium Hydroxide (Non-proprietary)

Mixture (gel), about 4% w/w Al_2O_3 in water. Net price 200 mL = 41p

Dose: hyperphosphataemia, 20–100 mL according to requirements of patient; antacid, see section 1.1.1

Note. The brand name NHS Aludrox® (Pfizer Consumer) is used for aluminium hydroxide mixture, net price 200 mL = 82p. For NHS Aludrox® tablets see preparations with magnesium, section 1.1.1

Alu-Cap® (3M)

Capsules, green/red, dried aluminium hydroxide 475 mg (low Na⁺). Net price 120-cap pack = £4.22

Dose: phosphate-binding agent in renal failure, 4–20 capsules daily in divided doses with meals; antacid, see section 1.1.1

CALCIUM CARBONATE

Indications: hyperphosphataemia

Cautions: see notes above; **interactions:** Appendix 1 (calcium salts)

Side-effects: hypercalcaemia

Calcichew®, section 9.5.1.1

Calcium-500, section 9.5.1.1

Titralac® (3M)

Tablets, calcium carbonate 420 mg (168 mg calcium or 4.2 mmol Ca^{2+}), glycine 180 mg. Net price 180-tab pack = £2.94

COUNSELLING. May be chewed, crushed or swallowed whole

Dose: calcium supplement, or phosphate-binding agent (with meals) in renal failure, according to the requirements of the patient

9.5.3   Fluoride

Availability of adequate fluoride confers significant resistance to dental caries. It is now considered that the topical action of fluoride on enamel and plaque is more important than the systemic effect.

Where the natural fluoride content of the drinking water is significantly less than 1 mg per litre (one part per million) artificial fluoridation is the most economical method of supplementing fluoride intake.

Daily administration of tablets or drops is a suitable alternative, but systemic fluoride supplements should not be prescribed without prior reference to the fluoride content of the local water supply; they are not advisable when the water contains more than 700 micrograms per litre (0.7 parts per million). In addition, the British Association for the Study of Community Dentistry now recommends[1] that infants need not receive fluoride supplements until the age of 6 months.

Use of dentifrices which incorporate sodium fluoride and/or monofluorophosphate is also a convenient source of fluoride.

Individuals who are either particularly caries prone or medically compromised may be given additional protection by use of fluoride rinses or by application of fluoride gels. Rinses may be used daily or weekly; daily use of a less concentrated rinse is more effective than weekly use of a more concentrated one. Gels must be applied on a regular basis under professional supervision; extreme caution is necessary to prevent the child from swallowing any excess. Less concentrated gels have recently become available for home use. Varnishes are also available and are particularly valuable for young or handicapped children since they adhere to the teeth and set in the presence of moisture.

SODIUM FLUORIDE

Note. Sodium fluoride 2.2 mg provides approx. 1 mg fluoride ion

Indications: prophylaxis of dental caries—see notes above

Contra-indications: not for areas where drinking water is fluoridated

Side-effects: occasional white flecks on teeth with recommended doses; rarely yellowish-brown discoloration if recommended doses are exceeded

Dose: expressed as fluoride ion (F⁻):

Water content less than 300 micrograms F⁻/litre (0.3 parts per million), CHILD up to 6 months none; 6 months–2 years 250 micrograms F⁻ daily, 2–4 years 500 micrograms F⁻ daily, over 4 years 1 mg F⁻ daily

Water content between 300 and 700 micrograms F⁻/litre (0.3–0.7 parts per million), CHILD up to 2 years none, 2–4 years 250 micrograms F⁻ daily, over 4 years 500 micrograms F⁻ daily

Water content above 700 micrograms F⁻/litre (0.7 parts per million), supplements not advised (see notes above)

---

1. The British Dental Association, The British Society of Paediatric Dentistry, The British Association for the Study of Community Dentistry and manufacturers of fluoride supplements are currently working together to establish consistent and simplified dosage instructions for fluoride supplements

Tablets

COUNSELLING. Tablets should be sucked or dissolved in the mouth and taken preferably in the evening

There are arrangements for health authorities to supply fluoride tablets in the course of pre-school dental schemes, and they may also be supplied in school dental schemes.

En-De-Kay® (Stafford-Miller)

Fluotabs 2–4 years, natural orange-flavoured, scored, sodium fluoride 1.1 mg (500 micrograms F⁻). Net price 200-tab pack = £1.83

Fluotabs 4+ years, natural orange-flavoured, scored, sodium fluoride 2.2 mg (1 mg F⁻). Net price 200-tab pack = £1.83

Fluor-a-day® (Dental Health)

Tablets, buff, sodium fluoride 1.1 mg (500 micrograms F⁻), net price 200-tab pack = £1.77; 2.2 mg (1 mg F⁻), 200-tab pack = £1.77

FluoriGard® (Colgate-Palmolive)

Tablets 0.5, purple, grape-flavoured, scored, sodium fluoride 1.1 mg (500 micrograms F⁻). Net price 200-tab pack = £1.82

Tablets 1.0, orange, orange-flavoured, scored, sodium fluoride 2.2 mg (1 mg F⁻). Net price 200-tab pack = £1.82

Oral drops

Note. Fluoride supplements not considered necessary below 6 months of age (see notes above)

En-De-Kay® (Stafford-Miller)

Fluodrops® (= paediatric drops), sugar-free, sodium fluoride 550 micrograms (250 micrograms F⁻)/0.15 mL. Net price 60 mL = £1.36

Note. Corresponds to Sodium Fluoride Oral Drops DPF 0.37% equivalent to sodium fluoride 80 micrograms (F⁻ 36 micrograms)/drop

FluoriGard® (Colgate-Palmolive)

Drops, sugar-free, sodium fluoride 275 micrograms (125 micrograms F⁻)/drop. Net price 30 mL = £1.62

Note. Corresponds to Sodium Fluoride Oral Drops DPF 0.84% equivalent to sodium fluoride 275 micrograms (F⁻ 125 micrograms)/drop

Mouthwashes

Rinse mouth for 1 minute and spit out

COUNSELLING. Avoid eating, drinking, or rinsing mouth for 15 minutes after use

En-De-Kay® (Stafford-Miller)

Daily fluoride mouthrinse (= mouthwash), blue, sodium fluoride 0.05%. Net price 250 mL = £1.45

CHILD 6 years and over, for *daily* use, rinse with 10 mL

PoM *Fluorinse* (= mouthwash), red, sodium fluoride 2%. Net price 100 mL = £3.07. Counselling, see above

CHILD 8 years and over, for *daily* use, dilute 5 drops to 10 mL of water; for *weekly* use, dilute 20 drops to 10 mL

FluoriGard® (Colgate-Palmolive)

Daily dental rinse (= mouthwash), blue, sodium fluoride 0.05%. Net price 500 mL = £2.73. Counselling, see above

CHILD 6 years and over, for *daily* use, rinse with 10 mL

Weekly dental rinse (= mouthwash), blue, sodium fluoride 0.2%. Net price 150 mL = £2.22. Counselling, see above

CHILD 6 years and over, for *weekly* use, rinse with 10 mL

9.5.4   Zinc

Oral zinc therapy should only be given when the[re] is good evidence of deficiency (hypoproteinaem[ia] spuriously lowers plasma-zinc concentration[s]). Zinc deficiency can occur in individuals on inad[e]quate diets, in malabsorption, with increased bo[dy] loss due to trauma, burns and protein-losing cond[i]tions, and during intravenous feeding. Therap[y] should continue until clinical improvement occu[rs] and be replaced by dietary measures unless there [is] severe malabsorption, metabolic disease, or conti[n]uing zinc loss. Side-effects of zinc salts are abd[o]minal pain and dyspepsia.

ZINC SALTS

Indications; Cautions; Side-effects: see note[s] above; **interactions:** Appendix 1 (zinc)

Solvazinc® (Thames)

Effervescent tablets, yellow-white, zinc sulpha[te] 200 mg (45 mg zinc). Net price 30 = £4.32. Labe[l] 13, 21

Dose: 1 tablet in water 1–3 times daily after foo[d]

Z Span® (Goldshield)

Spansule® (= capsules m/r), blue/clear, enclosi[ng] white and grey pellets, zinc sulphate mono[hy]drate 61.8 mg (22.5 mg zinc). Net price 30-ca[p] pack = £2.65. Label: 25

Dose: ADULT and CHILD over 12 years, suppl[e]ment, 1 capsule daily; deficiency (short-ter[m] treatment only) 1 capsule 3 times daily the[n] adjusted according to response; can be opene[d] and pellets sprinkled on cool food; not to b[e] chewed

9.6   Vitamins

9.6.1   Vitamin A
9.6.2   Vitamin B group
9.6.3   Vitamin C
9.6.4   Vitamin D
9.6.5   Vitamin E
9.6.6   Vitamin K
9.6.7   Multivitamin preparations

Vitamins are used for the prevention and treatme[nt] of specific deficiency states or where the diet [is] known to be inadequate; they may be prescribed [on] the NHS to prevent or treat deficiency but not a[s] dietary supplements.

Their use as general 'pick-me-ups' is of unprove[n] value and, in the case of preparations containi[ng] vitamin A or D, may actually be harmful if patien[ts] take more than the prescribed dose. The 'fad' f[or] mega-vitamin therapy with water-soluble vitamin[s] such as ascorbic acid and pyridoxine, is unscientif[ic] and can be harmful.

Dietary reference values for vitamins are avail[a]ble in the Department of Health publication:

Dietary Reference Values for Food Energy and Nutrien[ts] for the United Kingdom: Report of the Panel on Dieta[ry] Reference Values of the Committee on Medical Aspec[ts] of Food Policy. *Report on Health and Social Subjec[ts]* 41. London: HMSO, 1991

.6.1 Vitamin A

Deficiency of vitamin A (retinol) is associated with cular defects (particularly xerophthalmia) and an ncreased susceptibility to infections, but deficiency s rare in Britain (even in disorders of fat absorption).

Massive overdose can cause rough skin, dry hair, n enlarged liver, and a raised erythrocyte sedimenation rate and raised serum calcium and serum lkaline phosphatase concentrations.

In view of evidence suggesting that high levels of itamin A may cause birth defects, women who are or may become) pregnant are advised not to take itamin A supplements (including tablets and fishiver oil drops), except on the advice of a doctor or n antenatal clinic; nor should they eat liver or products such as liver paté or liver sausage.

VITAMIN A
(Retinol)
Indications; Cautions; Side-effects: see notes above
Dose: see notes above and under preparations

Vitamins A and D
Halibut-liver Oil (Non-proprietary)
Capsules, vitamin A 4000 units [also contains vitamin D]. Net price 20 = 18p
Available from Thornton & Ross
Vitamins A and D (Non-proprietary)
Capsules, vitamin A 4000 units, vitamin D 400 units. Net price 20 = 33p
Available from CP
IHS Halycitrol® (LAB)
Emulsion, vitamin A 4600 units, vitamin D 380 units/5 mL. Net price 114 mL = £1.29
Dose: 5 mL daily but see notes above

Vitamins A, D, and C for children
Children's Vitamin Drops (Houghs)
Oral drops, ascorbic acid (as sodium ascorbate) 20 mg, vitamin A 700 units, vitamin D 300 units/5 drops.
Recommended by Department of Health for routine supplementation in young children. Available direct to public under the Welfare Food Scheme from maternity and child health clinics and welfare food distribution centres; not available on prescription
Dose: CHILD 1 month–5 years, 5 drops daily
Note. The Department of Health recommends these drops for children aged 6 months to 2 years (preferably 5 years particularly in winter and early spring); some infants from 1 month of age may also benefit (for details see *Present Day Practice in Infant Feeding* 3rd Report)
Minadex® (Seven Seas)
Oral drops, ascorbic acid 15 mg, vitamin A 750 units, vitamin D 200 units/0.14 mL. Net price 25-mL pack with pipette = £1.28
Note. May contain arachis (peanut) oil
Dose: INFANT and CHILD under 5 years, 0.28 mL (upper level on graduated pipette) daily; INFANT fed on vitamin D-fortified milk, CHILD over 5 years and ADULT, 0.14 mL (lower level on graduated pipette) daily

Vitamin A injection
PoM Ro-A-Vit® (Cambridge)
Injection, vitamin A (retinol) 50 000 units (as palmitate)/mL. Net price 2-mL amp = £1.69
Dose: by deep intramuscular injection, deficiency, 100 000 units monthly, increased to weekly in acute deficiency states; courses no longer than 6 weeks with 2-week interval
Liver disease, 100 000 units every 2–4 months
INFANT under 1 year and CHILD 50 000 units monthly
Note. Contains polyethoxylated castor oil which has been associated with anaphylaxis; do **not** mix or dilute
Cautions: children, liver disease (specialist use), see also notes above

9.6.2 Vitamin B group

Deficiency of the B vitamins, other than deficiency of vitamin B_{12} (section 9.1.2) is rare in Britain and is usually treated by preparations containing thiamine (B_1), riboflavine (B_2), and nicotinamide, which is used in preference to nicotinic acid, as it does not cause vasodilatation. Other members (or substances traditionally classified as members) of the vitamin B complex such as aminobenzoic acid, biotin, choline, inositol, and pantothenic acid or panthenol may be included in vitamin B preparations but there is no evidence of their value.

The severe deficiency states Wernicke's encephalopathy and Korsakoff's psychosis, especially as seen in chronic alcoholism, are best treated by the parenteral administration of B vitamins (Pabrinex®); anaphylaxis has been reported with these preparations (see CSM advice, below).

As with other vitamins of the B group, pyridoxine (B_6) deficiency is rare, but it may occur during isoniazid therapy and is characterised by peripheral neuritis. High doses of pyridoxine are given in some metabolic disorders, such as hyperoxaluria, and it is also used in sideroblastic anaemia (section 9.1.3). Pyridoxine has been tried in a wide variety of other disorders, including the premenstrual syndrome, but there is little sound evidence to support the claims, and overdosage induces toxic effects.

RIBOFLAVINE
(Riboflavin, vitamin B_2)
Indications: see notes above

Preparations
Injections of vitamins B and C, see under Thiamine

Oral vitamin B complex preparations, see below

THIAMINE

(Vitamin B$_1$)

Indications: see notes above

Cautions: anaphylactic shock may occasionally follow injection (see CSM advice below)

Dose: mild chronic deficiency, 10–25 mg daily; severe deficiency, 200–300 mg daily

---

CSM advice

Since potentially serious allergic adverse reactions may occur during, or shortly after, administration, the CSM has recommended that:

1. Use be restricted to patients in whom parenteral treatment is essential;

2. Intravenous injections should be administered slowly (over 10 minutes);

3. Facilities for treating anaphylaxis should be available when administered.

Thiamine (Non-proprietary)

Tablets, thiamine hydrochloride 25 mg, net price 20 = 18p; 50 mg, 20 = 30p; 100 mg, 20 = 51p; 300 mg, 20 = 79p

Available from Roche (NHS Benerva®)

PoM **Pabrinex®** (Link)

Parenteral vitamins B and C for rapid correction of severe depletion or malabsorption (e.g in alcoholism, after acute infections, postoperatively, or in psychiatric states), maintenance of vitamins B and C in chronic intermittent haemodialysis

Dose: see CSM advice above

Coma or delirium from alcohol, from opioids, or from barbiturates, collapse following narcosis, by intravenous injection or infusion of *I/V High potency,* 2-3 pairs every 8 hours

Psychosis following narcosis or electroconvulsive therapy, toxicity from acute infections, by intravenous injection or infusion of *I/V High potency* or by deep intramuscular injection into the gluteal muscle of *I/M High potency,* 1 pair twice daily for up to 7 days

Haemodialysis, by intravenous infusion of *I/V High potency* (in sodium chloride intravenous infusion 0.9%) 1 pair every 2 weeks

I/M High potency injection, for intramuscular use only, ascorbic acid 500 mg, nicotinamide 160 mg, pyridoxine hydrochloride 50 mg, riboflavine 4 mg, thiamine hydrochloride 250 mg/7 mL. Net price 7 mL (in 2 amps) = £1.94

I/V High potency injection, for intravenous use only, ascorbic acid 500 mg, anhydrous glucose 1 g, nicotinamide 160 mg, pyridoxine hydrochloride 50 mg, riboflavine 4 mg, thiamine hydrochloride 250 mg/10 mL. Net price 10 mL (in 2 amps) = £1.74

Oral vitamin B complex preparations, see below

PYRIDOXINE HYDROCHLORIDE

(Vitamin B$_6$)

Indications: see under Dose

Cautions: **interactions:** Appendix 1 (vitamins)

Dose: deficiency states, 20–50 mg up to 3 time daily

Isoniazid neuropathy, prophylaxis 10 mg daily therapeutic, 50 mg three times daily

Idiopathic sideroblastic anaemia, 100–400 m daily in divided doses

Premenstrual syndrome, 50–100 mg daily (bu see notes above)

Pyridoxine (Non-proprietary)

Tablets, pyridoxine hydrochloride 10 mg, net pric 20 = 35p; 20 mg, 20 = 34p; 50 mg, 20 = 42p

Available from Cox, Hillcross, Roche Consumer Healt (NHS Benadon®)

NHS **Complement Continus®** (Seton)

Tablets, m/r, yellow, pyridoxine hydrochlorid 100 mg. Net price 28-tab pack = £1.99. Label: 25

Injections of vitamins B and C, see under Thiamin

NICOTINAMIDE

Indications: see notes above; acne vulgaris, se section 13.6.1

Nicotinamide (Non-proprietary)

Tablets, nicotinamide 50 mg. Net price 20 = 83p

Injections of vitamins B and C, see under Thiamin

NICOTINIC ACID

See section 2.12

FOLIC ACID

See section 9.1.2

CALCIUM FOLINATE

See section 8.1.3

VITAMIN B$_{12}$

See section 9.1.2

ORAL VITAMIN B COMPLEX PREPARATION

Note. Other multivitamin preparations are in section 9.6.7

Vitamin B Tablets, Compound, nicotinamide   15 mg riboflavine 1 mg, thiamine hydrochloride 1 mg. Ne price 20 = 7p

Dose: prophylactic, 1–2 tablets daily

Vitamin B Tablets, Compound, Strong, brown, f/c o s/c, nicotinamide 20 mg, pyridoxine hydrochloride 2 mg riboflavine 2 mg, thiamine hydrochloride 5 mg. Ne price 20 = 10p

Dose: treatment of vitamin-B deficiency, 1–2 tablets : times daily

NHS **Becosym®** (Roche Consumer Health)

Tablets, brown, f/c, vitamin B tablets, compound, strong Net price 20 = 31p

Forte tablets, brown, f/c, thiamine hydrochloride 15 mg riboflavine 15 mg, nicotinamide 50 mg, pyridoxin hydrochloride 10 mg. Net price 20 = 69p

NHS **Benerva Compound®** (Roche Consumer Health)

Tablets, yellow, vitamin B tablets, compound. Net pric 20 = 13p

NHS Vigranon B® (Wallace Mfg)
Syrup, thiamine hydrochloride 5 mg, riboflavine 2 mg, nicotinamide 20 mg, pyridoxine hydrochloride 2 mg, panthenol 3 mg/5 mL. Net price 150 mL = £1.74

OTHER COMPOUNDS

Potassium aminobenzoate has been used in the treatment of various disorders associated with excessive fibrosis such as scleroderma but its therapeutic value is **doubtful**.

Potaba® (Glenwood)
Capsules, red/white, potassium aminobenzoate 500 mg. Net price 20 = £1.42. Label: 21
Tablets, potassium aminobenzoate 500 mg. Net price 20 = £1.00. Label: 21
Envules® (= powder in sachets), potassium aminobenzoate 3 g. Net price 40 sachets = £15.37. Label: 13, 21
Dose: Peyronie's disease, scleroderma, 12 g daily in divided doses after food

9.6.3 Vitamin C
(Ascorbic acid)

Vitamin C therapy is essential in scurvy, but less florid manifestations of vitamin C deficiency are commonly found, especially in the elderly. It is rarely necessary to prescribe more than 100 mg daily except early in the treatment of scurvy.

Claims that vitamin C ameliorates colds or promotes wound healing have not been proved.

ASCORBIC ACID
Indications: prevention and treatment of scurvy
Dose: prophylactic, 25–75 mg daily; therapeutic, not less than 250 mg daily in divided doses

Ascorbic Acid (Non-proprietary)
Tablets, ascorbic acid 50 mg, net price 20 = 9p; 100 mg, 20 = 26p; 200 mg, 20 = 39p; 500 mg (label: 24), 20 = 71p
Available from APS, Cox, Roche Consumer Health (**NHS** Redoxon®)
Tablets, effervescent, ascorbic acid 1 g. Net price 10-tab pack = £1.14. Label: 13
Available from Roche Consumer Health (**NHS** Redoxon®)
Injection, ascorbic acid 100 mg/mL. Net price 5-mL amp = £2.28

For children's welfare vitamin drops containing vitamin C with A and D, see vitamin A

9.6.4 Vitamin D

Note. The term Vitamin D is used for a range of compounds which possess the property of preventing or curing rickets. They include ergocalciferol (calciferol, vitamin D_2), cholecalciferol (vitamin D_3), dihydrotachysterol, alfacalcidol (1α-hydroxycholecalciferol), and calcitriol (1,25-dihydroxycholecalciferol).

Simple vitamin D *deficiency*, which is not uncommon in Asians consuming unleavened bread and in the elderly living alone, can be prevented by taking an oral supplement of only 10 micrograms (400 units) of **ergocalciferol** (calciferol, vitamin D_2) daily. Since there is no plain tablet of this strength available **calcium and ergocalciferol tab-**lets can be given (although the calcium is unnecessary).

Vitamin D deficiency caused by *intestinal malabsorption* or *chronic liver disease* usually requires vitamin D in pharmacological doses, such as **calciferol tablets** up to 1 mg (40 000 units) daily; the hypocalcaemia of *hypoparathyroidism* often requires doses of up to 2.5 mg (100 000 units) daily in order to achieve normocalcaemia. The newer vitamin D derivatives, **alfacalcidol** and **calcitriol**, have a shorter duration of action, and therefore have the advantage that problems associated with hypercalcaemia due to excessive dosage are shorter lasting and easier to treat.

Vitamin D requires hydroxylation by the kidney to its active form therefore the hydroxylated derivatives **alfacalcidol** or **calcitriol** should be prescribed if patients with *severe renal impairment* require vitamin D therapy. Calcitriol is also licensed for the management of postmenopausal osteoporosis.

Important. All patients receiving pharmacological doses of vitamin D should have the plasma calcium concentration checked at intervals (initially weekly) and whenever nausea or vomiting are present. Breast milk from women taking pharmacological doses of vitamin D may cause hypercalcaemia if given to an infant.

ERGOCALCIFEROL
(Calciferol, Vitamin D_2)
Indications: see notes above
Cautions: take care to ensure correct dose in infants; monitor plasma calcium in patients receiving high doses and in renal impairment
Contra-indications: hypercalcaemia; metastatic calcification
Side-effects: symptoms of overdosage include anorexia, lassitude, nausea and vomiting, diarrhoea, weight loss, polyuria, sweating, headache, thirst, vertigo, and raised concentrations of calcium and phosphate in plasma and urine
Dose: see notes above

Daily supplements
Note. There is no plain vitamin D tablet available for treating simple deficiency (see notes above). Alternatives include vitamins capsules (see 9.6.7), preparations of vitamins A and D (see 9.6.1), and calcium and ergocalciferol tablets (see below).

Calcium and Ergocalciferol (Non-proprietary)
(Calcium and Vitamin D)
Tablets, calcium lactate 300 mg, calcium phosphate 150 mg (97 mg calcium or 2.4 mmol Ca^{2+}), ergocalciferol 10 micrograms (400 units). Net price 20 = 24p. Counselling, crush before administration or may be chewed

Calcichew® D3 (Shire)
Tablets (chewable), calcium carbonate 1.25 g (500 mg calcium or 12.6 mmol Ca^{2+}), cholecalciferol 5 micrograms (200 units). Net price 100-tab pack = £13.65. Label: 24
Additives: include aspartame

Calcichew® D3 Forte (Shire)

Tablets (chewable), calcium carbonate 1.25 g (500 mg calcium or 12.6 mmol Ca^{2+}), cholecalciferol 10 micrograms (400 units). Net price 100-tab pack = £16.50. Label: 24.
Additives: include aspartame

Pharmacological strengths (see notes above)

Calciferol (Non-proprietary)

Tablets, cholecalciferol or ergocalciferol 250 micrograms (10 000 units), net price 20 = £2.64; 1.25 mg (50 000 units) may also be available
Available from Norton
Note. The BP directs that when calciferol tablets qualified by a descriptor relating to strength (such as 'high strength') are prescribed or demanded, the intention of the prescriber or purchaser with respect to the strength expressed in micrograms or milligrams per tablet should be ascertained. To avoid **errors** arising from the use of such titles prescribers are required to **abandon** them and **specify strength required**

PoM *Injection,* cholecalciferol or ergocalciferol, 7.5 mg (300 000 units)/mL in oil. Net price 1-mL amp = £5.92, 2-mL amp = £7.07

ALFACALCIDOL
(1α-Hydroxycholecalciferol)

Indications: see notes above

Cautions; Contra-indications; Side-effects: see under Ergocalciferol

Dose: by mouth or by intravenous injection over 30 seconds, ADULT *and* CHILD over 20 kg, initially 1 microgram daily (elderly 500 nanograms), adjusted to avoid hypercalcaemia; maintenance, usually 0.25–1 microgram daily; NEONATE *and* PREMATURE INFANT initially 50–100 nanograms/kg daily, CHILD under 20 kg initially 50 nanograms/kg daily

PoM **AlfaD®** (Du Pont)

Capsules, alfacalcidol 250 nanograms (pink), net price 100-cap pack = £11.78; 1 microgram (orange), 30-cap pack = £10.53

PoM **One-Alpha®** (Leo)

Capsules, alfacalcidol 250 nanograms, net price 20 = £2.36; 1 microgram (brown), 20 = £7.02
Note. Contains sesame oil
Solution, sugar-free, alfacalcidol 200 nanograms/mL. Net price 60 mL = £15.19 (with oral syringe)
Injection, alfacalcidol 2 micrograms/mL, net price 0.5-mL amp = £2.43, 1-mL amp = £4.63
Note. Contains propylene glycol and should be used with caution in small premature infants

CALCITRIOL
(1,25-Dihydroxycholecalciferol)

Indications: see notes above
Cautions; Contra-indications; Side-effects: see under Ergocalciferol
Dose: see under preparations below

PoM **Calcijex®** (Abbott)

Injection, calcitriol 1 microgram/mL, net price 1-mL amp = £5.71; 2 micrograms/mL, 1-mL amp = £11.42
Dose: hypocalcaemia in dialysis patients with chronic renal failure, by intravenous injection (or injection through catheter) after haemodialysis, initially 500 nanograms (approx. 10 nanograms/kg) 3 times a week, increased if necessary in steps of 250–500 nanograms at intervals of 2–4 weeks; usual dose 0.5–3 micrograms 3 times a week; CHILD not established

PoM **Rocaltrol®** (Roche)

Capsules, calcitriol 250 nanograms (red/white), net price 20 = £4.31; 500 nanograms (red), 20 = £7.71
Dose: renal osteodystrophy, ADULT, initially 250 nanograms daily or on alternate days, increased if necessary in steps of 250 nanograms at intervals of 2–4 weeks; usual dose 0.5–1 micrograms daily; CHILD not established
Established postmenopausal osteoporosis, 250 nanograms twice daily (monitor plasma calcium and creatinine, see data sheet)

CHOLECALCIFEROL
(Vitamin D_3)

Indications; Cautions; Contra-indications; Side-effects: see under Ergocalciferol—alternative to ergocalciferol in calciferol tablets and injection

DIHYDROTACHYSTEROL

Indications; Cautions; Contra-indications; Side-effects: see under Ergocalciferol

AT 10® (Sanofi Winthrop)

Oral solution, dihydrotachysterol 250 micrograms/mL. Net price 15-mL dropper bottle = £21.27
Note. Contains arachis (peanut) oil
Dose: acute, chronic, and latent forms of hypocalcaemic tetany due to hypoparathyroidism, consult data sheet

9.6.5 Vitamin E
(Tocopherols)

The daily requirement of vitamin E has not been well defined but is probably about 3 to 15 mg daily. There is little evidence that oral supplements of vitamin E are essential in adults, even where there is fat malabsorption secondary to cholestasis. In young children with congenital cholestasis, abnormally low vitamin E concentrations may be found in association with neuromuscular abnormalities, which usually respond only to the parenteral administration of vitamin E.

Vitamin E has been tried for various other conditions but there is no scientific evidence of its value. High doses have been associated with adverse effects.

ALPHA TOCOPHERYL ACETATE

Indications: see notes above
Cautions: predisposition to thrombosis; increased risk of necrotising enterocolitis in premature infants weighing less than 1.5 kg

Side-effects: diarrhoea and abdominal pain with doses more than 1 g daily

Vitamin E Suspension (Cambridge)
Suspension, alpha tocopheryl acetate 500 mg/ 5 mL. Net price 100 mL = £9.52
Dose: malabsorption in cystic fibrosis, 100–200 mg daily; CHILD under 1 year 50 mg daily; 1 year and over, 100 mg daily
Malabsorption in abetalipoproteinaemia, ADULT and CHILD 50–100 mg/kg daily
Malabsorption in chronic cholestasis, INFANT 150–200 mg/kg daily
Note. Tablets containing tocopheryl acetate 50 mg and 200 mg available from Roche Consumer Health (Ephynal®)

9.6.6   Vitamin K

Vitamin K is necessary for the production of blood clotting factors and proteins necessary for the normal calcification of bone.

Because vitamin K is fat soluble, patients with *fat malabsorption,* especially in biliary obstruction or hepatic disease, may become deficient. For oral administration to prevent vitamin-K deficiency in malabsorption syndromes, a water-soluble preparation, **menadiol sodium phosphate** must be used; the usual dose is about 10 mg daily.

For *prophylaxis against vitamin K deficiency bleeding in infants* the Department of Health has advised that paediatricians and midwives and other health care professionals with responsibilities in this area of practice should establish locally agreed policies for each maternity service.

A report of an Expert Committee advising on the administration of vitamin K to infants has been published by the British Paediatric Association and is available from:

British Paediatric Association,
5 St Andrew's Place,
London NW1 4LB.

Oral coumarin *anticoagulants* act by interfering with vitamin K metabolism in the hepatic cells and their effects can be antagonised by giving vitamin K; for British Society for Haematology Guidelines, see section 2.8.2.

MENADIOL SODIUM PHOSPHATE

Indications; Dose: see notes above
Cautions: G6PD deficiency (see section 9.1.5) and vitamin E deficiency (risk of haemolysis); **interactions:** Appendix 1 (vitamins)
Contra-indications: neonates and infants, late pregnancy

Menadiol Phosphate (Non-proprietary)
Tablets, scored, menadiol sodium phosphate equivalent to 10 mg of menadiol phosphate. Net price 100-tab pack = £9.28

PHYTOMENADIONE

(Vitamin K₁)
Indications; Dose: see notes above

Cautions: intravenous injections should be given very slowly (see also below); **interactions:** Appendix 1 (vitamins)

Konakion® (Roche)
Tablets, s/c, phytomenadione 10 mg. Net price 25-tab pack = £4.62. To be chewed or allowed to dissolve slowly in the mouth (Label: 24)
PoM *Injection,* phytomenadione 2 mg/mL, net price 0.5-mL amp = 24p
Note. Contains polyethoxylated castor oil which has been associated with anaphylaxis; should not be diluted therefore **not** for intravenous infusion—for intramuscular or slow intravenous injection

Colloidal formulation
PoM Konakion® MM (Roche)
Injection, phytomenadione 10 mg/mL in a mixed micelles vehicle. Net price 1-mL amp = 45p
Additives: include glycocholic acid 54.6 mg/amp, lecithin
Cautions: reduce dose in elderly; liver impairment (glycocholic acid may displace bilirubin); reports of anaphylactoid reactions
Note. Konakion® MM may be administered by slow intravenous injection or by intravenous infusion in glucose 5% (see Appendix 6); **not** for intramuscular injection

PoM Konakion® MM Paediatric (Roche)
Injection, phytomenadione 10 mg/mL. Net price 0.2-mL amp = £1.62
Additives: include glycocholic acid 900 micrograms/amp, lecithin
Cautions: parenteral administration in premature infants of less than 2.5 kg (increased risk of kernicterus)
Note. Konakion® MM Paediatric may be administered *by mouth* or *by intramuscular injection* or *by intravenous injection*

9.6.7   Multivitamin preparations

Vitamins Capsules, ascorbic acid 15 mg, nicotinamide 7.5 mg, riboflavine 500 micrograms, thiamine hydrochloride 1 mg, vitamin A 2500 units, vitamin D 300 units. Net price 20 = 20p
Abidec® (W-L)
Drops, vitamins A, B group, C, and D. Net price 25 mL (with dropper) = £1.78
Dalivit® (Eastern)
Oral drops, vitamins A, B group, C, and D, net price 25 mL = £1.60, 50 mL = £2.85

VITAMIN AND MINERAL SUPPLEMENTS AND ADJUNCTS TO SYNTHETIC DIETS

Forceval® (Unigreg)
Capsules, brown/red, vitamins (ascorbic acid 60 mg, biotin 100 micrograms, cyanocobalamin 3 micrograms, folic acid 300 micrograms, nicotinamide 18 mg, pantothenic acid 4 mg, pyridoxine 2 mg, riboflavine 1.6 mg, thiamine 1.2 mg, vitamin A 2500 units, vitamin D₂ 400 units, vitamin E 10 mg, vitamin K₁ 70 micrograms), minerals and trace elements (calcium 100 mg, chromium 200 micrograms, copper 2 mg, iodine 140 micrograms, iron 12 mg, magnesium 30 mg, manganese 3 mg, molybdenum 250 micrograms, phosphorus 77 mg, potassium 4 mg, selenium 50 micrograms, zinc 15 mg). Net price 30-cap pack = £5.39, 45-cap pack = £7.70; 90-cap pack = £14.70
Dose: vitamin and mineral deficiency and as adjunct in synthetic diets, 1 capsule daily

---

Cautionary label wordings, see inside back cover

Junior capsules, brown, vitamins (ascorbic acid 25 mg, biotin 50 micrograms, cyanocobalamin 2 micrograms, folic acid 100 micrograms, nicotinamide 7.5 mg, pantothenic acid 2 mg, pyridoxine 1 mg, riboflavine 1 mg, thiamine 1.5 mg, vitamin A 1250 units, vitamin D_2 200 units, vitamin E 5 mg, vitamin K_1 25 micrograms), minerals and trace elements (chromium 50 micrograms, copper 1 mg, iodine 75 micrograms, iron 5 mg, magnesium 1 mg, manganese 1.25 mg, molybdenum 50 micrograms, selenium 25 micrograms, zinc 5 mg). Net price 30-cap pack = £4.05, 60-cap pack = £7.70

Dose: vitamin and mineral deficiency and as adjunct in synthetic diets, CHILD over 5 years, 2 capsules daily

Ketovite® (Paines & Byrne)

PoM *Tablets*, yellow, ascorbic acid 16.6 mg, riboflavine 1 mg, thiamine hydrochloride 1 mg, pyridoxine hydrochloride 330 micrograms, nicotinamide 3.3 mg, calcium pantothenate 1.16 mg, alpha tocopheryl acetate 5 mg, inositol 50 mg, biotin 170 micrograms, folic acid 250 micrograms, acetomenaphthone 500 micrograms. Net price 100-tab pack = £4.17

Dose: prevention of deficiency in disorders of carbohydrate or amino acid metabolism, 1 tablet 3 times daily; with Ketovite® Liquid as vitamin supplement with synthetic diets

Liquid, pink, sugar-free, vitamin A 2500 units, ergocalciferol 400 units, choline chloride 150 mg, cyanocobalamin 12.5 micrograms/5 mL. Net price 150-mL pack = £2.70

Dose: prevention of deficiency in disorders of carbohydrate or amino acid metabolism, 5 mL daily; with Ketovite® Tablets as vitamin supplement with synthetic diets

9.7   Bitters and tonics

Mixtures containing simple and aromatic bitters, such as alkaline gentian mixture, are traditional remedies for loss of appetite. All depend on suggestion.

Gentian Mixture, Acid, BP

Mixture, concentrated compound gentian infusion 10%, dilute hydrochloric acid 5% in a suitable vehicle. Extemporaneous preparations should be recently prepared according to the following formula: concentrated compound gentian infusion 1 mL, dilute hydrochloric acid 0.5 mL, double-strength chloroform water 5 mL, water to 10 mL

Dose: 10 mL 3 times daily in water before meals

Gentian Mixture, Alkaline, BP

(Alkaline Gentian Oral Solution)

Mixture, concentrated compound gentian infusion 10%, sodium bicarbonate 5% in a suitable vehicle. Extemporaneous preparations should be recently prepared according to the following formula: concentrated compound gentian infusion 1 mL, sodium bicarbonate 500 mg, double-strength chloroform water 5 mL, water to 10 mL

Dose: 10 mL 3 times daily in water before meals

NHS **Effico®** (Pharmax)

Tonic, green, thiamine hydrochloride 180 micrograms, nicotinamide 2.1 mg, caffeine 20.2 mg, compound gentian infusion 0.31 mL/5 mL. Net price 300-mL pack = £1.80, 500-mL pack = £2.43

NHS **Labiton®** (LAB)

Tonic, brown, thiamine hydrochloride 375 micrograms, caffeine 3.5 mg, kola nut dried extract 3.025 mg, alcohol 1.4 mL/5 mL. Net price 200 mL = £1.86

NHS **Metatone®** (W-L)

Tonic, thiamine hydrochloride 500 micrograms, calcium glycerophosphate 45.6 mg, manganese glycerophosphate 5.7 mg, potassium glycerophosphate 45.6 mg, sodium glycerophosphate 22.8 mg/5 mL. Net price 300 mL = £2.14

9.8   Metabolic disorders

This section covers drugs used in metabolic disorders and not readily classified elsewhere.

9.8.1   Wilson's disease, carnitine deficiency, and Gaucher's disease

WILSON'S DISEASE

Penicillamine (see also section 10.1.3) is used in Wilson's disease (hepatolenticular degeneration) to aid the elimination of copper ions. See below for other indications.

Trientine is used for the treatment of Wilson's disease only, in patients intolerant of penicillamine; it is **not** an alternative to penicillamine for rheumatoid arthritis or cystinuria.

PENICILLAMINE

Indications: see under Dose below

Cautions; Contra-indications; Side-effects: see section 10.1.3

Dose: Wilson's disease, 1.5–2 g daily in divided doses before food; max. 2 g daily for 1 year; maintenance 0.75–1 g daily; ELDERLY, 20 mg/kg daily in divided doses; CHILD, up to 20 mg/kg daily in divided doses, minimum 500 mg daily
Chronic active hepatitis (after disease controlled with corticosteroids), initially 500 mg daily in divided doses slowly increased over 3 months; usual maintenance dose 1.25 g daily; ELDERLY not recommended
Cystinuria, therapeutic, 1–3 g daily in divided doses before food, adjusted to maintain urinary cystine below 200 mg/litre. Prophylactic (maintain urinary cystine below 300 mg/litre) 0.5–1 g at bedtime; maintain adequate fluid intake (at least 3 litres daily); CHILD and ELDERLY minimum dose to maintain urinary cystine below 200 mg/litre
Severe active rheumatoid arthritis, see section 10.1.3
Copper and lead poisioning, see Emergency Treatment of Poisoning

Preparations

See section 10.1.3

TRIENTINE DIHYDROCHLORIDE

Indications: Wilson's disease in patients intolerant of penicillamine

Cautions: see notes above; pregnancy; **interactions:** Appendix 1 (trientine)

Side-effects: nausea; penicillamine-induced systemic lupus erythematosus may not resolve on transfer to trientine

Dose: 1.2–2.4 g daily in 2–4 divided doses before food

▼ PoM **Trientine Dihydrochloride Capsules,** trientine dihydrochloride 300 mg. Label: 6, 22
Available from K & K-Greeff
Note. The CSM has requested that in addition to the usual CSM reporting request special records should also be kept by the pharmacist

---

CARNITINE DEFICIENCY

Carnitine is available for the management of primary or secondary carnitine deficiency.

CARNITINE

Indications: primary and secondary carnitine deficiency

Cautions: renal impairment; pregnancy (but appropriate to use) and breast-feeding

Side-effects: nausea, vomiting, abdominal pain, diarrhoea, body odour; side-effects may be dose-related—monitor tolerance during first week and after any dose increase

Dose: by mouth, 1–3 g daily in divided doses (usual max. 3 g daily—higher doses occasionally required); CHILD (under 12 years, as Paediatric solution) 100 mg/kg daily (usual max. 3 g daily—higher doses occasionally required)

By intravenous injection over 2–3 minutes, ADULT and CHILD, according to requirement, 100 mg/kg daily (usual max. 3 g daily—higher doses occasionally required)

PoM **Carnitor**® (Shire)
Chewable tablets, L-carnitine 1 g. Net price 10-tab pack = £35.00
Oral liquid, L-carnitine 1 g/10-mL single-dose bottle. Net price 10 × 10-mL single-dose bottle = £35.00
Paediatric solution, L-carnitine 30%. Net price 20 mL = £21.00
Injection, L-carnitine 200 mg/mL. Net price 5-mL amp = £11.90

GAUCHER'S DISEASE

Alglucerase (Ceredase®, not on UK market) is administered by intravenous infusion as enzyme replacement therapy in Gaucher's disease, a familial disorder affecting principally the liver, spleen, bone marrow, and lymph nodes.

9.8.2 Acute porphyrias

The acute porphyrias (acute intermittent porphyria, variegate porphyria, hereditary coproporphyria and plumboporphyria) are hereditary disorders of haem biosynthesis; they have a prevalence of about 1 in 10 000 of the population.

Great care must be taken when prescribing for patients with acute porphyria since many drugs can induce acute porphyric crises. Since acute porphyrias are hereditary, relatives of affected individuals should be screened and advised about the potential danger of certain drugs.

Haem arginate (*Normosang*®, not on UK market) is administered by short intravenous infusion as haem replacement in moderate, severe or unremitting acute porphyria crises. It is available from Orphan Europe or Farillon. Supplies may be obtained outside office hours from the on-call pharmacist at:

University Hospital of Wales,
Cardiff   (01222) 747747

St. James's University Hospital,
Leeds   (01132) 433134
      or   (01132) 837010

King's College Hospital,
London   0171-737 4000
      or   0171-346 3347

The following list contains drugs on the UK market that have been classified as 'unsafe' in porphyria because they have been shown to be porphyrinogenic in animals or *in vitro*, or have been associated with acute attacks in patients.

Further information may be obtained from:
Welsh Drug Information Centre
University Hospital of Wales
Cardiff CF4 4XW
Telephone (01222) 742979

See next page for a list of drugs unsafe for use in acute porphyrias

---

Drugs unsafe for use in acute porphyrias

Note. Quite modest changes in chemical structure can lead to changes in porphyrinogenicity but where possible general statements have been made about groups of drugs; these should be checked first

Drug groups (please check **first**)

Amphetamines	Benzodiazepines[4]	Gold Salts	Mercury Compounds
Anabolic Steroids	Cephalosporins	Hormone Replacement	Progestogens
Antidepressants[1]	Contraceptives, steroid[5]	Therapy[5]	Sulphonamides[8]
Antihistamines[2]	Diuretics[6]	Menopausal Steroids[5]	Sulphonylureas[9]
Barbiturates[3]	Ergot Derivatives[7]		

Individual Drugs (please check groups above **first**)

Alcohol	Danazol	Lignocaine[14]	Phenoxybenzamine
Alcuronium	Dapsone	Lisinopril	Phenylbutazone
Aluminium-containing	Dexfenfluramine	Loxapine	Phenytoin
Antacids[10]	Dextropropoxyphene[13]	Mebeverine	Piroxicam
Aminoglutethimide	Diclofenac	Mefenamic Acid	Pivampicillin[16]
Amiodarone	Doxycycline	Meprobamate	Prilocaine
Azapropazone	Econazole	Methotrexate	Probenecid
Baclofen	Enflurane	Methyldopa	Pyrazinamide
Bromocriptine	Erythromycin	Metoclopramide	Ranitidine
Busulphan	Ethamsylate	Metyrapone	Rifampicin
Captopril	Ethionamide	Miconazole	Simvastatin
Carbamazepine	Ethosuximide	Mifepristone	Sulphinpyrazone
Carisoprodol	Etomidate	Minoxidil[15]	Sulpiride
Chloral Hydrate[11]	Fenfluramine	Nalidixic Acid	Tamoxifen
Chlorambucil	Flucloxacillin	Nifedipine	Theophylline[17]
Chloramphenicol	Flupenthixol	Nitrofurantoin	Thioridazine
Chloroform[12]	Griseofulvin	Orphenadrine	Tinidazole
Clonidine	Halothane	Oxybutynin	Triclofos[11]
Cocaine	Hydralazine	Oxycodone	Trimethoprim
Colistin	Hyoscine	Oxymetazoline	Valproate[5]
Cyclophosphamide	Isometheptene Mucate	Oxytetracycline	Verapamil
Cycloserine	Isoniazid	Pentazocine[13]	Zuclopenthixol
Cyclosporin	Ketoconazole		

1. Includes tricyclic (and related) and MAOIs.
2. Most antihistamines should be avoided but chlorpheniramine and cyclizine thought to be safe.
3. Includes methohexitone, primidone, and thiopentone.
4. Status epilepticus has been treated successfully with intravenous diazepam; temazepam is thought to be safe; where essential, seizure prophylaxis has been undertaken with clonazepam or valproate.
5. Includes both progestogen-only and combined (progestogen content probably more hazardous than oestrogen).
6. Acetazolamide, amiloride, bumetanide, cyclopenthiazide, ethacrynic acid, and triamterene have been used.
7. Includes ergometrine (oxytocin probably safe), lysuride and pergolide.

8. Includes co-trimoxazole and sulphasalazine.
9. Glipizide is thought to be safe
10. Absorption limited but magnesium-containing antacids preferable.
11. Although evidence of hazard is uncertain, manufacturer advises avoid
12. Small amounts in medicines probably safe.
13. Morphine, diamorphine, codeine, dihydrocodeine, and pethidine are thought to be safe.
14. Bupivacaine is thought to be safe.
15. May be used with caution if safer alternative not available.
16. Ampicillin and amoxycillin probably safe.
17. Includes aminophylline.

10: Drugs used in the treatment of

MUSCULOSKELETAL and JOINT DISEASES

In this chapter, drug treatment is discussed under the following headings:

10.1 Drugs used in rheumatic diseases and gout
10.2 Drugs used in neuromuscular disorders
10.3 Drugs for the relief of soft-tissue inflammation

For treatment of septic arthritis see section 5.1, table 1.

10.1 Drugs used in rheumatic diseases and gout

10.1.1 Non-steroidal anti-inflammatory drugs
10.1.2 Corticosteroids
10.1.3 Drugs which suppress the rheumatic disease process
10.1.4 Drugs for the treatment of gout

Most rheumatic diseases require symptomatic treatment to relieve pain. In *degenerative joint disease (osteoarthritis)* or for *soft-tissue lesions*, paracetamol (alone or with a low dose of an opioid analgesic—as in co-codamol 8/500 or co-dydramol 10/500) should be used first and can often give adequate pain relief. However, when pain and stiffness are due to *inflammatory rheumatic disease* treatment with a non-steroidal anti-inflammatory drug (NSAID) is indicated.

Drugs are also available which may affect the disease process itself and favourably influence the outcome. For *rheumatoid arthritis* these include penicillamine, gold salts, antimalarials (chloroquine and hydroxychloroquine), immunosuppressants (azathioprine, chlorambucil, cyclophosphamide, and methotrexate), and sulphasalazine—they are sometimes known as second-line or disease-modifying antirheumatic drugs (DMARDs); recent evidence has suggested that corticosteroids may also be able to reduce the rate of joint destruction. Drugs which may affect the disease process in *psoriatic arthritis* include gold salts, azathioprine, and methotrexate, and for *gout* they include uricosuric drugs and allopurinol.

10.1.1 Non-steroidal anti-inflammatory drugs (NSAIDs)

In *single doses* NSAIDs have analgesic activity comparable to that of paracetamol (see section 4.7.1), but paracetamol is preferred, particularly in the elderly (see also below).

In regular *full dosage* NSAIDs have both a lasting analgesic and an anti-inflammatory effect which makes them particularly useful for the treatment of continuous or regular pain associated with inflammation. Therefore, although paracetamol often gives adequate pain control in osteoarthritis (osteoarthrosis), NSAIDs are more appropriate than paracetamol or the opioid analgesics in the *inflammatory arthritides* (e.g. rheumatoid arthritis) and in some cases of *advanced osteoarthritis*. They may also be of benefit in the less well defined conditions of *back pain* and *soft-tissue disorders* (but in relation to the elderly see also below).

Differences in anti-inflammatory activity between different NSAIDs are small, but there is considerable variation in individual patient response. About 60% of patients will respond to any NSAID; of the others, those who do not respond to one may well respond to another. An analgesic effect should normally be obtained within a week, whereas an anti-inflammatory effect may not be achieved (or may not be clinically assessable) for up to three weeks. If appropriate responses are not obtained within these times, another NSAID should be tried.

The main differences between NSAIDs are in the incidence and type of side-effects. Before treatment is started the prescriber should weigh efficacy against possible side-effects.

ELDERLY AND NSAIDS. Owing to the *increased susceptibilty of the elderly* to the *side-effects of NSAIDs* the following recommendations are made:

for *osteoarthritis, soft-tissue lesions and back pain* first try measures such as weight reduction, warmth, exercise and use of a walking stick;

for *osteoarthritis, soft tissue lesions, back pain and rheumatoid arthritis* avoid giving an NSAID unless there is *definite evidence of inflammation* and *paracetamol* (alone or with a *low dose* of an opioid analgesic as in co-codamol 8/500 or co-dydramol 10/500) has failed adequately to relieve the pain;

where a paracetamol preparation has failed adequately to relieve the pain *add a very low dose of an NSAID* to the paracetamol preparation (starting with ibuprofen).

if an NSAID is considered necessary monitor the patient for gastro-intestinal bleeding for 4 weeks (and for a similar time on switching to another NSAID);

do **not** give two NSAIDs at the same time.

Ibuprofen is a propionic acid derivative with anti-inflammatory, analgesic, and antipyretic properties. It has fewer side-effects than other NSAIDs but its anti-inflammatory properties are weaker. Doses of 1.6 to 2.4 g daily are needed for rheumatoid arthritis and it is unsuitable for conditions where inflammation is prominent such as acute gout.

Other propionic acid derivatives:

Naproxen has emerged as one of the first choices as it combines good efficacy with a low incidence of side-effects (but more than ibuprofen, see CSM comment on next page) and administration is only twice daily.

Fenbufen is claimed to be associated with less gastro-intestinal bleeding, but there is a high risk of rashes (see p. 411).

Fenoprofen is as effective as naproxen, and **flurbiprofen** may be slightly more effective. Both are associated with slightly more gastro-intestinal side-effects than ibuprofen.

Ketoprofen has anti-inflammatory properties similar to ibuprofen and has more side-effects (see also CSM comment on next page).

Tiaprofenic acid is as effective as naproxen; it has more side-effects than ibuprofen (**important:** reports of severe cystitis, see CSM advice on p. 415).

Drugs with properties similar to those of propionic acid derivatives:

Azapropazone is similar in effect to naproxen; it has a tendency to cause rashes and is associated with an increased risk of severe gastro-intestinal toxicity (**important:** see CSM restrictions on p. 410).

Diclofenac has an action similar to that of naproxen; its side-effects are also similar.

Diflunisal is an aspirin derivative but its clinical effect more closely resembles that of the propionic acid derivatives than that of its parent compound. Its long duration of action allows twice-daily administration.

Etodolac is comparable in effect to naproxen; side-effects appear to be comparable to those of ibuprofen but long-term data are awaited.

Indomethacin has an action equal to or superior to that of naproxen, but with a high incidence of side-effects including headaches, dizziness, and gastro-intestinal disturbances (see also CSM comment below).

Mefenamic acid is a related analgesic but its anti-inflammatory properties are minor and side-effects differ in that diarrhoea and occasionally haemolytic anaemia may occur which necessitate discontinuation of treatment.

Nabumetone is comparable in effect to naproxen.

Phenylbutazone is a potent anti-inflammatory drug but because of occasional serious side-effects its use is limited to the hospital treatment of ankylosing spondylitis. In addition to its gastric side-effects it has two rare but dangerous side-effects. It causes fluid retention and, in predisposed patients, may precipitate cardiac failure. It also causes agranulocytosis (which may occur within the first few days of treatment) and aplastic anaemia. In ankylosing spondylitis prolonged administration may be necessary but it should not be used unless other drugs have failed.

Piroxicam is as effective as naproxen and has a prolonged duration of action which permits once-daily administration. It has more gastro-intestinal side-effects than ibuprofen, especially in the elderly (see also CSM comment below).

Sulindac is similar in tolerance to naproxen.

Tenoxicam is similar in activity and tolerance to naproxen. Its long half-life allows once-daily administration.

Tolmetin is comparable in effect to ibuprofen.

CAUTIONS and CONTRA-INDICATIONS. NSAIDs should be used with caution in the *elderly* (see also Elderly and NSAIDs, p. 407), in *allergic disorders* (they are **contra-indicated** in patients with a history of hypersensitivity to aspirin or any other NSAID—*which includes those* in whom attacks of *asthma, angioedema, urticaria or rhinitis* have been precipitated by aspirin or any other NSAID), and during *pregnancy*.

In patients with *renal, cardiac, or hepatic impairment* caution is required since the use of NSAIDs may result in deterioration of renal function (see also under Side-effects, below); the dose should be kept as **low as possible** and renal function should be **monitored**.

NSAIDs should not be given to patients with *active peptic ulceration*, see also **CSM advice** below. While it is preferable to avoid them in patients with current or previous gastro-intestinal ulceration, and to withdraw them if gastro-intestinal lesions develop, nevertheless patients with serious rheumatic diseases (e.g. rheumatoid arthritis) are usually dependent on NSAIDs for effective relief of pain and stiffness. Administration of histamine H_2-receptor blocking drugs (see section 1.3.1) or misoprostol (see section 1.3.4) may permit recommencement of a NSAID without further gastro-intestinal problems.

SIDE-EFFECTS. Side-effects are variable in severity and frequency. Gastro-intestinal discomfort, nausea, diarrhoea, and occasionally bleeding and ulceration occur; dyspepsia may be minimised by taking these drugs with food or milk. Other side-effects include hypersensitivity reactions (particularly angioedema, bronchospasm, and rashes), headache, dizziness, vertigo, hearing disturbances such as tinnitus, and haematuria. Blood disorders have also occurred. Fluid retention may occur (rarely precipitating congestive heart failure in elderly patients). Reversible acute renal failure may be provoked by NSAIDs especially in patients with pre-existing renal impairment (**important**, see also under Cautions above). Rarely, papillary necrosis or interstitial fibrosis associated with NSAIDs may lead to renal failure. Aseptic meningitis has been reported rarely with NSAIDs; patients with connective tissue disorders such as systemic lupus erythematosus may be especially susceptible. Hepatic damage is another rare side-effect.

Overdosage: see Emergency Treatment of Poisoning, p. 20

Recent evidence on the relative safety of 7 oral NSAIDs has indicated differences in the risks of serious upper gastro-intestinal side-effects. **Azapropazone** is associated with the *highest risk* (**important:** see also restrictions on p. 410) and **ibuprofen** with the *lowest*; **piroxicam**, **ketoprofen**, **indomethacin**, **naproxen** and **diclofenac** are associated with *intermediate risks* (possibly higher in the case of piroxicam). There are insufficient data to reach clear conclusions on other available oral NSAIDs.

Recommendations are that NSAIDs associated with low risk should *generally be preferred*, to start at the *lowest recommended dose, not to use more than one oral NSAID at a time*, and to remember that all NSAIDs are *contra-indicated* in patients with peptic ulceration.

Previous recommendations of the CSM have included the advice that in patients with a history of peptic ulcer disease and in the elderly, NSAIDs should be given only after other forms of treatment have been carefully considered.

CSM warning (asthma).

Any degree of worsening of asthma may be related to the ingestion of NSAIDs, either prescribed or (in the case of ibuprofen and others) purchased over the counter.

IBUPROFEN

Indications: pain and inflammation in rheumatic disease (including juvenile arthritis) and other musculoskeletal disorders; mild to moderate pain including dysmenorrhoea; postoperative analgesia; fever and pain in children see section 4.7.1

Cautions: history of gastro-intestinal disease (preferable to avoid, but see also notes above); allergic disorders (see also under contra-indications, below); elderly; pregnancy and breast-feeding (see Appendixes 4 and 5); cardiac, hepatic and renal impairment (**important:** see also notes above and Appendixes 2 and 3); coagulation defects; **interactions:** Appendix 1 (NSAIDs)

Contra-indications: gastro-intestinal ulceration or bleeding; history of hypersensitivity precipitated by aspirin or other NSAIDs (see also below)

HYPERSENSITIVITY. NSAIDs are **contra-indicated** in patients with a history of hypersensitivity to aspirin or any other NSAID—*which includes those* in whom attacks of *asthma, angioedema, urticaria or rhinitis* have been precipitated by aspirin or any other NSAID

Side-effects: gastro-intestinal discomfort—also nausea, diarrhoea and occasionally bleeding and ulceration (**important:** see also CSM advice above), hypersensitivity reactions—notably with bronchospasm, rashes, and angioedema (**important:** see also under Hypersensitivity, above); other side-effects associated with NSAIDs include fluid retention, headache, dizziness, vertigo, hearing disturbances such as tinnitus, photosensitivity, haematuria; blood disorders, reversible acute renal failure, renal papillary necrosis (or interstitial fibrosis), alveolitis, hepatic damage, pancreatitis, eye changes, and aseptic meningitis may also rarely occur; for fur-

ther details of these side-effects see also notes above

Dose: initially 1.2–1.8 g daily in 3–4 divided doses preferably after food; increased if necessary to max. of 2.4 g daily; maintenance dose of 0.6–1.2 g daily may be adequate; CHILD 20 mg/kg daily in divided doses (juvenile arthritis, up to 40 mg/kg daily), not recommended for children under 7 kg

PoM **Ibuprofen** (Non-proprietary)

Tablets, coated, ibuprofen 200 mg, net price 20 = 15p; 400 mg, 20 = 29p; 600 mg, 20 = 55p. Label: 21

Various strengths available from APS (Apsifen®), Ashbourne (Arthrofen®), Berk (Lidifen®), Cox, CP, DDSA (Ebufac®), Isis (Isisfen®), Kent, Lagap (Ibular®), Norton, Rima (Rimafen®), Upjohn (Motrin®, including an 800-mg strength)

Note. Proprietary brands of ibuprofen preparations are on sale to the public; brand names include Anadin® Ibuprofen, Cuprofen®, Hedex® Ibuprofen, Ibrufhalal®, Inoven®, Junifen®, Librofem®, Migrafen®, Novaprin®, Nurofen®, Pacifene®, PhorPain®, Proflex®, Relcofen®; compound proprietary preparations containing ibuprofen include Nurofen® Cold & Flu (ibuprofen, pseudoephedrine), Nurofen® Plus (ibuprofen, codeine), Lemsip® Power + (ibuprofen, pseudoephedrine)

PoM **Brufen**® (Knoll)

Tablets, all magenta, ibuprofen 200 mg (s/c), net price 20 = 58p; 400 mg (s/c), 20 = £1.17; 600 mg (f/c), 20 = £1.85. Label: 21

Syrup, orange, ibuprofen 100 mg/5 mL. Net price 500 mL = £7.34. Label: 21

Dose: 20 mg/kg daily in divided doses *or* 1–2 years 2.5 mL 3–4 times daily, 3–7 years 5 mL 3–4 times daily, 8–12 years 10 mL 3–4 times daily; not recommended for children weighing less than 7 kg; juvenile rheumatoid arthritis up to 40 mg/kg daily in divided doses

Granules, effervescent, ibuprofen 600 mg/sachet. Net price 20-sachet pack = £5.15. Label: 13, 21

Note. Contains sodium approx. 9 mmol/sachet

Junifen Sugar-Free® : see section 4.7.1

Topical preparations : section 10.3.2

Modified release

PoM **Brufen Retard**® (Knoll)

Tablets, m/r, f/c, ibuprofen 800 mg, net price 56-tab pack = £11.76. Label: 25, 27

Dose: 2 tablets daily as a single dose, preferably in the early evening, increased in severe cases to 3 tablets daily in 2 divided doses; CHILD not recommended

PoM **Fenbid**® (Goldshield)

Spansule® (= capsule m/r), maroon/pink, enclosing off-white pellets, ibuprofen 300 mg. Net price 120-cap pack = £9.64. Label: 25

Dose: 1–3 capsules every 12 hours; CHILD not recommended

With codeine

For an adverse comment on compound analgesic preparations, see p. 189. For details of the **side-effects, cautions**, and **contra-indications** of opioid analgesics, see p. 195 (**important:** the elderly are particularly susceptible to opioid side-effects).

PoM **Codafen Continus**® (Napp)

Tablets, white/pink, ibuprofen 300 mg (m/r), codeine phosphate 20 mg. Net price 112-tab pack = £12.57. Label: 2, 21, 25

Dose: 1–2 tablets every 12 hours; max. 3 tablets every 12 hours; CHILD not recommended

ACECLOFENAC

Indications: pain and inflammation in rheumatoid arthritis, osteoarthrosis and ankylosing spondylitis

Cautions; Contra-indications; Side-effects: see under Ibuprofen and notes above; avoid in porphyria (see section 9.8.2); **interactions:** Appendix 1 (NSAIDs)

Dose: 100 mg twice daily (reduce to 100 mg daily initially in hepatic impairment); CHILD not recommended

▼ PoM **Preservex®** (Bristol-Myers)
Tablets, f/c, aceclofenac 100 mg, net price 60-tab pack = £14.95. Label: 21

ACEMETACIN

(Glycolic acid ester of indomethacin)

Indications: pain and inflammation in rheumatic disease and other musculoskeletal disorders; postoperative analgesia

Cautions; Contra-indications; Side-effects: see under Indomethacin and notes above
DRIVING. Dizziness may affect performance of skilled tasks (e.g. driving)

Dose: 120 mg daily in divided doses with food, increased if necessary to 180 mg daily; CHILD not recommended

PoM **Emflex®** (Merck)
Capsules, yellow/orange, acemetacin 60 mg, net price 90-cap pack = £22.48. Label: 21, counselling, driving

AZAPROPAZONE

Indications: see under CSM restrictions, below
CSM RESTRICTIONS. CSM *has restricted* azapropazone to use in rheumatoid arthritis, ankylosing spondylitis and acute gout only when other NSAIDs have been tried and failed, *has* **contra-indicated** it in patients with a history of peptic ulceration, and *has reduced* the maximum daily dose to 600 mg for rheumatoid arthritis and ankylosing spondylitis in patients over 60

Cautions; Contra-indications; Side-effects: see under Ibuprofen and notes above; also specifically contra-indicated if history of peptic ulceration, inflammatory bowel disease or blood disorder; for specific restrictions and contra-indications relating to renal impairment see under Dose; photosensitivity, see CSM advice below; avoid in porphyria (see section 9.8.2); **important:** reports of serious enhancement of effect of warfarin; other **interactions:** Appendix 1 (NSAIDs)
PHOTOSENSITIVITY. CSM has reminded of need to advise patients taking azapropazone to avoid direct exposure to sunlight (or to use sunblock preparations)

Dose:
Rheumatoid arthritis and ankylosing spondylitis only, 1.2 g daily in 2 or 4 divided doses; in renal impairment or in elderly 300 mg twice daily, avoid altogether in severe renal impairment; CHILD not recommended
Acute gout (always ensure increased fluid intake), 1.8 g daily in divided doses until acute symptoms subside (usually by 4th day) *then* 1.2 g daily in divided doses until symptoms resolve—consider appropriate alternative therapy if they persist; in mild renal impairment or in elderly, 1.8 g daily for first 24 hours then 1.2 g daily in divided doses reducing to max. 600 mg daily in divided doses as soon as possible (preferably by 4th day) *then* continuing only until acute symptoms resolve—consider appropriate alternative therapy if they persist, and *avoid altogether for gout* in moderate to severe renal impairment and *avoid for gout in elderly* even in mild renal impairment; CHILD not recommended

PoM **Rheumox®** (Wyeth)
Capsules, orange, azapropazone 300 mg. Net price 20 = £2.86. Label: 11 (also photosensitivity counselling, see above), 21
Tablets, orange, f/c, scored, azapropazone 600 mg. Net price 20 = £4.98. Label: 11 (also photosensitivity counselling, see above), 21

DICLOFENAC SODIUM

Indications: pain and inflammation in rheumatic disease (including juvenile arthritis) and other musculoskeletal disorders; acute gout; postoperative pain, see section 15.1.4.2

Cautions; Contra-indications; Side-effects: see under Ibuprofen and notes above; porphyria (see section 9.8.2); suppositories may cause rectal irritation; special cautions for injection see section 15.1.4.2; **interactions:** Appendix 1 (NSAIDs)

Dose: by mouth, 75–150 mg daily in 2–3 divided doses, preferably after food
By deep intramuscular injection into the gluteal muscle, acute exacerbations and post-operative 75 mg once daily (twice daily in severe cases) for max. of 2 days
Ureteric colic, 75 mg then a further 75 mg after 30 minutes if necessary
By intravenous infusion, see section 15.1.4.2
By rectum in suppositories, 75–150 mg daily in divided doses
Max. total daily dose by any route 150 mg
CHILD 1–12 years, juvenile arthritis, *by mouth or by rectum,* 1–3 mg/kg daily in divided doses (25 mg e/c tablets, 12.5 mg and 25 mg suppositories only)

PoM **Diclofenac Sodium** (Non-proprietary)
Tablets, both e/c, diclofenac sodium 25 mg, net price 20 = 68p; 50 mg, 20 = £1.20. Label: 5, 25
Available from APS, Ashbourne (Diclozip®), Berk, Cox Eastern (Volraman®), Isis (Isclofen®, 50 mg), Ken (Enzed®), Lagap (Rhumalgan®), Norton, Opus (Lofensaid®), Pharmacia (Dicloflex®), Shire (Valenac®), Sterwin
Injection, diclofenac sodium 25 mg/mL. Net price 3-mL amp = 83p
Available from Antigen
Note. Licensed for intramuscular use

---

oM **Voltarol**® (Geigy)

Tablets, both e/c, diclofenac sodium 25 mg (yellow), net price 84-tab pack = £7.88; 50 mg (brown), 84-tab pack = £15.32. Label: 5, 25

Dispersible tablets, pink, diclofenac, equivalent to diclofenac sodium 50 mg, net price 21-tab pack = £5.15. Label: 13, 21

Note. Voltarol Dispersible tablets are more suitable for **short-term** use in acute conditions for which treatment required for no more than 3 months (no information on use beyond 3 months)

Injection, diclofenac sodium 25 mg/mL. Net price 3-mL amp = 83p

Suppositories, diclofenac sodium 12.5 mg, net price 10 = 72p; 25 mg, 10 = £1.28; 50 mg, 10 = £2.10; 100 mg, 10 = £3.76

Emulgel® gel, section 10.3.2

Modified release

oM **Diclomax SR**® (P-D)

Capsules, m/r, yellow, diclofenac sodium 75 mg. Net price 56-cap pack = £13.01. Label: 21, 25

Dose: 1 capsule 1–2 times daily *or* 2 capsules once daily, preferably with food; CHILD not recommended

oM **Diclomax Retard**® (P-D)

Capsules, m/r, diclofenac sodium 100 mg. Net price 28-tab pack = £9.36. Label: 21, 25

Dose: 1 capsule daily preferably with food; CHILD not recommended

oM **Motifene**® **75 mg** (Panpharma)

Capsules, e/c, m/r, diclofenac sodium 75 mg (enclosing e/c pellets containing diclofenac sodium 25 mg and m/r pellets containing diclofenac sodium 50 mg). Net price 56-cap pack = £14.99. Label: 25

Dose: 1 capsule 1-2 times daily; CHILD not recommended

oM **Voltarol**® **75 mg SR** (Geigy)

Tablets, m/r, pink, diclofenac sodium 75 mg. Net price 28-tab pack = £8.68; 56-tab pack = £17.35. Label: 21, 25

Dose: 75 mg 1–2 times daily preferably with food; CHILD not recommended

Note. Modified-release tablets containing diclofenac sodium 75 mg available from Lagap (*Rhumalgan*® *CR*), Trinity (*Volsaid*® *Retard*)

oM **Voltarol**® **Retard** (Geigy)

Tablets, m/r, red, diclofenac sodium 100 mg. Net price 28-tab pack = £12.72. Label: 21, 25

Dose: 1 tablet daily preferably with food; CHILD not recommended

Note. Modified-release tablets containing diclofenac sodium 100 mg available from APS, Berk (*Flamrase*® *SR*), Lagap (*Rhumalgan*® *CR*), Pharmacia (*Dicloflex*® *Retard*), Trinity (*Volsaid*® *Retard*)

With misoprostol

For prophylaxis against NSAID-induced gastroduodenal ulceration in patients requiring diclofenac for rheumatoid arthritis or osteoarthritis; cautions, contra-indications, and side-effects of misoprostol, see section 1.3.4

oM **Arthrotec**® (Searle)

Arthrotec® *50 tablets*, diclofenac sodium (in e/c core) 50 mg, misoprostol 200 micrograms. Net price 60-tab pack = £14.98; 140-tab pack = £34.94 (hosp. only). Label: 21, 25

Dose: 1 tablet 2–3 times daily with food; CHILD not recommended

Arthrotec® *75 tablets*, diclofenac sodium (in e/c core) 75 mg, misoprostol 200 micrograms. Net price 60-tab pack = £17.59. Label: 21, 25

Dose: 1 tablet twice daily with food; CHILD not recommended

DIFLUNISAL

Indications: pain and inflammation in rheumatic disease and other musculoskeletal disorders; mild to moderate pain including dysmenorrhoea

Cautions; Contra-indications; Side-effects: see under Ibuprofen and notes above; **interactions:** Appendix 1 (NSAIDs)

Dose: mild to moderate pain, initially 1 g, then 500 mg every 12 hours (increased to max. 500 mg every 8 hours if necessary)

Osteoarthrosis, rheumatoid arthritis, 0.5–1 g daily as a single daily dose *or* in 2 divided doses

Dysmenorrhoea, initially 1 g, then 500 mg every 12 hours

CHILD not recommended

PoM **Diflunisal** (Non-proprietary)

Tablets, coated, diflunisal 250 mg, net price 20 = £1.80; 500 mg, 20 = £3.61. Label: 21, 25, counselling, avoid aluminium hydroxide

Available from APS

PoM **Dolobid**® (Morson)

Tablets, both f/c, diflunisal 250 mg (peach), net price 20 = £1.80; 500 mg (orange), 20 = £3.61. Label: 21, 25, counselling, avoid aluminium hydroxide

ETODOLAC

Indications: pain and inflammation in rheumatoid arthritis and osteoarthrosis

Cautions; Contra-indications; Side-effects: see under Ibuprofen and notes above; **interactions:** Appendix 1 (NSAIDs)

Dose: 200 mg or 300 mg twice daily *or* 400 mg or 600 mg once daily; max. 600 mg daily; CHILD not recommended

PoM **Lodine**® (Wyeth)

Capsules, etodolac 200 mg (light- and dark-grey), net price 60-cap pack = £10.55; 300 mg (light-grey), 60-cap pack = £14.65. Label: 21

Tablets, brown, f/c, etodolac 200 mg. Net price 60-tab pack = £10.55. Label: 21

Modified release

PoM **Lodine SR**® (Wyeth)

Tablets, m/r, light-grey, etodolac 600 mg. Net price 30-tab pack = £15.50. Label : 25

Dose: 1 tablet daily; CHILD not recommended

FENBUFEN

Indications: pain and inflammation in rheumatic disease and other musculoskeletal disorders

Cautions; Contra-indications; Side-effects: see under Ibuprofen and notes above, but also high risk of rashes (discontinue immediately); erythema multiforme and Stevens-Johnson syndrome reported; also allergic interstitial lung disorders (may follow rashes); **interactions:** Appendix 1 (NSAIDs)

Dose: 300 mg in the morning and 600 mg at bedtime *or* 450 mg twice daily; CHILD under 14 years not recommended

PoM Lederfen® (Lederle)
Capsules, dark blue, fenbufen 300 mg. Net price 84-cap pack = £18.83. Label: 21
Note. Fenbufen capsules also available from APS, Ashbourne (Fenbuzip®), Cox, Hillcross, Norton

Tablets, both light blue, f/c, fenbufen 300 mg, net price 84-tab pack = £18.83; 450 mg, 56-tab pack = £18.83. Label: 21
Note. Fenbufen tablets also available from APS, Ashbourne (Fenbuzip®), Cox (450 mg), Hillcross, Kent, Norton

FENOPROFEN
Indications: pain and inflammation in rheumatic disease and other musculoskeletal disorders; mild to moderate pain
Cautions; Contra-indications; Side-effects: see under Ibuprofen and notes above; upper respiratory infection, nasopharyngitis, and cystitis also reported; **interactions:** Appendix 1 (NSAIDs)
Dose: 200–600 mg 3–4 times daily with food; max. 3 g daily; CHILD not recommended

PoM Fenopron® (Dista)
Tablets, both orange, fenoprofen (as calcium salt) 300 mg (*Fenopron®* 300), net price 100-tab pack = £9.45; 600 mg (*Fenopron®* 600, scored), 100-tab pack = £18.29. Label: 21
PoM Progesic® (Lilly)
Tablets, yellow, fenoprofen 200 mg (as calcium salt). Net price 100-tab pack = £16.63. Label: 21

FLURBIPROFEN
Indications: pain and inflammation in rheumatic disease and other musculoskeletal disorders; mild to moderate pain including dysmenorrhoea; post-operative analgesia
Cautions; Contra-indications; Side-effects: see under Ibuprofen and notes above; suppositories may cause rectal irritation; **interactions:** Appendix 1 (NSAIDs)
Dose: by mouth or by rectum in suppositories, 150–200 mg, daily in divided doses, increased in acute conditions to 300 mg daily
Dysmenorrhoea, initially 100 mg, then 50–100 mg every 4–6 hours; max. 300 mg daily
CHILD not recommended

PoM Froben® (Knoll)
Tablets, both yellow, s/c, flurbiprofen 50 mg, net price 20 = £1.65; 100 mg, 20 = £3.13. Label: 21
Note. Flurbiprofen tablets also available from APS, Cox, Du Pont, Kent, Lagap, Norton
Suppositories, flurbiprofen 100 mg. Net price 12 = £2.90

Modified release
PoM Froben SR® (Knoll)
Capsules, m/r, yellow, enclosing off-white beads, flurbiprofen 200 mg. Net price 30-cap pack = £10.88. Label: 21, 25
Dose: rheumatic disease, 1 capsule daily, preferably in the evening; CHILD not recommended

INDOMETHACIN
(Indometacin)
Indications: pain and moderate to severe inflammation in rheumatic disease and other acute musculoskeletal disorders; acute gout; dysmenorrhoea; closure of ductus arteriosus (section 7.1.1.1)
Cautions; Contra-indications: see under Ibuprofen and notes above; caution also in epilepsy, parkinsonism, psychiatric disturbances; during prolonged therapy ophthalmic and blood examinations are particularly advisable; avoid rectal administration in proctitis and haemorrhoids; **interactions:** Appendix 1 (NSAIDs)
DRIVING. Dizziness may affect performance of skilled tasks (e.g. driving)
Side-effects: see under Ibuprofen and notes above; frequently gastro-intestinal disturbances (including diarrhoea), headache, dizziness, and light headedness; gastro-intestinal ulceration and bleeding; rarely, drowsiness, confusion, insomnia, convulsions, psychiatric disturbances, depression, syncope, blood disorders (particularly thrombocytopenia), hypertension, hyperglycaemia, blurred vision, corneal deposits, peripheral neuropathy; suppositories may cause rectal irritation and occasional bleeding
Dose: by mouth, rheumatic disease, 50–200 mg daily in divided doses, with food; CHILD not recommended
Acute gout, 150–200 mg daily in divided doses
Dysmenorrhoea, up to 75 mg daily
By rectum in suppositories, 100 mg at night and in the morning if required; CHILD not recommended
Combined oral and rectal treatment, max. total daily dose 150–200 mg

PoM Indomethacin (Non-proprietary)
Capsules, indomethacin 25 mg, net price 20 = 21p; 50 mg, 20 = 47p. Label: 21, counselling, driving, see above
Available from APS, Ashbourne (Indomax®), Berk (Imbrilon®), Cox, Galen (Mobilan®), Kent, Morson (Indocid®), Norton, Rima (Rimacid®)
Suspension, sugar-free, indomethacin 25 mg/5 mL. Net price 200 mL = £3.12. Label: 21, counselling, driving, see above
Available from Morson (Indocid®)
Suppositories, indomethacin 100 mg. Net price 10 = £1.11. Counselling, driving, see above
Available from Berk (Imbrilon®), Cox, Morson (Indocid®), Norton

Modified release
PoM Indomethacin m/r preparations
Capsules, m/r, indomethacin 75 mg. Net price 20 = £3.34. Label: 21, 25, counselling, driving, see above
Dose: 1 capsule 1–2 times daily; CHILD not recommended
Available from Ashbourne (Indomax 75 SR®, 28-cap pack), Generics (Slo-Indo®), Hillcross (Rheumacin LA®), Pharmacia (Indomod®, 30-cap pack; also 25-mg strength), Lagap (Indolar SR®), Morson (Indocid-R®), Opus (Maximet SR®), Trinity (Artracin SR®)
Tablets, m/r, indomethacin 25 mg (*Flexin-25 Continus®,* green), net price 56-tab pack = £7.1

50 mg (*Flexin-LS Continus*®, red), 28-tab pack = £7.15; 75 mg (*Flexin Continus*®, yellow), 28-tab pack = £10.21. Label: 21, 25, counselling, driving, see above

Dose: initially 75 mg daily, adjusted in steps of 25–50 mg; range 25–200 mg daily in 1–2 divided doses; dysmenorrhoea, up to 75 mg daily; CHILD not recommended

Available from Napp

KETOPROFEN

Indications: pain and mild inflammation in rheumatic disease and other musculoskeletal disorders, and after orthopaedic surgery; acute gout; dysmenorrhoea

Cautions; Contra-indications; Side-effects: see under Ibuprofen and notes above; pain may occur at injection site (occasionally tissue damage); suppositories may cause rectal irritation; **interactions:** Appendix 1 (NSAIDs)

Dose: by mouth, rheumatic disease, 100–200 mg daily in 2–4 divided doses with food; CHILD not recommended

Pain and dysmenorrhoea, 50 mg up to 3 times daily; CHILD not recommended

By rectum in suppositories, rheumatic disease, 100 mg at bedtime; CHILD not recommended

Combined oral and rectal treatment, max. total daily dose 200 mg

By deep intramuscular injection into the gluteal muscle, 50–100 mg every 4 hours (max. 200 mg in 24 hours) for up to 3 days; CHILD not recommended

PoM **Alrheumat**® (Bayer)
Capsules, off-white, ketoprofen 50 mg. Net price 20 = £1.22. Label: 21

PoM **Orudis**® (Rhône-Poulenc Rorer)
Capsules, ketoprofen 50 mg (green/purple), net price 112-cap pack = £8.65; 100 mg (pink), 56-cap pack = £8.68. Label: 21
Suppositories, ketoprofen 100 mg. Net price 10 = £3.73

PoM **Oruvail**® (Rhône-Poulenc Rorer)
Injection, ketoprofen 50 mg /mL. Net price 2-mL amp = 73p
Gel, section 10.3.2

Modified release
PoM **Oruvail**® (Rhône-Poulenc Rorer)
Capsules, all m/r, enclosing white pellets, ketoprofen 100 mg (pink/purple), net price 56-cap pack = £16.30; 150 mg (pink), 28-cap pack = £9.31; 200 mg (pink/white), 28-cap pack = £16.25. Label: 21, 25
Dose: 100–200 mg once daily with food; CHILD not recommended

Note. Modified-release capsules containing ketoprofen 100 mg and 200 mg also available from APS (Ketovail®), Ashbourne (Ketozip XL®-200 mg), Du Pont (Ketoprofen CR®), Lagap (Larafen CR®-200 mg), Opus (Fenoket®-200 mg), Trinity (Ketocid®-200 mg)

KETOROLAC TROMETAMOL

See section 15.1.4.2

MEFENAMIC ACID

Indications: mild to moderate pain in rheumatoid arthritis (including juvenile arthritis), osteoarthrosis, and related conditions; dysmenorrhoea and menorrhagia

Cautions; Contra-indications: see under Ibuprofen and notes above; also specifically contra-indicated in inflammatory bowel disease; blood tests required during long-term treatment; porphyria (see section 9.8.2); **interactions:** Appendix 1 (NSAIDs)

Side-effects: see notes above; drowsiness; diarrhoea or rashes (withdraw treatment); thrombocytopenia, haemolytic anaemia; convulsions in overdosage

Dose: 500 mg 3 times daily preferably after food; CHILD over 6 months, 25 mg/kg daily in divided doses for not longer than 7 days, except in juvenile arthritis

PoM **Mefenamic Acid** (Non-proprietary)
Capsules, mefenamic acid 250 mg. Net price 20 = 59p. Label: 21
Available from APS, Ashbourne (Dysman 250®), Berk (Contraflam®), Cox, Kent, Lagap, Norton, Opus (Opustan 250®), P-D (Ponstan®), Sterwin, Trinity (Meflam 250®)

Tablets, mefenamic acid 500 mg, net price 20 = £1.77. Label: 21
Available from APS, Ashbourne (Dysman 500®), Berk, Cox, Norton, Opus (Opustan 500®), P-D (Ponstan Forte®), Trinity (Meflam 500®)
Paediatric oral suspension, mefenamic acid 50 mg/5 mL. Net price 125 mL = £3.37. Label: 21
Available from P-D (Ponstan®)

NABUMETONE

Indications: pain and inflammation in osteoarthrosis and rheumatoid arthritis

Cautions; Contra-indications; Side-effects: see under Ibuprofen and notes above; **interactions:** Appendix 1 (NSAIDs)

Dose: 1 g at night, in severe conditions 0.5–1 g in morning as well; elderly 0.5–1 g daily; CHILD not recommended

PoM **Relifex**® (Bencard)
Tablets, red, f/c, nabumetone 500 mg. Net price 56-tab pack = £18.11. Label: 21, 25
Suspension, sugar-free, nabumetone 500 mg/ 5 mL. Net price 300-mL pack = £25.22. Label: 21

NAPROXEN

Indications: pain and inflammation in rheumatic disease (including juvenile arthritis) and other musculoskeletal disorders; dysmenorrhoea; acute gout

Cautions; Contra-indications; Side-effects: see under Ibuprofen and notes above; suppositories may cause rectal irritation and occasional bleeding; **interactions:** Appendix 1 (NSAIDs)

Dose: *by mouth*, 0.5–1 g daily in 2 divided doses
or 1 g once daily; CHILD (over 5 years), juvenile
arthritis, 10 mg/kg daily in 2 divided doses

Acute musculoskeletal disorders and dysmenorrhoea, 500 mg initially, then 250 mg every 6–8
hours as required; max. dose after first day 1.25 g
daily; CHILD under 16 years not recommended

Acute gout, 750 mg initially, then 250 mg every 8
hours until attack has passed; CHILD under 16
years not recommended

By rectum in suppositories, 500 mg at bedtime; if
necessary 500 mg in morning as well; CHILD
under 16 years not recommended

PoM Naproxen (Non-proprietary)
Tablets, naproxen 250 mg, net price 20 = £1.71;
500 mg, 20 = £2.79. Label: 21
Available from APS, Ashbourne (Arthrosin®), Berk
(Timpron®), BHR (Prosaid®), Cox, CP (Arthroxen®),
Lagap (Laraflex®), Norton, Shire (Valrox®), Sterwin

PoM Naprosyn® (Roche)
Tablets, all scored, naproxen 250 mg (buff), net
price 20 = £2.43; 500 mg (buff), 56-tab pack =
£13.65. Label: 21
Tablets, all e/c, (*Naprosyn EC®*), naproxen
250 mg, net price 56-tab pack = £6.83; 375 mg,
56-tab pack = £10.24; 500 mg, 56-tab pack =
£13.65. Label: 5, 25
Suspension, orange, naproxen 125 mg/5 mL. Contains about 1.7 mmol Na⁺/5 mL. Net price 240 mL
= £5.09. Label: 21
Suppositories, naproxen 500 mg. Net price 10 =
£3.18

PoM Nycopren® (Nycomed)
Tablets, both e/c, naproxen 250 mg, net price 20 =
£2.07; 500 mg, 60-tab pack = £12.41. Label: 5, 25

PoM Synflex® (Roche)
Tablets, blue, naproxen sodium 275 mg. Net price
20 = £2.83. Label: 21
Note. 275 mg naproxen sodium ≡ 250 mg naproxen
Dose: musculoskeletal disorders, postoperative analgesia, 550 mg twice daily when necessary, preferably after
food; max. 1.1 g daily; CHILD under 16 years not recommended
Dysmenorrhoea, initially 550 mg then 275 mg every 6–8
hours as required; max. of 1.375 g on 1st day and 1.1 g
daily thereafter; CHILD under 16 years not recommended

Modified release
PoM Naprosyn® S/R (Roche)
Tablets, m/r, f/c, scored, naproxen 500 mg (as sodium salt), net price 56-tab pack = £15.29. Label:
25
Dose: rheumatic and musculoskeletal disorders, 1–2
tablets once daily; CHILD under 16 years not recommended

With misoprostol
For cautions, contra-indications, and side-effects of
misoprostol, see section 1.3.4
PoM Napratec® (Searle)
Combination pack, 56 yellow scored tablets,
naproxen 500 mg; 56 white scored tablets, miso-
prostol 200 micrograms. Net price = £19.80.
Label: 21
Dose: patients requiring naproxen for rheumatoid arth-
ritis, osteoarthritis, or ankylosing spondylitis, with

prophylaxis against NSAID-induced gastroduodena
ulceration, 1 naproxen 500-mg tablet and 1 misoprosto
200-microgram tablet taken together twice daily with
food; CHILD not recommended

PHENYLBUTAZONE

Indications: ankylosing spondylitis when other therapy i
unsuitable
Cautions: blood counts before and during treatment if fo
more than 7 days; elderly (reduce dose); breast-feeding
allergic disorders (see also under Contra-indications
below), withdraw treatment if acute pulmonary
syndrome including fever and dyspnoea occurs; may
aggravate systemic lupus erythematosus; see also notes
above; **interactions:** Appendix 1 (NSAIDs)
COUNSELLING. Warn patient to tell doctor immediately
if sore throat, mouth ulcers, bruising, fever, malaise
rash, or non-specific illness develops.
Contra-indications: cardiovascular disease, pulmonary
renal and hepatic impairment; pregnancy; history o
peptic ulceration, gastro-intestinal haemorrhage, o
blood disorders; history of hypersensitivity precipitate
by aspirin or other NSAIDs (see also below); porphyri
(see section 9.8.2); Sjögren's syndrome; thyroid disease
children under 14
HYPERSENSITIVITY. NSAIDs are **contra-indicated** i
patients with a history of hypersensitivity to aspirin o
any other NSAID—*which includes those in whom
attacks of asthma, angioedema, urticaria or rhiniti.
have been precipitated by aspirin or any other NSAID*
Side-effects: see notes above; parotitis, stomatitis, goitre
pancreatitis, hepatitis, nephritis, visual disturbances
rarely leucopenia, thrombocytopenia, agranulocytosis
aplastic anaemia, erythema multiforme (Stevens-John
son syndrome), toxic epidermal necrolysis (Lyell'
syndrome), pulmonary toxicity
Dose: initially 200 mg 2–3 times daily for 2 days, with o
after food, then reduced to minimum effective, usuall.
100 mg 2–3 times daily; CHILD under 14 years not rec
ommended

PoM Butacote® (Geigy)
Tablets, pale blue, e/c, s/c, phenylbutazone 100 mg, ne
price 20 = 40p (hosp. only). Label: 5, 21, 25, counsel
ling, blood disorder symptoms (see above)

PIROXICAM

Indications: pain and inflammation in rheumati
disease (including juvenile arthritis) and othe
musculoskeletal disorders; acute gout
Cautions; Contra-indications: see under Ibupro
fen and notes above; porphyria (see sectior
9.8.2); **interactions:** Appendix 1 (NSAIDs)
Side-effects: see under Ibuprofen and notes above
pain may occur at injection site (occasionally tis
sue damage); suppositories may cause rectal irri
tation and occasional bleeding
Dose: *by mouth or by rectum*, rheumatic disease
initially 20 mg daily, maintenance 10–30 mg
daily, in single or divided doses
CHILD (over 6 years) *by mouth*, juvenile arthritis
less than 15 kg, 5 mg daily; 16–25 kg, 10 mg; 26–
45 kg, 15 mg; over 46 kg, 20 mg
Acute musculoskeletal disorders, 40 mg daily ir
single or divided doses for 2 days, then 20 m.
daily for 7–14 days; CHILD not recommended
Acute gout, 40 mg initially, then 40 mg daily ir
single or divided doses for 4–6 days; CHILD nc
recommended
By deep intramuscular injection into glutea
muscle, for initial treatment of acute conditions

as dose by mouth (on short-term basis); CHILD not recommended

PoM Piroxicam (Non-proprietary)

Capsules, piroxicam 10 mg, net price 20 = £1.15; 20 mg, 20 = £2.31. Label: 21

Available from APS, Ashbourne (Pirozip®), Berk (Flamatrol®), Cox, Hillcross, Kent (Kentene®), Lagap (Larapam®), Norton, Opus (Piroflam®)

PoM Feldene® (Pfizer)

Capsules, piroxicam 10 mg (maroon/blue), net price 56-cap pack = £6.00; 20 mg (maroon), 28-cap pack = £6.00. Label: 21

Tablets, (Feldene Melt®), piroxicam 20 mg, net price 28-tab pack = £9.83. Label: 10 patient information leaflet, 21

Note. Feldene Melt® tablets can be taken by placing on tongue or by swallowing; contain aspartame equivalent to phenylalanine 140 micrograms/tablet (see section 9.4.1)

Dispersible tablets, piroxicam 10 mg (scored), net price 56-tab pack = £9.75; 20 mg, 28-tab pack = £9.75. Label: 13, 21

Note. Piroxicam dispersible tablets also available from Hillcross

Injection, piroxicam 20 mg/mL. Net price 1-mL amp = 70p

Suppositories, piroxicam 20 mg. Net price 10 = £5.20

Gel, section 10.3.2

SULINDAC

Indications: pain and inflammation in rheumatic disease and other musculoskeletal disorders; acute gout

Cautions; Contra-indications; Side-effects: see under Ibuprofen and notes above; also caution if history of renal stones and ensure adequate hydration; urine discoloration occasionally reported; **interactions:** Appendix 1 (NSAIDs)

Dose: 200 mg twice daily with food (may be reduced according to response); max. 400 mg daily; acute gout may respond within 7 days; limit treatment of peri-articular disorders to 7–10 days; CHILD not recommended

PoM Clinoril® (MSD)

Tablets, both yellow, scored, sulindac 100 mg, net price 20 = £2.24; 200 mg, 20 = £4.32. Label: 21

Note. Sulindac tablets also available from APS, Generics

TENOXICAM

Indications: pain and inflammation in rheumatic disease and other musculoskeletal disorders

Cautions; Contra-indications; Side-effects: see under Ibuprofen and notes above; **interactions:** Appendix 1 (NSAIDs)

Dose: by mouth, rheumatic disease, 20 mg daily; CHILD not recommended

Acute musculoskeletal disorders, 20 mg daily for 7 days; max. 14 days; CHILD not recommended

By intravenous or intramuscular injection, for initial treatment for 1–2 days, as dose by mouth; CHILD not recommended

PoM Mobiflex® (Roche)

Tablets, red-brown, f/c, tenoxicam 20 mg. Net price 28-tab pack = £14.10. Label: 21

Injection, powder for reconstitution, tenoxicam 20 mg. Net price per amp (with solvent) = 93p

TIAPROFENIC ACID

Indications: pain and inflammation in rheumatic disease and other musculoskeletal disorders

Cautions; Contra-indications; Side-effects: see under Ibuprofen and notes above; also contra-indicated in active bladder or prostate disease (or symptoms) and history of recurrent urinary tract disorders—if urinary symptoms develop discontinue immediately and perform urine tests and culture; see also CSM advice below; **interactions:** Appendix 1 (NSAIDs)

CSM ADVICE. Following reports of **severe cystitis** associated with tiaprofenic acid the CSM has recommended that tiaprofenic acid *should not be given* to patients with pre-existing urinary tract disorders and *should be stopped* if urinary symptoms develop. Patients *should be advised* to stop taking tiaprofenic acid and to report to their doctor promptly if they develop urinary tract symptoms (such as increased frequency, nocturia, urgency, pain on urinating, or blood in urine)

Dose: 600 mg daily in 2–3 divided doses; CHILD not recommended

PoM Surgam® (Roussel)

Tablets, tiaprofenic acid 200 mg, net price 84-tab pack = £15.89; 300 mg, 56-tab pack = £15.89. Label: 21

Note. Tiaprofenic acid tablets also available from Cox

Modified release

PoM Surgam SA® (Roussel)

Capsules, m/r, maroon/pink enclosing white pellets, tiaprofenic acid 300 mg. Net price 56-cap pack = £15.89. Label: 25

Dose: 2 capsules once daily; CHILD not recommended

TOLMETIN

Indications: pain and inflammation in rheumatic disease (including juvenile arthritis) and other musculoskeletal disorders

Cautions; Contra-indications; Side-effects: see under Ibuprofen and notes above; **interactions:** Appendix 1 (NSAIDs)

Dose: 0.6–1.8 g daily in 2–4 divided doses; max. 30 mg/kg daily up to 1.8 g

CHILD, juvenile arthritis, 20–25 mg/kg daily in 3–4 divided doses; max. 30 mg/kg daily up to 1.8 g

PoM Tolectin® (Cilag)

Capsules, tolmetin (as sodium salt) 200 mg (ivory/orange), net price 90-cap pack = £15.97; 400 mg (orange), 90 cap = £23.97. Label: 21

ASPIRIN AND THE SALICYLATES

Aspirin was the traditional first choice anti-inflammatory analgesic but most physicians now prefer to start treatment with another NSAID which may be better tolerated and more convenient for the patient.

Cautionary label wordings, see inside back cover

Prices are **net**, see p.1

In regular high dosage aspirin has about the same anti-inflammatory effect as other NSAIDs. The required dose for active inflammatory joint disease is at least 3.6 g daily. There is little anti-inflammatory effect with less than 3 g daily. Gastro-intestinal side-effects such as nausea, dyspepsia, and gastro-intestinal bleeding may occur with any dosage of aspirin but anti-inflammatory doses are associated with a much higher incidence of side-effects. Anti-inflammatory doses of aspirin may also cause mild chronic salicylate intoxication (salicylism) characterised by dizziness, tinnitus, and deafness; these symptoms may be controlled by reducing the dosage.

ASPIRIN
(Acetylsalicylic Acid)

Indications: pain and inflammation in rheumatic disease and other musculoskeletal disorders (including juvenile arthritis); see also section 4.7.1; antiplatelet, see section 2.9

Cautions: asthma, allergic disease, uncontrolled hypertension, hepatic or renal impairment (avoid if severe), dehydration, pregnancy (particularly at term) (see also Appendix 4), elderly; G6PD-deficiency (see section 9.1.5); **interactions:** Appendix 1 (aspirin)

REYE'S SYNDROME. Owing to an association with Reye's syndrome the CSM has recommended that aspirin-containing preparations should no longer be given to children under the age of 12 years, unless specifically indicated, e.g. for juvenile arthritis (Still's disease). It is **important** to advise families that aspirin is not a suitable medicine for children with minor illnesses.

Contra-indications: gastro-intestinal ulceration; children under 12 years (except for juvenile arthritis) and breast-feeding (association with Reye's syndrome, see above); haemophilia and other bleeding disorders; not for treatment of gout

HYPERSENSITIVITY. Aspirin and other NSAIDs are **contra-indicated** in patients with a history of hypersensitivity to aspirin or any other NSAID—*which includes those* in whom attacks of *asthma, angioedema, urticaria or rhinitis* have been precipitated by aspirin or any other NSAID

Side-effects: common with anti-inflammatory doses; gastro-intestinal discomfort or nausea, ulceration with occult bleeding (but occasionally major haemorrhage); also other haemorrhage (e.g. subconjunctival); hearing disturbances such as tinnitus (leading rarely to deafness), vertigo, mental confusion, hypersensitivity reactions (angioedema, bronchospasm and rashes); increased bleeding time; rarely oedema, myocarditis, blood disorders, particularly thrombocytopenia; overdosage: see Emergency Treatment of Poisoning, p. 20

Dose: 0.3–1 g every 4 hours; max. in acute conditions 8 g daily; CHILD, juvenile arthritis, up to 80 mg/kg daily in 5–6 divided doses, increased in acute exacerbations to 130 mg/kg. Doses should be taken after food

Note. High doses of aspirin are very rarely required and are now given under specialist supervision only, and with plasma monitoring (especially in children)

Preparations

See section 4.7.1

BENORYLATE
(Benorilate)

(Aspirin-paracetamol ester; 2 g benorylate is equivalent to approximately 1.15 g aspirin and 970 mg paracetamol)

Indications: pain and inflammation in rheumatic disease and other musculoskeletal disorders; mild to moderate pain; pyrexia

Cautions; Contra-indications; Side-effects: see under Aspirin (above) and Paracetamol (section 4.7.1)

Dose: rheumatic disease, 4–8 g daily divided into 2–3 doses; max. 6 g daily for elderly; CHILD not recommended

Mild to moderate pain, 2 g twice daily preferably after food; CHILD not recommended

Benoral® (Sanofi Winthrop)

Tablets, benorylate 750 mg. Net price 100-tab pack = £8.36. Label: 21, 31

Granules, benorylate 2 g/sachet. Net price 60 sachet-pack = £13.77. Label: 13, 21, 31

Suspension, sugar-free, benorylate 2 g/5 mL. Net price 300 mL = £11.86. Label: 21, 31

Note. Generic versions of benorylate tablets and suspension are available from various manufacturers

10.1.2   Corticosteroids

10.1.2.1 SYSTEMIC CORTICOSTEROIDS

The general actions and uses of the corticosteroids are described in section 6.3. Treatment with corticosteroids in rheumatic diseases should be reserved for specific indications, e.g. when other anti-inflammatory drugs are unsuccessful.

In severe, possibly life-threatening, situations a high initial dose of corticosteroid is given to induce remission and the dose then gradually reduced to the lowest maintenance dose that will control the disease or, if possible, discontinued altogether. A major problem is that relapse may occur as dosage reduction is made, particularly if this is carried out too rapidly. The tendency is therefore to increase and maintain dosage and consequently the patient becomes dependent on corticosteroids. For this reason pulse doses of corticosteroids (e.g. methylprednisolone (as sodium succinate) up to 1 g intravenously on three consecutive days) is in current use to suppress highly active inflammatory disease while longer term and slower acting medication is being commenced.

Prednisolone is used for most purposes; it has the advantage over the more potent corticosteroids (see section 6.3.2) of permitting finer dosage adjustments. To minimise side-effects the maintenance dose of prednisolone should be kept as low as possible, usually 7.5 mg daily and seldom exceeding 10 mg daily.

Polymyalgia rheumatica and *giant cell (temporal) arteritis* are always treated with corticosteroids. The usual initial dose of prednisolone in polymyalgia rheumatica is 10 to 15 mg daily and in giant cell arteritis 40 to 60 mg daily (the higher dose being used if visual symptoms occur). Treatment should be continued until remission of disease activity and doses then gradually reduced to a maintenance level of about 7.5–10 mg daily. Relapse is common if therapy is stopped within 3 years but most patients can discontinue treatment after approximately 3 to 6 years after which recurrences become rare.

Polyarteritis nodosa and *polymyositis* are usually treated with corticosteroids. An initial dose of 60 mg of prednisolone daily is often used and reduced to a maintenance dose of 10 to 15 mg daily.

Systemic lupus erythematosus is treated with corticosteroids when necessary using a similar dosage regimen to that for polyarteritis nodosa and polymyositis (above). Patients with pleurisy, pericarditis, or other systemic manifestations will respond to corticosteroids. It may then be possible to reduce the dosage; alternate-day treatment is sometimes adequate, and the drug may be gradually withdrawn. In some mild cases corticosteroid treatment may be stopped after a few months. Many mild cases of systemic lupus erythematosus do not require corticosteroid treatment. Alternative treatment with anti-inflammatory analgesics, and possibly chloroquine, should be considered.

Since effective doses of systemic corticosteroids may cause Cushing's syndrome these drugs should **not** be used to suppress symptoms of *rheumatoid arthritis* unless alternative anti-inflammatory drugs and drugs which may affect the disease process (section 10.1.3) have proved unsuccessful, with increasing disability due to the inflammatory process. Recent evidence has suggested that prednisolone 7.5 mg daily may substantially reduce the rate of joint destruction in moderate to severe rheumatoid arthritis of less than 2 years duration but this has yet to be confirmed in a long-term study. The reduction in joint destruction must be distinguished from mere symptomatic improvement (which lasts only 6 to 12 months at this dose) and care should be taken to avoid gradually increasing the dosage (see also above). The smallest effective dose should be used and should not exceed the equivalent of prednisolone 7.5 to 10 mg daily. Corticosteroids in low dosage may also be useful in the elderly patient, and similar nocturnal doses may relieve morning stiffness.

Ankylosing spondylitis should not be treated with long-term corticosteroids; rarely, pulse doses may be needed and may be useful in extremely active disease that does not respond to conventional treatment.

10.1.2.2 LOCAL CORTICOSTEROID INJECTIONS

Corticosteroids are injected locally for an anti-inflammatory effect. In inflammatory conditions of the joints, particularly in rheumatoid arthritis, they are given by *intra-articular injection* to relieve pain, increase mobility, and reduce deformity in one or a few joints. Full aseptic precautions are essential; infected areas should be avoided. Occasionally an acute inflammatory reaction develops after an intra-articular or soft-tissue injection of a cortico-

steroid. This may be a reaction to the microcrystalline suspension of the corticosteroid used, but must be distinguished from sepsis introduced into the injection site. An almost insoluble compound such as triamcinolone hexacetonide has a long-acting (depot) effect and is preferred for intra-articular injection.

Smaller amounts of corticosteroids may also be injected directly into soft tissues for the relief of inflammation in conditions such as *tennis* or *golfer's elbow* or *compression neuropathies*. In *tendinitis*, injections should be made into the tendon sheath and not directly into the tendon (due to the absence of a true tendon sheath, the Achilles tendon should not be injected). A soluble preparation (e.g. containing betamethasone or dexamethasone sodium phosphate) is preferred for injection into the carpal tunnel.

Cortisone acetate is **not** effective for local injection and hydrocortisone acetate or one of the synthetic analogues such as triamcinolone hexacetonide is generally used. The risk of necrosis and muscle wasting may be slightly increased with triamcinolone; flushing has been reported with intra-articular corticosteroid injections. Charcot-like arthropathies have also been reported (particularly following repeated intra-articular injections).

Corticosteroid injections are also injected into soft tissues for the treatment of skin lesions (see section 13.4).

LOCAL CORTICOSTEROID INJECTIONS

Indications: local inflammation of joints and soft tissues (for details, see individual data sheets)
Cautions; Contra-indications; Side-effects: see notes above (for details see also individual data sheets)
Dose: see under preparations

Dose calculated as dexamethasone sodium phosphate
PoM Dexamethasone (Organon)
Injection, dexamethasone sodium phosphate 5 mg/mL (≡ dexamethasone 4 mg/mL ≡ dexamethasone phosphate 4.8 mg/mL). Net price 1-mL amp = 83p; 2-mL vial = £1.27
   Dose: by intra-articular or intrasynovial injection (for details see data sheet), 0.4–4 mg (calculated as dexamethasone sodium phosphate) according to size; where appropriate may be repeated at intervals of 3–21 days according to response

Dose calculated as dexamethasone phosphate
PoM Decadron® (MSD)
Injection, dexamethasone phosphate 4 mg/mL (≡ dexamethasone 3.33 mg/mL ≡ dexamethasone sodium phosphate 4.17 mg/mL). Net price 2-mL vial = £1.76
   Dose: by intra-articular or intrasynovial injection (for details see data sheet), 0.4–4 mg (calculated as dexamethasone phosphate) according to size (*soft-tissue infiltration* 2–6 mg); where appropriate may be repeated at intervals of 3–21 days; also for *intralesional injection*
   Note. Injection containing Dexamethasone phosphate 4 mg/mL (as sodium phosphate) is also available from David Bull

---

Cautionary label wordings, see inside back cover

Hydrocortisone acetate

PoM Hydrocortistab® (Knoll)

Injection, (aqueous suspension), hydrocortisone acetate 25 mg/mL. Net price 1-mL amp = £1.05

> *Dose: by intra-articular or intrasynovial injection* (for details see data sheet), 5–50 mg according to size; where appropriate may be repeated at intervals of 21 days; not more than 3 joints should be treated on any one day; CHILD 5–30 mg (divided)

Methylprednisolone acetate

PoM Depo-Medrone® (Upjohn)

Injection (aqueous suspension), methylprednisolone acetate 40 mg/mL. Net price 1-mL vial = £2.70; 2-mL vial = £4.87; 3-mL vial = £7.05

> *Dose: by intra-articular or intrasynovial injection* (for details see data sheet), 4–80 mg, according to size; where appropriate may be repeated at intervals of 7–35 days; also for *intralesional injection*

PoM Depo-Medrone® with Lidocaine (Upjohn)

Injection (aqueous suspension), methylprednisolone acetate 40 mg, lignocaine hydrochloride 10 mg/mL. Net price 1-mL vial = £2.70; 2-mL vial = £4.87

> *Dose: by intra-articular or intrasynovial injection* (for details see data sheet), 4–80 mg, according to size; where appropriate may be repeated at intervals of 7–35 days

Prednisolone acetate

PoM Deltastab® (Knoll)

Injection (aqueous suspension), prednisolone acetate 25 mg/mL. Net price 1-mL amp = £1.05

> *Dose: by intra-articular or intrasynovial injection* (for details see data sheet), 5–25 mg according to size; not more than 3 joints should be treated on any one day; where appropriate may be repeated when relapse occurs

For *intramuscular injection*, see section 6.3.2

Triamcinolone acetonide

PoM Adcortyl® Intra-articular / Intradermal (Squibb)

Injection (aqueous suspension), triamcinolone acetonide 10 mg/mL. Net price 1-mL amp = £1.02; 5-mL vial = £4.14

> *Dose: by intra-articular injection or intrasynovial injection* (for details see data sheet), 2.5–15 mg according to size (for larger doses use *Kenalog®* instead); where appropriate may be repeated when relapse occurs
>
> *By intradermal injection*, (for details see data sheet): 2–3 mg; max. 5 mg at any one site (total max. 30 mg); where appropriate may be repeated at intervals of 1–2 weeks
>
> CHILD under 6 years not recommended

PoM Kenalog® Intra-articular / Intramuscular (Squibb)

Injection (aqueous suspension), triamcinolone acetonide 40 mg/mL. Net price 1-mL vial = £1.70

> *Dose: by intra-articular or intrasynovial injection*, (for details see data sheet), 5–40 mg according to size; total max. 80 mg (for doses below 5 mg use *Adcortyl®* Intra-articular/Intradermal instead); where appropriate may be repeated when relapse occurs; CHILD under 6 years not recommended

For *intramuscular injection*, see section 6.3.2

Triamcinolone hexacetonide

PoM Lederspan® (Lederle)

Injection (aqueous suspension), triamcinolone hexacetonide 5 mg/mL. Net price 5-mL vial = £2.85

> *Dose: by intralesional injection* (for details see data sheet), up to 500 micrograms/square inch of affected skin

Injection (aqueous suspension), triamcinolone hexacetonide 20 mg/mL. Net price 1-mL vial = £2.48; 5 mL vial = £9.65

> *Dose: by intra-articular or intrasynovial injection* (for details see data sheet), 2–30 mg according to size; where appropriate may be repeated at intervals of 21–28 days; for *intralesional injection*, see above

10.1.3   Drugs which suppress the rheumatic disease process

Certain drugs such as gold, penicillamine, hydroxychloroquine, chloroquine, immunosuppressants, and sulphasalazine may suppress the disease process in *rheumatoid arthritis*, as may gold and immunosuppressants in *psoriatic arthritis*. They are sometimes known as second-line or disease-modifying antirheumatic drugs (DMARDs). Unlike NSAIDs they do not produce an immediate therapeutic effect but require 4 to 6 months of treatment for a full response. If one of these drugs does not lead to objective benefit within 6 months, it should be discontinued.

These drugs may improve not only the symptoms and signs of inflammatory joint disease but also extra-articular manifestations such as vasculitis. They reduce the erythrocyte sedimentation rate and sometimes the titre of rheumatoid factor. Some (e.g. the immunosuppressants) may retard erosive damage as judged radiologically.

These drugs are used in rheumatoid arthritis where treatment with NSAIDs alone provides inadequate control. Since, in the first few months, the course of rheumatoid arthritis is unpredictable, it is usual to delay treatment for about 6 months depending on the progress of the disease, but treatment should be initiated if severe symptoms persist.

Penicillamine and immunosuppressants are also sometimes used in rheumatoid arthritis where there are troublesome extra-articular features such as vasculitis, and in patients who are taking excessive doses of corticosteroids. Where the response is satisfactory there is often a striking reduction in requirements of both corticosteroids and other drugs. Gold and penicillamine are effective in *palindromic rheumatism* and chloroquine is sometimes used to treat *systemic* and *discoid lupus erythematosus*.

JUVENILE ARTHRITIS. Gold, penicillamine, and related drugs may also be used to treat *juvenile arthritis* (Still's disease) when indications are similar.

GOLD

Gold may be given by intramuscular injection as sodium aurothiomalate or by mouth as auranofin.

Sodium aurothiomalate must be given by deep intramuscular injection and the area gently massaged. A test dose of 10 mg must be given followed by doses of 50 mg at weekly intervals until there is definite evidence of remission. Benefit is not to be expected until about 300 to 500 mg has been given; if there is no remission after 1 g has been given it should be discontinued. In patients who do respond, the interval between injections is then gradually increased to 4 weeks and treatment is continued for up to 5 years after complete remission. If relapse occurs dosage may be immediately increased to 50 mg weekly and only once control has been obtained again should the dosage be reduced. It is important to avoid complete relapse since second courses of gold are not usually effective. Children may be given 1 mg/kg weekly to a maximum of 50 mg weekly, the intervals being gradually increased to 4 weeks according to response; an initial test dose is given corresponding to one-tenth to one-fifth of the calculated dose.

Auranofin is given by mouth. If there is no response after 9 months treatment should be discontinued.

Gold therapy should be discontinued in the presence of blood disorders or proteinuria (associated with immune complex nephritis) which is repeatedly above 300 mg/litre without other cause (such as urinary-tract infection). Urine tests and full blood counts (including total and differential white cell and platelet counts) must therefore be performed before each intramuscular injection; in the case of oral treatment the urine and blood tests should be carried out monthly. Rashes with pruritus often occur after 2 to 6 months of intramuscular treatment and may necessitate discontinuation of treatment; the most common side-effect of oral therapy, diarrhoea with or without nausea or abdominal pain, may respond to bulking agents (such as bran) or temporary reduction in dosage.

SODIUM AUROTHIOMALATE

Indications: active progressive rheumatoid arthritis, juvenile arthritis

Cautions: see notes above; patients should report pruritus, metallic taste, fever, sore throat or tongue, buccal ulceration, purpura, epistaxis, bleeding gums, bruising, menorrhagia, diarrhoea; renal and hepatic impairment, elderly, history of urticaria, eczema, colitis, drugs which cause blood disorders; annual chest X-ray; **interactions:** Appendix 1 (gold)

Contra-indications: severe renal and hepatic disease (see notes above); history of blood disorders or bone marrow aplasia, exfoliative dermatitis, systemic lupus erythematosus, necrotising enterocolitis, pulmonary fibrosis; pregnancy and breast-feeding (see Appendixes 4 and 5); porphyria (see section 9.8.2)

Side-effects: severe reactions (occasionally fatal) in up to 5% of patients; mouth ulcers, skin reactions, proteinuria, blood disorders (sometimes sudden and fatal); rarely colitis, peripheral neuritis, pulmonary fibrosis, hepatotoxicity with cholestatic jaundice, alopecia

Dose: by deep intramuscular injection, administered on expert advice, see notes above

PoM Myocrisin® (Rhône-Poulenc Rorer)
Injection, sodium aurothiomalate 20 mg/mL, net price 0.5-mL (10-mg) amp = £1.51; 40 mg/mL, 0.5-mL (20-mg) amp = £2.19; 100 mg/mL, 0.5-mL (50-mg) amp = £4.46

AURANOFIN

Indications: active progressive rheumatoid arthritis when NSAIDs inadequate alone

Cautions; Contra-indications: see under Sodium Aurothiomalate; also caution in inflammatory bowel disease
BLOOD COUNTS. Withdraw if platelets fall below 100 000/mm³ or if signs and symptoms suggestive of thrombocytopenia occur, see also notes above

Side-effects: diarrhoea most common (reduced by bulking agents such as bran); see also under Sodium Aurothiomalate

Dose: administered on expert advice, 6 mg daily (initially in 2 divided doses then if tolerated as single dose), if response inadequate after 6 months, increase to 9 mg daily (in 3 divided doses), discontinue if no response after a further 3 months; CHILD not recommended
COUNSELLING. Warn patient to tell doctor immediately if sore throat, mouth ulcers, bruising, fever. malaise, rash, diarrhoea or non-specific illness develops

PoM Ridaura® (Bencard)
Tablets, pale yellow, f/c, auranofin 3 mg. Net price 60-tab pack = £28.00. Label: 21, counselling, blood disorder symptoms (see above)

PENICILLAMINE

Penicillamine has a similar action to gold, and more patients are able to continue treatment than with gold but side-effects occur frequently. An initial dose of 125 to 250 mg daily before food is given for 1 month, increased by this amount every 4 to 12 weeks until remission occurs. Penicillamine should be discontinued if there is no improvement within 1 year. The usual maintenance dose is 500 to 750 mg daily, but up to 1.5 g may rarely be required.

Patients should be warned not to expect improvement for at least 6 to 12 weeks after treatment is initiated. If remission has been sustained for 6 months, reduction of dosage by 125 to 250 mg every 12 weeks may be attempted.

Blood counts, including platelets, and urine examinations should be carried out every 1 or 2 weeks for the first 2 months then every 4 weeks to detect blood disorders and proteinuria (they should also be carried out in the week after any dose increase). A reduction in platelet count indicates that treatment with penicillamine should be stopped, subsequently re-introduced at a lower dosage level and then, if possible, gradually increased. Proteinuria, associated with immune complex nephritis, occurs in up to 30% of patients, but may resolve despite continuation of treatment; treatment may be continued provided that renal function tests remain normal, oedema is absent, and the 24-hour urinary excretion of protein does not exceed 2 g.

Nausea may occur but is not usually a problem provided that penicillamine is taken before food or on retiring and that low initial doses are used and only gradually increased. Loss of taste may occur about 6 weeks after treatment is started but usually returns 6 weeks later irrespective of whether or not treatment is discontinued; mineral supplements are not recommended. Rashes are a common side-effect. Those which occur in the first few months of treatment disappear when the drug is stopped and treatment may then be re-introduced at a lower dose level and gradually increased. Late rashes are more resistant and often necessitate discontinuation of treatment.

There is some evidence that patients who are hypersensitive to penicillin may have a higher risk of penicillamine reactions.

PENICILLAMINE

Indications: see notes above and under Dose

Cautions: see notes above; renal impairment (see Appendix 3), pregnancy (see Appendix 4); avoid concurrent gold, chloroquine, hydroxychloroquine, or immunosuppressive treatment; avoid oral iron within 2 hours of a dose; **interactions:** Appendix 1 (penicillamine)

BLOOD COUNTS and URINE TESTS. See notes above. Longer intervals may be adequate in cystinuria and Wilson's disease. Consider withdrawal if platelets fall below 120 000/mm³ or white blood cells below 2500/mm³ or if 3 successive falls within normal range (can restart at reduced dose when counts return to normal but permanent withdrawal necessary if recurrence of neutropenia or thrombocytopenia)

COUNSELLING. Warn patient to tell doctor immediately if sore throat, mouth ulcers, bruising, fever, malaise, rash, or non-specific illness develops.

Contra-indications: hypersensitivity (except in life-threatening situation when desensitisation may be attempted—see data sheet); lupus erythematosus

Side-effects: (see also notes above) initially nausea, anorexia, fever, and skin reactions; taste loss (mineral supplements not recommended); blood disorders including thrombocytopenia, neutropenia, agranulocytosis and aplastic anaemia; proteinuria, rarely haematuria (withdraw immediately); haemolytic anaemia, nephrotic syndrome, lupus erythematosus-like syndrome, myasthenia gravis-like syndrome, pemphigus, Goodpasture's syndrome, and Stevens-Johnson syndrome also reported; in non-rheumatoid conditions rheumatoid arthritis-like syndrome also reported; late rashes (reduce dose or withdraw treatment)

Dose: severe active rheumatoid arthritis, administered on expert advice, ADULT initially 125–250 mg daily before food for 1 month increased by similar amounts at intervals of not less than 4 weeks to usual maintenance of 500–750 mg daily in divided doses; max. 1.5 g daily; ELDERLY initially up to 125 mg daily before food for 1 month increased by similar amounts at intervals of not less than 4 weeks; max. 1 g daily; CHILD maintenance of 15–20 mg/kg daily (initial dose lower and increased at intervals of 4 weeks over a period of 3-6 months)

Wilson's disease, chronic active hepatitis, and cystinuria, see section 9.8

Copper and lead poisoning, see Emergency Treatment of Poisoning, p. 24

PoM **Penicillamine** (Non-proprietary)

Tablets, penicillamine 125 mg, net price 20 = £1.80; 250 mg, 20 = £3.43. Label: 6, 22, counselling, blood disorder symptoms (see above)

Available from APS, Cox, Evans, Hillcross, Norton

PoM **Distamine®** (Dista)

Tablets, all f/c, penicillamine 125 mg, net price 20 = £2.17; 250 mg, 20 = £3.74. Label: 6, 22, counselling, blood disorder symptoms (see above)

PoM **Pendramine®** (ASTA Medica)

Tablets, both scored, f/c, penicillamine 125 mg, net price 20 = £1.80; 250 mg, 20 = £3.27. Label: 6, 22, counselling, blood disorder symptoms (see above)

ANTIMALARIALS

Chloroquine and **hydroxychloroquine** have a similar action to, and are better tolerated than, gold or penicillamine; retinopathy is rare provided the doses given below are not exceeded.

These drugs should not be used for psoriatic arthritis. It should also be noted that it is difficult to distinguish ageing changes from drug-induced retinopathy in the elderly.

Mepacrine (see section 5.4.4) is sometimes used in discoid lupus erythematosus.

CHLOROQUINE

Indications: active rheumatoid arthritis (including juvenile arthritis), systemic and discoid lupus erythematosus; malaria, see section 5.4.1

Cautions: hepatic and renal impairment, pregnancy (but for malaria benefit outweighs risk, see Appendix 4, Antimalarials), porphyria, may exacerbate psoriasis, neurological disorders (especially history of epilepsy), may aggravate myasthenia gravis, severe gastro-intestinal disorders, G6PD deficiency (see section 9.1.5); elderly (see notes above); avoid concurrent hepatotoxic drugs—other **interactions:** Appendix 1 (chloroquine)

Advice of College of Ophthalmologists on long-term therapy.

1. Eye examination before long-term chloroquine or hydroxychloroquine to establish baseline;

2. Patient to stop taking and seek immediate advice from prescribing medical practitioner or general practitioner or ophthalmologist if any disturbance of vision noted;

3. Prescribing medical practitioner to be responsible for monitoring if considered necessary;

4. If monitoring considered necessary, *once monthly Amsler testing by patient* may detect premaculopathy (visual disturbance in absence of ophthalmoscopically visible macular changes—which is frequently reversible).

Ocular toxicity very unlikely with chloroquine phosphate not exceeding 4 mg/kg daily (= chloroquine base approx. 2.5 mg/kg daily) or hydroxychloroquine sulphate not exceeding 6.5 mg/kg daily.

To avoid excessive dosage in obese patients special care needed to *calculate on basis of lean body-weight.*

Side-effects: gastro-intestinal disturbances, headache; also convulsions, visual disturbances, irreversible retinal damage, corneal opacities, depigmentation or loss of hair, skin reactions (rashes, pruritus), ECG changes; rarely blood disorders (thrombocytopenia, agranulocytosis and aplastic anaemia), psychosis reported; *important:* very toxic in overdosage—immediate advice from poisons centres essential (see also p. 22)

Dose: administered on expert advice, chloroquine (base) 150 mg daily; max. 2.5 mg/kg daily, see recommendations above; CHILD, up to 3 mg/kg daily

Note. Chloroquine base 150 mg ≡ chloroquine sulphate 200 mg ≡ chloroquine phosphate 250 mg (approx.).

Preparations
See section 5.4.1

HYDROXYCHLOROQUINE SULPHATE

Indications: active rheumatoid arthritis (including juvenile arthritis), systemic and discoid lupus erythematosus

Cautions; Side-effects: see under Chloroquine and notes (above)

Dose: administered on expert advice, initially 400 mg daily in divided doses; maintenance 200–400 mg daily; max. 6.5 mg/kg daily, see recommendations above; CHILD, up to 6.5 mg/kg daily

PoM **Plaquenil**® (Sanofi Winthrop)
Tablets, orange, s/c, hydroxychloroquine sulphate 200 mg. Net price 56-tab pack = £18.88. Label: 5

IMMUNOSUPPRESSANTS

When used in *rheumatoid arthritis* **immunosuppressants** have a similar action to gold and are useful alternatives in cases that have failed to respond to gold, penicillamine, chloroquine, or hydroxychloroquine.

Azathioprine (see section 8.2.1) is usually chosen and is usually given in a dose of 1.5 to 2.5 mg/kg daily in divided doses. Blood counts are needed to detect possible neutropenia and/or thrombocytopenia which is usually resolved by reducing the dose. Nausea, vomiting, and diarrhoea may occur, usually starting early during the course of treatment, and may necessitate withdrawal of the drug; herpes zoster infection may also occur.

Methotrexate has also been shown to be effective. It is usually given in an initial dose of 2.5 mg by mouth once a week, increased slowly to a maximum of 15 mg once a week (occasionally 20 mg), subject to regular full blood counts (including differential white cell count and platelet count) and liver-function tests.

Cyclosporin has also been shown to be effective and is now also licensed for severe active rheumatoid arthritis when conventional therapy is inappropriate or ineffective.

Chlorambucil (see section 8.1.1) is another immunosuppressant which is used in rheumatoid arthritis [unlicensed indication]; a dose of 100 to 200 micrograms/kg daily is usually given initially. Regular blood counts including platelets should be carried out. **Cyclophosphamide** (see section 8.1.1) is more toxic but may be used at a dose of 1 to 1.5 mg/kg daily by mouth for rheumatoid arthritis with severe systemic manifestations [unlicensed indication]. Cyclophosphamide may also be given intravenously in a dose of 0.5 to 1 g (with prophylactic mesna) for *severe systemic rheumatoid arthritis* and for other connective tissue diseases (especially with active vasculitis), repeated initially at fortnightly then at monthly intervals (according to clinical response and haematological monitoring).

Immunosuppressants are also used in the management of severe cases of *systemic lupus erythematosus* and other connective tissue disorders. They are often given in conjunction with corticosteroids for patients with severe or progressive renal disease though the evidence for their benefit is doubtful. They may be used in cases of *polymyositis* which are resistant to corticosteroids. They are used for their corticosteroid-sparing effect in patients whose corticosteroid requirements are excessive. **Azathioprine** is usually used but **chlorambucil** is an alternative.

Azathioprine and methotrexate are used in the treatment of *psoriatic arthropathy* [unlicensed indication] for severe or progressive cases which are not controlled with anti-inflammatory drugs. There is an impression that **azathioprine** is the more effective for psoriatic arthritis and that **methotrexate** is the more effective for skin manifestations.

AZATHIOPRINE

Indications: see notes above; transplantation rejection, see section 8.2.1

Cautions; Contra-indications; Side-effects: see under Azathioprine, section 8.2.1

Dose: *by mouth,* initially, rarely more than 3 mg/kg daily, reduced according to response; maintenance 1–3 mg/kg daily; consider withdrawal if no improvement within 3 months

Preparations
See section 8.2.1

CYCLOSPORIN
(Ciclosporin)

Indications: severe active rheumatoid arthritis when conventional therapy inappropriate or ineffective; graft-versus-host disease, see section 8.2.2; atopic dermatitis and psoriasis, see section 13.5.2.

Cautions; Side-effects: see section 8.2.2
ADDITIONAL CAUTIONS IN RHEUMATOID ARTHRITIS. **Contra-indicated** in abnormal renal function, hypertension not under control (see also below), infections not under control, and malignancy. Measure serum creat-

inine at least twice before treatment and monitor every 2 weeks for first 3 months, then every 4 weeks (or more frequently if dose increased or concomitant NSAIDs introduced or increased (see also *interactions*: Appendix 1 (cyclosporin)), reducing dose if serum creatinine increases more than 30% above baseline in more than 1 measurement; if above 50%, reducing dose by 50% (even if within normal range) and discontinuing if reduction not successful within 1 month; monitor blood pressure (discontinue if hypertension develops that cannot be controlled by antihypertensive therapy); monitor hepatic function if concomitant NSAIDs given.

Dose: ADULT over 18 years *by mouth*, administered in accordance with expert advice initially, 2.5 mg/kg daily in 2 divided doses, if necessary increased gradually after 6 weeks to max. 4 mg/kg daily (discontinuing if response still insufficient after 3 months); dose adjusted according to response for maintenance and treatment reviewed after 6 months (continue only if benefits outweigh risks); CHILD and under 18 years, not recommended

IMPORTANT. For preparations and counselling and for advice on conversion between the preparations, see section 8.2.2

METHOTREXATE

Indications: severe active rheumatoid arthritis unresponsive to conventional therapy; malignant disease, see section 8.1.3; psoriasis, see section 13.5.2

Cautions; Contra-indications; Side-effects: see Methotrexate, section 13.5.2
PULMONARY TOXICITY. Pulmonary toxicity may be a special problem in rheumatoid arthritis (patient to contact doctor immediately if dyspnoea or cough). For other special warnings, including counselling advice relating to interaction with aspirin and NSAIDs, see Methotrexate, section 13.5.2.

Dose: by mouth, 7.5 mg once weekly (as a single dose *or* divided into 3 doses of 2.5 mg given at intervals of 12 hours), adjusted according to response; max. total weekly dose 20 mg

Preparations
See section 8.1.3

SULPHASALAZINE

Sulphasalazine has a beneficial effect in suppressing the inflammatory activity of rheumatoid arthritis. Side-effects include rashes, gastro-intestinal intolerance and, especially in patients with rheumatoid arthritis, occasional leucopenia, neutropenia, and thrombocytopenia. These haematological abnormalities occur usually in the first 3 to 6 months of treatment and are reversible on cessation of treatment. Close monitoring of full blood counts (including differential white cell count and platelet count) is necessary initially, and at monthly intervals during the first 3 months (liver function tests also being performed at monthly intervals for the first 3 months).

SULPHASALAZINE
(Sulfasalazine)

Indications: active rheumatoid arthritis; ulcerative colitis, see section 1.5 and notes above

Cautions; Contra-indications; Side-effects: see section 1.5 and notes above
The CSM has recommended that patients receiving sulphasalazine should be advised to report any unexplained bleeding, bruising, purpura, sore throat, fever or malaise that occurs during treatment. A blood count should be performed and the drug stopped immediately if there is suspicion of a blood dyscrasia.

Dose: by mouth, administered on expert advice, as enteric-coated tablets, initially 500 mg daily, increased by 500 mg at intervals of 1 week to a max. of 2–3 g daily in divided doses

PoM **Salazopyrin EN-Tabs**® (Pharmacia)
Tablets, e/c, yellow, f/c, sulphasalazine 500 mg. Net price 100-tab pack = £10.81. Label: 5, 14, 25, counselling, blood disorder symptoms (see CSM recommendation above), contact lenses may be stained

10.1.4   Drugs for treatment of gout

It is important to distinguish drugs used for the treatment of acute attacks of gout from those used in the long-term control of the disease. The latter exacerbate and prolong the acute manifestations if started during an attack.

ACUTE ATTACKS

Acute attacks of gout are usually treated with high doses of **NSAIDs** such as azapropazone (**important**: see CSM restrictions on p. 410), diclofenac, indomethacin, ketoprofen, naproxen, piroxicam, or sulindac (section 10.1.1). Colchicine is an alternative. Aspirin is *not* indicated in gout. Allopurinol and uricosurics are not effective in treating an acute attack and may prolong it indefinitely if started during the acute episode.

Colchicine is probably as effective as NSAIDs. Its use is limited by the development of toxicity at higher doses, but it is of value in patients with heart failure since, unlike NSAIDs, it does not induce fluid retention; moreover it can be given to patients receiving anticoagulants.

COLCHICINE

Indications: acute gout, short-term prophylaxis during initial therapy with allopurinol and uricosuric drugs

Cautions: elderly, gastro-intestinal disease, cardiac, hepatic and renal impairment; **interactions:** Appendix 1 (colchicine)

Contra-indications: pregnancy and breast-feeding

Side-effects: most common are nausea, vomiting, and abdominal pain; excessive doses may also cause profuse diarrhoea, gastro-intestinal haemorrhage, rashes, renal and hepatic damage. Rarely peripheral neuritis, myopathy, alopecia, and with prolonged treatment blood disorders

Dose: 1 mg initially, followed by 500 micrograms every 2–3 hours until relief of pain is obtained or vomiting or diarrhoea occurs, or until a total dose of 10 mg has been reached. The course should not be repeated within 3 days

Prevention of attacks during initial treatment with allopurinol or uricosuric drugs, 500 micrograms 2–3 times daily

PoM Colchicine (Non-proprietary)
Tablets, colchicine 500 micrograms, net price 20 = £3.07
Available from CP, Kent, Norton

INTERVAL TREATMENT

For long-term ('interval') control of gout the formation of uric acid from purines may be reduced with the **xanthine-oxidase inhibitor** allopurinol, or the **uricosuric drugs** probenecid or sulphinpyrazone may be used to increase the excretion of uric acid in the urine. Treatment should be continued indefinitely once the decision has been made to prevent further attacks of gout by correcting the hyperuricaemia. These drugs should never be started during an acute attack. The initiation of treatment may precipitate an acute attack therefore colchicine or an anti-inflammatory analgesic should be used as a prophylactic and continued for at least one month after the hyperuricaemia has been corrected (usually about 3 months of prophylaxis).

  Allopurinol is a convenient well tolerated drug which is now widely used. It is especially useful in patients with renal impairment or urate stones where uricosuric drugs cannot be used. It is usually given once daily, as the active metabolite of allopurinol has a long half-life, but doses over 300 mg daily should be divided. Allopurinol treatment should not be started until an acute attack of gout has completely subsided, as further attacks may be precipitated. It is well tolerated in most patients but may occasionally cause rashes. Allopurinol is *not* indicated for the treatment of asymptomatic hyperuricaemia.

  The uricosuric drugs include **probenecid** and **sulphinpyrazone**. They can be used instead of allopurinol, or in conjunction with it in cases that are resistant to treatment.

  If an acute attack develops in a patient taking allopurinol or a uricosuric the treatment should continue at the same dosage while the acute attack is treated in its own right.

  Aspirin and salicylates antagonise the uricosuric drugs; they do not antagonise allopurinol but are nevertheless *not* indicated in gout.

  Crystallisation of urate in the urine may occur with the uricosuric drugs and it is important to ensure that there is an adequate urine output especially in the first few weeks of treatment. As an additional precaution the urine may be rendered alkaline.

  The **NSAIDs** are described in section 10.1.1.

ALLOPURINOL

Indications: prophylaxis of gout and of uric acid and calcium oxalate renal stones
Cautions: administer prophylactic colchicine or NSAID (*not* aspirin or salicylates) until at least 1 month after hyperuricaemia corrected; ensure adequate fluid intake (2 litres/day); hepatic and renal impairment (see Appendix 3). In neoplastic conditions treatment with allopurinol (if required) should be commenced before cytotoxic drugs are given; **interactions:** Appendix 1 (allopurinol)
Contra-indications: not a treatment for acute gout but continue if attack develops when already receiving allopurinol, and treat attack separately (see notes above)
Side-effects: rashes (**withdraw** therapy; if rash mild re-introduce cautiously but **discontinue** immediately if recurrence—skin reactions associated with exfoliation, fever, lymphadenopathy, arthralgia, and eosinophilia, resembling Stevens-Johnson or Lyell's syndrome, occur rarely); gastro-intestinal disorders. Rarely malaise, headache, vertigo, drowsiness, taste disturbances, hypertension, symptomless xanthine deposits in muscle, alopecia, hepatotoxicity, paraesthesia and neuropathy
Dose: initially 100 mg daily as a single dose, after food, gradually increased over 1–3 weeks according to the plasma or urinary uric acid concentration, to about 300 mg daily; usual maintenance dose 200–600 mg, rarely 900 mg daily, divided into doses of not more than 300 mg; CHILD (in neoplastic conditions, enzyme disorders) 10–20 mg/kg daily

PoM Allopurinol (Non-proprietary)
Tablets, allopurinol 100 mg, net price 20 = 23p; 300 mg, 20 = 58p. Label: 8, 21, 27
Available from APS, Ashbourne (Xanthomax®), Berk (Caplenal®), Cox, CP, DDSA (Cosuric®), Kent, Norton, Rima (Rimapurinol®)
PoM Zyloric® (Wellcome)
Tablets, allopurinol 100 mg, net price 100-tab pack = £10.96; 300 mg, 28-tab pack = £7.86. Label: 8, 21, 27

PROBENECID
Indications: gout prophylaxis (to correct hyperuricaemia); reduction of tubular excretion of penicillins and certain cephalosporins, see section 5.1
Cautions: during initial gout therapy administer prophylactic colchicine or NSAID (*not* aspirin or salicylates), ensure adequate fluid intake (about 2 litres daily), render urine alkaline if uric acid overload is high; peptic ulceration, renal impairment (avoid if severe); transient false-positive Benedict's test; G6PD-deficiency (see section 9.1.5); **interactions:** Appendix 1 (probenecid)
Contra-indications: history of blood disorders, nephrolithiasis, porphyria (see section 9.8.2), acute gout attack; avoid aspirin and salicylates
Side-effects: infrequent; occasionally nausea and vomiting, urinary frequency, headache, flushing, dizziness, rashes; rarely hypersensitivity, nephrotic syndrome, hepatic necrosis, aplastic anaemia
Dose: uricosuric therapy, initially 250 mg twice daily after food, increased after a week to 500 mg twice daily then up to 2 g daily in 2–4 divided doses according to plasma-uric acid concentration and reduced for maintenance

---

Cautionary label wordings, see inside back cover   Prices are **net**, see p.1

PoM Benemid® (MSD)

Tablets, scored, probenecid 500 mg. Net price 20 =
66p. Label: 12, 21, 27

SULPHINPYRAZONE
(Sulfinpyrazone)

Indications: gout prophylaxis, hyperuricaemia

Cautions; Contra-indications: see under Probenecid; regular blood counts advisable; avoid in
hypersensitivity to NSAIDs; cardiac disease (may
cause salt and water retention); **interactions:**
Appendix 1 (sulphinpyrazone)

Side-effects: gastro-intestinal disturbances, occasionally allergic skin reactions, salt and water
retention; rarely blood disorders, gastro-intestinal ulceration and bleeding, acute renal failure,
raised liver enzymes, jaundice and hepatitis

Dose: initially 100–200 mg daily with food (or
milk) increasing over 2–3 weeks to 600 mg daily
(rarely 800 mg daily), continued until serum uric
acid concentration normal then reduced for maintenance (maintenance dose may be as low as
200 mg daily)

PoM Anturan® (Geigy)

Tablets, both yellow, s/c, sulphinpyrazone 100 mg,
net price 20 = 94p; 200 mg, 84-tab pack = £7.82.
Label: 12, 21

10.2   Drugs used in
neuromuscular disorders

10.2.1   Drugs which enhance
neuromuscular transmission

Anticholinesterases are used as first-line treatment
in *myasthenia gravis*.

Corticosteroids are only given concomitantly if
anticholinesterase treatment is failing.

Plasmapheresis may produce temporary remission in otherwise unresponsive patients.

ANTICHOLINESTERASES

Anticholinesterase drugs are used to enhance
neuromuscular transmission in voluntary and involuntary muscle in myasthenia gravis. They prolong
the action of acetylcholine by inhibiting the action
of the enzyme acetylcholinesterase. Excessive dosage of these drugs may impair neuromuscular transmission and precipitate 'cholinergic crises' by
causing a depolarising block. This may be difficult
to distinguish from a worsening myasthenic state.

Side-effects of anticholinesterases are due to their
parasympathomimetic action. Muscarinic effects
include increased sweating, salivary, and gastric
secretion, also increased gastro-intestinal and
uterine motility, and bradycardia. These effects are
antagonised by atropine.

Edrophonium has a very brief action and is
therefore used mainly for the diagnosis of myasthenia gravis. A single test-dose usually causes substantial improvement in muscle power (lasting
about 5 minutes) in patients with the disease (if respiration already impaired, *only* in conjunction with
someone skilled at intubation).

It can also be used to determine whether a patient
with myasthenia is receiving inadequate or excessive treatment with cholinergic drugs. If treatment
is excessive an injection of edrophonium will either
have no effect or will intensify symptoms (if respiration already impaired, *only* in conjunction with
someone skilled at intubation). Conversely, transient improvement may be seen if the patient is
being inadequately treated. The test is best performed just before the next dose of anticholinesterase.

Neostigmine produces a therapeutic effect for up
to 4 hours. Its pronounced muscarinic action is a
disadvantage, and simultaneous administration of
an antimuscarinic drug such as atropine or propantheline may be required to prevent colic, excessive
salivation, or diarrhoea. In severe disease neostigmine may be given every 2 hours. The maximum that most patients can tolerate is 180 mg daily.

Pyridostigmine is less powerful and slower in
action than neostigmine but it has a longer duration
of action. It is preferable to neostigmine because of
its smoother action and the need for less frequent
dosage. It is particularly preferred in patients whose
muscles are weak on wakening. It has a compara-
tively mild gastro-intestinal effect but an antimuscarinic drug may still be required. It is inadvisable
to exceed a daily dose of 720 mg.

Distigmine has the most protracted action but the
danger of a 'cholinergic crisis' caused by accumulation of the drug is greater than with shorter-acting
drugs.

Neostigmine and edrophonium are also used to
reverse the actions of the non-depolarising muscle
relaxants (see section 15.1.6).

NEOSTIGMINE

Indications: myasthenia gravis; other indications,
see section 15.1.6

Cautions: asthma (*extreme* caution), bradycardia,
recent myocardial infarction, epilepsy, hypotension, parkinsonism, vagotonia, peptic ulceration, renal impairment, pregnancy and breast-
feeding. Atropine or other antidote to muscarinic
effects may be necessary (particularly when neostigmine is given by injection), but it should not
be given routinely as it may mask signs of overdosage; **interactions:** Appendix 1 (parasympathomimetics)

Contra-indications: intestinal or urinary obstruction

Side-effects: nausea, vomiting, increased salivation, diarrhoea, abdominal cramps (more marked
with higher doses). Signs of overdosage are
increased gastro-intestinal discomfort, bronchial
secretions, and sweating, involuntary defaecation
and micturition, miosis, nystagmus, bradycardia,
hypotension, agitation, excessive dreaming, and
weakness eventually leading to fasciculation and
paralysis

Dose: by mouth, neostigmine bromide 15–30 mg at suitable intervals throughout day, total daily dose 75–300 mg (but see also notes above); NEONATE 1–5 mg every 4 hours, half an hour before feeds; CHILD up to 6 years initially 7.5 mg, 6–12 years initially 15 mg, usual total daily dose 15–90 mg

By subcutaneous or intramuscular injection, neostigmine methylsulphate 1–2.5 mg at suitable intervals throughout day (usual total daily dose 5–20 mg); NEONATE 50–250 micrograms every 4 hours half an hour before feeds; CHILD 200–500 micrograms as required

PoM Neostigmine Bromide (Non-proprietary) (Cambridge)
Tablets, scored, neostigmine bromide 15 mg. Net price 20 = 53p

PoM Prostigmin® (Roche)
Injection, neostigmine methylsulphate 2.5 mg/mL. Net price 1-mL amp = 16p

PoM Neostigmine (Non-proprietary)
Tablets, scored, neostigmine bromide 15 mg. Net price 20 = 53p
Available from Cambridge

DISTIGMINE BROMIDE

Indications: myasthenia gravis; urinary retention and other indications, see section 7.4.1

Cautions; Contra-indications; Side-effects: see under Neostigmine

Dose: initially 5 mg daily half an hour before breakfast, increased at intervals of 3–4 days if necessary to a max. of 20 mg daily; CHILD up to 10 mg daily according to age

Preparations
See section 7.4.1

EDROPHONIUM CHLORIDE

Indications: see under Dose and notes above; surgery, see section 15.1.6

Cautions; Contra-indications; Side-effects: see under Neostigmine; have resuscitation facilities; *extreme* caution in respiratory distress (see notes above) and in asthma

Note. Severe cholinergic reactions can be counteracted by injection of atropine sulphate (which should always be available)

Dose: diagnosis of myasthenia gravis, *by intravenous injection,* 2 mg followed after 30 seconds (if no adverse reaction has occurred) by 8 mg; in adults without suitable veins, *by intramuscular injection,* 10 mg

Detection of overdosage or underdosage of cholinergic drugs, *by intravenous injection,* 2 mg (best before next dose of anticholinesterase, see notes above)

CHILD *by intravenous injection* 20 micrograms/kg followed after 30 seconds (if no adverse reaction has occurred) by 80 micrograms/kg

PoM Camsilon¹® (Cambridge)
Injection, edrophonium chloride 10 mg/mL. Net price 1-mL amp = £1.01
1. Formerly Tensilon®

PYRIDOSTIGMINE BROMIDE

Indications: myasthenia gravis

Cautions; Contra-indications; Side-effects: see under Neostigmine; weaker muscarinic action

Dose: by mouth, 30–120 mg at suitable intervals throughout day, total daily dose 0.3–1.2 g (but see also notes above); NEONATE 5–10 mg every 4 hours, ½–1 hour before feeds; CHILD up to 6 years initially 30 mg, 6–12 years initially 60 mg, usual total daily dose 30–360 mg

PoM Mestinon® (Roche)
Tablets, scored, pyridostigmine bromide 60 mg. Net price 20 = £1.11

IMMUNOSUPPRESSANT THERAPY

Corticosteroids (see section 6.3) are established as treatment for myasthenia gravis where *thymectomy* is inadvisable or to reduce the risk of surgery beforehand. The initial dose may be high (up to 100 mg **prednisolone** daily) but most advise starting with a smaller dose (20 mg prednisolone daily) and gradually increasing it. There is grave risk of exacerbation of the myasthenia during the initial stages of therapy, particularly in the first 2-3 weeks, therefore inpatient supervision is essential. Improvement usually begins after about 2 weeks on the high-dose regimen. In some patients a prolonged remission may be induced, but often patients need a maintenance dose of 10–40 mg of prednisolone daily; alternate-day therapy is popular. Patients who need a corticosteroid may benefit from the addition of **azathioprine** (see section 8.2.1) in a dose of 2 mg/kg daily which may allow a reduction in corticosteroid dosage.

10.2.2   Skeletal muscle relaxants

Drugs described below are used for the relief of chronic muscle spasm or spasticity; they are not indicated for spasm associated with minor injuries. They act principally on the central nervous system with the exception of dantrolene which has a peripheral site of action. They differ in action from the muscle relaxants used in anaesthesia (see section 15.1.5) which block transmission at the neuromuscular junction.

The underlying cause of spasticity should be treated and any aggravating factors (e.g. pressure sores, infection) remedied. Skeletal muscle relaxants are effective in most forms of spasticity except the rare alpha variety. The major disadvantage of treatment with these drugs is that reduction in muscle tone can cause a loss of splinting action of the spastic leg and trunk muscles and sometimes lead to an increase in disability.

Dantrolene acts directly on skeletal muscle and produces fewer central adverse effects making it a drug of choice. The dose should be increased slowly.

Baclofen inhibits transmission at spinal level and also depresses the central nervous system. The dose should be increased slowly to avoid the major side-effects of sedation and hypotonia (other adverse events are uncommon).

Diazepam may also be used. Sedation and, occasionally, extensor hypotonus are disadvantages. Other benzodiazepines also have muscle-relaxant properties. Muscle-relaxant doses of benzodiazepines are similar to anxiolytic doses (see section 4.1.2).

BACLOFEN

Indications: chronic severe spasticity resulting from disorders such as multiple sclerosis or traumatic partial section of spinal cord

Cautions: psychiatric illness, cerebrovascular disease, elderly; diabetes mellitus; respiratory, hepatic or renal impairment; epilepsy ; history of peptic ulcer; hypertonic bladder sphincter; pregnancy (see Appendix 4); avoid abrupt withdrawal (may precipitate autonomic dysreflexia); porphyria (see section 9.8.2); **interactions:** Appendix 1 (muscle relaxants)

DRIVING. Drowsiness may affect performance of skilled tasks (e.g. driving); effects of alcohol enhanced

Contra-indications: peptic ulceration

Side-effects: frequently sedation, drowsiness, nausea; occasionally lightheadedness, lassitude, confusion, dizziness, ataxia, hallucinations, headache, euphoria, insomnia, depression, tremor, nystagmus, paraesthesias, convulsions, muscular pain and weakness, respiratory or cardiovascular depression, hypotension, dry mouth, gastro-intestinal and urinary disturbances; rarely visual disorders, taste alterations, increased sweating, rash, blood sugar changes, altered liver function tests, and paradoxical increase in spasticity

Dose: by mouth, 5 mg 3 times daily, preferably after food, gradually increased; max. 100 mg daily; CHILD 0.75–2 mg/kg daily (over 10 years, max. 2.5 mg/kg daily) *or* 2.5 mg 4 times daily increased gradually according to age to maintenance: 1–2 years 10–20 mg daily, 2–6 years 20–30 mg daily, 6–10 years 30–60 mg daily

By intrathecal injection, see preparation below

PoM **Baclofen** (Non-proprietary)
Tablets, baclofen 10 mg. Net price 20 = £1.12. Label: 2, 8
Available from APS, Ashbourne (Baclospas®), Berk, Cox, Lagap, Norton

PoM **Lioresal®** (Geigy)
Tablets, scored, baclofen 10 mg. Net price 20 = £2.15. Label: 2, 8
Additives: include gluten
Liquid, sugar-free, baclofen 5 mg/5 mL. Net price 300 mL = £7.46. Label: 2, 8

By intrathecal injection
PoM **Lioresal®**
Intrathecal injection, baclofen, 50 micrograms/mL, net price 1-mL amp (for test dose) = £2.50; 500 micrograms/mL, 20-mL amp (for use with implantable pump) = £55.55; 2 mg/mL, 5-mL amp (for use with implantable pump) = £55.55

Important: consult data sheet for full instructions on dose testing and titration–it is important that patients are monitored closely in an appropriately equipped and staffed environment during screening and immediately following pump implantation, and that resuscitation equipment is available for immediate use

Dose: by intrathecal injection, specialist use only, for ADULT over 18 years with severe chronic spasticity unresponsive to oral antispastic drugs (or where side-effects of oral therapy unacceptable), initial *test dose* (with resuscitation equipment to hand, see also above) 25–50 micrograms over at least 1 minute via catheter or lumbar puncture, increased in steps to max. 100 micrograms to determine appropriate dose *then* dose-titration phase, most often using infusion pump (implanted into chest wall or abdominal wall tissues in experienced centres only) to establish *appropriate maintenance dose* (ranging from 10 to 1200 micrograms daily; usual range 300–800 micrograms daily) retaining some spasticity to avoid sensation of paralysis; CHILD under 18 years, not recommended

DANTROLENE SODIUM

Indications: chronic severe spasticity of voluntary muscle

Cautions: impaired cardiac and pulmonary function; test liver function before and at intervals during therapy; therapeutic effect may take a few weeks to develop but if treatment is ineffective it should be discontinued after 4–6 weeks. Avoid when spasticity is useful, for example, locomotion; **interactions:** Appendix 1 (muscle relaxants).

DRIVING. Drowsiness may affect performance of skilled tasks (e.g. driving); effects of alcohol enhanced

Contra-indications: hepatic impairment (may cause severe liver damage); acute muscle spasm

Side-effects: transient drowsiness, dizziness, weakness, malaise, fatigue, diarrhoea (withdraw if severe, discontinue treatment if recurs on re-introduction), anorexia, nausea, headache, rash; less frequently constipation, dysphagia, speech and visual disturbances, confusion, nervousness, insomnia, depression, seizures, chills, fever, increased urinary frequency; rarely, tachycardia, erratic blood pressure, dyspnoea, haematuria, possible crystalluria, urinary incontinence or retention, pleural effusion, pericarditis, dose-related hepatotoxicity (occasionally fatal) may be more common in women over 30 especially those taking oestrogens

Dose: initially 25 mg daily, may be increased at weekly intervals to max. of 100 mg 4 times daily; usual dose 75 mg 3 times daily; CHILD not recommended

PoM **Dantrium®** (Procter & Gamble Pharm.)
Capsules, both orange/brown, dantrolene sodium 25 mg, net price 20 = £3.42; 100 mg, 20 = £11.97. Label: 2
Injection—see section 15.1.8

DIAZEPAM

Indications: muscle spasm of varied aetiology, including tetanus; other indications, see sections 4.1.2, 4.8, 15.1.4.1

Cautions; Contra-indications; Side-effects: see section 4.1.2; also hypotonia; special precautions for intravenous injection (see section 4.8.2)

Dose: by mouth, 2–15 mg daily in divided doses, increased if necessary in spastic conditions to 60 mg daily according to response

Cerebral spasticity in selected cases, CHILD 2–40 mg daily in divided doses

By intramuscular or by slow intravenous injection (into a large vein at a rate of not more than 5 mg/minute), in acute muscle spasm, 10 mg repeated if necessary after 4 hours

Note. Only use intramuscular route when oral and intravenous routes not possible; special precautions for intravenous injection see section 4.8.2

Tetanus, ADULT and CHILD, *by intravenous injection,* 100–300 micrograms/kg repeated every 1–4 hours; *by intravenous infusion (or by nasoduodenal tube),* 3–10 mg/kg over 24 hours, adjusted according to response

Preparations
See section 4.1.2

OTHER MUSCLE RELAXANTS

The clinical efficacy of carisoprodol, meprobamate (see section 4.1.2), methocarbamol, and orphenadrine as muscle relaxants is **not** well established although they have been included in compound analgesic preparations.

CARISOPRODOL

Indications: short-term symptomatic relief of muscle spasm (but see notes above)

Cautions; Contra-indications; Side-effects: see under Meprobamate, section 4.1.2. Drowsiness is common; avoid in porphyria (see section 9.8.2)

Dose: 350 mg 3 times daily; ELDERLY half adult dose or less

PoM **Carisoma**® (Pharmax)
Tablets, carisoprodol 125 mg, net price 100 = £7.43; 350 mg, 100 = £8.32. Label: 2

METHOCARBAMOL

Indications: short-term symptomatic relief of muscle spasm (but see notes above)

Cautions: hepatic and renal impairment (avoid injection in renal impairment); **interactions:** Appendix 1 (as for Anxiolytics and Hypnotics)

DRIVING. Drowsiness may affect performance of skilled tasks (e.g. driving); effects of alcohol enhanced

Contra-indications: coma or pre-coma, brain damage, epilepsy, myasthenia gravis

Side-effects: lassitude, light-headedness, dizziness, restlessness, anxiety, confusion, drowsiness, nausea, allergic rash or angioedema, convulsions

Dose: by mouth, 1.5 g 4 times daily (elderly 750 mg or less); may be reduced to 750 mg 3 times daily

By slow intravenous injection or by infusion, 1–3 g (max. rate 300 mg/min.); max. dose 3 g (elderly, 1.5 g) daily for 3 days

PoM **Robaxin**® (Shire)
750 Tablets, scored, methocarbamol 750 mg. Net price 20 = £2.30. Label: 2
Injection, methocarbamol 100 mg/mL in aqueous macrogol '300'. Net price 10-mL amp = £2.33
PoM **Robaxisal Forte**® : see section 4.7.1

ORPHENADRINE CITRATE

Indications: short-term symptomatic relief of muscle spasm (but see notes above)

Cautions: see under Benzhexol Hydrochloride, section 4.9.2. Avoid in children; porphyria (see section 9.8.2); reduce dose in elderly

Side-effects: dry mouth and other antimuscarinic side-effects; see also Orphenadrine Hydrochloride, section 4.9.2

Dose: by intramuscular or by slow intravenous injection (over 5 minutes), 60 mg repeated after 12 hours if necessary

PoM **Norflex**® (3M)
Injection, orphenadrine citrate 30 mg/mL. Net price 2-mL amp = 60p

NOCTURNAL LEG CRAMPS

Quinine salts (see section 5.4.1) 200 to 300 mg at bedtime are effective in relieving nocturnal leg cramps. Quinine should be stopped if there is no improvement within 4 weeks; if improvement occurs, it is given on a long-term basis but treatment should be interrupted at intervals of approximately 3 months to check if it is still required. It is important to bear in mind that quinine is very toxic in overdosage and that accidental fatalities have occurred in children (see also below).

QUININE

Indications; Dose: see notes above; malaria, see section 5.4.1

Cautions; Contra-indications; Side-effects: see section 5.4.1; **important:** very toxic in overdosage—immediate advice from poison centres essential (see also p. 22)

Preparations
See section 5.4.1

10.3   Drugs for the relief of soft-tissue inflammation

10.3.1   Enzymes
10.3.2   Rubefacients and other topical antirheumatics

10.3.1   Enzymes

Hyaluronidase is used to render the tissues more easily permeable to injected fluids, e.g. for introduction of fluids by subcutaneous infusion (termed hypodermoclysis).

HYALURONIDASE

Indications: enhance permeation of subcutaneous or intramuscular injections, local anaesthetics and subcutaneous infusions; promote resorption of excess fluids and blood

---

Cautionary label wordings, see inside back cover   Prices are **net**, see p.1

Cautions: infants or elderly (control speed and total volume and avoid overhydration especially in renal impairment)

Contra-indications: do not apply direct to cornea; avoid sites where infection or malignancy; not for anaesthesia in unexplained premature labour; not to be used to reduce swelling of bites or stings; not for intravenous administration

Side-effects: occasional severe allergy

Dose: With subcutaneous or intramuscular injection, 1500 units dissolved directly in solution to be injected (ensure compatibility)

With local anaesthetics, 1500 units mixed with local anaesthetic solution (ophthalmology, 15 units/mL)

Hypodermoclysis, 1500 units dissolved in 1 mL water for injections or 0.9% sodium chloride injection, administered before start of 500–1000 mL infusion fluid

Extravasation or haematoma, 1500 units dissolved in 1 mL water for injections or 0.9% sodium chloride injection, infiltrated into affected area (as soon as possible after extravasation)

PoM Hyalase® (CP)
Injection, powder for reconstitution, hyaluronidase (ovine). Net price 1500-unit amp = £6.91

10.3.2   Rubefacients and other topical antirheumatics

Rubefacients act by counter-irritation. Pain, whether superficial or deep-seated, is relieved by any method which itself produces irritation of the skin. Counter-irritation is comforting in painful lesions of the muscles, tendons, and joints, and in non-articular rheumatism. Rubefacients probably all act through the same essential mechanism and differ mainly in intensity and duration of action.

Topical **NSAIDs** (e.g. benzydamine, felbinac, ibuprofen, salicylamide) may provide some slight relief of pain in musculoskeletal conditions.

TOPICAL NSAIDs AND COUNTER-IRRITANTS

CAUTIONS. Apply with gentle massage only. Avoid contact with eyes, mucous membranes, and inflamed or broken skin; discontinue if rash develops. Hands should be washed immediately after use. Not for use with occlusive dressings. Topical application of large amounts may result in systemic effects including hypersensitivity and asthma (renal disease has also been reported). Not generally suitable for children. Patient packs carry a **warning** to avoid during **pregnancy** or **breast-feeding**.

HYPERSENSITIVITY. For NSAID hypersensitivity and asthma warning, see p. 409

PHOTOSENSITIVITY. Patients should be advised against excessive exposure to sunlight of area treated in order to avoid possibility of photosensitivity

Algesal® (Solvay)
Cream, diethylamine salicylate 10%. Net price 50 g = 75p. Apply three times daily

Balmosa® (Pharmax)
Cream, camphor 4%, capsicum oleoresin 0.035%, menthol 2%, methyl salicylate 4%. Net price 40 g = 68p

Difflam® (3M)
Cream, benzydamine hydrochloride 3%. Net price 15 g = £1.05 (hosp. only); 100 g = £7.00. Apply 3–6 times daily for up to 10 days

PoM Feldene® (Pfizer)
Gel, piroxicam 0.5%. Net price 60 g = £5.00; 112 g = £7.84 (also 7.5 g starter pack, hosp. only)
Apply 3–4 times daily; therapy should be reviewed after 4 weeks

Ibugel® (Dermal)
Gel, ibuprofen 5%. Net price 100 g = £6.53
Apply up to 3 times daily

Ibuspray® (Dermal)
Spray application, ibuprofen 5%. Net price 100-mL = £6.95. Label: 15
Apply 3-4 times daily

Intralgin® (3M)
Gel, benzocaine 2%, salicylamide 5% in an alcoholic vehicle. net price 50 g = 49p

Movelat® (Panpharma)
Cream, heparinoid 0.2%, salicylic acid 2%, thymol 0.1%. Net price 100 g = £4.14. Apply up to 4 times daily
Gel, heparinoid 0.2%, salicylic acid 2%. Net price 100 g = £4.14. Apply up to 4 times daily

PoM Oruvail® (Rhône-Poulenc Rorer)
Gel, ketoprofen 2.5%. Net price 100 g = £6.78
Apply 2–4 times daily for up to 7 days (usual recommended dose 15 g daily)

PoM Powergel® (Searle)
Gel, ketoprofen 2.5%. Net price 50 g = £3.25; 100 g = £6.25; Twinpack (2 × 50-g pack) = £6.50
Apply 2–3 times daily for up to max. 10 days

Proflex® (Zyma)
Cream, ibuprofen 5%. Net price 100 g = £6.50
Apply 3–4 times daily

Transvasin® (Seton)
Cream, ethyl nicotinate 2%, hexyl nicotinate 2%, thurfyl salicylate 14%. Net price 40 g = 89p; 80 g = £1.51
Apply at least twice daily
Spray application, hydroxyethyl salicylate 5%, diethylamine salicylate 5%, methyl nicotinate 1%. Net price 125 mL = £1.46

PoM Traxam® (Lederle)
Foam, felbinac 3.17%. Net price 100 g = £7.00. Label:15
Gel, felbinac 3%. Net price 100 g = £7.00
Apply 2–4 times daily; max. 25 g daily; therapy should be reviewed after 14 days
Note. Felbinac is an active metabolite of the NSAID fenbufen

PoM Voltarol Emulgel® (Geigy)
Gel, diclofenac diethylammonium salt 1.16% (equivalent to diclofenac sodium 1%). Net price 20 g (hosp. only) = £1.55; 100 g = £7.00. Apply 3–4 times daily; therapy should be reviewed after 14 days (or after 28 days for osteoarthritis)

For list of topical NSAIDs and counter–irritants on sale to the public see below

Topical NSAIDs and counter–irritants on sale to the public together with their significant ingredients include:

Algesal® (diethylamine salicylate), **Algipan Rub®** (capsicin, glycol salicylate, methyl nicotinate), **Balmosa®** (camphor, capsicum oleoresin, menthol methyl salicylate), **Bengués Balsam®** (menthol methyl salicylate), **BN Liniment®** (turpentine oil strong ammonia solution, ammonium chloride) **Boots Pain Relief Balm®** (ethyl nicotinate, glycol monosalicylate, nonylic acid vanillylamide), **Boots**

Pain Relief Embrocation® (camphor, turpentine oil)

Cremalgin® (capsicin, glycol salicylate, methyl nicotinate)

Deep Freeze Cold Gel® (menthol), **Deep Freeze Pain Relief Spray**® (dichlorodifluoromethane, trichlorofluoromethane), **Deep Heat Extra Strength**®, **Deep Heat Massage Liniment**®, **Deep Heat Maximum**®, **Deep Heat Pre–Sport Rub**® (menthol, methyl salicylate), **Deep Heat Rub**® (eucalyptus oil, menthol, methyl salicylate, turpentine oil), **Deep Heat Spray Relief**® (glycol salicylate, ethyl salicylate, methyl salicylate, methyl nicotinate), **Deep Relief**® (ibuprofen, menthol), **Difflam**® **Cream** (benzydamine), **Dubam Cream**® (methyl salicylate, menthol, cineole), **Dubam Spray**® (ethyl salicylate, methyl salicylate, glycol salicylate, methyl nicotinate)

Elliman's Universal Embrocation® (acetic acid, turpentine oil)

Fenbid® **Gel** (ibuprofen), **Fiery Jack Cream**® (capsicum oleoresin, diethylamine salicylate, glycol salicylate, methyl nicotinate), **Fiery Jack Ointment**® (capsicum oleoresin)

Goddard's White Oil Embrocation® (dilute acetic acid, dilute ammonia solution, turpentine oil)

Ibuleve®, **Ibuleve Sports Gel**® (ibuprofen), **Intralgin**® (benzocaine, salicylamide)

Lloyds Cream® (diethyl salicylate)

Movelat® **Relief Cream** (heparinoid, salicylic acid, thymol), **Movelat**® **Relief Gel** (heparinoid, salicylic acid)

Nasciodine® (camphor, iodine, menthol, methyl salicylate, turpentine oil), **Nella Red Oil**® (clove oil, mustard oil, methyl nicotinate)

Oruvail® **Gel** (ketoprofen 30-g tube; 100-g tube prescribable on NHS (PoM))

PR Freeze Spray® (dimethylether, dimethoxymethane), **PR Heat Spray**® (ethyl nicotinate, methyl salicylate, camphor); **Proflex**® (ibuprofen), **Proflex Pain Relief**® (ibuprofen)

Radian–B Muscle Lotion®, **Radian–B Heat Spray**® (ammonium salicylate, camphor, menthol, salicylic acid), **Radian–B Muscle Rub**® (camphor, capsicin, menthol, methyl salicylate), **Ralgex Cream**® (capsicin, glycol monosalicylate, methyl nicotinate), **Ralgex Freeze Spray**® (methoxymethane, glycol monosalicylate, isopentane), **Ralgex Low Odour Spray**® (glycol monosalicylate, methyl nicotinate), **Ralgex Spray**® (ethyl salicylate, methyl salicylate, glycol monosalicylate, methyl nicotinate), **Ralgex Stick**® (capsicin, ethyl salicylate, methyl salicylate, glycol salicylate, menthol)

Salonair® (benzyl nicotinate, camphor, glycol salicylate, menthol, methyl salicylate, squalane), **Salonpas Plasters**® (glycol salicylate, methyl salicylate)

Tiger Balm Red Extra Strength® (camphor, clove oil, cajuput oil, cinnamon oil, menthol, peppermint oil), **Tiger Balm**® (cajuput oil, camphor, clove oil, menthol, peppermint oil), **Transvasin Cream**® (ethyl nicotinate, hexyl nicotinate, thurfyl salicylate), **Transvasin Spray**® (diethylamine salicylate, hydroxyethyl salicylate, methyl nicotinate), **Traxam Pain Relief**® (felbinac)

Zam–Buk® (camphor, eucalyptus oil, thyme oil, colophony)

COUNTER-IRRITANT FOR POST-HERPETIC NEURALGIA

Axsain® (Euroderma)

Cream, capsaicin 0.075%. Net price 45 g = £15.04. For post-herpetic neuralgia (**important: after** lesions have healed), apply up to 3–4 times daily

---

POULTICES

Kaolin Poultice, heavy kaolin 52.7%, thymol 0.05%, boric acid 4.5%, peppermint oil 0.05%, methyl salicylate 0.2%, glycerol 42.5%. Net price 200 g = £1.91

Warm and apply directly or between layers of muslin; avoid application of overheated poultice

Kaolin Poultice K/L Pack® (K/L)

Kaolin poultice. Net price 4 × 100-g pouches = £5.19

11: Drugs acting on the

EYE

In this chapter, drug treatment is discussed under the following headings:

The entries in this chapter generally relate only to local eye treatment. Systemic indications and side-effects of many of the drugs are given elsewhere (see index).

11.1 Administration of drugs to the eye

EYE-DROPS AND EYE OINTMENTS. When administered in the form of eye-drops, drugs penetrate the globe, probably through the cornea. However, systemic effects, which are usually undesirable, may well arise from absorption of drugs into the general circulation via conjunctival vessels or from the nasal mucosa after the excess of the preparation has drained down through the tear ducts. For example, timolol (a beta-blocker), administered as eye-drops may induce bronchospasm or bradycardia in susceptible individuals.

Eye ointments are often applied to lid margins for blepharitis. They may also be used in the conjunctival sac for other conditions especially where a prolonged action is required.

When two different preparations in the form of eye-drops are required at the same time of day, for example pilocarpine and timolol in glaucoma, dilution and overflow may occur when one immediately follows the other. The patient should therefore leave an interval of a few minutes. At night, an eye ointment for the second drug will reduce the problem.

Generally it is inadvisable for patients to continue to wear contact lenses, particularly hydrophilic (soft) contact lenses when receiving eye-drops. For warnings relating to eye-drops and contact lenses, see section 11.9.

EYE LOTIONS. These are solutions for the irrigation of the conjunctival sac. They act mechanically to flush out irritants or foreign bodies as a first-aid treatment. Sterile sodium chloride 0.9% solution (section 11.8.2) is usually used. In emergency, tap water drawn freshly from the main (not stored water) will suffice.

OTHER PREPARATIONS. Subconjunctival injection may be used to administer anti-infective drugs, mydriatics, or corticosteroids for conditions not responding to topical therapy. The drug diffuses through the sclera to the anterior and posterior chambers and vitreous humour in higher concentration than can be achieved by absorption from eye-drops. However, because the dose-volume is limited (usually not more than 1 mL), this route is suitable only for drugs which are readily soluble.

Drugs such as antibiotics and corticosteroids may be administered systemically to treat an eye condition.

Suitable plastic devices which gradually release a specified amount of drug over a period of, say, 1 week are also used (e.g. Ocuserts®).

11.2 Control of microbial contamination

Preparations for the eye should be sterile when issued. Eye-drops in multiple-application containers are suitably preserved but care should be taken to avoid contamination of the contents during use.

Eye-drops in multiple-application containers for *domiciliary use* should not be used for more than 4 weeks after first opening (unless otherwise stated).

Eye-drops for use in *hospital wards* should be discarded 1 week after opening. Individual containers should be provided for each patient and when both eyes are being treated, a separate container should be used for each eye. Containers used before an operation should be discarded at the time of the operation and fresh containers supplied. A fresh supply should also be provided upon discharge from hospital; it may be acceptable in specialist ophthalmology units to issue on discharge eye-drop bottles that have been in use for the patient for less than 36 hours.

Eye-drops used in *out-patient departments* should be discarded at the end of each day. In clinics for eye diseases and in accident and emergency departments, where the dangers of infection are high, single-application packs should be used; if a multiple-application pack is used, it should be discarded after single use.

Diagnostic dyes (e.g. fluorescein) should be used only from single-application packs.

In *eye surgery* it is wise to use single-application containers. Preparations used during intra-ocular procedures and others that may penetrate into the anterior chamber must be isotonic and without preservatives and buffered if necessary to a neutral pH. Large volume intravenous infusion preparations are not suitable for this purpose. For all surgical procedures, a previously unopened container is used for each patient.

11.3 Anti-infective eye preparations

11.3.1 Antibacterials
11.3.2 Antifungals
11.3.3 Antivirals

EYE INFECTIONS. Most acute superficial eye infections can be treated topically. Blepharitis and conjunctivitis are often caused by staphylococci; keratitis and endophthalmitis may be bacterial, viral, or fungal.

Bacterial *blepharitis* is treated by application of an antibacterial eye ointment to the conjunctival sac or to the lid margins but systemic treatment may occasionally be required.

Acute *infective conjunctivitis* is treated with antibacterial eye-drops and eye ointment. A poor response might indicate viral or allergic conjunctivitis. *Gonococcal conjunctivitis* is treated with systemic and topical antibiotics.

Corneal ulcer and *keratitis* require specialist treatment and may call for subconjunctival or systemic administration of antibiotics.

Endophthalmitis is a medical emergency which also calls for specialist management and often requires parenteral, subconjunctival, or intraocular administration of antibiotics.

For reference to the treatment of *crab lice of the eyelashes*, see section 13.10.4

11.3.1 Antibacterials

Bacterial infections are generally treated topically with eye-drops and eye ointments.

Chloramphenicol has a broad spectrum of activity and is the drug of choice for *superficial eye infections*. Other antibiotics with a broad spectrum of activity include **framycetin**, **gentamicin**, and **neomycin**, and also **ciprofloxacin** and **ofloxacin**. Gentamicin and tobramycin (and possibly ciprofloxacin and ofloxacin) are effective for infections caused by *Pseudomonas aeruginosa*.

Ciprofloxacin eye-drops are licensed for *corneal ulcers*; intensive application (especially in the first 2 days) is required throughout the day and night.

Chlortetracycline is used in the treatment of *chlamydial infections* including *trachoma* (consult World Health Organization guidelines).

Fusidic acid is useful for staphylococcal infections.

Propamidine isethionate is of little value in bacterial infections but is specific for the rare but devastating condition of *acanthamoeba keratitis* (neomycin may be used as an adjunct).

WITH CORTICOSTEROIDS. Many antibiotic preparations also incorporate a corticosteroid but such mixtures should **not** be used unless a patient is under close specialist supervision. In particular they should not be prescribed for undiagnosed 'red eye' which is sometimes caused by the herpes simplex virus and may be difficult to diagnose (section 11.4).

ADMINISTRATION
Eye-drops. Apply at least every 2 hours then reduce frequency as infection is controlled and continue for 48 hours after healing.
Eye ointment. Apply *either* at night (if eye-drops used during the day) *or* 3–4 times daily (if eye ointment used alone).

CHLORAMPHENICOL

Indications; Administration: see notes above
Side-effects: transient stinging; rare reports of aplastic anaemia

PoM **Chloramphenicol** (Non-proprietary)
Eye-drops, chloramphenicol 0.5%. Net price 10 mL = 49p
Eye ointment, chloramphenicol 1%. Net price 4 g = 78p

PoM **Chloromycetin®** (P-D)
Ophthalmic ointment (= eye ointment), chloramphenicol 1%. Net price 4 g = 67p
Redidrops (= eye-drops), chloramphenicol 0.5%. Net price 5 mL = £1.10; 10 mL = £1.18
Additives: include phenylmercuric acetate

PoM **Sno Phenicol®** (Chauvin)
Eye-drops, chloramphenicol 0.5%, in a viscous vehicle. Net price 10 mL = £1.08
Additives: include chlorhexidine acetate

Single use
PoM **Minims® Chloramphenicol** (Chauvin)
Eye-drops, chloramphenicol 0.5%. Net price 20 × 0.5 mL = £4.92

CHLORTETRACYCLINE

Indications: local treatment of infections, including trachoma (see notes above)
Administration: see notes above

PoM **Aureomycin®** (Lederle)
Ophthalmic ointment (= eye ointment), chlortetracycline hydrochloride 1%. Net price 3.5 g = 92p

CIPROFLOXACIN

Indications: superficial bacterial infections, see notes above; corneal ulcers
Cautions; Side-effects: local burning and itching; lid margin crusting; not recommended for children under 12 years; caution in pregnancy and breast-feeding
Administration: superficial bacterial infection, see notes above
Corneal ulcer, apply throughout day and night, first day 2 drops every 15 minutes for 6 hours then every 30 minutes for the rest of the day, second day apply 2 drops every hour, third to fourteenth days apply 2 drops every 4 hours; if longer treatment required physician to decide frequency (max. duration of treatment 21 days)

▼ PoM **Ciloxan®** (Alcon)
Ophthalmic solution (= eye-drops), ciprofloxacin (as hydrochloride) 0.3%. Net price 5 mL = £4.94
Additives: include benzalkonium chloride

FRAMYCETIN SULPHATE

Indications; Administration: see notes above

PoM Soframycin® (Roussel)
Eye-drops, framycetin sulphate 0.5%. Net price 10 mL = £2.69
Additives: include phenylmercuric nitrate
Eye ointment, framycetin sulphate 0.5%. Net price 5 g = 88p

FUSIDIC ACID

Indications: see notes above

PoM Fucithalmic® (Leo)
Eye-drops, m/r, fusidic acid 1% in gel basis (liquifies on contact with eye). Net price 5 g = £2.19
Additives: include benzalkonium chloride
Apply twice daily

GENTAMICIN

Indications; Administration: see notes above

PoM Cidomycin® (Roussel)
Drops (for ear or eye), gentamicin 0.3% (as sulphate). Net price 8 mL = £1.31
Additives: include benzalkonium chloride, disodium edetate
Eye ointment, gentamicin 0.3% (as sulphate), net price 5 g = £1.97
PoM Garamycin® (Schering-Plough)
Drops (for ear or eye), gentamicin 0.3% (as sulphate). Net price 10 mL = £1.79
Additives: include benzalkonium chloride
PoM Genticin® (Roche)
Drops (for ear or eye), gentamicin 0.3% (as sulphate). Net price 10 mL = £2.00
Additives: include benzalkonium chloride

Single use
PoM Minims® Gentamicin (Chauvin)
Eye-drops, gentamicin 0.3% (as sulphate). Net price 20 × 0.5 mL = £5.75

NEOMYCIN SULPHATE

Indications; Administration: see notes above

PoM Neomycin (Non-proprietary)
Eye-drops, neomycin sulphate 0.5% (3500 units/mL). Net price 10 mL = £2.43
Available from Martindale
Eye ointment, neomycin sulphate 0.5% (3500 units/g). Net price 3 g = £1.00
Available from Martindale
PoM Neosporin® (Dominion)
Eye-drops, gramicidin 25 units, neomycin sulphate 1700 units, polymyxin B sulphate 5000 units/mL. Net price 5 mL = £5.36
Additives: include thiomersal
Apply 2–4 times daily or more frequently if required

Single use
PoM Minims® Neomycin Sulphate (Chauvin)
Eye-drops, neomycin sulphate 0.5%. Net price 20 × 0.5 mL = £5.75

OFLOXACIN

Indications; Administration: see notes above
Cautions; Side-effects: local irritation including photophobia; dizziness, numbness, nausea and headache reported; caution in pregnancy and avoid in breast-feeding

▼ **PoM Exocin®** (Allergan)
Ophthalmic solution (= eye-drops), ofloxacin 0.3%. Net price 5 mL = £2.27
Additives: include benzalkonium chloride

POLYMYXIN B SULPHATE

Indications; Administration: see notes above

PoM Polyfax® (Dominion)
Eye ointment, polymyxin B sulphate 10 000 units, bacitracin zinc 500 units/g. Net price 4 g = £3.41
PoM Polytrim® (Dominion)
Eye-drops, trimethoprim 0.1%, polymyxin B sulphate 10 000 units/mL. Net price 5 mL = £3.19
Additives: include thiomersal
Eye ointment, trimethoprim 0.5%, polymyxin B sulphate 10 000 units/g. Net price 4 g = £3.19

PROPAMIDINE ISETHIONATE

Indications: local treatment of infections (but see notes above)

Brolene® (Rhône-Poulenc Rorer)
Eye-drops, propamidine isethionate 0.1%. Net price 10 mL = £1.96
Apply 4 times daily
Note. Eye-drops containing propamidine isethionate 0.1% also available from Typharm (Golden Eye Drops)
Eye ointment, dibromopropamidine isethionate 0.15%. Net price 5 g = £2.08
Apply 1–2 times daily
Note. Eye ointment containing dibromopropamidine isethionate 0.15% also available from Typharm (Golden Eye Ointment)

TOBRAMYCIN

Indications; Administration: see notes above

PoM Tobralex® (Alcon)
Eye-drops, tobramycin 0.3%. Net price 5 mL = £1.39
Additives: include benzalkonium chloride

11.3.2   Antifungals

Fungal infections of the cornea are rare but tend to occur after agricultural injuries, especially in hot and humid climates. Orbital mycosis is rare, and when it occurs is usually due to direct spread of infection from the paranasal sinuses. Increasing age, debility, or immunosuppression by drugs, for example, following renal transplantation, may encourage fungal proliferation in many parts of the body. The spread of infection via the bloodstream occasionally produces a metastatic endophthalmitis.

    Prices are **net**, see p. 1

A wide range of fungi are capable of producing ocular mycosis and may be identified by appropriate laboratory procedures.

Antifungal preparations for the eye are not generally available. Treatment will normally be carried out at specialist centres, but requests for information about supplies of preparations not available commercially should be addressed to the District Pharmaceutical Officer (or equivalent in Scotland or Northern Ireland) or to Moorfields Eye Hospital, City Road, London EC1V 2PD (0171-253 3411).

1.3.3 Antivirals

Herpes simplex infections producing, for example, dendritic corneal ulcer can be treated with **aciclovir**.

ACICLOVIR

Indications: local treatment of herpes simplex infections

Administration: apply 5 times daily (continue for at least 3 days after complete healing)

PoM **Zovirax**® (Wellcome)
Eye ointment, aciclovir 3%. Net price 4.5 g = £10.67
Tablets and *injection*, see section 5.3
Cream, see section 13.10.3

1.4 Corticosteroids and other anti-inflammatory preparations

11.4.1 Corticosteroids
11.4.2 Other anti-inflammatory preparations

1.4.1 Corticosteroids

Corticosteroids administered topically, by subconjunctival injection, and systemically have an important place in treating uveitis and scleritis; they are also used to reduce post-operative inflammation following eye operations.

Topical corticosteroids should normally only be used under expert supervision; they should not be prescribed for undiagnosed 'red eye'. There are two main dangers from topical corticosteroids. First the 'red eye' may be caused by herpes simplex virus which produces a dendritic ulcer; corticosteroids aggravate the condition which may lead to loss of vision or even loss of the eye. Second, again arising from the use of eye-drop formulations, a 'steroid glaucoma' may be produced, after a few weeks treatment, in patients predisposed to chronic simple glaucoma. Use of a combination product containing a corticosteroid with an anti-infective is rarely justified.

Systemic corticosteroids can usefully be given on an alternate-day basis to minimise side-effects. The risk of producing glaucoma is not great, but 'steroid cataract' is a very high risk (75%) if more than 15 mg of prednisolone or equivalent is given daily for several years. The longer the duration, the greater is the risk. A dose of less then 10 mg per day is usually safe.

BETAMETHASONE

Indications: local treatment of inflammation (short-term)

Cautions; Side-effects: see notes above

Administration: apply eye-drops every 1–2 hours until controlled then reduce frequency, eye ointment 2–4 times daily or at night when used with eye-drops

PoM **Betnesol**® (Evans)
Drops (for ear, eye, or nose), betamethasone sodium phosphate 0.1%. Net price 10 mL = £1.31
Additives: include benzalkonium chloride
Eye ointment, betamethasone sodium phosphate 0.1%. Net price 3 g = 56p
PoM **Betnesol-N**® (Evans)
Drops (for ear, eye, or nose), see section 12.1.1
Eye ointment, betamethasone sodium phosphate 0.1%, neomycin sulphate 0.5%. Net price 3 g = 64p
PoM **Vista-Methasone**® (Martindale)
Drops (for ear, eye, or nose), betamethasone sodium phosphate 0.1%. Net price 5 mL = £1.15; 10 mL = £1.31
Additives: include benzalkonium chloride
PoM **Vista-Methasone N**® (Martindale)
Drops (for ear, eye, or nose), see section 12.1.1

CLOBETASONE BUTYRATE

Indications: local treatment of inflammation (short-term)

Cautions; Side-effects: see notes above; reduced tendency to raise intra-ocular pressure

Administration: apply eye-drops 4 times daily; severe conditions every 1–2 hours until controlled then reduce frequency

PoM **Cloburate**® (Dominion)
Eye-drops, clobetasone butyrate 0.1%. Net price 10 mL = £2.85
Additives: include benzalkonium chloride
PoM **Cloburate-N**® (Dominion)
Eye-drops, clobetasone butyrate 0.1%, neomycin sulphate 0.5%. Net price 10 mL = £3.20
Additives: include benzalkonium chloride

DEXAMETHASONE

Indications: local treatment of inflammation (short-term)

Cautions; Side-effects: see notes above

Administration: apply eye-drops 4–6 times daily; severe conditions every hour until controlled then reduce frequency

PoM **Maxidex**® (Alcon)
Eye-drops, dexamethasone 0.1%, hypromellose 0.5%. Net price 5 mL = £1.49; 10 mL = £2.95
Additives: include benzalkonium chloride
PoM **Maxitrol**® (Alcon)
Eye-drops, dexamethasone 0.1%, hypromellose 0.5%, neomycin 0.35% (as sulphate), polymyxin B sulphate 6000 units/mL. Net price 5 mL = £1.77
Additives: include benzalkonium chloride
Eye ointment, dexamethasone 0.1%, neomycin 0.35% (as sulphate), polymyxin B sulphate 6000 units/g. Net price 3.5 g = £1.52
Additives: include hydroxybenzoates
PoM **Sofradex**® (Roussel)
Drops and ointment (for ear or eye), see section 12.1.1

FLUOROMETHOLONE

Indications: local treatment of inflammation (short-term)

Cautions; Side-effects: see notes above; reduced tendency to raise intra-ocular pressure

Administration: apply eye-drops 2–4 times daily (initially every hour for 24–48 hours then reduce frequency)

PoM **FML**® (Allergen)

Ophthalmic suspension (= eye-drops), fluorometholone 0.1%, polyvinyl alcohol (Liquifilm®) 1.4%. Net price 5 mL = £1.79; 10 mL = £3.09

Additives: include benzalkonium chloride, disodium edetate, polysorbate 80

PoM **FML-Neo**® (Allergen)

Eye-drops, fluorometholone 0.1%, neomycin sulphate 0.5%, polyvinyl alcohol (Liquifilm®) 1.4%. Net price 5 mL = £2.08

Additives: include benzalkonium chloride, disodium edetate, polysorbate 80

HYDROCORTISONE ACETATE

Indications: local treatment of inflammation (short-term)

Cautions; Side-effects: see notes above

PoM **Hydrocortisone** (Non-proprietary)

Eye-drops, hydrocortisone acetate 1%. Net price 10 mL = £2.98

Available from Martindale

Eye ointment, hydrocortisone acetate 0.5%, net price 3 g = £1.59; 1%, 3 g = £1.62; 2.5%, 3 g = £1.35

Available from Martindale

PoM **Neo-Cortef**® (Dominion)

Drops and *ointment* (for ear or eye), see section 12.1.1

Note. Eye-drops containing hydrocortisone acetate 1.5% and neomycin sulphate 0.5% also available from Martindale

PREDNISOLONE

Indications: local treatment of inflammation (short-term)

Cautions; Side-effects: see notes above

Administration: apply eye-drops every 1–2 hours until controlled then reduce frequency

PoM **Pred Forte**® (Allergen)

Eye-drops, prednisolone acetate 1%. Net price 5 mL = £1.59; 10 mL = £3.19

Additives: include benzalkonium chloride, disodium edetate, polysorbate 80

Apply 2–4 times daily

PoM **Predsol**® (Evans)

Drops (for ear or eye), prednisolone sodium phosphate 0.5%. Net price 10 mL = £1.31

Additives: include benzalkonium chloride

PoM **Predsol-N**® (Evans)

Drops (for ear or eye), see section 12.1.1

Single use

PoM **Minims**® **Prednisolone** (Chauvin)

Eye-drops, prednisolone sodium phosphate 0.5%. Net price 20 × 0.5 mL = £5.75

11.4.2   Other anti-inflammatory preparations

Other preparations used for the topical treatment of inflammation and allergic conjunctivitis include antihistamines, lodoxamide, and sodium cromoglycate.

Topical preparations of **antihistamines** such as eye-drops containing antazoline sulphate (with xylometazoline hydrochloride as Otrivine-Antistin®) may be used for short-term treatment of allergic conjunctivitis. **Levocabastine**, a recently introduced antihistamine is also indicated for short-term treatment of allergic conjunctivitis.

Sodium cromoglycate eye-drops may be useful for vernal catarrh and other allergic forms of conjunctivitis. **Nedocromil sodium** eye-drops have recently been introduced for allergic conjunctivitis.

Lodoxamide eye-drops have been introduced for allergic conjunctival conditions including seasonal allergic conjunctivitis and vernal catarrh.

ANTAZOLINE

Indications: allergic conjunctivitis

Otrivine-Antistin® (CIBA Vision)

Eye-drops, antazoline sulphate 0.5%, xylometazoline hydrochloride 0.05%. Net price 10 mL = £2.13

Additives: include benzalkonium chloride, disodium edetate

Apply 2–3 times daily

LEVOCABASTINE

Indications: allergic conjunctivitis

Side-effects: local irritation, blurred vision, local oedema, urticaria; dyspnoea, headache, drowsiness

Administration: ADULT and CHILD over 9 years apply twice daily, increased if necessary to 3–4 times daily, discontinue if no improvement within 3 days; max. 4 weeks treatment per year

▼ PoM **Livostin**® (CIBA Vision)

Eye-drops, levocabastine 0.05% (as hydrochloride). Net price 4 mL = £8.49

Additives: include benzalkonium chloride disodium edetate, polysorbate 80

LODOXAMIDE

Indications: allergic conjunctivitis

Side-effects: mild transient burning, stinging, itching, and lachrymation

Administration: ADULT and CHILD over 4 years apply eye drops 4 times daily

PoM **Alomide**® (Galen)

Ophthalmic solution (= eye-drops), lodoxamide 0.1% (as trometamol). Net price 10 mL = £5.48

Additives: include benzalkonium chloride, disodium edetate

NEDOCROMIL SODIUM

Indications: allergic conjunctivitis

Administration: seasonal and perennial conjunctivitis, ADULT and CHILD over 6 years, apply
twice daily increased if necessary to 4 times
daily; max. 12 weeks treatment for seasonal allergic conjunctivitis

Vernal kerato-conjunctivitis, ADULT and CHILD
over 6 years, apply 4 times daily

▼ PoM **Rapitil**® (Fisons)
Eye-drops, nedocromil sodium 2%. Net price 5 mL
= £7.49
Additives: include benzalkonium chloride, disodium edetate

SODIUM CROMOGLYCATE

Indications: allergic conjunctivitis

Administration: apply eye-drops 4 times daily,
eye ointment 2–3 times daily

PoM ¹**Sodium Cromoglycate** (Non-proprietary)
Eye-drops, sodium cromoglycate 2%. Net price
13.5 mL = £2.50
Available from Baker Norton (Hay-Crom® Aqueous),
Dominion, Fisons (Opticrom® Aqueous), Novex (Vivid-
rin®)

Eye ointment, sodium cromoglycate 4%. Net price
5 g = £7.53
Available from Fisons (Opticrom®)

. Sodium cromoglycate 2% eye-drops and 4% eye ointment can be sold to the public (in max. pack sizes of
10 mL for eye-drops and 5 g for eye ointment) for treatment of acute seasonal (allergic) conjunctivitis; propri-
ary brands of eye-drops on sale to the public include Brol-
ze®, Clariteyes®, Hay-Crom® Hay Fever, Opticrom®
Allergy, and Optrex® Hayfever Allergy

11.5   Mydriatics and cycloplegics

Antimuscarinics dilate the pupil and paralyse the
ciliary muscle; they vary in potency and duration of
action. The relative potencies and durations of
action of the principal drugs, in ascending order,
are:

tropicamide (3 hours)
cyclopentolate, homatropine (all up to 24 hours)
atropine (7 days or longer)

Short-acting, relatively weak mydriatics, such as
tropicamide 0.5%, facilitate the examination of
the fundus of the eye. **Cyclopentolate 1%** or **atropine** are preferable for producing cycloplegia for
refraction in young children. Atropine 1% (in ointment form) is sometimes preferred for children
under 5 years of age. Atropine is also used for the
treatment of iridocyclitis mainly to prevent posterior synechiae, often with phenylephrine 10% eye-
drops (2.5% in children, elderly, and those with cardiac disease).

CAUTIONS AND SIDE-EFFECTS. Contact dermatitis is
not uncommon with the antimuscarinic mydriatic
drugs, especially atropine. In addition, toxic systemic reactions to atropine and cyclopentolate may
occur in the very young and the very old.

Cautionary label wordings, see inside back cover

Darkly pigmented iris is more resistant to pupillary dilatation and caution should be exercised to
avoid overdosage.

Mydriasis may precipitate acute closed-angle
('congestive') glaucoma in a few patients, usually
aged over 60 years, who are predisposed to the condition because of a shallow anterior chamber.

Interactions. Phenylephrine may interact with
systemically administered monoamine-oxidase
inhibitors; see also Appendix 1 (sympathomimetics).

DRIVING. Patients should be warned not to drive for
1 to 2 hours after mydriasis.

ANTIMUSCARINICS

ATROPINE SULPHATE

Indications: refraction procedures in young children; see also notes above

Cautions: action persistent, may precipitate glaucoma; see also notes above

PoM **Atropine** (Non-proprietary)
Eye-drops, atropine sulphate 0.5%, net price
10 mL = £1.82; 1%, 10 mL = 74p
Available from Martindale

Eye ointment, atropine sulphate 1%. Net price 3 g
= £2.03
Available from Martindale

PoM **Isopto Atropine**® (Alcon)
Eye-drops, atropine sulphate 1%, hypromellose
0.5%. Net price 5 mL = 99p
Additives: include benzalkonium chloride

Single use
PoM **Minims**® **Atropine Sulphate** (Chauvin)
Eye-drops, atropine sulphate 1%. Net price 20 ×
0.5 mL = £4.92

CYCLOPENTOLATE HYDROCHLORIDE

Indications: see notes above

Cautions: patients with raised intra-ocular pressure; see notes above

PoM **Mydrilate**® (Boehringer Ingelheim)
Eye-drops, cyclopentolate hydrochloride 0.5%, net
price 5 mL = 73p; 1%, 5 mL = 98p
Additives: include benzalkonium chloride

Single use
PoM **Minims**® **Cyclopentolate** (Chauvin)
Eye-drops, cyclopentolate hydrochloride 0.5 and
1%. Net price 20 × 0.5 mL (both) = £4.92

HOMATROPINE HYDROBROMIDE

Indications; Cautions: see notes above

PoM **Homatropine** (Non-proprietary)
Eye-drops, homatropine hydrobromide 1%, net
price 10 mL = £1.34; 2%, 10 mL = £1.36
Available from Martindale

Single use
PoM Minims® Homatropine Hydrobromide
(Chauvin)
Eye-drops, homatropine hydrobromide 2%. Net price 20 × 0.5 mL = £5.75

TROPICAMIDE
Indications; Cautions: see notes above

PoM Mydriacyl® (Alcon)
Eye-drops, tropicamide 0.5%, net price 5 mL = £1.36; 1%, 5 mL = £1.68
Additives: include benzalkonium chloride

Single use
PoM Minims® Tropicamide (Chauvin)
Eye-drops, tropicamide 0.5 and 1%. Net price 20 × 0.5 mL (both) = £5.75

SYMPATHOMIMETICS

ADRENALINE
Section 11.6

PHENYLEPHRINE HYDROCHLORIDE
Indications; Cautions: see notes above

Phenylephrine (Non-proprietary)
Eye-drops, phenylephrine hydrochloride 10%. Net price 10 mL = £2.66
Available from Martindale
See also under Hypromellose (section 11.8.1)

Single use
Minims® Phenylephrine Hydrochloride
(Chauvin)
Eye-drops, phenylephrine hydrochloride 2.5%, net price 20 × 0.5 mL = £5.75; 10%, 20 × 0.5 mL = £5.75

11.6   Treatment of glaucoma

An abnormally high intra-ocular pressure, glaucoma, may result in blindness. In virtually all cases, rise in pressure is due to reduced outflow of aqueous humour, the inflow remaining constant.

Glaucoma is treated by the application of eye-drops containing beta-blockers, miotics, or adrenaline (and guanethidine). Acetazolamide and dichlorphenamide are given by mouth and, in emergency or before surgery, mannitol may be given by intravenous infusion.

Probably the commonest condition is *chronic simple glaucoma* where the obstruction is in the trabecular meshwork. It is commonly first treated with a topical beta-blocker and other drugs added as necessary to control the intra-ocular pressure e.g. adrenaline or pilocarpine.

If supplementary topical treatment is required after *iridectomy* or a drainage operation in either open-angle or closed-angle glaucoma, a beta-

blocker is preferred to pilocarpine. This is because of the risk that posterior synechiae will be formed as a result of the miotic effect of pilocarpine, especially in closed-angle glaucoma. It is then also advantageous to utilise the mydriatic side-effect of adrenaline.

Apraclonidine (section 11.8.2) reduces the rate of production of aqueous humour. Eye-drops containing apraclonidine 1% are used to control post-operative intra-ocular pressure after anterior segment laser surgery; eye-drops containing apraclonidine 0.5% are used for a short term to delay laser treatment or surgery for glaucoma in patients not adequately controlled by another drug.

MIOTICS

The small pupil is an unfortunate side-effect of these drugs (except when pilocarpine is used temporarily prior to operation for *closed-angle glaucoma*). The key factor is the opening up of the inefficient drainage channels in the trabecular meshwork resulting from contraction or spasm of the ciliary muscle. This also produces accommodation spasm that may result in blurring of vision and browache (a particular disadvantage in patients under 40 years of age).

Pilocarpine has a duration of action of 3 to hours. **Physostigmine** is more potent; it is still used with pilocarpine but is not usually used alone. **Carbachol** is sometimes used to lower intra-ocular pressure, usually in conjunction with other miotic such as physostigmine.

Demecarium bromide (as *Tosmilen®*, Sinclair and **ecothiopate iodide** (as *Phospholine Iodide®* Dominion) are no longer on the UK market but are still available on a named-patient basis for use under expert supervision.

Generalised parasympathomimetic side effects such as sweating, bradycardia and intestinal colic may follow systemic absorption of these eye-drops other effects may include hypersalivation and bronchospasm.

CARBACHOL
Indications: see notes above
Administration: apply eye-drops up to 4 times daily

PoM Isopto Carbachol® (Alcon)
Eye-drops, carbachol 3%, hypromellose 1%. Net price 10 mL = £1.76
Additives: include benzalkonium chloride

PHYSOSTIGMINE SULPHATE
(Eserine)
Indications; Side-effects: see notes above
Administration: apply eye-drops 2–6 times daily

PoM Physostigmine (Non-proprietary)
Eye-drops, physostigmine sulphate 0.25%, net price 10 mL = £2.50; 0.5%, 10 mL = £2.74
May no longer be available

PILOCARPINE

Indications; Side-effects: see notes above
Administration: apply eye-drops 3–6 times daily

PoM Pilocarpine Hydrochloride (Non-proprietary)
Eye-drops, pilocarpine hydrochloride 0.5%, net price 10 mL = £1.03; 1%, 10 mL = 90p; 2%, 10 mL = £1.01; 3%, 10 mL = £1.19; 4%, 10 mL = £1.33
Available from APS, Martindale

PoM Isopto Carpine® (Alcon)
Eye-drops, all with hypromellose 0.5%; pilocarpine hydrochloride 0.5%, net price 10 mL = 73p; 1%, 10 mL = 81p; 2%, 10 mL = 90p; 3%, 10 mL = 97p; 4%, 10 mL = £1.04
Additives: include benzalkonium chloride

PoM Sno Pilo® (Chauvin)
Eye-drops, in a viscous vehicle, pilocarpine hydrochloride 1%, net price 10 mL = £1.04; 2%, 10 mL = £1.14; 4%, 10 mL = £1.36
Additives: include benzalkonium chloride

Single use
PoM Minims® Pilocarpine Nitrate (Chauvin)
Eye-drops, pilocarpine nitrate 1, 2, and 4%. Net price 20 × 0.5 mL (all) = £4.92

Modified release
PoM Ocusert® (Dominion)
Pilo-20 ocular insert, m/r, pilocarpine 20 micrograms released per hour for 1 week. Net price pack of 8 inserts = £35.08. Counselling, method of use
Pilo-40 ocular insert, m/r, pilocarpine 40 micrograms released per hour for 1 week. Net price pack of 8 inserts = £40.90. Counselling, method of use

ADRENALINE/GUANETHIDINE

Adrenaline probably acts both by reducing the rate of production of aqueous humour and by increasing the outflow through the trabecular meshwork. It is contra-indicated in closed-angle glaucoma because it is a mydriatic, unless an iridectomy has been carried out. Side-effects include severe smarting and redness of the eye; adrenaline should be used with caution in patients with hypertension and heart disease.

Dipivefrine is a prodrug of adrenaline. It is stated to pass more rapidly through the cornea and is then converted to the active form.

Guanethidine enhances and prolongs the effects of adrenaline. Prolonged use, particularly at the higher strengths may result in conjunctival fibrosis with secondary corneal changes; the conjunctiva and cornea should be examined at least every six months.

ADRENALINE

Indications; Contra-indications; Side-effects: see notes above
Administration: apply eye-drops 1–2 times daily

PoM Eppy® (Chauvin)
Eye-drops, adrenaline 1%. Net price 7.5 mL = £4.06
Additives: include benzalkonium chloride, also acetylcysteine as antioxant

PoM Simplene® (Chauvin)
Eye-drops, adrenaline, in a viscous vehicle, 0.5%, net price 7.5 mL = £3.45; 1%, 7.5 mL = £3.79
Additives: include benzalkonium chloride, also acetylcysteine as antioxant

DIPIVEFRINE HYDROCHLORIDE

Indications; Contra-indications; Side-effects: as for Adrenaline, see notes above
Administration: apply 1 drop twice daily

PoM Propine® (Allergan)
Eye-drops, dipivefrine hydrochloride 0.1%. Net price 5 mL = £3.99, 10 mL = £4.99, triple pack (3 × 5 mL) = £10.47
Additives: include benzalkonium chloride, disodium edetate

GUANETHIDINE MONOSULPHATE

Indications; Cautions: see notes above
Administration: apply eye-drops 1–2 times daily

PoM Ganda® (Chauvin)
Eye-drops '1 + 0.2', guanethidine monosulphate 1%, adrenaline 0.2% in a viscous vehicle. Net price 7.5 mL = £4.49
Additives: include benzalkonium chloride
Eye-drops '3 + 0.5', guanethidine monosulphate 3%, adrenaline 0.5% in a viscous vehicle. Net price 7.5 mL = £5.86
Additives: include benzalkonium chloride

BETA-BLOCKERS

Topical application of a beta-blocker to the eye reduces intra-ocular pressure effectively in *chronic simple glaucoma*, probably by reducing the rate of production of aqueous humour. Administration by mouth also reduces intra-ocular pressure but this route is not used since side-effects may be troublesome.

Beta-blockers used as eye-drops include **timolol** and, more recently, **betaxolol**, **carteolol**, **levobunolol**, and **metipranolol**.

CAUTIONS, CONTRA-INDICATIONS AND SIDE-EFFECTS. Systemic absorption may follow topical application therefore eye-drops containing a beta-blocker are contra-indicated in patients with bradycardia, heart block, or heart failure. **Important:** for a warning to avoid in asthma see CSM advice below. Consider also other cautions, contra-indications and side-effects of beta-blockers (p. 75). Local side-effects of eye-drops include transitory dry eyes and allergic blepharoconjunctivitis.

CSM advice. The CSM has advised that beta-blockers, even those with apparent cardioselectivity, should not be used in patients with asthma or a history of obstructive airways disease, unless no alternative treatment is available. In such cases the risk of inducing bronchospasm should be appreciated and appropriate precautions taken.

INTERACTIONS. Since systemic absorption may follow topical application the possibility of interactions, in particular, with drugs such as verapamil should be borne in mind. See also Appendix 1 (beta-blockers).

BETAXOLOL HYDROCHLORIDE

Indications; Cautions; Contra-indications; Side-effects: see notes above

Administration: apply eye-drops twice daily

PoM **Betoptic**® (Alcon)

Eye-drops, betaxolol 0.5% (as hydrochloride). Net price 5 mL = £5.17

Additives: include benzalkonium chloride

CARTEOLOL HYDROCHLORIDE

Indications; Cautions; Contra-indications; Side-effects: see notes above

Administration: apply eye-drops twice daily

PoM **Teoptic**® (CIBA Vision)

Eye-drops, carteolol hydrochloride 1%, net price 5 mL = £4.83; 3 × 5 mL = £12.32; 2%, 5 mL = £5.67; 3 × 5 mL = £14.46

Additives: include benzalkonium chloride

LEVOBUNOLOL HYDROCHLORIDE

Indications; Cautions; Contra-indications; Side-effects: see notes above

Administration: apply eye-drops once or twice daily

PoM **Betagan**® (Allergan)

Eye-drops, levobunolol hydrochloride 0.5%, polyvinyl alcohol (Liquifilm®) 1.4%. Net price 5-mL bottle with C Cap® = £4.88, triple pack (3 × 5 mL) = £12.45

Additives: include benzalkonium chloride, disodium edetate

Unit dose eye-drops, levobunolol hydrochloride 0.5%, polyvinyl alcohol (Liquifilm®) 1.4%. Net price 30 × 0.4 mL = £10.45

Additives: include disodium edetate

METIPRANOLOL

Indications; Cautions; Contra-indications; Side-effects: see notes above but in chronic open angle glaucoma **restricted** to patients allergic to preservatives or to those wearing soft contact lenses (in whom benzalkonium chloride should be avoided); granulomatous anterior uveitis reported (discontinue treatment)

Administration: apply eye-drops twice daily

PoM **Minims**® **Metipranolol** (Chauvin)

Eye-drops, metipranolol 0.1%, net price 20 × 0.5 mL = £10.19; 0.3%, 20 × 0.5 mL = £11.09

TIMOLOL MALEATE

Indications; Cautions; Contra-indications; Side effects: see notes above

Administration: apply eye-drops twice daily

PoM **Timoptol**® (MSD)

Eye-drops, in Ocumeter® metered-dose unit, timolol (as maleate) 0.25%, net price 5 mL = £5.1 0.5%, 5 mL = £5.82

Additives: include benzalkonium chloride

Unit dose eye-drops, timolol (as maleate) 0.25% net price 30 × 0.25 mL = £9.60; 0.5%, 30 0.25 mL = £10.97

PoM **Glaucol**® (Baker Norton)

Unit dose eye-drops, timolol (as maleate) 0.25% net price 30 unit-dose vials = £5.18; 0.5%, 3 unit-dose vials = £5.82

Modified release

▼ PoM **Timoptol**®**-LA** (MSD)

Ophthalmic gel-forming solution (= eye-drops m/r, timolol (as maleate) 0.25%, net pri 2.5 mL = £5.18; 0.5%, 2.5 mL = £5.82

Additives: include benzododecinium bromide

Apply eye drops once daily

CARBONIC ANHYDRASE INHIBITORS AND SYSTEMIC DRUGS

The side-effects of beta-blockers are probably suffi cient to prevent their being prescribed by the op thalmologist for administration by mouth. Hen **acetazolamide** will retain a significant place treatment. It inhibits carbonic anhydrase, th reducing the bicarbonate in aqueous humour ar the water secreted with it, resulting in a fall in t intra-ocular pressure. **Dichlorphenamide** has similar but more prolonged action. Both these dru have a diuretic action and a moderate incidence side-effects, giving rise, especially in the elderly, paraesthesia, hypokalaemia, lack of appetite, drov siness and depression; rashes and blood disorde occur rarely and renal calculi have been reported.

Acetazolamide by intramuscular or preferab intravenous injection is also useful in the pre-oper tive treatment of closed-angle glaucoma.

Dorzolamide, a topical carbonic anhydra inhibitor, is licensed for use in patients resistant beta-blockers or those in whom beta-blockers a contra-indicated. It is used alone or as an adjunct a topical beta-blocker. Side-effects similar to tho of systemic sulphonamides may occur and m require discontinuation if severe.

Intravenous hypertonic **mannitol**, or **glycerol** mouth, are useful short-term ocular hypotensi drugs.

ACETAZOLAMIDE

Indications; Side-effects: see notes above

Cautions: avoid in severe renal impairment; pregnancy; not generally recommended for prolonged administration but if given blood counts needed; **interactions:** Appendix 1 (acetazolamide)

Dose: by mouth or by intravenous injection, 0.25–1 g daily in divided doses

By intramuscular injection, as for intravenous injection but preferably avoided because of alkaline pH

PoM Diamox® (Storz)

Tablets, acetazolamide 250 mg. Net price 20 = £1.91. Label: 3

Sodium Parenteral (= injection), powder for reconstitution, acetazolamide (as sodium salt). Net price 500-mg vial = £14.76

PoM Diamox® SR (Storz)

Capsules, m/r, two-tone orange, enclosing orange f/c pellets, acetazolamide 250 mg. Net price 28-cap pack = £10.50. Label: 3, 25

Dose: 1–2 capsules daily

DICHLORPHENAMIDE

Indications; Cautions; Side-effects: see under Acetazolamide and notes above

Dose: initially 100–200 mg, then 100 mg every 12 hours, adjusted according to the patient's response

PoM Daranide® (MSD)

Tablets, yellow, scored, dichlorphenamide 50 mg. Net price 20 = 95p

DORZOLAMIDE

Indications: adjunct to beta-blockers or used alone in raised intra-ocular pressure in ocular hypertension, open-angle glaucoma, or pseudoexfoliative glaucoma in patients unresponsive to beta-blockers or if beta-blockers contra-indicated

Cautions: hepatic impairment; systemic absorption follows topical application

Contra-indications: severe renal impairment or hyperchloraemic acidosis; pregnancy and breast-feeding

Side-effects: bitter taste, burning, stinging and itching of the eye, blurred vision, tearing; eyelid inflammation and conjunctivitis (may be allergic); headache, nausea, asthenia; rarely rash and iridocyclitis; urolithiasis reported; see also notes above

Administration: used alone, apply 3 times daily; with topical beta-blocker, apply twice daily

▼ PoM **Trusopt®** (MSD)

Ophthalmic solution (= eye-drops), dorzolamide (as hydrochloride) 2%. Net price 5 mL = £9.31

Additives: include benzalkonium chloride

11.7   Local anaesthetics

Oxybuprocaine and amethocaine are probably the most widely used topical local anaesthetics. Proxymetacaine causes less initial stinging and is useful for children. Cocaine was formerly used in surgery; its toxicity to corneal epithelium was its main drawback. Oxybuprocaine or a combined preparation of lignocaine and fluorescein is used for tonometry. Lignocaine, with or without adrenaline, is injected into the eyelids for minor surgery, while retrobulbar or peribulbar injections are used for surgery of the globe itself.

AMETHOCAINE HYDROCHLORIDE

Indications: local anaesthetic

PoM Amethocaine (Non-proprietary)

Eye-drops, amethocaine hydrochloride 0.5%, net price, 10 mL = £3.07; 1%, 10 mL = £3.44

Available from Martindale

Single use

PoM Minims® Amethocaine Hydrochloride (Chauvin)

Eye-drops, amethocaine hydrochloride 0.5 and 1%. Net price 20 × 0.5 mL (both) = £5.75

LIGNOCAINE HYDROCHLORIDE

Indications: local anaesthetic

PoM Minims® Lignocaine and Fluorescein (Chauvin)

Eye-drops, lignocaine hydrochloride 4%, fluorescein sodium 0.25%. Net price 20 × 0.5 mL = £6.93

OXYBUPROCAINE HYDROCHLORIDE

Indications: local anaesthetic

PoM Minims® Benoxinate (Oxybuprocaine) Hydrochloride (Chauvin)

Eye-drops, oxybuprocaine hydrochloride 0.4%. Net price 20 × 0.5 mL = £4.92

PROXYMETACAINE HYDROCHLORIDE

Indications: local anaesthetic

PoM Ophthaine® (Squibb)

Eye-drops, proxymetacaine hydrochloride 0.5%. Net price 15 mL = £4.49

Additives: include benzalkonium chloride, chlorbutol

11.8 Miscellaneous ophthalmic preparations

11.8.1 Preparations for tear deficiency

Chronically sore eyes associated with reduced tear secretion, usually in cases of rheumatoid arthritis (Sjögren's syndrome), often respond to hypromellose eye-drops and mucolytic agents.

ACETYLCYSTEINE
Indications: tear deficiency, impaired or abnormal mucus production
Administration: apply eye-drops 3–4 times daily

PoM Ilube® (Alcon)
Eye-drops, acetylcysteine 5%, hypromellose 0.35%. Net price 10 mL = £4.63
Additives: include benzalkonium chloride, disodium edetate

CARBOMERS
(Polyacrylic acid)
Synthetic high molecular weight polymers of acrylic acid cross-linked with either allyl ethers of sucrose or allyl ethers of pentaerythritol
Indications: dry eyes including keratoconjunctivitis sicca, unstable tear film
Administration: apply 3–4 times daily or as required

Viscotears® (CIBA Vision)
Liquid gel (= eye-drops), carbomer 940 (polyacrylic acid) 0.2%. Net price 10 g = £2.95
Additives: include cetrimide, disodium edetate

HYDROXYETHYLCELLULOSE
Indications: tear deficiency

Minims® Artificial Tears (Chauvin)
Eye-drops, hydroxyethylcellulose 0.44%. Net price 20 × 0.5 mL = £5.75

HYPROMELLOSE
Indications: tear deficiency

Hypromellose (Non-proprietary)
Eye-drops, hypromellose 0.3%. Net price 10 mL = 52p
Available from CP, Martindale
Isopto Alkaline® (Alcon)
Eye-drops, hypromellose 1%. Net price 10 mL = 99p
Additives: include benzalkonium chloride
Isopto Plain® (Alcon)
Eye-drops, hypromellose 0.5%. Net price 10 mL = 85p
Additives: include benzalkonium chloride
Tears Naturale® (Alcon)
Eye-drops, dextran '70' 0.1%, hypromellose 0.3%. Net price 15 mL = £1.68
Additives: include benzalkonium chloride, disodium edetate

With phenylephrine
Isopto Frin® (Alcon)
Eye-drops, phenylephrine hydrochloride 0.12%, hypromellose 0.5%. Net price 10 mL = £1.14
Additives: include benzethonium chloride

LIQUID PARAFFIN
Indications: tear deficiency

Lacri-Lube® (Allergan)
Eye ointment, white soft paraffin, liquid paraffin. Net price 3.5 g = £1.99, 5 g = £2.59
Additives: include wool fat derivatives

POLYVINYL ALCOHOL
Indications: tear deficiency

Hypotears® (CIBA Vision)
Eye-drops, macrogol '8000' 2%, polyvinyl alcohol 1%. Net price 15 mL = £1.09
Additives: include benzalkonium chloride, disodium edetate
Liquifilm Tears® (Allergan)
Ophthalmic solution (= eye-drops), polyvinyl alcohol 1.4%. Net price 15 mL = £1.69
Additives: include benzalkonium chloride, disodium edetate
Preservative-free ophthalmic solution (= eye-drops), polyvinyl alcohol 1.4%, povidone 0.6%. Net price 30 × 0.4 mL = £5.60
Sno Tears® (Chauvin)
Eye-drops, polyvinyl alcohol 1.4%. Net price 10 mL = £1.10
Additives: include benzalkonium chloride, disodium edetate

11.8.2 Other preparations

Zinc sulphate is a traditional astringent which has been used in eye-drops for treatment of excessive lacrimation.

Simple eye ointment is a bland sterile preparation which may be used to soften crusts in blepharitis or as a bland lubricant at night.

Fluorescein sodium and **rose bengal** are used in diagnostic procedures and for locating damaged areas of the cornea due to injury or disease. Rose bengal is much more efficient for the diagnosis of conjunctival epithelial damage.

Certain eye-drops, e.g. benzylpenicillin, colistin, desferrioxamine, and trisodium edetate (see also section 9.5.1.2), may be prepared aseptically from material supplied for injection.

ACETYLCHOLINE CHLORIDE
Indications: cataract surgery, penetrating keratoplasty, iridectomy, and other anterior segment surgery requiring rapid complete miosis

PoM Miochol® (CIBA Vision)
Solution for intra-ocular irrigation, acetylcholine chloride 1%, mannitol 3% when reconstituted. Net price 2 mL-vial = £8.32

APRACLONIDINE

Note. Apraclonidine is a derivative of clonidine

Indications; Administration: control of intra-ocular pressure, see under preparations below

Cautions: history of angina, severe coronary insufficiency, recent myocardial infarction, cardiac failure, cerebrovascular disease, vasovagal attack, chronic renal failure; depression; pregnancy and breast-feeding; monitor intra-ocular pressure and visual fields; loss of effect may occur over time; suspend treatment if reduction in vision occurs in end-stage glaucoma; exaggerated reduction in intra-ocular pressure following peri-operative use should be closely monitored; **interactions:** Appendix 1 (apraclonidine)

DRIVING. Drowsiness may affect performance of skilled tasks (e.g. driving)

Contra-indications: history of severe or unstable and uncontrolled cardiovascular disease

Side-effects: dry mouth, taste disturbance; hyperaemia, ocular pruritus, discomfort and tearing (withdraw if ocular intolerance including oedema of lids and conjunctiva); headache, asthenia, dry nose; lid retraction, conjunctival blanching and mydriasis reported after peri-operative use; since absorption may follow topical application systemic effects (see Clonidine Hydrochloride, section 2.5.2) may occur

PoM **Iopidine**® (Alcon)

Ophthalmic solution (= eye-drops), apraclonidine 1% (as hydrochloride). Net price 12 × 2 single use 0.25-mL units = £81.90

Administration: control or prevention of postoperative elevation of intra-ocular pressure after anterior segment laser surgery, apply 1 drop 1 hour before laser procedure then 1 drop immediately after completion of procedure; CHILD not recommended

▼*Iopidine 0.5% ophthalmic solution* (= eye-drops), apraclonidine 0.5% (as hydrochloride). Net price 5 mL = £11.45

Administration: short-term adjunctive treatment of chronic glaucoma in patients not adequately controlled by another drug (see note below), apply 1 drop 3 times daily usually for max. 1 month; CHILD not recommended

Note. May not provide additional benefit if patient already using two drugs that suppress the production of aqueous humour

CHYMOTRYPSIN

Indications: zonulolysis in intracapsular cataract extraction

PoM **Zonulysin**® (Henleys)

Injection, powder for reconstitution, alphachymotrypsin 300 USP units (≡ 1.5 microkatals). Net price per vial (with diluent) = £9.47

DICLOFENAC SODIUM

Indications: inhibition of intraoperative miosis during cataract surgery (but does not possess intrinsic mydriatic properties); postoperative inflammation in cataract surgery; pain in corneal epithelial defects after photorefractive keratectomy

PoM **Voltarol**® **Ophtha** (CIBA Vision)

Eye-drops, diclofenac sodium 0.1%. Net price pack of 5 single-dose units = £4.99, 40 single-dose units = £39.90

FLURBIPROFEN SODIUM

Indications: inhibition of intraoperative miosis (but does not possess intrinsic mydriatic properties); anterior segment inflammation following postoperative and post-laser trabeculoplasty when corticosteroids contra-indicated

PoM **Ocufen**® (Allergan)

Ophthalmic solution (= eye-drops), flurbiprofen sodium 0.03%, polyvinyl alcohol (Liquifilm®) 1.4%. Net price 40 × 0.4 mL = £38.90

KETOROLAC TROMETAMOL

Indications: prophylaxis and reduction of inflammation and associated symptoms following ocular surgery

▼ PoM **Acular**® (Allergan)

Eye-drops, ketorolac trometamol 0.5%. Net price 5 mL = £6.99

PARAFFIN, YELLOW, SOFT

Indications: see notes above

Simple Eye Ointment, liquid paraffin 10%, wool fat 10%, in yellow soft paraffin. Net price 4 g = £2.09

Available from Martindale

SODIUM CHLORIDE

Indications: irrigation, including first-aid removal of harmful substances; intra-ocular or topical irrigation during surgical procedures

Sodium Chloride 0.9% Solutions

See section 13.11.1

Balanced Salt Solution

Solution (sterile), sodium chloride 0.64%, sodium acetate 0.39%, sodium citrate 0.17%, calcium chloride 0.048%, magnesium chloride 0.03%, potassium chloride 0.075%.

Available from Alcon (15 mL and 30 mL) and from CIBA Vision (*Iocare*®, 15 mL and 500 mL)

Single use

Minims® **Sodium Chloride** (Chauvin)

Eye-drops, sodium chloride 0.9%. Net price 20 × 0.5 mL = £4.92

Cautionary label wordings, see inside back cover   Prices are **net**, see p.1

SODIUM HYALURONATE

A visco-elastic polymer normally present in the aqueous and vitreous humour

Indications: used during surgical procedures on the eye

Side-effects: occasional hypersensitivity (avian origin); occasional transient rise in intra-ocular pressure

PoM **Healonid®** (Pharmacia)
Injection, sodium hyaluronate 10 mg/mL in disposable syringes, net price 0.5 mL = £44.87, 0.75 mL = £67.24

PoM **Ophthalin®** (CIBA Vision)
Injection, sodium hyaluronate 1% (10 mg/mL) in disposable syringe, net price 1 mL = £57.00

ZINC SULPHATE

Indications; Cautions: see notes above

Zinc Sulphate (Non-proprietary)
Eye-drops, zinc sulphate 0.25%. Net price 10 mL = £2.43
Available from Martindale, Rhône-Poulenc Rorer (Sootheye® with Autodrop®)

DIAGNOSTIC PREPARATIONS

FLUORESCEIN SODIUM

Indications: detection of lesions and foreign bodies

Minims® Fluorescein Sodium (Chauvin)
Eye-drops, fluorescein sodium 1 or 2%. Net price 20 × 0.5 mL (both) = £4.92

ROSE BENGAL

Indications: detection of lesions and foreign bodies

Minims® Rose Bengal (Chauvin)
Eye-drops, rose bengal 1%. Net price 20 × 0.5 mL = £5.75

11.9   Contact lenses

Note. Some recommendations in this section involve non-licensed indications.

For cosmetic reasons many people prefer to wear contact lenses rather than spectacles; contact lenses are also sometimes required for medical indications. Visual defects are corrected by either rigid ('hard' or gas permeable) lenses or soft (hydrogel) lenses; soft lenses are the most popular type, because they are the most comfortable, though they may not give the best vision. Lenses should usually be worn for a specified number of hours each day. Continuous (extended) wear involves much greater risks to eye health and is not recommended except where medically indicated.

Contact lenses require meticulous care. Poor compliance with directions for use, and with daily cleaning and disinfection, may result in complications which include ulcerative keratitis, conjunctival problems (such as purulent or papillary conjunctivitis).

Acanthamoeba keratitis, a sight-threatening condition, is associated with ineffective lens cleaning and disinfection or the use of contaminated lens cases. The condition is especially associated with the use of soft lenses (including disposable lenses). Acanthamoeba keratitis is treated by specialists with intensive use of polyhexanide (polyhexamethylene biguanide), propamidine isethionate, chlorhexidine and neomycin drops, sometimes in combination.

CONTACT LENSES AND DRUG TREATMENT. Special care is required in prescribing eye preparations for contact lens users. Some drugs and preservatives in eye preparations can accumulate in hydrogel lenses and may induce toxic reactions. Therefore, unless medically indicated, the lenses should be removed before instillation and not worn during the period of treatment. Alternatively, unpreserved drops can be used. Ointment preparations should never be used in conjunction with contact lens wear.

Many drugs given systemically can also have adverse effects on contact lens wear. These include oral contraceptives (particularly those with a higher oestrogen content), drugs which reduce blink rate (e.g. anxiolytics, hypnotics, antihistamines, and muscle relaxants), drugs which reduce tear production (e.g. antihistamines, antimuscarinics, phenothiazines and related drugs, some beta-blockers, diuretics, and tricyclic antidepressants), and drugs which increase lacrimation (including ephedrine and hydralazine). Other drugs that may affect contact lens wear are isotretinoin (may cause conjunctival inflammation), primidone (may cause ocular or eyelid oedema), aspirin (salicylic acid appears in tears and may be absorbed by contact lenses—leading to irritation), and rifampicin and sulphasalazine (may discolour lenses)

12: Drugs used in the treatment of diseases of the
EAR, NOSE, and OROPHARYNX

In this chapter, drug treatment is discussed under the following headings:

12.1 Drugs acting on the ear
12.2 Drugs acting on the nose
12.3 Drugs acting on the oropharynx

12.1 Drugs acting on the ear

12.1.1 Otitis externa
12.1.2 Otitis media
12.1.3 Removal of ear wax

12.1.1 Otitis externa

Otitis externa is an inflammatory reaction of the meatal skin. It is important to exclude an underlying chronic otitis media before treatment is commenced. Many cases recover after thorough cleansing of the external ear canal by suction, dry mopping, or gentle syringing. A frequent problem in resistant cases is the difficulty in applying lotions and ointments satisfactorily to the relatively inaccessible affected skin. The most effective method is to introduce a ribbon gauze dressing soaked with **corticosteroid** ear drops or with an astringent such as **aluminium acetate** solution. When this is not practical, the ear should be gently cleaned with a probe covered in cotton wool and the patient encouraged to lie with the affected ear uppermost for ten minutes after the canal has been filled with a liberal quantity of the appropriate solution.

If infection is present, a topical anti-infective which is not used systemically (such as **neomycin** or **clioquinol**) may be used, but for only about a week as excessive use may result in fungal infections; these may be difficult to treat and require expert advice. Sensitivity to the anti-infective or solvent may occur and resistance to antibacterials is a possibility with prolonged use. **Chloramphenicol** may also be used but the ear drops contain propylene glycol and cause sensitivity in about 10% of patients (the eye ointment can be used instead [unlicensed indication]). Solutions containing an anti-infective and a corticosteroid (such as Locorten-Vioform®) are used for treating cases where infection is present with inflammation and eczema. The CSM has warned that when otitis externa is treated topically with preparations containing aminoglycosides (e.g. neomycin, framycetin) or polymyxins in patients who have a perforation of the tympanic membrane (ear drum), there is an increased risk of drug-induced deafness. The CSM states that it is therefore important to ensure that there is no perforation in such patients before prescription of these preparations. However, many specialists do use these drops cautiously in patients with a perforation (see otitis media section 12.1.2).

An acute infection may cause severe pain and a systemic antibiotic is required with a simple analgesic such as paracetamol. When a resistant staphylococcal infection (a boil) is present in the external auditory meatus, **flucloxacillin** is the drug of choice (see section 5.1, table 1).

The skin of the pinna adjacent to the ear canal is often affected by eczema. Topical corticosteroid creams and ointments (see section 13.4) are then required, but prolonged use should be avoided.

ASTRINGENT PREPARATIONS

ALUMINIUM ACETATE
Indications: inflammation in otitis externa (see notes above)

Aluminium Acetate Ear drops (13%) consists of aluminium acetate solution, BP.
Insert into the meatus or apply on a gauze wick which should be kept saturated with the ear drops
Available from manufacturers of 'special order' products

Aluminium Acetate Ear drops (8%)
Prepared by diluting 8 parts of aluminium acetate solution, BP, with 5 parts of purified water, freshly boiled and cooled; it must be freshly prepared. Directions as above

---

ANTI-INFLAMMATORY PREPARATIONS

BETAMETHASONE SODIUM PHOSPHATE
Indications: eczematous inflammation in otitis externa (see notes above)
Cautions: avoid prolonged use
Contra-indications: untreated infection
Side-effects: local sensitivity reactions

PoM **Betnesol®** (Evans)
Drops (for ear, eye, or nose), betamethasone sodium phosphate 0.1%. Net price 10 mL = £1.31
Additives: include benzalkonium chloride
Ear, apply 2–3 drops every 2–3 hours; reduce frequency when relief obtained; *eye*, see section 11.4.1; *nose*, see section 12.2.1

PoM **Vista-Methasone®** (Martindale)
Drops (for ear, eye, or nose), betamethasone sodium phosphate 0.1%. Net price 5 mL = £1.15; 10 mL = £1.31
Additives: include benzalkonium chloride
Ear, apply 2–3 drops every 3–4 hours; reduce frequency when relief obtained; *eye*, see section 11.4.1; *nose*, see section 12.2.1

With antibacterial
PoM **Betnesol-N®** (Evans)
Drops (for ear, eye, or nose), betamethasone sodium phosphate 0.1%, neomycin sulphate 0.5%. Net price 10 mL = £1.35
Additives: include benzalkonium chloride
Ear, apply 2–3 drops 3–4 times daily; *eye*, see section 11.4.1; *nose*, section 12.2.3

PoM **Vista-Methasone N**® (Martindale)

Drops (for ear, eye, or nose), betamethasone sodium phosphate 0.1%, neomycin sulphate 0.5%. Net price 5 mL = £1.23; 10 mL = £1.35

Additives: include thiomersal

Ear, apply 2–3 drops every 3–4 hours; reduce frequency when relief obtained; *eye*, see section 11.4.1; *nose*, section 12.2.3

DEXAMETHASONE

Indications: eczematous inflammation in otitis externa (see notes above)

Cautions: avoid prolonged use

Contra-indications: untreated infection

Side-effects: local sensitivity reactions

With antibacterial

PoM **Otomize**® (Stafford-Miller)

Ear spray, dexamethasone 0.1%, neomycin sulphate 3250 units/mL, glacial acetic acid 2%. Net price 5-mL pump-action aerosol unit = £3.85

Apply 1 metered spray into the ear 3 times daily

PoM **Sofradex**® (Roussel)

Drops (for ear or eye), dexamethasone (as sodium metasulphobenzoate) 0.05%, framycetin sulphate 0.5%, gramicidin 0.005%. Net price 10 mL = £3.90

Ear, apply 2–3 drops 3–4 times daily; *eye*, see section 11.4.1

Ointment (for ear or eye), dexamethasone 0.05%, framycetin sulphate 0.5%, gramicidin 0.005%. Net price 5 g = £1.95

Ear, apply 1–2 times daily; *eye*, see section 11.4.1

FLUMETHASONE PIVALATE

Indications: eczematous inflammation in otitis externa (see notes above)

Cautions: avoid prolonged use

Contra-indications: untreated infection

Side-effects: local sensitivity reactions

With antibacterial

PoM **Locorten-Vioform**® (Zyma)

Ear drops, flumethasone pivalate 0.02%, clioquinol 1%. Net price 7.5 mL = £1.02

Apply 2–3 drops into the ear twice daily for up to 7–10 days; not recommended for child under 2 years

HYDROCORTISONE

Indications: eczematous inflammation in otitis externa (see notes above)

Cautions: avoid prolonged use

Contra-indications: untreated infection

Side-effects: local sensitivity reactions

With antibacterial

PoM **Gentisone HC**® (Roche)

Ear drops, hydrocortisone acetate 1%, gentamicin 0.3% (as sulphate). Net price 10 mL = £4.16

Additives: include benzalkonium chloride

Apply 2–4 drops into the ear 3–4 times daily and at night

PoM **Neo-Cortef**® (Dominion)

Drops (for ear or eye), hydrocortisone acetate 1.5%, neomycin sulphate 0.5%. Net price 10 mL = £4.30

Additives: include miripirium chloride (myristyl-gamma-picolinium chloride)

Ear, apply 2–3 drops 3–4 times daily; *eye*, see section 11.4.1

Ointment (for ear or eye), hydrocortisone acetate 1.5%, neomycin sulphate 0.5%. Net price 3.9 g = £1.60

Ear, apply 1–2 times daily; *eye*, see section 11.4.1

PoM **Otosporin**® (Wellcome)

Ear drops, hydrocortisone 1%, neomycin sulphate 3400 units, polymyxin B sulphate 10 000 units/mL. Net price 5 mL = £2.15; 10 mL = £4.30

Apply 3 drops into the ear 3–4 times daily

PREDNISOLONE SODIUM PHOSPHATE

Indications: eczematous inflammation in otitis externa (see notes above)

Cautions: avoid prolonged use

Contra-indications: untreated infection

Side-effects: local sensitivity reactions

PoM **Predsol**® (Evans)

Drops (for ear or eye), prednisolone sodium phosphate 0.5%. Net price 10 mL = £1.31

Additives: include benzalkonium chloride

Ear, apply 2–3 drops every 2–3 hours; reduce frequency when relief obtained; *eye*, see section 11.4.1

With antibacterial

PoM **Predsol-N**® (Evans)

Drops (for ear or eye), prednisolone sodium phosphate 0.5%, neomycin sulphate 0.5%. Net price 10 mL = £1.20

Additives: include benzalkonium chloride

Ear, apply 2–3 drops 3–4 times daily; *eye*, see section 11.4.1

TRIAMCINOLONE ACETONIDE

Indications: eczematous inflammation in otitis externa (see notes above)

Cautions: avoid prolonged use

Contra-indications: untreated infection

Side-effects: local sensitivity reactions

With antibacterial

PoM **Audicort**® (Lederle)

Ear drops, triamcinolone acetonide 0.1%, neomycin (as neomycin undecenoate) 0.35%. Net price 10 mL = £4.30

Apply 2–5 drops into the ear 3–4 times daily; CHILD not recommended

PoM **Tri-Adcortyl Otic**® (Squibb)

Ear ointment, triamcinolone acetonide 0.1%, gramicidin 0.025%, neomycin 0.25% (as sulphate), nystatin 100 000 units/g in Plastibase®. Net price 10 g = £1.58

Apply into the ear 2–4 times daily

ANTI-INFECTIVE PREPARATIONS

CHLORAMPHENICOL

Indications: bacterial infection in otitis externa (but see notes above)

Cautions: avoid prolonged use (see notes above)

Side-effects: high incidence of sensitivity reactions to vehicle

PoM **Chloramphenicol** (Non-proprietary)
Ear drops, chloramphenicol 5% in propylene glycol. Net price 10 mL = £1.35
Apply 2–3 drops into the ear 2–3 times daily

CLIOQUINOL

Indications: mild bacterial or fungal infections in otitis externa (see notes above)

Cautions: avoid prolonged use (see notes above)

Contra-indications: perforated tympanic membrane

Side-effects: local sensitivity; stains skin and clothing

With corticosteroid
PoM **Locorten-Vioform®**, see Flumethasone (p. 444)

CLOTRIMAZOLE

Indications: fungal infection in otitis externa (see notes above)

Side-effects: occasional local irritation or sensitivity

Canesten® (Baypharm)
Solution, clotrimazole 1% in polyethylene glycol (macrogol 400). Net price 20 mL = £2.32
Ear, apply 2–3 times daily continuing for at least 14 days after disappearance of infection; *skin,* see section 13.10.2

FRAMYCETIN SULPHATE

Indications; Cautions; Side-effects: see under Gentamicin

With corticosteroid
PoM **Sofradex®**, see Dexamethasone (p. 444)

GENTAMICIN

Indications: bacterial infection in otitis externa (see notes above)

Cautions; Contra-indications: avoid prolonged use; slight risk of ototoxicity increased if perforated eardrum (see notes above); pregnancy and breast-feeding

Side-effects: local sensitivity

PoM **Cidomycin®** (Roussel)
Drops (for ear or eye), gentamicin 0.3% (as sulphate). Net price 8 mL = £1.31
Additives: include benzalkonium chloride, disodium edetate
Ear, apply 2–4 drops 3–4 times daily and at night; *eye,* see section 11.3.1

PoM **Garamycin®** (Schering-Plough)
Drops (for ear or eye), gentamicin 0.3% (as sulphate). Net price 10 mL = £1.79
Additives: include benzalkonium chloride
Ear, apply 3–4 drops 3–4 times daily; reduce frequency when relief obtained; *eye,* see section 11.3.1

PoM **Genticin®** (Roche)
Drops (for ear or eye), gentamicin 0.3% (as sulphate). Net price 10 mL = £2.00
Additives: include benzalkonium chloride
Ear, apply 2–3 drops 3–4 times daily and at night; *eye,* see section 11.3.1

With corticosteroid
PoM **Gentisone HC®**, see Hydrocortisone (p. 444)

NEOMYCIN SULPHATE

Indications: bacterial infection in otitis externa (see notes above)

Cautions; Contra-indications: avoid prolonged use (see notes above); slight risk of ototoxicity increased if perforated eardrum (see notes above)

Side-effects: local sensitivity

With corticosteroid
PoM **Audicort®**, see Triamcinolone (p. 444)
PoM **Betnesol-N®**, see Betamethasone (p. 443)
PoM **Neo-Cortef®**, see Hydrocortisone (p. 444)
PoM **Otomize®**, see Dexamethasone (p. 444)
PoM **Otosporin®**, see Hydrocortisone (p. 444)
PoM **Predsol-N®**, see Prednisolone (p. 444)
PoM **Tri-Adcortyl Otic®**, see Triamcinolone (p. 444)
PoM **Vista-Methasone N®**, see Betamethasone (p. 444)

OTHER AURAL PREPARATIONS

Choline salicylate is a mild analgesic but it is of doubtful value when applied topically. There is no place for the use of local anaesthetics in ear drops.

NHS **Audax®** (Seton)
Ear drops, choline salicylate 20%, glycerol 12.6%. Net price 8 mL = £1.99

12.1.2 Otitis media

Acute otitis media is the commonest cause of severe pain in small children and recurrent attacks, especially in infants, are particularly distressing. *Otitis media with effusion* ('glue ear') is present in about 10% of the child population and in 90% of children with cleft palates; this condition should be referred to hospital because of the risk of permanent damage to middle ear function and impaired language development. Chronic otitis media is thought to be a legacy from untreated or resistant cases of otitis media with effusion.

Local treatment of *acute otitis media* is ineffective and there is no place for drops containing a local anaesthetic. Many attacks are viral in origin and need only treatment with a **simple analgesic** such as paracetamol for pain. Severe attacks of bacterial origin should be treated with **systemic antibiotics**; bacterial examination of any discharge is helpful in selecting the appropriate treatment (see section 5.1, table 1). Again, simple analgesics such as paracetamol are used to relieve pain. In *recurrent acute otitis media* a daily dose of a prophylactic antibiotic (trimethoprim or erythromycin) during the winter months can be tried.

The organisms recovered from patients with *chronic otitis media* are often opportunists living in the debris, keratin, and necrotic bone present in the middle ear and mastoid. Thorough cleansing with an aural suction tube may completely control infection of many years duration. Acute exacerbations of chronic infection may require systemic antibiotics (see section 5.1, table 1). A swab should be taken to determine the organism present and its antibiotic sensitivity. Unfortunately the culture often produces *Pseudomonas aeruginosa* and *Proteus* spp, sensitive only to parenteral antibiotics. Local debridement of the meatal and middle ear contents may then be followed by topical treatment with ribbon gauze dressings as for otitis externa (section 12.1.1). This is particularly true with infections in mastoid cavities when dusting powders can also be tried.

In the presence of a perforation, however, many specialists use ear drops containing **aminoglycosides** (e.g. neomycin) or **polymyxins**, if the otitis media has failed to settle with systemic antibiotics; it is considered that the pus in the middle ear associated with otitis media carries a higher risk of ototoxicity than the drops themselves.

12.1.3   Removal of ear wax

Wax is a normal bodily secretion which provides a protective film on the meatal skin and need only be removed if it causes deafness or interferes with a proper view of the ear drum. As a general rule syringing is best avoided in patients with a history of recurring otitis externa, a perforated ear drum, or previous ear surgery. A person who has hearing only in one ear should not have that ear syringed because even a very slight risk of damage is unacceptable in this situation.

Wax may be removed by syringing with warm water. If necessary, wax can be softened with simple remedies such as **olive oil** or **almond oil** before syringing. The patient should lie with the affected ear uppermost for 5 to 10 minutes after a generous amount of the solution has been introduced into the ear. Some proprietary preparations containing organic solvents can cause irritation of the meatal skin, and in most cases the simple remedies which are indicated above are just as effective and less likely to cause irritation. **Docusate sodium** is an ingredient in a number of proprietary preparations.

Almond Oil
 Allow to warm to room temperature before use
Olive Oil
 Allow to warm to room temperature before use
Sodium Bicarbonate Ear Drops, BP
 Ear drops, sodium bicarbonate 5%
  Extemporaneous preparations should be recently prepared according to the following formula: sodium bicarbonate 500 mg, glycerol 3 mL, freshly boiled and cooled purified water to 10 mL
Cerumol® (LAB)
 Ear drops, chlorbutol 5%, paradichlorobenzene 2%, arachis (peanut) oil 57.3%. Net price 11 mL = £1.15

Exterol® (Dermal)
 Ear drops, urea-hydrogen peroxide complex 5% in glycerol. Net price 8 mL = £1.89
Molcer® (Wallace Mfg)
 Ear drops, docusate sodium 5%. Net price 15 mL = £1.23
Otex® (DDD)
 Ear drops, urea hydrogen peroxide 5%. Net price 8 mL = £2.17
Waxsol® (Norgine)
 Ear drops, docusate sodium 0.5%. Net price 10 mL = 95p

12.2   Drugs acting on the nose

  12.2.1   Drugs used in nasal allergy
  12.2.2   Topical nasal decongestants
  12.2.3   Anti-infective nasal preparations

Rhinitis is often self-limiting and sinusitis is best treated with antibiotics (see section 5.1, table 1). There are few indications for the use of sprays and drops except in allergic rhinitis where topical preparations of corticosteroids or sodium cromoglycate have much to offer. Most other preparations contain sympathomimetic drugs which may damage the nasal cilia and their prolonged use causes mucosal oedema and severe nasal obstruction (rhinitis medicamentosa). Systemic nasal decongestants are of doubtful value (see section 3.10). Douching the nose with salt and water is **not** recommended for the treatment of chronic rhinitis. However some ENT departments use saline sniffs for a short period after endonasal surgery.

12.2.1   Drugs used in nasal allergy

Mild cases are controlled by **oral antihistamines** and **systemic nasal decongestants** (see sections 3.4.1 and 3.10). Many patients with severe symptoms can now expect relief from topical preparations of **corticosteroids** or **sodium cromoglycate**. Although sodium cromoglycate is less effective than a topical corticosteroid, it is often the first choice in children. Treatment should begin 2 to 3 weeks before the hay fever season commences and may have to be continued for months or even years in some patients. No significant side-effects have been reported. Very disabling symptoms occasionally justify the use of **systemic corticosteroids** for short periods (see section 6.3), for example in students taking important examinations. They may also be used at the beginning of a course of treatment with a corticosteroid spray to relieve severe mucosal oedema and allow the spray to penetrate the nasal cavity.

Azelastine is an antihistamine available as a nasal spray for allergic rhinitis. It is less effective than a topical corticosteroid but probably more effective than cromoglycate. **Levocabastine** is a new antihistamine also available as a nasal spray for allergic rhinitis.

AZELASTINE HYDROCHLORIDE
Indications: allergic rhinitis
Side-effects: irritation of nasal mucosa; taste disturbance

PoM **Rhinolast®** (ASTA Medica)

Aqueous nasal spray, azelastine hydrochloride 140 micrograms (0.14 mL)/metered spray. Net price 20 mL (with metered pump) = £12.48

Apply 140 micrograms (1 spray) into each nostril twice daily; CHILD not recommended

BECLOMETHASONE DIPROPIONATE
(Beclometasone Dipropionate)

Indications: prophylaxis and treatment of allergic and vasomotor rhinitis

Cautions: untreated nasal infection, prolonged use in children, previous treatment with corticosteroids by mouth

Side-effects: sneezing after administration; rarely dryness and irritation of nose and throat, epistaxis, taste disturbance; nasal septal perforation reported

PoM [1]**Beconase®** (A&H)

Aqueous nasal spray (aqueous suspension), beclomethasone dipropionate 50 micrograms/metered spray. Net price 200-spray unit with applicator = £5.01

ADULT and CHILD over 6 years, apply 100 micrograms (2 sprays) into each nostril twice daily *or* 50 micrograms (1 spray) into each nostril 3–4 times daily; max. total 400 micrograms (8 sprays) daily

1. Can be sold to the public for nasal administration (other than by aerosol) if supplied for the prevention and treatment of seasonal allergic rhinitis in adults and children over 12 years subject to max. single dose of 100 micrograms per nostril, max. daily dose of 200 micrograms per nostril, and a pack size limit of 200 doses; a proprietary brand (Beconase® Hayfever) is on sale to the public

BETAMETHASONE SODIUM PHOSPHATE

Indications; Cautions; Side-effects: see under Beclomethasone Dipropionate

PoM **Betnesol®** (Evans)

Drops (for ear, eye, or nose), betamethasone sodium phosphate 0.1%. Net price 10 mL = £1.31

Additives: include benzalkonium chloride

Nose, apply 2–3 drops into each nostril 2–3 times daily; *ear*, section 12.1.1; *eye*, see section 11.4.1

PoM **Vista-Methasone®** (Martindale)

Drops (for ear, eye, or nose), betamethasone sodium phosphate 0.1%. Net price 5 mL = £1.15, 10 mL = £1.31

Additives: include benzalkonium chloride

Nose, apply 2–3 drops into each nostril twice daily; *ear*, section 12.1.1; *eye*, see section 11.4.1

BUDESONIDE

Indications: prophylaxis and treatment of allergic and vasomotor rhinitis

Cautions: see under Beclomethasone Dipropionate; also patients with pulmonary tuberculosis

Side-effects: see under Beclomethasone Dipropionate

PoM **Rhinocort Aqua®** (Astra)

Nasal spray, budesonide 100 micrograms/metered spray. Net price 100-spray unit = £5.85

ADULT and CHILD over 12 years, apply 200 micrograms (2 sprays) into each nostril once daily in the morning *or* 100 micrograms (1 spray) into each nostril twice daily; when control achieved reduced to 100 micrograms (1 spray) into each nostril once daily

FLUNISOLIDE

Indications: prophylaxis and treatment of allergic rhinitis

Cautions: see under Beclomethasone Dipropionate; history of pulmonary tuberculosis

Side-effects: see under Beclomethasone Dipropionate

PoM [1]**Syntaris®** (Roche)

Aqueous nasal spray, flunisolide 25 micrograms/metered spray. Net price 240-spray unit with pump and applicator = £5.50

ADULT, apply 50 micrograms (2 sprays) into each nostril twice daily, increased if necessary to max. 3 times daily then reduced for maintenance; CHILD over 5 years initially 25 micrograms (1 spray) into each nostril up to 3 times daily for no longer than 4 weeks of continuous treatment

1. Flunisolide non-pressurised nasal spray can be sold to the public (in max. pack size of 240 metered units) for the prevention and treatment (in adults and children of not less than 12 years) of seasonal allergic rhinitis, including hayfever; max. adult dose 50 micrograms per nostril and max. daily dose 100 micrograms per nostril (children 12–16 years max. 25 micrograms per nostril and max. daily dose 75 micrograms per nostril); a proprietary brand (Syntaris® Hayfever) is on sale to the public

FLUTICASONE PROPIONATE

Indications: prophylaxis and treatment of allergic rhinitis

Cautions; Side-effects: see under Beclomethasone Dipropionate

PoM **Flixonase®** (A&H)

Aqueous nasal spray, fluticasone propionate 50 micrograms/metered spray. Net price 120-spray unit with applicator = £11.43

ADULT and CHILD over 12 years, apply 100 micrograms (2 sprays) into each nostril once daily, preferably in the morning, increased to twice daily if required; max. total 8 sprays daily; CHILD 4–11 years, 50 micrograms (1 spray) into each nostril once daily, increased to twice daily if required; max. total 4 sprays daily

LEVOCABASTINE

Indications: treatment of allergic rhinitis

Cautions: renal impairment (see Appendix 3)

Side-effects: nasal irritation; headache, fatigue, somnolence reported

▼ PoM **Livostin®** (CIBA Vision)

Aqueous nasal spray, levocabastine (as hydrochloride) 0.5%. Net price 10-mL spray pump = £8.90

Apply 2 sprays into each nostril twice daily for no more than 4 weeks, increased if necessary to 3-4 times daily; CHILD under 9 years not recommended

NEDOCROMIL SODIUM

Indications: prophylaxis and treatment of seasonal allergic rhinitis

Side-effects: mild nasal irritation; taste disturbance

PoM **Tilarin** ® (Fisons)

Aqueous nasal spray, nedocromil sodium 1%. Net price 15 mL = £7.90

ADULT and CHILD over 12 years, apply 1 spray into each nostril 4 times daily; CHILD under 12 years not recommended

SODIUM CROMOGLYCATE
(Sodium Cromoglicate)

Indications: prophylaxis of allergic rhinitis (see notes above)

Side-effects: local irritation; rarely transient bronchospasm

Rynacrom® (Fisons)

4% aqueous nasal spray, sodium cromoglycate 4% (5.2 mg/squeeze). Net price 22 mL with pump = £9.21

Additives: include benzalkonium chloride

ADULT and CHILD, apply 1 squeeze into each nostril 2–4 times daily

Rynacrom Compound® (Fisons)

Nasal spray, sodium cromoglycate 2% (2.6 mg/metered spray) and xylometazoline hydrochloride 0.025% (32.5 micrograms/metered spray). Net price 26 mL with pump = £6.83

Additives: include benzalkonium chloride

Apply 1 spray into each nostril 4 times daily

Note. A proprietary brand of sodium cromoglycate 2% and xylometazoline hydrochloride 0.025% (Resiston One®) is on sale to the public

Vividrin® (Novex)

Nasal spray, sodium cromoglycate 2%. Net price 15 mL = £5.45

Additives: include benzalkonium chloride

ADULT and CHILD, apply 1 spray into each nostril 4–6 times daily

12.2.2   Topical nasal decongestants

The nasal mucosa is sensitive to changes in the atmospheric temperature and humidity and these alone may cause slight nasal congestion. The nose and nasal sinuses produce a litre of mucus in 24 hours and much of this finds its way silently into the stomach via the nasopharynx. Slight changes in the nasal airway, accompanied by an awareness of mucus passing along the nasopharynx causes some patients to be inaccurately diagnosed as suffering from chronic sinusitis. These symptoms are particularly noticeable in the later stages of the common cold for which there is no effective treatment at the moment; the temptation to use nasal drops should be resisted. **Sodium chloride** 0.9% given as nasal drops may relieve nasal congestion by helping to liquefy mucous secretions.

Symptomatic relief from the nasal congestion associated with vasomotor rhinitis, nasal polypi, and the common cold can be obtained by the short-term use (usually not longer than 7 days) of decongestant nasal drops and sprays. These all contain sympathomimetic drugs which exert their effect by vasoconstriction of the mucosal blood vessels which in turn reduces the thickness of the nasal mucosa. They are of limited value as they can give rise to a rebound phenomenon as their effects wear off, due to a secondary vasodilatation with a subsequent temporary increase in nasal congestion. This in turn tempts the further use of the decongestant, leading to a vicious circle of events. **Ephedrine nasal drops** is the safest sympathomimetic preparation and can give relief for several hours. The more potent sympathomimetic drugs oxymetazoline, phenylephrine, and xylometazoline are more likely to cause a rebound effect. **All** of these preparations may cause a hypertensive crisis if used during treatment with a monoamine-oxidase inhibitor.

Non-allergic watery rhinorrhoea often responds well to treatment with **ipratropium bromide**.

Inhalations of **warm moist air** are useful in the treatment of symptoms of acute infective conditions, and the use of compounds containing volatile substances such as menthol and eucalyptus may encourage their use (see section 3.8). There is no evidence that nasal preparations containing antihistamines and anti-infective agents have any therapeutic effect.

Systemic nasal decongestants—see section 3.10.

SYMPATHOMIMETICS

EPHEDRINE HYDROCHLORIDE

Indications: nasal congestion

Cautions: avoid excessive or prolonged use; caution in infants under 3 months (no good evidence of value—if irritation occurs might narrow nasal passage); **interactions:** Appendix 1 (sympathomimetics)

Side-effects: local irritation; after excessive use tolerance with diminished effect, rebound congestion

Administration: see below

Ephedrine Nasal Drops, BP

Nasal drops, ephedrine hydrochloride in a suitable aqueous vehicle

Note. The BP directs that if no strength is specified 0.5% drops should be supplied; net price 10 mL = £1.07

Instil 1–2 drops into each nostril up to 3 or 4 times daily when required

XYLOMETAZOLINE HYDROCHLORIDE

Indications: nasal congestion

Cautions; Side-effects: see under Ephedrine Hydrochloride

Xylometazoline Nasal Drops, xylometazoline hydrochloride 0.1%, net price 10 mL = £1.35

Instil 2–3 drops into each nostril 2–3 times daily when required; max. duration 7 days; not recommended for children under 12 years

Xylometazoline Nasal Drops, Paediatric,

xylometazoline hydrochloride 0.05%, net price 10 mL = £1.35

CHILD over 3 months instil 1–2 drops into each nostril 1–2 times daily when required (not recommended for infants under 3 months of age, doctor's advice only under 2 years); max. duration 7 days

Note. The brand name NHSOtrivine® (Zyma) is used for xylometazoline adult nasal drops 0.1%, children's nasal drops 0.05%, and adult nasal spray 0.1%

Sympathomimetic nasal preparations on sale to the public (not prescribable on the NHS) include: **Afrazine**® (oxymetazoline), **Dristan**® (oxymetazoline), **Fenox**® (phenylephrine), **Otrivine**® (xylometazoline—prescribable in non-proprietary form as nasal drops, see above), **Sudafed**® nasal spray (oxymetazoline), **Vicks Sinex**® (oxymetazoline)

─────────────

ANTIMUSCARINIC

IPRATROPIUM BROMIDE

Indications: watery rhinorrhoea associated with perennial rhinitis

Cautions: see section 3.1.2; avoid spraying near eyes

Side-effects: dryness and irritation of nose, epistaxis

Administration: apply 20–40 micrograms (1–2 sprays) into affected nostril up to 4 times daily; not recommended for children under 12 years

PoM **Rinatec**® (Boehringer Ingelheim)
Nasal spray, ipratropium bromide 20 micrograms/metered spray. Net price 200-dose unit = £4.59

12.2.3 Anti-infective nasal preparations

There is **no** evidence that topical anti-infective nasal preparations have any therapeutic value; for elimination of nasal staphylococci, see below.

Systemic treatment of sinusitis—see section 5.1, table 1.

PoM **Betnesol-N**® (Evans)
Drops (for ear, eye, or nose), betamethasone sodium phosphate 0.1%, neomycin sulphate 0.5%. Net price 10 mL = £1.35
Additives: include benzalkonium chloride
Nose, apply 2–3 drops into nostril 2–3 times daily; *eye,* see section 11.4.1; *ear,* see section 12.1.1

PoM **Dexa-Rhinaspray**® (Boehringer Ingelheim)
Nasal inhalation, dexamethasone 21-isonicotinate 20 micrograms, neomycin sulphate 100 micrograms, tramazoline hydrochloride 120 micrograms/metered inhalation. Net price 125-dose unit = £1.95
Allergic rhinitis (but not recommended, see notes above), ADULT and CHILD over 12 years, apply 1 spray into each nostril 2–3 times daily; max. duration 14 days; CHILD 5-12 years 1 spray into each nostril up to twice daily; under 5 years not recommended

PoM **Locabiotal**® (Servier)
Aerosol spray, fusafungine 125 micrograms/metered inhalation. Net price 200-dose unit with nasal and oral adaptors = £1.55
Infection and inflammation of upper respiratory tract (but not recommended, see notes above), using nasal adaptor, ADULT and CHILD over 12 years, 3 sprays into each nostril 5 times daily for 7–10 days (withdraw if no improvement after 7 days); CHILD 3–5 years, 1 spray into each nostril 5 times daily; 6–12 years 2 sprays into each nostril 5 times daily
Note. May also be sprayed into mouth, using oral adaptor

PoM **Vista-Methasone N**® (Martindale)
Drops (for ear, eye, or nose), betamethasone sodium phosphate 0.1%, neomycin sulphate 0.5%. Net price 5 mL = £1.23, 10 mL = £1.35
Additives: include thiomersal
Nose, apply 2–3 drops into each nostril twice daily; *eye,* see section 11.4.1; *ear,* see section 12.1.1

─────────────

NASAL STAPHYLOCOCCI

Elimination of organisms such as staphylococci from the nasal vestibule can be achieved by the use of a cream containing **chlorhexidine and neomycin** (Naseptin®), but re-colonisation frequently occurs. Coagulase-positive staphylococci can be obtained from the noses of 40% of the population.

A nasal ointment containing **mupirocin** is also available; it should probably be kept in reserve for resistant cases. To avoid the development of resistance its use in hospital should, if possible, be avoided and it should not be used for longer than 10 days.

PoM **Bactroban Nasal**® (Beecham)
Nasal ointment, mupirocin 2% (as calcium salt) in white soft paraffin basis. Net price 3 g = £5.67
For eradication of nasal carriage of staphylococci, including methicillin-resistant *Staphylococcus aureus* (MRSA), apply 2–3 times daily to the inner surface of each nostril

PoM **Naseptin**® (Zeneca)
Cream, chlorhexidine hydrochloride 0.1%, neomycin sulphate 3250 units/g. Net price 15 g = 99p
Ingredients: include arachis (peanut) oil
For eradication of nasal carriage of staphylococci, apply to nostrils 4 times daily for 10 days; for preventing nasal carriage of staphylococci apply to nostrils twice daily

─────────────

12.3 Drugs acting on the oropharynx

12.3.1 Drugs for oral ulceration and inflammation
12.3.2 Oropharyngeal anti-infective drugs
12.3.3 Lozenges and sprays
12.3.4 Mouthwashes, gargles, and dentifrices
12.3.5 Treatment of dry mouth

12.3.1 Drugs for oral ulceration and inflammation

Ulceration of the oral mucosa may be caused by trauma (physical or chemical), recurrent aphthae, infections, carcinoma, dermatological disorders, nutritional deficiencies, gastro-intestinal disease, haematopoietic disorders, and drug therapy. It is important to establish the diagnosis in each case as the majority of these lesions require specific management in addition to local treatment. Patients with an unexplained mouth ulcer of more than 3 weeks' duration require urgent referral to hospital to exclude oral cancer. Local treatment aims at pro-

─────────────

Cautionary label wordings, see inside back cover

tecting the ulcerated area, or at relieving pain or reducing inflammation.

SIMPLE MOUTHWASHES. A **saline** or **compound thymol glycerin** mouthwash (see section 12.3.4) may relieve the pain of traumatic ulceration. The mouthwash is made up with warm water and used at frequent intervals until the discomfort and swelling subsides.

ANTISEPTIC MOUTHWASHES. Secondary bacterial infection may be a feature of any mucosal ulceration; it can increase discomfort and delay healing. Use of a **chlorhexidine** or **povidone-iodine** mouthwash (see section 12.3.4) is often beneficial and may accelerate healing of recurrent aphthae.

MECHANICAL PROTECTION. **Carmellose gelatin paste** may relieve some discomfort arising from ulceration by protecting the ulcer site. The paste adheres to the mucosa, but is difficult to apply effectively to some parts of the mouth.

CORTICOSTEROIDS. Topical corticosteroid therapy may be used for some forms of oral ulceration. In the case of aphthous ulcers it is most effective if applied in the 'prodromal' phase.

Thrush or other types of candidiasis are recognised complications of corticosteroid treatment.

Hydrocortisone lozenges are allowed to dissolve next to an ulcer and are useful in recurrent aphthae, erosive lichen planus, discoid lupus erythematosus, and benign mucous membrane pemphigoid.

Triamcinolone dental paste is designed to keep the corticosteroid in contact with the mucosa for long enough to permit penetration of the lesion, but is difficult for patients to apply properly.

Systemic corticosteroid therapy is reserved for severe conditions such as pemphigus vulgaris (see section 6.3.4).

LOCAL ANALGESICS. Local analgesics have a limited role in the management of oral ulceration. When applied topically their action is of a relatively short duration so that analgesia cannot be maintained continuously throughout the day. The main indication for a topical local analgesic is to relieve the pain of otherwise intractable oral ulceration particularly when it is due to major aphthae. For this purpose lignocaine 5% ointment or lozenges containing a local anaesthetic are applied to the ulcer. When local anaesthetics are used in the mouth care must be taken not to produce anaesthesia of the pharynx before meals as this might lead to choking.

Benzydamine mouthwash or spray may be useful in palliating the discomfort associated with a variety of ulcerative conditions. It has also been found to be effective in reducing the discomfort of post-irradiation mucositis. Some patients find the full-strength mouthwash causes some stinging and, for them, it should be diluted with an equal volume of water.

Choline salicylate dental gel has some analgesic action and may provide relief for recurrent aphthae, but excessive application or confinement under a denture irritates the mucosa and can itself cause ulceration. Benefit in teething may merely be due to pressure of application (comparable with biting a teething ring); excessive use can lead to salicylate poisoning.

OTHER PREPARATIONS. **Carbenoxolone** gel or mouthwash may be of some value. **Tetracycline** rinsed in the mouth may also be of value.

BENZYDAMINE HYDROCHLORIDE

Indications: painful inflammatory conditions of oropharynx

Side-effects: occasional numbness or stinging

Difflam® (3M)

Oral rinse, green, benzydamine hydrochloride 0.15%. Net price 300 mL = £4.10

Rinse or gargle, using 15 mL (diluted with water if stinging occurs) every 1½–3 hours as required, usually for not more than 7 days; not suitable for children aged 12 years or under

Spray, benzydamine hydrochloride 0.15%. Net price 30-mL unit = £3.57

ADULT, 4–8 puffs onto affected area every 1½–3 hours; CHILD under 6 years 1 puff per 4 kg to max. 4 puffs every 1½–3 hours; 6–12 years 4 puffs every 1½–3 hours

---

CARBENOXOLONE SODIUM

Indications: mild oral and perioral lesions

Bioral Gel® (Sterling Health)

Gel, carbenoxolone sodium 2% in adhesive basis Net price 5 g = £2.12

Apply after meals and at bedtime

PoM Bioplex® (Thames)

Mouthwash granules, carbenoxolone sodium 1% (20 mg/sachet). Net price 24 × 2-g sachets = £9.60

For mouth ulcers, rinse with 1 sachet in 30–50 mL of warm water 3 times daily and at bedtime

---

CARMELLOSE SODIUM

Indications: mechanical protection of oral and perioral lesions

Orabase® (ConvaTec)

Oral paste, carmellose sodium 16.58%, pectin 16.58%, gelatin 16.58%, in Plastibase®. Net price 30 g = £1.69; 100 g = £3.74

Apply a thin layer when necessary after meals

Orahesive® (ConvaTec)

Powder, carmellose sodium, pectin, gelatin, equal parts. Net price 25 g = £1.88

Sprinkle on the affected area

CORTICOSTEROIDS

Indications: oral and perioral lesions

Contra-indications: untreated oral infection

Side-effects: occasional exacerbation of local infection

PoM [1]**Adcortyl in Orabase**® (Squibb)

Oral paste, triamcinolone acetonide 0.1% in adhesive basis. Net price 10 g = £1.27

ADULT and CHILD, apply a thin layer 2–4 times daily; do not rub in; use limited to 5 days for children and short-term use also advised for elderly

1. A 5-g tube (Adcortyl® in Orabase for Mouth Ulcers) is on sale to the public for the treatment of common mouth ulcers for a treatment period not exceeding 5 days

Corlan® (Evans)

Pellets (= lozenges), hydrocortisone 2.5 mg (as sodium succinate). Net price 20 = £1.40

ADULT and CHILD, 1 lozenge 4 times daily, allowed to dissolve slowly in the mouth in contact with the ulcer; if ulcers recur rapidly treatment may be continued for a period at reduced dosage

LOCAL ANAESTHETICS

Indications: relief of pain in oral lesions
Cautions: avoid prolonged use; hypersensitivity

Preparations

Local anaesthetics are included in some mouth ulcer preparations, for details see below
Local anaesthetics are also included in some throat lozenges and sprays, see section 12.3.3

Teething gels
Teething gels containing local anaesthetics include: Anbesol®, Calgel®, Dentinox®, Rinstead®, Woodward's®, Ulc-Aid®

SALICYLATES

Indications: mild oral and perioral lesions
Cautions: frequent application, especially in children, may give rise to salicylate poisoning
Note. CSM warning on aspirin and Reye's syndrome does not apply to non-aspirin salicylates or to topical preparations such as teething gels

Choline salicylate
Choline Salicylate Dental Gel, BP

Oral gel, choline salicylate 8.7% in a flavoured gel basis
Available as Bonjela® (R&C), net price 15 g (sugar-free) = £1.38; Teejel® (Seton), 10 g = 96p

Apply ½-inch of gel with gentle massage not more often than every 3 hours; CHILD over 4 months ¼-inch of gel not more often than every 3 hours; max. 6 applications daily

Salicylic acid
Pyralvex® (Norgine)

Oral paint, brown, rhubarb extract (anthraquinone glycosides 0.5%), salicylic acid 1%. Net price 10 mL with brush = £1.41

Apply 3–4 times daily; CHILD under 12 years not recommended

TETRACYCLINE

Indications: severe recurrent aphthous ulceration; oral herpes (section 12.3.2)
Side-effects: fungal superinfection
For side-effects, cautions and contra-indications relating to systemic administration of tetracyclines see section 5.1.3

Local application
For preparation of a mouthwash, the contents of a 250-mg tetracycline capsule (see section 5.1.3) can be stirred

into a small amount of water, then held in the mouth for 2–3 minutes 3-4 times daily usually for 3 days; longer courses are sometimes used (but precautions may be required to avoid oral thrush); it should preferably not be swallowed [unlicensed indication]

Note. Tetracycline stains teeth; avoid in children under 12 years of age

The following list includes topical treatments for mouth ulcers on sale to the public, together with their significant ingredients:

Adcortyl® in **Orabase**® for Mouth Ulcers (triamcinolone acetonide), **Anbesol**® (cetylpyridinium, chlorocresol, lignocaine), **Bansor**® (cetrimide), **Bioral Gel**® (carbenoxolone), **Bonjela gel**® (choline salicylate), **Bonjela pastilles**® (aminacrine, lignocaine), **Frador**® (chlorbutol, menthol), **Medijel**® (aminacrine, lignocaine), **Oragard**® (cetylpyridinium, lignocaine), **Pyralvex**® (anthraquinone glycoside, salicylic acid), **Rinstead gel**® (benzocaine, chloroxylenol), **Rinstead pastilles**® (chloroxylenol, menthol), **Teejel**® (choline salicylate), **Ulc-Aid gel**® (cetylpyridinium, lignocaine), **Ulc-Aid lozenges**® (benzocaine, cetylpyridinium, tyrothricin)

12.3.2 Oropharyngeal anti-infective drugs

The most common cause of a sore throat is a viral infection which does not benefit from anti-infective treatment. Streptococcal sore throats require systemic **penicillin** therapy (see section 5.1, table 1). Acute ulcerative gingivitis (Vincent's infection) responds to systemic **metronidazole** 200 mg 3 times daily for 3 days (see section 5.1.11).

Preparations administered in the dental surgery for the local treatment of periodontal disease include gels of metronidazole (*Elyzol*®, Dumex) and of minocycline (*Dentomycin*®, Lederle).

FUNGAL INFECTIONS

Candida albicans may cause thrush and other forms of stomatitis which are sometimes a sequel to the use of broad-spectrum antibiotics or cytotoxics; withdrawing the causative drug may lead to rapid resolution. Otherwise, an antifungal drug may be effective.

Of the antifungal drugs used for mouth infections, **amphotericin** and **nystatin** are not absorbed from the gastro-intestinal tract and are used by local application in the mouth. **Miconazole** occupies an intermediate position since it is used by local application in the mouth but is also absorbed to the extent that care is needed to take account of *potential interactions*. **Fluconazole** is absorbed when taken by mouth and is available for oral administration (see section 5.2).

AMPHOTERICIN

Indications: oral and perioral fungal infections
Side-effects: mild gastro-intestinal disturbances reported

PoM Fungilin® (Squibb)

Lozenges, yellow, amphotericin 10 mg. Net price 60-lozenge pack = £3.95. Label: 9, 24, counselling, after food

Dissolve 1 lozenge slowly in the mouth 4 times daily, may require 10–15 days' treatment (continued for 48 hours after lesions have resolved); increase to 8 daily if infection severe

Oral suspension, yellow, sugar-free, amphotericin 100 mg/mL. Net price 12 mL with pipette = £2.31. Label: 9, counselling, use of pipette, hold in mouth, after food

Place 1 mL in the mouth after food and retain near lesions 4 times daily for 14 days (continued for 48 hours after lesions have resolved)

MICONAZOLE

Indications: oral fungal infections

Cautions: pregnancy; avoid in porphyria (see section 9.8.2); **interactions:** Appendix 1 (antifungals, imidazole and triazole)

Side-effects: mild gastro-intestinal disturbances reported

PoM ¹Daktarin® (Janssen)

Oral gel, sugar-free, miconazole 25 mg/mL. Net price 15-g tube = £2.04, 80-g tube = £5.00. Label: 9, counselling, hold in mouth, after food

Place 5–10 mL in the mouth after food and retain near lesions 4 times daily; CHILD under 2 years 2.5 mL twice daily, 2–6 years 5 mL twice daily, over 6 years 5 mL 4 times daily

Localised lesions, smear small amount of gel on affected area with clean finger

1. 15-g tube can be sold to the public

Tablets—see section 5.2

PoM Dumicoat® (Dumex)

Denture lacquer, miconazole 50 mg/g. Net price pack of 3 × 1-g bottles (with brushes and cleansing tissues) = £13.50. Label: 10 patient information leaflet

Candida-associated denture stomatitis, apply contents of 1 bottle to upper surface of upper denture after thorough cleansing, allow to dry, and replace; repeat twice at intervals of 1 week

NYSTATIN

Indications: oral and perioral fungal infections

Side-effects: oral irritation and sensitisation, nausea reported; see also section 5.2

Dose: (as pastilles or as suspension) 100 000 units 4 times daily after food, usually for 7 days (continued for 48 hours after lesions have resolved)

Note. Immunosuppressed patients may require higher doses (e.g. 500 000 units 4 times daily)

PoM Nystatin (Non-proprietary)

Oral suspension, nystatin 100 000 units/mL. Net price 30 mL = £2.00. Label: 9, counselling, hold in mouth, after food

Available from Lagap, Rosemont (Nystamont®, sugar-free)

PoM Nystan® (Squibb)

Pastilles, yellow/brown, nystatin 100 000 units. Net price 28-pastille pack = £3.24. Label: 9, 24, counselling, after food

Oral suspension, yellow, nystatin 100 000 units/mL. Net price 30 mL with pipette = £2.05. Label: 9, counselling, use of pipette, hold in mouth, after food

Oral suspension (sugar-free), nystatin 100 000 units/mL when reconstituted with water. Net price 24 mL with pipette = £1.67. Label: 9, counselling, use of pipette, hold in mouth, after food

VIRAL INFECTIONS

The management of herpes infections of the mouth is a soft diet, adequate fluid intake, analgesics as required, and the use of **chlorhexidine** mouthwash (section 12.3.4) to control plaque accumulation if toothbrushing is painful. In the case of severe herpetic stomatitis, systemic **aciclovir** is required (see section 5.3).

Herpes infections of the mouth may also respond to **tetracycline** (section 12.3.1) rinsed in the mouth.

Idoxuridine 0.1% paint has been superseded by more effective preparations.

ACICLOVIR
See section 5.3

TETRACYCLINE
Section 12.3.1

12.3.3 Lozenges and sprays

There is no convincing evidence that antiseptic lozenges and sprays have a beneficial action and they sometimes irritate and cause sore tongue and sore lips. Some of these preparations also contain local anaesthetics which relieve pain but may cause sensitisation.

The following list includes throat lozenges and sprays on sale to the public, together with their significant ingredients.

AAA® (benzocaine), **Bradosol®** (benzalkonium), **Bradosol Plus®** (domiphen, lignocaine), **Dequacaine®** (benzocaine, dequalinium), **Dequadin®** (dequalinium), **Eludril®** spray (amethocaine, chlorhexidine), **Famel®** pastilles (creosote, menthol), **Labosept®** (dequalinium), **Meggezones®** (menthol), **Mentholatum®** lozenges (amylmetacresol, menthol), **Merocaine®** (benzocaine, cetylpyridinium), **Merocets®** lozenges (cetylpyridinium), **Merothol®** lozenges (cetylpyridinium, menthol), **Strepsils®** (amylmetacresol, dichlorobenzyl alcohol), **Strepsils Dual Action®**(amylmetacresol, dichlorobenzyl alcohol, lignocaine), **TCP®** pastilles (phenols), **Tyrocane®** (benzocaine, cetylpyridinium, tyrothricin), **Tyrocane Junior®** (cetylpyridinium), **Tyrozets®** (benzocaine, tyrothricin), **Valda®** (menthol, thymol), **Vicks Ultra Chloraseptic®** (benzocaine)

12.3.4 Mouthwashes, gargles, and dentifrices

Mouthwashes have a mechanical cleansing action and freshen the mouth. Warm **compound sodium chloride mouthwash** or **compound thymol glycerin** is as useful as any.

Mouthwashes containing an oxidising agent, such as **hydrogen peroxide**, may be useful in the treatment of acute ulcerative gingivitis (Vincent's infection) as the organisms involved are anaerobes. It also has a mechanical cleansing effect due to frothing when in contact with oral debris. **Sodium perborate** is similar in effect to hydrogen peroxide.

There is evidence that **chlorhexidine** has a specific effect in inhibiting the formation of plaque on teeth. A chlorhexidine mouthwash may be useful as an adjunct to other oral hygiene measures in cases of oral infection or when toothbrushing is not possible.

There is no convincing evidence that gargles are effective.

CETYLPYRIDINIUM CHLORIDE

Indications: oral hygiene

Merocet® (Merrell)

Solution (= mouthwash or gargle), yellow, cetylpyridinium chloride 0.05%. Net price 200 mL = £1.72

To be used undiluted or diluted with an equal volume of warm water

CHLORHEXIDINE GLUCONATE

Indications: oral hygiene; plaque inhibition
Side-effects: idiosyncratic mucosal irritation; reversible brown staining of teeth

Chlorohex 2000® (Colgate-Palmolive)

Mouthwash, chlorhexidine gluconate 0.2% (mint-flavoured). Net price 300 mL = £2.20

Rinse the mouth with 10 mL for about 1 minute twice daily

Corsodyl® (SmithKline Beecham Healthcare)

Dental gel, chlorhexidine gluconate 1%. Net price 50 g = £1.10

Brush on the teeth once or twice daily

Mouthwash, chlorhexidine gluconate 0.2% (aniseed or mint-flavoured). Net price 300 mL = £1.67

Rinse the mouth with 10 mL for about 1 minute twice daily

Oral spray, chlorhexidine gluconate 0.2% (mint-flavoured). Net price 60 mL = £3.39

Apply as required to tooth and gingival surfaces using up to max. 12 actuations (approx. 0.14 mL/actutation) twice daily

Eludril® (Chefaro)

Mouthwash, chlorhexidine gluconate 0.1%, chlorbutol 0.5%. Net price 90 mL = £1.16; 250 mL = £2.35; 500 mL = £4.14

Use 10–15 mL in a third of a tumblerful of warm water 2–3 times daily

HEXETIDINE

Indications: oral hygiene

Oraldene® (Warner Wellcome)

Mouthwash or *gargle*, red, hexetidine 0.1%. Net price 100 mL = £1.13; 200 mL = £1.78

Use 15 mL undiluted 2–3 times daily

OXIDISING AGENTS

Indications: oral hygiene, see notes above

Hydrogen Peroxide Mouthwash, DPF, consists of Hydrogen Peroxide Solution 6% (≡approx. 20 volume) BP

Rinse the mouth for 2–3 minutes with 15 mL in half a tumblerful of warm water 2–3 times daily

Bocasan® (Oral B Labs)

Mouthwash, sodium perborate 68.6% (buffered). Net price 20 × 1.7-g sachet-pack = £1.75

Use 1 sachet in 30 mL of water 3 times daily after meals

Cautions: Do not use for longer than 7 days because of possible absorption of borate; not recommended in renal impairment or for children under 5 years

POVIDONE-IODINE

Indications: oral hygiene
Cautions: pregnancy; breast-feeding
Contra-indications: avoid regular use in patients with thyroid disorders or those receiving lithium therapy
Side-effects: idiosyncratic mucosal irritation and hypersensitivity reactions; may interfere with thyroid-function tests and with tests for occult blood

Betadine® (Seton)

Mouthwash or *gargle*, amber, povidone-iodine 1%. Net price 250 mL = £1.17

Adults and children over 6 years, up to 10 mL undiluted or diluted with an equal quantity of warm water for up to 30 seconds up to 4 times daily for up to 14 days

SODIUM CHLORIDE

Indications: oral hygiene, see notes above

Sodium Chloride Mouthwash, Compound, BP

Mouthwash, sodium bicarbonate 1%, sodium chloride 1.5% in a suitable vehicle with a peppermint flavour.

Extemporaneous preparations should be prepared according to the following formula: sodium chloride 1.5 g, sodium bicarbonate 1 g, concentrated peppermint emulsion 2.5 mL, double-strength chloroform water 50 mL, water to 100 mL.

To be diluted with an equal volume of warm water

THYMOL

Indications: oral hygiene, see notes above

Compound Thymol Glycerin, BP 1988, glycerol 10%, thymol 0.05% with colouring and flavouring

To be used undiluted or diluted with 3 volumes of warm water

Mouthwash Solution-tablets, consist of tablets which may contain antimicrobial, colouring, and flavouring agents in a suitable soluble effervescent basis to make a mouthwash suitable for dental purposes.

Dissolve 1 tablet in a tumblerful of warm water

12.3.5   Treatment of dry mouth

Xerostomia (dry mouth) may be caused by irradiation of the head and neck region, damage to or disease of the salivary glands, or by the administration of drugs with antimuscarinic (anticholinergic) side-effects (e.g. antispasmodics, tricyclic antidepressants, and some antipsychotics). Dry mouth may be relieved in many patients by simple measures such as frequent sips of cool drinks or sucking pieces of ice or sugar-free fruit pastilles.

An **artificial saliva** can provide useful relief of dry mouth. A properly balanced artificial saliva should be of a neutral pH and contain electrolytes (including fluoride) to correspond approximately to the composition of saliva. Of the proprietary preparations available, *Luborant®* is licensed for any condition giving rise to a dry mouth; *Saliva Orthana®*, *Salivace®*, *Saliveze®* and *Glandosane®* have ACBS approval for dry mouth associated only with radiotherapy or sicca syndrome. *Salivix®* pastilles, which act locally as salivary stimulants, are also available and have similar ACBS approval.

Pilocarpine tablets have been introduced recently, and are restricted to use in xerostomia following irradiation for head and neck cancer. They are effective only in patients who have some residual salivary gland function, and therefore should be withdrawn if there is no response.

LOCAL TREATMENT

Glandosane® (Fresenius)
Aerosol spray, carmellose sodium 500 mg, sorbitol 1.5 g, potassium chloride 60 mg, sodium chloride 42.2 mg, magnesium chloride 2.6 mg, calcium chloride 7.3 mg, and dipotassium hydrogen phosphate 17.1 mg/50 g. Net price 50-mL unit (neutral, lemon or peppermint flavoured) = £3.95
ACBS: patients suffering from dry mouth as a result of having (or having undergone) radiotherapy, or sicca syndrome, spray onto oral and pharyngeal mucosa as required

Luborant® (Antigen)
Oral spray, pink, sorbitol 1.8 g, carmellose sodium (sodium carboxymethylcellulose) 390 mg, dibasic potassium phosphate 48.23 mg, potassium chloride 37.5 mg, monobasic potassium phosphate 21.97 mg, calcium chloride 9.972 mg, magnesium chloride 3.528 mg, sodium fluoride 258 micrograms/60 mL, with preservatives and colouring agents. Net price 60-mL unit = £3.96
Saliva deficiency, 2–3 sprays onto oral mucosa up to 4 times daily, or as directed

Saliva Orthana® (Nycomed)
Oral spray, gastric mucin 3.5%, xylitol 2%, sodium fluoride 4.2 mg/litre, with preservatives and flavouring agents. Net price 50-mL bottle = £3.80; 450-mL refill = £25.10
Lozenges, mucin 65 mg, xylitol 59 mg, in a sorbitol basis. Net price 45-lozenge pack = £2.75
ACBS: patients suffering from dry mouth as a result of having (or having undergone) radiotherapy, or sicca syndrome, spray 2–3 times onto oral and pharyngeal mucosa, when required
Note. Saliva Orthana® lozenges do not contain fluoride

Salivace® (Penn)
Oral spray, carmellose sodium (sodium carboxymethylcellulose), xylitol, calcium chloride, dibasic potassium phosphate, sodium chloride, potassium chloride, and methyl hydroxybenzoate. Net price 100 mL = £4.95
ACBS: patients suffering from dry mouth as a result of having (or having undergone) radiotherapy, or sicca syndrome, 1–2 sprays onto oral mucosa as required

Saliveze® (Wyvern)
Oral spray, carmellose sodium (sodium carboxymethylcellulose), calcium chloride, magnesium chloride, potassium chloride, sodium chloride, and dibasic sodium phosphate. Net price 50-mL bottle (mint-flavoured) = £3.50
ACBS: patients suffering from dry mouth as a result of having (or having undergone) radiotherapy or sicca syndrome, 1 spray onto oral mucosa as required

Salivix® (Thames)
Pastilles, sugar-free, reddish-amber, acacia, malic acid and other ingredients. Net price 50-pastille pack = £2.65
ACBS: patients suffering from dry mouth as a result of having (or having undergone) radiotherapy, or sicca syndrome, suck 1 pastille when required

SYSTEMIC TREATMENT

PILOCARPINE HYDROCHLORIDE
Indications: alleviation of symptoms of salivary gland hypofunction in xerostomia following irradiation for head and neck cancer (see also notes above)
Cautions: close medical supervision in asthma (avoid if uncontrolled, see Contra-indications) and in cardiovascular disease; cholelithiasis or biliary tract disease, peptic ulcer, hepatic impairment (reduce initial dose), renal impairment; risk of increased urethral smooth muscle tone and renal colic; eye examinations before treatment (decreased visual acuity more likely at night and in patients with central lens changes); maintain adequate fluid intake to avoid dehydration associated with excessive sweating; cognitive or psychiatric disturbances; **interactions:** Appendix 1 (parasympathomimetics)
COUNSELLING. Blurred vision may affect ability to drive, particularly at night, and to perform hazardous activities in reduced lighting
Contra-indications: uncontrolled asthma and chronic obstructive airways disease (increased bronchial secretions and increased airways resistance); acute iritis, narrow-angle glaucoma; pregnancy and breast-feeding
Side-effects: sweating; also chills, diarrhoea, nausea, vomiting, lachrymation, abdominal pain, amblyopia, hypertension, constipation, abnormal vision (see Counselling), dizziness, rhinitis, asthenia, increased urinary frequency, headache, dyspepsia, vasodilatation, flushing; other possible side-effects include: respiratory distress, gastro-intestinal spasm, AV block, tachycardia, bradycardia, other arrhythmias, hypotension, shock, confusion, tremors
Dose: 5 mg 3 times daily with or immediately after meals (last dose always with evening meal); if dose tolerated but response not sufficient after 4-8 weeks, may be increased to max. 30 mg daily in divided doses (but associated with increased side-effects); discontinue if no improvement after 3 months; CHILD not recommended

▼ PoM **Salagen®** (Chiron)
Tablets, f/c, pilocarpine hydrochloride 5 mg. Net price 84-tab pack = £51.43. Label: 21, 27, counselling, driving

13: Drugs acting on the

SKIN

In this chapter, drug treatment is discussed under the following headings:

Suitable quantities of dermatological preparations to be prescribed for specific areas of the body are:

	Creams and Ointments	Lotions
Face	15 to 30g	100 mL
Both hands	25 to 50 g	200 mL
Scalp	50 to 100 g	200 mL
Both arms or both legs	100 to 200 g	200 mL
Trunk	400 g	500 mL
Groins and genitalia	15 to 25 g	100 mL

These amounts are usually suitable for an adult for twice daily application for 1 week. The recommendations do not apply to corticosteroid preparations—for suitable quantities of corticosteroid preparations see p. 460

ADDITIVES.The following additives in topical preparations may be associated with sensitisation, particularly of eczematous skin. Details of whether they are contained in preparations listed in the BNF are given after the preparation entry.

Most commonly	Less commonly	Rarely[2]
Wool fat and related substances[1]	Benzyl alcohol	Beeswax
Chlorocresol	Butylated hydroxyanisole	Edetic acid (EDTA)
Ethylenediamine	Butylated hydroxytoluene	Isopropyl palmitate
Fragrances	Hydroxybenz-oates (parabens)	
	Polysorbates	
	Propylene glycol	
	Sorbic acid	

1. Purified versions of wool fat have reduced the problem, but it remains significant
2. Non-dermatologists can reasonably disregard the substances in this category

13.1   Vehicles

Both vehicle and active ingredients are important in the treatment of skin conditions; it is being increasingly recognised that the vehicle alone may have more than a mere placebo effect. The vehicle affects the degree of hydration of the skin, has a mild anti-inflammatory effect, and aids the penetration of active drug in the preparation.

The vehicle may take the form of an *application, collodion, cream, dusting powder, lotion, ointment,* or *paste*:

Applications are usually viscous solutions, emulsions, or suspensions for application to the skin.

Collodions are painted on the skin and allowed to dry to leave a flexible film over the site of application.

Creams are emulsions of oil and water and are generally well absorbed into the skin. They may contain an antimicrobial preservative unless the active ingredient or basis has sufficient intrinsic bactericidal or fungicidal activity. Generally, creams are cosmetically more acceptable than ointments as they are less greasy and easier to apply.

Dusting powders are finely divided powders that contain one or more active ingredients with or without auxiliary substances. They are intended to be applied to skin for therapeutic, prophylactic or lubricant purposes. Dusting powder intended for large open wounds or severely injured skin should be sterile.

Lotions have a cooling effect and may be preferred to ointments or creams when it is intended to apply the preparation over a hairy area. *Shake lotions* (such as calamine lotion) containing insoluble powders and leave a deposit of inert powder on the skin surface.

Ointments are greasy preparations which are normally anhydrous and insoluble in water, and are more occlusive than creams. They are particularly suitable for chronic, dry lesions. The most commonly used ointment bases consist of soft paraffin or a combination of soft, liquid and hard paraffin. Some modern ointment bases have both *hydrophilic and lipophilic* properties; they may have occlusive properties on the skin surface, encourage hydration, and also be miscible with water; they often have a mild anti-inflammatory effect. *Water-soluble ointments* contain macrogols which are freely soluble in water and are therefore readily washed off; they have a limited but useful application in circumstances where ready removal is desirable.

Pastes are stiff preparations containing a high proportion of finely powdered solids such as zinc oxide and starch suspended in an ointment. They are used for circumscribed lesions such as those which occur in lichen simplex, chronic eczema, or psoriasis. They are less occlusive than ointments and can be used to protect inflamed, lichenified, or excoriated skin.

DILUTION. The BP directs that creams and ointments should **not** normally be diluted but that should dilution be necessary care should be taken, in particular, to prevent microbial contamination. The appropriate diluent should be used and heating should be avoided during mixing; excessive dilution may affect the stability of some creams. Diluted creams should normally be used within 2 weeks of their preparation.

13.2 Emollient and barrier preparations

13.2.1 Emollients
13.2.2 Barrier preparations
13.2.3 Dusting powders

BORDERLINE SUBSTANCES. The preparations marked 'ACBS' are regarded as drugs when prescribed in accordance with the advice of the Advisory Committee on Borderline Substances for the clinical conditions listed. Prescriptions issued in accordance with this advice and endorsed 'ACBS' will normally not be investigated. See Appendix 7 for listing by clinical condition.

13.2.1 Emollients

Emollients soothe, smooth and hydrate the skin and are indicated for all dry scaling disorders (such as ichthyosis). Their effects are short-lived and they should be applied frequently even after improvement occurs. They are useful in dry eczematous disorders, and to a lesser extent in psoriasis (section 13.5.2). Simple preparations such as **aqueous cream** are often as effective as the more complex proprietary formulations; in general, the choice depends on patient preference. Some ingredients may occasionally cause sensitisation, notably hydrous wool fat (lanolin) and this should be suspected if an eczematous reaction occurs.

Camphor, menthol, and phenol are intended to have a mild antipruritic effect when used in emollient preparations but there is no real evidence of efficacy. Calamine and zinc oxide may also be included as they are particularly useful in dry eczema. Thickening agents such as talc and kaolin may also be included. Preparations containing an antibacterial should be avoided unless infection is present (section 13.10).

Urea is employed as a hydrating agent. It is used in scaling conditions and may be useful in elderly patients. It is often used with other topical agents such as corticosteroids to enhance penetration.

Aqueous Cream, BP, emulsifying ointment 30%, phenoxyethanol 1% in freshly boiled and cooled purified water. Net price 100 g = 29p
Emulsifying Ointment, BP, emulsifying wax 30%, white soft paraffin 50%, liquid paraffin 20%. Net price 100 g = 31p
Hydrous Ointment, BP (oily cream), dried magnesium sulphate 0.5%, phenoxyethanol 1%, wool alcohols ointment 50%, in freshly boiled and cooled purified water. Net price 100 g = 39p
Paraffin, White Soft, BP (white petroleum jelly). Net price 100 g = 32p

Paraffin, Yellow Soft, BP (yellow petroleum jelly). Net price 100 g = 31p
Zinc Cream, BP, zinc oxide 32%, arachis (peanut) oil 32%, calcium hydroxide 0.045%, oleic acid 0.5%, wool fat 8%, in freshly boiled and cooled purified water. Net price 50 g = 24p
For napkin and urinary rash and eczematous conditions
Zinc Ointment, BP, zinc oxide 15%, in Simple Ointment BP 1988 (which contains wool fat 5%, hard paraffin 5%, cetostearyl alcohol 5%, white soft paraffin 85%. Net price 25 g = 13p
For napkin and urinary rash and eczematous conditions
Zinc and Castor Oil Ointment, BP, zinc oxide 7.5%, castor oil 50%, arachis (peanut) oil 30.5%, white beeswax 10%, cetostearyl alcohol 2%. Net price 25 g = 14p
For napkin and urinary rash
Alcoderm® (Novex)
Cream, containing liquid paraffin, cetyl alcohol, stearyl alcohol, sodium lauryl sulphate, carbomer, triethanolamine, sorbitan monostearate, sorbitol, spermaceti, silicone fluid. Net price 60 g = £2.40
For dry skin conditions
Additives: include hydroxybenzoates (parabens), isopropyl palmitate
Lotion, water-miscible, ingredients as above. Net price 120 mL = £2.86
For dry skin conditions
Aveeno® (Bioglan)
Cream, colloidal oatmeal, white oat fraction in emollient basis. Net price 100 mL = £3.43
ACBS: For endogenous and exogenous eczema, xeroderma, ichthyosis, and senile pruritus (pruritus of the elderly) associated with dry skin
Additives: include benzyl alcohol
Dermamist® (Yamanouchi)
Spray application, white soft paraffin 10% in a basis containing liquid paraffin, fractionated coconut oil. Net price 250-mL pressurised aerosol unit = £9.60
For dry skin conditions including eczema, ichthyosis, pruritus of the elderly
Caution: flammable
Additives: none as listed in section 13.1
Diprobase® (Schering-Plough)
Cream, cetomacrogol 2.25%, cetostearyl alcohol 7.2%, liquid paraffin 6%, white soft paraffin 15%, water-miscible basis used for Diprosone® cream. Net price 50 g = £1.61; 500-g dispenser = £6.92
For dry skin conditions
Additives: include chlorocresol
Ointment, liquid paraffin 5%, white soft paraffin 95%, basis used for Diprosone® ointment. Net price 50 g = £1.61
For dry skin conditions
Additives: none as listed in section 13.1
Dermalex® —section 13.10.5
Drapolene® —section 13.2.2
E45® (Crookes)
Cream, light liquid paraffin 12.6%, white soft paraffin 14.5%, hypoallergenic hydrous wool fat (hypoallergenic lanolin) 1% in self-emulsifying monostearin. Net price 50 g = £1.12; 125 g = £2.27; 500 g = £5.33
For dry skin conditions
Additives: include hydroxybenzoates (parabens)
Wash E45, soap substitute, zinc oxide 5% in an emollient basis. Net price 150 mL = £2.35
ACBS: for endogenous and exogenous eczema, xeroderma, ichthyosis and senile pruritus (pruritus of the elderly) associated with dry skin
Additives: include butylated hydroxytoluene

Hewletts Cream® (Kestrel)

Cream, hydrous wool fat 4%, zinc oxide 8%, arachis (peanut) oil, oleic acid, white soft paraffin. Net price 35 g = £1.19; 400 g = £4.85

For nursing hygiene and care of skin, and chapped hands
Additives: include fragrance

Humiderm® (ConvaTec)

Cream, pyrrolidone carboxylic acid 5% (as sodium salt). Net price 60 g = £3.71

For dry skin conditions
Additives: include hydroxybenzoates (parabens), propylene glycol

Hydromol® (Quinoderm Ltd)

Cream, arachis (peanut) oil 10%, isopropyl myristate 5%, liquid paraffin 10%, sodium pyrrolidone carboxylate 2.5%, sodium lactate 1%. Net price 50 g = £2.04; 100 g = £3.40; 500 g = £10.94.

For dry skin conditions
Additives: include hydroxybenzoates (parabens)

Kamillosan® (Norgine)

Ointment, chamomile extracts 10.5% in a basis containing wool fat. Net price 30 g = £1.50; 1.5 g sachets (hosp. only)

For napkin rash, sore nipples and chapped hands
Additives: include beeswax, hydroxybenzoates (parabens)

Keri® (Bristol-Myers)

Lotion, mineral oil 16%, with lanolin oil. Net price 190-mL pump pack = £3.56; 380-mL pump pack = £5.81.

For dry skin conditions and napkin rash
Additives: include hydroxybenzoates (parabens), propylene glycol, fragrance

Lacticare® (Stiefel)

Lotion, lactic acid 5%, sodium pyrrolidone carboxylate 2.5%. Net price 150 mL = £3.19.

For dry skin conditions
Additives: include isopropyl palmitate, fragrance

Lipobase® (Yamanouchi)

Cream, fatty cream basis used for Locoid Lipocream®. Net price 50 g = £2.05
Additives: include hydroxybenzoates (parabens)

Massé Breast Cream® (Cilag)

Cream (water-miscible), containing arachis (peanut) oil, cetyl alcohol, glycerol, glyceryl monostearate, wool fat, polysorbate 60, potassium hydroxide, sorbitan monostearate, stearic acid. Net price 28 g = £1.40.

For pre- and post-natal nipple care
Caution: contains arachis (peanut) oil which might expose infant to potential allergens
Additives: include hydroxybenzoates (parabens)

Morhulin® (Seton)

Ointment, cod-liver oil 11.4%, zinc oxide 38%, in a basis containing wool fat and paraffin. Net price 50 g = £1.02; 350 g = £4.90.

For minor wounds, varicose ulcers, and pressure sores
Additives: include wool fat derivative

Neutrogena® Dermatological Cream (Neutrogena)

Cream, glycerol 40% in an emollient basis. Net price 100 g = £3.67.

For dry skin conditions
Additives: include hydroxybenzoates (parabens)

Oilatum® (Stiefel)

Cream, arachis (peanut) oil 21%. Net price 40 g = £1.79; 80 g = £2.78

For dry skin conditions
Additives: include fragrance

Shower emollient (gel), light liquid paraffin 70%. Net price 65 g = £2.52; 125 g = £4.84

For dry skin conditions including dermatitis
Additives: include fragrance

Sudocrem® (Tosara)

Cream, benzyl alcohol 0.39%, benzyl benzoate 1.01%, benzyl cinnamate 0.15%, wool fat 4%, zinc oxide 15.25%. Net price 30 g = 74p; 60 g = 80p; 125 g = £1.33; 250 g = £2.38; 400 g = £3.48.

For napkin rash and pressure sores
Additives: include beeswax (synthetic), polysorbates, propylene glycol, fragrance

Ultrabase® (Schering Health)

Cream, water-miscible, containing liquid paraffin and white soft paraffin. Net price 50 g = £1.05; 500-g dispenser = £6.89.

For dry skin conditions
Additives: include hydroxybenzoates (parabens), disodium edetate, fragrance

Unguentum Merck® (Merck)

Cream (hydrophilic and lipophilic), cetostearyl alcohol, glyceryl monostearate, saturated neutral oil, liquid paraffin, white soft paraffin, propylene glycol, polysorbate '40', silicic acid, sorbic acid. Net price 50 g = £1.59; 100 g = £3.13; 200 mL dispenser = £6.19; 500 g = £9.55.

For dry skin conditions and napkin rash

Vaseline Dermacare® (Elida Gibbs)

Cream, dimethicone 1%, white soft paraffin 15%. Net price 150 mL = £2.11

ACBS: for endogenous and exogenous eczema, xeroderma, ichthyosis and senile pruritus (pruritus of the elderly) associated with dry skin
Additives: include hydroxybenzoates (parabens)

Lotion, dimethicone 1%, liquid paraffin 4%, white soft paraffin 5% in an emollient basis. Net price 75 mL = £1.18; 200 mL = £2.29

ACBS: as for Vaseline Dermacare® Cream
Additives: include disodium edetate, hydroxybenzoates (parabens), wool fat

Preparations containing urea

Aquadrate® (Procter & Gamble Pharm.)

Cream, urea 10%. Net price 30 g = £1.59; 100 g = £4.79

For dry scaling and itching skin, apply thinly and rub into area when required
Additives: none as listed in section 13.1

Calmurid® (Novex)

Cream, urea 10%, lactic acid 5%. Diluent aqueous cream, life of diluted cream 14 days. Net price 100 g = £4.75; 500-g dispenser = £21.48

For dry, scaling and itching skin, apply a thick layer for 3–5 minutes, massage into area, and remove excess, usually twice daily. Use half-strength cream for 1 week if stinging occurs
Additives: none as listed in section 13.1

Nutraplus® (Novex)

Cream, urea 10%. Net price 60 g = £2.62

For dry scaling and itching skin, apply 2–3 times daily
Additives: include hydroxybenzoates (parabens), propylene glycol

13.2.1.1 EMOLLIENT BATH ADDITIVES

Alpha Keri Bath® (Bristol-Myers)

Bath oil, liquid paraffin 91.7%, oil-soluble fraction of wool fat 3%. Net price 240 mL = £3.45; 480 mL = £6.43

For dry skin conditions including ichthyosis and pruritus of the elderly, add 10–20 mL /bath (infants 5 mL)
Additives: include fragrance

Aveeno® (Bioglan)

Aveeno® Bath oil, colloidal oatmeal, white oat fraction in emollient basis. Net price 250 mL = £3.66

ACBS: for endogenous and exogenous eczema, xeroderma, ichthyosis, and senile pruritus (pruritus of the elderly) associated with dry skin
Additives: include beeswax, fragrance

Aveeno Oilated® *Bath additive*, oatmeal, white oat fraction in emollient basis. Net price 10 × 50-g sachets = £6.30

ACBS: as for Aveeno® Bath oil; add 1 sachet/bath (infants half sachet)

Additives: none as listed in section 13.1

Aveeno Regular® *Bath additive*, oatmeal, white oat fraction in emollient basis. Net price 10 × 50-g sachets = £6.30

ACBS: as for Aveeno® Bath oil; add 1 sachet/bath (infants half sachet)

Additives: none as listed in section 13.1

Balneum® (Merck)

Balneum® *bath oil*, soya oil 84.75%. Net price 200 mL = £2.79; 500 mL = £6.06; 1 litre = £11.70

For dry skin conditions including those associated with dermatitis and eczema; add 20 mL/bath (infant 5mL)

Additives: include butylated hydroxytoluene, propylene glycol, fragrance

Balneum Plus® *bath oil*, soya oil 82.95%, mixed lauromacrogols 15%. Net price 500 mL = £8.33

For dry skin conditions including those associated with dermatitis and eczema where pruritus also experienced; add 20 mL/bath (infant 5 mL)

Additives: include butylated hydroxytoluene, propylene glycol, fragrance

Balneum with Tar®—section 13.5.2

Bath E45® (Crookes)

Bath oil, cetyl dimethicone 5%. Net price 150 mL = £2.35

ACBS: for endogenous and exogenous eczema, xeroderma, ichthyosis, and senile pruritus (pruritus of the elderly) associated with dry skin; add 15 mL/bath

Additives: include butylated hydroxyanisole

Diprobath® (Schering-Plough)

Bath additive, isopropyl myristate 39%, light liquid paraffin 46%. Net price 500 mL = £7.50

For dry skin conditions including dermatitis and eczema; add 25 mL/bath (infant 10 mL)

Additives: none as listed in section 13.1

Emmolate® (Bio-Medical)

Bath oil, acetylated wool alcohols 5%, liquid paraffin 65%. Net price 200 mL = £2.25

For contact dermatitis, dry skin conditions including ichthyosis and pruritus of the elderly; add 15–20 mL/ bath (infant and child 5–10 mL)

Additives: none as listed in section 13.1

Emulsiderm® (Dermal)

Liquid emulsion, liquid paraffin 25%, isopropyl myristate 25%, benzalkonium chloride 0.5%. Net price 300 mL (with 15-mL measure) = £4.33; 1 litre (with 30-mL measure) = £12.73

For dry skin conditions including eczema and ichthyosis; add 7–30 mL/bath

Additives: include polysorbate 60

Hydromol Emollient® (Quinoderm Ltd)

Bath additive, isopropyl myristate 13%, light liquid paraffin 37.8%. Net price 150 mL = £1.64; 350 mL = £3.06; 1 litre = £7.09

For dry skin conditions including eczema, ichthyosis and pruritus of the elderly; add 1–3 capfuls/bath (infant ½–2 capfuls)

Additives: none as listed in section 13.1

Oilatum® (Stiefel)

Oilatum Emollient® *bath additive* (emulsion), acetylated wool alcohols 5%, liquid paraffin 63.4%. Net price 250 mL = £2.75; 500 mL = £4.57

For dry skin conditions including dermatitis, pruritus of the elderly and ichthyosis; add 5–15 mL/bath (infant 2.5–10 mL)

Additives: include isopropyl palmitate, fragrance

Oilatum Plus® *bath additive*, benzalkonium chloride 6%, triclosan 2%, light liquid paraffin 52.5%. Net price 500 mL = £7.86

For topical treatment of eczema including eczema at risk from infection; add 1–2 capfuls/bath (infant over 6 months 1 mL)

Additives: include wool fat, isopropyl palmitate

13.2.2   Barrier preparations

Barrier preparations often contain water-repellent substances such as **dimethicone** or other silicones. They are used for areas around stomata (see also Appendix 9), sore areas in the elderly, bedsores, etc. They are no substitute for adequate nursing care, and it is doubtful if they are any more effective than the traditional compound **zinc ointments**.

NAPKIN RASH. Barrier creams and ointments are used to give protection against napkin rash which is usually a local dermatitis. The first line of treatment is to ensure that napkins are changed frequently, and that tightly fitting plastic pants are avoided. The rash may clear when left exposed to the air and a napkin rash preparation (see preparations below) may be helpful. If the rash is associated with a fungal infection, an antifungal cream such as clotrimazole cream (see section 13.10.2) is useful. A mild corticosteroid such as hydrocortisone may be useful but treatment should be limited to a week or less and it should be remembered that napkins and plastic pants may act as an occlusive dressing and increase absorption (for cautions, see hydrocortisone p. 461).

Conotrane® (Yamanouchi)

Cream, benzalkonium chloride 0.1%, dimethicone '350' 22%. Net price 100 g = 99p; 500 g = £3.74

For napkin and urinary rash and pressure sores

Additives: include fragrance

Drapolene® (Warner Wellcome)

Cream, benzalkonium chloride 0.01%, cetrimide 0.2% in a water-miscible basis. Net price 75 g = 98p; 150 g = £1.60; 350 g = £3.57; 500 g = £4.99

For napkin and urinary rash; minor wounds

Additives: include chlorocresol, wool fat

Metanium® (Roche)

Ointment, titanium dioxide 20%, titanium peroxide 5%, titanium salicylate 3%, titanium tannate 0.1%, in a silicone basis. Net price 25 g = £1.19

For napkin rash and related disorders

Additives: none as listed in section 13.1

Siopel® (Zeneca)

Barrier cream, dimethicone '1000' 10%, cetrimide 0.3%. Net price 50 g = 62p

For dermatoses, colostomy and ileostomy care, urinary rash, and related conditions

Additives: include butylated hydroxytoluene, hydroxybenzoates (parabens)

Sprilon® (Perstorp)

Spray application, dimethicone 1.04%, zinc oxide 12.5%, in a basis containing wool fat, wool alcohols, cetostearyl alcohol, dextran, white soft paraffin, liquid paraffin, propellants. Net price 115-g pressurised aerosol unit = £3.71

For urinary rash, pressure sores, and ileostomy

Caution: flammable

Vasogen® (Pharmax)

Barrier cream, dimethicone 20%, calamine 1.5%, zinc oxide 7.5%. Net price 50 g= 70p; 100 g = £1.20
For napkin and urinary rash, pressure sores, and pruritus ani

Additives: include hydroxybenzoates (parabens), wool fat

13.2.3 Dusting powders

Dusting powders are used in folds where friction may occur between opposing skin surfaces. They should not be applied in areas that are very moist as they tend to cake and abrade the skin. **Talc** acts as a lubricant powder but does not absorb moisture whereas **starch** is less lubricant but absorbs water. Other inert powders such as kaolin or zinc oxide may also be used in the formulation of dusting powders. See also section 13.11 for antiseptic dusting powders.

Talc Dusting Powder, BP, starch 10% in sterilised purified talc. Net price 100 g = 42p

Zinc, Starch and Talc Dusting-powder, BPC, zinc oxide 25%, starch 25%, sterilised purified talc 50%. Net price 50 g = 22p

ZeaSORB® (Stiefel)

Dusting powder, aldioxa 0.2%, chloroxylenol 0.5%, pulverised maize core 45%. Net price 50 g = £2.15
Additives: include fragrance

13.3 Topical local anaesthetics and antipruritics

Pruritus may be caused by systemic disease (such as drug hypersensitivity, obstructive jaundice, endocrine disease, and certain malignant diseases) as well as by skin disease (e.g. psoriasis, eczema, urticaria, and scabies). Where possible the underlying causes should be treated. There is no really effective topical antipruritic. **Calamine** preparations are widely prescribed for pruritus, and **emollient** preparations (section 13.2.1) may also be of value. **Crotamiton** does not appear to be any more effective than calamine. An emollient may be of value where the pruritus is associated with dry skin which is common in otherwise healthy elderly people).

Insect stings are also best treated with calamine preparations. Topical antihistamines and local anaesthetics may very occasionally cause sensitisation and are only marginally effective.

For preparations used in *pruritus ani,* see section 1.7.1.

CALAMINE

Indications: pruritus

Calamine Cream, Aqueous, BP, calamine 4%, zinc oxide 3%, liquid paraffin 20%, self-emulsifying glyceryl monostearate 5%, cetomacrogol emulsifying wax 5%, phenoxyethanol 0.5%, freshly boiled and cooled purified water 62.5%. Net price 100 mL = 52p

Calamine Lotion, BP, calamine 15%, zinc oxide 5%, glycerol 5%, bentonite 3%, sodium citrate 0.5%, liquefied phenol 0.5%, in freshly boiled and cooled purified water. Net price 200 mL = 62p

Calamine Lotion, Oily, BP1980, calamine 5%, arachis (peanut) oil 50%, oleic acid 0.5%, wool fat 1%, in calcium hydroxide solution. Net price 200 mL = 98p

CROTAMITON

Indications: pruritus (including pruritus after scabies), but see notes above
Cautions: avoid use near eyes and broken skin
Contra-indications: acute exudative dermatoses

Eurax® (Zyma)

Cream, crotamiton 10%. Net price 30 g = £1.91; 100 g = £3.25
Additives: include beeswax, hydroxybenzoates (parabens), fragrance

Lotion, crotamiton 10%. Net price 100 mL = £2.46
Additives: include propylene glycol, sorbic acid, fragrance

TOPICAL LOCAL ANAESTHETICS

Indications: relief of local pain, see notes above. See section 15.2 for use in surface anaesthesia
Cautions: occasionally cause hypersensitivity
Note. Topical local anaesthetic preparations may be absorbed, especially through mucosal surfaces, therefore excessive application should be avoided and they should preferably not be used for more than about 3 days; not generally suitable for young children

The following is a list of topical local anaesthetic preparations on sale to the public, together with their significant ingredients:
Anethaine® (amethocaine), **BurnEze®** (benzocaine), **Dermidex®** (lignocaine, alcloxa, cetrimide, chlorbutol), **Lanacane® cream** (benzocaine, chlorothymol, resorcinol), **Lanasting®** (lignocaine, benzyl alcohol), **Solarcaine®** (benzocaine, triclosan), **Wasp–Eze® spray** (benzocaine, mepyramine)

TOPICAL ANTIHISTAMINES

Indications: see notes above
Cautions: may cause hypersensitivity; avoid in eczema; photosensitivity (diphenhydramine); not recommended for longer than 3 days

The following is a list of topical antihistamine preparations on sale to the public, together with their significant ingredients:
Aller–Eze® cream (diphenhydramine), **Anthisan®** (mepyramine), **Caladryl®** (diphenhydramine, calamine, camphor), **R.B.C.®** (antazoline, calamine, camphor, cetrimide, menthol), **Wasp–Eze® ointment** (antazoline), **Wasp–Eze® spray** (mepyramine, benzocaine)

13.4 Topical corticosteroids

Topical corticosteroids are used for the treatment of inflammatory conditions of the skin other than those due to an infection, in particular the *eczematous disorders* (for further details see p. 466). Corticosteroids suppress various components of the inflammatory reaction while in use; they are in no sense curative, and when treatment is discontinued a rebound exacerbation of the condition may occur. They are indicated for the relief of symptoms and for the suppression of signs of the disorder when potentially less harmful measures are ineffective.

Topical corticosteroids are of no value in the treatment of *urticaria* and are **contra-indicated** in *rosacea* and in *ulcerative conditions* as they worsen the condition. They should not be used indiscriminately in *pruritus* (where they act by alleviating inflammation) and are **not** recommended for *acne vulgaris*.

Systemic or potent topical corticosteroids should be avoided or given only under specialist supervision *in psoriasis* because, although they may suppress the psoriasis in the short term, relapse or vigorous rebound occurs on withdrawal (sometimes precipitating severe pustular psoriasis). Topical use of potent corticosteroids on widespread psoriasis also inevitably leads to systemic as well as to local side-effects. It is reasonable, however, to prescribe a weaker corticosteroid (such as hydrocortisone) for short periods (perhaps up to 4 weeks) for *flexural* and *facial psoriasis* (**important:** not more potent than hydrocortisone 1% on the face). In the case of *scalp psoriasis* it is reasonable to use a more potent corticosteroid such as betamethasone or fluocinonide.

In general, the most potent topical corticosteroids should be reserved for recalcitrant dermatoses such as *chronic discoid lupus erythematosus, lichen simplex chronicus, hypertrophic lichen planus*, and *palmoplantar pustulosis*. With rare exceptions, potent corticosteroids should not be used on the face as they may precipitate a rosacea-like disorder and cause skin atrophy.

Intralesional corticosteroid injections (see section 10.1.2.2) are more effective than the very potent topical corticosteroid preparations and they should be reserved for severe cases where there are localised lesions (such as *keloid scars* or *hypertrophic lichen planus*) and topical treatment has failed. Their effects may last for several weeks or even months. Particular care is needed to inject accurately into the lesion in order to avoid severe skin atrophy and loss of pigmentation.

SIDE-EFFECTS. Unlike the *potent* and *very potent* groups, the *moderate* and *mild* groups are rarely associated with side-effects. The more potent the preparation the more care is required, as absorption through the skin can cause severe pituitary-adrenal-axis suppression and Cushing's syndrome (see section 6.3.2), both of which depend on the area of the body treated and the duration of the treatment. It must also be remembered that absorption is greatest from areas of thin skin, raw surfaces, and intertriginous areas, and is increased by occlusion.

Local side-effects include:
(a)   spread and worsening of untreated infection;
(b)   thinning of the skin which may be restored over a period of time after stopping although the original structure may never return;
(c)   irreversible striae atrophicae and telangiectasia;
(d)   contact dermatitis;
(e)   perioral dermatitis, an inflammatory papular disorder on the face of young women;
(f)   acne at the site of application in some patients;
(g)   mild depigmentation.

CHOICE OF FORMULATION. *Water-miscible* creams are suitable for moist or weeping lesions whereas *ointments* are generally chosen for dry, lichenified or scaly lesions or where a more occlusive effect is required. *Lotions* may be useful when minimal application to a large area is required or for the treatment of exudative lesions. *Occlusive polythene dressings* increase absorption, but also increase the risk of side-effects; they are therefore used only under supervision on a short-term basis for very thick areas of skin (such as the palms and soles). The *inclusion of urea* or *salicylic acid* increases the penetration of the corticosteroid.

TOPICAL CORTICOSTEROID POTENCIES

Potency	Examples
Mild	Hydrocortisone 1%
Moderately potent	Clobetasone butyrate 0.05%
Potent	Betamethasone 0.1% (as valerate)
	Hydrocortisone butyrate
Very potent	Clobetasol propionate 0.05%

The preparation containing the **least potent** drug at the lowest strength which is effective is the one of choice; dilution should be avoided whenever possible.

FREQUENCY OF APPLICATION. Corticosteroid preparations should normally be applied once or twice daily. It is not necessary to apply more frequently.

Suitable quantities of corticosteroid preparations to be prescribed for specific areas of the body are:

	Creams and Ointments
Face and neck	15 to 30 g
Both hands	15 to 30 g
Scalp	15 to 30 g
Both arms	30 to 60 g
Both legs	100 g
Trunk	100 g
Groins and genitalia	15 to 30 g

These amounts are usually suitable for an adult for twice daily application for 1 week

USE IN CHILDREN. Children, especially babies, are particularly susceptible to side-effects. The more potent corticosteroids are **contra-indicated** in infants under 1 year, and in general should be **avoided** in paediatric treatment or if necessary used with great care for short periods; a mild corticosteroid such as hydrocortisone 1% ointment or cream is useful for treating napkin rash (see section 13.2.2) and for atopic eczema in childhood (but see caution below).

COMPOUND PREPARATIONS. The advantages of including other substances (such as antibacterials or antifungals) with corticosteroids in topical preparations are debatable, but they may have a place where there is associated bacterial or fungal infection.

HYDROCORTISONE

Indications: mild inflammatory skin disorders such as eczemas (but for over-the-counter preparations, see next page); napkin rash, see notes above and section 13.2.2

Cautions: see notes above; also avoid prolonged use in infants and children (extreme caution in dermatoses of infancy including napkin rash—where possible treatment should be limited to 5–7 days), avoid prolonged use on the face (and keep away from eyes); more potent corticosteroids **contra-indicated** in infants under 1 year (see also notes above)

PSORIASIS. Risks of more potent corticosteroids in psoriasis include possibility of rebound relapse, development of generalised pustular psoriasis, and local and systemic toxicity, see also section 13.5.2; they are specifically **contra-indicated** in widespread plaque psoriasis

Contra-indications: untreated bacterial, fungal, or viral skin lesions; rosacea (acne rosacea), perioral dermatitis; not recommended for acne vulgaris (more potent corticosteroids specifically **contra-indicated**)

Side-effects: see notes above

Administration: apply thinly 1–2 times daily

PoM **Hydrocortisone** (Non-proprietary)

Cream, hydrocortisone 0.5%, net price, 15 g = 34p; 30 g = 60p; 1%, 15 g = 37p. Label: 28. Potency: mild

Ointment, hydrocortisone 0.5%, net price 15 g = 38p; 30 g = 60p; 1%, 15 g = 38p. Label: 28. Potency: mild

When hydrocortisone cream or ointment is prescribed and no strength is stated, the 1% strength should be supplied

Over–the–counter products. The following is a list of skin creams and ointments that contain hydrocortisone (alone or with other ingredients) that can be sold to the public: **Dermacort** (hydrocortisone 0.1%, cream), **Eurax Hc** (hydrocortisone 0.25%; crotamiton 10%, cream), **Hc45** (hydrocortisone acetate 1%, cream), **Lanacort** (hydrocortisone acetate 1%, cream and ointment), **Zenoxone** (hydrocortisone 1%, cream). They can be sold to the public for treatment of allergic contact dermatitis, irritant dermatitis, insect bite reactions and (more recently) mild to moderate eczema

Cautions: not for children under 10 years or in pregnancy, without medical advice

Contra-indications: eyes/face, anogenital region, broken or infected skin (including cold sores, acne, and athlete's foot)

Administration: apply sparingly over small area 1–2 times daily for max. of 1 week

Proprietary hydrocortisone preparations

Note. The following preparations are PoM; those on sale to the public (with restrictions) are specified above.

PoM **Cobadex** (Cox)

Cream, hydrocortisone 1%, dimethicone '350' 20%. Net price 20 g = £1.00. Label: 28. Potency: mild

Additives: include hydroxybenzoates (parabens), polysorbate 80, propylene glycol

PoM **Dioderm** (Dermal)

Cream, hydrocortisone 0.1%. Net price 30 g = £2.59. Label: 28. Potency: mild

Additives: include propylene glycol

Note. Although this contains only 0.1% hydrocortisone, the formulation is designed to provide a clinical activity comparable to that of Hydrocortisone Cream 1% BP

PoM **Efcortelan** (Glaxo)

Cream, hydrocortisone 0.5%, net price, 30 g = 60p; 1%, 30 g = 74p; 2.5%, 30 g = £1.66. Label: 28. Potency: mild

Additives: include chlorocresol

Ointment, hydrocortisone 0.5%, net price, 30 g = 60p; 1%, 30 g = 74p; 2.5%, 30 g = £1.66. Label: 28. Potency: mild

Additives: none as listed in section 13.1

PoM **Hydrocortisyl** (Roussel)

Cream, hydrocortisone 1%. Net price 15 g = 27p. Label: 28. Potency: mild

Additives: include chlorocresol

Ointment, hydrocortisone 1%. Net price 15 g = 27p. Label: 28. Potency: mild

Additives: include wool fat

PoM **Mildison** (Yamanouchi)

Lipocream, hydrocortisone 1%. Net price 30 g = £2.19. Label: 28. Potency: mild

Additives: include hydroxybenzoates (parabens)

Compound preparations

Note. Compound preparations with coal tar, section 13.5.2

PoM **Alphaderm** (Procter & Gamble Pharm.)

Cream, hydrocortisone 1%, urea 10%. Net price 30 g = £2.36; 100 g = £7.32. Label: 28. Potency: moderate

Additives: none as listed in section 13.1

PoM **Calmurid HC** (Novex)

Cream, hydrocortisone 1%, urea 10%, lactic acid 5%. Net price 30 g = £2.33; 100 g = £7.30. Label: 28. Potency: moderate

Additives: none as listed in section 13.1

Note. Manufacturer advises dilute to half-strength with aqueous cream for 1 week if stinging occurs then transfer to undiluted preparation (but see section 13.1 for advice to avoid dilution where possible)

PoM **Eurax-Hydrocortisone** (Zyma)

Cream, hydrocortisone 0.25%, crotamiton 10%. Net price 30 g = 91p. Label: 28. Potency: mild

Additives: include hydroxybenzoates (parabens), propylene glycol, fragrance

Note. A 15-g tube is on sale to the public for treatment of contact dermatitis and insect bites (Eurax Hc)

PoM **Hydrocal** (Bioglan)

Cream, hydrocortisone acetate 1%, in a basis containing calamine. Net price 100 g = £3.10. Label: 28. Potency: mild

Additives: include hydroxybenzoates (parabens), polysorbates

With antimicrobials

See notes above for comment on compound preparations

PoM **Canesten HC** (Baypharm)

Cream, hydrocortisone 1%, clotrimazole 1%. Net price 30 g = £2.25. Label: 28. Potency: mild

Additives: include benzyl alcohol

PoM **Daktacort** (Janssen)

Cream, hydrocortisone 1%, miconazole nitrate 2%. Net price 30 g = £2.24. Label: 28. Potency: mild

Additives: include butylated hydroxyanisole, disodium edetate

Ointment, hydrocortisone 1%, miconazole nitrate 2%. Net price 30 g = £2.25. Label: 28. Potency: mild

Additives: none as listed in section 13.1

PoM **Econacort** (Squibb)

Cream, hydrocortisone 1%, econazole nitrate 1%. Net price 30 g = £2.25. Label: 28. Potency: mild

Additives: include butylated hydroxyanisole

PoM Fucidin H® (Leo)

Cream, hydrocortisone acetate 1%, fusidic acid 2%. Net price 15 g = £3.22; 30 g = £5.55. Label: 28. Potency: mild

Additives: include butylated hydroxyanisole, potassium sorbate

Gel, hydrocortisone acetate 1%, fusidic acid 2%. Net price 15 g = £2.84; 30 g = £4.93. Label: 28. Potency: mild

Additives: include hydroxybenzoates (parabens), polysorbate 80

Ointment, hydrocortisone acetate 1%, sodium fusidate 2%. Net price 15 g = £2.63; 30 g = £4.56. Label: 28. Potency: mild

Additives: include wool fat

PoM Gregoderm® (Unigreg)

Ointment, hydrocortisone 1%, neomycin sulphate 0.4%, nystatin 100 000 units/g, polymyxin B sulphate 7250 units/g. Net price 15 g = £2.51. Label: 28. Potency: mild

Additives: none as listed in section 13.1

PoM Nystaform-HC® (Bayer)

Cream, hydrocortisone 0.5%, nystatin 100 000 units/g, chlorhexidine hydrochloride 1%. Net price 30 g = £2.66. Label: 28. Potency: mild

Additives: include benzyl alcohol, polysorbate '60'

Ointment, hydrocortisone 1%, nystatin 100 000 units/g, chlorhexidine acetate 1%. Net price 30 g = £2.66. Label: 28. Potency: mild

Additives: none as listed in section 13.1

PoM Quinocort® (Quinoderm Ltd)

Cream, hydrocortisone 1%, potassium hydroxyquinoline sulphate 0.5%. Net price 30 g = £1.56. Label: 28. Potency: mild

Additives: include edetic acid (EDTA), chlorocresol

PoM Terra-Cortril® (Pfizer)

Topical ointment, hydrocortisone 1%, oxytetracycline 3% (as hydrochloride). Net price 15 g = £1.01; 30 g = £1.82. Label: 28. Potency: mild

Additives: none as listed in section 13.1

PoM Terra-Cortril Nystatin® (Pfizer)

Cream, hydrocortisone 1%, nystatin 100 000 units/ g, oxytetracycline 3% (as calcium salt). Net price 30 g = £2.01. Label: 28. Potency: mild

Additives: include hydroxybenzoates (parabens), polysorbate, propylene glycol, fragrance

PoM Timodine® (R&C)

Cream, hydrocortisone 0.5%, nystatin 100 000 units/g, benzalkonium chloride solution 0.2%, dimethicone '350' 10%. Net price 30 g = £2.38. Label: 28. Potency: mild

Additives: include butylated hydroxyanisole, hydroxybenzoates (parabens), sorbic acid

PoM Vioform-Hydrocortisone® (Zyma)

Cream, hydrocortisone 1%, clioquinol 3%. Net price 30 g = £1.53. Label: 28. Potency: mild

Additives: none as listed in section 13.1

Ointment, hydrocortisone 1%, clioquinol 3%. Net price 30 g = £1.53. Label:28. Potency: mild

Additives: none as listed in section 13.1

Caution: stains clothing

HYDROCORTISONE BUTYRATE

Indications: severe inflammatory skin disorders such as eczemas unresponsive to less potent corticosteroids; psoriasis, see notes above

Cautions; Contra-indications; Side-effects: see under Hydrocortisone and notes above

Administration: apply thinly 1–2 times daily

PoM Locoid® (Yamanouchi)

Cream, hydrocortisone butyrate 0.1%. Net price 30 g = £2.27; 100 g = £6.95. Label: 28. Potency: potent

Additives: include hydroxybenzoates (parabens)

Lipocream, hydrocortisone butyrate 0.1%. Net price 30 g = £2.38; 100 g = £7.29. Label: 28. Potency: potent

Additives: include hydroxybenzoates (parabens)

Note. For bland cream basis see Lipobase®, section 13.2.1

Ointment, hydrocortisone butyrate 0.1%. Net price 30 g = £2.27; 100 g = £6.95. Label: 28. Potency: potent

Additives: none as listed in section 13.1

Scalp lotion, hydrocortisone butyrate 0.1%, in an aqueous isopropyl alcohol basis. Net price 30 ml = £3.20; 100 mL = £9.81. Label: 15, 28. Potency: potent

Additives: none as listed in section 13.1

PoM Locoid Crelo® (Yamanouchi)

Lotion (topical emulsion), hydrocortisone butyrate 0.1% in a water-miscible basis. Net price 100 g (with applicator) = £8.33. Label: 28. Potency: potent

Additives: include hydroxybenzoates (parabens), propylene glycol

With antimicrobials

See notes above for comment on compound preparations

PoM Locoid C® (Yamanouchi)

Cream, hydrocortisone butyrate 0.1%, chlorquinaldol 3%. Net price 30 g = £2.97. Label: 28. Potency: potent

Additives: none as listed in section 13.1

Caution: causes staining

Ointment, ingredients as for cream, in a greasy basis. Net price 30 g = £2.97. Label: 28. Potency: potent

Additives: none as listed in section 13.1

Caution: causes staining

ALCLOMETASONE DIPROPIONATE

Indications: inflammatory skin disorders such as eczemas

Cautions; Contra-indications; Side-effects: see under Hydrocortisone and notes above

Administration: apply thinly 1–2 times daily

PoM Modrasone® (Schering-Plough)

Cream, alclometasone dipropionate 0.05%. Net price 50 g = £2.95. Label: 28. Potency: moderate

Additives: include chlorocresol, propylene glycol

Ointment, alclometasone dipropionate 0.05%. Net price 50 g = £2.95. Label: 28. Potency: moderate

Additives: include beeswax, propylene glycol

BECLOMETHASONE DIPROPIONATE

Indications: severe inflammatory skin disorders such as eczemas unresponsive to less potent corticosteroids; psoriasis, see notes above

Cautions; Contra-indications; Side-effects: see under Hydrocortisone and notes above

Administration: apply thinly 1–2 times daily

PoM **Propaderm®** (Glaxo)

Cream, beclomethasone dipropionate 0.025%. Net price 30 g = £1.58. Label: 28. Potency: potent
Additives: include chlorocresol

Ointment, beclomethasone dipropionate 0.025%. Net price 30 g = £1.58. Label: 28. Potency: potent
Additives: include propylene glycol

BETAMETHASONE ESTERS

Indications: severe inflammatory skin disorders such as eczemas unresponsive to less potent corticosteroids; psoriasis, see notes above

Cautions; Contra-indications; Side-effects: see under Hydrocortisone and notes above. Application of more than 100 g per week of 0.1% preparation is likely to cause adrenal suppression

Administration: apply thinly 1–2 times daily

PoM **Betamethasone Valerate** (Non-proprietary)

Cream, betamethasone 0.1% (as valerate). Net price 30 g = £1.40. Label: 28. Potency: potent

Ointment, betamethasone 0.1% (as valerate). Net price 30 g = £1.40. Label: 28. Potency: potent

PoM **Betacap®** (Dermal)

Scalp application, betamethasone 0.1% (as valerate) in a water-miscible basis containing coconut oil derivative. Net price 100 mL = £4.42. Label: 15, 28. Potency: potent
Additives: none as listed in section 13.1

PoM **Betnovate®** (Glaxo)

Cream, betamethasone 0.1% (as valerate), in a water-miscible basis. Net price 30 g = £1.40; 100 g = £3.95. Label: 28. Potency: potent
Additives: include chlorocresol

Ointment, betamethasone 0.1% (as valerate), in an anhydrous paraffin basis. Net price 30 g = £1.40; 100 g = £3.95. Label: 28. Potency: potent
Additives: none as listed in section 13.1

Lotion, betamethasone 0.1% (as valerate). Net price 100 mL = £4.75. Label: 28. Potency: potent
Additives: include hydroxybenzoates (parabens)

Scalp application, betamethasone 0.1% (as valerate) in a water-miscible basis. Net price 100 mL = £5.18. Label: 15, 28. Potency: potent
Additives: none as listed in section 13.1

PoM **Betnovate-RD®** (Glaxo)

Cream, betamethasone 0.025% (as valerate) in a water-miscible basis (1 in 4 dilution of Betnovate® cream). Net price 100 g = £3.26. Label: 28. Potency: moderate
Additives: include chlorocresol

Ointment, betamethasone 0.025% (as valerate) in an anhydrous paraffin basis (1 in 4 dilution of Betnovate® ointment). Net price 100 g = £3.26. Label: 28. Potency: moderate
Additives: none as listed in section 13.1

PoM **Bettamousse®** (Evans)

Foam (= scalp application), betamethasone valerate 0.12% (≡ betamethasone 0.1%). Net price 100 g = £7.50. Label: 28. Potency: potent
Additives: include polysorbate 60, propylene glycol
Caution: flammable

PoM **Diprosone®** (Schering-Plough)

Cream, betamethasone 0.05% (as dipropionate). Net price 30 g = £2.51; 100 g = £7.12. Label: 28. Potency: potent
Additives: include chlorocresol

Ointment, betamethasone 0.05% (as dipropionate). Net price 30 g = £2.51; 100 g = £7.12. Label: 28. Potency: potent
Additives: none as listed in section 13.1

Lotion, betamethasone 0.05% (as dipropionate). Net price 30 mL = £3.17; 100 mL = £9.07. Label: 28. Potency: potent
Additives: none as listed in section 13.1

With salicylic acid
See notes above for comment on compound preparations

PoM **Diprosalic®** (Schering-Plough)

Ointment, betamethasone 0.05% (as dipropionate), salicylic acid 3%. Net price 30 g = £3.30; 100 g = £9.50. Label: 28. Potency: potent
Additives: none as listed in section 13.1
Apply thinly 1–2 times daily; max. 60 g per week

Scalp application, betamethasone 0.05% (as dipropionate), salicylic acid 2%, in an alcoholic basis. Net price 100 mL = £10.50. Label: 28. Potency: potent
Additives: include disodium edetate
Apply a few drops 1–2 times daily

With antimicrobials
See notes above for comment on compound preparations

PoM **Betnovate-C®** (Glaxo)

Cream, betamethasone 0.1% (as valerate), clioquinol 3%. Net price 30 g = £1.72. Label: 28. Potency: potent
Additives: include chlorocresol
Caution: stains clothing

Ointment, betamethasone 0.1% (as valerate), clioquinol 3%. Net price 30 g = £1.72. Label: 28. Potency: potent
Additives: none as listed in section 13.1
Caution: stains clothing

PoM **Betnovate-N®** (Glaxo)

Cream, betamethasone 0.1% (as valerate), neomycin sulphate 0.5%. Net price 30 g = £1.72; 100 g = £4.77. Label: 28. Potency: potent
Additives: include chlorocresol

Ointment, betamethasone 0.1% (as valerate), neomycin sulphate 0.5%. Net price 30 g = £1.72; 100 g = £4.77. Label: 28. Potency: potent
Additives: none as listed in section 13.1

PoM **Fucibet®** (Leo)

Cream, betamethasone 0.1% (as valerate), fusidic acid 2%. Net price 15 g = £3.74; 30 g = £6.32; 60 g = £12.64. Label: 28. Potency: potent
Additives: include chlorocresol

PoM **Lotriderm®** (Schering-Plough)

Cream, betamethasone 0.05% (as dipropionate), clotrimazole 1%. Net price 15 g = £3.40. Label: 28. Potency: potent
Additives: include benzyl alcohol, propylene glycol

BUDESONIDE

Indications: severe inflammatory skin disorders such as eczemas; psoriasis, see notes above

Cautions; Contra-indications; Side-effects: see under Hydrocortisone and notes above

Administration: apply thinly 1–2 times daily

PoM **Preferid**® (Yamanouchi)
Cream, budesonide 0.025%. Net price 30 g =
£2.27; 100 g = £6.95. Label: 28. Potency: potent
Additives: include sorbic acid
Ointment, budesonide 0.025%. Net price 30 g =
£2.27; 100 g = £6.95. Label: 28. Potency: potent
Additives: include white beeswax, propylene glycol

CLOBETASOL PROPIONATE

Indications: short-term treatment only of severe
resistant inflammatory skin disorders such as
recalcitrant eczemas unresponsive to less potent
corticosteroids; psoriasis, see notes above
Cautions; Contra-indications; Side-effects: see
under Hydrocortisone and notes above. Not more
than 50 g of 0.05% preparation should be applied
per week
Administration: apply thinly 1–2 times daily for
up to 4 weeks

PoM **Dermovate**® (Glaxo)
Cream, clobetasol propionate 0.05%. Net price
30 g = £2.56; 100 g = £7.52. Label: 28. Potency:
very potent
Additives: include beeswax (or beeswax substitute), chlorocresol,
propylene glycol
Ointment, clobetasol propionate 0.05%. Net price
30 g = £2.56; 100 g = £7.52. Label: 28. Potency:
very potent
Additives: include propylene glycol
Scalp application, clobetasol propionate 0.05%, in
a thickened alcoholic basis. Net price 30 mL =
£2.93; 100 mL = £9.91. Label: 15, 28. Potency:
very potent
Additives: none as listed insection 13.1

With antimicrobials
See notes above for comment on compound preparations
PoM **Dermovate-NN**® (Glaxo)
Cream, clobetasol propionate 0.05%, neomycin
sulphate 0.5%, nystatin 100 000 units/g. Net price
30 g = £3.50. Label: 28. Potency: very potent
Additives: include beeswax substitute
Ointment, ingredients as for cream, in a paraffin
basis. Net price 30 g = £3.50. Label: 28. Potency:
very potent
Additives: none as listed in section 13.1

CLOBETASONE BUTYRATE

Indications: eczemas and dermatitis of all types;
maintenance between courses of more potent corticosteroids
Cautions; Contra-indications; Side-effects: see
under Hydrocortisone and notes above
Administration: apply thinly 1–2 times daily

PoM **Eumovate**® (Glaxo)
Cream, clobetasone butyrate 0.05%. Net price 30 g
= £1.76; 100 g = £5.16. Label: 28. Potency: moderate
Additives: include beeswax substitute, chlorocresol
Ointment, clobetasone butyrate 0.05%. Net price
30 g = £1.76; 100 g = £5.16. Label: 28. Potency:
moderate
Additives: none as listed in section 13.1

With antimicrobials
See notes above for comment on compound preparations
PoM **Trimovate**® (Glaxo)
Cream, clobetasone butyrate 0.05%, oxytetra-
cycline 3% (as calcium salt), nystatin
100 000 units/g. Net price 30 g = £3.13. Label: 28.
Potency: moderate
Additives: include chlorocresol
Caution: stains clothing

DESOXYMETHASONE
(Desoximetasone)
Indications: severe acute inflammatory, allergic,
and chronic skin disorders; psoriasis, see notes
above
Cautions; Contra-indications; Side-effects: see
under Hydrocortisone and notes above
Administration: apply thinly 1–2 times daily

PoM **Stiedex**® (Stiefel)
LP Oily cream, desoxymethasone 0.05%. Net
price 30 g = £2.86; 100 g = £8.58. Label:28.
Potency: moderate
Additives: include edetic acid (EDTA), wool fat
Lotion, desoxymethasone 0.25%, salicylic acid
1%. Net price 50 mL = £8.05. Label: 28. Potency:
potent
Additives: include disodium edetate, propylene glycol

DIFLUCORTOLONE VALERATE

Indications: severe inflammatory skin disorders
such as eczemas unresponsive to less potent corticosteroids; high strength (0.3%), short-term treatment of severe exacerbations; psoriasis, see notes
above
Cautions; Contra-indications; Side-effects: see
under Hydrocortisone and notes above; not more
than 60 g of 0.3% applied per week
Administration: apply thinly 1–2 times daily for
up to 4 weeks (0.1% preparations) or 2 weeks
(0.3% preparations), reducing strength as condition responds

PoM **Nerisone**® (Schering Health)
Cream, diflucortolone valerate 0.1%. Net price
30 g = £1.59. Label: 28. Potency: potent
Additives: include disodium edetate, hydroxybenzoates
(parabens)
Oily cream, diflucortolone valerate 0.1%. Net
price 30 g = £2.56. Label: 28. Potency: potent
Additives: none as listed in section 13.1
Ointment, diflucortolone valerate 0.1%. Net price
30 g = £1.59. Label: 28. Potency: potent
Additives: none as listed in section 13.1
PoM **Nerisone Forte**® (Schering Health)
Oily cream, diflucortolone valerate 0.3%. Net
price 15 g = £2.09. Label: 28. Potency: very
potent
Additives: none as listed in section 13.1
Ointment, diflucortolone valerate 0.3%. Net price
15 g = £2.09. Label: 28. Potency: very potent
Additives: none as listed in section 13.1

FLUOCINOLONE ACETONIDE

Indications: inflammatory skin disorders such as eczemas, 0.0025–0.01% in milder conditions, 0.025% in severe conditions; psoriasis, see notes above

Cautions; Contra-indications; Side-effects: see under Hydrocortisone and notes above

Administration: apply thinly 1–2 times daily, reducing strength as condition responds

PoM **Synalar**® (Zeneca)
Cream, fluocinolone acetonide 0.025%. Net price 30 g = £1.37. Label: 28. Potency: potent
Additives: include benzyl alcohol, polysorbates, propylene glycol
Gel, fluocinolone acetonide 0.025%. Net price 30 g = £1.45. For use on scalp and other hairy areas. Label: 28. Potency: potent
Additives: include hydroxybenzoates (parabens), propylene glycol
Ointment, fluocinolone acetonide 0.025%. Net price 30 g = £1.37. Label: 28. Potency: potent
Additives: include propylene glycol, wool fat

PoM **Synalar 1 in 4 Dilution**® (Zeneca)
Cream, fluocinolone acetonide 0.00625%. Net price 50 g = £1.56. Label: 28. Potency: moderate
Additives: include benzyl alcohol, polysorbates, propylene glycol
Ointment, fluocinolone acetonide 0.00625%. Net price 50 g = £1.83. Label: 28. Potency: moderate
Additives: include propylene glycol, wool fat

PoM **Synalar 1 in 10 Dilution**® (Zeneca)
Cream, fluocinolone acetonide 0.0025%. Net price 50 g = £1.48. Label: 28. Potency: mild
Additives: include benzyl alcohol, polysorbates, propylene glycol

With antibacterials
See notes above for comment on compound preparations
PoM **Synalar C**® (Zeneca)
Cream, fluocinolone acetonide 0.025%, clioquinol 3%. Net price 15 g = 94p. Label: 28. Potency: potent
Additives: include disodium edetate, hydroxybenzoates (parabens), polysorbates, propylene glycol
Ointment, ingredients as for cream. Net price 15 g = 94p. Label: 28. Potency: potent.
Caution: stains clothing
Additives: include propylene glycol, wool fat

PoM **Synalar N**® (Zeneca)
Cream, fluocinolone acetonide 0.025%, neomycin sulphate 0.5%. Net price 30 g = £1.41. Label: 28. Potency: potent
Additives: include hydroxybenzoates (parabens), polysorbates, propylene glycol
Ointment, ingredients as for cream, in a greasy basis. Net price 30 g = £1.41. Label: 28. Potency: potent
Additives: include propylene glycol, wool fat

FLUOCINONIDE

Indications: severe inflammatory skin disorders such as eczemas unresponsive to less potent corticosteroids; psoriasis, see notes above

Cautions; Contra-indications; Side-effects: see under Hydrocortisone and notes above

Administration: apply thinly 1–2 times daily

PoM **Metosyn**® (Zeneca)
FAPG cream, fluocinonide 0.05%. Net price 25 g = £1.22; 100 g = £4.59. Label: 28. Potency: potent
Additives: include propylene glycol
Ointment, fluocinonide 0.05%. Net price 25 g = £1.22; 100 g = £4.59. Label: 28. Potency: potent
Additives: include propylene glycol, wool fat
Scalp lotion, fluocinonide 0.05% in a propylene glycol-alcohol basis. Net price 30 mL (with applicator) = £1.56. Label: 15, 28. Potency: potent
Additives: include propylene glycol

FLUOCORTOLONE

Indications: 0.25%—severe inflammatory skin disorders such as eczemas unresponsive to less potent corticosteroids; 0.1%—milder inflammatory skin disorders; psoriasis, see notes above

Cautions; Contra-indications; Side-effects: see under Hydrocortisone and notes above

Administration: apply thinly 1–2 times daily, reducing strength as condition responds

PoM **Ultralanum Plain**® (Schering Health)
Cream, fluocortolone hexanoate 0.25%, fluocortolone pivalate 0.25%. Net price 50 g = £2.95. Label: 28. Potency: moderate
Additives: include disodium edetate, hydroxybenzoates (parabens), fragrance
Ointment, fluocortolone 0.25%, fluocortolone hexanoate 0.25%. Net price 50 g = £2.95. Label: 28. Potency: moderate
Additives: include wool fat, fragrance

FLURANDRENOLONE
(Fludroxycortide)

Indications: inflammatory skin disorders such as eczemas

Cautions; Contra-indications; Side-effects: see under Hydrocortisone and notes above

Administration: apply thinly 1–2 times daily, reducing strength as condition responds

PoM **Haelan**® (Dista)
Cream, flurandrenolone 0.0125%. Net price 60 g = £3.26. Label: 28. Potency: moderate
Additives: include propylene glycol
Ointment, flurandrenolone 0.0125%. Net price 60 g = £3.26. Label: 28. Potency: moderate
Additives: include beeswax, polysorbate
NHS *Tape*, polythene adhesive film impregnated with flurandrenolone 4 micrograms/cm². Net price 7.5 cm × 50 cm = £4.05; 7.5 cm × 200 cm = £13.62
For chronic localised recalcitrant dermatoses (but not acute or weeping), cut tape to fit lesion, apply to clean, dry skin shorn of hair, usually for 12 of each 24 hours

FLUTICASONE PROPIONATE

Indications: inflammatory skin disorders such as dermatitis and eczemas unresponsive to less potent corticosteroids

Cautions; Contra-indications; Side-effects: see under Hydrocortisone and notes above

Administration: apply cream thinly once daily *or* ointment twice daily

▼ PoM **Cutivate®** (Glaxo)

Cream, fluticasone propionate 0.05%. Net price 15 g = £2.35; 50 g = £6.95. Label: 28. Potency: potent

Additives: include propylene glycol

Ointment, fluticasone propionate 0.005%. Net price 15 g = £2.35, 50 g = £6.95. Label: 28. Potency: potent

HALCINONIDE

Indications: short-term treatment only of severe resistant inflammatory skin disorders such as recalcitrant eczemas unresponsive to less potent corticosteroids; psoriasis, see notes above

Cautions; Contra-indications; Side-effects: see under Hydrocortisone and notes above

Administration: apply thinly 1–2 times daily

PoM **Halciderm Topical®** (Squibb)

Cream, halcinonide 0.1%. Net price 30 g = £3.40. Label: 28. Potency: very potent

Additives: include propylene glycol

MOMETASONE FUROATE

Indications: severe inflammatory skin disorders such as eczemas unresponsive to less potent corticosteroids; psoriasis, see notes above

Cautions; Contra-indications; Side-effects: see under Hydrocortisone and notes above

Administration: apply thinly once daily (to scalp in case of lotion)

PoM **Elocon®** (Schering-Plough)

Cream, mometasone furoate 0.1%. Net price 30 g = £4.88. Label: 28. Potency: potent

Additives: none as listed in section 13.1

Ointment, mometasone furoate 0.1%. Net price 30 g = £4.88. Label: 28. Potency: potent

Additives: none as listed in section 13.1

Lotion, mometasone furoate 0.1% in an aqueous isopropyl alcohol basis. Net price 30 mL = £4.88. Label: 28. Potency: potent

Additives: include propylene glycol

TRIAMCINOLONE ACETONIDE

Indications: severe inflammatory skin disorders such as eczemas unresponsive to less potent corticosteroids; psoriasis, see notes above

Cautions; Contra-indications; Side-effects: see under Hydrocortisone and notes above

Administration: apply thinly 1–2 times daily

PoM **Adcortyl®** (Squibb)

Cream, triamcinolone acetonide 0.1%. Net price 30 g = £1.59. Label: 28. Potency: potent

Additives: include benzyl alcohol, propylene glycol

Ointment, triamcinolone acetonide 0.1%. Net price 30 g = £1.59. Label: 28. Potency: potent

Additives: none as listed in section 13.1

With antimicrobials

See notes above for comment on compound preparations

PoM **Adcortyl with Graneodin®** (Squibb)

Cream, triamcinolone acetonide 0.1%, gramicidin 0.025%, neomycin 0.25% (as sulphate). Net price 25 g = £3.00. Label: 28. Potency: potent

Additives: include benzyl alcohol, propylene glycol

PoM **Aureocort®** (Lederle)

Ointment, triamcinolone acetonide 0.1%, chlortetracycline hydrochloride 3%, in an anhydrous greasy basis containing wool fat and white soft paraffin. Net price 15 g = £2.70. Label: 28. Potency: potent

Additives: include hydroxybenzoates (parabens), wool fat

Caution: stains clothing

PoM **Nystadermal®** (Squibb)

Cream, triamcinolone acetonide 0.1%, nystatin 100 000 units/g. Net price 15 g = £2.27. Label: 28. Potency: potent

Additives: include benzyl alcohol, propylene glycol, fragrance

PoM **Pevaryl TC®** (Cilag)

Cream, triamcinolone 0.1%, econazole nitrate 1%. Net price 15 g = £4.00. Label: 28. Potency: potent

Additives: include butylated hydroxyanisole, disodium edetate, benzoic acid

PoM **Tri-Adcortyl®** (Squibb)

Cream, triamcinolone acetonide 0.1%, gramicidin 0.025%, neomycin 0.25% (as sulphate), nystatin 100 000 units/g. Net price 30 g = £3.15. Label: 28. Potency: potent

Additives: include benzyl alcohol, ethylenediamine, propylene glycol, fragrance

Ointment, ingredients as for cream, in an ointment basis. Net price 30 g = £3.15. Label: 28. Potency: potent

Additives: none as listed in section 13.1

Note. Not recommended owing to presence of ethylenediamine in the cream and also because combination of antibiotic with antifungal not considered useful in either the cream or ointment

13.5   Preparations for eczema and psoriasis

13.5.1   Preparations for eczema
13.5.2   Preparations for psoriasis

13.5.1   Preparations for eczema

An eczematous disorder (dermatitis) is a cutaneous reaction characterised by inflammation and itching. Where possible, the cause (e.g. household detergent) should be established and removed; a patient with suspected contact dermatitis should be patch tested to establish the diagnosis. *Atopic eczema* is the most common form of eczema and usually requires regular application of an **emollient** (see section 13.2.1) with short courses of a **mild to moderate topical corticosteroid** (see section 13.4); the topical corticosteroid chosen should always be the least potent that is effective. In *mild to moderate atopic eczema* use of the topical corticosteroid should be restricted to periods of one to two weeks, in conjunction with regular use of an **emollient** (section 13.2.1). *Severe atopic eczema on the limbs or body* (or a flare-up of mild to moderate eczema) may require application of a **potent or moderately potent corticosteroid** for the first one to two weeks, followed by a **weaker preparation** as the condition improves; an **emollient** should also be used and, if itching is a major problem, consideration should be given to administration of an **antihistamine** by mouth and possibly of an **antibiotic** by mouth.

Dry, fissured, scaly lesions are treated with bland **emollients** (section 13.2.1) which are often all that is necessary to allay irritation and permit healing. Preparations such as **aqueous cream** or **emulsifying ointment** are used as soap substitutes and in the bath; addition of a bath oil may also be helpful.

Weeping eczemas may be treated with topical corticosteroid creams (section 13.4); they are, however, commonly secondarily infected. Wet dressings of **potassium permanganate** (0.01%) (section 13.11.6) are applied; if a large area is involved, potassium permanganate baths are taken. When necessary **topical antibacterials** are used (section 13.10.1) but those which are not given systemically should usually be chosen.

Ichthammol has a milder action than coal tar (see section 13.5.2) and is usually used in chronic lichenified forms of eczema. It can be applied conveniently to flexures of the limbs as **zinc paste and ichthammol bandage** (section 13.13.1).

Cyclosporin (section 13.5.2) is now available for *severe resistant atopic dermatitis*; its use calls for specialist care in a hospital context.

For comment on the role of **corticosteroids** in eczema see section 13.4. For comment on **gamolenic acid** see below.

COAL TAR

See section 13.5.2

ICHTHAMMOL

Indications: chronic lichenified eczema
Side-effects: skin irritation
Administration: apply 1–3 times daily

Ichthammol Ointment, BP 1980, ichthammol 10%, yellow soft paraffin 45%, wool fat 45%. Net price 25 g = 21p
Zinc and Ichthammol Cream, BP, ichthammol 5%, cetostearyl alcohol 3%, wool fat 10%, in zinc cream. Net price 100 g = 73p
Zinc Paste and Ichthammol Bandage, BP (Ichthopaste®, Icthaband®), see section 13.13.1

GAMOLENIC ACID

Gamolenic acid has been claimed to improve patients with atopic eczema. However, the evidence in favour of a useful therapeutic effect is poor.

GAMOLENIC ACID

Indications: see under preparations
Cautions: history of epilepsy, concomitant treatment with epileptogenic drugs e.g. phenothiazines; pregnancy
Side-effects: occasional nausea, indigestion, headache
Dose: see below

PoM **Epogam®** (Searle)
Capsules, gamolenic acid 40 mg in evening primrose oil. Net price 240-cap pack = £24.41. Counselling, see below
Additives: include vitamin E 10 mg as *in vivo* antoxidant
Dose: symptomatic relief of atopic eczema 4–6 capsules twice daily; CHILD 1–12 years, 2–4 capsules twice daily
Paediatric capsules, gamolenic acid 80 mg in evening primrose oil. Net price 60-cap pack = £15.41. Counselling, see below
Additives: include vitamin E 20 mg as *in vivo* antoxidant
Dose: symptomatic relief of atopic eczema, CHILD 1–12 years, 1–2 capsules twice daily
COUNSELLING. Capsules may be cut open and contents swallowed or taken on bread; paediatric capsules have 'snip-off' neck for convenience of administration

Mastalgia
(for advice see p. 326.)
PoM **Efamast®** (Searle)
Capsules, gamolenic acid 40 mg in evening primrose oil. Net price 224-cap pack = £23.72
Additives: include vitamin E 10 mg as *in vivo* antoxidant
Dose: symptomatic relief of cyclical and non-cyclical mastalgia, 3–4 capsules twice daily, usually for 8–12 weeks then stopped or continued at lower maintenance dose

13.5.2 Preparations for psoriasis

Psoriasis is characterised by epidermal thickening and scaling. It commonly affects extensor surfaces and the scalp. For mild conditions, treatment, other than reassurance and an **emollient**, may be unnecessary.

In more troublesome cases of psoriasis, local application of salicylic acid, coal tar, calcipotriol, or dithranol may have a beneficial effect.

Salicylic acid may be used in all hyperkeratotic and scaling conditions to enhance the rate of loss of surface scale. Preparations containing salicylic acid 2% are used initially and then gradually increased to concentrations of 3 to 6%. Side-effects are few but include irritation, or, when large areas are treated, salicylate toxicity (see p. 416 for details of symptoms and treatment).

Coal tar is more active than salicylic acid and has anti-inflammatory and antiscaling properties. It is used in psoriasis and occasionally in *chronic atopic eczema*. The formulation and strength chosen depends on patient acceptability and severity of the condition; the 'thicker' the patch of eczema or psoriasis the stronger the concentration of coal tar required. **Coal tar paste** or **zinc and coal tar paste** are generally suitable for most cases but are limited by their unpleasant appearance and smell and they may not be used on the face. Some of the newer preparations are less unsightly and may be preferred. Preparations such as Carbo-Dome® are suitable for treating the face. **Zinc paste and coal tar bandage** (section 13.13.1) is useful for treating the limbs. **Tar shampoos** are described in section 13.9. When lesions are extensive coal tar baths are useful. Combinations of coal tar with zinc or salicylic acid have no advantage over the simpler preparations. Preparations containing hydrocortisone and coal tar are useful in eczemas.

Dithranol is very effective in psoriasis. The preparation is applied carefully to the lesion, covered with a dressing, and left for one hour. Applications are preferably left on the skin overnight but short contact applications of 30 minutes to an hour are also effective and are more convenient; usual concentrations are 0.1–2% (**important:** if going above 0.1% the sensitivity of the skin must first be tested using 0.5%—further increases must be gradual). Dithranol must be used with caution as it can cause quite severe skin irritation (especially to perilesional skin). For this reason it must be applied only to the lesions and it is customary to start with low concentrations (e.g. 0.1%) and gradually build up (e.g. every 5 days) to the maximum concentration which produces a therapeutic effect without irritation. It should not be applied to flexural areas since burning may occur. Hands should be washed thoroughly after use. Some patients are intolerant to dithranol even in low concentrations; it is important to recognise them early in treatment because continued use can result in their psoriasis becoming unstable. Fair skin is more sensitive than dark skin. Proprietary preparations may be more convenient as they may cause less staining than dithranol paste. *Ingram's method* of applying dithranol is sometimes used in hospital. The patient soaks in a warm bath containing coal tar solution 1 in 800 and after drying is exposed to ultraviolet radiation B (UVB) to produce a slight erythema. **Dithranol paste** is applied to the lesions and the normal skin protected by applying talc and stockinette dressings. The procedure is repeated daily.

UVB phototherapy is also effective by itself in mild to moderate, guttate or chronic plaque psoriasis.

Calcipotriol is a vitamin D derivative that is now widely used for topical application for mild to moderate psoriasis affecting up to 40% of skin area; a scalp solution is now also available. Advantages are that it does not have an unpleasant smell and does not stain clothing. **Tacalcitol**, another vitamin D analogue, has been introduced recently for once-daily application in the treatment of plaque psoriasis.

PUVA, photochemotherapy using psoralens with long-wave ultraviolet irradiation (UVA), is an effective method of treating some patients with psoriasis. Special lamps are required, and a psoralen, generally methoxsalen [unlicensed] is given by mouth about 2 hours beforehand, to sensitise the skin to the effects of irradiation. A course of PUVA is usually given twice a week and may last for 4 to 6 weeks. Some centres use UVA after bathing in a solution of methoxsalen to avoid the systemic side-effects associated with administration by mouth; this is termed 'bath PUVA'. Treatment is only available in specialist centres; it has to be carefully regulated, owing to the short-term hazard of severe burning and the long-term hazards of cataract formation, accelerated ageing, and the development of skin cancer.

Acitretin is a retinoid given by mouth for the treatment of *severe resistant or complicated psoriasis* and some of the *congenital disorders of kerat-*

inisation including Darier's disease (keratosis follicularis). It is a metabolite of **etretinate** (which it has replaced). It should be prescribed **only** by, or under the supervision of, a consultant dermatologist and is available to hospitals (or specified retail pharmacies) **only**. It is a retinoid (a vitamin A derivative) with marked effects on keratinising epithelia. A therapeutic effect occurs after 2 to 4 weeks with maximum benefit after 4 to 6 weeks. Acitretin treats only manifestations not the ultimate causes of these diseases, but treatment should be limited to a period of 6 to 9 months with a 3- to 4-month rest period before repeating treatment. Most patients suffer from dryness and cracking of the lips. Other side-effects include a mild transient increase in the rate of hair fall (reversible on withdrawal), occasional generalised pruritus, paronychia, and nose bleeds. There is a tendency for the plasma lipids to rise in some patients. Acitretin is **teratogenic** and must be **avoided** in pregnancy. Contraceptive measures must be taken at least **1 month before** and during treatment by women who may become pregnant and for at least **two years after** a course of the drug.

An antimetabolite, usually **methotrexate**, may also be used for *severe resistant psoriasis*, but this must again always be done under hospital supervision, the dose being adjusted according to severity of the condition and in accordance with haematological and biochemical measurements; the usual dose is 10 to 25 mg of methotrexate once weekly, by mouth.

Cyclosporin is now also available for *severe resistant psoriasis* and once again its use calls for specialist care in a hospital context.

For comment on the limited role of **corticosteroids** in psoriasis, see section 13.4.

TOPICAL PREPARATIONS FOR PSORIASIS

CALCIPOTRIOL

Indications: see under Administration
Cautions: pregnancy; avoid use on face and inadvertent transfer to other body areas; wash hands thoroughly after application; risk of hypercalcaemia if more than 100 g weekly used (reported with less in generalised pustular or erythrodermic exfoliative psoriasis)
Contra-indications: disorders of calcium metabolism
Side-effects: local irritation; also dermatitis, pruritus, erythema, aggravation of psoriasis, photosensitivity; rarely facial or perioral dermatitis; hypercalcaemia (see Cautions)
Administration: cream or ointment, mild to moderate plaque psoriasis affecting up to 40% of skin area, apply twice daily; max. 100 g weekly (less with *scalp solution*, see below); CHILD not recommended

PoM **Dovonex®** (Leo)
Cream, calcipotriol 50 micrograms/g. Net price 30 g = £8.15; 60 g = £16.30; 120 g = £29.40
Additives: include disodium edetate

Ointment, calcipotriol 50 micrograms/g. Net price 30 g = £8.15; 60 g = £16.30; 120 g = £29.40
Additives: include disodium edetate, propylene glycol
Scalp solution, calcipotriol 50 micrograms/mL. Net price 60 mL = £22.28
Additives: include propylene glycol
Scalp psoriasis, apply to scalp twice daily; max. 60 mL weekly (may be less with cream or ointment, see below); CHILD not recommended
MAX. WHEN PREPARATIONS USED TOGETHER. Max. total calcipotriol 5 mg in any one week (e.g. *scalp solution* 60 mL with *cream* or *ointment* 30 g or *cream* or *ointment* 60 g with *scalp solution* 30 mL)

TACALCITOL

Indications: plaque psoriasis
Cautions: pregnancy; avoid use on scalp, contact with eyes and inadvertent transfer to other body areas; wash hands thoroughly after application; risk of hypercalcaemia in generalised pustular or erythrodermic exfoliative psoriasis; monitor plasma calcium if risk of hypercalcaemia or in renal impairment; may be degraded by UV light (including sunlight)
Contra-indications: disorders of calcium metabolism including hypercalcaemia (see Cautions)
Side-effects: local irritation including itching, erythema, burning, paraesthesia
Administration: apply daily preferably at bedtime; max. 5 g daily; usual max. duration 2 courses of 8 weeks per year; CHILD not recommended

▼ PoM **Curatoderm**® (Merck)
Ointment, tacalcitol (as monohydrate) 4 micrograms/g. Net price 30 g = £15.09; 60 g = £26.06
Additives: none as listed in section 13.1

COAL TAR

Indications: psoriasis and occasionally chronic atopic eczema
Cautions: avoid eyes, mucosa and broken or inflamed skin
Contra-indications: not for use in sore, acute, or pustular psoriasis or in presence of infection
Side-effects: skin irritation and acne-like eruptions, photosensitivity; stains skin, hair, and fabric
Administration: apply 1–3 times daily starting with low-strength preparations
Note. For shampoo preparations see section 13.9; impregnated dressings see section 13.13.1

Non-proprietary preparations
Supplies may be difficult to obtain—moreover some patients may find that the newer proprietary preparations are more pleasant to use
Calamine and Coal Tar Ointment, BP, calamine 12.5 g, strong coal tar solution 2.5 g, zinc oxide 12.5 g, hydrous wool fat 25 g, white soft paraffin 47.5 g
Apply 1–2 times daily
Coal Tar and Salicylic Acid Ointment, BP, coal tar 2 g, salicylic acid 2 g, emulsifying wax 11.4 g, white soft paraffin 19 g, coconut oil 54 g, polysorbate '80' 4 g, liquid paraffin 7.6 g
Apply 1–2 times daily

Coal Tar Paste, BP, strong coal tar solution 7.5%, in compound zinc paste
Apply 1–2 times daily .
Zinc and Coal Tar Paste, BP, zinc oxide 6%, coal tar 6%, emulsifying wax 5%, starch 38%, yellow soft paraffin 45%
Apply 1–2 times daily

Proprietary preparations
Alphosyl® (Stafford-Miller)
Cream, coal tar extract 5%, allantoin 2%, in a vanishing-cream basis. Net price 100 g = £2.44
Additives: include beeswax, hydroxybenzoates (parabens), isopropyl palmitate, propylene glycol
Psoriasis, apply to skin 2–4 times daily
Lotion, coal tar extract 5%, allantoin 2%. Net price 250 mL = £2.21
Additives: include isopropyl palmitate, propylene glycol
Psoriasis, apply to skin or scalp 2–4 times daily
Carbo-Dome® (Lagap)
Cream, coal tar solution 10%, in a water-miscible basis. Net price 30 g = £3.95; 100 g = £8.93
Additives: include beeswax, hydroxybenzoates (parabens)
Psoriasis, apply to skin 2–3 times daily
Clinitar® (Shire)
Cream, coal tar extract 1%. Net price 100 g = £5.37
Additives: include isopropyl palmitate, propylene glycol
Psoriasis and eczema, apply to skin 1–2 times daily
Cocois® (Bioglan)
Scalp ointment, coal tar solution 12%, salicylic acid 2%, precipitated sulphur 4%, in a coconut oil emollient basis. Net price 40 g (with applicator nozzle) = £4.71; 100 g = £8.85
Additives: none as listed in section 13.1
Scaly scalp disorders including psoriasis, eczema, seborrhoeic dermatitis and dandruff, apply to scalp once weekly as necessary (if severe use daily for first 3–7 days), shampoo off after 1 hour; CHILD 6–12 years, medical supervision required (not recommended under 6 years)
Gelcosal® (Quinoderm Ltd)
Gel, strong coal tar solution 5%, pine tar 5%, salicylic acid 2%. Net price 50 g = £3.12
Additives: none as listed in section 13.1
Psoriasis and chronic scaling dermatitis, apply to skin twice daily
Gelcotar® (Quinoderm Ltd)
Gel, strong coal tar solution 5%, pine tar 5%. Net price 50 g = £2.83; 500 g = £14.74
Additives: none as listed in section 13.1
Psoriasis and chronic dermatitis, apply to skin twice daily
Liquid, see section 13.9
Pragmatar® (Bioglan)
Cream, cetyl alcohol-coal tar distillate 4%, salicylic acid 3%, sulphur (precipitated) 3%. Net price 25 g = £2.40; 100 g = £7.75
Additives: include fragrance
Scaly skin disorders, apply thinly once daily; dandruff and other seborrhoeic conditions, apply to scalp once weekly or in severe cases daily. Dilute with a few drops of water before application to infants
Psoriderm® (Dermal)
Cream, coal tar 6%, lecithin 0.4%. Net price 225 mL = £3.24
Additives: include hydroxybenzoates (parabens), isopropyl palmitate, propylene glycol
Psoriasis, apply to skin or scalp twice daily
Scalp lotion—section 13.9
PsoriGel® (Novex)
Gel, coal tar solution USP 7.5% in an alcoholic emollient basis. Net price 100 g = £4.23
Additives: include propylene glycol
Psoriasis and eczema, apply to skin or scalp 1–2 times daily

Bath preparations
Coal Tar Solution, BP, coal tar 20%, polysorbate '80' 5%, in alcohol (96%). Net price 100 mL = 79p
Use 100 mL in a bath
Note. Strong Coal Tar Solution BP contains coal tar 40%

Balneum with Tar® (Merck)
Bath oil, coal tar distillate 30%, soya oil 55%. Net price 200 mL = £3.23.
Additives: none as listed in section 13.1
Psoriasis, eczema, pruritic dermatoses, and ichthyosis, use 1 measure (20 mL) in bath (infants 10 mL) and soak for 20 minutes

Pixol® (Thames)
Bath oil, coal tar solution 0.5%, cade oil 0.1%, pine tar 2%. Net price 150 mL = £2.16; 300 mL = £4.17.
Additives: include tetrasodium edetate, fragrance
Psoriasis, eczema, dermatitis, seborrhoea, and dandruff, use 20–30 mL in bath and soak for up to 20 minutes; scalp, apply 5–15 mL and rinse off after 2-3 minutes

Polytar Emollient® (Stiefel)
Bath additive, coal tar solution 2.5%, arachis (peanut) oil extract of coal tar 7.5%, tar 7.5%, cade oil 7.5%, liquid paraffin 35%. Net price 350 mL = £4.87.
Additives: include isopropyl palmitate
Psoriasis, eczema, atopic and pruritic dermatoses, use 2–4 capfuls (15–30 mL) in bath and soak for 20 minutes

Psoriderm® (Dermal)
Bath emulsion, coal tar 40%. Net price 200 mL = £2.88.
Additives: include polysorbate 20
Psoriasis, use 30 mL in a bath and soak for 5 minutes

With corticosteroids
PoM Alphosyl HC® (Stafford-Miller)
Cream, coal tar extract 5%, hydrocortisone 0.5%, allantoin 2%. Net price 30 g = £1.66; 100 g = £4.73. Label: 28. Potency: mild
Additives: include beeswax, hydroxybenzoates (parabens), isopropyl palmitate, wool fat
Psoriasis, apply thinly 1–2 times daily; CHILD under 5 years not recommended

PoM Carbo-Cort® (Lagap)
Cream, coal tar solution 3%, hydrocortisone 0.25%. Net price 30 g = £3.61. Label: 28. Potency: mild
Additives: include beeswax, hydroxybenzoates (parabens)
Chronic dermatoses including eczema, apply thinly 1–2 times daily

PoM Tarcortin® (Stafford-Miller)
Cream, coal tar extract 5%, hydrocortisone 0.5%. Net price 100 g = £3.08. Label: 28. Potency: mild
Additives: include hydroxybenzoates (parabens), isopropyl palmitate, propylene glycol, fragrance
Psoriasis, eczema, seborrhoea and dermatoses, apply to skin thinly 1–2 times daily

DITHRANOL

Indications: subacute and chronic psoriasis, see notes above

Cautions: avoid use near eyes and sensitive areas of skin; see also notes above

Contra-indications: hypersensitivity; acute and pustular psoriasis

Side-effects: local burning sensation and irritation; stains skin, hair, and fabrics

Administration: see notes above and under preparations

Note. Some of these dithranol preparations also contain coal tar or salicylic acid—for cautions and side-effects see under Coal Tar (above) or under Salicylic Acid

PoM * Dithranol Ointment, BP dithranol, in yellow soft paraffin; usual strengths 0.1–2%. Part of basis may be replaced by hard paraffin if a stiffer preparation is required. Label: 28
* PoM if dithranol content more than 1%, otherwise P

Dithranol Paste, BP, dithranol in zinc and salicylic acid (Lassar's) paste. Usual strengths 0.1–1% of dithranol. Label: 28

Dithrocream® (Dermal)
Cream, dithranol 0.1%, net price 50 g = £3.86; 0.25%, 50 g = £4.14; 0.5%, 50 g = £4.77; 1%, 50 g = £5.55; PoM 2%, 50 g = £6.95. Label: 28. For application to skin or scalp; 0.1–0.5% suitable for overnight treatment, 1–2% for max. 1 hour
Additives: include chlorocresol, salicylic acid

Psorin® (Thames)
Ointment, dithranol 0.11%, crude coal tar 1%, salicylic acid 1.6%. Net price 50 g = £5.30, 100 g = £10.50. Label: 28. For application to skin up to twice daily
Additives: include beeswax, wool fat
Scalp gel, dithranol 0.25%, salicylic acid 1.6% in gel basis containing methyl salicylate. Net price 50 g = £3.98. Label: 28. For application to scalp, initially apply on alternate days for 10–20 minutes; may be increased to daily application for max. 1 hour and then wash off
Additives: none as listed in section 13.1

SALICYLIC ACID

For coal tar preparations containing salicylic acid, see under Coal Tar p. 469; for dithranol preparations containing salicylic acid see under Dithranol, above

Indications: hyperkeratotic skin disorders

Cautions: see notes above; avoid broken or inflamed skin

SALICYLATE TOXICITY. If large areas of skin are treated, salicylate toxicity may be a hazard, for details of symptoms and treatment, see p. 416

Side-effects: sensitivity, excessive drying, irritation, systemic effects after widespread use (see under Cautions)

Salicylic Acid Collodion, BP —section 13.7

Salicylic Acid Ointment, BP, salicylic acid 2%, in wool alcohols ointment. Net price 25 g = 18p
Apply twice daily

Zinc and Salicylic Acid Paste, BP (Lassar's Paste), zinc oxide 24%, salicylic acid 2%, starch 24%, white soft paraffin 50%. Net price 25 g = 16p
Apply twice daily

ORAL RETINOIDS FOR PSORIASIS

ACITRETIN

Note. Acitretin is a metabolite of etretinate

Indications: severe extensive psoriasis resistant to other forms of therapy; palmoplantar pustular psoriasis; severe congenital ichthyosis; severe Darier's disease (keratosis follicularis)

Cautions: exclude pregnancy before starting—patients should avoid pregnancy at least 1 month before, during, and for at least 2 years after treatment, should avoid tetracycline, high doses of vitamin A (more than 4000–5000 units daily) and use of keratolytics, and should not donate blood during or for at least 1 year after stopping therapy (teratogenic risk); monitor hepatic function and plasma lipids at start, 1 month after initiating treatment, and then at intervals of 3 months; diabetes (can alter glucose tolerance—initial frequent blood glucose checks); radiographic assessment on long-term treatment; investigate atypical musculoskeletal symptoms; not recommended for children except under exceptional circumstances (premature epiphyseal closure reported); patients should avoid excessive exposure to sunlight and unsupervised use of sunlamps; **interactions:** Appendix 1 (retinoids)

Contra-indications: hepatic and renal impairment; pregnancy (**important teratogenic risk:** see Cautions and Appendix 4); breast-feeding

Side-effects: (mainly dose-related) dryness of mucous membranes (sometimes erosion), of skin (sometimes scaling, thinning, erythema especially of face, and pruritus), and of conjunctiva (sometimes conjunctivitis and decreased tolerance of contact lenses); other side-effects reported include palmoplantar exfoliation, epistaxis, epidermal fragility, paronychia, granulomatous lesions, reversible hair thinning and alopecia, myalgia and arthralgia, occasional nausea, headache, malaise, drowsiness and sweating; benign intracranial hypertension (**avoid** concomitant tetracyclines); photosensitivity, mood changes and blood disorders (including thrombocytopenia and anaemia) reported for etretinate, raised liver enzymes, rarely jaundice and hepatitis (**avoid** concomitant methotrexate); raised triglycerides; decreased night vision reported; skeletal hyperostosis and extraosseous calcification reported following long-term administration of etretinate (and premature epiphyseal closure in children, see Cautions)

Dose: administered in accordance with expert advice, initially 25–30 mg daily (Darier's disease 10 mg daily) for 2–4 weeks, then adjusted according to response, usually within range 25–50 mg daily (in some cases up to max. 75 mg daily) for further 6–8 weeks (in Darier's disease and ichthyosis not more than 50 mg daily for up to 6 months); CHILD (**important:** exceptional circumstances only, see Cautions), 500 micrograms/kg daily (occasionally up to 1 mg/kg daily to max. 35 mg daily for limited periods) with careful monitoring of musculoskeletal development

PoM Neotigason® (Roche)

Capsules, acitretin 10 mg (brown/white), net price 56-cap pack = £26.53; 25 mg (brown/yellow), 56-cap pack = £61.57 (**hosp. or specified retail pharmacy only**—see data sheet for details, specialist dermatological supervision). Label: 10 patient information leaflet, 21

ETRETINATE

Note. Etretinate is a derivative of tretinoin which is a form of vitamin A

Indications; Cautions; Contra-indications; Side-effects: see under Acitretin

TERATOGENIC RISK. It is **important** to bear in mind that pregnancy must continue to be **avoided** for **2 years** after stopping treatment (nor should blood be donated for 2 years after stopping)

PoM Tigason® (Roche)
Product discontinued

ORAL IMMUNOSUPPRESSANTS FOR PSORIASIS

CYCLOSPORIN
(Ciclosporin)

Indications: see under Dose; transplantation and graft-versus-host disease, see section 8.2.2

Cautions; Side-effects: see section 8.2.2

ADDITIONAL CAUTIONS IN ATOPIC DERMATITIS AND PSORIASIS. *Contra-indicated* in abnormal renal function, hypertension not under control (see also below), infections not under control, and malignancy (see also below). Dermatological and physical examination, including blood pressure and renal function measurements required at least twice before starting; discontinue if hypertension develops that cannot be controlled by dose reduction or antihypertensive therapy; avoid excessive exposure to sunlight and use of UVB or PUVA; *in atopic dermatitis,* also allow herpes simplex infections to clear before starting (if they occur during treatment withdraw if severe); *Staphylococcus aureus* skin infections not absolute contra-indication providing controlled (but avoid erythromycin unless no other alternative—see also **interactions:** Appendix 1 (cyclosporin)); monitor serum creatinine every 2 weeks throughout; *in psoriasis,* also exclude malignancies (including those of skin and cervix) before starting (biopsy any lesions not typical of psoriasis) and treat patients with malignant or pre-malignant conditions of skin only after appropriate treatment (and if no other option); monitor serum creatinine every 2 weeks for first 3 months then every 2 months (monthly if dose more than 2.5 mg/kg daily), reducing dose by 25–50% if increases more than 30% above baseline (even if within normal range) and discontinuing if reduction not successful within 1 month; also discontinue if lymphoproliferative disorder develops

Dose: ADULT over 16 years *by mouth,* administered in accordance with expert advice

Short-term treatment (max. 8 weeks) of severe atopic dermatitis where conventional therapy ineffective or inappropriate, initially 2.5 mg/kg daily in 2 divided doses, if good initial response not achieved within 2 weeks, increase rapidly to max. 5 mg/kg daily; initial dose of 5 mg/kg daily if very severe; CHILD under 16 years not recommended

Severe psoriasis where conventional therapy ineffective or inappropriate, initially 2.5 mg/kg daily in 2 divided doses, increased gradually to max. 5 mg/kg daily if no improvement within 1 month (discontinue if response still insufficient after 6 weeks); initial dose of 5 mg/kg daily justified if condition requires rapid improvement; CHILD under 16 years not recommended

IMPORTANT. For preparations and counselling and for advice on conversion between the preparations, see section 8.2.2

METHOTREXATE

Indications: severe uncontrolled psoriasis unresponsive to conventional therapy; malignant disease, see section 8.1.3; rheumatoid arthritis, see section 10.1.3

Cautions; Side-effects: methotrexate is an antime-tabolite with severe haematological, pulmonary, gastro-intestinal, and other toxicity for use only by specialists (see also notes above, section 8.1.3, and data sheet); investigations required before starting include complete haematological analy-sis, renal function tests (**contra-indicated** if sig-nificant impairment, see section 8.1.3 and Appendix 3), liver function tests (**contra-indi-cated** if abnormalities, see below and Appendix 2), followed by constant monitoring during treat-ment; also **contra-indicated** in pregnancy (fol-lowing administration to woman or man, avoid conception for **at least 6 months** after stopping) and breast-feeding (see Cytotoxic drugs, Appen-dixes 4 and 5) and immunodeficiency syndromes; also may decrease male or female fertility (effect appears to be reversible on discontinuation); extreme caution in peptic ulceration, ulcerative colitis, diarrhoea and ulcerative stomatitis (with-draw if stomatitis develops—may be first sign of gastro-intestinal toxicity); photosensitivity—lesions of psoriasis aggravated by UV radiation (skin ulceration reported); **interactions:** see below and Appendix 1 (methotrexate)

BLOOD COUNT. Haematopoietic suppression may occur abruptly (with apparently safe dosage); any profound drop in white cell or platelet count calls for immediate withdrawal of methotrexate and introduction of support-ive therapy

LIVER TOXICITY. Particular attention should be paid to the possible development of liver toxicity by carrying out liver function tests before starting methotrexate and every 2–4 months during therapy. Treatment should not be started or should be discontinued if any abnormality of liver function tests or liver biopsy is present or devel-ops during therapy. Abnormalities may return to normal within 2 weeks after which treatment may be recom-menced if judged appropriate

PULMONARY TOXICITY. May be special problem in rheu-matoid arthritis (patient to contact doctor immediately if dyspnoea or cough)

ASPIRIN and other NSAIDs. Concurrent administration of aspirin or other NSAIDs may reduce excretion of methotrexate and increase its toxicity. If aspirin or other NSAIDs are given concurrently the dose of metho-trexate should be carefully monitored. Patients should be advised to avoid self-medication with over-the-coun-ter aspirin or ibuprofen

Dose: by mouth, 10–25 mg once weekly, adjusted according to response; ELDERLY consider dose reduction (extreme caution); CHILD not recom-mended

IMPORTANT. Please note that the above dose is a **weekly** dose

Preparations

See section 8.1.3

13.6   Preparations for acne

13.6.1 Topical preparations for acne
13.6.2 Oral preparations for acne

The treatment of acne depends on whether it is pre-dominantly inflammatory or comedonal.

13.6.1   Topical preparations for acne

Significant comedonal acne responds well to topi-cal retinoids (see p. 473), whereas both comedones and inflamed lesions respond well to benzoyl per-oxide or azelaic acid (see below). Alternatively, topical application of an antibiotic such as erythro-mycin or clindamycin may be effective for inflammatory or comedonal acne. If topical prepa-rations prove inadequate oral preparations may be needed (see section 13.6.2).

BENZOYL PEROXIDE AND AZELAIC ACID

Both comedones and inflamed lesions respond well to **benzoyl peroxide** or **azelaic acid**. Benzoyl per-oxide and azelaic acid irritate the skin, but it is thought that irritation is associated with the thera-peutic effect; the scaling and redness often subsides with continued treatment.

BENZOYL PEROXIDE

Indications: acne vulgaris
Cautions: avoid contact with eyes, mouth, and mucous membranes; may bleach fabrics
Side-effects: skin irritation
Administration: apply 1–2 times daily, starting treatment with lower-strength preparations

Acetoxyl® (Stiefel)
Gel, benzoyl peroxide in an aqueous-acetone-gel basis, 2.5% (*'2.5' Gel*), net price 40 g = £1.08; 5% (*'5' Gel*), 40 g = £1.08
Additives: include propylene glycol

Acnecide® (Novex)
Gel, benzoyl peroxide, in an aqueous gel basis, 5% (*'5' Gel*), net price 60 g = £3.00; 10% (*'10' Gel*), 60 g = £3.30
Additives: include propylene glycol

Acnegel® (Stiefel)
Gel, benzoyl peroxide in an aqueous alcoholic basis, 5% net price 50 g = £1.38; 10% (*'Forte' Gel*), 50 g = £1.38
Additives: none as listed in section 13.1

Benoxyl® (Stiefel)
Cream, benzoyl peroxide, in a non-greasy basis, 5% (*'5' Cream*), net price 40 g = £1.51
Additives: include isopropyl palmitate, propylene glycol
Lotion, benzoyl peroxide, in a non-greasy basis, 5% (*'5' Lotion*), net price 30 mL = £1.45; 10% (*'10' Lotion*), 30 mL = £1.45
Additives: include isopropyl palmitate, propylene glycol

Nericur® (Schering Health)
Gel, benzoyl peroxide, in an aqueous gel basis, 5% (*'5' Gel*), net price 30 g = £1.45; 10% (*'10' Gel*), 30 g = £1.60
Additives: include propylene glycol

Panoxyl® (Stiefel)
Aquagel (= aqueous gel), benzoyl peroxide 2.5% (*'2.5' Aquagel*), net price 40 g = £1.76; 5% (*'5' Aquagel*), 40 g = £1.92; 10% (*'10' Aquagel*), 40 g = £2.07.
Additives: include propylene glycol
Gel, benzoyl peroxide, in an aqueous alcoholic basis, 5% (*'5' Gel*), net price 40 g = £1.51; 10% (*'10' Gel*), 40 g = £1.69
Additives: include fragrance

Wash, benzoyl peroxide, in a detergent basis, 10% ('10' Wash), net price 150 mL = £3.50
Additives: none as listed in section 13.1

With antimicrobials

Acnidazil® (Cilag)
Cream, benzoyl peroxide 5%, miconazole nitrate 2%. Net price 15 g = £2.21; 30 g = £3.40
Additives: include polysorbate 20, propylene glycol

PoM **Benzamycin®** (Bioglan)
Gel, pack for reconstitution, providing erythromycin 3% and benzoyl peroxide 5%. Net price per pack to provide 23.3 g = £8.31
Additives: include hydroxybenzoates (parabens)
Apply twice daily (very fair skin, initially once daily at night)

Quinoderm® (Quinoderm Ltd)
Cream, benzoyl peroxide 10%, potassium hydroxyquinoline sulphate 0.5%, in an astringent vanishing-cream basis. Net price 25 g = £1.24; 50 g = £1.86
Additives: include edetic acid (EDTA)
Cream 5, benzoyl peroxide 5%, potassium hydroxyquinoline sulphate 0.5%, in an astringent vanishing-cream basis. Net price 50 g = £1.69
Additives: include edetic acid (EDTA)
Lotio-gel 5%, benzoyl peroxide 5%, potassium hydroxyquinoline sulphate 0.5%, in an astringent creamy basis. Net price 30 mL = £1.47
Additives: include edetic acid (EDTA)

AZELAIC ACID

Indications: acne vulgaris
Cautions: pregnancy, breast-feeding; avoid contact with eyes
Side-effects: local irritation (reduce frequency or discontinue use temporarily); rarely photosensitisation

PoM **Skinoren®** (Schering Health)
Cream, azelaic acid 20%, net price 30 g = £5.00
Additives: include propylene glycol
Apply twice daily (sensitive skin, once daily for first week). Extended treatment may be required but manufacturer advises period of treatment should not exceed 6 months

TOPICAL ANTIBIOTICS FOR ACNE

Topical antibiotics are used for mild to moderately severe acne. Topical preparations of erythromycin, tetracycline, and clindamycin seem to be quite useful for many patients with the milder forms of acne; they can produce mild irritation of the skin but rarely sensitise.

Cross resistance, especially between erythromycin and clindamycin is an increasing problem. To avoid this:

when possible use non-antibiotic antimicrobials (such as benzoyl peroxide);

avoid concomitant treatment with different oral and topical antibiotics;

if a particular antibiotic is effective, use it for repeat courses.

Topical neomycin is not suitable owing to sensitisation.

ANTIBIOTICS

Indications: acne vulgaris
Cautions: Some manufacturers say alcoholic preparations are not suitable for use with benzoyl peroxide
DURATION OF TREATMENT. Usual max. duration of treatment 10–12 weeks to minimise problems with antibiotic resistance (but course may be repeated after interval of few weeks)

PoM **Benzamycin®** see under Benzoyl Peroxide above

PoM **Dalacin T®** (Upjohn)
Topical solution, clindamycin (as phosphate) 1%, in an aqueous alcoholic basis. Net price (both with applicator) 30 mL = £4.54; 50 mL = £7.57
Additives: include propylene glycol
Apply twice daily
Lotion, clindamycin (as phosphate) 1% in an aqueous basis. Net price 30 mL = £5.32; 50 mL = £8.87
Additives: include hydroxybenzoates (parabens)
Apply twice daily

PoM **Stiemycin®** (Stiefel)
Solution, erythromycin 2% in an alcoholic basis. Net price 50 mL = £9.00
Additives: include propylene glycol
Apply twice daily

PoM **Topicycline®** (Monmouth)
Solution, powder for reconstitution, tetracycline hydrochloride, 4-epitetracycline hydrochloride, providing tetracycline hydrochloride 2.2 mg/mL when reconstituted with solvent containing *n*-decyl methyl sulphoxide and citric acid in 40% alcohol. Net price per pack of powder and solvent to provide 70 mL = £7.70
Additives: none as listed in section 13.1
Apply twice daily

PoM **Zineryt®** (Yamanouchi)
Topical solution, powder for reconstitution, erythromycin 40 mg, zinc acetate 12 mg/mL when reconstituted with solvent containing ethanol. Net price per pack of powder and solvent to provide 30 mL = £8.04; 90 mL = £22.91
Additives: none as listed in section 13.1.
Apply twice daily

TOPICAL RETINOIDS FOR ACNE

Topical application of **tretinoin** (which is the acid form of vitamin A) or of its isomer **isotretinoin** is anticomedogenic. They are useful in treating acne but patients should be warned that some redness and skin peeling may occur after application for several days but settles with time. Isotretinoin is also given by mouth, see section 13.6.2 for **additional warnings**.

TRETINOIN

Note. Tretinoin is the acid form of vitamin A
Indications: see under preparatations below
Cautions: avoid contact with eyes, nostrils, mouth, and mucous membranes; do not use simultaneously with other peeling agents (can be alternated every 12 hours with benzoyl peroxide); do not use with ultra-violet lamps (and minimise exposure to sunlight)

Contra-indications: pregnancy, eczema, broken or sunburned skin; personal or family history of cutaneous epithelioma

Side-effects: irritation, erythema, peeling; changes in pigmentation, photosensitivity

Administration: see under preparations below

PoM Retin-A® (Cilag)

Cream, tretinoin 0.025%, net price 60 g = £6.03.
Acne vulgaris, for dry or fair skin, apply thinly 1–2 times daily
Additives: include butylated hydroxytoluene, sorbic acid

Gel, tretinoin 0.01%, net price 60 g = £6.03; 0.025%, 60 g = £6.03.
Acne vulgaris, (for severe acne, for initial treatment of acne, or for dark and oily skins), apply thinly 1–2 times daily
Additives: include butylated hydroxytoluene

Lotion, tretinoin 0.025%. Net price 100 mL = £6.94.
Acne vulgaris, for application to large areas such as the back, apply thinly 1–2 times daily
Additives: include butylated hydroxytoluene

Photodamage

Application of tretinoin 0.05% cream is reported to be associated with gradual improvement in photodamaged skin (usually within 3–4 months of starting)

PoM ¹Retinova® (Cilag)

Cream, tretinoin 0.05%, net price 20 g = £13.75.
For mottled hyperpigmentation, roughness and fine wrinkling of photodamaged skin due to chronic sun exposure, apply thinly at night, then reduce to 1–3 nights weekly
Additives: include fragrance

1. Currently prescribable but prescriptions may be sent to Health Authorities to investigate circumstances under which written.

ISOTRETINOIN

Note. Isotretinoin is an isomer of tretinoin
Indications; Cautions; Contra-indications; Side-effects: (after topical application **only**): see under Tretinoin and notes above
IMPORTANT. For **indications, cautions, contra-indications** and **side-effects** of isotretinoin **when given by mouth,** see p. 475.
Administration: apply thinly 1–2 times daily

PoM Isotrex® (Stiefel)

Gel, isotretinoin 0.05%. Net price 30 g = £6.96.
Label: 10 patient information leaflet
Additives: include butylated hydroxytoluene

TOPICAL CORTICOSTEROIDS FOR ACNE

Topical **corticosteroids** should **not** be used in acne.

CORTICOSTEROIDS

Indications: not recommended (see notes above)
Cautions; Contra-indications; Side-effects: section 13.4 and notes above

PoM Actinac® (Roussel)

Lotion (powder for reconstitution with solvent), chloramphenicol 40 mg, hydrocortisone acetate 40 mg, allantoin 24 mg, butoxyethyl nicotinate 24 mg, precipitated sulphur 320 mg/g. Discard after 21 days. Net price 2 × 6.25 g bottles powder with 2 × 20-mL bottles solvent = £9.30. Label: 28. Potency: mild
Additives: none as listed in section 13.1

OTHER TOPICAL PREPARATIONS FOR ACNE

Salicylic acid is of dubious value in acne and is no longer used although some preparations still have a role in seborrhoeic eczema. Preparations containing **sulphur** and **abrasive agents** are no longer considered beneficial in acne.

A topical preparation of **nicotinamide** has recently been made available for inflammatory acne.

ABRASIVE AGENTS

Indications: acne vulgaris (but see notes above)
Cautions: avoid contact with eyes; discontinue use temporarily if skin becomes irritated
Contra-indications: superficial venules, telangiectasia

Brasivol® (Stiefel)

Paste No. 1, aluminium oxide 38.09% in fine particles, in a soap-detergent basis; *Paste No. 2,* aluminium oxide 52.2% in medium particles, net price 75 g (both) = £2.49
Additives: include fragrance
Use instead of soap 1–3 times daily, starting with *No.1*

Ionax Scrub® (Novex)

Gel, polyethylene granules 21.9%, benzalkonium chloride 0.25% in a foaming aqueous alcoholic basis. Net price 60 g = £3.13
Additives: include propylene glycol
Use instead of soap 1–2 times daily

NICOTINAMIDE

Indications: see under preparation
Cautions: avoid contact with eyes and mucous membranes (including nose and mouth); reduce frequency of application if excessive dryness, irritation or peeling
Side-effects: dryness of skin; also pruritus, erythema, burning and irritation

Papulex® (Euroderma)

Gel, nicotinamide 4%. Net price 60 g = £7.98
Additives: none as listed in section 13.1
Inflammatory acne vulgaris, apply twice daily; reduce to once daily or on alternate days if irritation occurs

SALICYLIC ACID

Indications: acne vulgaris
Cautions: avoid contact with mouth, eyes, mucous membranes; systemic effects after excessive use (see section 10.1.1)
Side-effects: local irritation

Acnisal® (Euroderma)

Topical solution, salicylic acid 2% in a detergent basis.
Net price 177 mL = £4.13. Use up to 3 times daily
Additives: include benzyl alcohol, hydroxybenzoates (parabens)

SULPHUR

Cautions: avoid contact with eyes, mouth, and mucous membranes; causes skin irritation

With resorcinol

Prolonged application of resorcinol may interfere with thyroid function therefore not recommended

Eskamel® (Goldshield)

Cream, resorcinol 2%, sulphur 8%, in a non-greasy flesh-coloured basis. Net price 25 g = £2.17

Additives: include propylene glycol, fragrance

With salicylic acid

see above for cautions relating to salicylic acid

Salicylic Acid and Sulphur Cream, BP 1980, salicylic acid 2%, precipitated sulphur 2%, in aqueous cream

Salicylic Acid and Sulphur Ointment, BPC, salicylic acid 3%, precipitated sulphur 3%, in hydrous ointment (oily cream)

3.6.2   Oral preparations for acne

ORAL ANTIBIOTICS FOR ACNE

Systemic antibacterial treatment is useful. **Tetracycline** (see section 5.1.3), **erythromycin** (see section 5.1.5), and occasionally other antibacterials are used. The usual dosage regimen for tetracycline and erythromycin, is 500 mg twice daily for 3 months reduced to 250 mg twice daily for a further 3 months. If there is no improvement after the first 3 months the antibiotic should be changed. Maximum improvement usually occurs after four to six months but in the more severe cases treatment may need to be continued for two or more years.

As an alternative to tetracycline, **minocycline** (see section 5.1.3) offers less likelihood of bacterial resistance but may sometimes cause irreversible pigmentation; it is given in a dosage of 100 mg daily. **Doxycycline** may also be used in a dosage of 50 mg daily. Although **trimethoprim** is not licensed for acne it, too, is used in a dosage of 300 mg twice daily.

Concomitant use of different topical and systemic antibiotics is undesirable owing to the increased likelihood of the development of bacterial resistance.

ERYTHROMYCIN
See section 5.1.5

TETRACYCLINES
See section 5.1.3

HORMONE TREATMENT FOR ACNE

Cyproterone acetate with **ethinyloestradiol** (Dianette®) contains an anti-androgen. It is no more effective than an oral broad spectrum antibiotic but is useful in women who also wish to receive oral contraception.

Improvement of acne probably occurs because of decreased sebum secretion which is under androgen control. Some women with moderately severe hirsutism may also benefit as hair growth is also androgen-dependent. Its contra-indications include pregnancy and a predisposition to thrombosis.

CYPROTERONE ACETATE

Indications: see notes above; male hypersexuality, see section 6.4.2; prostate cancer, see section 8.3.4.2

Cautions; Contra-indications; Side-effects: see under Combined Oral Contraceptives (7.3.1)

With ethinyloestradiol

PoM **Dianette®** (Schering Health)

Tablets, beige, s/c, cyproterone acetate 2 mg, ethinyloestradiol 35 micrograms. Net price 21-tab pack = £5.52

Dose: 1 tablet daily for 21 days starting on 1st day of menstrual cycle and repeated after a 7-day interval, usually for several months; withdraw when acne or hirsutism completely resolved (repeat courses may be given if recurrence)

ORAL RETINOID FOR ACNE

Isotretinoin (Roaccutane®) is a retinoid used for the systemic treatment of nodulo-cystic and conglobate acne and severe acne which has failed to respond to an adequate course of a systemic antimicrobial agent. It is also useful in women with acne developing in the third or fourth decades of life, since this late onset acne is frequently resistant to antibiotics.

It acts primarily by greatly reducing sebum secretion. It should be prescribed **only** by, or under the supervision of, a consultant dermatologist, and is available to hospitals **only**. It is given in doses of 500 micrograms/kg/day for at least 16 weeks but doses may be adjusted if necessary after 4 weeks. Repeat courses are occasionally required. An exacerbation is common some 2–4 weeks after starting treatment but usually subsides after a few weeks.

Side-effects of isotretinoin include dry lips, sore eyes, nose bleeds, mild transient hair loss, and joint pains. The drug is **teratogenic** and must **not** be given to women who are pregnant or those who may become pregnant unless there is concomitant effective contraception and then only after detailed explanation by the physician. The contraceptive measures must continue for at least **one month** after ceasing treatment with the drug.

ISOTRETINOIN

Note. Isotretinoin is an isomer of tretinoin

Indications: see notes above

Cautions: exclude pregnancy before starting—pregnancy must be avoided at least 1 month before, during, and for at least 1 month after treatment; avoid donating blood during and for at least 1 month after treatment; monitor hepatic function and plasma lipids at start, 1 month after initiating treatment, then at intervals of 3 months; avoid tetracyclines, high doses of vitamin A (more than 4000–5000 units daily) and use of keratolytics during treatment; monitor blood glucose in diabetic patients, monitor for keratitis (especially in those with dry eye syndrome); **interactions:** Appendix 1 (retinoids)

Contra-indications: pregnancy (**important tera-togenic risk:** see Cautions and Appendix 4); breast-feeding; renal or hepatic impairment; hypervitaminosis A, hyperlipidaemia

Side-effects: (mainly dose-related) dryness of skin (with scaling, thinning, erythema, pruritus), epidermal fragility (trauma may cause blistering); rarely acne fulminans, facial hyperpigmentation; dryness of nasal mucosa (with mild epistaxis), of pharyngeal mucosa (with hoarseness), of conjunctiva (sometimes conjunctivitis), decreased tolerance to contact lenses and rarely keratitis; visual disturbances (papilloedema, optic neuritis, corneal opacities, cataracts, decreased night vision, photophobia, blurred vision)—expert referral and consider withdrawal; hair thinning (reversible on withdrawal) or (rarely) hirsutism; nausea, headache, malaise, drowsiness, sweating; benign intracranial hypertension (avoid concomitant tetracyclines); myalgia and arthralgia; raised serum creatinine concentrations reported; raised liver enzymes (rarely jaundice and hepatitis); raised plasma triglycerides and cholesterol (risk of pancreatitis if triglycerides above 8 g/litre); allergic vasculitis and granulomatous lesions reported, other side-effects reported include hearing deficiency, mood changes, convulsions, menstrual irregularities, hyperuricaemia, inflammatory bowel disease, paronychia and Gram-positive infections, bone changes (including early epiphyseal closure and skeletal hyperostosis following long-term administration), thrombocytopenia, thrombocytosis, neutropenia and anaemia, lymphadenopathy, and haematuria and proteinuria

Dose: initially 500 micrograms/kg daily (in 1–2 divided doses) with food for 4 weeks; if good response continue for further 8–12 weeks; if little response, up to 1 mg/kg daily for 8–12 weeks; if intolerant, reduce dose to 100–200 micrograms/kg daily

PoM **Roaccutane**® (Roche)
Capsules, isotretinoin 5 mg (red-violet/white), net price 56-cap pack = £19.08; 20 mg (red-violet/white), 56-cap pack = £54.98 (**hosp. or specified retail pharmacy only**—see data sheet for details, specialist dermatological supervision). Label: 10, patient information card, 21

13.7   Preparations for warts and calluses

The least destructive method possible should be chosen to treat these lesions as they are self-limiting (in patients who are not immunosuppressed) and all viral warts including those on the soles of the feet (verrucas) eventually disappear spontaneously.

Salicylic acid preparations act as keratolytics; they are useful but can cause considerable irritation of the treated area. They are suitable for the removal of *warts and calluses.* An ointment containing **podophyllum resin with salicylic acid** (*Posalfilin*®) is available for treating *plantar warts*

(for podophyllum preparations suitable for treating genital warts see next page).

Preparations containing **formaldehyde** and **glutaraldehyde** are also available.

SALICYLIC ACID

Indications: see under preparations
Cautions: protect surrounding skin and avoid broken skin; not suitable for application to face, and genital region, or large areas
Contra-indications: diabetes or if peripheral blood circulation impaired
Side-effects: skin irritation, see notes above
ADMINISTRATION. Instructions in proprietary packs generally incorporate advice to remove dead skin by gentle rubbing with a pumice stone and to cover with plaster after application (unless in collodion basis)

Salicylic Acid Collodion, BP, salicylic acid 12%, in flexible collodion. Label: 15. For warts and calluses, apply daily or on alternate days
Cuplex® (S&N Hlth.)
Gel, salicylic acid 11%, lactic acid 4%, copper acetate (= Cu²⁺ 0.0011%), in a collodion basis. Net price 5 g = £2.33. Label: 15. For plantar and mosaic warts, corns, and calluses, apply twice daily
Duofilm® (Stiefel)
Paint, salicylic acid 16.7%, lactic acid 16.7%, in flexible collodion. Net price 15 mL (with applicator) = £1.95. Label: 15. For plantar and mosaic warts, apply daily
Occlusal® (Euroderma)
Application, salicylic acid 26% in polyacrylic solution. Net price 10 mL (with applicator) = £2.41. Label : 15. For common and plantar warts, apply daily
Salactol® (Dermal)
Paint, salicylic acid 16.7%, lactic acid 16.7%, in flexible collodion. Net price 10 mL (with applicator) = £1.93. Label: 15. For warts, particularly plantar warts, verrucas, corns, and calluses, apply daily
Salatac® (Dermal)
Gel, salicylic acid 12%, lactic acid 4% in a collodion basis. Net price 8 g (with applicator) = £3.36. Label: 15. For warts, verrucas, corns, and calluses, apply daily
Verrugon® (Pickles)
Ointment, salicylic acid 50% in a paraffin basis. Net price 6 g = £1.62. For plantar warts, apply daily

With podophyllum
Posalfilin® (Norgine)
Ointment, podophyllum resin 20%, salicylic acid 25%. Net price 10 g = £3.12. For plantar warts, apply daily
Note. Owing to the salicylic acid content, not suitable for anogenital warts; owing to the podophyllum content also contra-indicated in pregnancy

FORMALDEHYDE

Indications: see under preparations
Cautions; Contra-indications; Side-effects: see under Salicylic Acid

Formaldehyde Lotion, formaldehyde solution, BP, 3 mL, water to 100 mL. For plantar warts, applied at night as a soak

Veracur® (Typharm)

Gel, formaldehyde 0.75% in a water-miscible gel basis. Net price 15 g = £1.45. For warts, particularly plantar warts, apply twice daily

GLUTARALDEHYDE

Indications: see under preparations

Cautions; Contra-indications; Side-effects: see under Salicylic Acid, stains skin brown

Glutarol® (Dermal)

Solution (= application), glutaraldehyde 10%. Net price 10 mL (with applicator) = £2.19. For warts, particularly plantar warts, apply twice daily

Verucasep® (Galen)

Gel, glutaraldehyde 10%. Net price 15 g = £1.95. For warts, particularly plantar warts, apply twice daily

GENITAL WARTS

Podophyllum preparations may be useful for *genital warts* but can cause considerable irritation of the treated area and can cause **severe toxicity** on excessive application (see Cautions below). They are contra-indicated in pregnancy. Preparations containing the major active constituent **podophyllotoxin** (*Condyline®* and *Warticon®*) are now also available for genital warts.

PODOPHYLLUM

Indications: see under preparations

Cautions: avoid normal skin and open wounds; keep away from face; very irritant to eyes; **important:** see also warnings below

Contra-indications: pregnancy and breast-feeding; children

Side-effects: see notes above

PoM **Podophyllin Paint, Compound, BP,** (podophyllum resin 15% in compound benzoin tincture), podophyllum resin 1.5 g, compound benzoin tincture to 10 mL; 5 mL to be dispensed unless otherwise directed. Label: 15

External genital warts, applied weekly in genitourinary clinic (or at a general practitioner's surgery by trained nurses after screening for other sexually transmitted diseases)

IMPORTANT. Should be allowed to stay on the treated area for not longer than 6 hours and then washed off. Care should be taken to avoid splashing the surrounding skin during application (which must be covered with soft paraffin as a protection). Where there are a large number of warts only a few should be treated at any one time as **severe toxicity** caused by absorption of podophyllin has been reported

Podophyllotoxin

PoM **Condyline®** (Nycomed)

Solution, podophyllotoxin 0.5% in alcoholic basis. Net price 3.5 mL (with applicators) = £14.49. Label: 15

Condylomata acuminata affecting the penis or the female external genitalia, apply twice daily for 3 consecutive days; treatment may be repeated at weekly intervals if necessary for a total of five 3-day treatment courses; direct medical supervision for lesions in the

female and for lesions greater than 4 cm² in the male; max. 50 single applications ('loops') per session (see leaflet)

PoM **Warticon®** (Perstorp)

Cream, podophyllotoxin 0.15%. Net price 5 g (with mirror) = £17.40

Condylomata acuminata affecting the penis or the female external genitalia, apply twice daily for 3 consecutive days; treatment may be repeated at weekly intervals if necessary for a total of four 3-day treatment courses; direct medical supervision for lesions greater than 4 cm²

Solution, podophyllotoxin 0.5% in alcoholic basis. Net price 3 mL (with applicators)— *Warticon®*[for men]; with applicators and mirror—*Warticon Fem®* [for women]) = £14.50. Label: 15

Condylomata acuminata affecting the penis or the female external genitalia, apply twice daily for 3 consecutive days; treatment may be repeated at weekly intervals if necessary for a total of four 3-day treatment courses; direct medical supervision for lesions greater than 4 cm²; max. 50 single applications ('loops') per session (see leaflet)

13.8 Sunscreens and camouflagers

13.8.1 Sunscreening preparations
13.8.2 Camouflaging preparations

13.8.1 Sunscreening preparations

Solar ultraviolet irradiation can be harmful to the skin. It is responsible for disorders such as *polymorphic light eruption, solar urticaria,* and the various *cutaneous porphyrias.* It also provokes (or at least aggravates) disorders such as *rosacea* and *lupus erythematosus.* It may also cause photosensitivity in patients taking some drugs such as demeclocycline, phenothiazines, or amiodarone. All these conditions (as well as *sunburn*) may occur after relatively short periods of exposure to the sun. Exposure over longer periods may cause more serious problems. Both *melanoma* and *non-melanoma skin cancer* are now thought to be caused in many instances by solar ultraviolet irradiation. It is now also believed that exposure to the sun causes the skin to wrinkle and develop other signs *associated with ageing.* Solar ultraviolet irradiation also provokes attacks of *recurrent herpes labialis* (although it is not known whether the effect of sunlight exposure is local or systemic).

Solar ultraviolet radiation is approximately 200–400 nm in wavelength. The medium wavelengths (280–310 nm, known as UVB) cause sunburn and contribute to the long-term changes responsible for skin cancer and ageing. The long wavelengths (310–400 nm, known as UVA) do not cause sunburn but are responsible for many *photosensitivity reactions* and *photodermatoses;* they also seem to contribute to long-term damage and to be involved in the pathogenesis of *skin cancer* and *photodamage.*

Sunscreen preparations contain substances that protect the skin against UVB and hence against sunburn. The sun protection factor (SPF, usually indicated in the preparation title) provides guidance on the degree of protection offered against UVB; it indicates the multiples of protection provided against burning, compared with unprotected skin; for example, an SPF of 8 should enable a person to remain 8 times longer in the sun without burning. Such preparations, however, do not prevent long-term damage associated with UVA, which might not become apparent for 10 to 20 years. Preparations that also contain reflective substances, such as titanium dioxide, provide the most effective protection against UVA. Some products now indicate the degree of protection offered against UVA with a star rating system. This system does not refer to an absolute measure but indicates the protection against UVA relative to protection against UVB for the same product. Four stars indicate that the product offers a balanced amount of UVA and UVB protection; products with three, two, or one star rating indicate that the protection offered is greater against UVB than UVA. However the usefulness of the star rating system remains controversial.

Some sunscreens, particularly aminobenzoates, may rarely cause photosensitivity reactions. Bergamot oil (which contains 5-methoxypsoralen) occasionally causes photosensitisation with subsequent pigmentation; it is suspected of increasing the incidence of skin cancers, but this has not been established.

BORDERLINE SUBSTANCES. The preparations marked 'ACBS' are regarded as drugs when prescribed for skin protection against ultraviolet radiation in abnormal cutaneous photosensitivity resulting from genetic disorders or photodermatoses, including those resulting from radiotherapy; chronic or recurrent herpes simplex labialis. Preparations with SPF less than 15 are no longer prescribable. See also Appendix 7.

Coppertone® (Scholl)

Ultrashade 23 lotion, (UVA and UVB protection; UVB-SPF23) ethylhexyl *p*-methoxycinnamate 7.5%, oxybenzone 3%, padimate-O 2.5%. Net price 150 mL = £4.46. ACBS

Additives: include hydroxybenzoates (parabens), wool fat, fragrance

Piz Buin® (Zyma)

Sunblock lotion, (UVA and UVB protection; UVB-SPF 20), ethylhexyl *p*-methoxycinnamate 7.5%, avobenzone 1.5%, titanium dioxide 3%. Net price 200 mL = £6.64. ACBS

Additives: include hydroxybenzoates (parabens), propylene glycol, fragrance

RoC® (RoC)

Total sunblock cream, (UVA and UVB protection; UVB-SPF 25), colourless or tinted, containing avobenzone, ethylhexyl *p*-methoxycinnamate. Net price 50 mL = £4.06. ACBS

Additives: include beeswax, hydroxybenzoates (parabens)

Spectraban® (Stiefel)

Lotion, (UVB protection; UVB-SPF 25) aminobenzoic acid 5%, padimate-O 3.2%, in an alcoholic basis. Net price 150 mL = £2.99. ACBS

Additives: include fragrance
Caution: flammable; stains clothing

Ultra lotion, (UVA and UVB protection; UVB SPF 28), water resistant, avobenzone 2%, oxybenzone 3%, padimate-O 8%, titanium dioxide 2%. Net price 150 mL = £5.19. ACBS

Additives: include benzyl alcohol, disodium edetate, sorbic acid, fragrance

Sun E45® (Crookes)

Lotion, (UVA and UVB protection; UVB-SPF 15) water resistant, titanium dioxide 2.4%, zinc oxide 10.5%. Net price 100 mL = £4.78. ACBS

Additives: include hydroxybenzoates (parabens)

Sunblock cream, (UVA and UVB protection; UVB-SPF 25), water resistant, titanium dioxide 5.2%, zinc oxide 12%. Net price 75 mL = £4.78. ACBS

Additives: include butylated hydroxytoluene, isopropyl palmitate

Uvistat® (Windsor)

Lipscreen, (UVA and UVB protection; UVB-SPF 15), ethylhexyl *p*-methoxycinnamate 3%, avobenzone 4%. Net price 5-g stick = £1.58. ACBS

Additives: include butylated hydroxyanisole, fragrance

Babysun cream (UVA and UVB protection; UVB-SPF 22), water-resistant, ethylhexyl *p*-methoxy cinnamate 7%, avobenzone 4%, titanium dioxide 4.5%. Net price 50 g = £3.63, 100 g = £5.10. ACBS

Additives: include disodium edetate, hydroxybenzoates (parabens), fragrance

Cream (UVA and UVB protection; UVB-SPF 27 but marketed as 'factor 20'), water-resistant, ethylhexyl *p*-methoxycinnamate 7%, avobenzone 4%, titanium dioxide 4.5%. Net price 50 g = £3.40, 100 g = £5.10. ACBS

Additives: include disodium edetate, hydroxybenzoates (parabens), fragrance

Lotion (UVA and UVB protection; UVB-SPF 25) tinted, water-resistant, methylbenzylidene camphor 6%, avobenzone 4%, titanium dioxide 4%. Net price 200 mL = £5.08. ACBS

Additives: include edetic acid (EDTA), hydroxybenzoates (parabens), fragrance

Ultrablock cream, (UVA and UVB protection; UVB-SPF 30), ethylhexyl *p*-methoxycinnamate 7.5%, avobenzone 4%, titanium dioxide 6.5%. Net price 50 g = £4.08. ACBS

Additives: include disodium edetate, hydroxybenzoates (parabens), fragrance

13.8.2   Camouflagers

Disfigurement of the skin can be very distressing to patients and have a marked psychological effect. In skilled hands, or with experience, these preparations can be very effective in concealing scars and birthmarks. The depigmented patches in vitiligo are also very disfiguring and camouflage creams are of great cosmetic value.

BORDERLINE SUBSTANCES. The preparations marked 'ACBS' are regarded as drugs when prescribed for postoperative scars and other deformities and as an adjunctive therapy in the relief of emotional disturbances due to disfiguring skin disease, such as vitiligo. See also Appendix 7.

Boots Covering Cream® (Boots)

Cream (2 shades). Net price 50 g = £1.64. ACBS
Additives: include hydroxybenzoates (parabens)

Covermark® (Cupharma)

Classic foundation (masking cream, 10 shades).
Net price 30 g = £11.23. ACBS
Additives: include beeswax, hydroxybenzoates (parabens), fragrance

Finishing powder. Net price 75 g = £9.50. ACBS
Additives: include beeswax, hydroxybenzoates (parabens), fragrance

Dermablend® (Baker Norton)

Cover creme. Net price 10.7 g (10 shades) = £6.25;
28.4 g (11 shades)= £10.55. ACBS
Additives: include beeswax, hydroxybenzoates (parabens)

Leg and body cover, (7 shades) Net price 64 g =
£9.35. ACBS
Additives: include beeswax, hydroxybenzoates (parabens)

Setting powder. Net price 28 g = £9.00. ACBS
Additives: include hydroxybenzoates (parabens)

Dermacolor® (Fox)

Camouflage creme, (30 shades). Net price 30 g =
£7.25. ACBS
Additives: include beeswax, wool fat, fragrance

Fixing powder, (5 shades). Net price 60 g = £5.88.
ACBS
Additives: include fragrance

Keromask® (Network Management)

Masking cream, (2 shades). Net price 15 mL =
£4.28. ACBS
Additives: include butylated hydroxyanisole, hydroxybenzoates (parabens), wool fat

Finishing powder. Net price 25 g = £4.28. ACBS
Additives: none as listed in section 13.1

Veil® (Blake)

Cover cream, (19 shades). Net price 19 g = £4.54;
44 g = £7.09; 70 g = £9.65. ACBS
Additives: include hydroxybenzoates (parabens), wool fat derivative

Finishing powder, translucent. Net price 35 g =
£4.54. ACBS
Additives: include butylated hydroxyanisole, hydroxybenzoates (parabens)

13.9 Shampoos and some other scalp preparations

Dandruff (*pityriasis capitis*) is believed to be
caused by follicular overgrowth with pityrosporum
yeasts; it often increases at puberty. The treatment
of choice is the frequent use of a mild detergent
shampoo generally once or twice weekly; this rids
the scalp of scale but does not have a therapeutic
effect in itself. Shampoos containing antimicrobial
agents such as **pyrithione zinc** have beneficial
effects and are on sale to the general public.
Shampoos containing **tar** extracts may be used
and they are also used in *psoriasis*, both as adjunctive treatment and for the removal of pastes etc.
Shampoos containing **selenium sulphide** are of no
more value than the other shampoos and should not
be used within 48 hours of applying hair colouring
or permanent waving preparations. **Ketoconazole**
is also useful as a shampoo (see section 13.10.2).

For more severe conditions, **corticosteroid** gels
and lotions (section 13.4), applied to the scalp may
be helpful.

Cradle cap in infants may be treated with **olive
oil** or **arachis oil** (ground-nut oil, peanut oil) applications before shampooing.

See also sections 13.5 (psoriasis and eczema),
13.10.4 (lice), and 13.10.2 (ringworm).

ADMINISTRATION. Shampoos should generally be
used once to three times weekly

Alphosyl 2 in 1® (Stafford-Miller)

Shampoo, alcoholic coal tar extract 5%. Net price
125 mL = £1.81; 250 mL = £3.43.

Baltar® (Merck)

Shampoo, coal tar distillate 1.5% in soap-free
basis. Net price 200 mL = £2.28; 500 mL = £4.48

Betadine® (Seton)

Scalp and skin cleanser—section 13.11.4

Shampoo solution, povidone-iodine 4%, in a surfactant solution. Net price 250 mL = £2.43.

Capasal® (Dermal)

Shampoo, coal tar 1%, coconut oil 1%, salicylic
acid 0.5%. Net price 250 mL = £4.83

Ceanel Concentrate® (Quinoderm Ltd)

Shampoo, cetrimide 10%, undecenoic acid 1%,
phenylethyl alcohol 7.5%. Net price 50 mL =
£1.07; 150 mL = £2.83; 500 mL = £8.33

Clinitar® (Shire)

Shampoo solution, coal tar extract 2%. Net price
100 g = £2.50

Cocois® —section 13.5.2

Gelcotar® (Quinoderm Ltd)

Liquid, strong coal tar solution 1.25%, cade oil
0.5%, in a shampoo basis. Net price 150 mL =
£1.41; 350 mL = £2.83

Gel, see section 13.5.2

Ionil T® (Novex)

Shampoo application, benzalkonium chloride
0.2%, coal tar solution 4.25%, salicylic acid 2%
in an alcoholic basis. Net price 200 mL = £2.56

Lenium® (Cilag)

Cream, selenium sulphide 2.5%. Net price 42 g =
94p; 100 g = £1.59

Meted® (Euroderma)

Shampoo, salicylic acid 3%, sulphur 5%. Net price
120 mL = £3.90

PoM **Nizoral®** shampoo—section 13.10.2

Pentrax® (Euroderma)

Shampoo, coal tar 4.3%. Net price 120 mL = £3.90

Pixol® —section 13.5.2

Polytar® (Stiefel)

Liquid, arachis (peanut) oil extract of crude coal
tar 0.3%, cade oil 0.3%, coal tar solution 0.1%,
oleyl alcohol 1%, tar 0.3%. Net price 250 mL =
£2.23

Polytar AF® (Stiefel)

Shampoo, arachis (peanut) oil extract of coal tar
0.3%, cade oil 0.3%, coal tar solution 0.1%, pine
tar 0.3%, pyrithione zinc 1%. Net price 150 mL =
£4.40.

Polytar Plus® (Stiefel)

Liquid, ingredients as Polytar® liquid with hydro-
lysed animal protein 3%. Net price 350 mL =
£3.29

Pragmatar® —section 13.5.2

Psoriderm® (Dermal)

Scalp lotion (= shampoo), coal tar 2.5%, lecithin 0.3%. Net price 250 mL = £4.85

Selsun® (Abbott)

Shampoo application, selenium sulphide 2.5%. Net price 50 mL = £1.16; 100 mL = £1.74; 150 mL = £2.37 (for adults and children over 5 years)

T/Gel® (Neutrogena)

Shampoo, coal tar extract 2%. Net price 125 mL = £2.80; 250 mL = £4.46

LITHIUM SUCCINATE

Topical application of **lithium succinate** in the form of an ointment has been shown to be effective in seborrhoeic dermatitis.

PoM Efalith® (Searle)

Ointment, lithium succinate 8%, zinc sulphate 0.05%. Net price 20 g = £12.19

Additives: include wool fat derivative

Seborrhoeic dermatitis (adults only), apply thinly twice daily initially, then reduce

Cautions: may exacerbate psoriasis

MALE-PATTERN BALDNESS

Topical application of **minoxidil** may stimulate limited hair growth in a small proportion of patients but only for as long as it is used.

MINOXIDIL

Indications: male-pattern baldness (men and women)

Cautions; Contra-indications; Side-effects: see section 2.5.1 (only about 1.4% absorbed); monitor hypertensive patients closely; avoid contact with eyes, mouth and mucous membranes, broken, infected, or inflamed skin; avoid inhalation of spray mist and use with topically applied drugs known to enhance absorption; local side-effects: irritant dermatitis, allergic contact dermatitis

Administration: ADULT aged 18–65 years, apply 1 mL twice daily to dry hair and scalp (discontinue if no improvement after 1 year)

NHS Regaine® (Upjohn)

Topical solution, minoxidil 2% in an aqueous alcoholic basis. Net price 60-mL bottle with applicators = £14.16

Additives: include propylene glycol

Cautions: flammable; wash hands after application

13.10   Anti-infective skin preparations

13.10.1 Antibacterial preparations
13.10.2 Antifungal preparations
13.10.3 Antiviral preparations
13.10.4 Parasiticidal preparations
13.10.5 Preparations for minor cuts and abrasions

13.10.1   Antibacterial preparations

13.10.1.1 Antibacterial preparations only used topically
13.10.1.2 Antibacterial preparations also used systemically

For many skin infections such as *erysipelas* and *cellulitis* systemic antibacterial treatment is the method of choice because the infection is too deeply sited for adequate penetration of topical preparations. For details of suitable treatment see section 5.1, table 1.

Impetigo may be treated by topical application of **fusidic acid** or **mupirocin** or, if widespread, with oral administration of **flucloxacillin** or **erythromycin** (see section 5.1, table 1). Mild antiseptics such as **povidone-iodine** (section 13.11.4) are used to soften crusts and exudate.

Although there are a great many antibacterial drugs presented in topical preparations some are potentially hazardous and frequently their use is not necessary if adequate hygienic measures can be taken. Moreover not all skin conditions that are oozing, crusted, or characterised by pustules are actually infected. Topical antibiotics should be **avoided** on *leg ulcers* unless used in short courses for defined infections; treatment of bacterial colonisation is generally inappropriate.

To minimise the development of resistant organisms it is advisable to limit the choice of antibiotics applied topically to those not used systemically. Unfortunately some of these, for example neomycin, may cause sensitisation, and there is cross-sensitivity with other aminoglycoside antibiotics, such as gentamicin. If *large areas of skin* are being treated, ototoxicity may also be a hazard with aminoglycoside antibiotics (and also with polymyxins), particularly in children, in the elderly, and in those with renal impairment. *Resistant organisms* are more common in hospitals, and whenever possible swabs for bacteriological examination should be taken before beginning treatment.

Mupirocin is not related to any other antibiotic in use; it is effective for skin infections, particularly those due to Gram positive organisms but it is not indicated for pseudomonal infection. Although *Staphylococcus aureus* strains with low level resistance to mupirocin are emerging, it is generally useful when there is resistant infection. To avoid the development of resistance it should not be used for longer than 10 days and its use in hospital should if possible be avoided.

Silver sulphadiazine is used in the treatment of infected burns.

FRAMYCETIN SULPHATE

Indications: bacterial skin infections

Cautions; Side-effects: sensitisation (see also notes above); large areas, see below

LARGE AREAS. If large areas of skin are being treated ototoxicity may be a hazard, particularly in children, in the elderly, and in those with renal impairment

PoM **Soframycin**® (Roussel)

Ointment, framycetin sulphate 1.5%, gramicidin 0.005%, in a wool fat and paraffin basis. Net price 15 g = £1.68

Additives: include wool fat

Superficial bacterial infection, apply up to 3 times daily (short-term use)

Sofra-Tulle® *see* Framycetin Gauze Dressing, section 13.13.6

MUPIROCIN

Indications: bacterial skin infections (see also notes above)

Administration: apply up to 3 times daily for up to 10 days

PoM **Bactroban**® (Beecham)

Ointment, mupirocin 2%. Net price 15 g = £4.71

Additives: none as listed in section 13.1

Note. Manufacturer advises: contains macrogol therefore caution in renal impairment; may sting

Nasal ointment, see section 12.2.3

NEOMYCIN SULPHATE

Indications: bacterial skin infections

Cautions; Side-effects: sensitisation (see also notes above); large areas, see below

LARGE AREAS. If large areas of skin are being treated ototoxicity may be a hazard, particularly in children, in the elderly, and in those with renal impairment

PoM **Neomycin Cream BPC**

Cream, neomycin sulphate 0.5%, cetomacrogol emulsifying ointment 30%, chlorocresol 0.1%, disodium edetate 0.01%, in freshly boiled and cooled purified water. Net price 15 g = 88p

Apply up to 3 times daily (short-term use)

PoM **Cicatrin**® (Wellcome)

Cream, neomycin sulphate 3300 units, bacitracin zinc 250 units, cysteine 2 mg, glycine 10 mg, threonine 1 mg/g. Net price 15 g = 90p; 30 g = £1.80

Additives: include wool fat derivative

Superficial bacterial infection of skin, apply up to 3 times daily; ADULT max. 60 g daily for 3 weeks; do not repeat for at least 3 months; CHILD reduced dose

Dusting powder, neomycin sulphate 3300 units, bacitracin zinc 250 units, cysteine 2 mg, glycine 10 mg, threonine 1 mg/g. Net price 15 g = 90p; 50 g = £3.00

Additives: none as listed in section 13.1

Superficial bacterial infection of skin, apply up to 3 times daily; ADULT max. 50 g daily for 4 weeks; do not repeat for at least 3 months; CHILD reduced dose

PoM **Graneodin**® (Squibb)

Ointment, neomycin sulphate 0.25%, gramicidin 0.025%. Net price 25 g = £1.47

Additives: none as listed in section 13.1

Superficial bacterial infection of skin, apply 2–4 times daily (for max. 7 days—possibly longer for sycosis barbae)

POLYMYXINS

(Includes colistin sulphate and polymyxin B sulphate)

Indications: bacterial skin infections

Cautions; Side-effects: sensitisation (see also notes above); large areas, see below

LARGE AREAS. If large areas of skin are being treated ototoxicity may be a hazard, particularly in children, in the elderly, and in those with renal impairment

PoM **Polyfax**® (Dominion)

Ointment, polymyxin B sulphate 10 000 units, bacitracin zinc 500 units/g. Net price 20 g = £4.84

Apply 3 times daily

PoM **Colomycin**® (Pharmax)

Powder, sterile, for making topical preparations (usually 1%), colistin sulphate. Net price 1 g vial = £19.24

SILVER SULPHADIAZINE

Indications: prophylaxis and treatment of infection in burn wounds; as an adjunct to short-term treatment of infection in leg ulcers and pressure sores; as an adjunct to prophylaxis of infection in skin graft donor sites and extensive abrasions; for conservative management of finger-tip injuries

Cautions: hepatic and renal impairment; G6PD deficiency; pregnancy and breast-feeding (avoid in late pregnancy and in neonate—see also Appendix 4); may inactivate enzymatic debriding agents therefore concomitant use may be inappropriate; for large amounts see also **interactions:** Appendix 1 (co-trimoxazole and sulphonamides)

LARGE AREAS. Plasma-sulphadiazine concentrations may approach therapeutic levels with *side-effects* and *interactions* as for sulphonamides (see section 5.1.8) if large areas of skin are treated. Owing to the association of sulphonamides with severe blood and skin disorders treatment should be stopped immediately if blood disorders or rashes develop—but leucopenia developing 2–3 days after starting treatment of burns patients is reported usually to be self-limiting and silver sulphadiazine need not usually be discontinued provided blood counts are monitored carefully to ensure return to normality within a few days. Argyria may also occur if large areas of skin are treated (or if application is prolonged).

Contra-indications: pregnancy and breast-feeding; sensitivity to sulphonamides; not recommended for neonates (see also Appendix 4)

Side-effects: allergic reactions including burning, itching and rashes; argyria reported following prolonged use; leucopenia reported (monitor blood levels)

PoM **Flamazine**® (S&N Hlth.)

Cream, silver sulphadiazine 1%. Net price 50 g = £4.30; 250 g = £11.52; 500 g = £20.40

Additives: include polysorbates, propylene glycol

In burns apply daily with sterile applicator or more frequently if volume of exudate large; in leg ulcers daily (or every 48 hours—not recommended for leg or pressure ulcers that are very exudative); in finger-tip injuries apply every 2–3 days—for details see data sheet

13.10.1.2 ANTIBACTERIAL PREPARATIONS ALSO USED SYSTEMICALLY

CHLORTETRACYCLINE HYDROCHLORIDE

Indications: bacterial skin infections (see notes above)

Cautions: see notes above; overgrowth with non-susceptible organisms; stains clothing

Side-effects: rarely local hypersensitivity reactions

Administration: apply 1 to 3 times daily

PoM **Aureomycin®** (Lederle)

Cream, chlortetracycline hydrochloride 3% (as chlortetracycline). Net price 30 g = £1.77

Additives: include chlorocresol

Ointment, chlortetracycline hydrochloride 3%. Net price 30 g = £1.77

Additives: include hydroxybenzoates (parabens), wool fat

FUSIDIC ACID

Indications: staphylococcal skin infections

Cautions: see notes above; avoid contact with eyes

Side-effects: rarely local hypersensitivity reactions

Administration: apply 3–4 times daily

PoM **Fucidin®** (Leo)

Cream, fusidic acid 2%. Net price 15 g = £2.87; 30 g = £4.84

Additives: include butylated hydroxyanisole

Gel, fusidic acid 2%. Net price 15 g = £2.48; 30 g = £4.29

Additives: include hydroxybenzoates (parabens), polysorbate 80

Ointment, sodium fusidate 2%. Net price 15 g = £2.34; 30 g = £3.97

Additives: include wool fat

PoM **Fucidin Intertulle®** *see* section 13.13.6

GENTAMICIN

Indications: bacterial skin infections

Cautions; Side-effects: sensitisation (see also notes above); large areas, see below

LARGE AREAS. If large areas of skin are being treated ototoxicity may be a hazard, particularly in children, in the elderly, and in those with renal impairment

Administration: apply 3–4 times daily

PoM **Cidomycin Topical®** (Roussel)

Cream, gentamicin 0.3% (as sulphate). Net price 15 g = £1.71; 30 g = £3.31

Additives: include hydroxybenzoates (parabens), propylene glycol

Ointment, gentamicin 0.3% (as sulphate). Net price 15 g = £1.71; 30 g = £3.31

Additives: none as listed in section 13.1

METRONIDAZOLE

Indications: see under preparations

Side-effects: local skin irritation

Rosacea

PoM **Metrogel®** (Sandoz)

Gel, metronidazole 0.75%. Net price 40 g = £17.36. Label: 10 patient information leaflet

Additives: include hydroxybenzoates (parabens), propylene glycol

Administration: acute inflammatory exacerbations of acne rosacea, apply thinly twice daily for 8–9 weeks; avoid contact with eyes

PoM **Rozex®** (Stafford-Miller)

Gel, metronidazole 0.75%. Net price 30 g = £12.00. Label: 10 patient information leaflet

Additives: include disodium edetate, hydroxybenzoates (parabens), propylene glycol

Administration: inflammatory papules, pustules and erythema of acne rosacea, apply thinly twice daily; avoid contact with eyes

Malodorous tumours

PoM **Anabact®** (ASTA Medica)

Gel, metronidazole 0.75%. Net price 15 g = £4.70; 30 g = £8.31

Additives: include hydroxybenzoates (parabens), propylene glycol

Administration: fungating malodorous tumours, apply to clean wound twice daily and cover with non-adherent dressing

PoM **Metrotop®** (Pharmacia)

Gel, metronidazole 0.8%. Net price 15 g = £4.95; 30 g = £8.75

Additives: none as listed in section 13.1

Administration: de-odourisation of fungating malodorous tumours, apply to clean wound 1 to 2 times daily and cover (flat wounds, apply liberally; cavities, smear on paraffin gauze and pack loosely); use tube once only

TETRACYCLINE HYDROCHLORIDE

Indications; Cautions; Side-effects: see under Chlortetracycline Hydrochloride

PoM **Achromycin Topical®** (Lederle)

Ointment, tetracycline hydrochloride 3%. Net price 30 g = £1.44

Additives: include hydroxybenzoates (parabens), wool fat

Apply 1–3 times daily

13.10.2   Antifungal preparations

Ideally skin scrapings should be examined to confirm diagnosis before treatment is begun. Widespread or intractable fungal infections are treated systemically (see section 5.2). Most localised infections are treated with the topical preparations described below.

Most ringworm infections, including tinea pedis, can be treated adequately with topical preparations. The imidazoles **clotrimazole**, **econazole**, **miconazole** and **sulconazole** are all effective and commonly used. Nail ringworm (tinea unguium) and scalp ringworm (*T. capitis*) are treated systemically (see section 5.2). **Amorolfine** is a newly introduced antifungal that differs chemically from other antifungals and has some activity against moulds. It is available as a cream for fungal skin infections and a lacquer for fungal nail infections. **Terbinafine** has also been recently introduced in the form of a cream; it is also available for systemic administration (see section 5.2). Combinations of imidazoles and weak corticosteroids may be of use in the treatment of eczematous intertrigo and, in the first few days only, of a severely inflamed patch of ringworm. **Compound benzoic acid ointment** (Whitfield's ointment) was also quite effective but was cosmetically less acceptable than the proprietary preparations and is rarely used. The **undecenoates** are less effective in treating ringworm infections.

Candidal skin infections may also be treated by topical application with the broad-spectrum antifungals, clotrimazole, econazole, and miconazole. Oral preparations of some antifungals are now also available (see section 5.2), but should preferably be reserved for those who are resistant to (or intolerant of) topical preparations. **Nystatin** preparations are also equally as effective in candidiasis although they are ineffective against infections due to dermatophyte fungi (tinea).

Lotions or sprays are generally chosen for application to large and hairy areas. Ointments are best avoided on moist surfaces because of their occlusive properties. Nail lacquers and paints may be effective for early fungal dystrophy of the nails and should be considered when up to 2 nails are affected (or where systemic therapy is contra-indicated). Dusting-powders have no place in the treatment of fungal infections, except for toiletry or cosmetic purposes, as they are therapeutically ineffective and may cause skin irritation.

AMOROLFINE

Indications: see under preparations
Cautions: pregnancy, breast-feeding; avoid eyes, ears, and mucous membranes
Side-effects: occasional transient burning sensation, erythema, pruritus

PoM **Loceryl**® (Roche)
Cream, amorolfine (as hydrochloride) 0.25%. Net price 20 g = £4.83. Label: 10 patient information leaflet
Additives: include disodium edetate
Administration: fungal skin infections, apply once daily after cleansing in the evening for at least 2–3 weeks (up to 6 weeks for foot mycosis) continuing for 3–5 days after lesions have healed
Nail lacquer, amorolfine (as hydrochloride) 5%. Net price 5-mL pack (with nail files, spatulas and cleansing swabs) = £34.38. Label: 10 patient information leaflet
Administration: fungal nail infections, apply to infected nails 1–2 times weekly after filing and cleansing; allow to dry (approx. 3 minutes); treat finger nails for 6 months, toe nails for 9–12 months (review at intervals of 3 months)

BENZOIC ACID

Indications: ringworm (tinea), but see notes above

Benzoic Acid Ointment, Compound, BP
(Whitfield's ointment), benzoic acid 6%, salicylic acid 3%, in emulsifying ointment
Apply twice daily

BENZOYL PEROXIDE

Indications: fungal skin infections, particularly tinea pedis

Quinoped® (Quinoderm Ltd)
Cream, benzoyl peroxide 5%, potassium hydroxyquinoline sulphate 0.5%, in an astringent basis. Net price 25 g = 96p
Additives: include edetic acid (EDTA)
Apply twice daily

CLOTRIMAZOLE

Indications: fungal skin infections
Side-effects: occasional skin irritation or sensitivity
Administration: apply 2–3 times daily continuing for 14 days after lesions have healed

Canesten® (Baypharm)
Cream, clotrimazole 1%. Net price 20 g = £1.77; 50 g = £4.15
Additives: include benzyl alcohol, polysorbate 60
Note. A generic version of clotrimazole 1% cream is available from APS, CP, Cox; proprietary brands on sale to the public include Canesten® AF and Mycil Gold®
Solution, clotrimazole 1% in macrogol 400 (polyethylene glycol 400). Net price 20 mL = £2.32. For hairy areas
Additives: none as listed in section 13.1
Spray, clotrimazole 1%, in 30% isopropyl alcohol. Net price 40-mL atomiser = £4.99. Label: 15. For large or hairy areas
Additives: include propylene glycol
Dusting powder, clotrimazole 1%. Net price 30 g = £1.52
Additives: none as listed in section 13.1
Masnoderm® (Dominion)
Cream, clotrimazole 1%. Net price 20 g = £1.54
Additives: include benzyl alcohol, polysorbates

ECONAZOLE NITRATE

Indications; Side-effects: see under Clotrimazole
Administration: apply 2–3 times daily continuing for 14 days after lesions have healed

Ecostatin® (Squibb)
Cream, econazole nitrate 1%. Net price 15 g = £1.49; 30 g = £2.75
Additives: include butylated hydroxyanisole, fragrance
Pevaryl® (Cilag)
Cream, econazole nitrate 1%. Net price 30 g = £2.65
Additives: include butylated hydroxyanisole, fragrance
Lotion, econazole nitrate 1%. Net price 30 mL = £3.33
Additives: include butylated hydroxyanisole, fragrance

KETOCONAZOLE

Indications; Side-effects: see under Clotrimazole

PoM **Nizoral®** (Janssen-Cilag)

NHS*Cream*, ketoconazole 2%. Net price 30 g = £3.81

Additives: include polysorbates, propylene glycol

Apply 1–2 times daily, continuing for a few days after lesions have healed

* except for seborrhoeic dermatitis and pityriasis versicolor and endorsed 'SLS' ('S2B' in Scotland)

Shampoo, ketoconazole 2%. Net price 120 mL = £8.75

Additives: none as listed in section 13.1

For seborrhoeic dermatitis and dandruff apply twice weekly for 2–4 weeks, for pityriasis versicolor once daily for max. 5 days; avoid for 2 weeks following topical corticosteroid treatment

Note. Can be sold to the public for the prevention and treatment of dandruff and seborrhoeic dermatitis of the scalp as a shampoo formulation containing ketoconazole max. 2%, in a pack containing max.120 mL and labelled to show a max. frequency of application of once every 3 days; a brand on sale to the public is Nizoral® Dandruff Shampoo (60-mL pack)

MICONAZOLE NITRATE

Indications; Side-effects: see under Clotrimazole
Administration: apply twice daily continuing for 10 days after lesions have healed; nail infections, apply daily under occlusive dressing

Daktarin® (Janssen)

Cream, miconazole nitrate 2%. Net price 30 g = £2.07

Additives: include butylated hydroxyanisole

Note. A generic version of miconazole nitrate 2% cream is available from APS, Hillcross

Dusting powder, miconazole nitrate 2%. Net price 20 g = £1.81

Additives: none as listed in section 13.1

Spray powder, miconazole nitrate 0.16%, in an aerosol basis. Net price 100 g = £1.81

Additives: none as listed in section 13.1

Twin pack, 1 × 30 g pack of cream miconazole nitrate 2%, with 1 × 30 g dusting-powder miconazole nitrate 2%. Net price = £3.80

NYSTATIN

Indications: skin infections due to *Candida* spp.
Administration: apply 2–4 times daily, continuing for 7 days after lesions have healed

PoM **Nystaform®** (Bayer)

Cream, nystatin 100 000 units/g, chlorhexidine hydrochloride 1%. Net price 30 g = £2.62

Additives: include benzyl alcohol, polysorbate 60

PoM **Nystan®** (Squibb)

Cream, nystatin 100 000 units/g. Net price 30 g = £2.18

Additives: include benzyl alcohol, propylene glycol, fragrance

Gel, nystatin 100 000 units/g. Net price 30 g = £2.66

Additives: include chlorocresol, fragrance

Ointment, nystatin 100 000 units/g, in Plastibase®. Net price 30 g = £1.75

Additives: none as listed in section 13.1

PoM **Tinaderm-M®** (Schering-Plough)

Cream, nystatin 100 000 units/g, tolnaftate 1%. Net price 20 g = £1.83. For *Candida* infections and tinea

Additives: include butylated hydroxytoluene, hydroxybenzoates (parabens), fragrance

SALICYLIC ACID

Indications: fungal skin infections, particularly tinea
Side-effects: hypersensitivity reactions

Phytex® (Pharmax)

Paint, salicylic acid 1.46% (total combined), tannic acid 4.89% and boric acid 3.12% (as borotannic complex), in a vehicle containing alcohol and ethyl acetate. Net price 25 mL (with brush) = £1.29. For fungal nail infections (onychomycosis)

Additives: none as listed in section 13.1

Apply twice daily

Caution: flammable; avoid in pregnancy and children under 5 years

SULCONAZOLE NITRATE

Indications; Side-effects: see under Clotrimazole
Cautions: avoid contact with eyes (lens changes in *animals* after high oral doses)

PoM **Exelderm®** (Zeneca)

Cream, sulconazole nitrate 1%. Net price 30 g = £3.00

Apply 1–2 times daily continuing for 2–3 weeks after lesions have healed

Additives: include polysorbates, propylene glycol

TERBINAFINE

Indications: fungal skin infections
Cautions: pregnancy, breast-feeding; avoid contact with eyes
Side-effects: redness, itching, or stinging; rarely allergic reactions (discontinue)

▼ PoM **Lamisil®** (Sandoz)

Cream, terbinafine hydrochloride 1%. Net price 15 g = £4.86; 30 g = £8.76

Apply thinly 1–2 times daily for up to 1 week in tinea pedis, 1–2 weeks in tinea corporis and tinea cruris, 2 weeks in cutaneous candidiasis and pityriasis versicolor; review after 2 weeks; CHILD not recommended

Additives: include benzyl alcohol, polysorbate 60

Tablets, see section 5.2

TIOCONAZOLE

Indications: see under preparations
Side-effects: local irritation, usually during first week of treatment; discontinue if sensitivity reaction develops

Trosyl® (Pfizer)

PoM *Nail solution*, tioconazole 28%. Net price 12 mL (with applicator brush) = £27.38

Additives: none as listed in section 13.1

Administration: fungal nail infections, apply to nails and surrounding skin twice daily for up to 6 months (may be extended to 12 months)

Cream, tioconazole 1%. Net price 15 g = £1.51; 30 g = £2.78

Additives: include benzyl alcohol, polysorbate 60
Administration: fungal skin infections, apply once or twice daily for 2–4 weeks (up to 6 weeks for foot mycosis)

UNDECENOATES
Indications: skin infections, particularly tinea pedis

Monphytol® (LAB)
Paint, methyl undecenoate 5%, propyl undecenoate 0.7%, salicylic acid 3%, methyl salicylate 25%, propyl salicylate 5%, chlorbutol 3%. Net price 18 mL (with brush) = £1.26. For fungal (particularly nail) infections
Additives: none as listed in section 13.1
Apply twice daily

Mycota® (Seton)
Cream, zinc undecenoate 20%, undecenoic acid 5%. Net price 25 g = 96p
Additives: include fragrance
Dusting powder, zinc undecenoate 20%, undecenoic acid 2%. Net price 70 g = £1.45
Additives: include fragrance
Spray application, undecenoic acid 2.5%, dichlorophen 0.25% (pressurised aerosol pack). Net price 100 mL = £1.56
Additives: include fragrance
Apply 1–2 times daily

13.10.3 Antiviral preparations

Aciclovir cream is indicated for the treatment of initial and recurrent labial and genital *herpes simplex infections*; treatment should begin as early as possible. Systemic treatment is necessary for buccal or vaginal infections; *herpes zoster (shingles)* also requires systemic treatment (for details of systemic use see section 5.3). **Penciclovir** cream has been introduced recently; it is indicated for the treatment of labial *herpes simplex infection*.

Idoxuridine solution (5% in dimethyl sulphoxide) is of little value.

ACICLOVIR
Indications: see notes above
Cautions: avoid contact with eyes and mucous membranes
Side-effects: transient stinging or burning; occasionally erythema or drying of the skin

PoM Zovirax® (Warner Wellcome)
Cream, aciclovir 5%. Net price 2 g = £5.29; 10 g = £15.94
Administration: apply to lesions every 4 hours (5 times daily) for 5 days, started at first sign of attack
Additives: include propylene glycol
Note. A 2-g tube and a pump pack are on sale to the public for the treatment of cold sores (Zovirax® Cold Sore Cream)
Eye ointment, see section 11.3.3
Tablets, see section 5.3

PENCICLOVIR
Indications: see notes above
Cautions; Side-effects: see under Aciclovir

▼ **PoM Vectavir®** (SmithKline Beecham)
Cream, penciclovir 1%. Net price 2 g = £4.20
Administration: Herpes labialis, apply to lesions every 2 hours during waking hours for 4 days, started as early as possible after first sign of attack; CHILD under 16 years, not recommended
Additives: include propylene glycol

IDOXURIDINE IN DIMETHYL SULPHOXIDE
Indications: of little value, see notes above
Cautions: avoid contact with the eyes, mucous membranes, and textiles; breast-feeding (may taste unpleasant)
Contra-indications: pregnancy (toxicity in *animal* studies); **not** to be used in mouth
Side-effects: stinging on application, changes in taste; overuse may cause maceration

PoM Herpid® (Yamanouchi)
Application, idoxuridine 5% in dimethyl sulphoxide. Net price 5 mL (with applicator) = £6.25
Administration: Herpes simplex or herpes zoster, apply to lesions 4 times daily for 4 days, starting at first sign of attack; CHILD under 12 years, not recommended

PoM Iduridin® (Ferring)
Application, idoxuridine 5% in dimethyl sulphoxide. Net price 5 mL (with applicator) = £5.88
Administration: Herpes simplex or herpes zoster, apply to lesions 4 times daily for 4 days, starting at first sign of attack; CHILD under 12 years, not recommended
Application, idoxuridine 40% in dimethyl sulphoxide. Net price 5 mL (with applicator) = £19.00; 20 mL with dropper = £39.00
Administration: Severe herpes zoster only, apply on plain lint and retain over affected area (dermatome), changing once every 24 hours for 4 days (**not** for herpes simplex); CHILD under 12 years, not recommended

PoM Virudox® (Bioglan)
Application, idoxuridine 5% in dimethyl sulphoxide. Net price 5 mL (with applicator) = £6.19
Administration: Herpes simplex or herpes zoster, apply to lesions 4 times daily for 4 days, starting at first sign of attack; CHILD under 12 years, not recommended

13.10.4 Parasiticidal preparations

Suitable quantities of parasiticidal preparations to be prescribed for specific areas of the body in adults are:

	Skin creams	Lotions	Cream rinses
Scalp (headlice)	—	50 mL	50–100 mL
Body (scabies)	30–60 g	100 mL	—
Body (crab lice)	30–60 g	100 mL	—

These amounts are usually suitable for an adult for single application.

SCABIES

Malathion and **permethrin** are indicated for *scabies (Sarcoptes scabiei)*.

Aqueous preparations are preferable to alcoholic lotions, which are not recommended owing to irritation of excoriated skin and the genitalia.

Lindane has recently been discontinued. Older preparations include benzyl benzoate, which is an irritant and should be avoided in children; monosulfiram, which was liable to induce disulfiram-like reactions with alcohol has been discontinued.

APPLICATION. Although acaricides have traditionally been applied after a hot bath, this is **not** necessary and there is even evidence that a hot bath may increase absorption into the bloodstream, removing them from their site of action on the skin.

All members of the affected household should be treated. Treatment should be applied to the whole body paying particular attention to the webs of the fingers and toes and brushing lotion under the ends of the nails. In the case of infants and young children (up to the age of about 2 years) application should be extended to the scalp, neck, face, and ears. Application may also need to be extended to the scalp, neck, face, and ears in the elderly, immunocompromised and those who have experienced treatment failure. Providing the application is done properly malathion and permethrin need only be applied once; in the case of benzyl benzoate up to three applications on consecutive days may be needed. It is important to warn users **not** to wash their hands since this would require re-application. Patients with hyperkeratotic (crusted or 'Norwegian') scabies may require two or three applications of acaricide on consecutive days to ensure that enough penetrates the skin crusts to kill all the mites.

ITCHING. The *itch of scabies* persists for some weeks after the infestation has been eliminated and antipruritic treatment may be required. Application of **crotamiton** can be used to control itching after treatment with more effective acaricides, but caution is necessary if the skin is excoriated—**calamine** is probably more suitable. Oral administration of a **sedative antihistamine** (see section 3.4.1) at night may also be useful.

HEAD LICE

Malathion and **carbaryl** are recommended for *head lice* (*Pediculus humanus capitis*). Both should generally be used as lotions in preference to shampoos, which are not in contact with the hair long enough and are normally diluted too much in use to be effective; aqueous formulations are preferred for asthmatic patients and small children, to avoid alcoholic fumes. A contact time of 12 hours or overnight treatment is recommended. A 2-hour treatment is no longer regarded as sufficient to ensure death of eggs.

Permethrin and **phenothrin** are pyrethroids, both of which can be effective but lice have developed resistance in some districts.

In general, treatment for head lice should preferably be repeated after 7 days to kill lice emerging from any eggs that might have survived the first application.

Most health districts operate a **rotating policy** for head lice treatment. In view of increasing resistance, however, if there is any doubt about the efficacy of a product, it may be appropriate to switch to another one.

A **head lice repellant** containing piperonal 2% (Rappell®) is on sale to the public.

CRAB LICE

Malathion and **carbaryl** are effective for *crab lice* (*Pthirus pubis*). Aqueous lotions should be applied to **all** parts of the body (not merely the groins and axillae) for 12 hours or overnight; a second treatment is preferable after 7 days to kill lice emerging from surviving eggs. Alcoholic lotions are not recommended (owing to irritation of excoriated skin and the genitalia).

Aqueous **malathion** lotion is effective for *crab lice of the eye lashes* (but does not have a product licence for this indication).

BENZYL BENZOATE

Benzyl benzoate is effective for *scabies* but is not a first-choice for *scabies* (see notes above).

BENZYL BENZOATE

Indications: see notes above and under preparations

Cautions: children (see notes above), avoid contact with eyes and mucous membranes; do not use on broken or secondarily infected skin; pregnancy and breast-feeding

Side-effects: skin irritation, burning sensation especially on genitalia and excoriations, occasionally rashes

Benzyl Benzoate Application, BP, benzyl benzoate 25% in an emulsion basis. Net price 500 mL = £2.36

Administration: scabies—apply 25% application over the whole body; repeat without bathing on the following day and wash off 24 hours later; a third application may be required in some cases

Note. Not recommended for children—dilution to reduce irritant effect also reduces efficacy (see notes above). Some manufacturers recommend application to the body but exclude the head and neck, but in case of the elderly, the immunocompromised and those who have experienced treatment failure, application may need to be extended to the scalp, neck, face, and ears

Available from CP, Norton, Rhône-Poulenc Rorer (Ascabiol®)

CARBARYL

Carbaryl is recommended for *head lice* and *crab lice* (see notes above). In the light of conclusions (based on experimental data in *animals*) it would be prudent to consider carbaryl as a potential human carcinogen, it has recently been restricted to prescription only use. The Department of Health has emphasised that the risk is a theoretical one and that any risk from the intermittent use of head lice preparations is likely to be exceedingly small.

CARBARYL

Indications: see notes above and under preparations

Cautions: avoid contact with eyes; do not use on broken or secondarily infected skin; alcoholic lotions **not** recommended for pediculosis in asthmatics or small children, or for crab lice (see notes above); do not use lotion more than once a week for 3 weeks at a time; children under 6 months, medical supervision required

Side-effects: skin irritation

Administration: lotion—apply to dry hair and rub into the hair and scalp or affected areas, allow to dry naturally, comb, and remove by washing 12 hours later (see also notes above); shampoo—shampoo in, leave on hair for 5 minutes, rinse, repeat, rinse, allow to dry, comb, repeat twice at intervals of 3 days

▸M Carylderm® (Seton)
Lotion, carbaryl 0.5%, in an alcoholic basis. Net price 55 mL = £2.10; 160 mL = £4.71. Label: 15. For crab lice and head lice (alcoholic, see notes above)

Shampoo, carbaryl 1%. Net price 100 mL = £3.13. For crab lice and head lice

▸M Clinicide® (De Witt)
Lotion, carbaryl 0.5% in an aqueous basis containing 10% alcohol. Net price 50 mL = £1.52. For crab lice and head lice

▸M Derbac® C (Seton)
Liquid (= lotion), carbaryl 1% in an aqueous basis. Net price 50 mL = £2.10; 200 mL = £5.33. For head lice

▸M Suleo-C® (Seton)
Lotion, carbaryl 0.5%, in an alcoholic basis. Net price 50 mL = £2.10; 200 mL = £5.33. Label: 15. For head lice (alcoholic, see notes above)

LINDANE

Lindane was formerly used for *scabies* and *crab lice.* It is no longer available.

LINDANE

Indications: see notes above

Cautions: avoid contact with eyes and mucous membranes; do not use on broken or secondarily infected skin; do not use more than twice for one course of treatment; pregnancy (see Appendix 4) and breast-feeding; children under 6 months, medical supervision required

Side-effects: skin irritation

Quellada®—product discontinued

MALATHION

Malathion is recommended for *scabies, head lice* and *crab lice* (for details see notes above).

MALATHION

Indications: see notes above and under preparations

Cautions: avoid contact with eyes; do not use on broken or secondarily infected skin; alcoholic lotions **not** recommended for pediculosis in asthmatics or small children, or for scabies or crab lice (see notes above); do not use lotion more than once a week for 3 weeks at a time; children under 6 months, medical supervision required

Side-effects: skin irritation

Administration: pediculosis—rub 0.5% lotion into dry hair, scalp, and affected area, comb, allow to dry naturally, remove by washing after 12 hours (see also notes above); apply 1% shampoo to hair for 5 minutes, rinse, repeat, rinse again, comb, repeat twice at intervals of 3 days

Scabies—apply 0.5% preparation over whole body, and wash off after 24 hours, see also notes above

Note. Manufacturer recommends application to the body but excludes the head and neck. In the case of young children, however, application may need to be extended to the scalp, neck, face, and ears. This extended application may also be necessary for the elderly, for the immunocompromised and for those who have experienced treatment failure

Derbac-M® (Seton)
Liquid, malathion 0.5% in an aqueous basis. Net price 50 mL = £1.93; 200 mL = £4.84. For crab lice, head lice and scabies

Prioderm® (Seton)
Lotion, malathion 0.5%, in an alcoholic basis. Net price 55 mL = £1.93; 160 mL = £4.27. Label: 15. For crab lice, head lice and scabies (alcoholic, see notes above)

Cream shampoo, malathion 1%. Net price 40 g = £2.14. For crab lice and head lice

Quellada M® (Stafford-Miller)
Liquid, malathion 0.5% in an aqueous basis. Net price 50 mL = £1.94; 200 mL = £4.84. For crab lice, head lice and scabies

Cream shampoo, malathion 1%. Net price 40 g = £2.14. For crab lice and head lice

Suleo-M® (Seton)
Lotion, malathion 0.5%, in an alcoholic basis. Net price 50 mL = £1.93; 200 mL = £4.84. Label: 15. For head lice (alcoholic, see notes above)

PERMETHRIN

Permethrin is effective for *scabies* and *head lice* (for details see notes above).

PERMETHRIN

Indications: see notes above and under preparations

Cautions: avoid contact with eyes; do not use on broken or secondarily infected skin; pregnancy and breast-feeding; children under 6 months, medical supervision required for cream rinse (head lice); children aged 2 months—2 years, medical supervision required for dermal cream (scabies)

Side-effects: pruritus, erythema, and stinging; rarely rashes and oedema

Lyclear® (Warner Wellcome)
Cream rinse, permethrin 1% in basis containing isopropyl alcohol 20%. Net price 59 mL = £2.14
Administration: head lice, apply to clean damp hair, leave on for 10 minutes, rinse and dry; not affected by chlorine in swimming pools

Dermal cream, permethrin 5%. Net price 30 g =
£5.50. Label: 10 patient information leaflet
Administration: scabies, apply over whole body and
wash off after 8–24 hours; CHILD apply over whole body
including face, neck, scalp and ears. If hands are washed
with soap and water within 8 hours of application, cream
should be reapplied
Note. Manufacturer recommends application to the body
but excludes the head and neck. In the case of young
children, however, application may need to be extended
to the scalp, neck, face, and ears. This extended application may also be necessary for the elderly, for the immunocompromised and for those who have experienced
treatment failure.
In larger patients one 30-g pack may not be enough
resulting in inadequate treatment.

PHENOTHRIN

Phenothrin is recommended for *head lice* and *crab
lice* (for details see notes above).

PHENOTHRIN
Indications: see notes above and under preparations
Cautions: avoid contact with eyes; do not use on
broken or secondarily infected skin; children
under 6 months, medical supervision required;
may cause wheezing in asthmatics
Side-effects: skin irritation

Full Marks® (Seton)
Lotion, phenothrin 0.2% in basis containing isopropyl alcohol 69.3%. Net price 55 mL = £1.93;
160 mL = £4.27. Label: 15
Administration: crab lice and head lice (alcoholic, see
above), apply to dry hair, allow to dry naturally; shampoo after 2 hours, comb while still wet

13.10.5   Preparations for minor cuts and abrasions

Some of the preparations listed are used in minor
burns, and abrasions. They are applied as necessary.
Preparations containing camphor, hydrargaphen,
and sulphonamides should be **avoided**. Preparations such as magnesium sulphate paste are also
listed but are now rarely used to treat carbuncles
and boils as these are best treated with antibiotics
(see section 5.1.1.2).

Cetrimide Cream, BP, cetrimide 0.5% in a suitable
water-miscible basis such as cetostearyl alcohol 5%,
liquid paraffin 50% in freshly boiled and cooled purified water. Net price 50 g = 66p
Chlorhexidine Cream, BP 1988, chlorhexidine
gluconate solution usually 5% (≡ chlorhexidine
gluconate 1%), cetomacrogol emulsifying wax 25%,
liquid paraffin 10%, in purified water, freshly boiled
and cooled
Proflavine Cream, BPC, proflavine hemisulphate 0.1%,
yellow beeswax 2.5%, chlorocresol 0.1%, liquid paraffin 67.3%, freshly boiled and cooled purified water
25%, wool fat 5%. Net price 100 mL = 88p
Caution: stains clothing
Anaflex® (Geistlich)
Cream, polynoxylin 10%, in a water-miscible
basis. Net price 50 g = £2.71

Betadine® (Seton)
Ointment, povidone-iodine 10%, in a water-misci-
ble basis. Net price 20 g = £1.45; 80 g = £2.92
Avoid in children under 2 years
Additives: none as listed in section 13.1
Brulidine® (Rhône-Poulenc Rorer)
Cream, dibromopropamidine isethionate 0.15%, in
a water-miscible basis. Net price 25 g = 89p
Additives: include hydroxybenzoates (parabens), fragrance
Cetavlex® (Zeneca)
Cream, cetrimide 0.5%, in a water-miscible basis.
Net price 50 g = 54p
Additives: include hydroxybenzoates (parabens)
Dermalex® (Sanofi Winthrop)
Skin lotion, allantoin 0.2%, hexachlorophane
0.5%, squalane 3% in an emulsion basis. Net
price 100 mL = £2.00; 250 mL = £5.22.
For prevention of pressure sores and prevention and
treatment of urinary rash. Avoid in children under 2
years, except under medical supervision
Additives: include butylated hydroxyanisole, edetic acid
hydroxybenzoates (parabens), wool fat, fragrance
Vesagex® (Rybar)
Cream, cetrimide 1%. Net price 500 g = £6.23
Additives: include chlorocresol, fragrance

Preparations for boils
Magnesium Sulphate Paste, BP, dried
magnesium sulphate 45 g, glycerol 55 g, phenol
500 mg. Net price 25 g = 50p; 50 g = 54p. Should
be stirred before use
Apply under dressing

COLLODION

Flexible collodion may be used to seal minor cuts
and wounds that have partially healed.

Collodion, Flexible, BP, castor oil 2.5%, colophony 2.5% in a collodion basis, prepared by dissolving pyroxylin (10%) in a mixture of 3
volumes of ether and 1 volume of alcohol (90%).
Net price 10 mL = 18p. Label: 15 (**important:
very highly inflammable**)

SURGICAL TISSUE ADHESIVE

Enbucrilate is used as a tissue adhesive for closure
of minor skin wounds and sealing sutured skin
wounds. Within 20 seconds of contact with tissue
moisture it polymerises with an exothermic reaction
into a firm adhesive bond. It must therefore be
applied very thinly (to avoid heat damage) and with
proper technique (poor alignment cannot be corrected). Contact with eyes, internal organs, blood
vessels, and nervous tissue should be **avoided**.

Histoacryl® (Davis & Geck)
Tissue adhesive, sterile, enbucrilate with blue dye.
Net price (single use) 500-mg vial = £9.60 (hosp.
use only)

13.11 Disinfectants and cleansers

13.11.1 Alcohols and saline
13.11.2 Chlorhexidine salts
13.11.3 Cationic surfactants and soaps
13.11.4 Chlorine and iodine
13.11.5 Phenolics
13.11.6 Astringents, oxidisers, and dyes
13.11.7 Desloughing agents

The choice of *cleanser* is an important factor in treating skin conditions. For example, scaling disorders are best treated with **emulsifying ointment** (section 13.2.1) or other cleansers that do not irritate the skin.

Sodium chloride solution 0.9% is suitable for general cleansing of skin and wounds.

Useful *disinfectants* for skin cleansing include **cetrimide** (which has useful detergent properties), **chlorhexidine** and **potassium permanganate solution** 1 in 10 000. **Povidone-iodine** is preferred to chlorinated solutions (such as dilute sodium hypochlorite solution) which are too irritant and are no longer recommended. Topical preparations of **hexachlorophane** should be used with caution in neonates and should **not** be used on large raw surfaces.

Astringent preparations, such as **potassium permanganate** solution are useful for oozing eczematous reactions (section 13.5.1). Silver nitrate lotion is now rarely used as it stains the skin black and may cause toxic effects if used for prolonged periods.

13.11.1 Alcohols and saline

ALCOHOL

Indications: skin preparation before injection
Cautions: flammable; avoid broken skin; patients have suffered severe burns when diathermy has been preceded by application of alcoholic skin disinfectants

Industrial Methylated Spirit, BP
Mixture of 19 volumes of ethanol (absolute alcohol) of an appropriate strength with 1 volume of approved wood naphtha and is Industrial Methylated Spirit of the quality known either as '66 OP' or as '74 OP'
Net price 100 mL = 18p. Label: 15

Surgical Spirit, BP, methyl salicylate 0.5 mL, diethyl phthalate 2%, castor oil 2.5%, in industrial methylated spirit. Net price 100 mL = 19p. Label: 15

SODIUM CHLORIDE

Indications: see notes above

Irriclens® (ConvaTec)
Solution in aerosol can, (sterile), sodium chloride 0.9%. Net price 240-mL can = £2.75

Normasol® (Seton)
Solution (sterile), sodium chloride 0.9%. Net price 25 × 25-mL sachet = £5.85; 6 × 100-mL sachet = £4.30
See also section 11.8.2

Sterac® Sodium Chloride (Galen)
Solution (sterile), sodium chloride 0.9%. Net price 150 mL = 83p

Sterijet® Sodium Chloride (Seton)
Solution (sterile), sodium chloride 0.9%. Net price 20 × 25-mL flexible ampoule = £6.20

Steripod® Sodium Chloride (Seton)
Steripod® sodium chloride 0.9% solution (sterile), sodium chloride 0.9%. Net price 25 × 20-mL sachet = £6.83

13.11.2 Chlorhexidine salts

CHLORHEXIDINE

Indications: see under preparations; bladder irrigation and catheter patency solutions (see section 7.4.4)
Cautions: avoid contact with eyes, brain, meninges and middle ear; not for use in body cavities; alcoholic solutions not suitable before diathermy
Side-effects: occasional sensitivity

Chlorhexidine 0.05% (Baxter)
2000 Solution (sterile), pink, chlorhexidine acetate 0.05%. Net price 1000 mL = 77p
For cleansing and disinfecting wounds and burns

CX Antiseptic Dusting Powder® (DePuy)
Dusting powder, sterile, chlorhexidine acetate 1%. Net price 15 g = £2.25
For skin disinfection and antisepsis
Note. Chlorhexidine Dusting Powder BP 1988 contains chlorhexidine hydrochloride 0.5% but no preparation is available commercially

Hibiscrub® (Zeneca)
Cleansing solution, red, chlorhexidine gluconate solution 20% (≡ 4% chlorhexidine gluconate), perfumed, in a surfactant solution. Net price 250 mL = £1.10; 500 mL = £1.61
Use instead of soap for pre-operative hand and skin preparation and for general hand and skin antisepsis

Hibisol® (Zeneca)
Solution, chlorhexidine gluconate solution 2.5% (≡ 0.5% chlorhexidine gluconate), in isopropyl alcohol 70% with emollients. Net price 500 mL = £1.68
To be used undiluted for hand and skin disinfection

Hibitane Obstetric® (Zeneca)
Cream, chlorhexidine gluconate solution 5% (≡ 1% chlorhexidine gluconate), in a pourable water-miscible basis. Net price 250 mL = 98p.
For use in obstetrics and gynaecology as an antiseptic and lubricant (for application to skin around vulva and perineum and to hands of midwife or doctor)

Phiso-med® (Sanofi Winthrop)
Solution, chlorhexidine gluconate 4% in an emulsion basis. Net price 150 mL = £4.64.
For use as a soap substitute in acne and seborrhoeic conditions; for bathing babies in maternity units (as 1 in 10 dilution) to prevent cross-infection and for pre-operative hand and skin preparation

Sterexidine® (Galen)
Solution (sterile), chlorhexidine gluconate 0.02%. Net price 150 mL = 83p
For disinfection and wound cleansing

Steripod® Chlorhexidine (Seton)
Steripod® Chlorhexidine solution, chlorhexidine gluconate solution 0.25% (≡ chlorhexidine gluconate 0.05%). Net price 25 × 20-mL vials = £6.83
For swabbing wounds and burns

Unisept® (Seton)
Solution (sterile), pink, chlorhexidine gluconate 0.05%. Net price 25 × 25-mL sachet = £5.85; 6 × 100-mL sachet = £4.30
For cleansing and disinfecting wounds and burns and swabbing in obstetrics

With cetrimide
Steripod® Chlorhexidine/Cetrimide (Seton)
Steripod® Chlorhexidine/Cetrimide solution, chlorhexidine gluconate solution 0.075% (≡ chlorhexidine gluconate 0.015%), cetrimide 0.15%. Net price 25 × 20-mL vials = £6.83
For cleansing and disinfecting wounds and burns

Tisept® (Seton)
Solution (sterile), yellow, chlorhexidine gluconate 0.015%, cetrimide 0.15%. Net price 25 × 25-mL sachet = £5.85; 6 × 100-mL sachet = £4.30
To be used undiluted for general skin disinfection and wound cleansing

Travasept 100® (Baxter)
Solution (sterile), yellow, chlorhexidine acetate 0.015%, cetrimide 0.15%. Net price 500 mL = 72p; 1000 = 77p
To be used undiluted in skin disinfection such as wound cleansing and obstetrics

CONCENTRATES

Hibitane 5% Concentrate® (Zeneca)
Solution, red, chlorhexidine gluconate solution 25% (≡ 5% chlorhexidine gluconate), in a perfumed aqueous solution. Net price 5 litres = £11.46
To be used diluted 1 in 10 (0.5%) with alcohol 70% for pre-operative skin preparation, or 1 in 100 (0.05%) with water for general skin disinfection
Note. Alcoholic solutions not suitable before diathermy (see Alcohol, above)

With cetrimide
Hibicet Hospital Concentrate® (Zeneca)
Solution, orange, chlorhexidine gluconate solution 7.5% (≡ chlorhexidine gluconate 1.5%), cetrimide 15%. Net price 5 litres = £8.54
To be used diluted 1 in 100 (1%) to 1 in 30 with water for skin disinfection and wound cleansing, and diluted 1 in 30 in alcohol 70% for pre-operative skin preparation
Note. Alcoholic solutions not suitable before diathermy (see Alcohol, above)

13.11.3   Cationic surfactants and soaps

BENZALKONIUM CHLORIDE
Indications: skin disinfection such as pre-operative skin preparation
Cautions: avoid contact with eyes

Roccal® (Sanofi Winthrop)
Solution, blue, benzalkonium chloride 1%. Net price 2.25 litres = £14.25
To be used diluted 1 in 10 to 1 in 200
Additives: include fragrance

Roccal Concentrate 10X® (Sanofi Winthrop)
Concentrate, blue, benzalkonium chloride 10%. Net price 2.25 litres = £58.49
For preparation of Roccal Solution with freshly boiled and cooled purified water
Additives: include fragrance

CETRIMIDE
Indications: skin disinfection
Cautions: avoid contact with eyes; avoid use in body cavities
Side-effects: skin irritation and occasionally sensitisation

Preparations
Ingredient of Hibicet Hospital Concentrate®, Steripod®, Tisept®, and Travasept®100, see above

SOFT SOAP
Indications: removal of adherent crusts

Soap Spirit, BP, soft soap 65% in alcohol (90%). Net price 100 mL = 40p

SUBSTITUTE SOAPS
See section 13.2.1 (emulsifying ointment); section 13.2.1.1 (emollient bath additives)

13.11.4   Chlorine and iodine

CHLORINATED SOLUTIONS
Cautions: bleaches fabric; irritant (protect surrounding tissues with soft paraffin)

Chlorinated Lime and Boric Acid Solution, BP,
(Eusol), chlorinated lime 1.25%, boric acid 1.25%, in purified water, freshly boiled and cooled. Contains not less than 0.25% available chlorine. It must be freshly prepared. Has been used undiluted for skin disinfection, particularly in wound and ulcer cleansing but no longer recommended (too irritant)

Chlorinated Soda Solution, Surgical, BPC,
(Dakin's Solution), boric acid, chlorinated lime, sodium carbonate, sufficient of each to provide a solution containing 0.5% of available chlorine in purified water, freshly boiled and cooled. Net price 500 mL = 74p. Has been used undiluted for cleansing wounds and ulcers but no longer recommended (too irritant)

Chlorasol® (Seton)
Solution (sterile), sodium hypochlorite, containing 0.3–0.4% available chlorine. Net price 25 × 25-mL sachets = £8.89
Irritant therefore no longer recommended

ODINE COMPOUNDS

Indications: skin disinfection

Cautions: pregnancy, breast-feeding; broken skin (see below); renal impairment (see Appendix 3)

LARGE OPEN WOUNDS. The application of povidone-iodine to large wounds or severe burns may produce systemic adverse effects such as metabolic acidosis, hypernatraemia and impairment of renal function.

Contra-indications: avoid regular use in patients with thyroid disorders or those receiving lithium therapy

Side-effects: rarely sensitivity; may interfere with thyroid function tests

Betadine® (Seton)

Antiseptic paint, povidone-iodine 10% in an alcoholic solution. Net price 8 mL (with applicator brush) = £1.06

Apply undiluted to minor wounds and infections, twice daily

Alcoholic solution, povidone-iodine 10%. Net price 500 mL = £2.00

To be applied undiluted in pre- and post-operative skin disinfection; CHILD not recommended for regular use in neonates (and contra-indicated in very low birthweight infants)

Note. Flammable—caution in procedures involving hot wire cautery and diathermy

Antiseptic solution, povidone-iodine 10% in aqueous solution. Net price 500 mL = £1.83

To be applied undiluted in pre- and post-operative skin disinfection; CHILD not recommended for regular use in neonates (and contra-indicated in very low birthweight infants)

Note. Not for body cavity irrigation

Dry powder spray, povidone-iodine 2.5% in a pressurised aerosol unit. Net price 150-g unit = £2.92

For skin disinfection, particularly minor wounds and infections; CHILD under 2 years not recommended

Note. Not for use in serous cavities

Scalp and skin cleanser solution, povidone-iodine 7.5%, in a surfactant basis. Net price 250 mL = £2.43

Use for seborrhoeic conditions of scalp and acne vulgaris of face and neck 1–2 times daily; CHILD under 2 years not recommended

Skin cleanser solution, povidone-iodine 4%, in a surfactant basis. Net price 250 mL = £2.24

For infective conditions of the skin. Retain on skin for 3–5 minutes before rinsing; repeat twice daily; CHILD under 2 years not recommended

Surgical scrub, povidone-iodine 7.5%, in a non-ionic surfactant basis. Net price 500 mL = £1.65

To be used as a pre-operative scrub for hands and skin; CHILD not recommended for regular use in neonates (and contra-indicated in very low birthweight infants)

Savlon® Dry Powder (Zyma)

Savlon® Dry powder spray, povidone-iodine 1.14% in a pressurised aerosol unit. Net price 50-mL unit = £1.82; 150-mL = £2.71

For minor wounds

13.11.5 Phenolics

HEXACHLOROPHANE

Hexachlorophene)

Indications: see under preparations (below)

Contra-indications: avoid use on badly burned or excoriated skin; pregnancy; children under 2 years except on medical advice

Side-effects: sensitivity; rarely photosensitivity

PoM Ster-Zac DC Skin Cleanser® (Houghs)

Cream, hexachlorophane 3%. Net price 150 mL = £1.13

Use 3–5 mL instead of soap as pre-operative scrub for hands

Additives: include chlorocresol, edetic acid (EDTA), propylene glycol, wool fat, fragrance

Ster-Zac Powder® (Houghs)

Dusting-powder, hexachlorophane 0.33%, zinc oxide 3%, talc 88.67%, starch 8% (sterile). Net price 30 g = 79p

Additives: include fragrance

Prevention of neonatal staphylococcal sepsis, after ligature of cord sprinkle on perineum, groin, front of abdomen, and axillas; after cutting cord and spraying with plastic dressing, powder stump and adjacent skin; after every napkin change powder stump, adjacent skin, perineum, groin, axillas, buttocks, and front of abdomen; continue until stump drops away and wound healed

Adjunct for treatment of recurrent furunculosis, powder daily area of skin normally subject to furunculosis

TRICLOSAN

Indications: skin disinfection

Cautions: avoid contact with eyes

Aquasept® (Houghs)

Skin cleanser, blue, triclosan 2%. Net price 28.5 mL = 33p; 100 mL = 90p; 250 mL = £1.10; 500 mL = £1.68

For disinfection and pre-operative hand preparation

Additives: include chlorocresol, edetic acid (EDTA), propylene glycol, fragrance

Manusept® (Houghs)

Antibacterial hand rub, triclosan 0.5%, isopropyl alcohol 70%. Net price 100 mL = 59p; 250 mL = £1.07; 500 mL = £1.56

For disinfection and pre-operative hand preparation

Additives: none as listed in section 13.1

Caution: flammable

Ster-Zac Bath Concentrate® (Houghs)

Solution, triclosan 2%. Net price 28.5 mL = 40p; 500 mL = £4.46

For staphylococcal skin infections; prevention of cross-infection use 1 sachet/bath

Additives: include edetic acid (EDTA)

13.11.6 Astringents, oxidisers, and dyes

ALUMINIUM ACETATE

Indications: exudative eczematous reactions and wounds

Aluminium Acetate Lotion, aluminium acetate solution 5 mL, purified water, freshly boiled and cooled, to 100 mL. It should be freshly prepared. To be used undiluted as a wet dressing

Note. Aluminium acetate solution (13%) for the preparation of aluminium acetate lotion (0.65%) is available from Martindale (special order)

CRYSTAL VIOLET
(Gentian violet; Methylrosanilium Chloride)
Indications: see below
Cautions: stains clothes and skin
Side-effects: mucosal ulcerations

Crystal Violet Paint, BP1980, crystal violet 0.5%, in purified water, freshly boiled and cooled. To be used undiluted
Note. Licensed for topical application on unbroken skin only; no longer recommended for application to mucous membranes or open wounds; restrictions do not apply to use for skin marking prior to surgery

HYDROGEN PEROXIDE
Indications: skin disinfection, particularly cleansing and deodorising wounds and ulcers
Cautions: large or deep wounds; avoid normal skin; bleaches fabric

Hydrogen Peroxide Solution, BP
Solution 6% (20 vols). Net price 100 mL = 21p
Solution 3% (10 vols). Net price 100 mL = 23p
Note. The BP directs that when hydrogen peroxide is prescribed, hydrogen peroxide solution 6% (20 vols) should be dispensed.
IMPORTANT. Strong solutions of hydrogen peroxide which contain 27% (90 vols) and 30% (100 vols) are only for the preparation of weaker solutions
Hioxyl® See Desloughing Agents (below)

POTASSIUM PERMANGANATE
Indications: cleansing and deodorising suppurating eczematous reactions and wounds
Cautions: irritant to mucous membranes; stains skin and clothing
Administration: wet dressings or baths, approx. 0.01% solution

Potassium Permanganate Solution, potassium permanganate 0.1% (1 in 1000) in water
To be diluted 1 in 10 to provide a 0.01% (1 in 10 000) solution
Permitabs® (Bioglan)
Solution tablets, for preparation of topical solution, potassium permanganate 400 mg. Net price 30-tab pack = £3.19
1 tablet dissolved in 4 litres of water provides a 0.01% (1 in 10 000) solution

13.11.7   Desloughing agents

Desloughing agents for ulcers are second-line treatment and the underlying causes should be treated. The main beneficial effect is removal of slough and clot and the ablation of local infection. Preparations which absorb or help promote the removal of exudate may also help (section 13.13.8). It should be noted that substances applied to an open area are easily absorbed and perilesional skin is easily sensitised. Gravitational dermatitis may be complicated by superimposed contact sensitivity to substances such as neomycin or lanolin. Enzyme preparations such as streptokinase-streptodornase or alternatively dextranomer (section 13.13.8) are designed for sloughing ulcers and may help.

Aserbine® (Forley)
Cream, benzoic acid 0.025%, malic acid 0.375% propylene glycol 1.75%, salicylic acid 0.006%. Net price 100 g = £1.17
Apply liberally to wound surface (best results with twice daily wound dressing but more frequent changes may be needed)
Additives: include hydroxybenzoates (parabens)
Solution, benzoic acid 0.15%, malic acid 2.25% propylene glycol 40%, salicylic acid 0.0375%. Net price 500 mL = £1.76
Use as wash before each application of cream (or use a wet dressing)
Additives: include fragrance
Hioxyl® (Quinoderm Ltd)
Cream, hydrogen peroxide (stabilised) 1.5%. Net price 25 g = £1.81; 100 g = £5.66
For leg ulcers and pressure sores
Additives: none as listed in section 13.1
Apply when necessary and if necessary cover with a dressing
PoM **Varidase Topical®** (Lederle)
Powder, streptokinase 100 000 units, streptodornase 25 000 units. For preparing solutions for topical use. Net price per vial = £7.80; with sterile physiological saline 20 mL (combi-pack) = £8.20
Additives: none as listed in section 13.1
Reconstitute with 20 mL sterile physiological saline (or water for injections) and apply as wet dressing 1–2 times daily; cover with semi-occlusive dressing; irrigate lesion thoroughly with physiological saline and remove loosened material before next application; also used to dissolve clots in the bladder or urinary catheters; *contra indicated:* active haemorrhage; *side-effects:* infrequent allergic reactions (reduced by careful and frequent removal of exudate and thorough irrigation with physiological saline); transient burning reported

13.12   Antiperspirants

Aluminium chloride is a potent antiperspirant used in the treatment of severe hyperhidrosis.

ALUMINIUM CHLORIDE
Indications: hyperhidrosis affecting axillae, hands or feet
Cautions: avoid contact with eyes or mouth; do not shave axilla or use depilatories within 12 hours of use
Side-effects: skin irritation
Administration: apply at night to dry skin, wash off on following morning, initially daily then reduce frequency as condition improves—do not apply within 1 hour of taking a bath

Anhydrol Forte® (Dermal)
Solution (= application), aluminium chloride hexahydrate 20% in an alcoholic basis. Net price 60-mL bottle with roll-on applicator = £2.82. Label: 15
Driclor® (Stiefel)
Application, aluminium chloride hexahydrate 20% in an alcoholic basis. Net price 60-mL bottle with roll on applicator = £2.82. Label: 15
Note. A 30-mL pack is on sale to the public (Driclor® Solution)

13.13 Wound management products

13.13.1 Bandages
13.13.2 Surgical adhesive tapes
13.13.3 Adhesive dressings
13.13.4 Surgical absorbents
13.13.5 Wound dressing pads
13.13.6 Tulle dressings
13.13.7 Vapour-permeable films and membranes
13.13.8 Gel and colloid dressings
13.13.9 Foam dressings
13.13.10 Elastic hosiery

13.13.1 Bandages

RETENTION BANDAGES

Non-stretch fabric retention bandages

Open-wove Bandage, BP 1988 (types 1, 2 and 3). Cotton cloth, plain weave, warp of cotton, weft of cotton, viscose, or combination, one continuous length. Type 1, 5 m (all): 2.5 cm, net price = 27p; 5 cm = 45p; 7.5 cm = 64p; 10 cm = 84p (most suppliers) 5 m × 5 cm supplied when size not stated
Uses: protection and retention of absorbent dressings; support for minor strains, sprains; securing splints
*Note.*Type 1 bandage formerly described as Open-Wove Bandage BPC 1973; Type 2 formerly described as 'medium quality'; Type 3 formerly described as 'hospital quality'

Triangular Calico Bandage, BP 1980. Unbleached calico rt. angle triangle. 90 cm × 90 cm × 1.27 m, net price = £1.02 (most suppliers)
Uses: sling

NHS Domette Bandage, BP 1988. Fabric, plain weave, cotton warp and wool weft (hospital quality also available, all colours). 5 m (all): 5 cm, net price = 54p; 7.5 cm = 81p; 10 cm = £1.08; 15 cm = £1.61 (Robert Bailey, Vernon-Carus)
Uses: protection and support where warmth required

Multiple Pack Dressing No. 1 (Drug Tariff). Contains absorbent cotton, absorbent cotton gauze type 13 light (sterile), open-wove bandages (banded). Net price per pack = £3.00

Multiple Pack Dressing No. 2 (Drug Tariff). As for No. 1 (above) but with larger quantities of cotton and cotton gauze and two sizes of bandages. Net price per pack = £5.03

Stretch fabric retention bandages

Cotton Conforming Bandage, BP 1988. Cotton fabric, plain weave, treated to impart some elasticity to warp and weft. 3.5 m (all):
type A, 5 cm, net price = 57p, 7.5 cm = 71p, 10 cm = 86p, 15 cm = £1.19 (S&N Hlth—*Crinx* ®)
type B, 5 cm = 58p, 7.5 cm = 75p, 10 cm = 91p, 15 cm = £1.20 (J&J—*Kling* ®)
Uses: retention of dressings in difficult positions (e.g. over joints)

Knitted Polyamide and Cellulose Contour Bandage, BP 1988. Fabric, knitted warp of polyamide filament, weft of cotton or viscose, fast edges, one continuous length. 4 m stretched (all): 5 cm = 18p, 7 cm = 23p, 10 cm = 25p, 15 cm = 44p (Parema—*K-Band* ®)

Polyamide and Cellulose Contour Bandage, BP 1988 (formerly Nylon and Viscose Stretch Bandage). Fabric, plain weave, warp of polyamide filament, weft of cotton or viscose, fast edges, one continuous length. 4 m stretched (all): Robinsons—*Stayform*® (5 cm = 30p,

7.5 cm = 38p, 10 cm = 43p, 15 cm = 73p); Seton—*Slinky*® (net price 5 cm = 37p, 7.5 cm = 52p, 10 cm = 63p, 15 cm = 89p); S&N Hlth—*Easifix* ® (5 cm = 30p, 7.5 cm = 37p, 10 cm = 43p, 15 cm = 73p)
Uses: retention of dressings

NHS Tubular Gauze Bandage, Seamless. Unbleached cotton yarn, positioned with applicators. 20 m roll (all): 00, net price = £2.10; 01 = £2.12; 12 = £2.85; 34 = £4.17; 56 = £5.76; 78 = £6.77; T1 = £9.70; T2 = £12.55 (Seton—*Tubegauz*®)
Uses: retention of dressings on limbs, abdomen, trunk

Elasticated Tubular Bandage, BP (formerly Elasticated Surgical Tubular Stockinette). Knitted fabric, elasticated threads of rubber-cored polyamide or polyester with cotton or cotton and viscose yarn, tubular. Lengths 50 cm and 1 m, various widths 6.25 cm–12 cm, (Seton—*Texagrip*®, JLB Textiles—*Textube*® (formerly called *Lastogrip*®); Salt—*Rediform* ®; S&N Hlth—*Tensogrip*®; Seton—*Tubigrip*®; Sigma—*Sigma ETB*®). Where no brand stated by prescriber, net price of stockinette supplied not to exceed: length 50 cm, 6.25 cm = 57p, 6.75 cm = 60p, 7.5 cm = 60p, 8.75 cm = 68p, 10 cm = 68p, 12 cm = 73p; length 1 m, 6.25 cm = £1.04, 6.75 cm = £1.09, 7.5 cm = £1.09, 8.75 cm = £1.14, 10 cm = £1.14, 12 cm = £1.40
Uses: retention of dressings on limbs, abdomen, trunk

Elasticated Surgical Tubular Stockinette, Foam padded (Drug Tariff specification 25). Fabric as for Elasticated Tubular Bandage with polyurethane foam lining. Heel, elbow, knee, small, net price = £2.27, medium = £2.46, large = £2.63; sacral, small, medium, and large (all) = £11.73 (Seton—*Tubipad*®)
Uses: relief of pressure and elimination of friction in relevant area; porosity of foam lining allows normal water loss from skin surface

Elasticated Viscose Stockinette (Drug Tariff specification 46). Lightweight plain-knitted elasticated tubular bandage. Length 1 m (all): net price 3.5 cm (small limb) = 71p; 5 cm (medium limb) = 75p; 7.5 cm (large limb) = 99p; 10.75 cm (OS limb, head, child trunk) = £1.59; 17.5 cm (adult trunk) = £2.00 (Seton—*Tubifast*®)
Uses: retention of dressings

Elastic Net Surgical Tubular Stockinette (Drug Tariff Specification 26). Lightweight elastic open-work net tubular fabric.
type A : arm/leg, 40 cm × 1.8 cm (size C), net price = 33p; thigh/head, 60 cm × 2.5 cm (size E) = 60p; trunk (adult), 60 cm × 4.5 cm (size F) = 88p; trunk (OS adult) 60 cm × 5.4 cm (size G) = £1.18 (Seton—*Netelast*®)
type B: *Setonet*® withdrawn
type C: *Macrofix*® withdrawn

Cotton Stockinette, Bleached, BP 1988 (formerly Cotton Surgical Tubular Stockinette). Knitted fabric, cotton yarn, tubular. 1 m × 2.5 cm, net price = 25p; 5 cm = 38p; 7.5 cm = 46p; 6 m × 10 cm = £3.15 (J&J, Seton)
Uses: 1 m lengths, basis (with wadding) for Plaster of Paris bandages etc. ; 6 m length, compression bandage

Ribbed Cotton and Viscose Surgical Tubular Stockinette, BP 1988. Knitted fabric of 1:1 ribbed structure, singles yarn spun from blend of two-thirds cotton and one-third viscose fibres, tubular. Length 5 m (all):
type A (lightweight): arm/leg (child), arm (adult) 5 cm, net price = £1.98; arm (OS adult), leg (adult) 7.5 cm = £2.58; leg (OS adult) 10 cm = £3.44; trunk (child) 15 cm = £4.94; trunk (adult) 20 cm = £5.69; trunk (OS adult) 25 cm = £6.83 (Seton)
type B (heavyweight): sizes as for type A, net price £1.91–£6.57 (Sallis—*Eesiban*®)
Drug Tariff specifies various combinations of sizes to provide sufficient material for part or full body coverage
Uses: protective dressings with tar-based and other non-steroid ointments

SUPPORT AND COMPRESSION BANDAGES

Non-adhesive woven extensible bandages

Crepe Bandage, BP 1988. Fabric, plain weave, warp of wool threads and crepe-twisted cotton threads, weft of cotton threads; stretch bandage. 4.5 m stretched (all): 5 cm, net price = 79p; 7.5 cm = £1.10; 10 cm = £1.46; 15 cm = £2.08 (most suppliers)
Uses: light support system for strains, sprains, compression over paste bandages for varicose veins

Cotton Crepe Bandage, BP 1988. Fabric, plain weave, warp of crepe-twisted cotton threads, weft of cotton and/or viscose threads; stretch bandage. 4.5 m stretched (all): 7.5 cm, net price = £2.51; 10 cm = £3.25; other sizes **NHS** (most suppliers)
Uses: light support system for strains, sprains, compression over paste bandages for varicose veins

NHS Cotton Stretch Bandage, BP 1988. Fabric, plain weave, warp of crepe-twisted cotton threads, weft of cotton threads; stretch bandage, lighter than cotton crepe. 4.5 m stretched (all): 5 cm, net price = 30p; 7.5 cm = 41p; 10 cm = 54p; 15 cm = 76p (most suppliers)
Uses: light support system for strains, sprains, compression over paste bandages for varicose veins

Cotton Suspensory Bandage (Drug Tariff). Type 1: cotton net bag with draw tapes and webbing waistband; net price small, medium, and large (all) = £1.36, extra large = £1.43. Type 2: cotton net bag with elastic edge and webbing waistband; small = £1.48, medium = £1.53, large = £1.59, extra large = £1.66. Type 3: cotton net bag with elastic edge and webbing waistband with elastic insertion; small, medium, and large (all) = £1.61; extra large = £1.67
Type supplied to be endorsed
Uses: support of scrotum

NHS Cotton and Rubber Elastic Bandage, BP. Fabric, plain weave, warp of combined cotton and rubber threads, weft of cotton threads (S&N Hlth)
Uses: provision of high compression and medium support

Heavy Cotton and Rubber Elastic Bandage, BP. Heavy version of above with one end folded as foot loop; fastener also supplied. 1.8 m unstretched × 7.5 cm, net price = £10.79 (Marlow, Seton, S&N Hlth—*Elastoweb*®).
Uses: provision of high even compression over large surface

Elastic Web Bandage, BP (also termed Blue Line Webbing). Characteristic fabric woven ribbon fashion, warp threads of cotton and rubber with mid-line threads coloured blue, weft threads of cotton or combined cotton and viscose; may be dyed skin colour; with or without foot loop. Per m (both) 7.5 cm, net price = 70p; 10 cm = £1.00; with foot loop (Drug Tariff specification 2a) 7.5 cm each = £4.02 (Marlow, Seton)
Uses: provision of support and high compression over large surface

Elastic Web Bandage without Foot Loop (also termed Red Line Webbing) (Drug Tariff specification 2b) (Scott-Curwen). Characteristic fabric woven ribbon fashion, warp threads of cotton and rubber with mid-line threads coloured red, weft threads of cotton or combined cotton and viscose. 7.5 cm × 2.75 m (2.5 m unstretched), net price = £3.18; 7.5 cm × 3.75 m (3.5 m unstretched) = £3.84
Uses: provision of support and high compression over large surfaces

High compression extensible bandages
(Drug Tariff specification 52)

PEC High Compression Bandage (Drug Tariff). Polyamide, elastane, and cotton compression (high) extensible bandage, 3.5 m unstretched (both): 7.5 cm, net price = £2.29; 10 cm = £2.96 (Seton—*Setopress*®)
Uses: high compression for varicose ulcers

VEC High Compression Bandage (Drug Tariff). Viscose, elastane, and cotton compression (high) extensible bandage, 3 m unstretched (both): 7.5 cm, net price = £2.29; 10 cm = £2.96 (S&N—*Tensopress*®)
Uses: high compression for varicose ulcers

High Compression Bandage (Drug Tariff). Cotton viscose, nylon, and Lycra® extensible bandage, 3 m (unstretched), 10 cm = £2.96 (ConvaTec—*SurePress*®) also available **NHS** *SurePress*® absorbent padding, net price 6 = £3.00
Uses: high compression for venous leg ulcers

Adhesive woven extensible bandages

Elastic Adhesive Bandage, BP. Woven fabric, elastic in warp (crepe-twisted cotton threads), weft of cotton and/or viscose threads spread with adhesive mass containing zinc oxide. 4.5 m stretched (all): 5 cm, net price = £2.95; 7.5 cm = £4.26; 10 cm = £5.67 (Robinsons—*Flexoplast*®; S&N Hlth—*Elastoplast*® Bandage). 7.5 cm width supplied when size not stated
Uses: compression for chronic leg ulcers; compression and support for fractured ribs, clavicles, swollen or sprained joints

NHS Half-spread Elastic Adhesive Bandage, BP 1988. Fabric as for elastic adhesive bandage but only partially spread with adhesive. (S&N Hlth)
Uses: compression for leg ulcers; compression and support for fractured ribs, clavicles, swollen/sprained joints

NHS Ventilated Elastic Adhesive Bandage, BP. Fabric as for elastic adhesive bandage but adhesive spread such that there are regular strips of unspread fabric along length. (S&N Hlth)
Uses: compression for leg ulcers; compression and support for fractured ribs, clavicles, swollen/sprained joints

NHS Extension strapping, BP. Woven fabric, elastic in weft, spread with adhesive mass containing zinc oxide, warp threads cotton and/or viscose, weft threads crepe-twisted cotton. (S&N Hlth)
Uses: support of light strains, joints and limbs removed from plaster casts, fractured ribs; traction bandaging

NHS Cohesive extensible bandages
These elastic bandages adhere to themselves and not to the patient's skin, which prevents slipping during use. 3M—*Coban*®, 4.5 m stretched (2.5, 5, 7.5, 10 and 15 cm); J&J—*Secure*® *Forte*, 4.5 m stretched (6, 8 and 10 cm); S&N Hlth—*Coplus*®, 6.3 m stretched (2.5, 3.8, 5, 7.5, 10 and 15 cm)
Uses: support of sprained joints

MEDICATED BANDAGES

Zinc Paste Bandage, BP. Cotton fabric, plain weave, impregnated with suitable paste containing zinc oxide; requires additional bandaging. Net price 6 m × 7.5 cm = £2.95 (Seton—*Steripaste*® (15%)); £2.90 (Seton—*Zincaband*® (15%)); £2.97 (S&N Hlth—*Viscopaste PB7*® (10%), *additives:* include hydroxybenzoates)

Zinc Paste and Calamine Bandage (Drug Tariff specification 5). Cotton fabric, plain weave, impregnated with suitable paste containing calamine and zinc oxide; requires additional bandaging. Net price 6 m × 7.5 cm = £2.99 (Seton—*Calaband*®)

Zinc Paste, Calamine, and Clioquinol Bandage, BP. Cotton fabric, plain weave, impregnated with suitable paste containing calamine, clioquinol, and zinc oxide; requires additional bandaging. Net price 6 m × 7.5 cm = £2.99 (Seton—*Quinaband*®, *additives:* include hydroxybenzoates)

Zinc Paste and Coal Tar Bandage, BP. Cotton fabric, plain weave, impregnated with a suitable paste containing coal tar and zinc oxide; requires additional bandaging. Net price 6 m × 7.5 cm = £2.90 (Seton—*Tarband*®, *additives: include* hydroxybenzoates; S&N Hlth—*Coltapaste*®, *additives: include* wool fat)
Uses: see section 13.5

Zinc Paste and Ichthammol Bandage, BP. Cotton fabric, plain weave, impregnated with suitable paste containing zinc oxide and ichthammol; requires additional bandaging. Net price 6 m × 7.5 cm = £2.90 (Seton—*Icthaband*®(15/2%), *additives: include* hydroxybenzoates; S&N Hlth—*Ichthopaste*®(6/2%), *additives:* none as listed in section 13.1)
Uses: see section 13.5

13.13.2   Surgical adhesive tapes

PERMEABLE ADHESIVE TAPES

Zinc Oxide Adhesive Tape, BP 1988. (Zinc Oxide Plaster). Fabric, plain weave, warp and weft of cotton and/or viscose, spread with an adhesive containing zinc oxide. 1.25 cm, net price 3 m = 53p, 5 m = 74p; 2.5 cm, 1 m = 34p, 3 m = 79p, 5 m = £1.07; 5 cm × 5 m = £1.82; 7.5 cm × 5 m = £2.76 (most suppliers)
Drug Tariff specifies 1 m × 2.5 cm supplied when size not stated
Uses: securing dressings and immobilising small areas

Permeable Woven Synthetic Adhesive Tape, BP 1988. Non-extensible closely woven fabric, spread with a polymeric adhesive. 5 m (both): 1.25 cm, net price = 63p; 2.5 cm = 92p; 5 cm = £1.60 (Beiersdorf—*Leukosilk*®)
Uses: securing dressings
For patients with skin reaction to other plasters and strapping, requiring use for long periods

Elastic Adhesive Tape, BP 1988 (Elastic Adhesive Plaster). Woven fabric, elastic in warp (crepe-twisted cotton threads), weft of cotton and/or viscose threads, spread with adhesive mass containing zinc oxide. 1.5 m stretched × 2.5 cm, net price = 72p; 4.5 m stretched × 2.5 cm = £1.35 (Robinsons—*Flexoplast*®; S&N—*Elastoplast*®).
Uses: securing dressings
For 5 cm width, see Elastic Adhesive Bandage, section 13.13.1

Permeable Non-woven Synthetic Adhesive Tape, BP 1988. Backing of paper-based or non-woven textile material spread with a polymeric adhesive mass. 5 m (all): BioDiagnostics—*Scanpor*® (net price 1.25 cm = 43p, 2.5 cm = 68p, 5 cm = £1.18); Beiersdorf—*Leukopor*® (1.25 cm = 56p, 2.5 cm = 85p, 5 cm = £1.51); 3M—*Micropore*® (1.25 cm = 58p, 2.5 cm = 88p, 5 cm = £1.63); S&N Hlth—*Hypal 2*® (1.25 cm = 58p, 2.5 cm = 88p, 5 cm = £1.63). Where no brand stated by prescriber, net price of tape supplied not to exceed 39p (1.25 cm), 63p (2.5 cm), £1.09 (5 cm)
Uses: securing dressings; skin closures for small incisions
For patients with skin reaction to other plasters and strapping, requiring use for long periods

OCCLUSIVE ADHESIVE TAPES

Impermeable Plastic Adhesive Tape, BP 1988. Extensible water-impermeable plastic film spread with an adhesive mass. 2.5 cm × 3 m, net price = £1.04; 5 m = £1.56; 5 cm × 5 m = £1.98; 7.5 cm × 5 m = £2.87 (Robinsons; Seton; S&N Hlth)
Uses: securing dressings; covering site of infection where exclusion of air, water, and water vapour is required

Impermeable Plastic Synthetic Adhesive Tape, BP 1988. Extensible water-impermeable plastic film spread with a polymeric adhesive mass. 5 m (both): net price, 2.5 cm = £1.47; 5 cm = £2.80 (3M—*Blenderm*®)
Uses: isolating wounds from external environment; covering sites where total exclusion of water and water vapour required; securing dressings and appliances

13.13.3   Adhesive dressings
(also termed Island dressings)

PERMEABLE ADHESIVE DRESSINGS

NHS **Elastic Adhesive Dressing, BP.** Wound dressing or dressing strip, pad attached to piece of extension plaster, leaving suitable adhesive margin; both pad and margin covered with suitable protector; pad may be dyed yellow and may be impregnated with suitable antiseptic (see below); extension plaster may be perforated or ventilated
Uses: general purpose wound dressing
Note. Permitted antiseptics are aminacrine hydrochloride, chlorhexidine hydrochloride (both 0.07–0.13%), chlorhexidine gluconate (0.11–0.20%); domiphen bromide (0.05–0.25%)

NHS **Permeable Plastic Wound Dressing, BP.** Consisting of an absorbent pad, which may be dyed and impregnated with a suitable antiseptic (see under Elastic Adhesive Dressing), attached to a piece of permeable plastic surgical adhesive tape, to leave a suitable adhesive margin; both pad and margin covered with suitable protector (most suppliers)
Uses: general purpose wound dressing, permeable to air and water

VAPOUR-PERMEABLE (SEMIPERMEABLE) ADHESIVE DRESSINGS

Vapour-permeable Waterproof Plastic Wound Dressing, BP (former Drug Tariff title: Semipermeable Waterproof Plastic Wound Dressing). Consists of absorbent pad, may be dyed and impregnated with suitable antiseptic (see under Elastic Adhesive Dressing), attached to piece of semipermeable waterproof surgical adhesive tape, to leave suitable adhesive margin; both pad and margin covered with suitable protector. 8.5 cm × 6 cm, net price = 30p (S&N Hlth—*Elastoplast Airstrip*®)
Uses: general purpose waterproof wound dressing, permeable to air and water vapour

OCCLUSIVE ADHESIVE DRESSINGS

NHS **Impermeable Plastic Wound Dressing, BP.** Consists of absorbent pad, may be dyed and impregnated with suitable antiseptic (see under Elastic Adhesive Dressing), attached to piece of impermeable plastic surgical adhesive tape, to leave suitable adhesive margin; both pad and margin covered with suitable protector (most suppliers)
Uses: protective covering for wounds requiring an occlusive dressing

13.13.4   Surgical absorbents

Absorbent Cotton, BP. Carded cotton fibres of not less than 10 mm average staple length, available in rolls and balls. 25 g, net price = 53p; 100 g = £1.23; 500 g = £4.23

(most suppliers). 25-g pack to be supplied when weight not stated

Uses: general purpose cleansing and swabbing, pre-operative skin preparation, application of medicaments; supplementary absorbent pad to absorb excess wound exudate

Absorbent Cotton, Hospital Quality. As for absorbent cotton but lower quality materials, shorter staple length etc. 100 g, net price = 88p; 500 g = £2.84 (most suppliers)

Drug Tariff specifies to be supplied only where specifically ordered

Uses: suitable only as general purpose absorbent, for swabbing, and routine cleansing of incontinent patients; not for wound cleansing

Gauze and Cotton Tissue, BP 1988. Consists of absorbent cotton enclosed in absorbent cotton gauze type 12 or absorbent cotton and viscose gauze type 2. 500 g, net price = £5.48 (most suppliers, including Robinsons—*Gamgee Tissue*® (blue label))

Uses: absorbent and protective pad, as burns dressing on non-adherent layer

Gauze and Cotton Tissue (Drug Tariff specification 14). Similar to above. 500 g, net price = £4.01 (most suppliers, including Robinsons—*Gamgee Tissue*® (pink label))

Drug Tariff specifies to be supplied only where specifically ordered

Uses: absorbent and protective pad, as burns dressing on non-adherent layer

Absorbent Lint, BPC. Cotton cloth of plain weave with nap raised on one side from warp yarns. 25 g, net price = 71p; 100 g = £2.14; 500 g = £8.99 (most suppliers). 25-g pack supplied where no quantity stated

Uses: external absorbent protective dressing

Absorbent Cotton Gauze, BP 1988. Cotton fabric of plain weave, in rolls and as swabs (see below), usually Type 13 light, sterile. 90 cm (all) ×1 m, net price = 83p; 3 m = £1.76; 5 m = £2.75; 10 m = £5.34 (most suppliers). 1-m packet supplied when no size stated

Uses: pre-operative preparation, for cleansing and swabbing

Note. Drug Tariff also includes unsterilised absorbent cotton gauze, 25 m roll, net price = £12.05

Cellulose Wadding, BP 1988. Delignified wood pulp bleached white, in multiple laminate form. 500 g, net price = £2.22 (most suppliers, including Robinsons—*Cellosene*®)

Uses: absorbing large volumes of fluid

Gauze and Cellulose Wadding Tissue, BP 1988. Consists of thick layer of cellulose wadding enclosed in absorbent cotton gauze type 12 or absorbent cotton and viscose gauze type 2. 500 g, net price = £2.98 (most suppliers)

Uses: absorbing large volumes of fluid

NHS Absorbent Muslin, BP 1988. Fabric of plain weave, warp threads of cotton, weft threads of cotton and/or viscose

Uses: wet dressing, soaked in 0.9% sterile sodium chloride solution

NHS Absorbent Cotton Ribbon Gauze, BP. Cotton fabric of plain weave in ribbon form with fast selvedge edges

Uses: post-surgery cavity packing for sinus, dental, throat cavities etc.

Absorbent Cotton and Viscose Ribbon Gauze, BP. Woven fabric in ribbon form with fast selvedge edges, warp threads of cotton, weft threads of viscose or combined cotton and viscose yarn, sterile. 5 m (both) × 1.25 cm, net price = 63p; 2.5 cm = 70p

Uses: post-surgery cavity packing for sinus, dental, throat cavities etc.

Gauze Swab, BP 1988. Consists of absorbent cotton gauze type 13 light or absorbent cotton and viscose gauze type 1 folded into squares or rectangles of 8-ply with no cut edges exposed. Sterile, 7.5 cm square, net price 5-pad packet = 29p; non-sterile, 10 cm square 100-pad packet = £4.98 (most suppliers)

Filmated Gauze Swab, BP 1988. As for Gauze Swab, but with thin layer of Absorbent Cotton enclosed within. Non-sterile, 10 cm × 10 cm, net price 100-pad packet = £6.20 (Vernon-Carus—*Cotfil*®)

Uses: general swabbing and cleansing

Non-woven Fabric Swab (Drug Tariff specification 28). Consists of non-woven fabric folded 4-ply; alternative to gauze swabs, type 13 light. Sterile, 7.5 cm square, net price 5-pad packet = 20p; non-sterile, 10 cm square, 100-pad packet = £2.34 (J & J—*Topper 8*®); 100-pad pack = £2.34 (CliniMed)

Uses: general purpose swabbing and cleansing; absorbs more quickly than gauze

Filmated Non-woven Fabric Swab (Drug Tariff specification 29). Film of viscose fibres enclosed within non-woven viscose fabric folded 8-ply. Non-sterile, 10 cm square, net price 100-pad packet = £5.07 (J & J—*Regal*®)

Uses: general purpose swabbing and cleansing

13.13.5   Wound dressing pads

Perforated Film Absorbent Dressing (Drug Tariff specification 9). Low-adherence dressing consisting of 3 layers; wound-facing layer, film of poly-(ethylene terephthalate) perforated in regular pattern; absorbent middle layer of type 1 consists of non-woven bleached cotton and viscose fibres or mixture of these with poly-acrylonitrile fibres; in type 2 (NHS) middle layer consists of bleached cotton fibres; backing layer of type 1 is apertured non-woven cellulose material; in type 2, the backing layer is identical with wound-facing layer; in type 3 outer layer comprises sleeve of film of poly(ethylmethylacrylate) perforated in regular pattern, forming wound-facing layer on side without join and backing layer on side with join (absorbent middle layer consists of bleached cotton fibres or viscose fibres or mixture of these sandwiched between two layers of apertured non-woven cellulose material); in type 4 wound-facing layer is similar to that in type 1 (absorbent middle layer consists of bleached cotton fibres and backing layer identical with wound-facing layer).

Type 1, 5 cm × 5 cm, net price, each = 13p; 10 cm × 10 cm = 20p; 20 cm × 10 cm = 40p (S&N Hlth—*Melolin*®).

Type 3, 5 cm × 5 cm, net price, each = 11p; 10 cm × 10 cm = 19p; 20 cm × 10 cm = 36p (J&J—*Release*®)

Type 4, 5 cm × 5 cm, net price, each = 10p; 10 cm × 10 cm = 17p; 20 cm × 10 cm = 33p (Robinson—*Skintact*®)

Where size not stated, 5 cm size supplied

Uses: dressing for post-operative and low exudate wounds; low adherence property and low absorption capacity

Knitted Viscose Primary Dressing, BP. Warp knitted fabric manufactured from a bright viscose monofilament. 9.5 cm × 9.5 cm (all): net price = 28p (J&J—*N-A Dressing*®); net price = 24p (S&N—*Tricotex*®); silicone-coated, net price = 28p (J&J—*N-A Ultra*®)

Uses: low adherence wound contact layer for use on ulcerative and other granulating wounds with superimposed absorbent pad

Sterile Dressing Pack (Drug Tariff specification 10; Scottish, 16). Contains gauze and cotton tissue pad, gauze swabs, absorbent cotton balls, absorbent paper towel, water repellent inner wrapper. Net price per pack = 69p

---

Sterile Dressing Pack with Non-woven Pads (Drug Tariff specification 35). Contains non-woven fabric covered dressing pad (*Surgipad®*), non-woven fabric swabs (*Topper 8®*), absorbent cotton wool balls, absorbent paper towel, water repellent inner wrapper. Net price per pack = 74p

NHS Ete®. Wound pad of rayon wadding with rayon silk wound contact layer stitched in chequered pattern (Molnlycke)

Uses: leg wounds, decubitus ulcers, minor burns, donor sites

NHS Melolite®. Absorbent fabric pad covered on both sides by polyethylene net (S&N Hlth)

Uses: primary dressing over clean sutured wounds, lacerations, and abrasions

NHS Mesorb®. Cellulose wadding pad with gauze wound contact layer and non-woven repellent backing (Molnlycke)

Uses: post-operative dressing for heavily exuding wounds

NHS Perfron®. Absorbent pad consisting of alternate layers of absorbent cotton and crepe cellulose tissue, in sleeve of non-woven viscose fabric with coating of polypropylene (J&J)

Uses: low adherence pad for heavily exuding wounds; laminate structure delays strike through

NHS * Surgipad®. Absorbent pad of absorbent cotton and viscose in sleeve of non-woven viscose fabric (J&J)

Uses: for heavily exuding wounds requiring frequent dressing changes

* Except in Sterile Dressing Pack with Non-woven Pads

Charcoal cloth dressings

Uses: to deodorise discharging, infected, malodorous wounds and ulcers

NHS Actisorb Plus®. Knitted fabric of activated charcoal, with one-way stretch, with silver residues, within spun-bonded nylon sleeve. Net price (each) 10.5 cm × 10.5 cm = £2.48 (J&J)

NHS Carbonet®. Activated charcoal dressing. 10 cm × 10 cm, net price, each = £2.20 (S&N Hlth)

NHS Carbosorb®. Outer cover of non-woven polyester-nylon fabric, activated charcoal cloth layer bonded to outer cover and semipermeable polyurethane film contact layer (Seton)

NHS CliniSorb® Odour Control Dressings. Layer of activated charcoal cloth between viscose rayon with outer polyamide coating. Net price 10 cm × 10 cm, 10 = £13.20; 10 cm × 20 cm, 10 = £17.60; 15 cm × 25 cm, 10 = £28.60 (CliniMed)

NHS Lyofoam C®. Lyofoam sheet with layer of activated charcoal cloth and additional outer envelope of polyurethane foam. 10 cm × 10 cm, net price, each = £2.10; 15 cm × 20 cm = £4.65; 25 cm × 10 cm = £3.91 (Seton)

Medicated viscose dressing

Povidone-iodine Fabric Dressing (Drug Tariff specification 43). Knitted viscose primary dressing impregnated with povidone-iodine ointment 10%, 5 cm × 5 cm, net price, each = 25p; 9.5 cm × 9.5 cm = 38p (J&J—*Inadine®*)

Uses: wound contact layer for abrasions and superficial burns; max. 4 dressings at same time

13.13.6   Tulle dressings

Non-medicated tulle dressings

Paraffin Gauze Dressing, BP (Tulle Gras). Fabric of leno weave, weft and warp threads of cotton and/or viscose yarn, impregnated with white or yellow soft paraffin; sterile. 10 cm × 10 cm, net price, each = 30p; pack

of 10 pieces = £2.10 (most suppliers including Seton—*Paratulle®*; Roussel—*Unitulle®*; S&N Hlth—*Jelonet®*)

Uses: treatment of abrasions, burns, and other injuries of skin, and ulcerative conditions; post-operatively as penile and vaginal dressing and for sinus packing; heavier loading for skin graft transfer

Medicated tulle dressings

Chlorhexidine Gauze Dressing, BP. Fabric of leno weave, weft and warp threads of cotton and/or viscose yarn, impregnated with ointment containing chlorhexidine acetate; sterile. 5 cm × 5 cm, net price each = 21p; 10 cm × 10 cm = 45p (Seton—*Serotulle®*; Roussel—*Clorhexitulle®*; S&N Hlth—*Bactigras®*)

PoM Framycetin Gauze Dressing, BP. Fabric of leno weave, weft and warp threads of cotton, impregnated with ointment containing framycetin sulphate 1% in white soft paraffin containing 10% wool fat; sterile. 10 cm × 10 cm, net price each = 23p; **NHS** 10 cm × 30 cm, 10 = £8.24 (Roussel—*Sofra-Tulle ®*)

Cautions: large areas (risk of ototoxicity); see also cautions in section 13.10.1

Uses: wide range of infected lesions

PoM Sodium Fusidate Gauze Dressing, BP. Leno weave cotton gauze impregnated with ointment containing sodium fusidate 2% in white soft paraffin and wool fat. 10 cm × 10 cm, net price = 22p (Leo—*Fucidin Intertulle®*)

13.13.7   Vapour-permeable films and membranes

Vapour-permeable Adhesive Film Dressing, BP.
(Semi-permeable Adhesive Dressing) Sterile, extensible, waterproof, water vapour-permeable polyurethane film coated with synthetic adhesive mass; transparent. Supplied in single-use pieces. Type 1: 10 cm × 12 cm, net price = £1.18 (S&N Hlth—*Opsite® Flexigrid*), Type 2: 10 cm × 12 cm, net price = £1.21 (3M—*Tegaderm®*). Type 3: 10.2 cm × 12.7 cm, net price = £1.28 (J&J—*Bioclusive®*); Type 4, 7.5 cm × 10 cm, net price each = 64p; 10 cm × 14 cm, each = £1.09 (Beiersdorf—*Cutifilm®*)

Uses: post-operative dressing, donor sites, IV sites, superficial decubitus ulcers, amputation stumps, stoma care; protective cover to prevent skin breakdown

NHS Arglaes®, Sterile, semi-permeable, self-adhesive, clear, controlled release polyurethane film dressing containing silver. Net price 6 cm × 8 cm, 1 = 99p; 10 cm × 12 cm, 1 = £1.99; 15 cm × 25 cm, 1 = £3.99 (Maersk)

Uses: flat moist wounds including cuts and abrasions; burns and scalds; superficial pressure areas; surgical wounds

NHS Omiderm®. Sterile, water-vapour permeable polyurethane film (plain and meshed versions). Net price 5 cm × 7 cm, 20 = £24.79; 8 cm × 10 cm, 20 = £43.81; meshed, 20 = £58.70; 18 cm × 10 cm, 10 = £58.70; meshed, 10 = £58.70; 60 cm × 10 cm, 10 = £147.21; 21 cm × 31 cm, 5 = £75.36; meshed, 5 = £100.98; meshed, 23 cm × 39 cm, 4 = £119.87 (Omni Triage)

Uses: ulcers; donor sites; superficial and partial thickness burns; meshed: donor sites, skin grafts

NHS Spyroflex®. (formerly Flexipore 6000) Sterile, semipermeable, polyurethane membrane with hydrophilic adhesive. Net price 10 cm × 10 cm, 25 = £46.25; 20 cm × 20 cm, 10 = £68.40; 10 cm × 30 cm, 15 cm × 20 cm, 10 = £51.50; 20 cm × 30 cm, 5 = £51.50 (ConvaTec).

Uses: minor trauma, skin closure (alternative to skin sutures)

13.13.8   Gel and colloid dressings

Occlusive or semi-occlusive dressings which adhere to dry skin and interact with moisture in the wound to form a gel; may remain on a wound for up to 7 days.

Hydrogels

NHS Bard Absorption Dressing®. A dry polysaccharide derivative in flake form which is mixed with water and applied directly into the wound. 60-g pack
Uses: treatment of wounds and ulcers

Debrisan® (DrugTariff title: Dextranomer Paste Pad Dressing (Sterile), Drug Tariff specification 49). Spherical beads of dextranomer packed in plastic castors, paste or pads. Beads sprinkled onto cleansed wound and covered with a suitable non-woven, adhesive, semi-occlusive covering, or sterile dressing. Alternatively paste or pad is applied and covered in similar manner. Beads, net price 60 g = £29.01; paste, 6 × 10 g = £29.93; pads, 7 × 3 g = £16.09 (Pharmacia)
Uses: debriding agent to remove necrotic tissue

NHS Fibracol®. Calcium alginate with collagen matrix. Net price 5 cm × 5 cm each = 98p; 9.5 cm × 9.5 cm = £1.50; 10 cm × 20 cm = £3.60 (J & J)
Uses: small size for foot ulcers, pressure sores and toe nail beds; large size for moderate to heavily exuding wounds, leg ulcers, pressure sores

NHS Geliperm®. Gel sheets, wet form and tubed granulated gel. Granulate, 20 g, 6 tubes = £19.92, 50 g, 6 tubes = £49.80. Wet, 10 cm × 10 cm, net price, 20 sheets = £42.90, 12 cm × 13 cm, 6 sheets = £29.26; 12 cm × 26 cm, 6 sheets = £52.36 (Geistlich)
Uses: wound and ulcer dressing, burns, donor sites

Intrasite® Gel (formerly Scherisorb®) Drug Tariff specification 50. A ready-mixed hydrogel containing modified carboxymethylcellulose polymer applied directly into the wound. 15-g sachet, net price = £1.81 (S&N Hlth)

PoM Iodosorb®. Powder, microbeads of cadexomer iodine (modified starch gel containing iodine 0.9%). Net price 3-g sachet = £1.93; also Iodosorb® Ointment, 4 × 10 g = £18.05; 2 × 20 g = £18.05; also **PoM** Iodoflex® Paste, 5 × 5-g units = £20.40; 3 × 10-g units = £24.50; 2 × 17-g = £25.84 (Perstorp)
Uses: for venous leg ulcers and pressure sores apply 3 mm layer to wound surface and renew daily (3 times weekly for ointment or paste) or when saturated with exudate
Cautions; Contra-indications: avoid in thyroid disorders, in those receiving lithium or sulphonylureas, and in pregnancy and breast-feeding; caution in patients with past history of thyroid disorders; iodine may be absorbed particularly if large wounds treated

NHS Kaltocarb®. Dressing in 3 layers: wound-facing layer of calcium alginate fibre; absorbent middle layer of activated charcoal cloth; backing layer of bonded polyester and viscose non-woven material. Net price 7.5 cm × 12 cm, 25 = £51.48; 15 cm × 15 cm, 15 = £67.80 (ConvaTec)
Uses: discharging infected malodorous wounds and ulcers

Kaltogel®. (Alginate Dressing, Sterile, BP, type A) Calcium sodium alginate fibre, highly absorbent, quick gelling dressing, net price 5 cm × 5 cm, each = 70p; 10 cm × 10 cm = £1.45 (ConvaTec)
Uses: moderately to heavily exuding wounds including leg ulcers, pressure sores, fungating lesions

Kaltostat® (Alginate Dressing, Sterile, BP, type C). Calcium alginate fibre, flat non-woven pads, 5 cm × 5 cm, net price, each = 72p; 7.5 cm × 12 cm = £1.57; other sizes (**NHS**) 10 cm × 20 cm, 25 = £92.75; 15 cm × 25 cm, 25 = £160.00; 30 cm × 60 cm, 5 = £123.40; wound packing, 2 g, 25 = £82.00; also (**NHS**) Kaltostat Fortex®, 10 cm × 10 cm, 10 = £31.40 (ConvaTec)
Uses: haemostatic

Sorbsan® (Alginate Dressing, Sterile, BP, type A). Calcium alginate fibre, highly absorbent, flat non-woven pads, 5 cm × 5 cm, net price, each = 87p; 10 cm × 10 cm = £1.54; other sizes (**NHS**) 10 cm × 20 cm, 5 = £22.00 surgical packing 30 cm, 5 = £24.50; ribbon, 40 cm (+12.5-cm probe), 5 = £16.50; also (bonded to a secondary absorbent viscose pad) Sorbsan® Plus (**NHS**) 7.5 cm × 10 cm, 5 = £11.50; 10 cm × 15 cm, 5 = £22.50 (Maersk)
Uses: heavily to moderately exuding wounds

NHS Sorbsan® SA. Calcium alginate fibre, highly absorbent flat non-woven pads for wound contact bonded to adhesive semi-permeable polyurethane foam. Net price 9 cm × 11 cm, 5 = £11.00 (Maersk)
Uses: moderately to lightly exuding shallow wounds

Tegagen® (formerly Tegagel®) (Alginate Dressing, Sterile, BP, type B). Net price each 5 cm × 5 cm = 72p 10 cm × 10 cm = £1.50
Uses: for leg ulcers, pressure sores, second degree burns, post-operative wounds, fungating carcinomas

Tielle®. (Drug Tariff title: Polyurethane Foam Film Dressing with Adhesive Margin, Drug Tariff specification 47, type 3). Semi-permeable, foamed gel with non-woven wicking layer and polyurethane backing layer. Net price 11 cm × 11 cm = £1.92; 15 cm × 20 cm = £3.99; 18 cm × 18 cm = £3.99 (J&J)
Uses: light to moderately exuding wounds, leg ulcers

NHS Vigilon®. Semi-permeable hydrogel sheets on polyethylene mesh support. Sterile, 3 in × 6 in, net price 10 = £66.25, 4 in × 4 in, 10 = £66.25; non-sterile, 4 in × 4 in, 10 = £46.20, 13 in × 24 in, 2 = £80.35 (Seton)

Hydrocolloids

NHS Biofilm S®. Hydrocolloid dressing with polyurethane-polyester backing; also in powder form for direct application into wound: 10 cm × 10 cm, net price 10 = £16.50; 20 cm × 20 cm, 5 = £28.50; Biofilm® powder, 10 sachets = £18.20 (CliniMed)

Comfeel® . Soft elastic pad consisting of carmellose (carboxymethylcellulose) sodium particles embedded in adhesive mass; smooth outer layer and polyurethane film backing; available as sheets, powder in plastic blister units and paste for direct application into the wound. Ulcer dressing, 10 cm × 10 cm, net price each = £2.11 15 cm × 15 cm = £4.19; 20 cm × 20 cm = £6.28. Comfeel® Alginate (Alginate Dressing, Sterile, type C), 4 cm × 6 cm = 69p; 10 cm × 10 cm = £1.44 Comfeel® Plus Contour Dressing, 6 cm × 8 cm, 1 = £1.67; 9 cm × 11 cm, 1 = £2.89; Comfeel® Plus Ulcer Dressing, 10 cm × 10 cm = £2.11; 15 cm × 15 cm = £4.19; 20 cm × 20 cm = £6.28; other sizes (**NHS**): 4 cm × 6 cm, 30 = £30.30; transparent dressing, 5 cm × 7 cm 10 = £12.10; 9 cm × 14 cm, 10 = £35.50; 15 cm × 20 cm 5 = £39.80; powder 6 g, 10 = £33.70; paste 12-g sachet 10 = £13.00; 50 g, 10 = £49.80; **NHS** Comfeel® Alginate Filler, 2 g, 6 = £21.78; **NHS** Comfeel® Pressure Relief, 7 cm × 7 cm, 10 = £34.90; 10 cm × 10 cm, 10 £34.90; 15 cm × 15 cm, 10 = £72.00 (Coloplast)

Dermasorb®. Sterile hydrocolloid/alginate dressing . Net price 35 cm spirals, 10 = £40.00 (ConvaTec)
Uses: For treatment of deep wounds and ulcers

NHS Dermiflex®. Hydrocolloid dressing bonded to PVC foam 10.2 cm × 10.2 cm, net price, each = £1.95 (J&J)

Granuflex® Hydrocolloid wound contact layer bonded to plastic foam layer, with outer semipermeable polyurethane film. 10 cm × 10 cm, net price each = £2.12 15 cm × 15 cm = £3.99; 15 cm × 20 cm = £4.35; 20 cm 20 cm, 1 = £9.99; **NHS** 20 cm × 30 cm, 5 = £55.75; Duoderm® Extra Thin (formerly Granuflex® ExtraThin 7.5 cm × 7.5 cm, 1 = 60p; 10 cm × 10 cm, 1 = £1.00 (**NHS**),15 cm × 15 cm, 1 = £2.65; 5 cm × 10 cm, 1 = 69p 5 cm × 20 cm, 1 = £1.38; also Granuflex® Compression Bandage (**NHS**), 10 cm × 6.5 m (stretched), 6 = £32.64 also Granuflex® Paste (**NHS**), net price 30 g = £2.68 also, Granuflex® Bordered Dressing, 10 cm × 10 cm, 1

£2.50; 10 cm × 13 cm, 1 = £2.95; 15 cm × 18 cm, 1 = £4.60; also (NHS), 6 cm × 6 cm, 5 = £7.38; 15 cm × 15 cm, 5 = £30.98; triangular dressing, 10 cm × 13 cm, 5 = £15.61; 15 cm × 18 cm, 5 = £26.55; also GranuGel®, net price 15 g = £1.75 (ConvaTec)

Uses: chronic ulcers, pressure sores, open wounds, debridement of wounds; powders, gel, and pastes used with sheet dressings to fill deep or heavily exuding wounds

Tegasorb®. Hydrocolloid dressing 10 cm × 12 cm (oval), net price each = £2.01; 13 cm × 15 cm (oval), 1 = £3.79; 10 cm × 10 cm, (square) 1 = £2.05; 15 cm × 15 cm, (square) 1 = £3.97 (3M)

Uses: chronic wounds such as leg ulcers and pressure sores

Keloid dressing

NHS Cica-Care®. Soft, self-adhesive, semi-occlusive silicone gel sheet with backing. Net price, 15 cm × 12 cm, 1 sheet = £21.00 (S&N Hlth)

Uses: temporary management of both existing and new hypertrophic and keloid scars; also for temporary prophylaxis of hypertrophic or keloid scarring in closed wounds

13.13.9   Foam dressings

Polyurethane Foam Dressing, BP. Absorbent foam dressing of low adherence; sterile. 7.5 cm × 7.5 cm, net price, each = 83p; 10 cm × 10 cm, each = 99p; 10 cm × 17.5 cm, each = £1.54; 15 cm × 20 cm, each = £2.08; other sizes (NHS) 10 cm × 25 cm, 35 = £58.05; 25 cm × 30 cm, each = £3.91 (Seton—*Lyofoam®*)

Uses: treatment of burns, decubitus ulcers, donor sites, granulating wounds

Lyofoam Extra®. Extra absorbent polyurethane foam dressing, non-adhesive. Net price 10 cm × 10 cm, 1 = £1.69; 17.5 cm x 10 cm, 1 = £2.85; 20 cm × 15 cm, 1 = £3.70; 25 cm x 10 cm, 1 = £3.45; (NHS) 30 cm × 25 cm, 1 = £12.00 (Seton)

Uses: treatment of heavily exuding wounds

NHS Cavi-Care®. Soft, conforming cavity wound dressing prepared by mixing thoroughly for 15 seconds immediately before use and allowing to expand its volume within the cavity. Net price 20 g = £8.03 (S&N Hlth)

Uses: in the management of open post-operative granulating cavity wounds (with no underlying tracts or sinuses) such as pilonidal sinus excision, dehisced surgical wounds, hydradenitis, suppurativa wounds, peri-anal wounds, perineal wounds, pressure sores

Allevyn®. (Drug Tariff title: Polyurethane Foam Film Dressing, Drug Tariff specification 47, type 2) Hydrophilic polyurethane dressing; foam sheets with trilaminate structure, non-adherent wound contact layer, foam based central layer, bacteria and waterproof outer layer. 5 cm × 5 cm, each = 95p; 10 cm × 10 cm, each = £1.90; 10 cm × 20 cm, each = £3.03; 20 cm × 20 cm, each = £5.06; also Allevyn® Adhesive (Drug Tariff title: Polyurethane Foam Film Dressing with Adhesive Margin, Drug Tariff specification 47, type 4), 7.5 cm × 7.5 cm = £1.12; 12.5 cm × 12.5 cm = £2.02; 17.5 cm × 17.5 cm = £3.98; 22.5 cm × 22.5 cm = £5.79; **NHS**Allevyn® Cavity, circular (5 and 10 cm), tubular (2.5 cm × 9 cm and 4 cm × 12 cm) (S&N Hlth)

Uses: treatment of light to moderately exuding wounds

Spyrosorb® (Drug Tariff title: Polyurethane Foam Film Dressing, Drug Tariff specification 47, type 1). Sterile, semipermeable, absorbent polyurethane membrane with polyurethane film and hydrophilic adhesive. Net price 10 cm × 10 cm, 5 = £9.90; 20 cm × 20 cm, 5 = £28.25 (ConvaTec).

Uses: light to moderately exuding wounds

13.13.10   Elastic hosiery

Before elastic hosiery can be dispensed, the quantity (single or pair), article (including accessories), and compression class (I, II or III) must be specified by the prescriber; all dispensed articles must state on the packaging that they conform with Drug Tariff technical specification No. 40, for further details see Drug Tariff.

Graduated compression hosiery

Class 1 Light Support

Hosiery, compression at ankle 14–17 mm Hg, thigh length or below knee with knitted in heel. Net price per pair, circular knit (standard), thigh length = £5.96, below knee = £5.44; light weight elastic net (made-to-measure), thigh length = £15.96, below knee = £12.46

Uses: superficial or early varices, varicosis during pregnancy

Class 2 Medium Support

Hosiery, compression at ankle 18–24 mm Hg, thigh length or below knee with knitted in heel. Net price per pair, circular knit (standard), thigh length = £8.86, below knee = £7.96, (made-to-measure), thigh length = £29.60, below knee = £18.52; net (made-to-measure), thigh length = £15.96, below knee = £12.46; flat bed (made-to-measure, only with closed heel and open toe), thigh length = £29.60, below knee = £18.52

Uses: varices of medium severity, ulcer treatment and prophylaxis, mild oedema, varicosis during pregnancy

Class 3 Strong Support

Hosiery, compression at ankle 25–35 mm Hg, thigh length or below knee with open or knitted in heel. Net price per pair, circular knit (standard), thigh length = £10.50, below knee = £9.02, (made-to-measure) thigh length = £29.60, below knee = £18.52; one way stretch (made-to-measure, only with open heel and open toe), thigh length = £29.60, below knee = £18.52

Uses: gross varices, post thrombotic venous insufficiency, gross oedema, ulcer treatment and prophylaxis

Accessories

Suspender, for thigh stockings, net price = 52p, belt (specification 13), = £3.97, fitted (additional price) = 52p

Anklets

Class 2 Medium Support

Anklets, compression 18–24 mm Hg, circular knit (standard and made-to-measure), net price per pair = £5.22; flat bed (standard and made-to-measure) = £10.84; net (made-to-measure) = £10.26

Uses: soft tissue support

Class 3 Strong Support

Anklets, compression 25–35 mm Hg, circular knit (standard and made-to-measure), net price per pair = £7.28; one way stretch (standard and made-to-measure) = £7.28

Uses: soft tissue support

Kneecaps

Class 2 Medium Support

Kneecaps, circular knit (standard and made-to-measure), net price per pair = £5.22; flat bed (standard and made-to-measure) = £10.84; net (made-to-measure) = £8.52

Uses: soft tissue support

Class 3 Strong Support

Kneecaps, circular knit (standard and made-to-measure), net price per pair = £6.96; one way stretch (standard and made-to-measure) = £6.96

Uses: soft tissue support

13.14   Topical circulatory preparations

These preparations are used to improve circulation in conditions such as bruising, superficial thrombophlebitis, chilblains and varicose veins but are of little value. Chilblains are best managed by avoidance of exposure to cold; neither systemic nor topical vasodilator therapy is established as being effective. Sclerotherapy of varicose veins is described in section 2.13.

Rubefacients are described in section 10.3.2.

Hirudoid® (Panpharma)

Cream, heparinoid 0.3% in a vanishing-cream basis. Net price 50 g = £1.35

Additives: include hydroxybenzoates (parabens)

Gel, heparinoid 0.3%. Net price 50 g = £1.35

Additives: include propylene glycol, fragrance

Apply up to 4 times daily in superficial soft-tissue injuries and superficial thrombophlebitis

Lasonil® (Bayer)

Ointment, heparinoid 50 units, hyaluronidase 150 units/g. Net price 14 g = 38p; 40 g = £1.08

Additives: include wool fat derivative

Apply 2–3 times daily in superficial soft-tissue injuries

14: Immunological products and
VACCINES

In this chapter, immunisation is discussed under the following headings:

14.1 Active immunity

Vaccines may consist of:

1. a *live attenuated* form of a virus (e.g. rubella or measles vaccine) or bacteria (e.g. BCG vaccine)
2. *inactivated* preparations of the virus (e.g. influenza vaccine) or bacteria (e.g. whole cell typhoid vaccine), or
3. *extracts of* or *detoxified exotoxins* produced by a micro-organism (e.g. tetanus vaccine).

They stimulate production of antibodies and other components of the immune mechanism.

For **live attenuated** vaccines, immunisation is generally achieved with a single dose (but 3 doses are required with oral poliomyelitis and oral typhoid vaccines). Live attenuated vaccines usually produce a durable immunity but not always as long as that of the natural infection. When two live virus vaccines are required (and are not available as a combined preparation) they should be given either simultaneously at different sites or with an interval of at least 3 weeks.

Inactivated vaccines may require a primary series of injections of vaccine to produce adequate antibody response and in most cases reinforcing or 'booster' injections are required; the duration of immunity varies from months to many years.

Extracts of or **detoxified exotoxins** are more immunogenic if adsorbed onto an adjuvant (such as aluminium hydroxide). They require a primary series of injections followed by reinforcing doses.

> Guidelines in this chapter reflect those in the handbook *Immunisation against Infectious Disease*, which in turn reflects the advice of the Joint Committee on Vaccination and Immunisation (JCVI). Copies can be obtained from:
>
> HMSO Publications Centre
>
> PO Box 276, London SW8 5DT
>
> Telephone orders, 0171-873 9090.

SIDE-EFFECTS. Some vaccines (e.g. poliomyelitis) produce very few reactions, while others (e.g. measles and rubella) may produce a very mild form of the disease. Some vaccines may produce discomfort at the site of injection and mild fever and malaise. Occasionally there are more serious untoward reactions and these should always be reported to the CSM. Anaphylactic reactions are very rare but can be fatal (see section 3.4.3 for management). For full details of side-effects, the manufacturer's data sheet should always be consulted.

CONTRA-INDICATIONS. Most vaccines have some basic contra-indication to their use, and the manufacturer's data sheet should always be consulted. In general, vaccination should be postponed if the subject is suffering from an *acute illness*. Minor infections without fever or systemic upset are not contra-indications.

Some viral vaccines contain small quantities of antibiotics such as neomycin or polymyxin (or both); such vaccines may need to be withheld from individuals who are *sensitive to the antibiotic*. *Hypersensitivity to egg* contra-indicates influenza vaccine (residual egg protein present) and, if evidence of previous anaphylactic reaction, also MMR and yellow fever vaccines.

Live vaccines should not be routinely administered to *pregnant women* because of possible harm to the fetus but where there is a significant risk of exposure (e.g. to poliomyelitis or yellow fever), the need for vaccination outweighs any possible risk to the fetus. Live vaccines should not be given to individuals with *impaired immune response*, whether caused by disease (for special reference to *AIDS*, see below) or as a result of radiotherapy or treatment with high doses of corticosteroids or other immunosuppressive drugs[1,2]. They should not be given to those suffering from *malignant conditions* such as leukaemia and tumours of the reticuloendothelial system[2].

The intramuscular route should not be used in patients with bleeding disorders such as haemophilia or thrombocytopenia.

VACCINES AND AIDS. The Department of Health has advised that HIV-positive subjects with or without symptoms can receive the following live vaccines:

measles[2] (or MMR), mumps, poliomyelitis[3], rubella;

and the following inactivated vaccines:

cholera, diphtheria, haemophilus influenzae type b, hepatitis A, hepatitis B, influenza, meningococcal, pertussis, pneumococcal, poliomyelitis[3], tetanus, typhoid (injection).

HIV-positive subjects should **not** receive:

BCG, yellow fever[4], typhoid (oral)

Note. The above advice differs from that for other immunocompromised patients.

1. Live vaccines should be postponed until at least 3 months after stopping corticosteroids and 6 months after stopping chemotherapy.
2. Consideration should be given to use of normal immunoglobulin after exposure to measles (see p. 515) and to varicella-zoster immunoglobulin after exposure to chickenpox or herpes zoster (see p. 516).
3. Virus may be excreted for longer periods than in normal subjects; contacts should be warned of this and need for washing hands after changing a vaccinated infant's nappies; HIV-positive contacts are at greater risk than normal contacts. For HIV-positive symptomatic subjects inactivated poliomyelitis vaccine can be used at discretion of clinician.
4. Because insufficient evidence of safety.

Immunisation programmes

Vaccines for the childhood immunisation programme should be obtained **via local Health Authorities** or (in England only) **direct from Farillon**—not available on FP10 prescription (since not available to pharmacies).

Age	Vaccine	Interval	Notes
During the first year of life	DTPer/Vac/Ads *and* Haemophilus influenzae b *and* Pol/Vac (Oral)	3 doses[1] at intervals of 4 weeks	The first doses should be given at 2 months of age Pertussis and unimmunised older children, see p. 510 BCG and neonates at risk, see p. 503
During the second year of life	Meas/Mump/Rub (MMR) Vac (Live)		At 12–15 months of age
	Haemophilus influenzae b		One dose at 13 months–4 years of age if not previously immunised (over 4 years, see p. 506)
At school entry or entry to nursery school	DT/Vac/Ads *and* Pol/Vac (Oral) *and* Meas/Mump/Rub (MMR) Vac (Live)[2]	Preferable to allow an interval of at least 3 years after completing basic course	
Between 10th and 14th birthdays	BCG	Leave an interval of not less than 3 weeks between BCG and rubella immunisation	For tuberculin-negative children. For tuberculin-negative contacts at any age
Between 10th and 14th birthdays (girls only)	Rub/Vac (Live)		See MR vaccine, (both sexes), p. 510
On leaving school or before employment or further education	Pol/Vac (Oral) *and* DT/Vac/Ads (Adult)		DT/Vac/Ads (Adult) is for adults and children *over 10 years*
Adult life	Pol/Vac (Oral) if previously unimmunised	3 doses at intervals of 4 weeks	No adult should remain unimmunised; reinforcing doses for travellers where polio endemic and for health care workers in possible contact with polio
	Rub/Vac (Live) for susceptible women of child-bearing age		Women of child-bearing age should be tested for rubella antibodies and if sero-negative offered rubella immunisation. Pregnancy must be excluded, but see also p. 513
	Tet/Vac/Ads if previously unimmunised	For previously unimmunised adults: 2 doses at an interval of 4 weeks followed by a third dose 4 weeks later	A reinforcing dose 10 years after primary course and again 10 years later maintains a satisfactory level of protection; give DT/Vac/Ads (Adult) if diphtheria cover also needed
	Hepatitis A and B, Influenza, Pneumococcal		All for individuals (adults or children) in high-risk groups, see under individual vaccines

1. If the pertussis component has been omitted from earlier immunisations 3 doses of pertussis vaccine can be given at monthly intervals to provide protection. Where the basic course against diphtheria and tetanus is incomplete triple vaccine may be used to begin or complete the course against whooping-cough so that the infant is not given more injections than necessary.

2. Measles/mumps/rubella (MMR) vaccine can be given at the time of the reinforcing dose of diphtheria/tetanus vaccine and poliomyelitis vaccine; because the diphtheria/tetanus vaccine can be more painful, measles/mumps/rubella vaccine should be injected first; the diphtheria/tetanus should then be given with a separate syringe and needle in the opposite limb (or a second appointment can be made).

14.2   Passive immunity

Immunity with immediate protection against certain infective organisms can be obtained by injecting preparations made from the plasma of immune individuals with adequate levels of antibody to the disease for which protection is sought (see under Immunoglobulins, section 14.5). This passive immunity lasts only a few weeks; where necessary passive immunisation can be repeated.

Antibodies of human origin are usually termed *immunoglobulins*. The term *antiserum* is applied to material prepared in animals. Because of serum sickness and other allergic-type reactions that may follow injections of antisera, this therapy has been replaced wherever possible by the use of immunoglobulins. Reactions are theoretically possible after injection of human immunoglobulins but reports of such reactions are very rare.

14.3   Storage and use

Care must be taken to store all vaccines and other immunological products under the conditions recommended in the manufacturer's leaflet, otherwise the preparation may become denatured and totally ineffective. **Refrigerated storage** is usually necessary; many vaccines need to be stored at 2–8°C and not allowed to freeze. Opened multidose vials which have not been fully used should be discarded *within one hour* if no preservative is present (most live virus vaccines) or *within 3 hours* or at the end of a session (when vaccines containing a preservative are used but also including oral poliomyelitis vaccine).

Particular attention must be paid to the instructions on the use of diluents and ampoules of vaccine should always be *adequately shaken* before use to ensure uniformity of the material to be injected.

Note. The Department of Health has advised *against the use of jet guns* for vaccination owing to the risk of transmitting blood-borne infections, such as HIV.

14.4   Vaccines and antisera

AVAILABILITY.   Anthrax, rabies, and yellow fever vaccines, botulism antitoxin, and snake venom antitoxin are available from local designated holding centres. Details of names, addresses, and telephone numbers of holding centres are given in:

The Health Service Supply Purchasing Guide, section D pp. 1101–1109

For antivenom, see Emergency Treatment of Poisoning, p. 26

Enquiries for vaccines not available commercially can also be made to

Department of Health
Room 715
133–155 Waterloo Road
London SE1 8UG
telephone 0171-972 4476/7

In Scotland information about availability of vaccines can be obtained from the Chief Administrative Pharmaceutical Officer of the local Health Board. In Wales enquiries should be directed to the Welsh Office, Cathays Park, Cardiff CF1 3NQ, telephone 01222 825111, extn 4658 and in Northern Ireland to the Department of Health and Social Services, Dundonald House, Belfast BT4 3SB, telephone 01232 520000.

For further details of availability, see under individual vaccines.

ANTHRAX VACCINE

Anthrax vaccine is available for anyone subject to heavy exposure to anthrax, such as those exposed to infected hides and carcasses and to imported bone-meal, fishmeal, and feeding stuffs. The vaccine is the alum precipitate of an antigen from *Bacillus anthracis* and, following the primary course of injections, reinforcing doses should be given at about yearly intervals.

PoM Anthrax Vaccine

Dose: initial course 3 doses of 0.5 mL by intramuscular injection at intervals of 3 weeks followed by a 4th dose after an interval of 6 months
Reinforcing doses: 0.5 mL annually
Available from Public Health Laboratory Service

BCG VACCINES

BCG (Bacillus Calmette-Guérin) is a live attenuated strain derived from *Mycobacterium bovis* which stimulates the development of hypersensitivity to *M. tuberculosis*. BCG vaccine should be given intradermally by operators skilled in the technique (see below).

Within 2–6 weeks a small swelling appears at the injection site which progresses to a papule or to a benign ulcer about 10 mm in diameter and heals in 6–12 weeks. A dry dressing may be used if the ulcer discharges, but air should **not** be excluded.

The CSM has reported that serious reactions with BCG are uncommon and most often consist of prolonged ulceration or subcutaneous abscess formation due to faulty injection technique.

BCG is recommended for the following groups if **successful** BCG immunisation has not previously been carried out and they are negative for tuberculoprotein hypersensitivity:

contacts of those with active respiratory tuberculosis (immigrants in whose communities there is a high incidence of tuberculosis may be regarded as contacts—newborn infants need not be tested for sensitivity but should be immunised without delay);

health service staff (including medical students, hospital medical staff, nurses, and anybody who comes into contact with patients, including physiotherapists and radiographers, technical staff in pathology departments and any others considered to be at special risk because of the likelihood of contact with infective patients or their sputum; particularly important to test staff in maternity and paediatric departments);

children between their tenth and fourteenth birthdays (see schedule, section 14.1);

veterinary and other staff who handle animal species known to be susceptible to tuberculosis;

those travelling to countries with a high incidence of tuberculosis (section 14.6)

Apart from newborn infants any person being considered for BCG immunisation must first be given a skin test for hypersensitivity to tuberculoprotein (see under Diagnostic agents, below).

It is recommended that an interval of at least 3 weeks should be allowed between the administration of a live virus vaccine and BCG. However, when BCG is given to infants, there is no need to delay the primary immunisations, including poliomyelitis.

See section 14.1 for general contra-indications. BCG is also contra-indicated in subjects with generalised septic skin conditions (in the case of eczema, a vaccination site free from lesions should be chosen).

Intradermal
PoM **Bacillus Calmette-Guérin Vaccine.**
BCG Vaccine, Dried Tub/Vac/BCG. A freeze-dried preparation of live bacteria of a strain derived from the bacillus of Calmette and Guérin.

Dose: 0.1 mL (INFANT under 3 months 0.05 mL) by intradermal injection

Available from District Health Authorities or (in England only) direct from Farillon

INTRADERMAL INJECTION TECHNIQUE. After swabbing with spirit and allowing to dry, skin is stretched between thumb and forefinger and needle (size 25G or 26G) inserted (bevel upwards) for about 2 mm into superficial layers of dermis (almost parallel with surface). Needle should be short with short bevel (can usually be seen through epidermis during insertion). Raised blanched bleb showing tips of hair follicles is sign of correct injection; 7 mm bleb ≡ 0.1 mL injection; if considerable resistance not felt, needle is removed and reinserted before giving more vaccine.

Injection site is at insertion of deltoid muscle onto humerus (sites higher on arm more likely to lead to keloid formation); tip of shoulder should be **avoided**; for cosmetic reasons, upper and lateral surface of thigh may be preferred and this is an acceptable alternative.

PoM **Bacillus Calmette-Guérin Vaccine, Isoniazid-Resistant.** A freeze-dried preparation of live bacteria of an isoniazid-resistant strain derived from the bacillus of Calmette and Guérin.

Dose: 0.1 mL (INFANT under 3 months 0.05 mL) by intradermal injection; for active immunisation of tuberculosis contacts receiving prophylactic treatment with isoniazid—but **no longer recommended**.

Available from Evans (special order)

Percutaneous

The percutaneous multiple puncture technique is an acceptable alternative **only** for young infants in whom the technique of intradermal injection may be difficult (18–20 puncture points are required)

PoM **Bacillus Calmette-Guérin Vaccine, Percutaneous** Tub/Vac/BCG(Perc). A preparation of live bacteria of a strain derived from the bacillus of Calmette and Guérin (**important:** this preparation must **not** be confused with the intradermal preparation)

Dose: about 0.03 mL by percutaneous administration but only recommended as an alternative for infants, see notes above

Available from District Health Authorities or (in England only) direct from Farillon

DIAGNOSTIC AGENTS. In the *Mantoux test* the initial diagnostic dose in patients in whom tuberculosis is suspected (or who are known to be hypersensitive to tuberculin) is 1 unit of tuberculin PPD in 0.1 mL by intradermal injection and in subsequent tests 10 and finally 100 units in 0.1 mL may be given. For routine pre-BCG skin-testing the 10-unit dose of tuberculin PPD is used. In the *Heaf test* (multiple puncture) a solution containing 100 000 units in 1 mL is used.

PoM **Tuberculin PPD.** Prepared from the heat treated products of growth and lysis of the appropriate species of mycobacterium, and containing 100 000 units/mL. Net price 1-mL amp = £5.89. Also available diluted 1 in 100 (1000 units/mL), 1 in 1000 (100 units/mL), and 1 in 10 000 (10 units/mL). Net price 1 mL (all) = £2.22

Available from District Health Authorities or (in England only) direct from Farillon

BOTULISM ANTITOXIN

A trivalent botulism antitoxin is available for the post-exposure prophylaxis of botulism and for the treatment of persons thought to be suffering from botulism. It specifically neutralises the toxins produced by *Clostridium botulinum* types A, B, and E. It is not effective against infantile botulism as the toxin (type A) is seldom, if ever, found in the blood in this type of infection.

Hypersensitivity reactions are a problem. It is essential to read the contra-indications, warnings, and details of sensitivity tests on the package insert. Prior to treatment checks should be made regarding previous administration of any antitoxin and history of any allergic condition, e.g. asthma, hay fever, etc. All patients should be tested for sensitivity (diluting the antitoxin if history of allergy).

PoM **Botulism Antitoxin.** A preparation containing the specific antitoxic globulins that have the power of neutralising the toxins formed by types A, B, and E of *Clostridium botulinum*.

Note. The BP title Botulinum Antitoxin is not used because the preparation currently available has a higher phenol content (0.45% against 0.25%).

Dose: prophylaxis, 20 mL by intramuscular injection as soon as possible after exposure; treatment, 20 mL by slow intravenous infusion followed by 10 mL 2–4 hours later if necessary, and further doses at intervals of 12–24 hours.

Available from local designated centres. For supplies outside working hours apply to Department of Health Duty Officer, telephone 0171-210 5371

CHOLERA VACCINE

Cholera vaccine contains heat-killed Inaba and Ogawa sub-types of *Vibrio cholerae*, Serovar O1. Cholera vaccine provides little protection and cannot control the spread of the disease. The Department of Health has therefore advised that:

immunisation against cholera is no longer a legal requirement for entry into any foreign country and should not be required of any traveller. However, border officials in some countries may still ask people travelling from endemic or epidemic areas for evidence of immunisation. Travellers who are likely to cross borders from such areas, especially overland, should therefore be advised to have the vaccine here before travel rather than risk injections abroad. For this purpose one injection is sufficient.

Travellers to a country where cholera exists should be warned that attention to food and water and personal hygiene is **essential**, even after vaccination.

PoM **Cholera Vaccine** Cho/Vac. Net price 1.5-mL vial = £4.51

Dose: first dose, as specified on the label, usually 0.5 mL by deep subcutaneous or intramuscular injection; second dose, after at least a week and preferably 4 weeks, 1 mL; reinforcing dose every 6 months on continued exposure; CHILD 1–5 years 0.1 mL, second dose 0.3 mL, 5–10 years 0.3 mL, second dose 0.5 mL

Note. For purposes of **providing a certificate for travellers** the Department of Health has recommended that **one injection is sufficient**, see notes above. If it is required to give the full course, adverse reactions can be minimised by giving the second and subsequent doses intradermally in a volume of 0.2 mL (0.1 mL at two separate sites) if the subcutaneous dose is more than 0.5 mL, and 0.1 mL if the subcutaneous dose is 0.5 mL or less.

Available from Evans

DIPHTHERIA VACCINES

Protection against diphtheria is essentially due to antitoxin, the production of which is stimulated by vaccines prepared from the toxin of *Corynebacterium diphtheriae*. These are more effective and cause fewer reactions if adsorbed onto a mineral carrier. Adsorbed diphtheria vaccines are recommended for the routine immunisation of babies and given in the form of a triple vaccine, **adsorbed diphtheria, tetanus, and pertussis vaccine**. A dose of poliomyelitis vaccine, live (oral) is generally given at the same time as each of the doses of

the triple vaccine (see schedule, section 14.1). Adsorbed diphtheria and tetanus vaccine is used in place of the triple vaccine when immunisation against pertussis is contra-indicated.

A reinforcing dose of **adsorbed diphtheria and tetanus vaccine** is recommended at school entry (4–5 years of age). This should preferably be given after an interval of at least 3 years from the last dose of the basic course. A further reinforcing dose is now recommended at school leaving; for this purpose **adsorbed diphtheria and tetanus vaccine for adults and adolescents** (a special low-dose version combined in a single injection with tetanus vaccine) has been developed.

Other reinforcing doses of diphtheria vaccine are not recommended as a routine except in the case of those who work in units where there is a potentially high risk of infection such as those employed in infectious disease units or microbiology laboratories. A low-dose vaccine, **adsorbed diphtheria vaccine for adults**, is available for this purpose.

The Chief Medical Officer has issued a warning on diphtheria in the former USSR. *Previously immunised* travellers require a booster dose if they are to live or work with local residents and their primary immunisation was more than 10 years ago. *Unimmunised travellers* require a full course of 3 doses at monthly intervals (**important:** adults and children *over 10 years* requiring either a primary course or a booster should be given a **low-dose** vaccine—those also requiring tetanus cover can be given the special low-dose version combined with tetanus vaccine).

See section 14.1 for general contra-indications.

Diphtheria vaccines for children

IMPORTANT. Not recommended for persons *aged 10 years or over* (use diphtheria vaccines for adults and adolescents instead)

With tetanus and pertussis (triple vaccine)

PoM **Adsorbed Diphtheria, Tetanus, and Pertussis Vaccine** DTPer/Vac/Ads.   Prepared from diphtheria formol toxoid, tetanus formol toxoid, and pertussis vaccine adsorbed on a mineral carrier.

Dose: primary immunisation of children, 0.5 mL by intramuscular or deep subcutaneous injection at 2 months followed by second dose after 4 weeks and third dose after another 4 weeks (see schedule, section 14.1)

Available from District Health Authorities or (in England only) direct from Farillon as Pasteur Mérieux brand or Evans (Trivax-AD®) brand

Note. The manufacturer of HibTiter® (Haemophilus influenzae type b vaccine) has recommmended that only Trivax-AD® brand of adsorbed diphtheria, tetanus and pertussis vaccine can be administered in the same syringe as HibTiter®

The manufacturer of ACT-HIB® (Haemophilus influenzae type b vaccine) has recommended that a single dose vial may be reconstituted with 0.5 mL of Pasteur Mérieux brand of adsorbed diphtheria, tetanus and pertussis vaccine. A pack containing both vaccines is available as ACT-HIB®DTP

With tetanus

PoM **Adsorbed Diphtheria and Tetanus Vaccine** DT/Vac/Ads. Prepared from diphtheria formol toxoid and tetanus formol toxoid adsorbed on a mineral carrier.

Dose: primary immunisation of children omitting pertussis component, 0.5 mL by intramuscular or deep subcutaneous injection at 2 months followed by second dose after 4 weeks and third dose after another 4 weeks (see schedule, section 14.1); reinforcement at school entry, 0.5 mL (see schedule, section 14.1)

Available from District Health Authorities or (in England only) direct from Farillon as Evans brand or Pasteur Mérieux brand

Single antigen

PoM **Adsorbed Diphtheria Vaccine** Dip/Vac/ Ads. Prepared from diphtheria formol toxoid adsorbed on a mineral carrier. Net price 0.5-mL amp = £1.12

Note. Used only for contacts of a diphtheria case or carrier; *immunised children under 10 years* are given one dose of 0.5 mL by intramuscular or by deep subcutaneous injection, *unimmunised children under 10 years* are given three doses of 0.5 mL with an interval of 4 weeks between first and second doses and another 4 weeks between second and third; *adults and children over 10 years* must be given diphtheria vaccine for adults, adsorbed (see below).

Available from District Health Authorities or (in England only) direct from Farillon

Diphtheria vaccines for adults and adolescents

IMPORTANT. Also for use in children aged *10 years or over*

The small quantity of diphtheria toxoid present in the preparations below is sufficient to recall immunity in individuals previously immunised against diphtheria but whose immunity may have diminished with time; it is insufficient to cause the serious reactions that may occur when diphtheria vaccine of conventional formulation is used in an individual who is already immune. The low dose vaccine must be used when immunising adults and children *over 10 years*; for school leavers a low-dose version combined in a single injection with tetanus vaccine is available (see notes above).

With tetanus

PoM **Adsorbed Diphtheria and Tetanus Vaccine for Adults and Adolescents** DT/ Vac/Ads (Adult). Prepared from diphtheria formol toxoid and tetanus formol toxoid adsorbed on a mineral carrier.

Dose: primary immunisation in *patients over 10 years*, three doses each of 0.5 mL by intramuscular or deep subcutaneous injection separated by intervals of 4 weeks; reinforcement, 0.5 mL after 10 years

Available from District Health Authorities or (in England only) direct from Farillon as Pasteur Mérieux brand (also known as Diftavax®)

Single antigen

PoM **Adsorbed Diphtheria Vaccine for Adults and Adolescents** Dip/Vac/Ads (Adult). Prepared from diphtheria formol toxoid adsorbed on a mineral carrier.

Dose: primary immunisation in *patients over 10 years*, three doses each of 0.5 mL by intramuscular or deep subcutaneous injection separated by intervals of 1 month; reinforcement, 0.5 mL

Note. Unimmunised adults and children *over 10 years* who are contacts of a diphtheria case or carrier are given the primary immunisation course; immunised adults and children *over 10 years* are given the reinforcement dose.

Available from District Health Authorities or (in England only) direct from Farillon

---

DIPHTHERIA ANTITOXIN

Diphtheria antitoxin is used for passive immunisation; it is prepared in horses therefore reactions are common after administration.

It is now only used in suspected cases of diphtheria (without waiting for bacteriological confirmation); tests for hypersensitivity should be first carried out.

It is no longer used for prophylaxis because of the risk of hypersensitivity; unimmunised contacts should be promptly investigated and given erythromycin prophylaxis (see section 5.1, table 2) and vaccine (see notes above).

PoM **Diphtheria Antitoxin** Dip/Ser.

Dose: prophylactic 500 to 2000 units by intramuscular injection (but **not** used, see notes above); therapeutic 10 000 to 30 000 units increased to 40 000 to 100 000 units in severe cases; doses of up to 30 000 units should be given intramuscularly but for those over 40 000 units a portion is given intramuscularly followed by the bulk of the dose intravenously after an interval of ½–2 hours

Note. Children require the same dose as adults, depending on the severity of the case.

Available from Pasteur Mérieux on a named patient basis or stocks may be held by hospital pharmacies

HAEMOPHILUS INFLUENZAE TYPE B VACCINE

Haemophilus influenzae type b vaccine (Hib) is given in a course of 3 doses at monthly intervals usually at the same time as routine childhood immunisation against diphtheria, tetanus, pertussis and poliomyelitis (see schedule, section 14.1) in infants from 2 months of age. Children under 13 months of age who have already commenced or completed their primary routine immunisation should still receive 3 doses of Hib vaccine at monthly intervals. Children over 13 months of age are at lower risk of infection, and the vaccine is effective after a single dose. The risk of infection falls sharply after the age of 4 years therefore the vaccine is not normally required for children over 4 years. However, it may be given to those over 4 years who are considered to be at increased risk of invasive Haemophilus influenzae type b disease (such as those with sickle cell disease, those receiving treatment for malignancy, and those without a spleen). Side-effects reported include fever, headache, malaise, irritability, prolonged crying, loss of appetite, vomiting, diarrhoea, and rash (including urticaria); convulsions, erythema multiforme, and

---

ansient cyanosis of the lower limbs have been ported.

See section 14.1 for general contra-indications

oM Haemophilus influenzae type b

Hib)

Capsular conjugated polysaccharide vaccine

Dose: 0.5 mL by intramuscular or deep subcutaneous injection in a different limb from other concurrently administered vaccines; for primary immunisation 3 doses are required at intervals of 1 month (see schedule, section 14.1)

Available from District Health Authorities or (in England only) direct from Farillon—Pasteur Mérieux (ACT-HIB®) brand; Lederle (HibTITER®) brand may be supplied in Wales. Either ACT-HIB® or HibTITER® may be used to complete a course started with the other

Note. The manufacturer of HibTITER® (Haemophilus influenzae type b vaccine) has recommmended that only Trivax-AD® brand of adsorbed diphtheria, tetanus and pertussis vaccine can be administered in the same syringe as HibTITER®

The manufacturer of ACT-HIB® (Haemophilus influenzae type b vaccine) has recommended that a single dose vial may be reconstituted with 0.5 mL of Pasteur Mérieux brand of adsorbed diphtheria, tetanus and pertusis vaccine. A pack containing both vaccines is available as ACT-HIB®DTP

HEPATITIS A VACCINE

Hepatitis A vaccine is prepared from formaldehyde-inactivated hepatitis A virus grown in human diploid cells. The vaccine is an alternative to human normal immunoglobulin for frequent travellers to moderate to high risk areas or those who stay for more than 3 months.

Protection against hepatitis A should be considered for those travelling to destinations outside Northern and Western Europe, North America, Australia and New Zealand. Travellers to high-risk areas who require immunisation less than two weeks before departure may be given the single-dose vaccine plus normal immunoglobulin at a different injection site. Administration of human normal immunoglobulin at the same time as the vaccine, at different injection sites, does not affect rate of seroconversion but the level of antibody may be reduced. In the UK some occupational groups such as sewage workers may be at risk from infection.

Side-effects, usually mild, include transient soreness, erythema, and induration at the injection site. Less common effects include fever, malaise, fatigue, headache, nausea, and loss of appetite. The CSM has reported that *Havrix®* provides safe and effective immunisation against hepatitis A, and that to date the only issues identified by spontaneous reporting are occasional generalised rashes and very rare neurological reactions (that are not necessarily caused by the vaccine).

See section 14.1 for general contra-indications.

▼ PoM **Avaxim®** (Pasteur Mérieux)

A suspension of formaldehyde-inactivated hepatitis A virus (GBM grown in human diploid cells) 320 antigen units/mL adsorbed onto aluminium hydroxide. Net price 0.5-mL prefilled syringe = £21.60

Dose: by intramuscular injection (see note below), 0.5 mL as a single dose; booster dose 0.5 mL 6 months following the initial dose; further booster doses, 0.5 mL every 10 years; CHILD under 16 years, not recommended
Note. The deltoid region is the preferred site of injection. The subcutaneous route may be used for patients with haemophilia

PoM **Havrix®** (SmithKline Beecham)
Product discontinued
Note. Patients who have received a course of Havrix® (720 ELISA units/mL) vaccine and who require a booster, should receive a single dose of Havrix Monodose® (1440 ELISA units/mL)

PoM **Havrix® Junior** (SmithKline Beecham)
Product discontinued
Note. Patients who have already started a course of Havrix® Junior (720 ELISA units/mL) vaccine (now discontinued) would need to continue to receive it both to complete the primary course and for the booster—contact the company

PoM **Havrix Monodose®** (SmithKline Beecham)

A suspension of formaldehyde-inactivated hepatitis A virus (HM 175 grown in human diploid cells) 1440 ELISA units/mL adsorbed onto aluminium hydroxide. Net price 1-mL prefilled syringe = £21.60; 0.5-mL prefilled syringe (Havrix® Junior Monodose®) = £16.39

Dose: by intramuscular injection (see note below), 1 mL as a single dose; booster dose, 1 mL 6–12 months following the initial dose; CHILD 1–15 years 0.5 mL
Note. The deltoid region is the preferred site of injection in adults. The subcutaneous route may be used for patients with haemophilia

HEPATITIS B VACCINE

Hepatitis B vaccine contains inactivated hepatitis B virus surface antigen (HBsAg) adsorbed on aluminium hydroxide adjuvant. It is made biosynthetically using recombinant DNA technology. The vaccine is used in individuals at high risk of contracting hepatitis B.

In the UK, high-risk groups include:
parenteral drug abusers;
individuals who frequently change sexual partners;
close family contacts of a case or carrier;
infants born to mothers who have had acute hepatitis B during pregnancy or who are hepatitis B carriers. Active immunisation is started immediately after delivery; if the hepatitis B occurred during pregnancy or the mother is a carrier who is e antigen positive or without anti-e antibody, *hepatitis B immunoglobulin* (see p. 516) is given at the same time as the vaccine;
haemophiliacs, those receiving regular blood transfusions or blood products, and relatives responsible for the administration of such products;
patients with chronic renal failure;
health care personnel who have direct contact with blood or blood-stained body fluids or with patients' tissues;
trainee health care workers;
other occupational risk groups such as morticians and embalmers;
staff and clients of residential accommodation for the mentally handicapped;

inmates of custodial institutions, who will be in custody for at least 6 months and those in custody for shorter periods who belong to other risk groups;

those travelling to areas of high prevalence who intend to seek employment as health care workers or who plan to remain there for lengthy periods and who may therefore be at increased risk of acquiring infection as the result of medical or dental procedures carried out in those countries.

Short-term tourists or business travellers are not generally at increased risk of infection but may place themselves at risk by their sexual behaviour when abroad.

It should be borne in mind that immunisation takes up to 6 months to confer adequate protection; the duration of immunity is thought to last for 3 to 5 years.

More detailed guidance is given in the memorandum *Immunisation against Infectious Disease* . Immunisation does not eliminate the need for commonsense precautions for avoiding the risk of infection from known carriers by the routes of infection which have been clearly established, see *Guidance for Clinical Health Care Workers: Protection against Infection with HIV and Hepatitis Viruses* and *Protecting Health Care Workers* and *Patients from Hepatitis B*. Accidental inoculation of hepatitis B virus-infected blood into a wound, incision, needle-prick, or abrasion may lead to infection, whereas it is unlikely that indirect exposure to a carrier will do so.

Specific **hepatitis B immunoglobulin** ('HBIG') is available for use with the vaccine in those accidentally infected and in infants (section 14.5).

See section 14.1 for general contra-indications.

PoM Engerix B® (SmithKline Beecham)

A suspension of hepatitis B surface antigen (rby, prepared from yeast cells by recombinant DNA technique) 20 micrograms/mL adsorbed onto aluminium hydroxide. Net price 0.5 mL (paediatric) vial = £8.96; 1-mL vial = £11.95; 1-mL prefilled syringe = £12.13

Dose: by intramuscular injection (see note below), 3 doses of 1 mL (20 micrograms), the second 1 month and the third 6 months after the first dose; more rapid (e.g. for travellers), third dose 2 months after first dose with booster at 12 months; CHILD birth to 12 years 3 doses of 0.5 mL (10 micrograms); INFANTS born to HBsAg-positive mothers, 3 doses of 0.5 mL (10 micrograms), first dose at birth with hepatitis B immunoglobulin injection (separate site)

Note. The deltoid muscle is the preferred site of injection in adults; the anterolateral thigh is the preferred site in infants and children; the buttock must not be used because vaccine efficacy may be reduced. The subcutaneous route is used for patients with haemophilia.

▼ PoM H-B-Vax® II (Pasteur Mérieux)

A suspension of hepatitis B surface antigen (prepared from yeast cells by recombinant DNA technique) 10 micrograms/mL adsorbed onto aluminium hydroxide. Net price 1-mL vial = £11.95

Dose: by intramuscular injection (see note below) doses of 1 mL (10 micrograms), the second 1 month a the third 6 months after the first dose; CHILD birth to years 3 doses of 0.5 mL (5 micrograms); INFANTS born HBsAg-positive mothers, 3 doses of 0.5 m (5 micrograms), first dose at birth with hepatitis immunoglobulin injection (separate site)

Note. The deltoid muscle is the preferred site of injection adults; the anterolateral thigh is the preferred site infants and children; the buttock must not be us because vaccine efficacy may be reduced. The subcu neous route is used for patients with haemophilia.

INFLUENZA VACCINES

While most viruses are antigenically stable, t influenza viruses A and B (especially A) are co stantly altering their antigenic structure as indicat by changes in the haemagglutinins (H) and ne raminidases (N) on the surface of the viruses. It essential that influenza vaccines in use contain t H and N components of the prevalent strain strains. Every year the World Health Organizati recommends which strains should be included.

The recommended strains are grown in the alla toic cavity of chick embryos (therefore **contr indicated** in those hypersensitive to eggs).

Since **influenza vaccines** will not control ep demics they are recommended *only for persons high risk*. Immunisation is strongly recommend for those of all ages, especially the elderly, with t following conditions:

chronic respiratory disease, including asthma;
chronic heart disease;
chronic renal failure;
diabetes mellitus, and other endocrine disorders;
immunosuppression due to disease or treatment.

Influenza vaccination is also recommended for res dents of nursing homes, residential homes for t elderly, and other long-stay facilities.

In non-pandemic years immunisation is not re ommended for Health Service staff, except f those at high risk (owing to medical disorders).

Interactions: Appendix 1 (influenza vaccine).

See section 14.1 for general contra-indications.

PoM Inactivated Influenza Vaccine (Split Virion) (Pasteur Mérieux)

Inactivated influenza vaccine (split virion) F Vac/Split. Net price 0.5-mL disposable syringe £5.10

Dose: 0.5 mL by deep subcutaneous or intramuscul injection; CHILD 6–47 months, 0.25 mL repeated on after 4–6 weeks; 4–12 years, 0.5 mL repeated once af 4–6 weeks; single doses are appropriate for childr who have already been immunised

PoM Fluarix® (SmithKline Beecham)

Inactivated influenza vaccine (split virion) F Vac/Split. Net price 0.5-mL disposable syringe £5.18

Dose: 0.5 mL by deep subcutaneous or intramuscul injection; CHILD 6 months to 6 years, 0.25 mL repeat once after 4-6 weeks; single doses are appropriate children who have already been immunised

PoM **Fluvirin®** (Evans)

Inactivated influenza vaccine (surface antigen) Flu/Vac/SA. Net price 0.5-mL disposable syringe = £5.09

Dose: 0.5 mL by deep subcutaneous or intramuscular injection; CHILD 4–13 years, 0.5 mL repeated once after 4–6 weeks; single doses are appropriate for children who have already been immunised

PoM **Fluzone®** (Servier)

Inactivated influenza vaccine (split virion) Flu/Vac/Split. Net price 0.5-mL disposable syringe = £5.18

Dose: 0.5 mL by deep subcutaneous or intramuscular injection; CHILD 6 months to 3 years, 0.25 mL repeated once after 4–6 weeks; 4–13 years, 0.5 mL repeated once after 4–6 weeks; single doses are appropriate for children who have already been immunised

PoM **Influvac Sub-unit®** (Solvay)

Inactivated influenza vaccine (surface antigen) Flu/Vac/SA. Net price 0.5-mL disposable syringe = £5.08

Dose: 0.5 mL by deep subcutaneous or intramuscular injection; CHILD 6 months–4 years, 0.25 mL repeated once after 4–6 weeks; 4–13 years, 0.5 mL repeated once after 4–6 weeks; single doses are appropriate for children who have already been immunised

MEASLES VACCINE

Measles vaccine has been replaced by a combined measles/mumps/rubella vaccine (MMR vaccine) for all eligible children.

Administration of a measles-containing vaccine to children may be associated with a mild measles-like syndrome with a measles-like rash and pyrexia about a week after injection. Much less commonly, convulsions and, very rarely, encephalitis have been reported. Convulsions in infants are much less frequently associated with measles vaccines than with other conditions leading to febrile episodes.

MMR vaccine may be used in the control of outbreaks of measles (see under MMR vaccine, below).

Single antigen vaccine

Available from Evans and Pasteur Mérieux on a named-patient basis

Combined vaccines, see under MMR and MR vaccines

MMR VACCINE

A combined **measles/mumps/rubella vaccine** (MMR vaccine) has been introduced with the aim of eliminating rubella (and congenital rubella syndrome), measles, and mumps. Health authorities have an obligation to ensure that every child has received MMR vaccine by entry to primary school, unless there is a valid contra-indication (see below) or parental refusal.

MMR vaccine has replaced measles vaccine for children of both sexes and should be given irrespec-

tive of previous measles, mumps or rubella infection (or measles vaccination).

The first dose of MMR vaccine is given to children aged 12–15 months. From 1 October 1996 a second (booster) dose is to be given at 3–5 years, at the same time as routine pre-school boosters of diphtheria, tetanus and polio vaccines.

MMR vaccine may also be used in the control of outbreaks of measles and should be offered to susceptible children within 3 days of exposure to infection (**important:** MMR vaccine is not suitable for prophylaxis following exposure to mumps or rubella since the antibody response to the mumps and rubella components is too slow for effective prophylaxis).

Children with partially or totally impaired immune responsiveness should not receive live vaccines (for advice on AIDS see section 14.1). If they have been exposed to measles infection they should be given immunoglobulin (section 14.5).

As with measles vaccine, malaise, fever and/or a rash may occur with MMR vaccine, most commonly about a week after immunisation and lasting about 2 to 3 days. Leaflets are available to provide parents with advice for reducing fever (including the use of paracetamol). Parotid swelling occasionally occurs, usually in the third week. Post-vaccination meningoencephalitis was reported (rarely and with complete recovery) following immunisation with MMR vaccine containing Urabe mumps vaccine, which has now been discontinued; the rate using Jeryl Lynn mumps vaccine is very much lower. Children with post-vaccination symptoms are not infectious.

Contra-indications to MMR include:

children with untreated malignant disease or altered immunity, and those receiving immunosuppressive drugs or radiotherapy, or high-dose corticosteroids;

children who have received another live vaccine by injection within 3 weeks;

children with allergies to neomycin or kanamycin, or a history of anaphylactic reaction to egg (see also below);

children with acute febrile illness (vaccination should be deferred);

if given to adult women, pregnancy should be avoided for 1 month (as for rubella vaccine);

should not be given within 3 months of an immunoglobulin injection.

It should be noted that:

children with a personal or close family history of convulsions should be given MMR vaccine, provided the parents understand that there may be a febrile response; immunoglobulin must not be given with MMR vaccine since the immune response to rubella and mumps may be inhibited; doctors should seek specialist paediatric advice rather than refuse vaccination;

allergy to egg is only a contra-indication if the child has had an anaphylactic reaction to food containing egg (dislike of egg or refusal to eat is not a contra-indication).

PoM **MMR Vaccine**

Live measles, mumps, and rubella vaccine

Dose: 0.5 mL by deep subcutaneous or by intramuscular injection

Available from District Health Authorities or (in England only) direct from Farillon as MMR II® (Pasteur Mérieux)

MR VACCINE

The Joint Committee on Vaccination and Immunisation recommended that all school children in school forms aged 5 up to 16 years should be immunised in a school-based campaign. The vaccine recommended was measles/rubella (MR) vaccine. During November 1994, school-based immunisation programmes were set up to provide the highest possible levels of coverage with MR vaccine. All children were invited for immunisation, irrespective of history of measles, rubella disease, previous measles or rubella immunisation, or previous MMR immunisation. For those that were already immune, re-immunisation provided a booster; for those that were still susceptible, it provided protection. The provision of rubella vaccine in this campaign allowed the discontinuation of the previous school rubella immunisation programme. Therefore, from September 1994, single antigen rubella vaccine no longer needs to be given to girls at around 11 years of age.

PoM MR Vaccine

Live measles and rubella vaccine

Dose: 0.5 mL by deep subcutaneous or by intramuscular injection

Available from Farillon (to District Health Authorities only) as Pasteur Mérieux brand or SmithKline Beecham (Eolarix®) brand

MENINGOCOCCAL POLYSACCHARIDE VACCINE

Meningococcal polysaccharide vaccine is indicated for areas of the world where the risk of acquiring meningococcal infection is much higher than in the UK, particularly for travellers proposing to travel 'rough'; travellers with asplenia (or severe dysfunction of the spleen) also particularly require protection.

These areas include New Delhi, Nepal, Mecca (see below), and the meningitis belt of Africa, which encompasses southern sub-Saharan parts of Senegal, Mali, Niger, Chad, and Sudan; all of Gambia, Guinea, Togo, and Benin; South-west Ethiopia; northern parts of Sierra Leone, Liberia, Ivory Coast, Nigeria, Cameroon, Central African Republic, Uganda, and Kenya.

Saudi Arabia requires vaccination of pilgrims to Mecca during the Haj annual pilgrimage; this may apply to others visiting Saudi Arabia in the months leading up to August.

For advice on the immunisation of *close contacts* of disease cases of Group A and Group C meningococcal meningitis in the UK and on the role of the vaccine in the control of *local outbreaks*, see the memorandum *Immunisation against Infectious Disease*.

See section 14.1 for general contra-indications.

PoM AC Vax® (SmithKline Beecham)

Meningococcal polysaccharide vaccine, Neimen/Vac. Prepared from *Neisseria meningitidis* (meningococcus) groups A and C. Net price single-dose vial (with diluent) = £6.86

Dose: ADULT and CHILD aged 2 months and over, 0.5 mL by deep subcutaneous or intramuscular injection

PoM Mengivac (A+C)® (Pasteur Mérieux)

Meningococcal polysaccharide vaccine, Neimen Vac. Prepared from *Neisseria meningitidis* (meningococcus) groups A and C. Net price single-dose vial (with syringe containing diluent) = £6.69

Dose: ADULT and CHILD aged over 18 months, 0.5 mL by deep subcutaneous or intramuscular injection

Note. The lower age range for AC Vax® and Mengivac (A+C)® differ; in the case of Mengivac (A+C)® the data sheet states that young children and infants respond less well to the vaccine than older children and adults, with little response to the Group C polysaccharide under 18 months of age and a poor response to Group A polysaccharide under 3 months of age. Additionally, protection in infants under 18 months of age is of shorter duration

MUMPS VACCINE

Mumps vaccine consists of a live attenuated strain of virus grown in chick-embryo tissue culture.

See under MMR vaccine and section 14.1 for contra-indications.

PoM Mumpsvax® (Pasteur Mérieux)

Mumps vaccine (Jeryl Lynn strain). Net price single-dose vial (with diluent) = £4.00

Dose: ADULT and CHILD over 1 year, 0.5 mL by subcutaneous injection

Combined vaccines
With measles and rubella
See MMR Vaccine

PERTUSSIS VACCINE

(Whooping-cough vaccine)

Pertussis vaccine is usually given combined with diphtheria and tetanus vaccine (in triple vaccine) starting at 2 months of age (see section 14.1).

With some vaccines available in the early 1960s *persistent screaming and collapse* were reported but these reactions are rarely observed with the vaccines now available. *Convulsions and encephalopathy* have been reported as rare complications, but such conditions may arise from other causes and be falsely attributed to the vaccine. Neurological complications *after whooping cough itself* are considerably more common than after the vaccine.

As with any other elective immunisation procedure it is advisable to postpone vaccination if the child is suffering from any acute illness, until fully recovered. Minor infections without fever or systemic upset are not reasons to delay immunisation. Immunisation should not be carried out in children who have a history of severe local or general reaction to a preceding dose; the following reactions should be regarded as severe:

Local—an extensive area of redness and swelling which becomes indurated and involves most of the antero-lateral surface of the thigh or a major part of the circumference of the upper arm.

General—fever equal to or more than 39.5°C within 48 hours of vaccine, anaphylaxis, bronchospasm, laryngeal oedema, generalised collapse, prolonged unresponsiveness, prolonged inconsolable screaming, and convulsions occurring within 72 hours.

A personal or family history of allergy is **not** a contra-indication to immunisation against whooping cough; nor are stable neurological conditions such as cerebral palsy or spina bifida.

Children with problem histories. When there is a personal or family history of *febrile* convulsions, there is an increased risk of these occurring after pertussis immunisation. In such children, immunisation is *recommended* but advice on the *prevention of fever* (see p. 503) should be given at the time of immunisation.

In a recent British study, children with a family history of epilepsy were immunised with pertussis vaccine without any significant adverse events. These childrens' developmental progress has been normal. In children with a close family history (first degree relatives) of *idiopathic epilepsy*, there may be a risk of developing a similar condition, irrespective of vaccine. Immunisation is *recommended* for these children.

Where there is a *still evolving neurological problem*, immunisation should be *deferred* until the condition is stable. When there has been a documented history of *cerebral damage in the neonatal period*, immunisation should be *carried out unless there is evidence of an evolving neurological abnormality*. If immunisation is to be deferred, this should be stated on the neonatal discharge summary. Where there is doubt, appropriate advice should be sought from a consultant paediatrician, district immunisation co-ordinator or consultant in public health medicine *rather than withholding vaccine*.

Older children. There is no contra-indication to administration of pertussis vaccine to unimmunised older children in order to protect infants and siblings. Since a course of 3 injections is required to protect against pertussis, vaccine cannot be used to control an outbreak.

▼ PoM **Acellular Pertussis Vaccine, APV**
(Lederle)
Unlicensed single-antigen acellular pertussis vaccine (APV) has been made available by the Department of Health under Crown Immunity only for completion of immunisation against pertussis in those children whose course of pertussis vaccine was not given (or not completed) as part of their triple vaccine course
Dose: 0.5 mL by intramuscular or deep subcutaneous injection, 3 doses at intervals of 1 month
Available from Farillon on a named-patient basis
Note. Should be ordered only when required for use
Combined vaccine (*pertussis, tetanus, and diphtheria*), see under Diphtheria vaccines

PNEUMOCOCCAL VACCINE
A polyvalent **pneumococcal polysaccharide vaccine** is available for the immunisation of persons (over the age of 2 years) for whom the risk of contracting pneumococcal pneumonia is unusually high or dangerous. For example in patients with:
Homozygous sickle cell disease;
Asplenia or severe dysfunction of the spleen;
Chronic renal disease or nephrotic syndrome;
Immunodeficiency or immunosuppression due to disease or treatment, including HIV infection;
Chronic heart disease;
Chronic lung disease;
Chronic liver disease including cirrhosis;
Diabetes mellitus.

Where possible, the vaccine should be given at least two weeks before splenectomy (together with advice about increased risk of pneumococcal infection) and before chemotherapy. Prophylactic antibiotic therapy against pneumococcal infection should not be stopped after immunisation. The vaccine is effective in a single dose if the types of pneumonia in the community are reflected in the polysaccharides contained in the vaccine. It should not be given in pregnancy, or when breast-feeding, or when there is infection. Hypersensitivity reactions may occur.

REVACCINATION. Routine revaccination of adults is not recommended owing to the possibility of an increased incidence of adverse reactions; nor should those who have previously received the 14-valent vaccine (Pneumovax®) be routinely revaccinated with the 23-valent vaccine (Pneumovax®II). Revaccination is however recommended for *adults with chronic conditions which increase the risk of fatal pneumococcal infection* (and who did not have a serious or severe reaction to the previous vaccination) and for those shown to have *a rapid decline in pneumococcal antibody levels* (e.g. those with nephrotic syndrome, renal failure or who are transplant recipients); the revaccination is recommended 4 or more years after the 14-valent vaccine (Pneumovax®) and 6 or more years after the 23-valent vaccine (Pneumovax®II).
Revaccination after 3–5 years (not sooner) should be considered for children at highest risk of pneumococcal infection (e.g. with asplenia, sickle-cell disease, or nephrotic syndrome) who would be 10 years or less at revaccination.

IMPORTANT. Not for intradermal injection which may cause severe local reactions
See section 14.1 for general contra-indications.

PoM **Pneumovax® II** (Pasteur Mérieux)
Polysaccharide from each of 23 capsular types of pneumococcus. Net price 0.5-mL vial = £9.94
Dose: 0.5 mL by subcutaneous or intramuscular injection; CHILD under 2 years, not recommended (suboptimal response and also safety and efficacy not established)

POLIOMYELITIS VACCINES
There are two types of poliomyelitis vaccine, poliomyelitis vaccine, live (oral) (Sabin) and poliomyelitis vaccine, inactivated (Salk). The oral vaccine, consisting of a mixture of attenuated strains of virus types 1, 2, and 3 is at present generally used in the UK.

INITIAL COURSE. **Poliomyelitis vaccine, live (oral)** is given on 3 occasions, usually at the same time as routine immunisation against diphtheria, tetanus, pertussis, and haemophilus influenzae b (see schedule, section 14.1). The initial course of 3 doses should also be given to all unimmunised adults.

REINFORCEMENT. A reinforcing dose of oral poliomyelitis vaccine is recommended at school entry at which time children should also receive a reinforcing dose of diphtheria and tetanus vaccine, and a dose of MMR vaccine if this has not already been given. Oral poliomyelitis vaccine is also recommended at school leaving.

Vaccine-associated poliomyelitis and poliomyelitis in contacts of vaccinees are both rare. In England and Wales there is an annual average of 1 recipient and 1 contact case in relation to over 2 million doses of oral vaccine. The need for strict personal hygiene must be stressed; the contacts of a recently vaccinated baby should be advised of the necessity for personal hygiene, particularly of the need to wash their hands after changing the baby's napkins.

Contra-indications to the use of oral poliomyelitis vaccine include vomiting and diarrhoea, and immunodeficiency disorders (or household contacts of patients with immunodeficiency disorders). See section 14.1 for further contra-indications.

Poliomyelitis vaccine (inactivated) may be used for those in whom poliomyelitis vaccine (oral) is contra-indicated because of immunosuppressive disorders (for advice on AIDS see section 14.1).

TRAVELLERS. Travellers to areas other than Australia, New Zealand, Northern and Western Europe, and North America should be given a full course of oral poliomyelitis vaccine if they have not been immunised in the past. Those who have not received immunisation within the last 10 years should be given a booster dose of oral poliomyelitis vaccine.

Live (oral) (Sabin)

PoM Poliomyelitis Vaccine, Live (Oral) Pol/Vac (Oral)[1]. A suspension of suitable live attenuated strains of poliomyelitis virus, types 1, 2, and 3. Available in single-dose and 10-dose containers

Dose: 3 drops from a multidose container or the total contents of a single-dose container; for primary immunisation 3 doses are required (see schedule, section 14.1)

Available from District Health Authorities or (in England and Scotland only) direct from Farillon

1. BP permits code OPV for vaccine in single doses provided it also appears on pack.

Note. Poliomyelitis vaccine loses potency once the container has been opened, therefore any vaccine remaining at the end of an immunisation session should be discarded; whenever possible sessions should be arranged to avoid undue wastage.

Inactivated (Salk)

PoM Poliomyelitis Vaccine, Inactivated Pol/Vac (Inact). An inactivated suspension of suitable strains of poliomyelitis virus, types 1, 2, and 3.

Dose: 0.5 mL or as stated on the label by deep subcutaneous or intramuscular injection; for primary immunisation 3 doses are required at intervals of 4 weeks

Available (in England and Scotland only) direct from Farillon; Wales—Welsh Health Common Services Authority, telephone 01222 500500; Northern Ireland—Central Services Agency, Belfast, telephone 01232 324431

Note. Should be ordered one dose at a time (on a named-patient basis) and only when required for use

RABIES VACCINE

A human diploid cell **rabies vaccine** is now in use. It should be offered prophylactically to those at high risk—those working in quarantine stations, animal handlers, veterinary surgeons, and field workers who may be exposed to bites of possibly infected wild animals.

The Department of Health has advised that for *prophylactic use* the vaccine produces a good antibody response when given in a 3-dose schedule on days 0, 7, and 28, with a reinforcing dose every 2–3 years to those at continued risk.

For *post-exposure treatment of previously immunised patients* two reinforcing doses are needed (one on day 0 and one on day 3–7). Rabies immunoglobulin is not needed for those who have been fully immunised.

For *post-exposure treatment of previously unimmunised patients* (or those whose prophylaxis is possibly inadequate) a course of injections should be started as soon as possible after exposure (days 0, 3, 7, 14, 30, and 90). The course may be discontinued if it is proved that the patient was not at risk. There are no specific contra-indications to this diploid cell vaccine and its use should be considered whenever a patient has been attacked by an animal in a country where rabies is endemic, even if there is no direct evidence of rabies in the attacking animal. **Rabies immunoglobulin** (section 14.5) should also be considered on day 0.

Staff in attendance on a patient who is highly suspected of, or known to be suffering from, rabies should be offered immunisation. Four intradermal doses of 0.1 mL of human diploid cell vaccine (Pasteur Mérieux) given on the same day at different sites (ensuring correct intradermal technique) has been suggested for this purpose [unlicensed route].

Advice on post-exposure immunisation and treatment of rabies is available from the Virus Reference Laboratory, Central Public Health Laboratory, Colindale, London NW9 5HT, tel 0181-200 4400.

PoM Rabies Vaccine BP Pasteur Mérieux (Pasteur Mérieux)

Freeze-dried inactivated Wistar rabies virus strain PM/WI 38 1503-3M cultivated in human diploid cells. Single-dose vial with syringe containing diluent

IMPORTANT. Studies have shown that when this vaccine is injected into the gluteal region there is a poor response. Concomitant administration of chloroquine may also affect the antibody response. Because of the potential consequences of inadequately treated rabies exposure and because there is no indication that fetal abnormalities have been associated with rabies vaccination, pregnancy is **not** considered a contra-indication to post-exposure prophylaxis. If there is substantial risk of exposure to rabies, pre-exposure prophylaxis may also be indicated during pregnancy

Dose: prophylactic, 1 mL by deep subcutaneous or intramuscular injection in the deltoid region, on days 0, 7, and 28; also further reinforcing doses every 2–3 years to those at continued risk

Note. This replaces the previous schedule which involved giving a second dose after 1 month and a third after 6–12 months. If this full course was not given it is still probable that in most cases 2 doses conferred protection provided they were given *1 month apart.* Subjects who have received 2 injections 1 month apart and also remain at continued risk should receive a reinforcing dose 6–12 months later, followed by further reinforcing doses at intervals of 2–3 years

Post-exposure, see notes above

Staff in attendance, see notes above

Also available from local designated centres (special workers and post-exposure treatment)

RUBELLA VACCINE

The selective policy of protecting women of child-bearing age from the risks of rubella (German measles) in pregnancy has been extended to a policy of eliminating the circulation of rubella among young children. The existing rubella immunisation policy is therefore being reinforced by the mass immunisation of children of both sexes, using combined measles, mumps, and rubella vaccine (MMR vaccine).

Rubella vaccine is recommended for *prepubertal girls between their tenth and fourteenth birthdays* (unless there is documented evidence that they have received MMR) [**Important:** but see also MR vaccine, p. 510] and for *seronegative women of child-bearing age* (see schedule, section 14.1) as well as those who might put pregnant women at risk of infection (e.g. nurses and doctors in obstetric units).

Rubella vaccine may conveniently be offered to previously *unimmunised and seronegative post-partum women*. Immunising susceptible post-partum women a few days after delivery is important as far as the overall reduction of congenital abnormalities in the UK is concerned, for about 60% of these abnormalities occur in the babies of multiparous women.

PREGNANCY. Rubella immunisation should be avoided in early pregnancy, and women of child-bearing age should be advised not to become pregnant within 1 month of immunisation. However, despite active surveillance in the UK, the USA, and Germany, no case of congenital rubella syndrome has been reported following inadvertent immunisation shortly before or during pregnancy. There is thus no evidence that the vaccine is teratogenic, and termination of pregnancy following inadvertent immunisation should not be routinely recommended; potential parents should be given this information before making a decision about termination.

See section 14.1 for general contra-indications.

PoM **Rubella Vaccine, Live** Rub/Vac (Live).
Prepared from Wistar RA 27/3 strain propagated in human diploid cells

Dose: 0.5 mL by deep subcutaneous or by intramuscular injection (see schedule, section 14.1 and notes above)

Available from District Health Authorities or (in England only) direct from Farillon as Evans brand (also known as *Almevax*®). SmithKline Beecham brand (*Ervevax*®) also available

Combined vaccines, see under MMR and MR vaccines

SMALLPOX VACCINE

Smallpox vaccination is no longer required routinely in the UK and other countries because global eradication of smallpox has now been achieved. Workers in laboratories where pox viruses (such as vaccinia) are handled, and others whose work involves an identifiable risk of exposure to pox virus, should be advised of the possible risk and vaccination should be considered. Detailed guidance for laboratory staff has been prepared by the Advisory Committee on Dangerous Pathogens and the Advisory Committee on Genetic Manipulation. There is no requirement for smallpox vaccination of travellers.

PoM **Smallpox Vaccine.** Consists of a suspension of live vaccinia virus grown in the skin of living animals, supplied in freeze-dried form with diluent

Advice on the need for vaccination and on contra-indications should be obtained from the Virus Reference Laboratory, Central Public Health Laboratory, Colindale (0181-200 4400) who will also supply the vaccine on a named-patient basis (free of charge)

TETANUS VACCINES
(Tetanus toxoids)

Tetanus vaccines stimulate the production of the protective antitoxin. In general, adsorption on aluminium hydroxide, aluminium phosphate, or calcium phosphate improves antigenicity. Adsorbed tetanus vaccine is offered routinely to babies in combination with adsorbed diphtheria vaccine (DT/Vac/Ads) and more usually also combined with killed *Bordetella pertussis* organisms as a triple vaccine, adsorbed diphtheria, tetanus, and pertussis vaccine (DT Per/Vac/Ads), see schedule, section 14.1.

In children, the triple vaccine not only gives protection against tetanus in childhood but also gives the basic immunity for subsequent reinforcing doses of tetanus vaccine at school entry and at school leaving (combined with low-dose adsorbed diphtheria vaccine) and also when a potentially tetanus-contaminated injury has been received. Normally, tetanus vaccine should not be given unless more than 10 years have elapsed since the last reinforcing dose because of the possibility that hypersensitivity reactions may develop.

Active immunisation is important for persons in older age groups who may never have had a routine or complete course of immunisation when younger. In these persons a course of adsorbed tetanus vaccine may be given. Very rarely, tetanus has developed after abdominal surgery; patients awaiting elective surgery should be asked about tetanus immunisation and immunised if necessary.

See section 14.1 for general contra-indications.

For serious, potentially contaminated wounds tetanus immunoglobulin injection (section 14.5) should be selectively used in addition to wound toilet, adsorbed tetanus vaccine (in separate site), and benzylpenicillin or another appropriate antibiotic (e.g. co-amoxiclav).

Single antigen vaccines

The BP directs that when Tetanus Vaccine is prescribed or demanded and the form is not stated, Adsorbed Tetanus Vaccine may be dispensed or supplied.

PoM Adsorbed Tetanus Vaccine Tet/Vac/Ads.
Prepared from tetanus formol toxoid with a mineral carrier (aluminium hydroxide).
Dose: 0.5 mL or as stated on the label, by intramuscular or deep subcutaneous injection followed after 4 weeks by a second dose and after a further 4 weeks by a third
Note. This dose reflects the guidelines of the Joint Committee on Vaccination and Immunisation, see *Immunisation against Infectious Disease*
Available from Evans (net price 0.5-mL amp = 71p, and as **Clostet**®, net price 0.5-mL single-dose syringe = £1.40), Pasteur Mérieux (net price 0.5-mL amp = 55p; 0.5-mL single-dose syringe = £1.20; 5-mL vial = £2.80), and from Servier (net price 0.5-mL amp = 62p; 0.5-mL syringe = £1.36)

Combined vaccines, see Diphtheria Vaccines

TYPHOID VACCINES

There are now three types of typhoid vaccine available, two given by injection and a third given by mouth. **None** of these typhoid vaccines is a substitute for personal hygiene (see section 14.6).

The original **typhoid vaccine, a whole cell** vaccine is normally given in 2 doses at intervals of 4–6 weeks for primary immunisation, with reinforcing doses about every 3 years on continued exposure. Local reactions to this vaccine, which consist of swelling, pain, and tenderness appear about 2–3 hours after *intramuscular or deep subcutaneous injection.* Systemic reactions, which consist of fever, malaise, and headache, may also occur and usually last for about 36 hours after injection. If severe reactions are experienced after the first dose *intradermal injection* may be preferred for the second dose and for subsequent boosters, as these reactions are virtually absent when the intradermal route is used.

A capsular **polysaccharide typhoid vaccine** is now available for single dose administration by *intramuscular or deep subcutaneous injection* with a reinforcing dose every 3 years on continued exposure. Local reactions, including pain, swelling or erythema, may appear 48–72 hours after administration.

An **oral typhoid vaccine** is now also available. It is a **live attenuated** vaccine contained in an enteric-coated capsule. It is taken *by mouth* as three doses of one capsule on alternate days, providing protection 7–10 days after the last dose. Protection may persist for up to 3 years in those constantly (or repeatedly) exposed to *S. typhi*, but occasional travellers require a repeat course at intervals of 1 year. Oral typhoid vaccine is **contra-indicated** in individuals who are immunosuppressed (whether due to disease or its treatment) and is inactivated by concomitant administration of *antibiotics* or *sulphonamides*. Administration of a dose of oral typhoid vaccine should be coordinated so that *mefloquine* is not taken for at least 12 hours before or after a dose (vaccination with oral typhoid vaccine should preferably be completed at least 3 days before the first dose of mefloquine).

For general contra-indications to vaccines, see section 14.1.

Whole cell vaccine for injection

PoM Typhoid Vaccine Typhoid/Vac. A suspension of killed *Salmonella typhi* organisms. Net price 1.5-mL vial = £4.11
Dose: 0.5 mL by deep subcutaneous or intramuscular injection, second dose 0.5 mL after 4–6 weeks; CHILD 1–10 years, 0.25 mL; under 12 months, not recommended
Note. The Department of Health recommends that second dose and subsequent boosters can be given intradermally, in a volume of 0.1 mL, to reduce adverse reactions
Available from Evans

Polysaccharide vaccine for injection

PoM Typhim Vi® (Pasteur Mérieux)
Vi capsular polysaccharide typhoid vaccine, 50 micrograms/mL virulence polysaccharide antigen of *Salmonella typhi*. Net price 0.5-mL single-dose prefilled syringe = £10.68
Dose: 0.5 mL by deep subcutaneous or intramuscular injection; CHILD under 18 months, may show suboptimal response

Live oral vaccine

▼ **PoM Vivotif**® (Evans)
Capsules, e/c, live attenuated *Salmonella typhi* (Ty 21a). Net price 3-cap pack = £14.85. Label: 23, 25, C, administration
Dose: ADULT and CHILD over 6 years, 1 capsule on days 1, 3, and 5; under 6 years, not recommended
COUNSELLING. Swallow as soon as possible after placing in mouth with a cold or lukewarm drink; it is important to store in refrigerator

YELLOW FEVER VACCINE

Yellow fever vaccine consists of a live attenuated yellow fever virus (17D strain) grown in developing chick embryos. Infants under 9 months of age should only be vaccinated if the risk of yellow fever is unavoidable since there is a small risk of encephalitis. The vaccine should not be given to those with impaired immune responsiveness, or who have had an anaphylactic reaction to egg; it should not be given during pregnancy (but where there is a significant risk of exposure the need for immunisation outweighs any risk to the fetus). See section 14.1 for further contra-indications. Reactions are few. The immunity which probably lasts for life is officially accepted for 10 years starting from 10 days after primary immunisation and for a further 10 years immediately after revaccination.

PoM Yellow Fever Vaccine, Live Yel/Vac. A suspension of chick embryo proteins containing attenuated 17D strain virus
Dose: 0.5 mL by subcutaneous injection
Available (only to designated Yellow Fever Vaccination centres) as **Arilvax**® (Evans)

14.5 Immunoglobulins

Human immunoglobulins have replaced immunoglobulins of animal origin (antisera) which were frequently associated with hypersensitivity. Injection of immunoglobulins produces immediate protection lasting for several weeks.

The two types of human immunoglobulin preparation are **normal immunoglobulin** and **specific immunoglobulins**.

Further information about immunoglobulins is included in *Immunisation against Infectious Disease* (see section 14.1).

AVAILABILITY. **Normal immunoglobulin** is now only available from the *Public Health Laboratory Service* laboratories for contacts and the control of outbreaks. It is available commercially for other purposes.

Specific immunoglobulins are available from the *Public Health Laboratory Service* laboratories and *Regional Blood Transfusion Centres* in England and Wales with the exception of **tetanus immunoglobulin** which is distributed through *Regional Blood Transfusion Centres* to hospital pharmacies or blood transfusion departments and is also available to general medical practitioners. **Rabies immunoglobulin** is available from the *Central Public Health Laboratory, London*. The large amounts of **hepatitis B immunoglobulin** required by transplant centres should be obtained commercially.

In Scotland all immunoglobulins are available from the *Blood Transfusion Service*. Tetanus immunoglobulin is distributed by the *Blood Transfusion Service* to hospitals and general medical practitioners on demand.

NORMAL IMMUNOGLOBULIN
(Gamma Globulin)

Human **normal immunoglobulin** ('HNIG') is prepared from pools of at least 1000 donations of human plasma; it contains antibody to measles, mumps, varicella, hepatitis A, and other viruses that are currently prevalent in the general population.

CAUTIONS and SIDE-EFFECTS. Side-effects of immunoglobulins include malaise, chills, fever, and rarely anaphylaxis. Human normal immunoglobulin is **contra-indicated** in patients with known class specific antibody to immunoglobulin A (IgA).

Normal immunoglobulin may **interfere with the immune response to live virus vaccines** which should therefore only be given **at least 3 weeks before or 3 months after** an injection of normal immunoglobulin (this does not apply to yellow fever vaccine since normal immunoglobulin does not contain antibody to this virus). For travellers, if there is insufficient time, the recommended interval may have to be ignored.

INTRAMUSCULAR

Normal immunoglobulin is administered by intramuscular injection for the protection of susceptible contacts against **hepatitis A** virus (infectious hepatitis), **measles** and, to a lesser extent, **rubella**.

HEPATITIS A. Control of hepatitis A depends on good hygiene and many studies have also shown the value of normal immunoglobulin in the prevention and control of outbreaks of this disease. It is recommended for controlling infection in contacts in closed institutions and also, under certain conditions, in school and home contacts and for travellers going to areas where the disease is highly endemic (all countries excluding Northern and Western Europe, North America, Australia, and New Zealand). Alternatively, **hepatitis A vaccine** (see p. 507) may be used for those aged 16 years or over visiting such countries frequently or who stay for longer than 3 months.

MEASLES. Normal immunoglobulin may be given for prophylaxis in children with compromised immunity (and in adults with compromised immunity who have no measles antibodies); it should be given as soon as possible after contact with measles. It should also be given to children under 12 months with recent severe illness for whom measles should be avoided; MMR vaccine should then be given (after an interval of **at least** 3 months) at around the usual age.

RUBELLA. Immunoglobulin after exposure does **not** prevent infection in non-immune contacts and is **not** recommended for protection of pregnant women exposed to rubella. It may however reduce the likelihood of a clinical attack which may possibly reduce the risk to the fetus. It should only be used when termination of pregnancy would be unacceptable when it should be given as soon as possible after exposure. Serological follow-up of recipients is essential. For routine prophylaxis, see **Rubella Vaccine** (p. 513).

REPLACEMENT THERAPY. Normal immunoglobulin may also be given intramuscularly for replacement therapy, but intravenous formulations (see next column) are normally preferred.

For intramuscular use

PoM Human Normal Immunoglobulin Human normal immunoglobulin injection. 250-mg vial; 750-mg vial

Dose: by deep intramuscular injection, Hepatitis A travel prophylaxis (2 months or less abroad), 250 mg; CHILD under 10 years 125 mg; longer travel prophylaxis (3–5 months abroad) and to control outbreaks, 500 mg; CHILD under 10 years 250 mg

Measles prophylaxis, CHILD under 1 year 250 mg, 1–2 years 500 mg, 3 years and over 750 mg; to allow attenuated attack, CHILD under 1 year 100 mg, 1 year and over 250 mg

Rubella in pregnancy, prevention of clinical attack, 750 mg

Available from BPL and SNBTS and from Public Health Laboratory Service (for contacts and control of outbreaks only, see above)

PoM Gammabulin® (Immuno)

Human normal immunoglobulin injection. Net price 2-mL vial = £3.12; 5-mL vial = £6.35; 10-mL vial = £10.70

Dose: see below

PoM **Kabiglobulin®** (Pharmacia)
Human normal immunoglobulin injection 16%.
Net price 2-mL amp = £2.78; 5-mL amp = £6.00
Dose: see below
Note. Doses for Gammabulin® and Kabiglobulin® are
expressed in terms of volume:
Dose: by intramuscular injection,
Hepatitis A prophylaxis, ADULT and CHILD 0.02–
0.04 mL/kg; greater exposure risk, 0.06–0.12 mL/kg
Measles prophylaxis, 0.2 mL/kg; to allow attenuated
attack, 0.04 mL/kg
Rubella in pregnancy, prevention of clinical attack,
20 mL
Antibody deficiency syndromes, see data sheet

INTRAVENOUS

Special formulations for intravenous administration
are available for replacement therapy for patients
with congenital agammaglobulinaemia and hypo-
gammaglobulinaemia, for the treatment of idiopathic thrombocytopenic purpura and Kawasaki
syndrome, and for the prophylaxis of infection following bone marrow transplantation.

For intravenous use
PoM **Normal Immunoglobulin for
Intravenous Use**
Available as: *Alphaglobin®* (2.5 g, 5 g, 10 g—
Alpha), *Endobulin®* (1 g, 2.5 g, 5 g, 10 g—
Immuno); *Gamimune-N®* (500 mg, 2.5 g, 5 g—
Cutter); Human Immunoglobulin (3 g—SNBTS);
Sandoglobulin® (1 g, 3 g, 6 g—Sandoz); *Vigam®S*
(2.5 g, 5 g—BPL)

SPECIFIC IMMUNOGLOBULINS

Specific immunoglobulins are prepared by pooling
the plasma of selected donors with high levels of
the specific antibody required.
   Although a hepatitis B vaccine is now available
for those at high risk of infection, specific **hepatitis
B immunoglobulin** ('HBIG') is available for use in
association with the vaccine for the prevention of
infection in laboratory and other personnel who
have accidentally become contaminated with hepatitis B virus, and in infants born to mothers who
have become infected with this virus in pregnancy
or who are high-risk carriers.
   Following exposure to a rabid animal, specific
rabies immunoglobulin of human origin should be
injected at the site of the bite and also given intramuscularly. Rabies vaccine should also be given.
   Tetanus immunoglobulin of human origin
('HTIG') should be used selectively in addition to
wound toilet, vaccine, and benzylpenicillin (or
another appropriate antibiotic e.g. co-amoxiclav)
for the more seriously contaminated wounds; it is
rarely required for those with an established immunity in whom protection may be achieved by a reinforcing dose of vaccine if considered advisable.
The administration of tetanus immunoglobulin
should be considered for patients not known to have
received active immunisation (a) whose wound was
sustained more than 6 hours before treatment was
received and (b) with puncture wounds or wounds
potentially heavily contaminated with tetanus

spores, septic, or with much devitalised tissue. A
dose of adsorbed tetanus vaccine should be given at
the same time as the tetanus immunoglobulin and
the course of vaccine subsequently completed.
   Varicella-zoster immunoglobulin (VZIG) is
indicated in *immunosuppressed patients at risk*,
including those who within 3 months of contact
have been on high-dose corticosteroid therapy (e.g.
prednisolone 2 mg/kg daily for more than one
week), *infants at risk*, and in *pregnant women at
risk*. (**Important:** for full details consult *Immunisation against Infectious Diseases* . It should also
be noted that **varicella vaccine** is available on a
named-patient basis from *SmithKline Beecham* or
Pasteur Mérieux).
   Cytomegalovirus immunoglobulin (available
on a named-patient basis from *Alpha* as *Alpha-
globin CMV®*) is indicated for prophylaxis in
patients receiving immunosuppressive treatment

Hepatitis B
PoM **Hepatitis B Immunoglobulin** (Antihepatitis B
Immunoglobulin). See notes above
   Dose: by intramuscular injection (as soon as possible
   after exposure), ADULT 500 units; CHILD under 4 years
   200 units, 5–9 years 300 units; NEONATE 200 units as
   soon as possible after birth; for full details see *Immunisation against Infectious Diseases*
   Available from Public Health Laboratory Service (except
   for Transplant Centres, see p. 515), also available from
   BPL and SNBTS

Rabies
PoM **Rabies Immunoglobulin** (Antirabies
Immunoglobulin Injection). See notes above
   Dose: 20 units/kg, half by intramuscular injection and
   half by infiltration around wound
   Available from Public Health Laboratory Service (also
   from BPL and SNBTS)

Tetanus
PoM **Tetanus Immunoglobulin** (Antitetanus
Immunoglobulin Injection). See notes above
   Dose: by intramuscular injection, prophylactic
   250 units, increased to 500 units if more than 24 hours
   have elapsed or there is risk of heavy contamination
   Therapeutic, 150 units/kg (multiple sites)
   Available from BPL and SNBTS
PoM **Tetabulin®** (Immuno)
Tetanus immunoglobulin injection. Net price 250 unit
prefilled syringe = £15.50
   Dose: by intramuscular injection, prophylactic,
   250 units, increased to 500 units if wound older than 12
   hours or if risk of heavy contamination or if patient
   weighs more than 90 kg; second dose of 250 units given
   after 3–4 weeks if patient immunosuppressed or if active
   immunisation with tetanus vaccine contra-indicated
   Therapeutic, 30–300 units/kg
PoM **Tetanus Immunoglobulin for
Intravenous Use.** Used for proven or suspected
clinical tetanus
   Dose: by intravenous infusion, 5000–10 000 units
   Available from SNBTS (2500-unit vial) on a named
   patient basis

Varicella-Zoster

PoM **Varicella-Zoster Immunoglobulin** (Anti-varicella-zoster Immunoglobulin) See notes above

Dose: by deep intramuscular injection, prophylaxis (as soon as possible—not later than 10 days after exposure), CHILD up to 5 years 250 mg, 6–10 years 500 mg, 11–14 years 750 mg, over 15 years 1 g; second dose required if further exposure occurs after 3 weeks

Note. No evidence that effective in treatment of severe disease—**aciclovir** (see section 5.3) should be used. An *intravenous preparation* of **normal immunoglobulin** (see Intravenous Therapy, p. 516) may be used to provide an immediate source of antibody.

Available from Public Health Laboratory Service (also from BPL and SNBTS)

ANTI-D (Rh$_0$) IMMUNOGLOBULIN

Anti-D immunoglobulin is available to prevent a rhesus-negative mother from forming antibodies to fetal rhesus-positive cells which may pass into the maternal circulation during childbirth or abortion. It should be injected within 72 hours of the birth or abortion but even if a longer period has elapsed it may still give protection and should be administered. The objective is to protect any subsequent child from the hazard of haemolytic disease of the newborn.

> **Joint Committee on Vaccination and Immunisation recommendation on live vaccines.**
>
> *Rubella vaccine* may be administered in the postpartum period simultaneously with anti-D (Rh$_0$) immunoglobulin injection providing separate syringes are used and the products are administered into contralateral limbs. A blood test should be done not sooner than 8 weeks later to ensure that rubella antibodies have been produced. If blood transfusion was necessary vaccination should be delayed for 3 months.
>
> *MMR vaccine* should not be given within 3 months of an injection of anti-D (Rh$_0$) immunoglobulin injection.

PoM **Anti-D (Rh$_0$) Immunoglobulin Injection.**

Available from Regional Blood Transfusion Centres and from BPL and SNBTS

Dose: by deep intramuscular injection, to rhesus-negative woman for prevention of Rh$_0$(D) sensitisation:

Following abortion or birth of rhesus-positive infant, 500 units immediately or within 72 hours; for transplacental bleed in excess of 4–5 mL fetal red cells, extra 100–125 units per mL fetal red cells

Following any potentially sensitising episode (e.g. stillbirth, amniocentesis) up to 20 weeks' gestation 250 units per episode (after 20 weeks, 500 units) immediately or within 72 hours

Following Rh$_0$(D) incompatible blood transfusion, 125 units per mL transfused rhesus-positive red cells

Note. The above doses reflect recommendations of the Standing Medical Advisory Committee on Haemolytic Disease of the Newborn.

Antenatal prophylaxis, 500 units may be given at weeks 28 and 34 of pregnancy; a further dose is still needed immediately or within 72 hours of delivery

PoM **Partobulin**® (Immuno)

Anti-D (Rh$_0$) immunoglobulin injection 1250 units/mL, net price 1-mL prefilled syringe = £16.48

Dose: by intramuscular injection, to rhesus-negative woman for prevention of Rh$_0$(D) sensitisation:

Following abortion, miscarriage or birth of rhesus-positive infant, 1250 units immediately or within 72 hours; for transplacental bleed in excess of 25 mL fetal blood (1% of fetal erythrocytes), 5000 units (*or* 50 units per mL fetal blood)

Following any potentially sensitising episode (e.g. amniocentesis) 1250 units immediately or within 72 hours

Following Rh$_0$(D) incompatible blood transfusion, at least 50–100 units per mL transfused rhesus-positive red cells

Antenatal prophylaxis, 1250 units may be given at weeks 28 and 34 of pregnancy; a further dose is still needed immediately or within 72 hours of delivery

INTERFERONS

INTERFERON ALFA

See section 8.2.4

INTERFERON BETA

See section 8.2.4

INTERFERON GAMMA-1b

(Immune interferon)

Indications: adjunct to antibiotics to reduce frequency of serious infection in patients with chronic granulomatous disease

Cautions: severe hepatic or renal impairment; seizure disorders or compromised central nervous system function; pre-existing cardiac disease (including ischaemia, congestive heart failure, and arrhythmias); monitor before and during treatment: haematological tests (including full blood count, differential white cell count, and platelet count), blood chemistry tests (including renal and liver function tests) and urinalysis

DRIVING. May impair ability to drive or operate machinery; effects may be enhanced by alcohol

Side-effects: fever, headache, chills, myalgia, fatigue; nausea, vomiting, arthralgia, rashes and injection-site reactions reported

▼ PoM **Immukin**® (Boehringer Ingelheim)

Injection, recombinant human interferon gamma-1b 200 micrograms/mL. Net price 0.5-mL vial = £88.00

Dose: by subcutaneous injection, 50 micrograms/m^2 3 times a week; patients with body surface area of 0.5 m^2 or less, 1.5 micrograms/kg 3 times a week; not yet recommended for children under 6 months

14.6   International travel

Note. For advice on **malaria chemoprophylaxis**, see section 5.4.1.

No particular immunisation is required for travellers to the United States, Europe, Australia, or New Zealand although all travellers should have immunity to tetanus and poliomyelitis (and childhood immunisations should be up to date). In Non-European areas surrounding the Mediterranean, in Africa, the Middle East, Asia, and South America, certain special precautions are required.

Long-term travellers to areas that have a high incidence of **poliomyelitis** or **tuberculosis** should be immunised with the appropriate vaccine; in the case of poliomyelitis previously immunised adults may be given a reinforcing dose of oral poliomyelitis vaccine. BCG immunisation is recommended for travellers proposing to stay for longer than one month (or in close contact with the local population) in Asia, Africa, or Central and South America; it should preferably be given three months or more before departure.

International Certificates of vaccination against **yellow fever** (see p. 514) are still required for travel to much of Africa and South America.

Immunisation against **meningococcal meningitis** is recommended for a number of areas of the world (for details, see p. 510).

Overland travellers to Asia and Africa and others at high risk may be given normal immunoglobulin injection (see p. 515) for protection against **hepatitis A**; hepatitis A vaccine (see p. 507) is preferable for frequent travellers and those planning to go for more than 3–5 months. If immunoglobulin is to be given, it is preferable to complete any active immunisation 4 weeks beforehand; an interval of 2 weeks is acceptable provided the immunoglobulin is given just before departure. If time is short, it can be given with any vaccine (including polio).

Typhoid vaccine is indicated for travellers to those countries where typhoid is endemic but is no substitute for personal precautions. Food should be freshly prepared and hot, avoiding uncooked vegetables (including green salads); only fruits which can be peeled should be eaten. Only suitable bottled water, or tap water that has been boiled, or treated with sterilising tablets should be used for drinking purposes. This advice also applies to cholera and other diarrhoeal diseases (including travellers' diarrhoea).

Cholera vaccine is no substitute for personal hygiene and has little value in preventing infections. For current advice, see p. 505

For advice on **diphtheria vaccine** and the former USSR, see p. 505. Advice about **Japanese** and **tick-borne encephalitis** is included in *Health Information for Overseas Travel*, see below.

Information on health advice for travellers

The Department of Health booklet, *Health Advice For Travellers* (code: T5) includes information on immunisation requirements (or recommendations) around the world. The booklet can be obtained from travel agents, post-offices or by telephoning 0800 555 777 (24-hour service).

The Department of Health handbook, *Health Information for Overseas Travel*, which draws together essential information *for doctors* regarding health advice for travellers, can be obtained from

HMSO Publications Centre,
PO Box 276, London SW8 5DT
Telephone orders, 0171 873 9090

Immunisation requirements change from time to time, and information on the current requirements for any particular country may be obtained from:

Communicable Disease Surveillance Centre Travel Unit, 61 Colindale Avenue, London NW9 5EQ, telephone 0181-200 6868 (for health care professionals only)

Communicable Diseases (Scotland) Unit, Ruchill Hospital, Bilslend Drive, Glasgow G20 9NB, telephone 0141-946 7120

Scottish Office Department of Health, Public Health Policy Unit, St. Andrew's House, Edinburgh EH1 3DG, telephone 0131-556 8400

Welsh Office, Cathays Park, Cardiff CF1 3NQ, telephone 01222 825111

Department of Health and Social Services, Dundonald House, Upper Newtownards Road, Belfast BT4 3SB, telephone 01232 520000

or from the embassy or legation of the appropriate country.

15: Drugs used in
ANAESTHESIA

This chapter describes briefly drugs used in anaesthesia; the reader is referred to other sources for
more detailed information. The chapter is divided
into two sections:

15.1   General anaesthesia
15.2   Local anaesthesia

15.1   General anaesthesia

15.1.1   Intravenous anaesthetics
15.1.2   Inhalational anaesthetics
15.1.3   Antimuscarinic drugs
15.1.4   Sedative and analgesic peri-operative
          drugs
15.1.5   Muscle relaxants
15.1.6   Anticholinesterases used in anaesthesia
15.1.7   Antagonists for central and respiratory
          depression
15.1.8   Drugs for malignant hyperthermia

Note. The drugs in section 15.1 should be used only
by experienced personnel and where adequate resuscitative equipment is available.

ANAESTHESIA AND DRIVING. Patients given sedatives and analgesics during minor outpatient procedures should be very carefully warned about the
risk of driving afterwards. For intravenous benzodiazepines and for a short general anaesthetic the
risk extends to **at least 24 hours** after administration. Responsible persons should be available to
take patients home. The dangers of taking **alcohol**
should also be emphasised.

MODERN ANAESTHETIC TECHNIQUE. It is now common practice to administer several drugs with different actions to produce a state of surgical
anaesthesia with minimal risk of toxic effects. An
intravenous anaesthetic is usually used for induction, followed by maintenance with inhalational
anaesthetics, perhaps supplemented by other drugs
administered intravenously. Specific drugs are often
used to produce muscular relaxation. These drugs
interfere with spontaneous respiration so intermittent positive pressure ventilation by manual or
mechanical means is commonly employed.

For certain procedures controlled hypotension
may be required. Labetalol (see section 2.4), sodium nitroprusside (see section 2.5.1) and glyceryl
trinitrate (see section 2.6.1) are used.

Beta-blockers (see section 2.4), adenosine, amiodarone (see section 2.3.2) or verapamil (see section
2.6.2) may be used to control arrhythmias during
anaesthesia.

Glyceryl trinitrate (see section 2.6.1) is also used
to control hypertension, particularly postoperatively.

GAS CYLINDERS

Each gas cylinder bears a label with the name of the
gas contained in the cylinder. The name or chemical
symbol of the gas is stencilled in paint on the shoulder of the cylinder; the letters are not less than 9 mm
high on cylinders up to and including 80 mm diameter, not less than 12 mm high on cylinders over 80 mm
and up to and including 105 mm diameter, and 19 mm
high on cylinders above 105 mm diameter. The name
or chemical symbol of the gas is also clearly and
indelibly stamped on the cylinder valve.

The colours applied to the valve end of the cylinder
extend down the cylinder to the shoulder; in the case
of mixed gases the colours for the individual gases
are applied in four segments, two for each colour. See
table below.

Gas cylinders should be stored in a cool well-venti-
lated room, free from materials of a flammable
nature.

No lubricant of any description should be used.

Name of gas	Symbol	Colour of cylinder body	Colour of valve end where different from body
Oxygen	O_2	Black	White
Nitrous oxide	N_2O	Blue	—
Cyclopropane[1]	C_3H_6	Orange	—
Carbon dioxide	CO_2	Grey	—
Ethylene	C_2H_4	Violet	—
Helium	He	Brown	—
Nitrogen	N_2	Grey	Black
Oxygen and carbon dioxide mixture	$O_2 + CO_2$	Black	White and Grey
Oxygen and helium mixture	$O_2 + He$	Black	White and Brown
Oxygen and nitrous oxide mixture	$O_2 + N_2O$	Blue	Blue and White
Air (medical)	AIR	Grey	White and Black

British Standard 1319:1976; Medical gas cylinders, valves and yoke connections. The colours used for gas cylinders
comply with specifications in British Standards 4800 and 5252.
1. Cyclopropane is no longer manufactured in the UK.

SURGERY AND LONG-TERM MEDICATION. The risk of stopping long-term medication before surgery is often greater than the risk of continuing it during surgery. This applies particularly to corticosteroids, since patients with adrenal atrophy (see section 6.3.2) may experience a precipitous fall in blood pressure unless corticosteroid cover is provided during anaesthesia and in the immediate postoperative period. Anaesthetists must therefore know whether a patient is, or has been, taking corticosteroids. Other drugs that should not normally be stopped before surgery include analgesics, anti-epileptics, antiparkinsonian drugs, bronchodilators, cardiovascular drugs, glaucoma drugs, and thyroid or antithyroid drugs. Although it is preferable to discontinue oral anticoagulants electively before operation, this is not possible in patients requiring long-term treatment (e.g. for valve prostheses). The haematologist or physician should be consulted for further advice. For general advice on surgery in diabetic patients see section 6.1.1.

Drugs that should be stopped before surgery include combined oral contraceptives (discontinue 4 weeks before major elective surgery with adequate alternative contraceptive arrangements—see Surgery, section 7.3.1 for details); hormone replacement therapy, however, does not normally need to be stopped (see section 6.4.1.1). In view of their hazardous interactions MAOIs should normally be stopped 2 weeks before surgery. Tricyclic antidepressants need not be stopped, but there may be an increased risk of arrhythmias and hypotension (and dangerous interaction with vasopressor drugs), therefore the anaesthetist should be informed if they are not. Lithium should be stopped 2 days before major surgery but the normal dose can be continued for minor surgery (with careful monitoring of fluids and electrolytes). To avoid withdrawal symptoms antidepressants need to be withdrawn gradually (see section 4.3).

It is vital that the anaesthetist should know of **all** drugs that a patient is (or has been) taking.

15.1.1   Intravenous anaesthetics

Intravenous anaesthetics may be used alone to produce anaesthesia for short surgical procedures but are more commonly used for induction only. Intravenous anaesthetics nearly all produce their effect in one arm-brain circulation time and can cause apnoea and hypotension, and so adequate resuscitative facilities **must** be available. They are **contraindicated** if the anaesthetist is not confident of being able to maintain the airway (e.g. in the presence of a tumour in the pharynx or larynx). Extreme care is required in surgery of the mouth, pharynx, or larynx and in patients with acute cardiovascular failure (shock) or fixed cardiac output.

Individual requirements vary considerably and the recommended dosage is only a guide. Smaller dosage is indicated in ill, shocked, or debilitated patients, while robust individuals may require more. To facilitate tracheal intubation, induction is followed by a neuromuscular blocking drug (section 15.1.5).

TOTAL INTRAVENOUS ANAESTHESIA. This is a technique in which major surgery is carried out with all anaesthetic drugs given intravenously. Respiration is controlled, the lungs being inflated with oxygen-enriched air. Muscle relaxants are used to provide relaxation and prevent reflex muscle movements. The main problem to be overcome is the assessment of depth of anaesthesia.

ANAESTHESIA AND DRIVING. See previous page.

BARBITURATES

Thiopentone sodium is a widely used intravenous anaesthetic, but has no analgesic properties. Induction is generally smooth and rapid, but owing to its narrow therapeutic margin, overdosage with cardiorespiratory depression may occur. The solution is highly alkaline and therefore irritant on misplaced injection outside the vein; arterial injection is particularly dangerous.

Awakening from a moderate dose of thiopentone is rapid due to redistribution of the drug in the whole body tissues. Metabolism is, however, slow and some sedative effects may persist for 24 hours. Repeated doses have a cumulative effect.

Methohexitone sodium is less irritant to tissues than thiopentone. Recovery is marginally more rapid than in the case of thiopentone, but induction is less smooth with an incidence of hiccup, tremor, involuntary movements, and pain on injection.

Both thiopentone and methohexitone are **contraindicated** in porphyria (see section 9.8.2).

METHOHEXITONE SODIUM
(Methohexital)

Indications: induction and maintenance of anaesthesia for short procedures; with other anaesthetics for more prolonged anaesthesia

Cautions; Contra-indications; Side-effects: avoid or reduce dose in liver disease; see also under Thiopentone Sodium and notes above

Dose: by intravenous injection, usually as a 1% solution, 50–120 mg according to response at rate of 10 mg in 5 seconds; maintenance, 20–40 mg (2–4 mL of 1% solution) every 4–7 minutes; CHILD induction approx. 1 mg/kg

PoM **Brietal Sodium®** (Lilly)

Injection, powder for reconstitution, methohexitone sodium, net price 100 mg in 10-mL vial = £1.14; 500 mg in 50-mL vial = £2.95

Note. The 100-mg strength may not be available at present

THIOPENTONE SODIUM
(Thiopental Sodium)

Indications: induction of general anaesthesia; anaesthesia of short duration

Cautions; Contra-indications; Side-effects: see notes above; reduce induction dose in severe liver disease; avoid in porphyria (see section 9.8.2); **interactions:** Appendix 1 (anaesthetics, general)

Dose: by intravenous injection, in fit premedicated adults, initially 100–150 mg (4–6 mL of 2.5% solution) over 10–15 seconds, followed by further quantity if necessary according to response after 30–60 seconds; *or* up to 4 mg/kg; CHILD induction 2–7 mg/kg

PoM **Intraval Sodium**® (Rhône-Poulenc Rorer)
Injection 2.5%, powder for reconstitution, thiopentone sodium. Net price 500-mg amp = £1.23 (with water for injections £1.66); 2.5-g vial = £4.58 (with water for injections £5.36)

OTHER INTRAVENOUS ANAESTHETICS

Etomidate is an induction agent associated with rapid recovery without hangover effect. It causes less hypotension than other drugs used for induction. There is a high incidence of extraneous muscle movement and of pain on injection; these effects can be minimised by premedication with an opioid analgesic and the use of larger veins. There is evidence that repeated doses of etomidate have an undesirable suppressant effect on adrenocortical function.

Propofol is associated with rapid recovery without hangover effect and is very widely used. There is sometimes pain on intravenous injection, but significant extraneous muscle movements do not occur. The CSM have received reports of convulsions, anaphylaxis, and delayed recovery from anaesthesia after propofol administration; since some of the convulsions are delayed the CSM has advised special caution after day surgery. Propofol has been associated with bradycardia, occasionally profound; intravenous administration of an antimuscarinic may be necessary to prevent this.

Ketamine can be given by the intravenous or the intramuscular route, and has good analgesic properties when used in sub-anaesthetic dosage. The maximum effect occurs after more than one arm-brain circulation time. Muscle tone is increased. There is cardiovascular stimulation and arterial pressure may rise with tachycardia. The main disadvantage is the high incidence of hallucinations and other transient psychotic sequelae, though it is believed that these are much less significant in children. The incidence can be reduced when drugs such as diazepam are also used. Ketamine is **contra-indicated** in patients with hypertension and is best avoided in those prone to hallucinations. It is used mainly for paediatric anaesthesia, particularly when repeated administrations are required. Recovery is relatively slow.

ETOMIDATE

Indications: induction of anaesthesia
Cautions; Contra-indications; Side-effects: see notes above; porphyria (see section 9.8.2); **interactions:** Appendix 1 (anaesthetics, general)
Dose: by slow intravenous injection, 300 micrograms/kg; high-risk patients, 100 micrograms/kg/minute until anaesthetised (about 3 minutes)

PoM **Hypnomidate**® (Janssen)
Injection, etomidate 2 mg/mL in propylene glycol 35%. Net price 10-mL amp = £1.58

KETAMINE

Indications: induction and maintenance of anaesthesia
Cautions; Contra-indications; Side-effects: see notes above; **interactions:** Appendix 1 (anaesthetics, general)
Dose: by intramuscular injection, short procedures, initially 6.5–13 mg/kg (10 mg/kg usually produces 12–25 minutes of surgical anaesthesia) Diagnostic manoeuvres and procedures not involving intense pain, initially 4 mg/kg
By intravenous injection over at least 60 seconds, short procedures, initially 1–4.5 mg/kg (2 mg/kg usually produces 5–10 minutes of surgical anaesthesia)
By intravenous infusion of a solution containing 1 mg/mL, longer procedures, induction, total dose of 0.5–2 mg/kg; maintenance (using microdrip infusion), 10–45 micrograms/kg/minute, rate adjusted according to response

PoM **Ketalar**® (P-D)
Injection, ketamine (as hydrochloride) 10 mg/mL, net price 20-mL vial = £3.52; 50 mg/mL, 10-mL vial = £7.31; 100 mg/mL, 5-mL vial = £6.71

PROPOFOL

Indications: induction and maintenance of general anaesthesia; sedation of ventilated patients receiving intensive care, for up to 3 days
Cautions; Contra-indications; Side-effects: see notes above; monitor blood lipid concentrations in patients at risk of fat overload; contra-indicated if history of propofol allergy (see CSM warning above); bacterial contamination (see below); **interactions:** Appendix 1 (anaesthetics, general)
BACTERIAL CONTAMINATION. In order to eliminate the **risk of infection** from bacterial contamination **strict aseptic technique** must be used when drawing-up propofol emulsion
Dose: induction, *by intravenous injection*, 2–2.5 mg/kg (less in those over 55 years) at a rate of 20–40 mg every 10 seconds (lower end of range in those over 55 years); CHILD over 3 years 2.5 mg/kg adjusted as necessary
Maintenance, *by intravenous infusion*, 4–12 mg/kg/hour *or by intravenous injection*, 25–50 mg repeated according to response; CHILD over 3 years 9–15 mg/kg/hour
Sedation during intensive care (with assisted ventilation), *by intravenous infusion*, 0.3–4 mg/kg/hour for up to 3 days; CHILD not recommended
Sedation for surgical and diagnostic procedures, initially *by intravenous injection*, 0.5–1 mg/kg over 1–5 minutes; maintenance, *by intravenous infusion*, 1.5–4.5 mg/kg/hour (in addition, if rapid increase in depth of sedation required, *by intravenous injection*, 10–20 mg); those over 55 years may require lower dose; CHILD not recommended

PoM **Diprivan**® (Zeneca)
Injection (emulsion), propofol 10 mg/mL, net price 20-mL amp = £3.88, 50-mL vial = £9.70, 100-mL vial = £19.40

15.1.2   Inhalational anaesthetics

Inhalational anaesthetics may be gases or volatile liquids. They can be used both for induction and maintenance of anaesthesia and may also be used following induction with an intravenous anaesthetic (section 15.1.1).

Gaseous anaesthetics require suitable equipment for storage and administration. They may be supplied via hospital pipelines or from metal cylinders. *Volatile liquid anaesthetics* are administered using calibrated vaporisers, using air, oxygen, or nitrous oxide–oxygen mixtures as the carrier gas. It should be noted that they can all trigger malignant hyperthermia.

To prevent hypoxia inhalational anaesthetics must be given with concentrations of oxygen greater than in air.

ANAESTHESIA AND DRIVING. See section 15.1.

VOLATILE LIQUID ANAESTHETICS

Halothane is a volatile liquid anaesthetic. Its advantages are that it is potent, induction is smooth, the vapour is non-irritant, pleasant to inhale, and seldom induces coughing or breath-holding. Despite these advantages, however, halothane is much less widely used than previously owing to its association with *severe hepatotoxicity* (**important:** see CSM advice, below).

Halothane causes cardiorespiratory depression. Respiratory depression results in elevation of arterial carbon dioxide tension and perhaps ventricular arrhythmias. Halothane also depresses the cardiac muscle fibres and may cause bradycardia. The result is diminished cardiac output and fall of arterial pressure. Adrenaline infiltrations should be avoided in patients anaesthetised with halothane as ventricular arrhythmias may result.

Halothane produces moderate muscle relaxation, but this may be inadequate for major abdominal surgery and specific muscle relaxants are then used.

CSM advice (halothane hepatotoxicity). In a publication on findings confirming that *severe hepatotoxicity* can follow halothane anaesthesia the CSM has reported that this occurs more frequently after repeated exposures to halothane and has a high mortality. The risk of severe hepatotoxicity appears to be increased by repeated exposures within a short time interval, but even after a long interval (sometimes of several years) susceptible patients have been reported to develop jaundice. Since there is no reliable way of identifying susceptible patients the CSM recommends the following precautions prior to use of halothane:

1. a careful anaesthetic history should be taken to determine previous exposure and previous reactions to halothane;

2. repeated exposure to halothane within a period of **at least** 3 months should be **avoided** unless there are **overriding** clinical circumstances;

3. a history of unexplained jaundice or pyrexia in a patient following exposure to halothane is an absolute **contra-indication** to its future use in that patient.

Enflurane is a volatile anaesthetic similar to halothane, but less potent, about twice the concentration being necessary for induction and maintenance.

Enflurane is a powerful cardiorespiratory depressant. Shallow respiration is likely to result in a rise of arterial carbon dioxide tension, but ventricular arrhythmias are uncommon and it is probably safe to use adrenaline infiltrations. Myocardial depression may result in a fall in cardiac output and in arterial hypotension. Enflurane may cause EEG changes and special caution is needed in those liable to have susceptibility to epileptic seizures.

Enflurane is usually given to supplement nitrous oxide–oxygen mixtures.

Isoflurane is an isomer of enflurane. It has a potency intermediate between that of halothane and enflurane, and even less of an inhaled dose is metabolised than with enflurane. Heart rhythm is generally stable during isoflurane anaesthesia, but heart-rate may rise, particularly in younger patients. Systemic arterial pressure may fall, due to a decrease in systemic vascular resistance and with less decrease in cardiac output than occurs with halothane. Respiration is depressed. Muscle relaxation is produced and muscle relaxant drugs potentiated.

Desflurane is a newly introduced rapid acting volatile liquid anaesthetic. It is reported to have about one-fifth the potency of isoflurane. Owing to limited experience it is not recommended in neurosurgical patients; owing to frequent occurrence of cough, breath-holding, apnoea, laryngospasm and increased secretions it is not recommended for induction in children.

Sevoflurane is a newly introduced rapid acting volatile liquid anaesthetic. Patients may require early postoperative pain relief as emergence and recovery are particularly rapid.

DESFLURANE

Indications; Cautions; Contra-indications; Side-effects: see notes above; **interactions:** Appendix 1 (anaesthetics, general)

IMPORTANT. Desflurane has been reported to interact with dry carbon dioxide absorbents to form carbon monoxide—to minimise risk, carbon dioxide absorbents should **not** be allowed to dry out

Dose: using a specifically designed calibrated vaporiser, *induction*, 4–11%; CHILD not recommended for induction

Maintenance, 2–6% in nitrous oxide; 2.5–8.5% in oxygen or oxygen-enriched air

▼ PoM **Suprane**® (Pharmacia)
Desflurane. Net price 240 mL = £46.50

ENFLURANE

Indications; Cautions; Side-effects: see notes above; porphyria (see section 9.8.2); caution is needed in epilepsy; **interactions:** Appendix 1 (anaesthetics, general)

IMPORTANT. Enflurane has been reported to interact with dry carbon dioxide absorbents to form carbon monoxide—to minimise risk, carbon dioxide absorbents should **not** be allowed to dry out

---

Dose: using a specifically calibrated vaporiser, *induction*, increased gradually from 0.4% to max. of 4.5% in air, oxygen, or nitrous oxide–oxygen, according to response
Maintenance, 0.5–3% in nitrous oxide–oxygen

Enflurane (Abbott)
Enflurane. Net price 250 mL = £34.00

HALOTHANE

Indications; Cautions; Contra-indications; Side-effects: see notes above (**important:** CSM advice see also notes above); porphyria (see section 9.8.2); **interactions:** Appendix 1 (anaesthetics, general)
Dose: using a specifically calibrated vaporiser, *induction*, increased gradually to 2–4% in oxygen or nitrous oxide–oxygen; CHILD 1.5–2%
Maintenance, 0.5–2%

Halothane (Rhône-Poulenc Rorer)
Halothane. Net price 250 mL = £10.23
Fluothane® (Zeneca)
Halothane. Net price 250 mL = £16.36

ISOFLURANE

Indications; Cautions; Side-effects: see notes above; **interactions:** Appendix 1 (anaesthetics, general)
IMPORTANT. Isoflurane has been reported to interact with dry carbon dioxide absorbents to form carbon monoxide—to minimise risk, carbon dioxide absorbents should **not** be allowed to dry out
Dose: using a specifically calibrated vaporiser, *induction*, increased gradually from 0.5% to 3%, in oxygen or nitrous oxide–oxygen
Maintenance, 1–2.5% in nitrous oxide–oxygen; an additional 0.5–1% may be required when given with oxygen alone; caesarean section, 0.5–0.75% in nitrous oxide–oxygen

Isoflurane (Abbott)
Isoflurane. Net price 100 mL = £39.00

SEVOFLURANE

Indications; Cautions; Contra-indications; Side-effects: see notes above; agitation occurs frequently in children; **interactions:** Appendix 1 (anaesthetics, general)
IMPORTANT. No interaction with dry carbon dioxide absorbents to form carbon monoxide reported, but to minimise possible risk, carbon dioxide absorbents should **not** be allowed to dry out
Dose: using a specifically calibrated vaporiser, *induction*, up to 5% in oxygen or nitrous oxide–oxygen; CHILD up to 7%
Maintenance, 0.5–3%

▼ PoM **Sevoflurane** (Abbott)
Sevoflurane. Net price 100 mL = £49.20

NITROUS OXIDE

Nitrous oxide is used for maintenance of anaesthesia and, in sub-anaesthetic concentrations, for analgesia. For *anaesthesia* it is commonly used in a concentration of 50 to 70% in oxygen as part of a balanced technique in association with other inhalational or intravenous agents. Nitrous oxide is unsatisfactory as a sole anaesthetic owing to lack of potency, but is useful as part of a sequence of drugs since it allows a significant reduction in dosage.

A mixture of nitrous oxide and oxygen containing 50% of each gas (Entonox®) is used to produce *analgesia without loss of consciousness*. Self-administration using a demand valve is popular and may be appropriate in obstetric practice, for changing painful dressings, as an aid to postoperative physiotherapy, and in emergency ambulances.

Nitrous oxide may have a deleterious effect if used in patients with an air-containing closed space since nitrous oxide diffuses into such a space with a resulting increase in pressure. This effect may be dangerous in the presence of a pneumothorax which may enlarge to compromise respiration.

Exposure of patients to nitrous oxide for prolonged periods, either by continuous or by intermittent administration, may result in megaloblastic anaemia due to interference with the action of vitamin B_{12}. For the same reason, exposure of anaesthetists and theatre staff to nitrous oxide should be minimised. Depression of white cell formation may also occur.

NITROUS OXIDE

Indications; Cautions; Side-effects: see notes above; **interactions:** Appendix 1 (anaesthetics, general)
Dose: using a suitable anaesthetic apparatus, a mixture with 25–30% oxygen for *maintenance* of light anaesthesia
Analgesic, as a mixture with 50% oxygen, according to the patient's needs

15.1.3 Antimuscarinic drugs

Antimuscarinic premedication drugs are used (less commonly nowadays) to dry bronchial and salivary secretions which are increased by intubation and some inhalational anaesthetics. They are also used before or with neostigmine (section 15.1.6) to prevent bradycardia, excessive salivation, and other muscarinic actions of neostigmine. They are also used to prevent bradycardia and hypotension associated with agents such as halothane, propofol, and suxamethonium.

Atropine is now rarely used for premedication but still has an emergency role in the treatment of vagotonic side-effects. For its role in acute arrhythmias after myocardial infarction, see section 2.3.1; see also cardiopulmonary resuscitation algorithm, section 2.7.3.

Hyoscine effectively reduces secretions and also provides a degree of amnesia, sedation and anti-emesis. Unlike atropine it may produce bradycardia rather than tachycardia. In some patients, especially the elderly, hyoscine may cause the central anticholinergic syndrome (excitement, ataxia, hallucinations, behavioural abnormalities, and drowsiness).

Glycopyrronium produces good drying of salivary secretions. When given intravenously it produces less tachycardia than atropine. It is widely used with neostigmine for reversal of non-depolarising muscle relaxants (section 15.1.5).

Phenothiazines have too little drying activity to be effective when used alone.

ATROPINE SULPHATE

Indications: drying secretions, reversal of excessive bradycardia; with neostigmine for reversal of competitive neuromuscular block; other indications, see sections 1.2, 2.3.1, 11.5

Cautions: cardiovascular disease; see also section 1.2; **interactions:** Appendix 1 (antimuscarinics)

Side-effects: tachycardia; see also section 1.2

Dose: premedication, *by intravenous injection,* 300–600 micrograms immediately before induction of anaesthesia, and in incremental doses of 100 micrograms for the treatment of bradycardia

By intramuscular injection, 300–600 micrograms 30–60 minutes before induction; CHILD 20 micrograms/kg

For control of muscarinic side-effects of neostigmine in reversal of competitive neuromuscular block, *by intravenous injection,* 0.6–1.2 mg

Arrhythmias after myocardial infarction, see section 2.3.1; see also cardiopulmonary resuscitation algorithm, section 2.7.3

PoM **Atropine** (Non-proprietary)
Injection, atropine sulphate 600 micrograms/mL. Net price 1-mL amp = 35p
Note. Other strengths also available

PoM **Min-I-Jet® Atropine Sulphate** (IMS)
Injection, atropine sulphate 100 micrograms/mL, net price 5-mL disposable syringe = £3.78, 10-mL disposable syringe = £4.24, 30-mL disposable syringe = £7.75
Note. A 10-mL prefilled syringe containing atropine sulphate 300 micrograms/mL is also available from Aurum; net price 10-mL disposable syringe = £4.32

CD **Morphine and Atropine Injection,** see under Morphine Salts (section 15.1.4.3)

GLYCOPYRRONIUM BROMIDE

Indications; Cautions; Side-effects: see under Atropine Sulphate

Dose: premedication, *by intramuscular or intravenous injection,* 200–400 micrograms, *or* 4–5 micrograms/kg to a max. of 400 micrograms; CHILD, *by intramuscular or intravenous injection,* 4–8 micrograms/kg to a max. of 200 micrograms; intra-operative use, *by intravenous injection,* as for premedication

For control of muscarinic side-effects of neostigmine in reversal of competitive neuromuscular block, *by intravenous injection,* 10–15 micrograms/kg with 50 micrograms/kg neostigmine; CHILD, 10 micrograms/kg with 50 micrograms/kg neostigmine

PoM **Robinul®** (Anpharm)
Injection, glycopyrronium bromide 200 micrograms/mL. Net price 1-mL amp = 32p; 3-mL amp = 53p
Available as a generic from Antigen

PoM **Robinul-Neostigmine®,** see under Neostigmine Methylsulphate (section 15.1.6)

HYOSCINE HYDROBROMIDE
(Scopolamine Hydrobromide)

Indications: drying secretions, amnesia; other indications, see section 4.6

Cautions; Side-effects: see under Atropine Sulphate; may slow heart; avoid in the elderly (see notes above); porphyria (see section 9.8.2)

Dose: premedication, *by subcutaneous or intramuscular injection,* 200–600 micrograms 30–60 minutes before induction of anaesthesia, usually with papaveretum

PoM **Hyoscine** (Non-proprietary)
Injection, hyoscine hydrobromide 400 micrograms/mL, net price 1-mL amp = £2.76; 600 micrograms/mL, 1-mL amp = £2.34

CD **Papaveretum and Hyoscine Injection,** see under Papaveretum (section 15.1.4.3)

15.1.4   Sedative and analgesic peri-operative drugs

15.1.4.1 Anxiolytics and neuroleptics
15.1.4.2 Non-opioid analgesics
15.1.4.3 Opioid analgesics

These drugs are given to allay the apprehension of the patient in the pre-operative period (including the night before operation), to relieve pain and discomfort when present, and to augment the action of subsequent anaesthetic agents. A number of the drugs used also provide some degree of pre-operative amnesia. The choice will vary with the individual patient, the nature of the operative procedure, the anaesthetic to be used and other prevailing circumstances such as outpatients, obstetrics, recovery facilities etc. The choice would also vary in elective and emergency operations.

PREMEDICATION IN CHILDREN. Oral or rectal administration is preferred to injections where possible but is not altogether satisfactory. Oral **trimeprazine** is still used but when given alone it may cause postoperative restlessness when pain is present. An alternative is **diazepam**. Some anaesthetists prefer the use of adult regimens, with dosage on a weight basis. (For guidelines on dose calculation in children, see Prescribing for Children, p. 11.)

Atropine or hyoscine is often given orally to children, but may be given intravenously immediately before induction.

ANAESTHESIA AND DRIVING. See section 15.1.

15.1.4.1 ANXIOLYTICS AND NEUROLEPTICS

Anxiolytic benzodiazepines are widely used whereas neuroleptics (e.g. chlorpromazine) are now rarely used.

BENZODIAZEPINES

Oral premedication with benzodiazepines is increasing in popularity, a short-acting oral benzodiazepine now being the most common premedicant.

Benzodiazepines are also of particular value for the production of light sedation during unpleasant procedures or during operations under local anaesthesia (including dentistry). The resultant amnesia is such that the patient is unlikely to have any unpleasant memories of the procedure (however, benzodiazepines, particularly when used for deep sedation, can sometimes induce sexual fantasies).

Diazepam is relatively insoluble in water and preparations formulated in organic solvents are painful on intravenous injection and followed by a high incidence of venous thrombosis (which may not be noticed until a week after the injection); they are also painful on intramuscular injection, and absorption from the injection site is erratic. An emulsion preparation for intravenous injection is less irritant and is followed by a negligible incidence of venous thrombosis; it is not suitable for intramuscular injection. Diazepam is also available as a rectal solution.

Benzodiazepines are also of particular value for sedation of patients in intensive care units, particularly those having assisted ventilation. Since they have no analgesic action they are often given in conjunction with opioid analgesics.

Benzodiazepines may on occasion cause marked respiratory depression and facilities for treatment of this are essential.

Diazepam is used to produce light sedation with amnesia. The 'sleep' dose shows too great an individual variation to recommend it for induction of anaesthesia. It is a long-acting drug with active metabolites, and a second period of drowsiness can occur 4–6 hours after its administration.

Temazepam is given by mouth and has a shorter action and a relatively more rapid onset than diazepam by mouth. Used as a premedicant, anxiolytic and sedative effects are produced which continue for one and a half hours. After this period patients are usually fully alert but there may be residual drowsiness. It has proved useful as a premedicant in inpatient and day-case surgery.

Lorazepam produces more prolonged sedation than temazepam. In addition amnesia is commonplace. It is used as a premedicant the night before major surgery. A further, smaller, dose may be required the following morning if any delay in starting surgery is anticipated. Alternatively the first dose may be given in the early morning of the day of operation.

Midazolam is a water-soluble benzodiazepine which is often used in preference to diazepam. Recovery is faster than with diazepam. The incidence of side-effects is low but the CSM has received reports of respiratory depression (sometimes associated with severe hypotension) following intravenous administration. It is also associated with some major interactions (see below).

DIAZEPAM

Indications: premedication; sedation with amnesia, and in conjunction with local anaesthesia; other indications, see sections 4.1.2, 4.8.2, 10.2.2

Cautions; Contra-indications; Side-effects: see notes above and sections 4.1.2, 4.8.2

Dose: by mouth, 5 mg at night, 5 mg on waking, and 5 mg 2 hours before minor or dental surgery

By intravenous injection, into a large vein 10–20 mg over 2–4 minutes as sedative cover for minor surgical and medical procedures; premedication 100–200 micrograms/kg

By rectum in solution, ADULT and CHILD over 3 years 10 mg; CHILD 1–3 years and ELDERLY 5 mg

Preparations
See section 4.1.2

LORAZEPAM

Indications: sedation with amnesia; as pre-medication; other indications, see sections 4.1.2, 4.8.2

Cautions; Contra-indications; Side-effects: see under Diazepam

Dose: by mouth, 2–3 mg the night before operation; 2–4 mg 1–2 hours before operation

By slow intravenous injection, preferably diluted with an equal volume of sodium chloride intravenous infusion 0.9% or water for injections, 50 micrograms/kg 30–45 minutes before operation

By intramuscular injection, diluted as above, 50 micrograms/kg 1–1½ hours before operation

PoM **Ativan**® (Wyeth)
Injection, lorazepam 4 mg/mL. Net price 1-mL amp = 40p
Tablets, see section 4.1.2

MIDAZOLAM

Indications: sedation with amnesia, and in conjunction with local anaesthesia; premedication, induction

Cautions; Contra-indications; Side-effects: see under Diazepam; see notes above for CSM warning; **important:** profound sedation with erythromycin and possibly other drugs, see **interactions:** Appendix 1 (anxiolytics and hypnotics)

Dose: sedation, *by intravenous injection* over 30 seconds, 2 mg (elderly 1–1.5 mg) followed after 2 minutes by increments of 0.5–1 mg if sedation not adequate; usual range 2.5–7.5 mg (about 70 micrograms/kg), elderly 1–2 mg

Premedication, *by intramuscular injection*, 70–100 micrograms/kg 30–60 minutes before surgery; usual dose 5 mg (2.5 mg in elderly)

Induction, *by slow intravenous injection*, 200–300 micrograms/kg (elderly 100–200 micrograms/kg); CHILD over 7 years, 150 micrograms/kg

Sedation of patients receiving intensive care, *by intravenous infusion*, initially 30–300 micrograms/kg given over 5 minutes, then 30–200 micrograms/kg/hour; reduce dose (or omit initial dose) in hypovolaemia, vasoconstriction, or hypothermia; low doses may be adequate if opioid analgesic also used; avoid abrupt withdrawal after prolonged administration (safety after more than 14 days not established)

PoM **Hypnovel**® (Roche)
Injection, midazolam (as hydrochloride) 2 mg/mL, net price 5-mL amp = £1.01; 5 mg/mL, 2-mL amp = 85p

TEMAZEPAM
Indications: premedication before minor surgery; anxiety before investigatory procedures; hypnotic, see section 4.1.1
Cautions; Contra-indications; Side-effects: see under Diazepam
Dose: *by mouth*, premedication, 20–40 mg (elderly, 10–20 mg) 1 hour before operation; CHILD 1 mg/kg (max. 30 mg)

Preparations
See section 4.1.1

CHLORMETHIAZOLE

Chlormethiazole is licensed for use as an intravenous infusion to maintain sleep during surgery carried out under regional anaesthesia, but is no longer in current use for this purpose.

CHLORMETHIAZOLE
(Clomethiazole)
Indications: sedative during regional anaesthesia (but see also notes above); other indications, see sections 4.1.1, 4.8.2, 4.10
Cautions; Contra-indications; Side-effects: see section 4.10
Dose: *by intravenous infusion*, as a 0.8% solution of chlormethiazole edisylate, induction 25 mL (200 mg)/minute for 1–2 minutes; maintenance 1–4 mL (8–32 mg)/minute
IMPORTANT. See special cautions for intravenous infusion, section 4.10

Preparations
See section 4.10

PHENOTHIAZINES AND RELATED

Neuroleptics such as **chlorpromazine** and **droperidol** are rarely used in the UK for premedication although chlorpromazine is licensed to prevent shivering in induction of hypothermia, it is no longer in current use for this purpose. **Trimeprazine** is used as a premedicant for children.

CHLORPROMAZINE HYDROCHLORIDE
Indications: see under Dose (but see also notes above); other indications, see section 4.2.1
Cautions; Contra-indications; Side-effects: see section 4.2.1
Dose: induction of hypothermia (to prevent shivering), *by deep intramuscular injection*, 25–50 mg every 6–8 hours; CHILD 1–12 years, initially 0.5–1 mg/kg, followed by maintenance 500 micrograms/kg every 4–6 hours

Preparations
See section 4.2.1

DROPERIDOL
Indications: anti-emetic, pre-operative sedation; other indications, see section 4.2.1
Cautions; Contra-indications; Side-effects: see section 4.2.1
Dose: premedication, *by intramuscular injection*, up to 10 mg 60 minutes before operation; CHILD 200–500 micrograms/kg
Neuroleptanalgesia, *by intravenous injection*, 5–15 mg at induction with an opioid analgesic; CHILD 200–300 micrograms/kg

PoM **Droleptan**® (Janssen)
Injection, droperidol 5 mg/mL. Net price 2-mL amp = 90p

PROMETHAZINE HYDROCHLORIDE
Indications: pre-operative sedative and antimuscarinic; anti-emetic, see section 4.6; other indications, see sections 3.4.1, 3.4.3
Cautions; Contra-indications; Side-effects: see section 4.6
Dose: premedication, *by mouth*, CHILD under 2 years not recommended, 2–5 years 15–20 mg, 5–10 years 20–25 mg
By deep intramuscular injection, 25–50 mg 1 hour before operation; CHILD 5–10 years, 6.25–12.5 mg

Preparations
See sections 3.4.1 and 15.1.4.3 (with pethidine)

TRIMEPRAZINE TARTRATE
(Alimemazine Tartrate)
Indications: pre-operative sedation, anti-emetic; other indications, see section 3.4.1
Cautions; Contra-indications; Side-effects: see notes above and section 3.4.1
Dose: *by mouth*, premedication, CHILD 2–7 years, up to 2 mg/kg 1–2 hours before operation

Preparations
See section 3.4.1

15.1.4.2 NON-OPIOID ANALGESICS

As NSAIDs do not depress respiration, do not impair gastro-intestinal motility, and do not cause dependence, they may be useful alternatives (or adjuncts) to the use of opioids for the relief of postoperative pain. They may be inadequate for the relief of severe pain.

Diclofenac, ketoprofen (section 10.1.1), and **ketorolac** can be given by injection as well as by mouth. Intramuscular injections of diclofenac and ketoprofen are given deep into the gluteal muscle to minimise pain and tissue damage; diclofenac can also be given by intravenous infusion for the treatment or prevention of postoperative pain. Ketorolac is less irritant on intramuscular injection but pain has been reported; it can also be given by intravenous injection.

DICLOFENAC SODIUM

Indications: postoperative pain; other indications see section 10.1.1

Cautions; Contra-indications; Side-effects: see section 10.1.1

INTRAVENOUS USE. Additional contra-indications include concomitant NSAID or anticoagulant use (including low-dose heparin), history of haemorrhagic diathesis, history of confirmed or suspected cerebrovascular bleeding, operations with high risk of haemorrhage, history of asthma, moderate or severe renal impairment, hypovolaemia, dehydration

Dose: *by deep intramuscular injection* into the gluteal muscle, 75 mg once daily (twice daily in severe cases) for max. 2 days

By intravenous infusion (in hospital setting), 75 mg over 30–120 minutes repeated if necessary after 4–6 hours for max. 2 days

Prevention of postoperative pain, initially after surgery 25–50 mg over 15–60 minutes then 5 mg/ hour for max. 2 days

By rectum, as suppositories, 75–150 mg daily in divided doses

Max. total daily dose by any route 150 mg

Preparations

See section 10.1.1

KETOPROFEN

Indications; Cautions; Contra-indications; Side-effects: see p. 413

KETOROLAC TROMETAMOL

Indications: short-term management of moderate to severe acute postoperative pain

Cautions: reduce dose in elderly and in those weighing less than 50 kg; reduce dose and monitor in mild renal impairment (avoid if moderate or severe, see also Appendix 3 and section 10.1.1); heart failure, hepatic impairment and other conditions leading to reduction in blood volume or in renal blood flow (including those taking diuretics); cardiac decompensation, hypertension or similar conditions (fluid retention and oedema reported); do not give with anticoagulants (including low-dose heparin), oxpentifylline, probenecid, lithium salts, or other NSAIDs; other **interactions:** Appendix 1 (NSAIDs) GASTRO-INTESTINAL EFFECTS. Elderly and debilitated more prone to risk of gastro-intestinal effects (risk increases with increased dose and duration); see also under Contra-indications and Side-effects below

Contra-indications: history of hypersensitivity to aspirin or any other NSAID (severe anaphylactic reactions reported), history of asthma, complete or partial syndrome of nasal polyps, angioedema or bronchospasm; history of peptic ulceration or gastro-intestinal bleeding; haemorrhagic diatheses (including coagulation disorders) and operations with high risk of haemorrhage or incomplete haemostasis; confirmed or suspected cerebrovascular bleeding; moderate or severe renal impairment; hypovolaemia or dehydration; pregnancy (including labour and delivery) and breast-feeding

Side-effects: side-effects reported include anaphylaxis (with rash, bronchospasm, laryngeal oedema and hypotension), fluid retention (see Cautions), nausea, dyspepsia, abdominal discomfort, bowel changes, peptic ulceration, gastro-intestinal bleeding (elderly at greater risk, see also above), pancreatitis, drowsiness, dizziness, headache, sweating, dry mouth, excessive thirst, mental and sensory changes, convulsions, myalgia, aseptic meningitis, hyponatraemia, hyperkalaemia, raised blood urea and creatinine, urinary symptoms and acute renal failure, flushing or pallor, bradycardia, hypertension, purpura, thrombocytopenia, inhibition of platelet aggregation and prolonged bleeding time, dyspnoea and pulmonary oedema, skin reactions (some severe, including Stevens-Johnson and Lyell's syndromes), postoperative wound haemorrhage, haematoma, epistaxis, oedema, liver function changes (discontinue if clinical symptoms); pain at injection site; for general side-effects of NSAIDs, see also section 10.1.1

Dose: *by mouth,* PATIENT over 16 years, 10 mg every 4–6 hours (ELDERLY every 6–8 hours); max. 40 mg daily; max. duration of treatment 7 days; CHILD under 16 years, not recommended

By intramuscular injection or by intravenous injection over not less than 15 seconds, PATIENT over 16 years, initially 10 mg, then 10–30 mg every 4–6 hours when required (every 2 hours in initial postoperative period); max. 90 mg daily (ELDERLY and patients weighing less than 50 kg max. 60 mg daily); max. duration of treatment 2 days by either route; CHILD under 16 years, not recommended

Note. Pain relief may not occur upwards of 30 minutes after intravenous or intramuscular injection. When converting from parenteral to oral administration, total combined dose on the day of converting should not exceed 90 mg (60 mg in the elderly and patients weighing less than 50 kg) of which the oral component should not exceed 40 mg; patients should be converted to oral route as soon as possible

PoM **Toradol**® (Roche)
Tablets, ivory, f/c, ketorolac trometamol 10 mg, net price 20-tab pack = £6.52. Label: 17, 21
Injection, ketorolac trometamol 10 mg/mL, net price 1-mL amp = £1.06; 30 mg/mL, 1-mL amp = £1.28

15.1.4.3 OPIOID ANALGESICS

Opioid analgesics were formerly commonly used as premedicants given intramuscularly about an hour before operation, usually combined with an antisialogogue. Sometimes they were combined with a phenothiazine or droperidol. The main side-effects of opioid analgesics are respiratory depression, cardiovascular depression, and nausea and vomiting. The principal advantages were that opioid analgesics provided analgesia persisting into the operative period giving a reduced chance of awareness during anaesthesia with full doses of muscle relaxants. Nowadays anaesthetists are more likely to give potent opioids by the intravenous route at induction. For **patient controlled analgesia** (PCA) consult **hospital protocols.**

INTRA-OPERATIVE ANALGESIA. Many of the conventional opioid analgesics are used to supplement general anaesthesia, usually in combination with nitrous oxide–oxygen and a muscle relaxant. Pethidine was the first to be used for this purpose but other drugs now available include alfentanil, fentanyl, meptazinol, nalbuphine, and phenoperidine.

Small doses of opioids given immediately before or with induction will reduce the induction dose and this is a popular technique in poor-risk patients. **Alfentanil** and **fentanyl** are particularly useful in this respect because of their rapid onset of action. Alfentanil may be preferable for short operations because of its brief duration of action; for long procedures it can be given as a continuous infusion.

Repeated intra-operative doses of analgesics should be given with care, since not only may the respiratory depression persist into the postoperative period but it may become apparent for the first time postoperatively when the patient is away from immediate nursing attention. The specific opioid antagonist, naloxone (section 15.1.7), will immediately reverse this respiratory depression but the dose may have to be repeated. It is important to bear in mind that in clinical doses it will also reverse most of the analgesia—*careful titration* is necessary to *avoid* this. An alternative approach is to use the specific respiratory stimulant, doxapram (section 15.1.7), which can be given in an infusion and which will not affect the opioid analgesia. The use of intra-operative opioids should be borne in mind when prescribing postoperative analgesics. In many instances they will delay the need for the first dose but caution is necessary since there may be some residual respiratory depression potentiated by the postoperative analgesic.

Fentanyl may produce severe respiratory depression, especially in patients with decreased respiratory function or when other respiratory depressant drugs have been given. Respiratory depression may be treated by artificial ventilation or be reversed by naloxone or doxapram (see above). Alfentanil may also cause severe respiratory depression, especially when other respiratory depressant drugs have already been given; this may be reversed with naloxone.

Meptazinol can be used for analgesia during or after operation. It is associated with nausea and vomiting, but is claimed to have a reduced incidence of respiratory depression.

For general notes on analgesics, see section 4.7.

ALFENTANIL

Indications: analgesia especially during short operative procedure and outpatient surgery; enhancement of anaesthesia; analgesia and suppression of respiratory activity in patients receiving intensive care with assisted ventilation, for up to 4 days

Cautions; Contra-indications; Side-effects: see section 4.7.2 and notes above

Dose: by intravenous injection, spontaneous respiration, ADULT, initially up to 500 micrograms over 30 seconds; supplemental, 250 micrograms

With assisted ventilation, ADULT and CHILD, initially 30–50 micrograms/kg; supplemental, 15 micrograms/kg

By intravenous infusion, with assisted ventilation, ADULT and CHILD, initially 50–100 micrograms/kg over 10 minutes *or* as a bolus, followed by maintenance of 0.5–1 micrograms/kg/minute

Analgesia and suppression of respiratory activity during intensive care, with assisted ventilation, *by intravenous infusion,* initially 2 mg/hour (approx. 30 micrograms/kg/hour) subsequently adjusted according to response (usual range 0.5–10 mg/hour); more rapid initial control may be obtained with an intravenous dose of 5 mg given in divided portions over 10 minutes (slowing if hypotension or bradycardia occur); additional doses of 0.5–1 mg may be given by intravenous injection during short painful procedures

CD Rapifen® (Janssen)

Injection, alfentanil 500 micrograms (as hydrochloride)/mL. Net price 2-mL amp = 72p; 10-mL amp = £3.31

Intensive care injection, alfentanil 5 mg (as hydrochloride)/mL. To be diluted before use. Net price 1-mL amp = £2.65

BUPRENORPHINE

Indications: peri-operative analgesia; premedication; analgesia in other situations, see section 4.7.2

Cautions; Contra-indications; Side-effects: see section 4.7.2; effects only partially reversed by naloxone

Dose: pain, *by slow intravenous injection,* 300–450 micrograms

Premedication, *by sublingual administration,* 400 micrograms

By intramuscular injection, 300 micrograms

Preparations
See section 4.7.2

FENTANYL

Indications: analgesia during operation, enhancement of anaesthesia; respiratory depressant in assisted respiration

Cautions; Contra-indications; Side-effects: see section 4.7.2 and notes above

Dose: by intravenous injection, with spontaneous respiration, 50–200 micrograms, then 50 micrograms as required; CHILD 3–5 micrograms/kg, then 1 microgram/kg as required

With assisted ventilation, 0.3–3.5 mg, then 100–200 micrograms as required; CHILD 15 micrograms/kg, then 1–3 micrograms/kg as required

▼ **CD Durogesic®**: see section 4.7.2
CD Sublimaze® (Janssen)
Injection, fentanyl 50 micrograms (as citrate)/mL. Net price 2-mL amp = 24p; 10-mL amp = £1.17
Available as a generic from Antigen, David Bull

MEPTAZINOL
See section 4.7.2

MORPHINE SULPHATE
Indications: analgesia during and after operation; enhancement of anaesthesia; pre-operative sedation; analgesia in other situations, see section 4.7.2

Cautions; Contra-indications; Side-effects: see section 4.7.2 and notes above

Dose: by subcutaneous or intramuscular injection, up to 10 mg 1–1½ hours before operation; CHILD, *by intramuscular injection*, 150 micrograms/kg. See also section 4.7.2 for analgesia

CD Morphine Sulphate Injection, morphine sulphate, 10 mg/mL. Net price 1-mL amp = 54p; other strengths see section 4.7.2

CD Morphine and Atropine Injection, morphine sulphate 10 mg, atropine sulphate 600 micrograms/mL. Net price 1-mL amp = £1.86
Dose: premedication, by subcutaneous injection, 0.5–1 mL

NALBUPHINE HYDROCHLORIDE
Indications: peri-operative analgesia; premedication; analgesia in other situations, see section 4.7.2

Cautions; Contra-indications; Side-effects: see section 4.7.2 and notes above; also caution in ambulant patients (impairment of mental and physical ability)

Dose: acute pain, *by subcutaneous, intramuscular, or intravenous injection*, 10–20 mg, adjusted according to response; CHILD up to 300 micrograms/kg repeated once or twice as necessary. See also section 4.7.2 for analgesia
Premedication, *by subcutaneous, intramuscular, or intravenous injection*, 100–200 micrograms/kg
Induction, *by intravenous injection*, 0.3–1 mg/kg over 10–15 minutes
Intra-operative analgesia, *by intravenous injection*, 250–500 micrograms/kg at 30-minute intervals

PoM Nubain® (Du Pont)
Injection, nalbuphine hydrochloride 10 mg/mL. Net price 1-mL amp = 73p; 2-mL amp = £1.13

PAPAVERETUM
IMPORTANT. Do **not** confuse with papaverine (see section 7.4.5)

A mixture of 253 parts of morphine hydrochloride, 23 parts of papaverine hydrochloride and 20 parts of codeine hydrochloride

REFORMULATION. *BP 1993, Addendum 1994*, includes the following explanation concerning the reformulation of papaveretum: *papaveretum injection* contains the three alkaloids *morphine, papaverine* and *codeine*; in reformulating the injection to remove *noscapine*, the amounts of the other three alkaloids have been maintained; thus the total amount of material per mL has decreased. Before reformulation the *lower strength injection* (which provides *the equivalent of 5 mg of the major component, morphine*) contained 10 mg per mL of the four-component material; it now contains 7.7 mg *of papaveretum per mL*. Likewise, before reformulation the *higher strength injection* (which provides *the equivalent of 10 mg of morphine*) contained 20 mg per mL of the four-component material; it now contains *15.4 mg of papaveretum per mL*.

The **CSM** has advised that to avoid confusion the figures of 7.7 mg/mL or 15.4 mg/mL should be used for prescribing purposes.

Indications: postoperative analgesia; premedication

Cautions; Contra-indications; Side-effects: see section 4.7.2 and notes above

Dose: by subcutaneous, intramuscular, or intravenous injection, 7.7–15.4 mg repeated every 4 hours if necessary (ELDERLY initially 7.7 mg); CHILD up to 1 month 115.5 micrograms/kg, 1–12 months 115.5–154 micrograms/kg, 1–12 years 154–231 micrograms/kg

INTRAVENOUS DOSE. In general the intravenous dose should be quarter to half corresponding subcutaneous or intramuscular dose.

CD Papaveretum (Non-proprietary)
Injection, papaveretum 7.7 mg/mL (providing the equivalent of 5 mg of anhydrous morphine/mL), net price 1-mL amp = 71p; 15.4 mg/mL (providing the equivalent of 10 mg of anhydrous morphine/mL), 1-mL amp = 81p
Available from Martindale
Note. The name Omnopon® was formerly used for papaveretum preparations.

With hyoscine
CD Papaveretum and Hyoscine Injection, papaveretum 15.4 mg (providing the equivalent of 10 mg of anhydrous morphine), hyoscine hydrobromide 400 micrograms/mL. Net price 1-mL amp = 83p
Dose: premedication, by subcutaneous or intramuscular injection, 0.5–1 mL

PETHIDINE HYDROCHLORIDE
Indications: peri-operative analgesia, enhancement of anaesthesia, for basal narcosis with phenothiazines; premedication; analgesia in other situations, see section 4.7.2

Cautions; Contra-indications; Side-effects: convulsions may occur with excessive doses; see section 4.7.2 and notes above

Dose: premedication, *by intramuscular injection*, 25–100 mg 1 hour before operation; CHILD 0.5–2 mg/kg

Adjunct to nitrous oxide–oxygen, *by slow intravenous injection*, 10–25 mg repeated when required

See also section 4.7.2 for analgesia

CD Pethidine (Non-proprietary)
Injection, pethidine hydrochloride 50 mg/mL, net price 1-mL amp = 31p; 2-mL amp = 32p; 10 mg/mL, 5-mL amp = 97p; 10-mL amp = £1.02
Various strengths available from Martindale, Roche
Tablets, see section 4.7.2

With promethazine
CD Pamergan P100® (Martindale)
Injection, pethidine hydrochloride 50 mg, promethazine hydrochloride 25 mg/mL. Net price 2-mL amp = 69p
Dose: premedication, 2 mL by intramuscular injection 1–1½ hours before operation; CHILD, by intramuscular injection, 8–12 years 0.75 mL, 13–16 years 1 mL

PHENOPERIDINE HYDROCHLORIDE
Indications: analgesia during operation, enhancement of anaesthetics; respiratory depressant in prolonged assisted respiration
Cautions; Contra-indications; Side-effects: see under Pethidine Hydrochloride and Fentanyl. Doses above 1 mg cause respiratory depression and require assisted ventilation
Dose: by intravenous injection, with spontaneous respiration, up to 1 mg, then 500 micrograms every 40–60 minutes as required; CHILD 30–50 micrograms/kg
With assisted ventilation, 2–5mg, then 1 mg as required; CHILD 100–150 micrograms/kg

CD Operidine® (Janssen)
Injection, phenoperidine hydrochloride 1 mg/mL. Net price 2-mL amp = 76p; 10-mL amp = £3.95

TRAMADOL HYDROCHLORIDE
See section 4.7.2

15.1.5   Muscle relaxants
Muscle relaxants used in anaesthesia are also known as **neuromuscular blocking drugs**. By specific blockade of the neuromuscular junction they enable light levels of anaesthesia to be employed with adequate relaxation of the muscles of the abdomen and diaphragm. They also relax the vocal cords and allow the passage of a tracheal tube. Their action differs from the muscle relaxants acting on the spinal cord or brain which are used in musculoskeletal disorders (see section 10.2.2).

Patients who have received a muscle relaxant should **always** have their respiration assisted or controlled until the drug has been inactivated or antagonised (section 15.1.6).

NON-DEPOLARISING MUSCLE RELAXANTS

Drugs of this group (also known as competitive muscle relaxants) cause blockade by competing with acetylcholine at the receptor site at the neuromuscular junction. These drugs are best suited to the production of paralysis of long duration. They have a slower, less complete action than suxamethonium. They may be used during surgical operations and for patients receiving long-term ventilation in intensive care units. Their action may be reversed with anticholinesterases such as neostigmine (section 15.1.6)—patients with myasthenia gravis have an increased susceptibility.

Atracurium and **vecuronium** are much more widely employed than the other muscle relaxants, atracurium because of its non-enzymatic elimination and vecuronium because it has the fewest side-effects.

Atracurium has a duration of action of 15 to 35 minutes. Histamine release may occur. The drug is without vagolytic or sympatholytic properties. It has an advantage over other non-depolarising muscle relaxants in patients with renal or hepatic impairment, as it is degraded by non-enzymatic Hofmann elimination and ester hydrolysis, which is independent of liver and kidney function. It is non-cumulative on repeated dosage. Its action is reversed by neostigmine.

Vecuronium has a duration of action of 20 to 30 minutes. Large doses may have a cumulative effect. The drug does not generally cause histamine release, sympathetic blockade, or vagolytic effects.

Pancuronium does not cause ganglionic blockade or significant changes in blood pressure and may therefore be favoured when it is important to maintain cardiac output.

Gallamine causes undesirable tachycardia by its vagolytic action. It should be avoided in patients with severe renal disease.

Mivacurium has a duration of action of about 15 minutes. Histamine release may occur particularly on rapid injection. It does not cause significant vagolytic effects. More prolonged muscle paralysis may occur in patients with low or atypical plasma pseudocholinesterase enzymes.

Rocuronium is a new competitive muscle relaxant reported to act within 1–2 minutes and to have a duration of action of 30 to 40 minutes. It is reported to be virtually free of cardiovascular effects.

Cisatracurium, a recently introduced muscle relaxant, is a single isomer of atracurium which is a mixture of several isomers. It undergoes non-enzymatic elimination similar to atracurium. Cisatracurium lacks the histamine releasing potential of atracurium and thus provides greater cardiovascular stability.

ATRACURIUM BESYLATE
(Atracurium Besilate)
Indications: non-depolarising muscle relaxant of short to medium duration

Cautions; Contra-indications; Side-effects: see notes above; **interactions:** Appendix 1 (muscle relaxants)

Dose: by intravenous injection, ADULT and CHILD over 1 month initially 300–600 micrograms/kg, then 100–200 micrograms/kg as required

By intravenous infusion, 5–10 micrograms/kg/minute (300–600 micrograms/kg/hour)

PoM **Tracrium**® (Wellcome)

Injection, atracurium besylate 10 mg/mL. Net price 2.5-mL amp = £1.86; 5-mL amp = £3.38; 25-mL amp = £14.53

CISATRACURIUM

Indications: non-depolarising muscle relaxant of medium duration

Cautions; Contra-indications; Side-effects: see notes above; **interactions:** Appendix 1 (muscle relaxants)

Dose: by intravenous injection, intubation, 150 micrograms/kg; maintenance, 30 micrograms/kg approximately every 20 minutes

CHILD over 2 years, initially, 100 micrograms/kg; maintenance, 20 micrograms/kg approximately every 9 minutes

By intravenous infusion, ADULT and CHILD over 2 years, initially, 3 micrograms/kg/minute, *then after stabilisation,* 1–2 micrograms/kg/minute; dose reduced by up to 40% with enflurane or isoflurane

CHILD under 2 years not recommended

▼ PoM **Nimbex**® (GlaxoWellcome)

Injection, cisatracurium (as besylate) 2 mg/mL, net price 2.5-mL amp = £2.30, 10-mL amp = £8.50

Forte injection, cisatracurium (as besylate) 5 mg/mL, net price 30-mL vial = £35.00

GALLAMINE TRIETHIODIDE

Indications: non-depolarising muscle relaxant of medium duration

Cautions; Contra-indications; Side-effects: see notes above; reduce dose in renal impairment (avoid if severe); **interactions:** Appendix 1 (muscle relaxants)

Dose: by intravenous injection, 80–120 mg, then 20–40 mg as required; NEONATE, 600 micrograms/kg; CHILD, 1.5 mg/kg

PoM **Flaxedil**® (Rhône-Poulenc Rorer)

Injection, gallamine triethiodide 40 mg/mL. Net price 2-mL amp = 72p

---

MIVACURIUM CHLORIDE

Indications: non-depolarising muscle relaxant of short duration

Cautions; Contra-indications; Side-effects: see notes above; **interactions:** Appendix 1 (muscle relaxants)

Dose: by intravenous injection, 70–250 micrograms/kg; maintenance 100 micrograms/kg every 15 minutes; CHILD 2–6 months initially 150 micrograms/kg, 7 months–12 years initially 200 micrograms/kg; maintenance (CHILD 2 months–12 years) 100 micrograms/kg every 6–9 minutes

Note. Doses up to 150 micrograms/kg may be given over 5–15 seconds, higher doses should be given over 30 seconds. In patients with asthma, cardiovascular disease or those who are sensitive to falls in arterial blood pressure give over 60 seconds

By intravenous infusion, maintenance of block, 8–10 micrograms/kg/minute, adjusted if necessary every 3 minutes by 1 microgram/kg/minute to usual dose of 6–7 micrograms/kg/minute; CHILD 2 months–12 years, usual dose 11–14 micrograms/kg/minute

PoM **Mivacron**® (Wellcome)

Injection, mivacurium 2 mg/mL (as chloride), net price 5-mL amp = £2.86; 10-mL amp = £4.62

PANCURONIUM BROMIDE

Indications: non-depolarising muscle relaxant of medium duration

Cautions; Contra-indications; Side-effects: see notes above; caution in hepatic impairment; reduce dose in renal impairment; **interactions:** Appendix 1 (muscle relaxants)

Dose: by intravenous injection, initially for intubation 50–100 micrograms/kg then 10–20 micrograms/kg as required; CHILD initially 60–100 micrograms/kg, then 10–20 micrograms/kg, NEONATE 30–40 micrograms/kg initially then 10–20 micrograms/kg

Intensive care, *by intravenous injection,* 60 micrograms/kg every 1–1½ hours

PoM **Pavulon**® (Organon-Teknika)

Injection, pancuronium bromide 2 mg/mL. Net price 2-mL amp = 66p

Available as a generic from David Bull

ROCURONIUM BROMIDE

Indications: non-depolarising muscle relaxant of medium duration

Cautions; Contra-indications; Side-effects: see notes above; caution in hepatic and renal impairment; **interactions:** Appendix 1 (muscle relaxants)

Dose: by intravenous injection, intubation, 600 micrograms/kg; maintenance, 150 micrograms/kg

By intravenous infusion, 300–600 micrograms/kg/hour (after initial intravenous injection of 600 micrograms/kg)

CHILD similar sensitivity to adults; INFANT under 1 month not recommended

▼ PoM **Esmeron**® (Organon-Teknika)

Injection, rocuronium bromide 10 mg/mL, net price 5-mL amp = £5.33, 10-mL amp = £10.67

VECURONIUM BROMIDE

Indications: non-depolarising muscle relaxant of short to medium duration

Cautions; Contra-indications; Side-effects: see notes above; reduce dose in renal impairment; **interactions:** Appendix 1 (muscle relaxants)

Dose: by intravenous injection, intubation, 80–100 micrograms/kg; maintenance 20–30 micrograms/kg according to response; NEONATE and INFANT up to 4 months, initially 10–20 micrograms/kg then incremental doses to achieve response; CHILD over 5 months, as adult dose (up to 1 year onset more rapid and high intubation dose may not be required)

By intravenous infusion, 50–80 micrograms/kg/hour (after initial intravenous injection of 40–100 micrograms/kg)

PoM Norcuron® (Organon-Teknika)
Injection, powder for reconstitution, vecuronium bromide. Net price 10-mg vial = £4.23 (with water for injections)

DEPOLARISING MUSCLE RELAXANTS

Suxamethonium is the only commonly used drug of this group. With a 5-minute duration of action it is ideal for passage of a tracheal tube but may be used in repeated dosage for longer procedures.

It acts by mimicking acetylcholine at the neuromuscular junction but hydrolysis is much slower than for acetylcholine; depolarisation is therefore prolonged and neuromuscular blockade results.

It produces rapid, complete, and predictable paralysis, and recovery is spontaneous. Unlike the non-depolarising muscle relaxants its action cannot be reversed.

Suxamethonium should be given after induction of anaesthesia because paralysis is usually preceded by painful muscle fasciculation. There is a transient rise in plasma potassium and creatine phosphokinase and there may be muscle pains postoperatively. Hypersensitivity (or a previous anaphylactic reaction) is an important contra-indication to suxamethonium; it is also contra-indicated in severe liver disease and in burned patients. Premedication with atropine is desirable.

Prolonged muscle paralysis may occur in patients with low or atypical plasma pseudocholinesterase enzymes. Prolonged paralysis may also occur in **dual block**, which occurs after repeated doses of suxamethonium have been used and is caused by the development of a non-depolarising block following the primary depolarising block. Assisted ventilation should be continued until muscle function is restored.

SUXAMETHONIUM CHLORIDE

Indications: depolarising muscle relaxant of short duration

Cautions; Contra-indications; Side-effects: see notes above; **interactions:** Appendix 1 (muscle relaxants)

Dose: by intravenous injection, ADULT 600 micrograms/kg (range 0.3–1.1 mg/kg depending on degree of relaxation required); usual range 20–100 mg; INFANT under 1 year, 2 mg/kg; CHILD 1–12 years, 1–2 mg/kg

By intravenous infusion, as a 0.1% solution, 2–5 mg/minute (2–5 mL/minute)

PoM Suxamethonium Chloride (Non-proprietary)
Injection, suxamethonium chloride 50 mg/mL
Available from Antigen net price 2-mL amp = 24p, Evans (Scoline® net price 2-mL amp = 31p), Wellcome (Anectine® net price 2-mL amp = 73p)

15.1.6   Anticholinesterases used in anaesthesia

Anticholinesterases reverse the effects of the non-depolarising (competitive) muscle relaxant drugs such as pancuronium but they prolong the action of the depolarising muscle relaxant drug suxamethonium.

Edrophonium has a transient action.

Neostigmine has a longer duration of action than edrophonium. It is the specific drug for reversal of non-depolarising (competitive) blockade. It acts within one minute of intravenous injection and lasts for 20 to 30 minutes; a second dose may then be necessary. Atropine or glycopyrronium (section 15.1.3) should be given before or with neostigmine in order to prevent bradycardia, excessive salivation, and other muscarinic actions of neostigmine.

EDROPHONIUM CHLORIDE

Indications: see under Dose

Cautions; Contra-indications; Side-effects: see section 10.2.1 and notes above. Atropine should also be given

Dose: brief reversal of non-depolarising neuromuscular blockade, *by intravenous injection* over several minutes, 500–700 micrograms/kg (after or with atropine sulphate 600 micrograms)
Diagnosis of myasthenia gravis, section 10.2.1

PoM Camsilon[1]® (Cambridge)
Injection, edrophonium chloride 10 mg/mL. Net price 1-mL amp = £1.01
1. Formerly Tensilon®

NEOSTIGMINE METHYLSULPHATE

Indications: see under Dose

Cautions; Contra-indications; Side-effects: see section 10.2.1 and notes above. Atropine should also be given

Dose: reversal of non-depolarising neuromuscular blockade, *by intravenous injection* over 1 minute, 50–70 micrograms/kg (max. 5 mg) after or with atropine sulphate 0.6–1.2 mg
Myasthenia gravis, see section 10.2.1

PoM Prostigmin® (Roche)
Injection, neostigmine methylsulphate 2.5 mg/mL. Net price 1-mL amp = 16p

With glycopyrronium
PoM Robinul-Neostigmine® (Anpharm)
Injection, neostigmine methylsulphate 2.5 mg, glycopyrronium bromide 500 micrograms/mL. Net price 1-mL amp = 53p

> *Dose:* by intravenous injection over 10–30 seconds, 1–2 mL *or* 0.02 mL/kg; CHILD 0.02 mL/kg (*or* 0.2 mL/kg of a 1 in 10 dilution using water for injections or sodium chloride injection 0.9%)

15.1.7 Antagonists for central and respiratory depression

The opioid antagonist **naloxone** can be used to reverse respiratory depression caused by opioid analgesics (**important:** unless the dosage is adjusted with considerable care, analgesia may also be reversed). **Doxapram** is a respiratory stimulant which does not reverse the other effects of opioid analgesics.

Flumazenil is a benzodiazepine antagonist for the reversal of the central sedative effects of benzodiazepines after anaesthetic and similar procedures. Flumazenil has a shorter half-life than that of diazepam and midazolam (and there is a risk that patients may become resedated).

DOXAPRAM HYDROCHLORIDE

Indications: see under Dose

Cautions: give with oxygen in severe irreversible airways obstruction or severely decreased lung compliance (because of increased work load of breathing); give with beta$_2$-adrenoceptor stimulant in bronchoconstriction; hypertension (avoid if severe), impaired cardiac reserve; hepatic impairment, pregnancy (compelling reasons only); **interactions:** Appendix 1 (doxapram)

Contra-indications: severe hypertension, status asthmaticus, coronary artery disease, thyrotoxicosis, epilepsy, physical obstruction of respiratory tract

Side-effects: moderate increase in blood pressure and heart rate; dizziness, perineal warmth; side-effects reported in postoperative period (causal effect not established) include muscle fasiculation, hyperactivity, sweating, confusion, hallucinations, cough, dyspnoea, laryngospasm, bronchospasm, sinus tachycardia, bradycardia, extrasystoles, nausea, vomiting and salivation

Dose: postoperative respiratory depression, *by intravenous injection* over at least 30 seconds, 1–1.5 mg/kg repeated if necessary after intervals of 1 hour *or* alternatively *by intravenous infusion*, 2–3 mg/minute adjusted according to response; CHILD not recommended

Acute respiratory failure, *by intravenous infusion*, 1.5–4 mg/minute adjusted according to response (given concurrently with oxygen and whenever possible monitor with frequent measurement of blood gas tensions); CHILD not recommended

PoM Dopram® (Anpharm)
Injection, doxapram hydrochloride 20 mg/mL. Net price 5-mL amp = £1.07
Intravenous infusion, doxapram hydrochloride 2 mg/mL in glucose 5%. Net price 500-mL bottle = £11.17

FLUMAZENIL

Indications: reversal of sedative effects of benzodiazepines in anaesthetic, intensive care, and diagnostic procedures

Cautions: short-acting (repeat doses may be necessary—benzodiazepine effects may persist for at least 24 hours); benzodiazepine dependence (may precipitate withdrawal symptoms); ensure neuromuscular blockade cleared before giving; avoid rapid injection in high-risk or anxious patients and following major surgery; hepatic impairment; severe head injury (rapid reversal of benzodiazepine sedation may increase risk of raised intracranial pressure); elderly, children, pregnancy and breast-feeding

Contra-indications: epileptics who have received prolonged benzodiazepine therapy

Side-effects: nausea, vomiting, and flushing; if wakening too rapid, agitation, anxiety, and fear; transient increase in blood pressure and heart-rate in intensive care patients; very rarely convulsions (particularly in epileptics)

Dose: by intravenous injection, 200 micrograms over 15 seconds, then 100 micrograms at 60-second intervals if required; usual dose range, 300–600 micrograms; max. total dose 1 mg (2 mg in intensive care); question aetiology if no response to repeated doses

By intravenous infusion, if drowsiness recurs after injection, 100–400 micrograms/hour, adjusted according to level of arousal

PoM Anexate® (Roche)
Injection, flumazenil 100 micrograms/mL. Net price 5-mL amp = £16.32

NALOXONE HYDROCHLORIDE

Indications: reversal of opioid-induced respiratory depression

Cautions: cardiovascular disease or those receiving cardiotoxic drugs (serious adverse cardiovascular effects reported); physical dependence on opioids (precipitates withdrawal); pain (see also under Titration of Dose, below); has short duration of action

TITRATION OF DOSE. When used postoperatively, the dose should be titrated for each patient in order to obtain optimum respiratory response while maintaining **adequate** analgesia

Side-effects: nausea and vomiting reported; tachycardia and fibrillation also reported

Dose: by intravenous injection, 100–200 micrograms (1.5–3 micrograms/kg); if response inadequate, increments of 100 micrograms every 2 minutes; further doses *by intramuscular injection* after 1–2 hours if required

CHILD, by intravenous injection, 10 micrograms/kg; subsequent dose of 100 micrograms/kg if no response; if intravenous route not possible, may be given in divided doses by *intramuscular or subcutaneous injection*

NEONATE, *by subcutaneous, intramuscular, or intravenous injection,* 10 micrograms/kg, repeated every 2 to 3 minutes *or* 200 micrograms (60 micrograms/kg) *by intramuscular injection* as a single dose at birth (onset of action slower)

PoM **Naloxone** (Non-proprietary)

Injection, naloxone hydrochloride 20 micrograms/mL. Net price 2-mL amp = 67p

Injection, naloxone hydrochloride 400 micrograms/mL—see under Emergency Treatment of Poisoning p. 22

PoM **Narcan**® —see under Emergency Treatment of Poisoning p. 22

PoM **Narcan Neonatal**® (Du Pont)

Injection, naloxone hydrochloride 20 micrograms/mL. Net price 2-mL amp = £3.48

15.1.8   Drugs for malignant hyperthermia

Dantrolene is used in the treatment of malignant hyperthermia which is a rare but potentially lethal complication of anaesthesia. It is characterised by a rapid rise in temperature, increasing muscle rigidity, tachycardia, and acidosis and can be triggered off by volatile anaesthetics, and suxamethonium. Dantrolene acts on skeletal muscle by interfering with calcium efflux in the muscle cell and stopping the contractile process. Known trigger agents should be avoided during anaesthesia.

DANTROLENE SODIUM

Indications: malignant hyperthermia

Cautions: avoid extravasation; **interactions:** Appendix 1 (muscle relaxants)

Dose: *by rapid intravenous injection*, 1 mg/kg, repeated as required to a cumulative max. of 10 mg/kg

PoM **Dantrium Intravenous**® (Procter & Gamble Pharm.)

Injection, powder for reconstitution, dantrolene sodium. Net price 20-mg vial = £22.52 (hosp. only)

15.2   Local anaesthesia

The use of local anaesthetics by injection or by application to mucous membranes to produce local analgesia is discussed in this section.

See also section 1.7 (colon and rectum), section 11.7 (eye), section 12.3 (oropharynx), and section 13.3 (skin).

USE OF LOCAL ANAESTHETICS. Local anaesthetic drugs act by causing a reversible block to conduction along nerve fibres. The drugs used vary widely in their potency, toxicity, duration of action, stability, solubility in water, and ability to penetrate mucous membranes. These variations determine their suitability for use by various routes, e.g. topical (surface), infiltration, plexus, epidural (extradural) or spinal block.

ADMINISTRATION. In estimating the safe dosage of these drugs it is important to take account of the rate at which they are *absorbed and excreted* as well as their potency. The patient's *age, weight, physique*, and *clinical condition*, the *degree of vas-*

cularity of the area to which the drug is to be applied, and the *duration of administration* are other factors which must be taken into account.

Local anaesthetics do not rely on the circulation to transport them to their sites of action, but uptake into the general circulation is important in terminating their action. Following most regional anaesthetic procedures, maximum arterial plasma concentrations of anaesthetic develop within about 10 to 25 minutes, so **careful surveillance** for toxic effects is necessary during the first 30 minutes after injection. Great care must be taken to avoid accidental intravascular injection.

Epidural anaesthesia is commonly used during surgery, often combined with general anaesthesia, because of its protective effect against the stress response of surgery. It is often used when good postoperative pain relief is essential (e.g. aortic aneurysm surgery or major gut surgery).

TOXICITY. Toxic effects associated with the local anaesthetics are usually a result of excessively high plasma concentrations, and systemic effects whether associated with acute or cumulative overdose or with accidental intravascular injection. Hypersensitivity reactions occur mainly with the ester-type local anaesthetics such as amethocaine, benzocaine, cocaine, and procaine; reactions are less frequent with the amide types such as lignocaine, bupivacaine, and prilocaine.

Toxicity may occur with repeated dosages due to accumulation of the drug, and reducing doses should therefore be given. Toxic effects may also occur if the injection is too rapid. Local anaesthetics should **not** be injected into inflamed or infected tissues nor should they be applied to the traumatised urethra. Under these conditions the drug may be so rapidly absorbed that a systemic rather than a local reaction is produced.

USE OF VASOCONSTRICTORS. Most local anaesthetics, with the exception of cocaine, cause dilatation of blood vessels. The addition of a vasoconstrictor such as **adrenaline** diminishes local blood flow, slows the rate of absorption of the local anaesthetic, and prolongs its local effect. Care is necessary when using adrenaline for this purpose because, in excess, it may produce ischaemic necrosis.

Adrenaline should **not** be added to injections used in digits and appendages. When adrenaline is included the final concentration should be 1 in 200 000 (5 micrograms/mL). In dental surgery, up to 1 in 80 000 (12.5 micrograms/mL) of adrenaline is used with local anaesthetics. There is no justification for using higher concentrations.

The total dose of adrenaline should **not** exceed 500 micrograms and it is essential to not exceed a concentration of 1 in 200 000 (5 micrograms/mL) if more than 50 mL of the mixture is to be injected. For general cautions associated with the use of adrenaline, see section 2.7.3. For drug interactions, see Appendix 1 (sympathomimetics).

LIGNOCAINE

Lignocaine is effectively absorbed from mucous membranes and is a useful surface anaesthetic in concentrations of 2 to 4%. Except for surface anaesthesia, solutions should not usually exceed 1% in strength. The duration of the block (with adrenaline) is about 1½ hours.

LIGNOCAINE HYDROCHLORIDE
(Lidocaine Hydrochloride)

Indications: see under Dose; also dental anaesthesia (see next page); ventricular arrhythmias (section 2.3.2)

Cautions: epilepsy, hepatic or respiratory impairment, impaired cardiac conduction, bradycardia; porphyria (see section 9.8.2); reduce dose in elderly or debilitated; resuscitative equipment should be available; see section 2.3.2 for effects on heart; **interactions:** Appendix 1 (lignocaine)

Contra-indications: hypovolaemia, complete heart block; do not use solutions containing adrenaline for anaesthesia in appendages

Side-effects: CNS effects include confusion, respiratory depression and convulsions; hypotension and bradycardia (may lead to cardiac arrest); hypersensitivity reported; see also notes above

Dose: infiltration anaesthesia, *by injection*, according to patient's weight and nature of procedure, max. 200 mg (or 500 mg if given in solutions containing adrenaline)—see also Administration on p. 534 and see also **important** warning below

Intravenous regional anaesthesia and nerve blocks, seek expert advice

Surface anaesthesia, usual strengths 2–4%, see preparations below

Important: the licensed doses stated above may not be appropriate in some settings and expert advice should be sought

Lignocaine hydrochloride injections

PoM **Lignocaine** (Non-proprietary)

Injection 0.5%, lignocaine hydrochloride 5 mg/mL, net price 10-mL amp = 22p

Injection 1%, lignocaine hydrochloride 10 mg/mL, net price 2-mL amp = 11p; 5-mL amp = 16p; 10-mL amp = 35p; 20-mL amp = 40p

Injection 2%, lignocaine hydrochloride 20 mg/mL, net price 2-mL amp = 17p; 5-mL amp = 19p

PoM **Min-I-Jet® Lignocaine Hydrochloride with Adrenaline** (IMS)

Injection 0.5% with adrenaline 1 in 200 000, lignocaine hydrochloride 5 mg/mL, adrenaline 1 in 200 000 (5 micrograms/mL). Net price 5-mL disposable syringe = £3.88

PoM **Xylocaine®** (Astra)

Injection 0.5%, anhydrous lignocaine hydrochloride 5 mg/mL. Net price 20-mL vial = 65p

Injection 0.5% with adrenaline 1 in 200 000, anhydrous lignocaine hydrochloride 5 mg/mL, adrenaline 1 in 200 000 (5 micrograms/mL). Net price 20-mL vial = 67p

Injection 1%, anhydrous lignocaine hydrochloride 10 mg/mL. Net price 20-mL vial = 67p

Injection 1% with adrenaline 1 in 200 000, anhydrous lignocaine hydrochloride 10 mg/mL, adrenaline 1 in 200 000 (5 micrograms/mL). Net price 20-mL vial = 69p

Injection 2%, anhydrous lignocaine hydrochloride 20 mg/mL. Net price 20-mL vial = 71p

Injection 2% with adrenaline 1 in 200 000, anhydrous lignocaine hydrochloride 20 mg/mL, adrenaline 1 in 200 000 (5 micrograms/mL). Net price 20-mL vial = 73p

Lignocaine injections for dental use

Note. Consult expert dental sources for specific advice in relation to dose of lignocaine for dental anaesthesia

A large variety of lignocaine injections, plain or with adrenaline or noradrenaline, is also available in dental cartridges under the names **Lignospan®**, **Lignostab A®**, **Xylocaine®**, and **Xylotox®**.

Lignocaine for surface anaesthesia

Important. Rapid and extensive absorption may result in systemic side-effects

PoM **Emla®** (Astra)

Drug Tariff cream, lignocaine 2.5%, prilocaine 2.5%. Net price 5-g tube = £1.73

Surgical pack cream, lignocaine 2.5%, prilocaine 2.5%. Net price 30-g tube = £10.25

Premedication pack cream, lignocaine 2.5%, prilocaine 2.5%. Net price 10 × 5-g tube with 25 occlusive dressings = £19.50

Anaesthesia before e.g. venepuncture (not for infants), apply a thick layer under an occlusive dressing 1–5 hours before procedure; split skin grafting, apply a thick layer under an occlusive dressing 2–5 hours before procedure; genital warts (not for children), apply up to 10 g 5–10 minutes before removal

Cautions: not for wounds, mucous membranes (except genital warts in adults) or atopic dermatitis; avoid use near eyes or middle ear; although systemic absorption is low, caution in anaemia, or congenital or acquired methaemoglobinaemia (see also Prilocaine, p. 536); *side-effects* include transient paleness, redness, and oedema; **contra-indicated** in infants under 1 year

Instillagel® (CliniFlex)

Gel, lignocaine 2%, chlorhexidine gluconate solution 0.25%, in a sterile lubricant basis in disposable syringe. Net price 6-mL syringe = £1.44; 11-mL syringe = £1.61

Dose: 6–11 mL into urethra

PoM **Laryng-O-Jet®** (IMS)

Jet spray 4% (disposable kit for laryngotracheal anaesthesia), lignocaine hydrochloride 40 mg/mL. Net price per unit (4-mL vial and disposable sterile cannula with cover and vial injector) = £4.55

Dose: usually 160 mg (4 mL) as a single dose instilled as jet spray into lumen of larynx and trachea (reduce dose according to size, age and condition of patient); max. 200 mg (5 mL)

Caution: may be rapidly and almost completely absorbed from respiratory tract and systemic side-effects may occur; extreme caution if mucosa has been traumatised or if sepsis present

Xylocaine® (Astra)

Antiseptic gel, anhydrous lignocaine hydrochloride 2%, chlorhexidine gluconate solution 0.25% in a sterile lubricant basis. Net price 20 g = £1.06; 20-g single-use syringe (Accordion®) = 98p

Dose: into urethra, men 10 mL followed by 3–5 mL; women 5–10 mL

Gel, anhydrous lignocaine hydrochloride 2%, in a sterile lubricant water-miscible basis. Net price 20 g = 76p; 20-g single-use syringe (Accordion®) = 98p

Additives: include hydroxybenzoates (parabens)
Dose:
Into urethra, men 10 mL, followed by further 10 mL (total of up to 40 mL for cystoscopy); women 5–10 mL
Endoscopy, 10–20 mL
Endotracheal intubation, 5 mL applied to surface of tube (avoid introducing gel into lumen)

Ointment, lignocaine 5% in a water-miscible basis. Net price 15 g = 80p

Additives: include propylene glycol
Dose: max. 35 g in 24 hours

Spray (= pump spray), lignocaine 10% (100 mg/g) supplying 10 mg lignocaine/dose; 500 spray doses per container. Net price 50-mL bottle = £3.13

Dose: dental practice, 1–5 doses; maxillary sinus puncture, 3 doses; during delivery in obstetrics, up to 20 doses; procedures in pharynx, larynx, and trachea, up to 20 doses

Topical 4%, anhydrous lignocaine hydrochloride 40 mg/mL. Net price 30-mL bottle = £1.21

Additives: include hydroxybenzoates (parabens)
Dose: bronchoscopy, 2–3 mL with suitable spray; biopsy in mouth, 3–4 mL with suitable spray *or* swab (with adrenaline if necessary); max. 7.5 mL

BUPIVACAINE

The great advantage of bupivacaine over other local anaesthetics is its longer duration of action. It has a slow onset of action, taking up to 30 minutes for full effect. It is often used in lumbar epidural blockade and is particularly suitable for continuous epidural analgesia in labour. It is **contra-indicated** in intravenous regional anaesthesia (Bier's block). It is the principal drug for spinal anaesthesia in the UK.

BUPIVACAINE HYDROCHLORIDE

Indications: see under Dose
Cautions; Contra-indications; Side-effects: see under Lignocaine Hydrochloride and notes above; avoid accidental intravascular injection; myocardial depression may be more severe and more resistant to treatment; contra-indicated in intravenous regional anaesthesia (Bier's block); **interactions:** Appendix 1 (bupivacaine)
Dose: adjusted according to patient's weight and nature of procedure—**important**: see also under Administration, above
Local infiltration, 0.25% (up to 60 mL)
Peripheral nerve block, 0.25% (max. 60 mL), 0.375% (max. 40 mL), 0.5% (max. 30 mL)

Epidural block,
Surgery, *lumbar*, 0.5–0.75% (max. 20 mL of either)
caudal, 0.5% (max. 30 mL)
Labour, *lumbar*, 0.25–0.5% (max. 12 mL of either)
caudal, but rarely used, 0.25% (max. 20 mL), 0.375% (max. 20 mL), 0.5% (max. 20 mL)

Note. 0.75% **contra-indicated** for epidural use in obstetrics.

Important: the licensed doses stated above may not be appropriate in some settings and expert advice should be sought

PoM Marcain Heavy® (Astra)

Injection, anhydrous bupivacaine hydrochloride 5 mg, glucose 80 mg/mL. Net price 4-mL amp = 98p

Dose: spinal anaesthesia, 2–4 mL

PoM Marcain® (Astra)

Injection, anhydrous bupivacaine hydrochloride 2.5 mg/mL (*Marcain®* 0.25%), net price 10-mL Polyamp® = £1.11; 3.75 mg/mL (*Marcain®* 0.375%), 10-mL Polyamp® = £1.22; 5 mg/mL (*Marcain®* 0.5%), 10-mL Polyamp® = £1.27; 7.5 mg/mL (*Marcain®* 0.75%), 10-mL Polyamp® = £1.90.

Note. Bupivacaine hydrochloride injection 0.25% and 0.5% also available from Antigen, David Bull

PoM Marcain with Adrenaline® (Astra)

Injection 0.25%, bupivacaine hydrochloride 2.5 mg/mL, adrenaline 1 in 200 000. Net price 10-mL amp = £1.40

Injection 0.5%, bupivacaine hydrochloride 5 mg/mL, adrenaline 1 in 200 000. Net price 10-mL amp = £1.23

PRILOCAINE

Prilocaine is a local anaesthetic of low toxicity which is similar to lignocaine. If used in high doses, methaemoglobinaemia may occur which can be treated with intravenous injection of methylene blue 1% using a dose of 1 mg/kg.

PRILOCAINE HYDROCHLORIDE

Indications: infiltration, intravenous regional anaesthesia, nerve block; also dental anaesthesia
Cautions; Contra-indications; Side-effects: see under Lignocaine Hydrochloride and notes above; caution in renal impairment; avoid in anaemia or congenital or acquired methaemoglobinaemia
Dose: adjusted according to site of operation and response of patient, to max. 400 mg used alone, or 600 mg if used with felypressin

PoM Citanest® (Astra)

Injection 0.5%, prilocaine hydrochloride 5 mg/mL. Net price 20-mL multidose vial = 71p; 50-mL multidose vial = 99p; 50-mL single dose vial = £1.27

Injection 1%, prilocaine hydrochloride 10 mg/mL. Net price 20-mL multidose vial = 73p; 50-mL multidose vial = £1.03

Injection 2%, prilocaine hydrochloride 20 mg/mL.
Net price 10-mL single dose vial = 73p

Injection 4%, prilocaine hydrochloride 40 mg/mL.
Net price 2-mL cartridge = 18p

℞oM **Citanest with Octapressin®** (Astra)

Injection 3%, prilocaine hydrochloride 30 mg/mL,
felypressin 0.03 unit/mL. For dental use. Net
price 2-mL cartridge and self-aspirating cartridge
(both) = 18p

PROCAINE

Procaine is now seldom used. It is as potent an anaesthetic
as lignocaine but has a shorter duration of action. It provides less intense analgesia because it has less tendency to
spread through the tissues. It is poorly absorbed from
mucous membranes and is of no value as a surface anaesthetic. When used for infiltration or regional anaesthesia,
adrenaline 1 in 200 000 is generally added. Its metabolite
para-aminobenzoic acid inhibits the action of the sulphonamides.

PROCAINE HYDROCHLORIDE

Indications: local anaesthesia by infiltration and regional
routes (but see notes above)

Cautions; Side-effects: see notes above

Dose: adjusted according to site of operation and
patient's response

By injection, up to 1 g (200 mL of 0.5% solution or
100 mL of 1%) with adrenaline 1 in 200 000

℞oM **Procaine Injection,** procaine hydrochloride 2%
(20 mg/mL) in sodium chloride intravenous infusion.
Net price 2-mL amp = 68p

AMETHOCAINE

Amethocaine is an effective local anaesthetic for
topical application; a 4% gel is indicated for anaesthesia prior to venepuncture or venous cannulation.
It is rapidly absorbed from mucous membranes and
should **never** be applied to inflamed, traumatised,
or highly vascular surfaces. It should **never** be used
to provide anaesthesia for bronchoscopy or cystoscopy, as lignocaine is a safer alternative. It is used
in ophthalmology (see section 11.7) and in skin
preparations (see section 13.3). Hypersensitivity to
amethocaine has been reported.

AMETHOCAINE
(Tetracaine)

Indications: see under preparation below

Cautions; Contra-indications; Side-effects: see
notes above; side-effects include erythema,
oedema and pruritus

Important. Rapid and extensive absorption may result
in systemic side-effects (see also notes above)

Ametop® (S&N Hlth.)

Gel, amethocaine 4%. Net price 1.5-g tube = £1.20

Dose: apply contents of tube to site of venepuncture or
venous cannulation and cover with occlusive dressing;
remove gel and dressing after 30 minutes for venepuncture and after 45 minutes for venous cannulation; PRE-
MATURE INFANT and INFANT under 1 month not recommended

OTHER LOCAL ANAESTHETICS

Benzocaine is a local anaesthetic of low potency
and toxicity. It is an ingredient of some proprietary
throat lozenges (see section 12.3.3).

Mepivacaine is a local anaesthetic used in dentistry. It is available in dental cartridges with or
without adrenaline as *Scandonest®*.

Cocaine readily penetrates mucous membranes
and is an effective surface anaesthetic with an
intense vasoconstrictor action. However, apart from
its use in otolaryngology (see below), it has now
been replaced by less toxic alternatives. It has
marked sympathomimetic activity and should
never be given by injection because of its toxicity.
As a result of its intense stimulant effect on the central nervous system it is a drug of addiction. Cocaine is still used in otolaryngology and is applied to
the nasal mucosa in concentrations of 4 to 10%
(40–100 mg/mL). The maximum total dose recommended for application to the nasal mucosa in fit
adults is a total of 1.5 mg/kg, which is equivalent to
a total topical dose of approximately 100 mg for an
adult male. It should be used only by those skilled
in the precautions needed to *minimise absorption*
and the *consequent risk of arrhythmias*. Although
cocaine interacts with other drugs liable to induce
arrhythmias, including adrenaline, some otolaryn-
gologists consider that combined use of topical cocaine with topical adrenaline (in the form of a paste
or a solution), improves the operative field and may
possibly reduce absorption. Cocaine is a mydriatic
as well as a local anaesthetic but owing to corneal
toxicity it is now little used in ophthalmology (see
section 11.7). Cocaine should be avoided in porphyria (see section 9.8.2).

Appendix 1: Interactions

Two or more drugs given at the same time may exert their effects independently or may interact. The interaction may be potentiation or antagonism of one drug by another, or occasionally some other effect. Adverse drug interactions should be reported to the CSM as for other adverse drug reactions.

Drug interactions may be **pharmacodynamic** or **pharmacokinetic**.

PHARMACODYNAMIC INTERACTIONS

These are interactions between drugs which have similar or antagonistic pharmacological effects or side-effects. They may be due to competition at receptor sites, or occur between drugs acting on the same physiological system. They are usually predictable from a knowledge of the pharmacology of the interacting drugs; in general, those demonstrated with one drug are likely to occur with related drugs. They occur to a greater or lesser extent in most patients who receive the interacting drugs.

PHARMACOKINETIC INTERACTIONS

These occur when one drug alters the absorption, distribution, metabolism, or excretion of another, thus increasing or reducing the amount of drug available to produce its pharmacological effects. They are not easily predicted and many of them affect only a small proportion of patients taking the combination of drugs. Pharmacokinetic interactions occurring with one drug cannot be assumed to occur with related drugs unless their pharmacokinetic properties are known to be similar.

Pharmacokinetic interactions are of several types:

AFFECTING ABSORPTION. The rate of absorption or the total amount absorbed can both be altered by drug interactions. Delayed absorption is rarely of clinical importance unless high peak plasma concentrations are required (e.g. when giving an analgesic). Reduction in the total amount absorbed, however, may result in ineffective therapy.

DUE TO CHANGES IN PROTEIN BINDING. To a variable extent most drugs are loosely bound to plasma proteins. Protein-binding sites are non-specific and one drug can displace another thereby increasing its proportion free to diffuse from plasma to its site of action. This only produces a detectable increase in effect if it is an extensively bound drug (more than 90%) that is not widely distributed throughout the body. Even so displacement rarely produces more than transient potentiation because this increased concentration of free drug results in an increased rate of elimination.

Displacement from protein binding plays a part in the potentiation of warfarin by phenylbutazone,

sulphonamides, and tolbutamide but the importance of these interactions is due mainly to the fact that warfarin metabolism is also inhibited.

AFFECTING METABOLISM. Many drugs are metabolised in the liver. Induction of the hepatic microsomal enzyme system by one drug can gradually increase the rate of metabolism of another, resulting in lower plasma concentrations and a reduced effect. On withdrawal of the inducer plasma concentrations increase and toxicity may occur. Barbiturates, griseofulvin, most antiepileptics, and rifampicin are the most important enzyme inducers in man. Drugs affected include warfarin and the oral contraceptives.

Conversely when one drug inhibits the metabolism of another higher plasma concentrations are produced, rapidly resulting in an increased effect with risk of toxicity. Some drugs which potentiate warfarin and phenytoin do so by this mechanism.

AFFECTING RENAL EXCRETION. Drugs are eliminated through the kidney both by glomerular filtration and by active tubular secretion. Competition occurs between those which share active transport mechanisms in the proximal tubule. Thus probenecid delays the excretion of many drugs including penicillins, some cephalosporins, indomethacin, and dapsone; aspirin may increase the toxicity of methotrexate by a similar mechanism.

RELATIVE IMPORTANCE OF INTERACTIONS

Many drug interactions are harmless and many of those which are potentially harmful only occur in a small proportion of patients; moreover, the severity of an interaction varies from one patient to another. Drugs with a small therapeutic ratio (e.g. phenytoin) and those which require careful control of dosage (e.g. anticoagulants, antihypertensives, and antidiabetics) are most often involved.

Patients at increased risk from drug interactions include the elderly and those with impaired renal or liver function.

HAZARDOUS INTERACTIONS. The symbol • has been placed against interactions that are **potentially hazardous** and where combined administration of the drugs involved should be **avoided** (or only undertaken with caution and appropriate monitoring).

Interactions that have no symbol do not usually have serious consequences.

List of drug interactions

The following is an alphabetical list of drugs and their interactions; to avoid excessive cross-referencing each drug or group is listed twice: in the alphabetical list and also against the drug or group with which it interacts; changes in the interactions lists since BNF No. 31 (March 1996) are <u>underlined</u>.

For explanation of symbol ● see previous page

Acamprosate
Note. Concomitant administration does not affect pharmacokinetics of alcohol; also no interaction demonstrated with diazepam, disulfiram or imipramine

Acarbose *see* Antidiabetics

ACE Inhibitors
Alcohol: enhanced hypotensive effect

Aldesleukin: enhanced hypotensive effect

Allopurinol: increased risk of toxicity with *captopril*, especially in renal impairment

● Anaesthetics: enhanced hypotensive effect

● Analgesics: antagonism of hypotensive effect and increased risk of renal damage with *NSAIDs*; hyperkalaemia with *indomethacin and possibly other NSAIDs*

Antacids: absorption of *fosinopril* reduced

Anti-arrhythmics: *procainamide* increases risk of toxicity with *captopril*, especially in renal impairment

Antibacterials: absorption of *tetracyclines* reduced by *quinapril* (tablets contain magnesium carbonate excipient)

Antidepressants: enhanced hypotensive effect

Antidiabetics: hypoglycaemic effect possibly enhanced

other Antihypertensives: enhanced hypotensive effect

Antipsychotics: severe postural hypotension with *chlorpromazine and possibly other phenothiazines*

Anxiolytics and Hypnotics: enhanced hypotensive effect

Beta-blockers: enhanced hypotensive effect

Calcium-channel Blockers: enhanced hypotensive effect

Cardiac Glycosides: plasma concentration of *digoxin* possibly increased by *captopril*

Corticosteroids: antagonism of hypotensive effect

● Cyclosporin: increased risk of hyperkalaemia

● Diuretics: enhanced hypotensive effect (can be extreme); hyperkalaemia with *potassium-sparing diuretics*

Dopaminergics: *levodopa* enhances hypotensive effect

● Epoetin: increased risk of hyperkalaemia

● Lithium: *ACE inhibitors* reduce excretion of *lithium* (increased plasma-lithium concentration)

Muscle Relaxants: *baclofen* enhances hypotensive effect

Nitrates: enhance hypotensive effect

Oestrogens and Progestogens: *oestrogens and combined oral contraceptives* antagonise hypotensive effect

● Potassium Salts: hyperkalaemia

Sympathomimetics: *see* Sympathomimetics (main list)

Ulcer-healing Drugs: *carbenoxolone* antagonises hypotensive effect

Uricosurics: *probenecid* reduces excretion of *captopril*

Acebutolol *see* Beta-blockers

Aceclofenac *see* NSAIDs

Acemetacin *see* NSAIDs

Acetazolamide *see* Diuretics (carbonic anhydrase inhibitor)

Aciclovir and Famciclovir
other Antivirals: extreme lethargy reported on administration of *zidovudine* with *intravenous aciclovir*

Aciclovir and Famciclovir (*continued*)
Mycophenolate Mofetil: higher plasma concentrations of *aciclovir* and of *mycophenolate mofetil* on concomitant administration

Uricosurics: *probenecid* reduces *aciclovir* and possibly *famciclovir* excretion (increased plasma concentrations and risk of toxicity)

Acitretin *see* Retinoids

Acrivastine *see* Antihistamines

Acrosoxacin *see* 4-Quinolones

Adenosine
Note. Possibility of interaction with drugs tending impair cardiac conduction

● Antiplatelet Drugs: effect enhanced and extended b *dipyridamole* (**important** risk of toxicity)

Theophylline: antagonism of anti-arrhythmic effect

Adrenaline *see* Sympathomimetics

Adrenergic Neurone Blockers
Alcohol: enhanced hypotensive effect

● Anaesthetics: enhanced hypotensive effect

Analgesics: *NSAIDs* antagonise hypotensive effect

Anti-arrhythmics: increased risk of myocardial depression with *bretylium*

Antidepressants: *tricyclics* antagonise hypotensive effect

other Antihypertensives: enhanced hypotensive effect

Antipsychotics: *phenothiazines* enhance hypotensiv effect (antagonism of hypotensive effect with higher doses of *chlorpromazine*)

Anxiolytics and Hypnotics: enhanced hypotensive effect

Beta-blockers: enhanced hypotensive effect

Calcium-channel Blockers: enhanced hypotensive effect

Corticosteroids: antagonism of hypotensive effect

Diuretics: enhanced hypotensive effect

Dopaminergics: *levodopa* enhances hypotensive effect

Nitrates: enhance hypotensive effect

Oestrogens and Progestogens: *oestrogens and combined oral contraceptives* antagonise hypotensive effect

Pizotifen: antagonism of hypotensive effect

● Sympathomimetics: *some anorectics, some cough an cold remedies (e.g. ephedrine)*, and *methylphenidate* antagonise hypotensive effect

Ulcer-healing Drugs: *carbenoxolone* antagonises hypotensive effect

Alcohol
ACE Inhibitors: enhanced hypotensive effect

Analgesics: sedative and hypotensive effect of *opioi analgesics* enhanced

Antibacterials: disulfiram-like reaction with *cephamandole, metronidazole, and tinidazole*

● Anticoagulants: *see* Warfarin

● Antidepressants: sedative effect of *tricyclics (and related)* enhanced; *tyramine contained in some alcoholic and dealcoholised beverages* interacts with *MAOIs* (hypertension crisis)—but if no tyramine, enhanced hypotensive effect

Antidiabetics: enhanced hypoglycaemic effect; flushing with *chlorpropamide* (in susceptible subjects); increased risk of lactic acidosis with *metformin*

Antiepileptics: CNS side-effects of *carbamazepine* possibly enhanced

Antihistamines: enhanced sedative effect

Antihypertensives: enhanced hypotensive effect; sedative effect of *indoramin* enhanced

Alcohol (*continued*)

Antimuscarinics: sedative effect of *hyoscine* enhanced

Antipsychotics: enhanced sedative effect

Anxiolytics and Hypnotics: enhanced sedative effect

Barbiturates and Primidone: enhanced sedative effect

Beta-blockers: enhanced hypotensive effect

Cytotoxics: disulfiram-like reaction with *procarbazine*

Dopaminergics: reduced tolerance to *bromocriptine*

Lofexidine: enhanced sedative effect

Muscle Relaxants: *baclofen* enhances sedative effect

Nabilone: enhanced sedative effect

Nitrates: enhanced hypotensive effect

Retinoids: *etretinate* formed from *acitretin* in presence of *alcohol*

Aldesleukin

Antihypertensives: enhanced hypotensive effect

Alendronic Acid *see* Bisphosphonates

Alfentanil *see* Opioid Analgesics

Alfuzosin *see* Alpha-blockers

Allopurinol

ACE Inhibitors: increased risk of toxicity with *captopril*, especially in renal impairment

Anticoagulants: effects of *nicoumalone and warfarin* possibly enhanced

Cyclosporin: plasma-cyclosporin concentration possibly increased (risk of nephrotoxicity)

• Cytotoxics: effects of *azathioprine* (*see also* p. 362) *and mercaptopurine* enhanced with increased toxicity

Alpha-blockers

ACE Inhibitors: enhanced hypotensive effect

Alcohol: enhanced hypotensive effect; sedative effect of *indoramin* enhanced

Aldesleukin: enhanced hypotensive effect

• Anaesthetics: enhanced hypotensive effect

Analgesics: *NSAIDs* antagonise hypotensive effect

• Antidepressants: enhanced hypotensive effect; manufacturer of *indoramin* advises avoid *MAOIs*

other Antihypertensives: additive hypotensive effect

Antipsychotics: enhanced hypotensive effect

Anxiolytics and Hypnotics: enhanced hypotensive and sedative effect

• Beta-blockers: enhanced hypotensive effect; increased risk of first-dose hypotensive effect of *post-synaptic alpha-blockers such as prazosin*

• Calcium-channel Blockers: enhanced hypotensive effect; increased risk of first-dose hypotensive effect of *post-synaptic alpha-blockers such as prazosin*

Corticosteroids : antagonism of hypotensive effect

• Diuretics: enhanced hypotensive effect; increased risk of first-dose hypotensive effect of *post-synaptic alpha-blockers such as prazosin*

Dopaminergics: *levodopa* enhances hypotensive effect

Muscle Relaxants: *baclofen* enhances hypotensive effect

Nitrates: enhanced hypotensive effect

Oestrogens and Progestogens: *oestrogens and combined oral contraceptives* antagonise hypotensive effect

Ulcer-healing Drugs: *carbenoxolone* antagonises hypotensive effect

Alprazolam *see* Anxiolytics and Hypnotics

Aluminium Hydroxide *see* Antacids and Adsorbents

Amantadine

Antihypertensives: *methyldopa* and *metirosine* have extrapyramidal side-effects

Antimuscarinics: increased antimuscarinic side-effects

Antipsychotics: all have extrapyramidal side-effects

Metoclopramide and Domperidone: have extrapyramidal side-effects

Tetrabenazine: has extrapyramidal side-effects

Amifostine

Note. Limited information available—rapid clearance from plasma minimises risk of interactions; possibility of interactions with antihypertensives and other drugs which potentiate hypotension

Amikacin *see* Aminoglycosides

Amiloride *see* Diuretics (potassium-sparing)

Aminoglutethimide

• Anticoagulants: metabolism of *nicoumalone and warfarin* accelerated (reduced anticoagulant effect)

Antidiabetics: manufacturer advises metabolism of *oral antidiabetics* possibly accelerated

Cardiac Glycosides: metabolism of *digitoxin only* accelerated (reduced effect)

Corticosteroids: metabolism of *corticosteroids* accelerated (reduced effect)

Diuretics: increased risk of hyponatraemia

other Hormone Antagonists: plasma concentration of *tamoxifen* reduced

Oestrogens and Progestogens: *aminoglutethimide* reduces plasma concentration of *medroxyprogesterone*

Theophylline: metabolism of *theophylline* accelerated (reduced effect)

Aminoglycosides

other Antibacterials: increased risk of nephrotoxicity with *colistin*; increased risk of ototoxicity and nephrotoxicity with *capreomycin* and *vancomycin*

• Anticoagulants: *see* Phenindione and Warfarin

Antidiabetics: *neomycin* possibly enhances hypoglycaemic effect of *acarbose* and increases severity of gastro-intestinal effects

Antifungals: increased risk of nephrotoxicity with *amphotericin*

Bisphosphonates: increased risk of hypocalcaemia

• Botulinum Toxin: neuromuscular block enhanced (risk of toxicity)

• Cyclosporin: increased risk of nephrotoxicity

• Cytotoxics: increased risk of nephrotoxicity and possibly of ototoxicity with *cisplatin*

• Diuretics: increased risk of ototoxicity with *loop diuretics* (*see also* p. 244)

• Muscle Relaxants: effect of *non-depolarising muscle relaxants* enhanced

• Parasympathomimetics: antagonism of effect of *neostigmine and pyridostigmine*

Aminophylline *see* Theophylline

Amiodarone

Note. Amiodarone has a long half-life; there is a potential for drug interactions to occur for several weeks (or even months) after treatment with it has been stopped

• *other* Anti-arrhythmics: additive effect with *disopyramide, flecainide, procainamide, and quinidine* (increased risk of ventricular arrhythmias); increased plasma concentrations of *flecainide and procainamide*; increased myocardial depression with any anti-arrhythmic

• Anticoagulants: metabolism of *nicoumalone and warfarin* inhibited (enhanced anticoagulant effect)

• Antidepressants: increased risk of ventricular arrhythmias with *tricyclics*

• Antiepileptics: metabolism of *phenytoin* inhibited (increased plasma concentration)

• Antihistamines: increased risk of ventricular arrhythmias with *astemizole* and *terfenadine*

Amiodarone (*continued*)
- Antimalarials: increased risk of ventricular arrhythmias with *halofantrine*
- Antipsychotics: increased risk of ventricular arrhythmias with *phenothiazines*
- Beta-blockers: increased risk of bradycardia, AV block, and myocardial depression; increased risk of ventricular arrhythmias associated with *sotalol*
- Calcium-channel Blockers: *diltiazem and verapamil* increase risk of bradycardia, AV block, and myocardial depression
- Cardiac Glycosides: increased plasma concentration of *digoxin* (halve digoxin maintenance dose)

Cyclosporin: plasma concentration of cyclosporin possibly increased

Diuretics: toxicity increased if hypokalaemia occurs with *acetazolamide, loop diuretics, and thiazides*

Thyroxine: for concomitant use see p. 69

Ulcer-healing Drugs: *cimetidine* increases plasma concentrations of *amiodarone*

Amitriptyline see Antidepressants, Tricyclic
Amlodipine see Calcium-channel Blockers
Amoxapine see Antidepressants, Tricyclic
Amoxycillin see Penicillins
Amphetamines see Sympathomimetics
Amphotericin (*see also* Cautions section 5.2)
Antibacterials: increased risk of nephrotoxicity with *aminoglycosides*

other Antifungals: antagonises *miconazole*
- Cardiac Glycosides: increased toxicity if hypokalaemia occurs
- Cyclosporin: increased risk of nephrotoxicity

Diuretics: increased risk of hypokalaemia with *loop diuretics* and *thiazides*
Ampicillin see Penicillins
Amylobarbitone see Barbiturates and Primidone
Anabolic Steroids
- Anticoagulants: anticoagulant effect of *nicoumalone, phenindione, and warfarin* enhanced
Anaesthetics, General (*see also* Surgery and Long-term Medication, section 15.1)
- ACE Inhibitors: enhanced hypotensive effect
Antibacterials: possible potentiation of *isoniazid* hepatotoxicity; effect of *thiopentone* enhanced by *sulphonamides*
Antidepressants: risk of arrhythmias and hypotension increased with *tricyclics; MAOIs, see* section 15.1
- Antihypertensives: enhanced hypotensive effect
- Antipsychotics: enhanced hypotensive effect
Anxiolytics and Hypnotics: enhanced sedative effect
- Beta-blockers: enhanced hypotensive effect
- Calcium-channel Blockers: enhanced hypotensive effect and AV delay with *verapamil*; hypotensive effect of *dihydropyridines* enhanced by *isoflurane*
- Dopaminergics: risk of arrhythmias if *volatile liquid anaesthetics such as halothane* given with *levodopa*

Oxytocin: oxytocic effect possibly reduced by *volatile anaesthetics* (also enhanced hypotensive effect and risk of arrhythmias)
- Sympathomimetics: risk of arrhythmias if *adrenaline or isoprenaline* given with *volatile liquid anaesthetics such as halothane*

Theophylline: increased risk of arrhythmias with *halothane*
Anaesthetics, Local see Bupivacaine, Lignocaine
Analgesics see Aspirin, Nefopam, NSAIDs, Opioid Analgesics, and Paracetamol
Anion-exchange Resins see Cholestyramine and Colestipol
Antacids and Adsorbents
ACE Inhibitors: *antacids* reduce absorption of *fosinopril*

Analgesics: excretion of *aspirin* increased in alkaline urine; *antacids* reduce absorption of *diflunisal*

Antacids and Adsorbents (*continued*)
Anti-arrhythmics: excretion of *quinidine* reduced in alkaline urine (may occasionally increase plasma concentrations)

Antibacterials: *antacids* reduce absorption of *azithromycin, cefpodoxime, ciprofloxacin, isoniazid, nitrofurantoin, norfloxacin, ofloxacin, pivampicillin, rifampicin, and most tetracyclines*

Antiepileptics: *antacids* reduce absorption of *gabapentin* and *phenytoin*

Antifungals: *antacids* reduce absorption of *itraconazole* and *ketoconazole*

Antiplatelet Drugs: *dipyridamole* patient information leaflet advises avoidance of *antacids*

Antimalarials: *antacids* reduce absorption of *chloroquine and hydroxychloroquine*

Antipsychotics: *antacids* reduce absorption of *phenothiazines*

Bisphosphonates: *antacids* reduce absorption

Iron: *magnesium trisilicate* reduces absorption of *oral iron*

Lithium: *sodium bicarbonate* increases excretion (reduced plasma-lithium concentration)

Mycophenolate Mofetil: *antacids* reduce absorption of *mycophenolate mofetil*

Penicillamine: *antacids* reduce absorption
Antazoline see Antihistamines
Anti-arrhythmics see Adenosine; Amiodarone; Disopyramide; Flecainide; Lignocaine; Mexiletine; Moracizine; Procainamide; Propafenone; Quinidine; Tocainide
Anticholinergics see Antimuscarinics
Anticholinesterases see Parasympathomimetics
Anticoagulants see Heparin, Phenindione, and Warfarin
Antidepressants see Antidepressants, SSRI; Antidepressants, Tricyclic; MAOIs; Mianserin; Moclobemide; Nefazodone; Trazodone; Tryptophan; Venlafaxine; Viloxazine
Antidepressants, SSRI
Alcohol: effects possibly enhanced
Anti-arrhythmics: plasma-flecainide concentration increased by *fluoxetine*
- Anticoagulants: effect of *nicoumalone and warfarin* possibly enhanced
- *other* Antidepressants: CNS effects of *MAOIs* increased (risk of toxicity); *SSRI* should not be started until 2 weeks after stopping *MAOI*; conversely, *MAOI* should not be started until at least 1 week after *SSRI* has been stopped (at least 5 weeks for *fluoxetine*, at least 2 weeks for *paroxetine* and *sertraline*); *moclobemide see* p. 177; plasma concentrations of some *tricyclics* increased; agitation and nausea with *tryptophan*
- Antiepileptics: antagonism (convulsive threshold lowered); plasma concentration of *carbamazepine* increased by *fluoxetine* and *fluvoxamine*; plasma concentration of *phenytoin* increased by *fluoxetine* and *fluvoxamine*; *phenytoin and possibly other antiepileptics* reduce plasma concentration of *paroxetine*
- Antipsychotics: plasma concentration of *clozapine* possibly increased by *fluvoxamine*; plasma concentration of *haloperidol* increased by *fluoxetine*

Anxiolytics and Hypnotics: plasma concentration of some *benzodiazepines* increased by *fluvoxamine*
- Barbiturates and Primidone: *see under* Antiepileptics, above

Beta-blockers: plasma concentration of *propranolol* increased by *fluvoxamine*
- Dopaminergics: hypertension and CNS excitation with *fluoxetine* and *selegiline*
- Lithium: increased risk of CNS effects (lithium toxicity reported)
- Sumatriptan: risk of CNS effects (lithium toxicity reported)

Antidepressants, SSRI (*continued*)
- Theophylline: plasma-theophylline concentration increased by *fluvoxamine* (**important:** see p. 128)

Antidepressants, Tricyclic
- Alcohol: enhanced sedative effect

  Anaesthetics: risk of arrhythmias and hypotension increased

  Analgesics: possibly increased side-effects with *nefopam*
- Anti-arrhythmics: increased risk of ventricular arrhythmias with drugs which prolong QT interval

  Antibacterials: plasma concentrations of some *tricyclics* reduced by *rifampicin* (reduced antidepressant effect)
- *other* Antidepressants: CNS excitation and hypertension with *MAOIs; tricyclic or related antidepressant* should not be started until 2 weeks after stopping *MAOI;* conversely, *MAOI* should not be started until at least 1 week after *tricyclic or related antidepressant; moclobemide* see p. 177; plasma concentrations of some *tricyclics* increased by *SSRIs*
- Antiepileptics: antagonism (convulsive threshold lowered); plasma concentrations of some *tricyclics* reduced (reduced antidepressant effect)

  Antihistamines: increased antimuscarinic and sedative effects; increased risk of ventricular arrhythmias with *astemizole* and *terfenadine*

  Antihypertensives: in general, hypotensive effect enhanced, but antagonism of effect of *adrenergic neurone blockers* and of *clonidine* (and increased risk of hypertension on clonidine withdrawal); possible risk of hypotension with *tricyclics* and *apraclonidine*
- Antimalarials: increased risk of ventricular arrhythmias with *halofantrine*

  Antimuscarinics: increased antimuscarinic side-effects

  Antipsychotics: increased plasma concentrations of *tricyclic antidepressants* and increased antimuscarinic side-effects with *phenothiazines*

  Anxiolytics and Hypnotics: enhanced sedative effect
- Barbiturates and Primidone: *see under* Antiepileptics, above
- Beta-blockers: risk of ventricular arrhythmias associated with *sotalol* increased

  Calcium-channel Blockers: *diltiazem* and *verapamil* increase plasma concentration of *imipramine* and possibly *other tricyclics*

  Disulfiram: inhibition of metabolism of *tricyclics* (increased plasma concentrations and increased disulfiram reaction reported with *alcohol with amitriptyline*)

  Diuretics: increased risk of postural hypotension

  Muscle Relaxants: enhanced muscle relaxant effect of *baclofen*

  Nitrates: reduced effect of *sublingual nitrates* (owing to dry mouth)

  Oestrogens and Progestogens: *oral contraceptives* antagonise antidepressant effect (but side-effects may be increased due to increased plasma concentrations of *tricyclics*)
- Sympathomimetics: hypertension and arrhythmias with *adrenaline* (but local anaesthetics with adrenaline appear to be safe); hypertension with *noradrenaline*

  Thyroxine: manufacturer of *lofepramine* advises avoid *thyroxine*

  Ulcer-healing Drugs: plasma concentrations of *amitriptyline, desipramine, doxepin, imipramine, nortriptyline,* and probably *other tricyclics* increased by *cimetidine* (inhibition of metabolism)

Antidiabetics
  Note. Includes Acarbose; Insulin; Metformin; Sulphonyl-ureas

  ACE Inhibitors: possibly enhance hypoglycaemic effect

Antidiabetics (*continued*)
  Alcohol: enhanced hypoglycaemic effect; flushing with *chlorpropamide* (in susceptible subjects); risk of lactic acidosis with *metformin*
- Analgesics: *azapropazone, phenylbutazone* and possibly *other NSAIDs* enhance effect of *sulphonylureas*

  Anion-exchange Resins: *cholestyramine* enhances hypoglycaemic effect of *acarbose*
- Antibacterials: *chloramphenicol, co-trimoxazole, 4-quinolones, sulphonamides,* and *trimethoprim* enhance effect of *sulphonylureas; neomycin* possibly enhances hypoglycaemic effect of *acarbose* and increases severity of gastro-intestinal effects; *rifamycins* reduce effect of *sulphonylureas* (accelerates metabolism)

  Antidepressants: *MAOIs* enhance hypoglycaemic effect

  Antiepileptics: *plasma-phenytoin* concentration transiently increased by *tolbutamide* (possibility of toxicity)
- Antifungals: *fluconazole* and *miconazole* increase plasma concentrations of *sulphonylureas*

  Antihistamines: depressed thrombocyte count with concomitant use of *oral antidiabetics* (notably biguanides) and *ketotifen*

  Antihypertensives: hypoglycaemic effect antagonised by *diazoxide*

  Antipsychotics: *phenothiazines* possibly antagonise hypoglycaemic effect of *sulphonylureas*

  Beta-blockers: enhanced hypoglycaemic effect (and masking of warning signs such as tremor)

  Calcium-channel Blockers: *nifedipine* may occasionally impair glucose tolerance

  Clofibrate Group: may improve glucose tolerance and have an additive effect

  Corticosteroids: antagonism of hypoglycaemic effect

  Diuretics: hypoglycaemic effect antagonised by *loop and thiazide diuretics; chlorpropamide* increases risk of hyponatraemia with *thiazides in combination with potassium-sparing diuretics*

  Hormone Antagonists: manufacturer advises metabolism of *oral antidiabetics* possibly accelerated by *aminoglutethimide; octreotide* may reduce *insulin and antidiabetic drug* requirements in diabetes mellitus

  Lithium: may occasionally impair glucose tolerance

  Oestrogens and Progestogens: *oral contraceptives* antagonise hypoglycaemic effect

  Pancreatin: hypoglycaemic effect of *acarbose* reduced by *pancreatin*

  Ulcer-healing Drugs: *cimetidine* inhibits renal excretion of *metformin* (increased plasma-metformin concentrations); *cimetidine* and *ranitidine* enhance hypoglycaemic effect of *sulphonylureas*
- Uricosurics: *sulphinpyrazone* enhances effect of *sulphonylureas*

Antiepileptics *see* Carbamazepine; Chlormethiazole; Clonazepam; Ethosuximide; Gabapentin; Lamotrigine; Phenytoin; Topiramate; Valproate; Vigabatrin and p. 203

Antifungals *see* Amphotericin; Antifungals, Imidazole and Triazole; Griseofulvin; Terbinafine

Antifungals, Imidazole and Triazole
  Note. Imidazole antifungals include ketoconazole and miconazole; triazoles include fluconazole and itraconazole

  Antacids and Adsorbents: *antacids* reduce absorption of *itraconazole* and *ketoconazole*
- Antibacterials: *rifampicin* accelerates metabolism of *fluconazole, itraconazole* and *ketoconazole* (reduced plasma concentration); plasma concentration of *rifabutin* increased by *fluconazole* (risk of uveitis)

Antifungals, Imidazole and Triazole (*continued*)
- Anticoagulants: effect of *nicoumalone* and *warfarin* enhanced by *fluconazole, itraconazole, ketoconazole,* and *miconazole* (note: oral gel absorbed)
- Antidiabetics: plasma concentrations of *sulphonylurea*s increased by *fluconazole* and *miconazole*
- Antiepileptics: effect of *phenytoin* enhanced by *fluconazole* and *miconazole*; plasma concentrations of *itraconazole* and *ketoconazole* reduced by *phenytoin*

  other Antifungals: *amphotericin* antagonises effect of *miconazole*
- Antihistamines: *itraconazole, ketoconazole* and possibly *other* imidazoles (and triazoles) inhibit *astemizole* and *terfenadine* metabolism (cardiac toxicity reported); manufacturer advises possibility of increased plasma-loratadine concentration with *ketoconazole*

  Antimuscarinics: reduced absorption of *ketoconazole*
- Anxiolytics and Hypnotics: plasma concentration of *midazolam* increased by *itraconazole, ketoconazole,* and possibly *fluconazole* (prolonged sedative effect)
- Cardiac Glycosides: plasma concentration of *digoxin* increased by *itraconazole*
- Cisapride: *fluconazole, itraconazole, ketoconazole* and *miconazole* inhibit metabolism (increased plasma-cisapride concentration—ventricular arrhythmias reported)
- Cyclosporin: metabolism inhibited by *itraconazole, ketoconazole* and possibly *fluconazole* and *miconazole* (increased plasma-cyclosporin concentration)

  Cytotoxics: *ketoconazole* possibly inhibits metabolism of *paclitaxel; see also* Docetaxel

  Lipid-lowering Drugs: *itraconazole* increases risk of myopathy with *simvastatin*

  Oestrogens and Progestogens: anecdotal reports of contraceptive failure with *fluconazole, itraconazole, ketoconazole* and possibly others
- Theophylline: plasma-theophylline concentration possibly increased by *fluconazole*

  Ulcer-healing Drugs: *histamine H₂- antagonists* reduce absorption of *itraconazole* and *ketoconazole; omeprazole* reduces absorption of *ketoconazole* and possibly *itraconazole; sucralfate* reduces absorption of *ketoconazole*

Antihistamines

Note. Sedative interactions apply to a lesser extent to the non-sedative antihistamines, and they do not appear to potentiate the effects of alcohol. Do not generally apply to antihistamines used for topical action (including inhalation)

Alcohol: enhanced sedative effect
- Anti-arrhythmics: increased risk of ventricular arrhythmias with *astemizole* and *terfenadine*
- Antibacterials: metabolism of *astemizole* and *terfenadine* inhibited by *clarithromycin* and *erythromycin* (risk of hazardous arrhythmias, *see* p. 138); manufacturer advises possibility of increased plasma-loratadine concentration with *erythromycin*
- Antidepressants: *MAOIs* and *tricyclics* increase antimuscarinic and sedative effects; *tricyclics* increase risk of ventricular arrhythmias with *astemizole* and *terfenadine*

  Antidiabetics: depressed thrombocyte count with concomitant use of *oral antidiabetics* (notably biguanides) and *ketotifen*
- Antifungals: *itraconazole, ketoconazole* and possibly *other imidazoles* (and triazoles) inhibit *astemizole* and *terfenadine* metabolism (cardiac toxicity reported) ; manufacturer advises possibility of increased plasma-loratadine concentration with *ketoconazole*

Antihistamines (*continued*)
- *other* Antihistamines: concomitant use of *astemizole* and *terfenadine* **not** recommended (risk of hazardous arrhythmias, *see* p. 138)
- Antimalarials: *halofantrine* and *quinine* increase risk of ventricular arrhythmias with *astemizole* and *terfenadine*

  Antimuscarinics: increased antimuscarinic side-effects
- Antipsychotics: increased risk of ventricular arrhythmias with *astemizole* and *terfenadine*

  Anxiolytics and Hypnotics: enhanced sedative effect
- Beta-blockers: *sotalol* increases risk of ventricular arrhythmias with *astemizole* and *terfenadine*

  Betahistine: antagonism (theoretical)

  Cytotoxics: *see* Docetaxel
- Diuretics: hypokalaemia increases risk of ventricular arrhythmias with *astemizole* and *terfenadine*

  Ulcer-healing Drugs: manufacturer advises possibility of increased plasma-loratadine concentration with *cimetidine*

Antihypertensives *see* individual drugs or groups

Antimalarials *see* individual drugs

Antimuscarinics

Note. Many drugs have antimuscarinic effects; concomitant use of two or more such drugs can increase side-effects such as dry mouth, urine retention, and constipation; concomitant use can also lead to confusion in the elderly; interactions do not generally apply to antimuscarinics used by inhalation

Alcohol: sedative effect of *hyoscine* enhanced

Analgesics: increased antimuscarinic effects with *nefopam*

Anti-arrhythmics: increased antimuscarinic effects with *disopyramide; atropine* delays absorption of *mexiletine*

Antidepressants: increased antimuscarinic side-effects with *tricyclics and MAOIs*

Antifungals: reduced absorption of *ketoconazole*

Antihistamines: increased antimuscarinic side-effects

Antipsychotics: increased antimuscarinic side-effects of *phenothiazines* (but reduced plasma concentrations)

Cisapride: antagonism of gastro-intestinal effect

Dopaminergics: increased antimuscarinic side-effects with *amantadine*

Metoclopramide and Domperidone: *antimuscarinics such as propantheline* antagonise gastro-intestinal effects

Nitrates: reduced effect of *sublingual nitrates* (failure to dissolve under tongue owing to dry mouth)

Parasympathomimetics: antagonism of effect

Antiplatelet Drugs *see* Aspirin and Dipyridamole

Antipsychotics

Note. Increased risk of toxicity with myelosuppressive drugs—clozapine in particular should not be used concurrently with drugs associated with a substantial potential for causing agranulocytosis, such as carbamazepine, co-trimoxazole, chloramphenicol, sulphonamides, pyrazolone analgesics such as azapropazone, penicillamine, or cytotoxics; also avoid clozapine with long-acting depot antipsychotics (have myelosuppressive potential)

ACE Inhibitors: severe postural hypotension with *chlorpromazine* and possibly *other phenothiazines*

Alcohol: enhanced sedative effect
- Anaesthetics: enhanced hypotensive effect

  Analgesics: enhanced sedative and hypotensive effect with *opioid analgesics*

  Antacids: reduced absorption of *phenothiazines*
- Anti-arrhythmics: increased risk of ventricular arrhythmias with drugs which prolong QT interval

  Antibacterials: *erythromycin* possibly increases plasma concentration of *clozapine* (possible increased risk of convulsions); *rifampicin* accelerates metabolism of *haloperidol* (reduced plasma-haloperidol concentration)

Antipsychotics (*continued*)
- Antidepressants: increased plasma concentrations and increased antimuscarinic effects notably on administration of *tricyclics* with *phenothiazines; fluvoxamine* possibly increases plasma concentration of *clozapine; fluoxetine* increases plasma concentration of *haloperidol; oxypertine* causes CNS excitation and hypertension with *MAOIs; clozapine* possibly enhances central effects of *MAOIs*

Antidiabetics: hypoglycaemic effect of *sulphonylureas* possibly antagonised
- Antiepileptics: antagonism (convulsive threshold lowered); *carbamazepine* accelerates metabolism of *haloperidol* (reduced plasma concentration); *phenytoin* accelerates metabolism of *clozapine*

Antihistamines: increased risk of ventricular arrhythmias with *astemizole* and *terfenadine*

Antihypertensives: enhanced hypotensive effect; higher doses of *chlorpromazine* antagonise hypotensive effect of *adrenergic neurone blockers*; increased risk of extrapyramidal effects on administration of *methyldopa* and *metirosine*
- Antimalarials: increased risk of ventricular arrhythmias with *halofantrine*

Antimuscarinics: antimuscarinic side-effects of *phenothiazines* increased (but reduced plasma concentrations)

Anxiolytics and Hypnotics: enhanced sedative effect
- Beta-blockers: *phenothiazines* increase risk of ventricular arrhythmias with *sotalol; propranolol* increases plasma concentration of *chlorpromazine*

Calcium-channel Blockers: enhanced hypotensive effect

Desferrioxamine: manufacturer advises avoid *prochlorperazine* (also *methotrimeprazine* on theoretical grounds)

Diuretics: hypokalaemia increases risk of ventricular arrhythmias with *pimozide*

Dopaminergics: antagonism of hypoprolactinaemic and antiparkinsonian effects of *bromocriptine*; antagonism of effect of *apomorphine, levodopa, lysuride,* and *pergolide*

Lithium: increased risk of extrapyramidal effects and possibility of neurotoxicity with *clozapine, haloperidol* and *phenothiazines*

Metoclopramide and Domperidone: increased risk of extrapyramidal effects with *metoclopramide*

Sympathomimetics: antagonise pressor action

Tetrabenazine: increased risk of extrapyramidal effects

Ulcer-healing Drugs: *cimetidine* may enhance effects of *chlorpromazine, clozapine,* and possibly *other antipsychotics*

Antivirals *see* Aciclovir and Famciclovir; Ganciclovir; Valaciclovir; Zalcitabine; Zidovudine

Anxiolytics and Hypnotics
Alcohol: enhanced sedative effect

Anaesthetics: enhanced sedative effect

Analgesics: *opioid analgesics* enhance sedative effect
- Antibacterials: *erythromycin* inhibits metabolism of *midazolam* (increased plasma-midazolam concentration, with profound sedation) and *zopiclone; isoniazid* inhibits metabolism of *diazepam; rifampicin* increases metabolism of *diazepam* and possibly *other benzodiazepines*

Anticoagulants: *chloral hydrate* and *triclofos* may transiently enhance anticoagulant effect of *nicoumalone and warfarin*

Antidepressants: enhanced sedative effect; manufacturer contra-indicates *buspirone* with *MAOIs*; plasma concentrations of some *benzodiazepines* increased by *fluvoxamine*

Anxiolytics and Hypnotics (*continued*)
Antiepileptics: metabolism of *clonazepam* accelerated (reduced effect); plasma-phenytoin concentrations increased or decreased by *diazepam* and possibly *other benzodiazepines*
- Antifungals: *itraconazole, ketoconazole,* and possibly *fluconazole* increase plasma concentration of *midazolam* (prolonged sedative effect)

Antihistamines: enhanced sedative effect

Antihypertensives: enhanced hypotensive effect; enhanced sedative effect with *alpha-blockers* and possibly *moxonidine*

Antipsychotics: enhanced sedative effect

Calcium-channel Blockers: *diltiazem* and *verapamil* inhibit metabolism of *midazolam* (increased plasma-midazolam concentration, with increased sedation)

Disulfiram: metabolism of *benzodiazepines* inhibited, with enhanced sedative effect (*temazepam* toxicity reported)

Dopaminergics: *benzodiazepines* occasionally antagonise effect of *levodopa*

Lofexidine: enhanced sedative effect

Muscle Relaxants: *baclofen* enhances sedative effect

Nabilone: enhanced sedative effect

Ulcer-healing Drugs: *cimetidine* inhibits metabolism of *benzodiazepines and chlormethiazole* (increased plasma concentrations); *omeprazole* inhibits metabolism of *diazepam* (increased plasma concentrations)

Apomorphine
Antipsychotics: antagonism of effects

Appetite Suppressants *see* Sympathomimetics

Apraclonidine
Antidepressants: possible risk of hypotension with *tricyclics*

Sympathomimetics: possible risk of hypertension with *adrenaline* and *noradrenaline*

Aspirin
other Analgesics: avoid concomitant administration of *other NSAIDs* (increased side-effects)

Antacids and Adsorbents: excretion of *aspirin* increased in alkaline urine
- Anticoagulants: increased risk of bleeding due to antiplatelet effect

Antiepileptics: enhancement of effect of *phenytoin* and *valproate*

Corticosteroids: increased risk of gastro-intestinal bleeding and ulceration
- Cytotoxics: reduced excretion of *methotrexate* (increased toxicity)

Diuretics: antagonism of diuretic effect of *spironolactone;* reduced excretion of *acetazolamide* (risk of toxicity)

Metoclopramide and Domperidone: *metoclopramide* enhances effect of *aspirin* (increased rate of absorption)

Mifepristone: manufacturer recommends avoid *aspirin* until 8–12 days after *mifepristone*

Uricosurics: effect of *probenecid and sulphinpyrazone* reduced

Astemizole *see* Antihistamines
Atenolol *see* Beta-blockers
Atovaquone
Antibacterials: plasma-atovaquone concentration reduced by *rifampicin*

Anticoagulants: anticoagulant effect of *warfarin* possibly enhanced

Metoclopramide and Domperidone: plasma-atovaquone concentration reduced by *metoclopramide*

Atracurium *see* Muscle Relaxants (non-depolarising)
Atropine *see* Antimuscarinics
Auranofin *see* Gold
Azapropazone *see* NSAIDs
Azatadine *see* Antihistamines

Azathioprine
- Allopurinol: enhancement of effect with increased toxicity (*see also* p. 362)
- Antibacterials: manufacturer reports interaction with *rifampicin* (transplants possibly rejected)

Azelastine *see* Antihistamines
Azithromycin *see* Erythromycin and other Macrolides
Azlocillin *see* Penicillins
Aztreonam
- Anticoagulants: anticoagulant effect of *nicoumalone and warfarin* possibly enhanced

Bacampicillin *see* Penicillins
Baclofen *see* Muscle Relaxants
Bambuterol *see* Sympathomimetics, Beta₂

Barbiturates and Primidone
  Alcohol: enhanced sedative effect
  Anti-arrhythmics: metabolism of *disopyramide and quinidine* increased (reduced plasma concentrations)
  Antibacterials: metabolism of *chloramphenicol, doxycycline, and metronidazole* accelerated (reduced effect); *sulphonamides* enhance effect of *thiopentone*
- Anticoagulants: metabolism of *nicoumalone and warfarin* accelerated (reduced anticoagulant effect)
- Antidepressants: antagonism of anticonvulsant effect (convulsive threshold lowered); metabolism of *mianserin and tricyclics* accelerated (reduced plasma concentrations)
- Antiepileptics: concomitant administration of *phenobarbitone or primidone* with other antiepileptics may enhance toxicity without a corresponding increase in antiepileptic effect; moreover interactions can complicate monitoring of treatment; interactions include enhanced effects, increased sedation, and reductions in plasma concentrations; for further details see p. 203
  Antifungals: *phenobarbitone* accelerates metabolism of *griseofulvin* (reduced effect)
- Antipsychotics: antagonism of anticonvulsant effect (convulsive threshold lowered)
- Calcium-channel Blockers: effect of *diltiazem, felodipine, isradipine, verapamil* and probably *nicardipine* and *nifedipine* reduced
  Cardiac Glycosides: metabolism of *digitoxin only* accelerated (reduced effect)
- Corticosteroids: metabolism of *corticosteroids* accelerated (reduced effect)
- Cyclosporin: metabolism of *cyclosporin* accelerated (reduced effect)
  Hormone antagonists: metabolism of *toremifene* possibly accelerated
- Oestrogens and Progestogens: metabolism of *gestrinone, tibolone,* and *oral contraceptives* accelerated (reduced contraceptive effect, **important:** see p. 337)
  Theophylline: metabolism of *theophylline* accelerated (reduced effect)
  Thyroxine: metabolism of thyroxine accelerated (may increase thyroxine requirements in hypothyroidism)
  Vitamins: *vitamin D* requirements possibly increased

Beclomethasone *see* Corticosteroids
Belladonna Alkaloids *see* Antimuscarinics
Bendrofluazide *see* Diuretics (thiazide)
Benorylate *see* Aspirin *and* Paracetamol
Benperidol *see* Antipsychotics
Benzhexol *see* Antimuscarinics
Benzodiazepines *see* Anxiolytics and Hypnotics
Benzthiazide *see* Diuretics (thiazide)
Benztropine *see* Antimuscarinics
Benzylpenicillin *see* Penicillins

Beta-blockers
  Note. Since systemic absorption may follow topical application of beta-blockers to the eye the possibility of interactions, in particular, with drugs such as verapamil should be borne in mind
  ACE Inhibitors: enhanced hypotensive effect

Beta-blockers (*continued*)
  Alcohol: enhanced hypotensive effect
  Aldesleukin: enhanced hypotensive effect
- Anaesthetics: enhanced hypotensive effect; increased risk of *bupivacaine* toxicity with *propranolol*
  Analgesics: *NSAIDs* antagonise hypotensive effect
- Anti-arrhythmics: increased risk of myocardial depression and bradycardia; with *amiodarone* increased risk of bradycardia and AV block; increased risk of *lignocaine* toxicity with *propranolol*; *propafenone* increases plasma concentration of *metoprolol* and *propranolol*; risk of ventricular arrhythmias associated with *sotalol* increased by *amiodarone, disopyramide, procainamide,* and *quinidine*
  Antibacterials: *rifampicin* accelerates metabolism of *bisoprolol* and *propranolol* (reduced plasma concentration)
- Antidepressants: *fluvoxamine* increases plasma concentration of *propranolol*; risk of ventricular arrhythmias associated with *sotalol* increased by *tricyclics*
  Antidiabetics: enhanced hypoglycaemic effect (and masking of warning signs such as tremor)
- Antihistamines: risk of ventricular arrhythmias associated with *sotalol* increased by *astemizole* and *terfenadine*
- Antihypertensives: enhanced hypotensive effect; increased risk of withdrawal hypertension with *clonidine*; increased risk of first-dose hypotensive effect with *post-synaptic alpha-blockers such as prazosin*
- Antimalarials: risk of ventricular arrhythmias associated with *sotalol* increased by *halofantrine*; increased risk of bradycardia with *mefloquine*
- Antipsychotics: risk of ventricular arrhythmias associated with *sotalol* increased by *phenothiazines*; plasma concentration of *chlorpromazine* increased by *propranolol*
  Anxiolytics and Hypnotics: enhanced hypotensive effect
- Calcium-channel Blockers: increased risk of bradycardia and AV block with *diltiazem*; severe hypotension and heart failure occasionally with *nifedipine* (but useful combination, see p. 95); asystole, severe hypotension, and heart failure with *verapamil* (see p. 98)
  Cardiac Glycosides: increased AV block and bradycardia
  Corticosteroids: antagonism of hypotensive effect
  Diuretics: enhanced hypotensive effect; risk of ventricular arrhythmias associated with *sotalol* increased by hypokalaemia
  Ergotamine: increased peripheral vasoconstriction
  Muscle Relaxants: *propranolol* enhances effect
  Oestrogens and Progestogens: *oestrogens* and *combined oral contraceptives* antagonise hypotensive effect
  Parasympathomimetics: risk of arrhythmias possibly increased by *pilocarpine*; *propranolol* antagonises effect of *neostigmine and pyridostigmine*
- Sympathomimetics: severe hypertension with *adrenaline and noradrenaline (especially with non-selective beta-blockers)*; severe hypertension also possible with *sympathomimetics in anorectics and cough and cold remedies*
  Theophylline: *beta-blockers* should be avoided on pharmacological grounds (bronchospasm)
  Thyroxine: metabolism of *propranolol* accelerated (reduced effect)
  Ulcer-healing Drugs: plasma concentrations of *labetalol and propranolol* increased by *cimetidine*; hypotensive effect antagonised by *carbenoxolone*
  Xamoterol: antagonism of effect of *xamoterol* and reduction in beta-blockade

Betahistine
  Antihistamines: antagonism (theoretical)

Betamethasone see Corticosteroids
Betaxolol see Beta-blockers
Bethanechol see Parasympathomimetics
Bethanidine see Adrenergic Neurone Blockers
Bezafibrate see Clofibrate Group
Bicalutamide
  Anticoagulants: effect of *warfarin* possibly enhanced
Biperiden see Antimuscarinics
Bismuth Chelate see Tripotassium Dicitratobismuth-
  ate
Bisoprolol see Beta-blockers
Bisphosphonates
  Analgesics: bioavailability of *tiludronic acid*
    increased by *indomethacin*
  Antacids: reduced absorption
  Antibacterials: increased risk of hypocalcaemia with
    aminoglycosides
  Calcium Salts: reduced absorption
  Iron: reduced absorption
Botulinum Toxin
  Antibacterials: effects enhanced by *aminoglycosides*
    and *spectinomycin* (risk of toxicity)
  Muscle Relaxants: effects enhanced by *non-
    depolarising muscle relaxants*
Bretylium see Adrenergic Neurone Blockers
Bromazepam see Anxiolytics and Hypnotics
Bromocriptine and Cabergoline
  Alcohol: reduced tolerance to *bromocriptine*
  Antibacterials: *erythromycin* and possibly *other
    macrolides* increase plasma concentration
    (increased risk of toxicity)
  Antipsychotics: antagonism of hypoprolactinaemic
    effect (and antiparkinsonian effect of
    bromocriptine)
  Metoclopramide and Domperidone: antagonise
    hypoprolactinaemic effect
  Sympathomimetics: increased risk of toxicity with
    bromocriptine and *isometheptene* or
    phenylpropanolamine
Brompheniramine see Antihistamines
Buclizine see Antihistamines
Budesonide see Corticosteroids
Bumetanide see Diuretics (loop)
Bupivacaine
  Anti-arrhythmics: increased myocardial depression
  Beta-blockers: increased risk of *bupivacaine* toxicity
    with *propranolol*
Buprenorphine see Opioid Analgesics
Buspirone see Anxiolytics and Hypnotics
Butobarbitone see Barbiturates and Primidone
Cabergoline see Bromocriptine and Cabergoline
Calcium Salts
  Antibacterials: reduced absorption of *tetracyclines*
  Bisphosphonates: reduced absorption
  Cardiac Glycosides: large intravenous doses of
    calcium can precipitate arrhythmias
  Diuretics: increased risk of hypercalcaemia with
    thiazides
Calcium-channel Blockers
  Note. Grapefruit juice possibly increases plasma concen-
  tration of dihydropyridine calcium-channel blockers
  ACE Inhibitors: enhanced hypotensive effect
  Aldesleukin: enhanced hypotensive effect
  Anaesthetics: *verapamil* increases hypotensive effect
    of *general anaesthetics* and risk of AV delay;
    isoflurane enhances hypotensive effect of
    dihydropyridines
  Anti-arrhythmics: *amiodarone-induced* risk of
    bradycardia, AV block, and myocardial depression
    increased by *diltiazem and verapamil*; plasma-
    concentration of *quinidine* reduced by *nifedipine*;
    increased risk of myocardial depression and
    asystole if *verapamil* given with *disopyramide* and
    flecainide; with *verapamil* raised plasma
    concentration of *quinidine* (extreme hypotension
    may occur)

Calcium-channel Blockers (*continued*)
  Antibacterials: *erythromycin* possibly inhibits
    metabolism of *felodipine* (increased plasma
    concentration); *rifampicin* increases metabolism of
    diltiazem, nifedipine, verapamil and possibly
    isradipine (reduced plasma concentrations)
  Antidepressants: *diltiazem* and *verapamil* increase
    plasma concentration of *imipramine and possibly
    other tricyclics*
  Antidiabetics: *nifedipine* may occasionally impair
    glucose tolerance
  Antiepileptics: effect of *carbamazepine* enhanced by
    diltiazem and verapamil; diltiazem and nifedipine
    increase plasma concentration of *phenytoin*; effect
    of *felodipine and isradipine* and probably
    nicardipine and nifedipine reduced by
    *carbamazepine, phenobarbitone, phenytoin, and
    primidone*; effect of *diltiazem and verapamil*
    reduced by *phenobarbitone and phenytoin*
  Antihypertensives: enhanced hypotensive effect;
    increased risk of first-dose hypotensive effect of
    post-synaptic alpha-blockers such as prazosin
  Antimalarials: possible increased risk of bradycardia
    with some *calcium-channel blockers* and
    mefloquine
  Antipsychotics: enhanced hypotensive effect
  Anxiolytics and Hypnotics: *diltiazem* and *verapamil*
    inhibit metabolism of *midazolam* (increased
    plasma-midazolam concentration, with increased
    sedation)
  Barbiturates and Primidone: *see under* Antiepileptics,
    above
  Beta-blockers: increased risk of bradycardia and AV
    block with *diltiazem;* occasionally severe
    hypotension and heart failure with *nifedipine* (but
    useful combination, see p. 95); asystole, severe
    hypotension, and heart failure with *verapamil* (see
    p. 98)
  other Calcium-channel Blockers: clearance of
    nifedipine reduced by *diltiazem* (increased plasma-
    nifedipine concentration)
  Cardiac Glycosides: plasma concentration of *digoxin*
    increased by *diltiazem, nicardipine, verapamil* and
    possibly *nifedipine*; increased AV block and
    bradycardia with *verapamil*
  Cyclosporin: plasma-cyclosporin concentrations
    increased by *diltiazem, nicardipine, and verapamil;*
    possibly increases plasma concentration of
    nifedipine
  Diuretics: enhanced hypotensive effect
  Lithium: neurotoxicity may occur without increased
    plasma-lithium concentrations in patients given
    diltiazem and verapamil
  Muscle Relaxants: *nifedipine* and *verapamil* enhance
    effect of *non-depolarising muscle relaxants;*
    hypotension, myocardial depression, and
    hyperkalaemia with *verapamil* and intravenous
    dantrolene
  Sympathomimetics: see Sympathomimetics (main
    list)
  Theophylline: *diltiazem, verapamil* and possibly *other
    calcium-channel blockers* enhance effect
    (increased plasma-theophylline concentration)
  Ulcer-healing Drugs: *cimetidine* inhibits metabolism
    of *some calcium-channel blockers* (increased
    plasma concentrations)
Cannrenoate see Diuretics (*as for* spironolactone)
Capreomycin
  other Antibacterials: increased risk of nephrotoxicity
    with *colistin*; increased risk of nephrotoxicity and
    ototoxicity with *aminoglycosides and vancomycin*
  Cytotoxics: increased risk of nephrotoxicity and
    ototoxicity with *cisplatin*
Captopril see ACE Inhibitors
Carbachol see Parasympathomimetics

Carbamazepine

Alcohol: CNS side-effects of *carbamazepine* possibly enhanced

- Analgesics: *dextropropoxyphene* enhances effect of *carbamazepine;* effect of *tramadol* decreased by *carbamazepine*
- Antibacterials: metabolism of *doxycycline* accelerated (reduced effect); plasma-carbamazepine concentration increased by *clarithromycin, erythromycin* and *isoniazid* (also isoniazid hepatotoxicity possibly increased)
- Anticoagulants: metabolism of *nicoumalone and warfarin* accelerated (reduced anticoagulant effect)
- Antidepressants: antagonism of anticonvulsant effect (convulsive threshold lowered); plasma concentration of *carbamazepine* increased by *fluoxetine, fluvoxamine,* and *viloxazine;* metabolism of *mianserin* and *tricyclics* accelerated (reduced plasma concentrations); manufacturer advises avoid with *MAOIs* or within 2 weeks of *MAOIs*
- *other* Antiepileptics: concomitant administration of *two or more antiepileptics* may enhance toxicity without a corresponding increase in antiepileptic effect; moreover interactions between individual antiepileptics can complicate monitoring of treatment; interactions include enhanced effects, increased sedation, and reductions in plasma concentrations; for further details, see p. 203
- Antimalarials: *chloroquine* and *mefloquine* antagonise anticonvulsant effect
- Antipsychotics: antagonism of anticonvulsant effect (convulsive threshold lowered); metabolism of *haloperidol* accelerated (reduced plasma-haloperidol concentration)
- Calcium-channel Blockers: *diltiazem and verapamil* enhance effect of *carbamazepine;* effect of *felodipine, isradipine* and probably *nicardipine* and *nifedipine* reduced

Cardiac Glycosides: metabolism of *digitoxin only* accelerated (reduced effect)

- Corticosteroids: metabolism accelerated (reduced effect)
- Cyclosporin: metabolism accelerated (reduced plasma-cyclosporin concentration)

Diuretics: increased risk of hyponatraemia

- Hormone Antagonists: *danazol* inhibits metabolism of *carbamazepine* (enhanced effect); metabolism of *toremifene* possibly accelerated

Lithium: neurotoxicity may occur without increased plasma-lithium concentration

Muscle Relaxants: effect of *non-depolarising muscle relaxants* antagonised (recovery from neuromuscular blockade accelerated)

- Oestrogens and Progestogens: *carbamazepine* accelerates metabolism of *oral contraceptives* (reduced contraceptive effect, **important:** see p. 337) and of *gestrinone and tibolone*

Retinoids: plasma concentration possibly reduced by *isotretinoin*

Theophylline: metabolism of *theophylline* accelerated (reduced effect)

Thyroxine: metabolism accelerated (may increase thyroxine requirements in hypothyroidism)

- Ulcer-healing Drugs: metabolism inhibited by *cimetidine* (increased plasma-carbamazepine concentration)

Vitamins: *carbamazepine* possibly increases *vitamin D* requirements

Carbenicillin *see* Penicillins

Carbenoxolone

Note. Interactions do not apply to small amounts used topically on oral mucosa

Antihypertensives: antagonism of hypotensive effect

Cardiac Glycosides: toxicity increased if hypokalaemia occurs

Corticosteroids: increased risk of hypokalaemia

Carbenoxolone (*continued*)

Diuretics: antagonism of diuretic effect; increased risk of hypokalaemia with *acetazolamide, thiazides, and loop diuretics;* inhibition of ulcer healing with *amiloride and spironolactone*

Carbonic Anhydrase Inhibitors *see* Diuretics

Cardiac Glycosides

ACE Inhibitors: *captopril* possibly increases plasma concentration of *digoxin*

Analgesics: *NSAIDs* may exacerbate heart failure, reduce GFR and increase plasma-cardiac glycoside concentrations

Anion-exchange Resins: absorption reduced by *cholestyramine and colestipol*

- Anti-arrhythmics: plasma concentration of *digoxin* increased by *amiodarone, propafenone,* and *quinidine* (halve maintenance dose of digoxin)

Antibacterials: *erythromycin* and possibly *other macrolides* enhance effect of *digoxin; rifamycins* accelerate metabolism of *digitoxin only* (reduced effect)

Antiepileptics: metabolism of *digitoxin only* accelerated (reduced effect)

- Antifungals: increased toxicity if hypokalaemia occurs with *amphotericin;* plasma concentration of *digoxin* increased by *itraconazole*
- Antimalarials: *quinine* (includes use of quinine for cramp) and possibly *chloroquine* and *hydroxychloroquine* raises plasma concentration of *digoxin* (halve maintenance dose of digoxin); possible increased risk of bradycardia with *mefloquine*

Barbiturates and Primidone: *see under* Antiepileptics above

Beta-blockers: increased AV block and bradycardia

Calcium Salts: large intravenous doses of *calcium* can precipitate arrhythmias

- Calcium-channel Blockers: plasma concentration of *digoxin* increased by *diltiazem, nicardipine, verapamil* and possibly *nifedipine;* increased AV block and bradycardia with *verapamil*

Corticosteroids: increased risk of hypokalaemia

- Diuretics: increased toxicity if hypokalaemia occurs with *acetazolamide, loop diuretics, and thiazides;* effects of *digoxin* enhanced by *spironolactone*

Hormone Antagonists: *aminoglutethimide* accelerates metabolism of *digitoxin only* (reduced effect)

Muscle Relaxants: arrhythmias with *suxamethonium*

Ulcer-healing Drugs: increased toxicity if hypokalaemia occurs with *carbenoxolone;* plasma concentration of *digoxin* possibly increased by *proton pump inhibitors;* absorption possibly reduced by *sucralfate*

Carisoprodol *see* Anxiolytics and Hypnotics

Carteolol *see* Beta-blockers

Carvedilol *see* Beta-blockers

Cefaclor *see* Cephalosporins

Cefadroxil *see* Cephalosporins

Cefixime *see* Cephalosporins

Cefodizime *see* Cephalosporins

Cefotaxime *see* Cephalosporins

Cefoxitin *see* Cephalosporins

Cefpirome *see* Cephalosporins

Cefpodoxime *see* Cephalosporins

Ceftazidime *see* Cephalosporins

Ceftibuten *see* Cephalosporins

Ceftizoxime *see* Cephalosporins

Ceftriaxone *see* Cephalosporins

Cefuroxime *see* Cephalosporins

Celiprolol *see* Beta-blockers

Cephalexin *see* Cephalosporins

Cephalosporins

Alcohol: disulfiram-like reaction with *cephamandole*

Antacids and Adsorbents: *antacids* reduce absorption of *cefpodoxime*

Cephalosporins (*continued*)
- Anticoagulants: anticoagulant effect of *warfarin and nicoumalone* enhanced by *cephamandole* and possibly others

  Ulcer-healing Drugs: *histamine H_2-antagonists* reduce absorption of *cefpodoxime*

  Uricosurics: excretion of *cephalosporins* reduced by *probenecid* (increased plasma concentrations)

Cephamandole *see* Cephalosporins

Cephazolin *see* Cephalosporins

Cephradine *see* Cephalosporins

Cetirizine *see* Antihistamines

Chloral *see* Anxiolytics and Hypnotics

Chloramphenicol

  other Antibacterials: *rifampicin* accelerates metabolism (reduced chloramphenicol-plasma concentration)
- Anticoagulants: anticoagulant effect of *nicoumalone and warfarin* enhanced
- Antidiabetics: effect of *sulphonylureas* enhanced
- Antiepileptics: metabolism accelerated by *phenobarbitone* (reduced chloramphenicol-plasma concentration); increased plasma concentration of *phenytoin* (risk of toxicity)
- Barbiturates and Primidone: *see under* Antiepileptics, above

Chlordiazepoxide *see* Anxiolytics and Hypnotics

Chlormethiazole *see* Anxiolytics and Hypnotics

Chloroquine and Hydroxychloroquine

  Antacids: reduced absorption
- Antiepileptics: antagonism of anticonvulsant effect

  other Antimalarials: increased risk of convulsions with *mefloquine;* increased risk of arrhythmias with *halofantrine* (**important:** see also CSM advice under Halofantrine, p. 276)
- Cardiac Glycosides: *chloroquine* and *hydroxychloroquine* possibly increase plasma concentration of *digoxin*
- Cyclosporin: *chloroquine* increases plasma-cyclosporin concentration (increased risk of toxicity)

  Parasympathomimetics: *chloroquine* and *hydroxychloroquine* have potential to increase symptoms of myasthenia gravis and thus diminish effect of *neostigmine* and *pyridostigmine*

  Ulcer-healing Drugs: *cimetidine* inhibits metabolism of *chloroquine* (increased plasma concentration)

  Vaccines: *see* Rabies Vaccine p. 512

Chlorothiazide *see* Diuretics (thiazide)

Chlorpheniramine *see* Antihistamines

Chlorpromazine *see* Antipsychotics

Chlorpropamide *see* Antidiabetics (sulphonylurea)

Chlortetracycline *see* Tetracyclines

Chlorthalidone *see* Diuretics (thiazide-related)

Cholestyramine and Colestipol

  Note. Other drugs should be taken at least 1 hour before or 4–6 hours after cholestyramine or colestipol to reduce possible interference with absorption

  Analgesics: reduced absorption of *paracetamol* and *phenylbutazone*

  Antibacterials: antagonism of effect of oral *vancomycin*
- Anticoagulants: anticoagulant effect of *nicoumalone, phenindione, and warfarin* may be enhanced or reduced

  Antidiabetics: hypoglycaemic effect of *acarbose* enhanced by *cholestyramine*

  Antiepileptics: absorption of *valproate* possibly reduced

  Cardiac Glycosides: reduced absorption

  Diuretics: reduced absorption of *thiazides* (give at least 2 hours apart)

  Mycophenolate Mofetil: absorption of *mycophenolate mofetil* reduced

  Thyroxine: reduced absorption

Cholinergics *see* Parasympathomimetics

Cilastatin [ingredient] *see Primaxin®*

Cilazapril *see* ACE Inhibitors

Cimetidine *see* Histamine H_2-antagonists

Cinnarizine *see* Antihistamines

Cinoxacin *see* 4-Quinolones

Ciprofibrate *see* Clofibrate Group

Ciprofloxacin *see* 4-Quinolones

Cisapride

  Analgesics: *opioid analgesics* possibly antagonise effect on gastro-intestinal motility
- Antibacterials: *clarithromycin* and *erythromycin* possibly inhibit metabolism of *cisapride* (risk of ventricular arrhythmias)

  Anticoagulants: effect of *oral anticoagulants* possibly enhanced
- Antifungals: *fluconazole, itraconazole, ketoconazole* and *miconazole* inhibit metabolism of *cisapride* (increased plasma concentration—ventricular arrhythmias reported)

  Antimuscarinics: antagonism of effect on gastro-intestinal motility

Cisatracurium *see* Muscle Relaxants (non-depolarising)

Cisplatin
- Antibacterials: *aminoglycosides and capreomycin* increase risk of nephrotoxicity and possibly of ototoxicity

  Diuretics: increased risk of nephrotoxicity and ototoxicity

Citalopram *see* Antidepressants, SSRI

Cladribine

  Note. Increased risk of myelosuppression with other *myelosuppressive drugs*

Clarithromycin *see* Erythromycin and other Macrolides

Clemastine *see* Antihistamines

Clindamycin

  Muscle Relaxants: enhancement of effect of *non-depolarising muscle relaxants*

  Parasympathomimetics: antagonism of effect of *neostigmine and pyridostigmine*

Clobazam *see* Anxiolytics and Hypnotics

Clodronate Sodium *see* Bisphosphonates

Clofibrate Group
- Anticoagulants: enhancement of effect of *nicoumalone, phenindione, and warfarin*

  Antidiabetics: may improve glucose tolerance and have additive effect

  other Lipid-lowering Drugs: increased risk of myopathy with *statins*

Clomipramine *see* Antidepressants, Tricyclic

Clonazepam (general sedative interactions *as for* Anxiolytics and Hypnotics)

Clonidine (for general hypotensive interactions *see also* Hydralazine)
- Antidepressants: *tricyclics* antagonise hypotensive effect and also increase risk of rebound hypertension on *clonidine* withdrawal
- Beta-blockers: increased risk of hypertension on *clonidine* withdrawal

Clopamide *see* Diuretics (thiazide)

Clorazepate *see* Anxiolytics and Hypnotics

Cloxacillin *see* Penicillins

Clozapine *see* Antipsychotics

Co-amoxiclav *see* Penicillins

Co-beneldopa *see* Levodopa

Co-careldopa *see* Levodopa

Codeine *see* Opioid Analgesics

Co-fluampicil *see* Penicillins

Colchicine
- Cyclosporin: possibly increases risk of nephrotoxicity and myotoxicity (increased plasma-cyclosporin concentration)

Cold and Cough Remedies *see* Antihistamines and Sympathomimetics

Colestipol *see* Cholestyramine and Colestipol

Colistin (other interactions *as for* Aminoglycosides)
Muscle Relaxants: enhanced muscle relaxant effect

Contraceptives, Oral
Note. Also covers oestrogens taken alone; in case of hormone replacement therapy low dose unlikely to induce interactions

ACE Inhibitors: *oestrogens* and *combined oral contraceptives* antagonise hypotensive effect

- Antibacterials: *rifamycins* accelerate metabolism of both *combined and progestogen-only oral contraceptives* (reduced contraceptive effect, **important:** see p. 337); when *broad-spectrum antibiotics such as ampicillin and tetracycline* given with *combined oral contraceptives* possibility of reduced contraceptive effect (risk probably small, but see p. 337)

- Anticoagulants: antagonism of anticoagulant effect of *nicoumalone, phenindione, and warfarin*

Antidepressants: antagonism of antidepressant effect has been reported, but side-effects of *tricyclics* may be increased due to higher plasma concentrations

Antidiabetics: antagonism of hypoglycaemic effect

- Antiepileptics: *carbamazepine, phenobarbitone, phenytoin, primidone* and *topiramate* accelerate metabolism (reduced effect of both combined and progestogen-only contraceptives, **important:** see p. 337)

- Antifungals: *griseofulvin* accelerates metabolism (reduced contraceptive effect, **important:** see p. 337); anecdotal reports of contraceptive failure with *fluconazole, itraconazole, ketoconazole* and possibly others

Antihypertensives: *combined oral contraceptives* antagonise hypotensive effect

- Barbiturates and Primidone: *see under* Antiepileptics, above

Beta-blockers: *oestrogens* and *combined oral contraceptives* antagonise hypotensive effect

Cyclosporin: increased plasma-cyclosporin concentration

Diuretics: *combined oral contraceptives* antagonise diuretic effect

Theophylline: *combined oral contraceptives* delay excretion (increased plasma-theophylline concentration)

Ulcer-healing drugs: manufacturer advises *lansoprazole* possibly accelerates metabolism

Corticosteroids
Note. Do not generally apply to corticosteroids used for topical action (including inhalation)

Analgesics: increased risk of gastro-intestinal bleeding and ulceration with *aspirin* and *NSAIDs*

- Antibacterials: *rifamycins* accelerate metabolism of *corticosteroids* (reduced effect)

Antidiabetics: antagonism of hypoglycaemic effect

- Antiepileptics: *carbamazepine, phenobarbitone, phenytoin, and primidone* accelerate metabolism of *corticosteroids* (reduced effect)

Antihypertensives: antagonism of hypotensive effect

- Barbiturates and Primidone: *see under* Antiepileptics, above

Cardiac Glycosides: increased toxicity if hypokalaemia occurs with *corticosteroids*

- Cyclosporin: plasma-cyclosporin concentration increased by high-dose *methylprednisolone*; *cyclosporin* increases plasma concentration of *prednisolone*

Diuretics: antagonism of diuretic effect; *acetazolamide, loop diuretics, and thiazides* increase risk of hypokalaemia

Hormone Antagonists: *aminoglutethimide* accelerates metabolism of *corticosteroids* (reduced effect)

Sympathomimetics *see* Sympathomimetics, Beta$_2$ (main list)

Ulcer-healing Drugs: *carbenoxolone* increases risk of hypokalaemia

Vaccines: see p. 501

Co-trimoxazole and Sulphonamides
Anaesthetics: effect of *thiopentone* enhanced

- Anticoagulants: effect of *nicoumalone and warfarin* enhanced

- Antidiabetics: effect of *sulphonylureas* enhanced

- Antiepileptics: antifolate effect and plasma concentration of *phenytoin* increased by *co-trimoxazole* and possibly *other sulphonamides*

- Antimalarials: increased risk of antifolate effect with *pyrimethamine* (includes *Fansidar*® and *Maloprim*®)

- Cyclosporin: increased risk of nephrotoxicity; plasma-cyclosporin concentration possibly reduced by *sulphadiazine*

Cytotoxics: antifolate effect of *methotrexate* increased by *co-trimoxazole*

Potassium Aminobenzoate: inhibits effect of *sulphonamides*

Cyclizine *see* Antihistamines

Cyclobarbitone *see* Barbiturates

Cyclopenthiazide *see* Diuretics (thiazide)

Cyclopentolate *see* Antimuscarinics

Cyclophosphamide and Ifosfamide

- Anticoagulants: *ifosfamide* possibly enhances effect of *warfarin*

Muscle Relaxants: *cyclophosphamide* enhances effect of *suxamethonium*

Cycloserine
other Antibacterials: increased CNS toxicity with *isoniazid*

- Antiepileptics: increased plasma concentration of *phenytoin* (risk of toxicity)

Cyclosporin
Note. Grapefruit juice increases plasma-cyclosporin concentration (risk of toxicity)

- ACE Inhibitors: increased risk of hyperkalaemia

Allopurinol: possibly increases plasma-cyclosporin concentration (risk of toxicity)

- Analgesics: increased risk of nephrotoxicity with *NSAIDs*; *cyclosporin* increases plasma concentration of *diclofenac* (halve diclofenac dose)

Anti-arrhythmics: *amiodarone* and *propafenone* possibly increase plasma-cyclosporin concentration

- Antibacterials: *aminoglycosides, co-trimoxazole (and trimethoprim alone),* and *4-quinolones* increase risk of nephrotoxicity; *doxycycline* possibly increases plasma-cyclosporin concentration; *erythromycin* and possibly *other macrolides* increase plasma-cyclosporin concentration; *rifampicin, intravenous sulphadimidine, intravenous trimethoprim* (and possibly *sulphadiazine*) reduce plasma-cyclosporin concentration

- Antiepileptics: *carbamazepine, phenobarbitone, phenytoin, and primidone* accelerate metabolism (reduced plasma-cyclosporin concentration)

- Antifungals: *amphotericin* increases risk of nephrotoxicity; *griseofulvin* possibly reduces plasma-cyclosporin concentration; *itraconazole, ketoconazole,* and possibly *fluconazole* and *miconazole* inhibit metabolism (increased plasma-cyclosporin concentration)

- Antimalarials: *chloroquine* increases plasma-cyclosporin concentration (risk of toxicity)

- Barbiturates and Primidone: *see under* Antiepileptics above

- Calcium-channel Blockers: *diltiazem, nicardipine, and verapamil* increase plasma-cyclosporin concentration; *cyclosporin* possibly increases plasma concentration of *nifedipine*

- Colchicine: possibly increases risk of nephrotoxicity and myotoxicity (increased plasma-cyclosporin concentration)

Cyclosporin (*continued*)

Corticosteroids: *high-dose methylprednisolone* increases plasma-cyclosporin concentration; *cyclosporin* increases plasma concentration of *prednisolone*

Cytotoxics: increased risk of neurotoxicity with *doxorubicin*; increased risk of nephrotoxicity with *melphalan*; increased toxicity with *methotrexate; see also* Docetaxel

Diuretics: *potassium-sparing diuretics* increase risk of hyperkalaemia

Hormone Antagonists: *danazol* inhibits metabolism (increased plasma-cyclosporin concentration); *octreotide* reduces absorption (reduced plasma-cyclosporin concentration)

Lipid-lowering Drugs: increased risk of myopathy with *statins*

Oestrogens and Progestogens: *progestogens* inhibit metabolism (increased plasma-cyclosporin concentration)

Potassium Salts: increased risk of hyperkalaemia

Ulcer-healing Drugs: *cimetidine* possibly increases plasma-cyclosporin concentration

Vaccines: *see* p. 501

Cyproheptadine *see* Antihistamines

Cytotoxics *see under* individual drugs

Dalteparin *see* Heparin

Danazol

Anticoagulants: effect of *nicoumalone and warfarin* enhanced (inhibits metabolism)

Antiepileptics: inhibits metabolism of *carbamazepine* (increased plasma-carbamazepine concentration)

Cyclosporin: inhibits metabolism (increased plasma-cyclosporin concentration)

Dantrolene *see* Muscle Relaxants

Dapsone

Antibacterials: plasma concentration reduced by *rifamycins*

Probenecid: *dapsone* excretion reduced (increased risk of side-effects)

Debrisoquine *see* Adrenergic Neurone Blockers

Demecarium *see* Parasympathomimetics

Demeclocycline *see* Tetracyclines

Desferrioxamine

Antipsychotics: manufacturer advises avoid *prochlorperazine* (also *methotrimeprazine* on theoretical grounds)

Desflurane *see* Anaesthetics, General (volatile liquid)

Desipramine *see* Antidepressants, Tricyclic

Desogestrel *see* Progestogens

Dexamethasone *see* Corticosteroids

Dexamphetamine *see* Sympathomimetics

Dexfenfluramine *see* Sympathomimetics

Dextromoramide *see* Opioid Analgesics

Dextropropoxyphene *see* Opioid Analgesics

Diamorphine *see* Opioid Analgesics

Diazepam *see* Anxiolytics and Hypnotics

Diazoxide (general hypotensive interactions *as for* Hydralazine)

Antidiabetics: antagonism of hypoglycaemic effect

Dichlorphenamide *see* Diuretics (carbonic anhydrase inhibitor)

Diclofenac *see* NSAIDs

Dicyclomine *see* Antimuscarinics

Diflunisal *see* NSAIDs

Digitoxin *see* Cardiac Glycosides

Digoxin *see* Cardiac Glycosides

Dihydrocodeine *see* Opioid Analgesics

Dihydroergotamine *see* Ergotamine

Diltiazem *see* Calcium-channel Blockers

Dimenhydrinate *see* Antihistamines

Diphenhydramine *see* Antihistamines

Diphenylpyraline *see* Antihistamines

Diphenoxylate *see* Opioid Analgesics

Dipipanone *see* Opioid Analgesics

Dipivefrine *see* Sympathomimetics (*as for* adrenaline)

Dipyridamole

Antacids: patient information leaflet advises avoidance of *antacids*

• Anti-arrhythmics: effect of *adenosine* enhanced and extended (**important** risk of toxicity)

• Anticoagulants: enhanced effect due to antiplatelet action of *dipyridamole*

Cytotoxics: efficacy of *fludarabine* possibly reduced

Disodium Etidronate *see* Bisphosphonates

Disodium Pamidronate *see* Bisphosphonates

Disopyramide

• *other* Anti-arrhythmics: *amiodarone* increases risk of ventricular arrhythmias; increased myocardial depression with any *anti-arrhythmic*

• Antibacterials: plasma concentration of *disopyramide* reduced by *rifampicin* but increased by *erythromycin* (risk of toxicity)

Antiepileptics: plasma concentration of *disopyramide* reduced by *phenobarbitone, phenytoin, and primidone*

• Antihistamines: increased risk of ventricular arrhythmias with *astemizole* and *terfenadine*

• Antimalarials: increased risk of ventricular arrhythmias with *halofantrine*

Antimuscarinics: increased antimuscarinic side-effects

• Antipsychotics: increased risk of ventricular arrhythmias with *phenothiazines*

Barbiturates and Primidone: *see under* Antiepileptics, above

• Beta-blockers: increased myocardial depression; increased risk of ventricular arrhythmias associated with *sotalol*

• Calcium-channel blockers: increased myocardial depression with *verapamil*

• Diuretics: cardiac toxicity of *disopyramide* increased if hypokalaemia occurs with *acetazolamide, loop diuretics,* and *thiazides*

Nitrates: reduced effect of *sublingual nitrates* (failure to dissolve under tongue owing to dry mouth)

Distigmine *see* Parasympathomimetics

Disulfiram

Alcohol: disulfiram reaction (*see* section 4.10)

Antibacterials: psychotic reaction with *metronidazole* reported

• Anticoagulants: effect of *nicoumalone and warfarin* enhanced

Antidepressants: inhibition of metabolism of *tricyclic antidepressants* (increased plasma concentrations); increased disulfiram reaction with alcohol reported if *amitriptyline* also taken

• Antiepileptics: inhibition of metabolism of *phenytoin* (increased risk of toxicity)

Anxiolytics and Hypnotics: inhibition of metabolism of *benzodiazepines,* with enhanced sedative effect (*temazepam* toxicity reported)

Theophylline: inhibition of metabolism (increased risk of toxicity)

Diuretics

• ACE Inhibitors: enhanced hypotensive effect (can be extreme); risk of hyperkalaemia with *potassium-sparing diuretics*

Analgesics: *diuretics* increase risk of nephrotoxicity of *NSAIDs; NSAIDs notably indomethacin* antagonise diuretic effect; *indomethacin and possibly other NSAIDs* increase risk of hyperkalaemia with *potassium-sparing diuretics*; occasional reports of decreased renal function when *indomethacin* given with *triamterene*; diuretic effect of *spironolactone* antagonised by *aspirin*; *aspirin* reduces excretion of *acetazolamide* (risk of toxicity)

Anion-exchange Resins: *cholestyramine and colestipol* reduce absorption of *thiazides* (give at least 2 hours apart)

Diuretics (*continued*)

- Anti-arrhythmics: toxicity of *amiodarone, disopyramide, flecainide, and quinidine* increased if hypokalaemia occurs; action of *lignocaine, mexiletine, and tocainide* antagonised by hypokalaemia; *acetazolamide* reduces excretion of *quinidine* (increased plasma concentration)
- Antibacterials: *loop diuretics* increase ototoxicity of *aminoglycosides* (*see also* section 5.1.4), *colistin, and vancomycin*

  Antidepressants: increased risk of postural hypotension with *tricyclics*

  Antidiabetics: hypoglycaemic effect antagonised by *loop and thiazide diuretics; chlorpropamide* increases risk of hyponatraemia associated with *thiazides in combination with potassium-sparing diuretics*

  Antiepileptics: increased risk of hyponatraemia with *carbamazepine; carbonic anhydrase inhibitors* possibly increase risk of osteomalacia with *antiepileptics* such as *phenytoin*

  Antifungals: increased risk of hypokalaemia if *loop diuretics* and *thiazides* given with *amphotericin*
- Antihistamines: hypokalaemia increases risk of ventricular arrhythmias with *astemizole* and *terfenadine*
- Antihypertensives: enhanced hypotensive effect; increased risk of first-dose hypotensive effect of post-synaptic *alpha-blockers such as prazosin;* increased risk of hypokalaemia with *indapamide*

  Antimalarials: electrolyte disturbances increase risk of ventricular arrhythmias with *halofantrine*

  Antipsychotics: in hypokalaemia increased risk of ventricular arrhythmias with *pimozide*

  Beta-blockers: enhanced hypotensive effect; in hypokalaemia increased risk of ventricular arrhythmias with *sotalol*

  Calcium Salts: risk of hypercalcaemia with *thiazides*

  Calcium-channel Blockers: enhanced hypotensive effect
- Cardiac Glycosides: increased toxicity if hypokal- aemia occurs with *acetazolamide, loop diuretics, and thiazides;* effect enhanced by *spironolactone*

  Corticosteroids: increased risk of hypokalaemia with *acetazolamide, loop diuretics, and thiazides;* antagonism of diuretic effect
- Cyclosporin: increased risk of hyperkalaemia with *potassium-sparing diuretics*

  Cytotoxics: increased risk of nephrotoxicity and ototoxicity with *cisplatin*

  other Diuretics: increased risk of hypokalaemia if *acetazolamide, loop diuretics or thiazides* given together; profound diuresis possible if *metolazone* given with *frusemide* (p. 62)

  Hormone Antagonists: increased risk of hyponatraemia with *aminoglutethimide; thiazides* increase risk of hypercalcaemia with *toremifene; trilostane* increases risk of hyperkalaemia with *potassium-sparing diuretics*
- Lithium: lithium excretion reduced by *loop diuretics, potassium-sparing diuretics and thiazides* (increased plasma-lithium concentration and risk of toxicity—*loop diuretics* safer than *thiazides*); lithium excretion increased by *acetazolamide*

  Oestrogens and Progestogens: *oestrogens and combined oral contraceptives* antagonise diuretic effect
- Potassium Salts: hyperkalaemia with *potassium-sparing diuretics*

  Sympathomimetics: increased risk of hypokalaemia if *acetazolamide, loop diuretics, and thiazides* given with high doses of *bambuterol, eformoterol, feno- terol, pirbuterol, reproterol, rimiterol, ritodrine, salbutamol, salmeterol, terbutaline, and tulo- buterol;* see also CSM advice, p. 122

Diuretics (*continued*)

  Ulcer-healing Drugs: increased risk of hypokalaemia if *acetazolamide, loop diuretics, and thiazides* given with *carbenoxolone; carbenoxolone* antago- nises diuretic effect; *amiloride and spironolactone* antagonise ulcer-healing effect of *carbenoxolone*

  Vitamins: increased risk of hypercalcaemia if *thiazides* given with *vitamin D*

Dobutamine *see* Sympathomimetics

Docetaxel

  Note. No formal clinical studies but *in-vitro* studies sug- gest possible interaction with cyclosporin, erythromycin ketoconazole, terfenadine, — consult product literature

Domperidone

  Analgesics: *opioid analgesics* antagonise effect on gastro-intestinal activity

  Antimuscarinics: antagonism of effect on gastro- intestinal activity

  Dopaminergics: antagonism of hypoprolactinaemic effect of *bromocriptine*

Dopamine *see* Sympathomimetics

Dopaminergics *see* Amantadine, Bromocriptine and Cabergoline, Levodopa, and Lysuride

Dopexamine *see* Sympathomimetics

Dorzolamide *see* Diuretics (carbonic anhydrase inhibitor)

  Note. Since systemic absorption may follow topical application of dorzolamide to the eye, the possibility of interactions should be borne in mind

Dothiepin *see* Antidepressants, Tricyclic

Doxapram

  Sympathomimetics: risk of hypertension

  Theophylline: increased CNS stimulation

Doxazosin *see* Alpha-blockers (post-synaptic)

Doxepin *see* Antidepressants, Tricyclic

Doxorubicin

- Cyclosporin: increased risk of neurotoxicity

Doxycycline *see* Tetracyclines

Doxylamine *see* Antihistamines

Droperidol *see* Antipsychotics

Dydrogesterone *see* Progestogens

Ecothiopate *see* Parasympathomimetics

Edrophonium *see* Parasympathomimetics

Eformoterol *see* Sympathomimetics, Beta$_2$

Enalapril *see* ACE Inhibitors

Enflurane *see* Anaesthetics, General (volatile liquid)

Enoxaparin *see* Heparin

Ephedrine *see* Sympathomimetics

Epoetin

- ACE Inhibitors: increased risk of hyperkalaemia

Ergotamine

- Antibacterials: ergotism with *erythromycin* and possibly *azithromycin*

  Beta-blockers: increased peripheral vasconstriction
- Sumatriptan: increased risk of vasospasm (see section 4.7.4.1)

Erythromycin and other Macrolides

  Note. Interactions do not apply to small amounts used topically

  Analgesics: plasma concentration of *alfentanil* increased by *erythromycin*

  Antacids and Adsorbents: *antacids* reduce absorption of *azithromycin*
- Anti-arrhythmics: plasma concentration of *disopyramide* increased by *erythromycin* (risk of toxicity)
- *other* Antibacterials: *clarithromycin* and possibly *other macrolides* increase plasma concentration of *rifabutin* (risk of uveitis)
- Anticoagulants: effect of *nicoumalone and warfarin* enhanced by *erythromycin* and possibly enhanced by some *other macrolides*
- Antiepileptics: *clarithromycin* and *erythromycin* inhibit metabolism of *carbamazepine* (increased plasma-carbamazepine concentration)

Erythromycin and other Macrolides (*continued*)

- Antihistamines: *clarithromycin* and *erythromycin* inhibit metabolism of *astemizole* and *terfenadine* (risk of hazardous arrhythmias, see p. 138); manufacturer advises possibility of increased plasma-loratadine concentration with *erythromycin*

  Antipsychotics: *erythromycin* possibly increases plasma concentration of *clozapine* (possible increased risk of convulsions)

  Antivirals: *clarithromycin tablets* reduce absorption of *zidovudine*

  Anxiolytics and Hypnotics: *erythromycin* inhibits metabolism of *midazolam* (increased plasma-midazolam concentration, with profound sedation) and *zopiclone*

  Calcium-channel Blockers: *erythromycin* possibly inhibits metabolism of *felodipine* (increased plasma concentration)

  Cardiac Glycosides: effect of *digoxin* enhanced by *erythromycin* and possibly enhanced by *other macrolides*

  Cisapride: *clarithromycin* and *erythromycin* possibly inhibit metabolism of *cisapride* (risk of ventricular arrhythmias)

- Cyclosporin: *erythromycin* and possibly *other macrolides* inhibit metabolism (increased plasma-cyclosporin concentration)

  Cytotoxics: *see* Docetaxel

  Dopaminergics: plasma concentration of *bromocriptine* and *cabergoline* increased by *erythromycin*

- Ergotamine: ergotism reported

  Tacrolimus *see* Tacrolimus, p. 564

- Theophylline: *clarithromycin* and *erythromycin* inhibit metabolism (increased plasma-theophylline concentration) (if erythromycin given by mouth, also decreased plasma-erythromycin concentration)

  Ulcer-healing Drugs: *cimetidine* increases plasma-erythromycin concentration (increased risk of toxicity, including deafness)

Erythropoietin *see* Epoetin

Esmolol *see* Beta-blockers

Ethacrynic Acid *see* Diuretics (loop)

Ethinyloestradiol *see* Contraceptives, Oral

Ethosuximide

- Antibacterials: *isoniazid* increases plasma concentrations (increased risk of toxicity)

- Antidepressants: antagonism (convulsive threshold lowered)

- *other* Antiepileptics: concomitant administration of two or more antiepileptics may enhance toxicity without a corresponding increase in antiepileptic effect; moreover interactions between individual antiepileptics can complicate monitoring of treatment; interactions include enhanced effects, increased sedation, and reductions in plasma concentrations; for further details, see p. 203

- Antipsychotics: antagonism (convulsive threshold lowered)

Ethynodiol *see* Progestogens

Etidronate Disodium *see* Bisphosphonates

Etodolac *see* NSAIDs

Etomidate *see* Anaesthetics, General

Famciclovir *see* Aciclovir and Famciclovir

Famotidine *see* Histamine H$_2$-antagonists

Fansidar® contains Sulfadoxine and Pyrimethamine

Felodipine *see* Calcium-channel Blockers

Fenbufen *see* NSAIDs

Fenfluramine *see* Sympathomimetics

Fenofibrate *see* Clofibrate Group

Fenoprofen *see* NSAIDs

Fenoterol *see* Sympathomimetics, Beta$_2$

Fentanyl *see* Opioid Analgesics

Ferrous Salts *see* Iron

Filgrastim

Note. Use not recommended in period from 24 hours before to 24 hours after chemotherapy—for further details consult product literature

Finasteride

Note. No clinically important interactions reported

Flavoxate *see* Antimuscarinics

Flecainide

- *other* Anti-arrhythmics: *amiodarone* increases plasma-flecainide concentration (and increases risk of ventricular arrhythmias); increased myocardial depression with any *anti-arrhythmic*

- Antidepressants: *fluoxetine* increases plasma-flecainide concentration; increased risk of arrhythmias with *tricyclics*

- Antihistamines: increased risk of ventricular arrhythmias with *astemizole* and *terfenadine*

- Antimalarials: *quinine* increases plasma concentration of *flecainide*; increased risk of arrhythmias with *halofantrine* (**important:** see p. 276)

- Beta-blockers: increased myocardial depression and bradycardia

- Calcium-channel Blockers: increased myocardial depression and asystole with *verapamil*

- Diuretics: toxicity increased if hypokalaemia occurs

  Ulcer-healing Drugs: *cimetidine* inhibits metabolism of *flecainide* (increased plasma-flecainide concentration)

Flucloxacillin *see* Penicillins

Fluconazole *see* Antifungals, Imidazole and Triazole

Fludarabine

  Antiplatelet Drugs: efficacy possibly reduced by *dipyridamole*

- *other* Cytotoxics: increased pulmonary toxicity with *pentostatin* (unacceptably high incidence of fatalities)

Fludrocortisone *see* Corticosteroids

Flunisolide *see* Corticosteroids

Flunitrazepam *see* Anxiolytics and Hypnotics

Fluorouracil

  Antibacterials: *metronidazole* inhibits metabolism (increased toxicity)

  Ulcer-healing Drugs: *cimetidine* inhibits metabolism (increased plasma-fluorouracil concentration)

Fluoxetine *see* Antidepressants, SSRI

Flupenthixol *see* Antipsychotics

Fluphenazine *see* Antipsychotics

Flurazepam *see* Anxiolytics and Hypnotics

Flurbiprofen *see* NSAIDs

Flutamide

- Anticoagulants: effect of *warfarin* enhanced

Fluticasone *see* Corticosteroids

Fluvastatin *see* Statins

Fluvoxamine *see* Antidepressants, SSRI

Folic Acid *see* Vitamins

Fosfomycin

  Metoclopramide and Domperidone: reduced plasma and urine concentrations with *metoclopramide*

Fosinopril *see* ACE Inhibitors

Framycetin *see* Aminoglycosides

Frusemide *see* Diuretics (loop)

Gabapentin

  Antacids and Adsorbents: *antacids* reduce absorption

  other Antiepileptics: none demonstrated with *carbamazepine, phenobarbitone, phenytoin,* or *valproate*

Gallamine *see* Muscle Relaxants (non-depolarising)

Ganciclovir

Note. Increased risk of myelosuppression with other *myelosuppressive drugs*—consult data sheet

- Antibacterials: increased toxicity with *Primaxin®* (convulsions reported)

- *other* Antivirals: profound myelosuppression with *zidovudine* (see also p. 270)

Ganciclovir (*continued*)
  Uricosurics: *probenecid* possibly reduces renal
    excretion (increased plasma half-life)
Gemfibrozil *see* Clofibrate Group
Gentamicin *see* Aminoglycosides
Gestodene *see* Progestogens
Gestrinone
  Antibacterials: *rifampicin* accelerates metabolism
    (reduced plasma concentration)
  Antiepileptics: *carbamazepine, phenobarbitone,
    phenytoin, and primidone* accelerate metabolism
    (reduced plasma concentration)
  Barbiturates and Primidone: *see under* Antiepileptics,
    above
Gestronol *see* Progestogens
Glibenclamide *see* Antidiabetics (sulphonylurea)
Gliclazide *see* Antidiabetics (sulphonylurea)
Glipizide *see* Antidiabetics (sulphonylurea)
Gliquidone *see* Antidiabetics (sulphonylurea)
Glyceryl Trinitrate (general hypotensive interactions
    as for Hydralazine)
  Anti-arrhythmics: *disopyramide* may reduce effect of
    sublingual nitrates (owing to dry mouth)
• Anticoagulants: excretion of *heparin* increased by
    glyceryl trinitrate infusion (reduced anticoagulant
    effect)
  Antidepressants: *tricyclics* may reduce effect of
    sublingual nitrates (owing to dry mouth)
  Antimuscarinics: *antimuscarinics such as atropine
    and propantheline* may reduce effect of *sublingual
    nitrates* (owing to dry mouth)
Gold
  Note. Increased risk of toxicity with other nephrotoxic
    and myelosuppressive drugs
Griseofulvin
• Anticoagulants: metabolism of *nicoumalone and
    warfarin* accelerated (reduced anticoagulant effect)
  Antiepileptics: metabolism accelerated by
    phenobarbitone (reduced effect)
  Barbiturates and Primidone: *see under* Antiepileptics,
    above
  Cyclosporin: plasma-cyclosporin concentration
    possibly reduced
• Oestrogens and Progestogens: metabolism of *oral
    contraceptives* accelerated (reduced contraceptive
    effect, **important:** see p. 337)
Guanethidine *see* Adrenergic Neurone Blockers
Guar Gum
  Antibacterials: absorption of
    phenoxymethylpenicillin reduced
Halofantrine
• Anti-arrhythmics: increased risk of ventricular
    arrhythmias with drugs which prolong QT interval
• Antidepressants: increased risk of ventricular
    arrhythmias with *tricyclics*
• Antihistamines: increased risk of ventricular
    arrhythmias with *astemizole* and *terfenadine*
• *other* Antimalarials: increased risk of arrhythmias
    with *chloroquine, mefloquine* and *quinine*
    (**important:** see also CSM advice under
    Halofantrine, p. 276)
• Antipsychotics: increased risk of ventricular
    arrhythmias with *phenothiazines*
• Beta-blockers: increased risk of ventricular
    arrhythmias with *sotalol*
• Diuretics: increased risk of ventricular arrhythmias if
    electrolyte disturbances occur
Haloperidol *see* Antipsychotics
Halothane *see* Anaesthetics, General (volatile liquid)
Heparin
• Analgesics: *aspirin* enhances anticoagulant effect;
    increased risk of haemorrhage with *ketorolac*, see
    p. 527
  Antiplatelet Drugs: *aspirin and dipyridamole*
    enhance anticoagulant effect
• Nitrates: *glyceryl trinitrate infusion* increases
    excretion (reduced anticoagulant effect)

Hexamine
  Potassium Citrate: urine should be acid
Histamine H$_1$-antagonists *see* Antihistamines
Histamine H$_2$-antagonists
  Analgesics: *cimetidine* inhibits metabolism of *opioid
    analgesics notably pethidine* (increased plasma
    concentrations); *cimetidine* possibly increases
    plasma concentration of *azapropazone*
  Anthelmintics: *cimetidine* possibly inhibits
    metabolism of *mebendazole* (increased plasma
    concentration)
• Anti-arrhythmics: *cimetidine* increases plasma
    concentrations of *amiodarone, flecainide,
    lignocaine, procainamide, propafenone, quinidine*,
    and possibly *moracizine*
  Antibacterials: absorption of *cefpodoxime* reduced;
    cimetidine increases plasma-erythromycin
    concentration (increased risk of toxicity, including
    deafness); *rifampicin* accelerates metabolism of
    cimetidine (reduced plasma-cimetidine
    concentration); *cimetidine* inhibits metabolism of
    metronidazole (increased plasma-metronidazole
    concentration)
• Anticoagulants: *cimetidine* enhances anticoagulant
    effect of *nicoumalone and warfarin* (inhibits
    metabolism)
  Antidepressants: *cimetidine* inhibits metabolism of
    *amitriptyline, desipramine, doxepin, imipramine,
    moclobemide, and nortriptyline* (increased plasma
    concentrations)
  Antidiabetics: *cimetidine* inhibits renal excretion of
    metformin (increased plasma concentration);
    cimetidine and *ranitidine* enhance hypoglycaemic
    effect of *sulphonylureas*
• Antiepileptics: *cimetidine* inhibits metabolism of
    carbamazepine, phenytoin, and valproate
    (increased plasma concentrations)
  Antifungals: absorption of *itraconazole and
    ketoconazole* reduced; plasma concentration of
    terbinafine increased by *cimetidine*
  Antihistamines: ; manufacturer advises possibility of
    increased plasma-loratadine concentration with
    cimetidine
  Antimalarials: *cimetidine* inhibits metabolism of
    chloroquine and quinine (increased plasma
    concentrations)
  Antipsychotics: *cimetidine* possibly enhances effect
    of *chlorpromazine, clozapine, and possibly other
    antipsychotics*
  Anxiolytics and Hypnotics: *cimetidine* inhibits
    metabolism of *benzodiazepines and
    chlormethiazole* (increased plasma concentrations)
  Beta-blockers: *cimetidine* inhibits metabolism of
    beta-blockers such as labetalol and propranolol
    (increased plasma concentrations)
  Calcium-channel Blockers: *cimetidine* inhibits
    metabolism of *some calcium-channel blockers*
    (increased plasma concentrations)
• Cyclosporin: *cimetidine* possibly increases plasma-
    cyclosporin concentration
  Cytotoxics: *cimetidine* increases plasma
    concentration of *fluorouracil*
  Hormone Antagonists: *octreotide* possibly delays
    absorption of *cimetidine*
• Theophylline: *cimetidine* inhibits metabolism
    (increased plasma-theophylline concentration)
Homatropine *see* Antimuscarinics
Hormone Antagonists *see* Aminoglutethimide;
    Danazol; Tamoxifen; Trilostane
Hydralazine
  ACE Inhibitors: enhanced hypotensive effect
  Alcohol: enhanced hypotensive effect
  Aldesleukin: enhanced hypotensive effect
• Anaesthetics: enhanced hypotensive effect
  Analgesics: *NSAIDs* antagonise hypotensive effect
  Antidepressants: enhanced hypotensive effect
  other Antihypertensives: additive hypotensive effect

Hydralazine (*continued*)

Antipsychotics: enhanced hypotensive effect

Anxiolytics and Hypnotics: enhanced hypotensive effect

Beta-blockers: enhanced hypotensive effect

Calcium-channel Blockers: enhanced hypotensive effect

Corticosteroids: antagonism of hypotensive effect

Diuretics: enhanced hypotensive effect

Dopaminergics: *levodopa* enhances hypotensive effect

Muscle Relaxants: *baclofen* enhances hypotensive effect

Nitrates: enhanced hypotensive effect

Oestrogens and Progestogens: *oestrogens and combined oral contraceptives* antagonise hypotensive effect

Ulcer-healing Drugs: *carbenoxolone* antagonises hypotensive effect

Hydrochlorothiazide *see* Diuretics (thiazide)

Hydrocortisone *see* Corticosteroids

Hydroflumethiazide *see* Diuretics (thiazide)

Hydroxychloroquine *see* Chloroquine and Hydroxychloroquine

Hydroxyprogesterone *see* Progestogens

Hydroxyzine *see* Antihistamines

Hyoscine *see* Antimuscarinics (for general sedative interactions *see also* Antihistamines)

Hypnotics *see* Anxiolytics and Hypnotics

Ibuprofen *see* NSAIDs

Ifosfamide *see* Cyclophosphamide and Ifosfamide

Imipenem *see* Primaxin®

Immunoglobulins

Note. For advice on immunoglobulins and live virus vaccines, see under Normal Immunoglobulin section 14.5

Imipramine *see* Antidepressants, Tricyclic

Indapamide *see* Diuretics (thiazide-related)

Indomethacin *see* NSAIDs

Indoramin *see* Alpha-blockers

Influenza Vaccine

Anticoagulants: effect of *warfarin* occasionally enhanced

Antiepileptics: effect of *phenytoin* enhanced

Theophylline: effect occasionally enhanced

Insulin *see* Antidiabetics

Interferons

Note. Consult product literature for interactions of interferon beta and gamma

Theophylline: *interferon alfa* inhibits metabolism of *theophylline* (enhanced effect)

Ipratropium *see* Antimuscarinics

Iron

Antacids: *magnesium trisilicate* reduces absorption of *oral iron*

Antibacterials: *tetracyclines* reduce absorption of *oral iron* (and *vice versa*); absorption of *ciprofloxacin, norfloxacin,* and *ofloxacin* reduced by *oral iron*

Bisphosphonates: reduced absorption

Dopaminergics: absorption of *levodopa* may be reduced

Penicillamine: reduced absorption of *penicillamine*

Trientine: reduced absorption of *oral iron*

Zinc: reduced absorption of *oral iron* (and *vice versa*)

Isocarboxazid *see* MAOIs

Isoflurane *see* Anaesthetics, General (volatile liquid)

Isometheptene *see* Sympathomimetics

Isoniazid

Anaesthetics: hepatotoxicity possibly potentiated by *isoflurane*

Antacids and Adsorbents: *antacids* reduce absorption

other Antibacterials: increased CNS toxicity with *cycloserine*

• Antiepileptics: metabolism of *carbamazepine, ethosuximide, and phenytoin* inhibited (enhanced effect); also, with *carbamazepine,* isoniazid hepatotoxicity possibly increased

Isoniazid (*continued*)

Anxiolytics and Hypnotics: metabolism of *diazepam* inhibited

Theophylline: *isoniazid* possibly increases plasma *theophylline* concentration

Isoprenaline *see* Sympathomimetics

Isosorbide Dinitrate *see* Glyceryl Trinitrate

Isosorbide Mononitrate *see* Glyceryl Trinitrate

Isotretinoin *see* Retinoids

Isradipine *see* Calcium-channel Blockers

Itraconazole *see* Antifungals, Imidazole and Triazole

Kanamycin *see* Aminoglycosides

Kaolin *see* Antacids and Adsorbents

Ketamine *see* Anaesthetics, General

Ketoconazole *see* Antifungals, Imidazole and Triazole

Ketoprofen *see* NSAIDs

Ketorolac *see* NSAIDs and p. 527

Ketotifen *see* Antihistamines

Labetalol *see* Beta-blockers

Lacidipine *see* Calcium-channel Blockers

Lamotrigine

• *other* Antiepileptics: concomitant administration of *two or more antiepileptics* may enhance toxicity without a corresponding increase in antiepileptic effect; moreover interactions between individual antiepileptics can complicate monitoring of treatment; interactions include enhanced effects, increased sedation, and reductions in plasma concentrations; for further details, see p. 203

Lansoprazole *see* Proton Pump Inhibitors

Lenograstim

Note. Use not recommended from 1 day before until 24 hours after chemotherapy—for further details consult data sheet

Levobunolol *see* Beta-blockers

Levocabastine *see* Antihistamines

Levodopa

• Anaesthetics: risk of arrhythmias with *volatile liquid anaesthetics such as halothane*

• Antidepressants: hypertensive crisis with *MAOIs* (including *moclobemide*)—avoid for at least 2 weeks after stopping MAOI

Antihypertensives: enhanced hypotensive effect

Antipsychotics: antagonism of effect

Anxiolytics and Hypnotics: occasional antagonism of effect by *chlordiazepoxide, diazepam, lorazepam and possibly other benzodiazepines*

Iron: absorption of *levodopa* may be reduced

Metoclopramide and Domperidone: levodopa-plasma concentrations increased by *metoclopramide*

Vitamins: effect of *levodopa* antagonised by *pyridoxine* unless a *dopa decarboxylase inhibitor* also given

Levonorgestrel *see* Progestogens

Lignocaine

other Anti-arrhythmics: increased myocardial depression

Beta-blockers: increased risk of myocardial depression; increased risk of *lignocaine* toxicity with *propranolol*

Diuretics: effect of *lignocaine* antagonised by hypokalaemia with *acetazolamide, loop diuretics, and thiazides*

Ulcer-healing Drugs: *cimetidine* inhibits metabolism of *lignocaine* (increased risk of toxicity)

Lipid-lowering Drugs *see* Cholestyramine and Colestipol; Clofibrate Group; Nicotinic Acid; Statins

Lisinopril *see* ACE Inhibitors

Lithium

• ACE Inhibitors: *lithium* excretion reduced (increased plasma-lithium concentration)

• Analgesics: *NSAIDs* reduce excretion of *lithium* (possibility of toxicity)—*ketorolac,* see p. 527

Lithium (*continued*)

Antacids and Adsorbents: *sodium bicarbonate* increases excretion of *lithium* (reduced plasma-lithium concentrations)

Antibacterials: *lithium* toxicity reported with *metronidazole* and *spectinomycin*

• Antidepressants: *SSRIs* increase risk of CNS effects (lithium toxicity reported)

Antidiabetics: *lithium* may occasionally impair glucose tolerance

Antiepileptics: neurotoxicity may occur with *carbamazepine and phenytoin* without increased plasma-lithium concentration

• Antihypertensives: neurotoxicity may occur with *methyldopa* without increased plasma-lithium concentration

Antipsychotics: increased risk of extrapyramidal effects and possibility of neurotoxicity (notably with *haloperidol*)

Calcium-channel Blockers: neurotoxicity may occur with *diltiazem and verapamil* without increased plasma-lithium concentration

• Diuretics: *lithium* excretion reduced by *loop diuretics, potassium-sparing diuretics, and thiazides* (increased plasma-lithium concentration and risk of toxicity—*loop diuretics safer than thiazides); lithium* excretion increased by *acetazolamide*

Metoclopramide and Domperidone: increased risk of extrapyramidal effects and possibility of neurotoxicity with *metoclopramide*

Muscle Relaxants: muscle relaxant effect enhanced; *baclofen* possibly aggravates hyperkinesis

Parasympathomimetics: *lithium* antagonises effect of *neostigmine and pyridostigmine*

• Sumatriptan: risk of CNS toxicity

Theophylline: *lithium* excretion increased (reduced plasma-lithium concentration)

Lofepramine *see* Antidepressants, Tricyclic

Lofexidine

Alcohol: enhanced sedative effect

Anxiolytics and Hypnotics: enhanced sedative effect

Loprazolam *see* Anxiolytics and Hypnotics

Loratadine *see* Antihistamines

Lorazepam *see* Anxiolytics and Hypnotics

Lormetazepam *see* Anxiolytics and Hypnotics

Losartan as for ACE Inhibitors

Loxapine *see* Antipsychotics

Lymecycline *see* Tetracyclines

Lysuride

Antipsychotics: antagonism of effect

Macrolides *see* Erythromycin and other Macrolides

Magnesium Salts (*see also* Antacids and Adsorbents)

Muscle Relaxants: effect of *non-depolarising muscle relaxants* enhanced by *parenteral magnesium salts*

Magnesium Trisilicate *see* Antacids and Adsorbents

Maloprim® contains Dapsone and Pyrimethamine

MAOIs

Note. For interactions of reversible MAO-A inhibitors (RIMAs) see Moclobemide, and for interactions of MAO-B inhibitors see Selegiline

• Alcohol: some *alcoholic and dealcoholised beverages contain tyramine* which interacts with *MAOIs* (hypertensive crisis)—but if no tyramine, enhanced hypotensive effect; foods, *see* MAOI card, section 4.3.2

• Analgesics: CNS excitation or depression (hypertension or hypotension) with *pethidine and possibly other opioid analgesics;* manufacturer advises avoid *nefopam*

Anaesthetics: *see* section 15.1

• Anorectics: *see* Sympathomimetics, below

MAOIs (*continued*)

• *other* Antidepressants: enhancement of CNS effects and toxicity with *other MAOIs* (avoid for at least a week after stopping *previous MAOIs* then start with reduced dose); increased risk of toxicity with *nefazodone* (**important:** if MAOIs discontinued shortly before, *initiate nefazodone cautiously* with *gradual dose increase*); CNS excitation and hypertension with most *tricyclics and related antidepressants* (avoid for at least 2 weeeks after stopping MAOI, and avoid MAOI for at least 1 week after stopping tricyclic); enhancement of CNS effects and toxicity possible with *SSRIs* (avoid for at least 2 weeks after stopping MAOI, and avoid MAOI for at least 1 week after stopping SSRI—*fluoxetine* for at least 5 weeks and *paroxetine* and *sertraline* for at least 2 weeks); CNS excitation and confusion with *tryptophan* (reduce tryptophan dose); enhancement of CNS effects and toxicity possible with *venlafaxine* (avoid for at least 2 weeks after stopping MAOI, and avoid MAOI for at least 1 week after stopping venlafaxine)

Antidiabetics: effect of *insulin, metformin, and sulphonylureas* enhanced

• Antiepileptics: antagonism of anticonvulsant effect (convulsive threshold lowered); manufacturer advises avoid *carbamazepine* with or within 2 weeks of *MAOIs*

• Antihypertensives: hypotensive effect enhanced; manufacturer advises avoidance of *indoramin*

Antihistamines: increased antimuscarinic and sedative effects

Antimuscarinics: increased side-effects

• Antipsychotics: CNS excitation and hypertension with *oxypertine; clozapine* possibly enhances central effects

Anxiolytics and Hypnotics: manufacturer advises avoidance of *buspirone*

• Barbiturates and Primidone: *see under* Antiepileptics, above

• Dopaminergics: hypertensive crisis with *levodopa* (avoid for at least 2 weeks after stopping MAOI); hypotension with *selegiline*

• Sumatriptan: risk of CNS toxicity

• Sympathomimetics: hypertensive crisis with *sympathomimetics such as dexamphetamine and other amphetamines, dexfenfluramine, dopamine, dopexamine, ephedrine, fenfluramine, isometh-eptene, methylphenidate, pemoline, phentermine, phenylephrine, phenylpropanolamine, and pseudo-ephedrine*

• Tetrabenazine: CNS excitation and hypertension

Maprotiline *see* Antidepressants, Tricyclic

Mebendazole

Ulcer-healing Drugs: metabolism possibly inhibited by *cimetidine* (increased plasma-mebendazole concentration)

Medroxyprogesterone *see* Progestogens

Mefenamic Acid *see* NSAIDs

Mefloquine

• Antiepileptics: antagonism of anticonvulsant effect

other Antimalarials: increased risk of convulsions with *chloroquine* and *quinine*, but should not prevent use of intravenous quinine in severe cases; for full precautions see footnote on p. 272 (also applies to *quinidine*); increased risk of ventricular arrhythmias with *halofantrine* (**important:** see also CSM advice under Halofantrine, p. 276)

Beta-blockers: possible increased risk of bradycardia

Calcium-channel Blockers: possible increased risk of bradycardia with some *calcium-channel blockers*

Cardiac Glycosides: possible increased risk of bradycardia with *digoxin*

Vaccines: *see* Typhoid Vaccine, p. 514

Mefruside *see* Diuretics (thiazide)

Megestrol see Progestogens

Melphalan

Antibacterials: increased toxicity with *nalidixic acid*

● Cyclosporin: increased risk of nephrotoxicity

Mepacrine

Antimalarials: increased plasma concentration of *primaquine* (risk of toxicity)

Meprobamate see Anxiolytics and Hypnotics

Meptazinol see Opioid Analgesics

Mequitazine see Antihistamines

Mercaptopurine

● Allopurinol: enhancement of effect (increased toxicity)

Mestranol see Contraceptives, Oral

Metaraminol see Sympathomimetics (*as* noradrenaline)

Metformin see Antidiabetics

Methadone see Opioid Analgesics

Methocarbamol see Muscle Relaxants

Methohexitone see Anaesthetics, General

Methotrexate

● Analgesics: excretion reduced by *aspirin, azapropazone, diclofenac, indomethacin, ketoprofen, naproxen, phenylbutazone, and probably other NSAIDs* (increased risk of toxicity)

● Antibacterials: antifolate effect increased by *co-trimoxazole and trimethoprim*; excretion reduced by penicillins (increased risk of toxicity)

Antiepileptics: *phenytoin* increases antifolate effect

Antimalarials: antifolate effect increased by *pyrimethamine* (ingredient of *Fansidar®* and *Maloprim®*)

● Cyclosporin: increased toxicity

● Retinoids: plasma concentration of *methotrexate* increased by *acitretin* (also increased risk of hepatotoxicity)

● Uricosurics: excretion reduced by *probenecid* (increased risk of toxicity)

Methotrimeprazine see Antipsychotics

Methoxamine see Sympathomimetics (*as* noradrenaline)

Methyldopa

Alcohol: enhanced hypotensive effect

● Anaesthetics: enhanced hypotensive effect

Analgesics: *NSAIDs* antagonise hypotensive effect

other Antihypertensives: enhanced hypotensive effect

Antipsychotics: increased risk of extrapyramidal effects; enhanced hypotensive effect

Anxiolytics and Hypnotics: enhanced hypotensive effect

Beta-blockers: enhanced hypotensive effect

Calcium-channel Blockers: enhanced hypotensive effect

Corticosteroids: antagonism of hypotensive effect

Diuretics: enhanced hypotensive effect

Dopaminergics: antagonism of antiparkinsonian effect; *levodopa* enhances hypotensive effect

● Lithium: neurotoxicity may occur without increased plasma-lithium concentration

Nitrates: enhance hypotensive effect

Oestrogens and Progestogens: *oestrogens and combined oral contraceptives* antagonise hypotensive effect

Sympathomimetics: see Sympathomimetics (main list)

Ulcer-healing Drugs: *carbenoxolone* antagonises hypotensive effect

Methylphenidate see Sympathomimetics

Methylphenobarbitone see Barbiturates

Methylprednisolone see Corticosteroids

Metipranolol see Beta-blockers

Metirosine

Antipsychotics: increased risk of extrapyramidal effects

Dopaminergics: antagonism

Metoclopramide

Analgesics: increased absorption of *aspirin and paracetamol* (enhanced effect); *opioid analgesics* antagonise effect on gastro-intestinal activity

Antibacterials: reduced plasma and urine concentrations of *fosfomycin*

Antimuscarinics: antagonism of effect on gastro-intestinal activity

Antipsychotics: increased risk of extrapyramidal effects

Atovaquone: plasma concentration reduced by *metoclopramide*

Dopaminergics: antagonism of hypoprolactinaemic effect of *bromocriptine*; increased plasma concentration of *levodopa*; antagonism of antiparkinsonian effects of *pergolide*

Lithium: increased risk of extrapyramidal effects and possibility of neurotoxicity

Tetrabenazine: increased risk of extrapyramidal effects

Metolazone see Diuretics (thiazide-related)

Metoprolol see Beta-blockers

Metronidazole

Alcohol: disulfiram-like reaction

● Anticoagulants: effect of *nicoumalone and warfarin* enhanced

● Antiepileptics: *metronidazole* inhibits metabolism of *phenytoin* (increased plasma-phenytoin concentration); *phenobarbitone* accelerates metabolism of *metronidazole* (reduced plasma-metronidazole concentration)

● Barbiturates and Primidone: *see under* Antiepileptics, above

Cytotoxics: *metronidazole* inhibits metabolism of *fluorouracil* (increased toxicity)

Disulfiram: psychotic reactions reported

Lithium: increased toxicity reported

Ulcer-healing Drugs: *cimetidine* inhibits metabolism (increased plasma-metronidazole concentration)

Mexiletine

Analgesics: *opioid analgesics* delay absorption

● *other* Anti-arrhythmics: increased myocardial depression with any combination of *anti-arrhythmics*

Antibacterials: *rifampicin* accelerates metabolism (reduced plasma-mexiletine concentration)

Antiepileptics: *phenytoin* accelerates metabolism (reduced plasma-mexiletine concentration)

Antimuscarinics: *atropine* delays absorption

Diuretics: action of *mexiletine* antagonised by hypokalaemia due to *acetazolamide, loop diuretics, and thiazides*

Theophylline: plasma-theophylline concentration increased

Mianserin

Alcohol: enhanced effect

other Antidepressants: as for Antidepressants, Tricyclic

● Antiepileptics: antagonism (convulsive threshold lowered); metabolism accelerated by *carbamazepine, phenobarbitone, and phenytoin* (reduced plasma-mianserin concentration)

Anxiolytics and Hypnotics: enhanced effect

● Barbiturates and Primidone: *see under* Antiepileptics, above

Miconazole see Antifungals, Imidazole and Triazole

Midazolam see Anxiolytics and Hypnotics

Mifepristone

Analgesics: manufacturer recommends avoid *aspirin* and *NSAIDs* until 8–12 days after *mifepristone* administration

Minocycline see Tetracyclines

Minoxidil see Hydralazine for general hypotensive interactions

Mivacurium see Muscle Relaxants (non-depolarising)

Moclobemide

Note. Moclobemide is a reversible MAO-A inhibitor (RIMA), see also p. 177

- Analgesics: CNS excitation or depression (hypertension or hypotension) with *codeine*, *pethidine*, and possibly *fentanyl*, *morphine*, and *other opioid analgesics*; effects of *ibuprofen* and possibly *other NSAIDs* enhanced
- Anorectics: as for MAOIs (see main list)
- *other* Antidepressants: see p. 177
- Dopaminergics: hypertensive crisis with *levodopa*
- Sumatriptan: risk of CNS toxicity
- Sympathomimetics: as for MAOIs (see main list)
  Ulcer-healing Drugs: *cimetidine* inhibits metabolism (increased plasma-moclobemide concentration)

Moexipril *see* ACE Inhibitors

Monoamine-oxidase Inhibitors *see* MAOIs, Moclobemide, and Selegiline

Moracizine

other Anti-arrhythmics: increased myocardial depression with any *anti-arrhythmic*

Theophylline: metabolism of *theophylline* accelerated (reduced effect)

Ulcer-healing Drugs: *cimetidine* possibly increases plasma-moracizine concentration

Morphine *see* Opioid Analgesics

Moxonidine

other Antihypertensives: enhanced hypotensive effect

Anxiolytics and Hypnotics: sedative effect of *benzodiazepines* possibly enhanced

Muscle Relaxants

ACE Inhibitors: enhanced hypotensive effect with *baclofen*

Alcohol: enhanced sedative effect with *baclofen*

Analgesics: *ibuprofen* and possibly *other NSAIDs* reduce excretion of *baclofen* (increased risk of toxicity)

- Anti-arrhythmics: *procainamide* and *quinidine* enhance muscle relaxant effect
- Antibacterials: effect of *non-depolarising muscle relaxants* enhanced by *aminoglycosides, azlocillin, clindamycin and colistin*

Antidepressants: *tricyclics* enhance muscle relaxant effect of *baclofen*

Antiepileptics: effect of *non-depolarising muscle relaxants* antagonised by *carbamazepine* and *phenytoin* (recovery from neuromuscular blockade accelerated)

Antihypertensives: enhanced hypotensive effect with *baclofen*

Anxiolytics and Hypnotics: enhanced sedative effect with *baclofen*

Beta-blockers: *propranolol* enhances muscle relaxant effect

- Botulinum Toxin: neuromuscular block enhanced by *non-depolarising muscle relaxants* (risk of toxicity)

Calcium-channel Blockers: *nifedipine* and *verapamil* enhance effect of *non-depolarising muscle relaxants*; hypotension, myocardial depression, and hyperkalaemia reported with intravenous *dantrolene* and *verapamil*

Cardiac Glycosides: arrhythmias if *suxamethonium* given with *digoxin*

Cytotoxics: *cyclophosphamide and thiotepa* enhance effect of *suxamethonium*

Lithium: *lithium* enhances muscle relaxant effect; *baclofen* possibly aggravates hyperkinesis

Magnesium Salts: *parenteral magnesium* enhances effect of *non-depolarising muscle relaxants*

Parasympathomimetics: *demecarium* and *ecothiopate* eye-drops, and *neostigmine, and pyridostigmine* enhance effect of *suxamethonium* but antagonise effect of *non-depolarising muscle relaxants*

Sympathomimetics: *bambuterol* enhances effect of *suxamethonium*

Mycophenolate Mofetil

Anion-exchange Resins: *cholestyramine* reduces absorption

Antacids and Adsorbents: *antacids* reduce absorption

Antivirals: higher plasma concentrations of *mycophenolate mofetil* and of *aciclovir* on concomitant administration

Nabilone

Alcohol: sedative effect of *nabilone* enhanced

Anxiolytics and Hypnotics: enhanced sedative effect

Nabumetone *see* NSAIDs

Nadolol *see* Beta-blockers

Nalbuphine *see* Opioid Analgesics

Nalidixic Acid *see* 4-Quinolones

Nandrolone *see* Anabolic Steroids

Naproxen *see* NSAIDs

Nefazodone

Note. Although interactions with alcohol, antipsychotics, and lithium have not been reported, caution should be observed on concomitant use with nefazodone

Antidepressants: increased risk of toxicity with *MAOIs* (**important:** if MAOIs discontinued shortly before, *initiate cautiously* with *gradual dosage increase*)

Antihypertensives: hypotensive effect possibly enhanced

Anxiolytics and Hypnotics: possibly enhanced sedative effect with *benzodiazepines*

Nefopam

- Antidepressants: manufacturer recommends avoid *MAOIs;* possibly increased side-effects with *tricyclics*

Antimuscarinics: increased side-effects

Neomycin *see* Aminoglycosides

Neostigmine *see* Parasympathomimetics

Netilmicin *see* Aminoglycosides

Nicardipine *see* Calcium-channel Blockers

Nicorandil

Note. Interactions not observed with beta-blockers, digoxin, rifampicin, cimetidine, nicoumalone, calcium-channel blockers, or frusemide; possibility of hypotensive interaction with vasodilators, tricyclics, or alcohol

Nicotine and **Tobacco**

Theophylline: *tobacco smoking* increases metabolism (reduced plasma-theophylline concentration)

Nicotinic Acid

Note. Interactions apply to lipid-lowering doses of nicotinic acid

- *other* Lipid-lowering Drugs: increased risk of myopathy with *statins*

Nicoumalone *see* Warfarin and other Coumarins

Nifedipine *see* Calcium-channel Blockers

Nimodipine *see* Calcium-channel Blockers

Nitrates *see* Glyceryl Trinitrate

Nitrazepam *see* Anxiolytics and Hypnotics

Nitrofurantoin

Antacids and Adsorbents: *magnesium trisilicate* reduces absorption

Uricosurics: *probenecid* reduces excretion of *nitrofurantoin* (risk of toxicity)

Nitroprusside *as for* Hydralazine

Nitrous Oxide *see* Anaesthetics

Nizatidine *see* Histamine H_2-antagonists

Noradrenaline *see* Sympathomimetics

Norethisterone *see* Progestogens

Norfloxacin *see* 4-Quinolones

Norgestimate *see* Progestogens

Norgestrel *see* Progestogens

Nortriptyline *see* Antidepressants, Tricyclic

NSAIDs (*see also* Aspirin)

Note. Interactions do not generally apply to topical NSAIDS

- ACE Inhibitors: antagonism of hypotensive effect; increased risk of renal damage and increased risk of hyperkalaemia on administration with *indomethacin* and possibly *other NSAIDs*

NSAIDs (*continued*)
- *other* Analgesics: avoid concomitant administration of two or more *NSAIDs* (increased side-effects); *ketorolac*, see p. 527

  Anion-exchange Resins: *cholestyramine* reduces absorption of *phenylbutazone*

  Antacids and Adsorbents: *antacids* reduce absorption of *diflunisal*

  Antibacterials: *NSAIDs* possibly increase risk of convulsions with *4-quinolones*
- Anticoagulants: *see* Warfarin; increased risk of haemorrhage with *ketorolac* and all *anticoagulants* (including low-dose heparin), see p. 527

  Antidepressants: *moclobemide* enhances effect of *ibuprofen* and possibly *other NSAIDs*
- Antidiabetics: effect of *sulphonylureas* enhanced by *azapropazone*, *phenylbutazone* and possibly *other NSAIDs*
- Antiepileptics: effect of *phenytoin* enhanced by *azapropazone* and *phenylbutazone*

  Antihypertensives: antagonism of hypotensive effect

  Beta-blockers: antagonism of hypotensive effect

  Bisphosphonates: bioavailability of *tiludronic acid* increased by *indomethacin*

  Cardiac Glycosides: *NSAIDs* may exacerbate heart failure, reduce GFR, and increase plasma-cardiac glycoside concentration

  Corticosteroids: increased risk of gastro-intestinal bleeding and ulceration
- Cyclosporin: increased risk of nephrotoxicity; *cyclosporin* increases plasma concentration of *diclofenac* (halve diclofenac dose)
- Cytotoxics: excretion of *methotrexate* reduced by *aspirin*, *azapropazone*, *diclofenac*, *indomethacin*, *ketoprofen*, *naproxen*, *phenylbutazone* and *probably other NSAIDs* (increased risk of toxicity)

  Diuretics: risk of nephrotoxicity of *NSAIDs* increased; *NSAIDs* notably *indomethacin* antagonise diuretic effect; *indomethacin and possibly other NSAIDs* increase risk of hyperkalaemia with *potassium-sparing diuretics*; occasional reports of decreased renal function when *indomethacin* given with *triamterene*
- Lithium: excretion of *lithium* reduced by *azapropazone*, *diclofenac*, *ibuprofen*, *indomethacin*, *ketorolac* (see p. 527), *mefenamic acid*, *naproxen*, *phenylbutazone*, *piroxicam*, *and probably other NSAIDs* (possibility of toxicity)

  Mifepristone: manufacturer recommends avoid *aspirin* and *NSAIDs* until 8–12 days after *mifepristone* administration

  Muscle Relaxants: *ibuprofen* and *possibly other NSAIDs* reduce excretion of *baclofen* (increased risk of toxicity)

  Thyroxine: false low total plasma-thyroxine concentration with *phenylbutazone*

  Ulcer-healing Drugs: plasma concentration of *azapropazone* possibly increased by *cimetidine*
- Uricosurics: *probenecid* delays excretion of *indomethacin*, *ketoprofen*, *ketorolac* (see p. 527), *and naproxen* (raised plasma concentrations)
- Vasodilators: risk of ketorolac-associated bleeding increased by *oxpentifylline*, see p. 527

Octreotide

  Antidiabetics: reduces *insulin and antidiabetic drug* requirements in diabetes mellitus

  Cyclosporin: absorption of *cyclosporin* reduced (reduced plasma concentration)

  Ulcer-healing Drugs: absorption of *cimetidine* possibly delayed

Oestrogens *see* Contraceptives, Oral

Ofloxacin *see* 4-Quinolones

Omeprazole *see* Proton Pump Inhibitors

Opioid Analgesics

  Alcohol: enhanced sedative and hypotensive effect

  Anti-arrhythmics: delayed absorption of *mexiletine*

Opioid Analgesics (*continued*)

  Antibacterials: *rifampicin* accelerates metabolism of *methadone* (reduced effect); *erythromycin* increases plasma concentration of *alfentanil;* manufacturer of *ciprofloxacin* advises avoid premedication with *opioid analgesics* (reduced plasma-ciprofloxacin concentration)
- Anticoagulants: *dextropropoxyphene* may enhance effect of *nicoumalone and warfarin*
- Antidepressants: CNS excitation or depression (hypertension or hypotension) if *pethidine and possibly other opioid analgesics* given to patients receiving *MAOIs* (including *moclobemide*)
- Antiepileptics: *dextropropoxyphene* enhances effect of *carbamazepine*; effect of *tramadol* decreased by *carbamazepine*

  Antipsychotics: enhanced sedative and hypotensive effect

  Antivirals: *methadone* possibly increases plasma concentration of *zidovudine*

  Anxiolytics and Hypnotics: enhanced sedative effect

  Cisapride: possible antagonism of gastro-intestinal effect
- Dopaminergics: hyperpyrexia and CNS toxicity reported with *selegiline*

  Metoclopramide and Domperidone: antagonism of gastro-intestinal effects

  Ulcer-healing Drugs: *cimetidine* inhibits metabolism of opioid analgesics notably *pethidine* (increased plasma concentration)

Orciprenaline *see* Sympathomimetics

Orphenadrine *see* Antimuscarinics

Oxazepam *see* Anxiolytics and Hypnotics

Oxitropium *see* Antimuscarinics

Oxpentifylline
- Analgesics: increased risk of bleeding with *ketorolac*, see p. 527

Oxprenolol *see* Beta-blockers

Oxybutynin *see* Antimuscarinics

Oxymetazoline *see* Sympathomimetics

Oxypertine *see* Antipsychotics

Oxytetracycline *see* Tetracyclines

Oxytocin

  Anaesthetics: *inhalational anaesthetics* possibly reduce oxytocic effect (also enhanced hypotensive effect and risk of arrhythmias)

  Prostaglandins: uterotonic effect potentiated

  Sympathomimetics: enhancement of vasopressor effect of *vasoconstrictor sympathomimetics*

Paclitaxel

  Antifungals: *ketoconazole* possibly inhibits metabolism of *paclitaxel*

Pamidronate Sodium *see* Bisphosphonates

Pancreatin

  Antidiabetics: hypoglycaemic effect of *acarbose* reduced

Pancuronium *see* Muscle Relaxants (non-depolarising)

Papaveretum *see* Opioid Analgesics

Paracetamol

  Anion-exchange Resins: *cholestyramine* reduces absorption of *paracetamol*

  Anticoagulants: prolonged regular use of *paracetamol* possibly enhances *warfarin*

  Metoclopramide and Domperidone: *metoclopramide* accelerates absorption of *paracetamol* (enhanced effect)

Parasympathomimetics

  Anti-arrhythmics: *procainamide, quinidine* and possibly *propafenone* antagonise effect of *neostigmine and pyridostigmine*
- Antibacterials: *aminoglycosides, clindamycin and colistin* antagonise effect of *neostigmine and pyridostigmine*

Parasympathomimetics (*continued*)

Antimalarials; *chloroquine* and *hydroxychloroquine* have potential to increase symptoms of myasthenia gravis and thus diminish effect of *neostigmine* and *pyridostigmine*

Antimuscarinics: antagonism of effect

Beta-blockers: risk of arrhythmias possibly increased by *pilocarpine*; *propranolol* antagonises effect of *neostigmine* and *pyridostigmine*

Lithium: antagonism of effect of *neostigmine and pyridostigmine*

Muscle Relaxants: *demecarium and ecothiopate eye-drops, and neostigmine and pyridostigmine* enhance effect of *suxamethonium*, but antagonise effect of *non-depolarising muscle relaxants*

Paroxetine *see* Antidepressants, SSRI
Pemoline *see* Sympathomimetics
Penicillamine

Antacids: reduced absorption of *penicillamine*
Iron: reduced absorption of *penicillamine*
Zinc: reduced absorption of *penicillamine*

Penicillins

Antacids: reduced absorption of *pivampicillin*
Anticoagulants: *see* Phenindione and Warfarin
- Cytotoxics: reduced excretion of *methotrexate* (increased risk of toxicity)
Guar Gum: reduced absorption of *phenoxymethylpenicillin*
Muscle Relaxants: effects of *non-depolarising muscle relaxants* enhanced by *azlocillin*
Oestrogens and Progestogens: *see* Contraceptives, Oral
Uricosurics: excretion of *penicillins* reduced by *probenecid*

Pentaerythritol Tetranitrate *see* Glyceryl Trinitrate
Pentazocine *see* Opioid Analgesics
Pentostatin
- *other* Cytotoxics: increases pulmonary toxicity of *fludarabine* (unacceptably high incidence of fatalities)

Pergolide

Antipsychotics: antagonism of effect
Metoclopramide and Domperidone: *metoclopramide* antagonises effect

Pericyazine *see* Antipsychotics
Perindopril *see* ACE Inhibitors
Perphenazine *see* Antipsychotics
Pethidine *see* Opioid Analgesics
Phenazocine *see* Opioid Analgesics
Phenelzine *see* MAOIs
Phenindamine *see* Antihistamines
Phenindione

Note. Change in patient's clinical condition, particularly associated with liver disease, intercurrent illness, or drug administration, necessitates more frequent testing. Major changes in diet (especially involving vegetables) and in alcohol consumption may also affect anticoagulant control

- Anabolic Steroids: anticoagulant effect enhanced by *oxymetholone, stanozolol and others*
- Analgesics: anticoagulant effect enhanced by *aspirin*; increased risk of haemorrhage with *ketorolac*, see p. 527
Anion-exchange Resins: anticoagulant effect enhanced or reduced by *cholestyramine*
Antibacterials: although studies have failed to demonstrate interaction common experience in anticoagulant clinics is that INR can be altered by course of *oral broad-spectrum antibiotic such as ampicillin* (may also apply to antibiotics given for local action on gut such as *neomycin*)
- Antiplatelet Drugs: anticoagulant effect enhanced by *aspirin and dipyridamole*
- Clofibrate Group: enhanced anticoagulant effect
- Oestrogens and Progestogens: anticoagulant effect antagonised by *oral contraceptives*
- Thyroxine: enhanced anticoagulant effect

Phenindione (*continued*)

- Vitamins: anticoagulant effect antagonised by *vitamin K* (present in some enteral feeds)

Pheniramine *see* Antihistamines
Phenobarbitone *see* Barbiturates
Phenoperidine *see* Opioid Analgesics
Phenothiazines *see* Antipsychotics
Phenoxymethylpenicillin *see* Penicillins
Phentermine *see* Sympathomimetics
Phentolamine *see* Alpha-blockers
Phenylbutazone *see* NSAIDs
Phenylephrine *see* Sympathomimetics
Phenylpropanolamine *see* Sympathomimetics
Phenytoin

- Analgesics: plasma-phenytoin concentration increased by *aspirin, azapropazone, and phenylbutazone*
Antacids: reduced *phenytoin* absorption
- Anti-arrhythmics: *amiodarone* increases plasma-phenytoin concentration; *phenytoin* reduces plasma concentrations of *disopyramide, mexiletine, and quinidine*
- Antibacterials: plasma-phenytoin concentration increased by *chloramphenicol, cycloserine, isoniazid, and metronidazole*; plasma-phenytoin concentration and antifolate effect increased by *co-trimoxazole* and *trimethoprim* and possibly *other sulphonamides*; plasma-phenytoin concentration reduced by *rifamycins*; plasma concentration of *doxycycline* reduced by *phenytoin*
- Anticoagulants: metabolism of *nicoumalone and warfarin* accelerated (possibility of reduced anticoagulant effect, but enhancement also reported)
- Antidepressants: antagonism of anticonvulsant effect (convulsive threshold lowered); *fluoxetine, fluvoxamine*, and *viloxazine* increase plasma-phenytoin concentration; *phenytoin* reduces plasma concentrations of *mianserin, paroxetine, and tricyclics*
Antidiabetics: plasma-phenytoin concentration transiently increased by *tolbutamide* (possibility of toxicity)
- *other* Antiepileptics: concomitant administration of *two or more antiepileptics* may enhance toxicity without a corresponding increase in antiepileptic effect; moreover interactions between individual antiepileptics can complicate monitoring of treatment; interactions include enhanced effects, increased sedation, and reductions in plasma concentrations; for further details see p. 203
- Antifungals: plasma-phenytoin concentration increased by *fluconazole and miconazole*; plasma concentration of *itraconazole and ketoconazole* reduced
- Antimalarials: antagonism of anticonvulsant effect; increased risk of antifolate effect with *pyrimethamine* (includes *Fansidar®* and *Maloprim®*)
Antiplatelet Drugs: plasma-phenytoin concentration increased by *aspirin*
- Antipsychotics: antagonism of anticonvulsant effect (convulsive threshold lowered); *phenytoin* accelerates metabolism of *clozapine*
Antivirals: plasma-phenytoin concentrations increased or decreased by *zidovudine*
Anxiolytics and Hypnotics: *diazepam* and possibly *other benzodiazepines* increase or decrease plasma-phenytoin concentration
- Calcium-channel Blockers: *diltiazem* and *nifedipine* increase plasma concentration of *phenytoin*; effect of *felodipine, isradipine* and probably *diltiazem, nicardipine, nifedipine*, and *verapamil* reduced
Cardiac Glycosides: metabolism of *digitoxin only* accelerated (reduced effect)
- Corticosteroids: metabolism of *corticosteroids* accelerated (reduced effect)

Phenytoin (*continued*)
  Cyclosporin: metabolism of *cyclosporin* accelerated (reduced plasma concentration)
  Cytotoxics: reduced absorption of *phenytoin*; increased antifolate effect with *methotrexate*
  Disulfiram: plasma-phenytoin concentration increased
  Diuretics: increased risk of osteomalacia with *carbonic anhydrase inhibitors*
  Food: some *enteral foods* may interfere with absorption of *phenytoin*
  Hormone Antagonists: metabolism of *toremifene* possibly accelerated
  Lithium: neurotoxicity may occur without increased plasma-lithium concentration
  Muscle Relaxants: effect of *non-depolarising muscle relaxants* antagonised (recovery from neuromuscular blockade accelerated)
  Oestrogens and Progestogens: metabolism of *gestrinone, tibolone,* and *oral contraceptives* accelerated (reduced contraceptive effect, **important:** see p. 337)
  Sympathomimetics: plasma-phenytoin concentration increased by *methylphenidate*
  Theophylline: metabolism of *theophylline* accelerated (reduced plasma-theophylline concentration)
  Thyroxine: metabolism of *thyroxine* accelerated (may increase thyroxine requirements in hypothyroidism)
  Ulcer-healing Drugs: *cimetidine* inhibits metabolism (increased plasma-phenytoin concentration); *sucralfate* reduces absorption; *omeprazole* enhances effect of *phenytoin* (interaction with *lansoprazole* possibly differs)
  Uricosurics: plasma-phenytoin concentration increased by *sulphinpyrazone*
  Vaccines: effect enhanced by *influenza vaccine*
  Vitamins: plasma-phenytoin concentration occasionally reduced by *folic acid; vitamin D* requirements possibly increased
Physostigmine *see* Parasympathomimetics
Phytomenadione *see* Vitamins (Vitamin K)
Pilocarpine *see* Parasympathomimetics
Pimozide *see* Antipsychotics (CSM: *see also* p. 164)
Pindolol *see* Beta-blockers
Piperacillin *see* Penicillins
Piperazine Oestrone Sulphate *see* Contraceptives, Oral
Pipothiazine *see* Antipsychotics
Pirbuterol *see* Sympathomimetics, Beta$_2$
Piretanide *see* Diuretics (loop)
Piroxicam *see* NSAIDs
Pivampicillin *see* Penicillins
Pizotifen
  Antihypertensives: hypotensive effect of *adrenergic neurone blockers* antagonised
Pivmecillinam *see* Antimuscarinics
Polymyxins *see* Colistin
Polythiazide *see* Diuretics (thiazides)
Potassium Aminobenzoate
  Antibacterials: effect of *sulphonamides* inhibited
Potassium Salts (includes Salt Substitutes)
  ACE Inhibitors: hyperkalaemia
  Cyclosporin: increased risk of hyperkalaemia
  Diuretics: hyperkalaemia with *potassium-sparing diuretics*
Pravastatin *see* Statins
Prazosin *see* Alpha-blockers (post-synaptic)
Prednisolone *see* Corticosteroids
Prednisone *see* Corticosteroids
Primaquine
  Mepacrine: increased plasma concentration of *primaquine* (risk of toxicity)
Primaxin®
  Antivirals: increased toxicity with *ganciclovir* (convulsions reported)

Primidone *see* Barbiturates and Primidone
Probenecid
  ACE Inhibitors: reduced excretion of *captopril*
• Analgesics: *aspirin* antagonises effect; excretion of *indomethacin, ketoprofen, ketorolac* (see p. 527), *and naproxen* delayed (increased plasma concentrations)
  Antibacterials: reduced excretion of *cephalosporins, cinoxacin, ciprofloxacin, dapsone, nalidixic acid, nitrofurantoin, norfloxacin,* and *penicillins* (increased plasma-concentrations); antagonism by *pyrazinamide*
  Antivirals: reduced excretion of *aciclovir, zidovudine,* and possibly *famciclovir* and *ganciclovir* (increased plasma concentrations and risk of toxicity)
• Cytotoxics: reduced excretion of *methotrexate* (increased risk of toxicity)
Procainamide
  ACE Inhibitors: increased risk of toxicity with *captopril*, especially in renal impairment
• other Anti-arrhythmics: *amiodarone* increases procainamide-plasma concentrations; increased myocardial depression with *any anti-arrhythmic*
  Antibacterials: *trimethoprim* increases plasma concentration of *procainamide*
• Antidepressants: increased risk of ventricular arrhythmias with *tricyclics*
• Antihistamines: increased risk of ventricular arrhythmias with *astemizole* and *terfenadine*
• Antimalarials: increased risk of ventricular arrhythmias with *halofantrine*
• Antipsychotics: increased risk of ventricular arrhythmias with *phenothiazines*
• Beta-blockers: increased risk of ventricular arrhythmias associated with *sotalol*
• Muscle Relaxants: muscle relaxant effect enhanced
  Parasympathomimetics: antagonism of effect of *neostigmine* and *pyridostigmine*
• Ulcer-healing Drugs: *cimetidine* inhibits excretion (increased plasma-procainamide concentration)
Procaine Penicillin *see* Penicillins
Procarbazine
  Alcohol: disulfiram-like reaction
Prochlorperazine *see* Antipsychotics
Procyclidine *see* Antimuscarinics
Progesterone *see* Progestogens
Progestogens (*see also* Contraceptives, Oral)
  Antibacterials: metabolism accelerated by *rifamycins* (reduced effect)
• Cyclosporin: increased plasma-cyclosporin concentration (inhibition of metabolism)
  Hormone Antagonists: *aminoglutethimide* reduces plasma concentration of *medroxyprogesterone*
Proguanil
• Anticoagulants: effect of *warfarin* possibly enhanced
Promazine *see* Antipsychotics
Promethazine *see* Antihistamines
Propafenone
  other Anti-arrhythmics: *quinidine* increases plasma concentration of *propafenone*; increased myocardial depression with any *anti-arrhythmic*
• Antibacterials: *rifampicin* reduces plasma concentration of *propafenone* (reduced effect)
• Anticoagulants: increased plasma concentration of *warfarin and nicoumalone* (enhanced effect)
• Antidepressants: increased risk of arrhythmias with *tricyclics*
• Antihistamines: increased risk of ventricular arrhythmias with *astemizole* and *terfenadine*
  Beta-blockers: increased plasma concentration of *metoprolol* and *propranolol*
• Cardiac Glycosides: increased plasma concentrations of *digoxin* (halve maintenance dose of digoxin)
  Cyclosporin: plasma-cyclosporin concentration possibly increased
  Parasympathomimetics: possible antagonism of effect of *neostigmine* and *pyridostigmine*

Propafenone (*continued*)
Theophylline: increased plasma-theophylline concentration
• Ulcer-healing Drugs: *cimetidine* increases plasma-propafenone concentration
Propantheline *see* Antimuscarinics
Propofol *see* Anaesthetics, General
Propranolol *see* Beta-Blockers
Prostaglandins
Oxytocin: uterotonic effect enhanced
Proton Pump Inhibitors
• Anticoagulants: effects of *warfarin* enhanced by *omeprazole*; interaction with *lansoprazole* possibly differs
• Antiepileptics: effects of *phenytoin* enhanced by *omeprazole*; interaction with *lansoprazole* possibly differs
Antifungals: absorption of *ketoconazole* and possibly *itraconazole* reduced
Anxiolytics and Hypnotics: metabolism of *diazepam* inhibited by *omeprazole* (increased effect possible)
Cardiac Glycosides: plasma concentration of *digoxin* possibly increased
Oestrogens and Progestogens: manufacturer advises that *lansoprazole* possibly accelerates metabolism of *oral contraceptives*
Protriptyline *see* Antidepressants, Tricyclic
Pseudoephedrine *see* Sympathomimetics
Pyrazinamide
Uricosurics: antagonism of effect of *probenecid and sulphinpyrazone*
Pyridostigmine *see* Parasympathomimetics
Pyridoxine *see* Vitamins
Pyrimethamine
• Antibacterials: increased antifolate effect with *co-trimoxazole* and *trimethoprim*
Antiepileptics: increased antifolate effect with *phenytoin*
Cytotoxics: increased antifolate effect with *methotrexate*
Quinagolide
Note. No interactions reported; theoretical possibility of reduced effect with dopamine antagonists (eg phenothiazines)
Quinalbarbitone *see* Barbiturates and Primidone
Quinapril *see* ACE Inhibitors
Quinidine
Antacids: reduced excretion in alkaline urine (plasma-quinidine concentration occasionally increased)
• *other* Anti-arrhythmics: *amiodarone* increases plasma-quinidine concentrations (and increases risk of ventricular arrhythmias); plasma concentration of *propafenone* increased; increased myocardial depression with *any anti-arrhythmic*
Antibacterials: *rifamycins* accelerate metabolism (reduced plasma-quinidine concentration)
Anticoagulants: effect of *nicoumalone and warfarin* may be enhanced
• Antidepressants: increased risk of ventricular arrhythmias with *tricyclics*
Antiepileptics: *phenobarbitone, phenytoin, and primidone* accelerate metabolism (reduced plasma-quinidine concentration)
• Antihistamines: increased risk of ventricular arrhythmias with *astemizole* and *terfenadine*
• Antimalarials: increased risk of ventricular arrhythmias with *halofantrine*
• Antipsychotics: increased risk of ventricular arrhythmias with *phenothiazines*
Barbiturates and Primidone: *see under* Antiepileptics, above
• Beta-blockers: increased risk of ventricular arrhythmias associated with *sotalol*

Quinidine (*continued*)
• Calcium-channel Blockers: *nifedipine* reduces plasma-quinidine concentration; *verapamil* increases plasma-quinidine concentration (possibility of extreme hypotension)
• Cardiac Glycosides: plasma concentration of *digoxin* increased (halve digoxin maintenance dose)
• Diuretics: *acetazolamide* reduces excretion (plasma-quinidine concentration occasionally increased); quinidine toxicity increased if hypokalaemia occurs with *acetazolamide, loop diuretics, and thiazides*
• Muscle Relaxants: muscle relaxant effect enhanced
Parasympathomimetics: antagonism of effect of *neostigmine and pyridostigmine*
• Ulcer-healing Drugs: *cimetidine* inhibits metabolism (increased plasma-quinidine concentration)
Quinine
Anti-arrhythmics: plasma concentration of *flecainide* increased
• Antihistamines: increased risk of ventricular arrhythmias with *astemizole* and *terfenadine*
• *other* Antimalarials: *see* Halofantrine, Mefloquine
• Cardiac Glycosides: plasma concentration of *digoxin* increased (halve digoxin maintenance dose); includes use of quinine for cramps
Ulcer-healing Drugs: *cimetidine* inhibits metabolism (increased plasma-quinine concentration)
4-Quinolones
Analgesics: possible increased risk of convulsions with *NSAIDs*; manufacturer of *ciprofloxacin* advises avoid premedication with *opioid analgesics* (reduced plasma ciprofloxacin concentration)
Antacids and Adsorbents: *antacids* reduce absorption of *ciprofloxacin, norfloxacin* and *ofloxacin*
• Anticoagulants: anticoagulant effect of *nicoumalone and warfarin* enhanced by *ciprofloxacin, nalidixic acid, norfloxacin* and *ofloxacin*
• Antidiabetics: effect of *sulphonylureas* enhanced
• Cyclosporin: increased risk of nephrotoxicity
Cytotoxics: toxicity of *melphalan* increased by *nalidixic acid*
Iron: absorption of *ciprofloxacin, norfloxacin,* and *ofloxacin* reduced by *oral iron*
• Theophylline: *ciprofloxacin* and *norfloxacin* increase plasma-theophylline concentration
Ulcer-healing Drugs: *sucralfate* reduces absorption of *ciprofloxacin, norfloxacin,* and *ofloxacin*
Uricosurics: *probenecid* reduces excretion of *cinoxacin, ciprofloxacin, nalidixic acid* and *norfloxacin*
Zinc Salts: *zinc* reduces absorption of *ciprofloxacin* and *norfloxacin*
Rabies Vaccine *see* p. 512
Ramipril *see* ACE Inhibitors
Ranitidine *see* Histamine H_2-antagonists
Ranitidine Bismuth Citrate *see* Histamine H_2-antagonists
Reproterol *see* Sympathomimetics, Beta$_2$
Retinoids
Alcohol: etretinate formed from *acitretin* in presence of *alcohol*
Antibacterials: possible increased risk of benign intracranial hypertension with *tetracyclines* and *acitretin and isotretinoin*
• Anticoagulants: *acitretin* possibly reduces anticoagulant effect of *warfarin*
Antiepileptics: plasma concentration of *carbamazepine* possibly reduced by *isotretinoin*
• Cytotoxics: *acitretin* increases plasma concentration of *methotrexate* (also increased risk of hepatotoxicity)
Rifabutin *see* Rifamycins
Rifampicin *see* Rifamycins

Rifamycins

Analgesics: metabolism of *methadone* accelerated (reduced effect)

Antacids: reduced absorption of *rifampicin*

- Anti-arrhythmics: metabolism accelerated—reduced plasma concentrations of *disopyramide, mexiletine, propafenone, and quinidine*
- *other* Antibacterials: metabolism of *chloramphenicol* accelerated by *rifampicin* (reduced plasma concentration); plasma concentration of *dapsone* reduced; plasma concentration of *rifabutin* increased by *clarithromycin* and possibly *other macrolides* (risk of uveitis)
- Anticoagulants: metabolism of *nicoumalone and warfarin* accelerated (reduced anticoagulant effect)

Antidepressants: metabolism of some *tricyclics* accelerated by *rifampicin* (reduced plasma concentration)

- Antidiabetics: metabolism of *chlorpropamide, tolbutamide and possibly other sulphonylureas* accelerated (reduced effect)
- Antiepileptics: metabolism of *phenytoin* accelerated (reduced plasma concentration)
- Antifungals: metabolism of *fluconazole, itraconazole and ketoconazole* accelerated by *rifampicin* (reduced plasma concentrations); plasma concentration of *terbinafine* reduced by *rifampicin*; plasma concentration of *rifabutin* increased by *fluconazole* (risk of uveitis)

Antipsychotics: metabolism of *haloperidol* accelerated by *rifampicin* (reduced plasma concentration)

Anxiolytics and Hypnotics: metabolism of *diazepam* and possibly *other benzodiazepines* accelerated (reduced plasma concentration)

Atovaquone: plasma concentration reduced by *rifampicin*

Beta-blockers: metabolism of *bisoprolol* and *propranolol* accelerated by *rifampicin* (reduced plasma concentration)

Calcium-channel Blockers: metabolism of *diltiazem, nifedipine, and verapamil and possibly isradipine* accelerated by *rifampicin* (reduced plasma concentration)

Cardiac Glycosides: metabolism of *digitoxin only* accelerated (reduced effect)

- Corticosteroids: metabolism of *corticosteroids* accelerated (reduced effect)
- Cyclosporin: metabolism accelerated (reduced plasma-cyclosporin concentration)
- Cytotoxics: manufacturer reports interaction with *azathioprine* (transplants possibly rejected)

Lipid-lowering Drugs: metabolism of *fluvastatin* accelerated (reduced effect)

- Oestrogens and Progestogens: metabolism accelerated (contraceptive effect of *both combined and progestogen-only oral contraceptives* reduced, **important:** see p. 337)

Theophylline: metabolism accelerated by *rifampicin* (reduced plasma-theophylline concentration)

Thyroxine: metabolism of *thyroxine* accelerated by *rifampicin* (may increase requirements in hypothyroidism)

Ulcer-healing Drugs: metabolism of *cimetidine* accelerated by *rifampicin* (reduced plasma concentration)

Riluzole

Note. No clinical data available but since riluzole extensively metabolised by the liver, possibility of interactions with a number of drugs — consult product literature for details

Rimiterol *see* Sympathomimetics, Beta$_2$

Risperidone *see* Antipsychotics

Ritodrine *see* Sympathomimetics, Sympathomimetics, Beta$_2$, and p. 332

Rocuronium *see* Muscle Relaxants (non-depolarising)

Rowachol®

Anticoagulants: effect of *nicoumalone and warfarin* possibly reduced

Salbutamol *see* Sympathomimetics, Beta$_2$

Salmeterol *see* Sympathomimetics, Beta$_2$

Salt Substitutes *see* Potassium Salts

Selegiline

Note. Selegiline is an MAO-B inhibitor

- Analgesics: hyperpyrexia and CNS toxicity with *pethidine*
- Antidepressants: hypertension and CNS excitation with *fluoxetine*; hypotension with *MAOIs*

Sermorelin

Note. Avoid preparations which affect release of growth hormone, see p. 318

Sertraline *see* Antidepressants, SSRI

Sevoflurane *see* Anaesthetics, General (volatile liquid)

Simvastatin *see* Statins

Sodium Aurothiomalate *see* Gold

Sodium Bicarbonate *see* Antacids and Adsorbents

Sodium Clodronate *see* Bisphosphonates

Sodium Valproate *see* Valproate

Sotalol *see* Beta-blockers

Spectinomycin

- Botulinum Toxin: neuromuscular block enhanced (risk of toxicity)

Lithium: increased toxicity reported

Spironolactone *see* Diuretics (potassium-sparing)

Stanozolol *see* Anabolic Steroids

Statins

Antibacterials: metabolism of *fluvastatin* accelerated by *rifampicin* (reduced effect)

- Anticoagulants: effect of *nicoumalone and warfarin* enhanced by *simvastatin*

Antifungals: *itraconazole* increases risk of myopathy with *simvastatin*

- Cyclosporin: increased risk of myopathy
- *other* Lipid-lowering Drugs: increased risk of myopathy with *clofibrate group* and nicotinic acid

Streptomycin *see* Aminoglycosides

Sucralfate

Antibacterials: reduced absorption of *ciprofloxacin, norfloxacin, ofloxacin,* and *tetracycline*

- Anticoagulants: absorption of *warfarin* possibly reduced
- Antiepileptics: reduced absorption of *phenytoin*

Antifungals: reduced absorption of *ketoconazole*

Cardiac Glycosides: absorption of *cardiac glycosides* possibly reduced

Thyroxine: reduced absorption of *thyroxine*

Sulfadoxine *see* Co-trimoxazole and Sulphonamides

Sulfametopyrazine *see* Co-trimoxazole and Sulphonamides

Sulindac *see* NSAIDs

Sulphadiazine *see* Co-trimoxazole and Sulphonamides

Sulphadimidine *see* Co-trimoxazole and Sulphonamides

Sulphinpyrazone

Analgesics: *aspirin* antagonises uricosuric effect

Antibacterials: *pyrazinamide* antagonises effect

- Anticoagulants: anticoagulant effect of *nicoumalone and warfarin* enhanced
- Antidiabetics: effect of *sulphonylureas* enhanced
- Antiepileptics: plasma concentration of *phenytoin* increased

Theophylline: plasma-theophylline concentration reduced

Sulphonamides *see* Co-trimoxazole and Sulphonamides

Sulphonylureas *see* Antidiabetics

Sulpiride *see* Antipsychotics

Sumatriptan

- Antidepressants: risk of CNS toxicity with *MAOIs* (including *moclobemide*) and *SSRIs*
- Ergotamine: increased risk of vasospasm (see p. 201)
- Lithium: risk of CNS toxicity

Suxamethonium *see* Muscle Relaxants
Sympathomimetics (*see below* for Beta₂-Sympathomimetics)
- Anaesthetics: risk of arrhythmias if *adrenaline and isoprenaline* given with volatile liquid anaesthetics
- Antidepressants: with *tricyclics* administration of *adrenaline and noradrenaline* may cause hypertension and arrhythmias (but local anaesthetics with adrenaline appear to be safe); with *MAOIs* administration of inotropics such as *dopamine* and *dopexamine* may cause hypertensive crisis; also with *MAOIs* administration of *dexamphetamine and other amphetamines, dexfenfluramine, ephedrine, fenfluramine, isometheptene, methylphenidate, pemoline, phentermine, phenylephrine, phenylpropanolamine, and pseudoephedrine* may cause hypertensive crisis (these drugs are contained in anorectics or cold and cough remedies)

Antiepileptics: *methylphenidate* increases plasma concentration of *phenytoin* and possibly of *phenobarbitone* and *primidone*

Antihypertensives: sympathomimetics in *anorectics and cold and cough remedies (see* above) antagonise hypotensive effect of *adrenergic neurone blockers;* possible risk of hypertension with *apraclonidine* and *adrenaline* or *noradrenaline;* hypotensive effect of some other antihypertensives may be enhanced by *dexfenfluramine and fenfluramine*

Barbiturates and Primidone: *see under* Antiepileptics, above
- Beta-blockers: severe hypertension with *adrenaline and noradrenaline* (especially with non-selective beta-blockers); severe hypertension also possible with sympathomimetics in *anorectics and cold and cough remedies, see* above
- Dopaminergics: increased risk of toxicity when *isometheptene* or *phenylpropanolamine* given with *bromocriptine*

Doxapram: risk of hypertension

Oxytocin: hypertension with *vasoconstrictor sympathomimetics*
- *other* Sympathomimetics: *dopexamine* possibly potentiates effect of *adrenaline* and *noradrenaline*

Sympathomimetics, Beta₂
Corticosteroids: increased risk of hypokalaemia if high doses of *corticosteroids* given with high doses of *bambuterol, eformoterol, fenoterol, pirbuterol, reproterol, rimiterol, ritodrine, salbutamol, salmeterol, terbutaline* and *tulobuterol; see also* CSM advice, p. 122

Diuretics: increased risk of hypokalaemia if *acetazolamide, loop diuretics,* and *thiazides* given with high doses of *bambuterol, eformoterol, fenoterol, pirbuterol, reproterol, rimiterol, ritodrine, salbutamol, salmeterol, terbutaline, and tulobuterol; see also* CSM advice, p. 122

Muscle Relaxants: effect of *suxamethonium* enhanced by *bambuterol*

Theophylline: increased risk of hypokalaemia if given with high doses of *bambuterol, eformoterol, fenoterol, pirbuterol, reproterol, rimiterol, ritodrine, salbutamol, salmeterol, terbutaline, and tulobuterol; see also* CSM advice. p. 122

Tacrolimus
Note. Clinical data are limited but since tacrolimus is extensively metabolised by the liver it may be affected by a number of drugs (e.g. erythromycin) and may in turn interfere with a number of drugs (e.g. oral contraceptives) — consult product literature for details

Tamoxifen
- Anticoagulants: anticoagulant effect of *nicoumalone and warfarin* enhanced

other Hormone Antagonists: *aminoglutethimide* reduces plasma-tamoxifen concentration

Tamsulosin *see* Alpha-blockers (post-synaptic)

Temazepam *see* Anxiolytics and Hypnotics
Temocillin *see* Penicillins
Tenoxicam *see* NSAIDs
Terazosin *see* Alpha-blockers (post-synaptic)
Terbinafine
Antibacterials: plasma concentration reduced by *rifampicin*

Ulcer-healing Drugs: plasma concentration increased by *cimetidine*
Terbutaline *see* Sympathomimetics, Beta₂
Terfenadine *see* Antihistamines
Tetrabenazine (general extrapyramidal interactions *as for* Antipsychotics)
- Antidepressants: CNS excitation and hypertension with *MAOIs*

Tetracyclines
ACE Inhibitors: *quinapril* reduces absorption (tablets contain magnesium carbonate excipient)

Antacids: reduced absorption

Anticoagulants: *see* Phenindione and Warfarin

Antiepileptics: *carbamazepine, phenobarbitone, phenytoin, and primidone* increase metabolism of *doxycycline* (reduced plasma concentration)

Barbiturates and Primidone: *see under* Antiepileptics, above

Calcium Salts: reduced absorption of *tetracyclines*
- Cyclosporin: *doxycycline* possibly increases plasma-cyclosporin concentration

Dairy products: reduced absorption (except *doxycycline* and *minocycline*)

Iron: absorption of *oral iron* reduced by *tetracyclines* and *vice versa*

Oestrogens and Progestogens: *see* Contraceptives, Oral (main list)

Retinoids: possible increased risk of benign intracranial hypertension with *tetracyclines* and *acitretin* and *isotretinoin*

Ulcer-healing Drugs: *tripotassium dicitrato-bismuthate* and *sucralfate* reduce absorption

Zinc Salts: reduced absorption (and *vice versa*)
Theophylline
Anaesthetics: increased risk of arrhythmias with *halothane*

Anthelmintics: *thiabendazole* may increase plasma-theophylline concentration

Anti-arrhythmics: antagonism of anti-arrhythmic effect of *adenosine;* plasma-theophylline concentration increased by *mexiletine* and *propafenone;* plasma-theophylline concentration reduced by *moracizine*
- Antibacterials: plasma-theophylline concentration increased by *ciprofloxacin, clarithromycin, erythromycin* (if erythromycin given by mouth, also decreased plasma-erythromycin concentration), and *norfloxacin* and possibly increased by *isoniazid;* plasma-theophylline concentration reduced by *rifampicin*
- Antidepressants: plasma-theophylline concentration increased by *fluvoxamine* (**important:** see p. 128) and *viloxazine*

Antiepileptics: plasma-theophylline concentration reduced by *carbamazepine, phenobarbitone, phenytoin, and primidone*
- Antifungals: plasma-theophylline concentration possibly increased by *fluconazole*

Barbiturates and Primidone: *see under* Antiepileptics, above

Beta-blockers: should be avoided on pharmacological grounds (bronchospasm)
- Calcium-channel Blockers: plasma-theophylline concentration increased by *diltiazem, verapamil,* and possibly *other calcium-channel blockers*

Disulfiram: increases plasma-theophylline concentration

Doxapram: increased CNS stimulation

Hormone Antagonists: plasma-theophylline concentration reduced by *aminoglutethimide*

Theophylline (*continued*)
   Interferons: plasma-theophylline concentration
      increased by *interferon alfa*
   Lithium: *lithium* excretion accelerated (reduced
      plasma-lithium concentration)
   Nicotine and Tobacco: plasma-theophylline
      concentration reduced by *tobacco smoking*
   Oestrogens and Progestogens: plasma-theophylline
      concentration increased by *combined oral
      contraceptives*
   Sympathomimetics: increased risk of hypokalaemia
      if *theophylline* given with high doses of *bambuter-
      ol, eformoterol, fenoterol, pirbuterol, reproterol,
      rimiterol, ritodrine, salbutamol, salmeterol, terbut-
      aline, and tulobuterol; see also* CSM advice, p. 122
 • Ulcer-healing Drugs: plasma-theophylline
      concentration increased by *cimetidine*
   Uricosurics: plasma-theophylline concentration
      reduced by *sulphinpyrazone*
   Vaccines: plasma-theophylline concentration
      occasionally increased by *influenza vaccine*
Thiabendazole
   Theophylline: plasma concentration may be
      increased
Thiazides *see* Diuretics
Thiopentone *see* Anaesthetics, General
Thioridazine *see* Antipsychotics
Thiotepa
   Muscle Relaxants: effect of *suxamethonium*
      enhanced
Thyroxine
   Analgesics: false low total plasma-thyroxine
      concentration with *phenylbutazone*
   Anion-exchange Resins: *cholestyramine* reduces
      absorption of *thyroxine*
   Anti-arrhythmics: for use with *amiodarone*, see p. 69
   Antibacterials: *rifampicin* accelerates metabolism of
      thyroxine (may increase requirements in
      hypothyroidism)
 • Anticoagulants: effect of *nicoumalone, phenindione,
      and warfarin* enhanced
   Antidepressants: manufacturer of *lofepramine*
      advises avoid *thyroxine*
   Antiepileptics: *carbamazepine, phenobarbitone,
      phenytoin, and primidone* accelerate metabolism of
      thyroxine (may increase requirements in
      hypothyroidism)
   Barbiturates and Primidone: *see under* Antiepileptics,
      above
   Beta-blockers: metabolism of *propranolol*
      accelerated (reduced effect)
   Ulcer-healing Drugs: *sucralfate* reduces absorption
      of *thyroxine*
Tiaprofenic Acid *see* NSAIDs
Tibolone
   Antibacterials: *rifampicin* accelerates metabolism
      (reduced plasma concentration)
   Antiepileptics: *carbamazepine, phenobarbitone,
      phenytoin, and primidone* accelerate metabolism
      (reduced plasma concentration)
   Barbiturates and Primidone: *see under* Antiepileptics,
      above
Ticarcillin *see* Penicillins
Tiludronic Acid *see* Bisphosphonates
Timolol *see* Beta-blockers
Tinidazole
   Alcohol: disulfiram-like reaction
Tinzaparin *see* Heparin
Tobramycin *see* Aminoglycosides
Tocainide
   other Anti-arrhythmics: increased myocardial
      depression with any anti-arrhythmic
   Beta-blockers: increased risk of bradycardia and
      myocardial depression
   Diuretics: effect of *tocainide* antagonised by
      hypokalaemia with *acetazolamide, loop diuretics,
      and thiazides*

Tolazamide *see* Antidiabetics (sulphonylurea)
Tolbutamide *see* Antidiabetics (sulphonylurea)
Tolmetin *see* NSAIDs
Topiramate
 • *other* Antiepileptics: concomitant administration of
      two or more antiepileptics may enhance toxicity
      without a corresponding increase in antiepileptic
      effect; moreover, interactions between individual
      antiepileptics can complicate monitoring of
      treatment; interactions include enhanced effects,
      increased sedation, and reductions in plasma
      concentrations; for further details, see p. 203
   Oestrogens and Progestogens: metabolism of *oral
      contraceptives* accelerated (reduced contraceptive
      effect, **important:** see p. 337)
Torasemide *see* Diuretics (loop)
Toremifene
 • Anticoagulants: anticoagulant effect of *nicoumalone*
      and *warfarin* possibly enhanced
   Antiepileptics: metabolism possibly accelerated by
      carbamazepine, phenobarbitone and *phenytoin*
      (reduced plasma-toremifene concentration)
   Diuretics: increased risk of hypercalcaemia with
      thiazides
Tramadol *see* Opioid Analgesics
Trandolapril *see* ACE Inhibitors
Tranylcypromine *see* MAOIs
Trazodone
   Alcohol: enhanced sedative effect
 • *other* Antidepressants: as for Antidepressants,
      Tricyclic
 • Antiepileptics: antagonism of anticonvulsant effect
   Anxiolytics and Hypnotics: enhanced sedative effect
Triamcinolone *see* Corticosteroids
Triamterene *see* Diuretics (potassium-sparing)
Triclofos *see* Anxiolytics and Hypnotics
Trientine
   Iron: absorption of *oral iron* reduced
Trifluoperazine *see* Antipsychotics
Trilostane
   Diuretics: increased risk of hyperkalaemia with
      potassium-sparing diuretics
Trimeprazine *see* Antihistamines
Trimethoprim
   Anti-arrhythmics: plasma concentration of
      procainamide increased
   Anticoagulants: effect of *nicoumalone* and *warfarin*
      possibly enhanced
   Antidiabetics: effect of *sulphonylureas* enhanced
   Antiepileptics: plasma concentration and antifolate
      effect of *phenytoin* increased
 • Antimalarials: increased risk of antifolate effect with
      pyrimethamine (ingredient of *Fansidar®* and
      Maloprim®)
 • Cyclosporin: increased risk of nephrotoxicity;
      plasma-cyclosporin concentration possibly reduced
      by *intravenous trimethoprim*
   Cytotoxics: antifolate effect of *methotrexate*
      increased
Trimipramine *see* Antidepressants, Tricyclic
Tripotassium Dicitratobismuthate
   Antibacterials: reduced absorption of *tetracyclines*
Triprolidine *see* Antihistamines
Tropicamide *see* Antimuscarinics
Tryptophan
 • *other* Antidepressants: CNS excitation and confusion
      with *MAOIs* (reduce tryptophan dose); agitation
      and nausea with *fluoxetine, fluvoxamine,
      paroxetine, and sertraline*
Tulobuterol *see* Sympathomimetics, Beta₂
Typhoid Vaccine *see* p. 514
Ulcer-healing Drugs *see* individual drugs
Uricosurics *see* individual drugs

Vaccines *see* Influenza Vaccine (p. 555), Rabies Vaccine (p. 512), Typhoid Vaccine (p. 514)

Note. For a general warning on *live vaccines* and *high doses of corticosteroids* or *other immunosuppressive drugs*, see section 14.1; for advice on *live vaccines* and *immunoglobulins*, see under Normal Immunoglobulin, section 14.5

Valaciclovir *see* Aciclovir and Famciclovir

Note. Interactions as for aciclovir

Valproate

Analgesics: *aspirin* enhances effect

Anion-exchange resins: *cholestyramine* possibly reduces absorption

Anticoagulants: anticoagulant effect of *nicoumalone* and *warfarin* possibly increased

- Antidepressants: antagonism of anticonvulsant effect (convulsive threshold lowered)
- *other* Antiepileptics: concomitant administration of *two or more antiepileptics* may enhance toxicity without a corresponding increase in antiepileptic effect; moreover, interactions between individual antiepileptics can complicate monitoring of treatment; interactions include enhanced effects, increased sedation, and reductions in plasma concentrations; for further details, see p. 203
- Antimalarials: *chloroquine* and *mefloquine* antagonise anticonvulsant effect
- Antipsychotics: antagonism of anticonvulsant effect (convulsive threshold lowered)

Ulcer-healing Drugs: *cimetidine* inhibits metabolism (increased plasma-valproate concentration)

Vancomycin

Anion-exchange Resins: antagonism of *oral vancomycin* by *cholestyramine*

other Antibacterials: increased risk of ototoxicity and nephrotoxicity with *aminoglycosides and capreomycin*

Diuretics: increased risk of ototoxicity with *loop diuretics*

Vecuronium *see* Muscle Relaxants (non-depolarising)

Venlafaxine

- *other* Antidepressants: CNS effects of *MAOIs* increased (risk of toxicity); *venlafaxine* should not be started until 2 weeks after stopping *MAOI*; conversely, *MAOI* should not be started until at least 1 week after stopping *venlafaxine*

Verapamil *see* Calcium-channel Blockers

Vigabatrin

- *other* Antiepileptics: concomitant administration of *two or more antiepileptics* may enhance toxicity without a corresponding increase in antiepileptic effect; moreover, interactions between individual antiepileptics can complicate monitoring of treatment; interactions include enhanced effects, increased sedation, and reductions in plasma concentrations; for further details, see p. 203

Viloxazine

- *other* Antidepressants: as for Antidepressants, Tricyclic
- Antiepileptics: increased plasma concentrations of *carbamazepine* and *phenytoin*

Theophylline: increased plasma-theophylline concentration

Vitamins

- Anticoagulants: anticoagulant effect of *nicoumalone, phenindione,* and *warfarin* antagonised by *vitamin K* (present in some enteral feeds)

Antiepileptics: *folic acid* occasionally reduces plasma-phenytoin concentration; *vitamin D* requirements possibly increased by *carbamazepine, phenobarbitone, phenytoin,* and *primidone*

Barbiturates and Primidone: *see under* Antiepileptics, above

Diuretics: increased risk of hypercalcaemia if *thiazides* given with *vitamin D*

Vitamins (*continued*)

Dopaminergics: effect of *levodopa* antagonised by *pyridoxine* (unless a dopa decarboxylase inhibitor also given)

Warfarin and other Coumarins

Note. Change in patient's clinical condition, particularly associated with liver disease, intercurrent illness, or drug administration, necessitates more frequent testing. Major changes in diet (especially involving vegetables) and in alcohol consumption may also affect warfarin control

- Alcohol: enhanced anticoagulant effect with large amounts (see also above)

Allopurinol: anticoagulant effect possibly enhanced

- Anabolic Steroids: *oxymetholone, stanozolol and others* enhance anticoagulant effect
- Analgesics: *aspirin* increases risk of bleeding due to antiplatelet effect; anticoagulant effect seriously enhanced by *azapropazone (see also* p. 410*)* and *phenylbutazone,* and possibly enhanced by *diclofenac, diflunisal, flurbiprofen, mefenamic acid, piroxicam, sulindac,* and possibly other *NSAIDs*; anticoagulant effect possibly also enhanced by *dextropropoxyphene* and by prolonged regular use of *paracetamol*; increased risk of haemorrhage with *ketorolac,* see p. 527
- Anion-exchange Resins: *cholestyramine* may enhance or reduce anticoagulant effect
- Anti-arrhythmics: *amiodarone and propafenone* enhance anticoagulant effect; *quinidine* may enhance anticoagulant effect
- Antibacterials: anticoagulant effect reduced by *rifamycins*; anticoagulant effect enhanced by *cephamandole, chloramphenicol, ciprofloxacin, co-trimoxazole, erythromycin, metronidazole, ofloxacin,* and *sulphonamides*; anticoagulant effect possibly also enhanced by *azithromycin, aztreonam, clarithromycin, nalidixic acid, neomycin, norfloxacin, tetracyclines,* and *trimethoprim*; although studies have failed to demonstrate interaction, common experience in anticoagulant clinics is that INR can be altered following course of oral *broad-spectrum antibiotic, such as ampicillin* (may also apply to antibiotics given for local action on gut such as *neomycin*)
- Antidepressants: *SSRIs* possibly enhance anticoagulant effect
- Antiepileptics: reduced anticoagulant effect with *carbamazepine, phenobarbitone,* and *primidone*; anticoagulant effect possibly increased by *valproate*; both reduced and enhanced effects reported with *phenytoin*
- Antifungals: anticoagulant effect reduced by *griseofulvin*; anticoagulant effect enhanced by *fluconazole, itraconazole, ketoconazole,* and *miconazole* (note: oral gel absorbed)
- Antimalarials: anticoagulant effect possibly enhanced by *proguanil*
- Antiplatelet Drugs: *aspirin and dipyridamole* increase risk of bleeding due to antiplatelet effect

Anxiolytics and Hypnotics: *chloral* and *triclofos* may transiently enhance anticoagulant effect

Atovaquone: anticoagulant effect possibly enhanced

- Barbiturates and Primidone: anticoagulant effect reduced

Cisapride: effect of *oral anticoagulants* possibly enhanced

- Cytotoxics: anticoagulant effect possibly enhanced by *ifosfamide*
- Disulfiram: enhanced anticoagulant effect
- Hormone Antagonists: *aminoglutethimide* reduces anticoagulant effect; *danazol, flutamide, tamoxifen* and possibly *bicalutamide* and *toremifene* enhance anticoagulant effect
- Lipid-lowering Drugs: *clofibrate group* and *simvastatin* enhance anticoagulant effect
- Oestrogens and Progestogens: *oral contraceptives* reduce anticoagulant effect

Warfarin and other Coumarins (*continued*)
* Retinoids: *acitretin* possibly reduces anticoagulant effect
  Rowachol®: possibly reduced anticoagulant effect
* Thyroxine: enhanced anticoagulant effect
* Ulcer-healing Drugs: *sucralfate* possibly reduces anticoagulant effect (reduced absorption); *cimetidine and omeprazole* enhance anticoagulant effect
* Uricosurics: *sulphinpyrazone* enhances anticoagulant effect
  Vaccines: *influenza vaccine* occasionally enhances anticoagulant effect
* Vitamins: *vitamin K* reduces anticoagulant effect; major changes in diet (especially involving vegetables) may affect control; *vitamin K* also present in some enteral feeds

Xamoterol
Beta-blockers: antagonism of effect of *xamoterol* and reduction in beta-blockade

Xipamide *see* Diuretics (thiazide-related)

Xylometazoline *see* Sympathomimetics

Zalcitabine
Note. Clinical data limited. Avoid use with other drugs which have potential to cause peripheral neuropathy—for further details consult product literature

Zidovudine
Note. Increased risk of toxicity with nephrotoxic and myelosuppressive drugs—for further details consult product literature
Analgesics: *methadone* possibly increases plasma-zidovudine concentration
Antibacterials: *clarithromycin tablets* reduce absorption of *zidovudine*
Antiepileptics: plasma-phenytoin concentrations increased or decreased
* *other* Antivirals: extreme lethargy reported on administration of *intravenous aciclovir*; profound myelosuppression with *ganciclovir* (see also p. 270)
Uricosurics: *probenecid* increases plasma-zidovudine concentration and risk of toxicity

Zinc
Antibacterials: reduced absorption of *ciprofloxacin* and *norfloxacin*; *tetracyclines* reduce absorption of *zinc* (and *vice versa*)
Iron: reduced absorption of *oral iron* (and *vice versa*)
Penicillamine: reduced absorption of *penicillamine*

Zolpidem *see* Anxiolytics and Hypnotics

Zopiclone *see* Anxiolytics and Hypnotics

Zuclopenthixol *see* Antipsychotics

Appendix 2: Liver Disease

Liver disease may alter the response to drugs in several ways as indicated below, and drug prescribing should be kept to a minimum in all patients with severe liver disease. The main problems occur in patients with jaundice, ascites, or evidence of encephalopathy.

IMPAIRED DRUG METABOLISM. Metabolism by the liver is the main route of elimination for many drugs, but the hepatic reserve appears to be large and liver disease has to be severe before important changes in drug metabolism occur. Routine liver-function tests are a poor guide to the capacity of the liver to metabolise drugs, and in the individual patient it is not possible to predict the extent to which the metabolism of a particular drug may be impaired.

A few drugs, e.g. rifampicin and fusidic acid, are excreted in the bile unchanged and may accumulate in patients with intrahepatic or extrahepatic obstructive jaundice.

HYPOPROTEINAEMIA. The hypoalbuminaemia in severe liver disease is associated with reduced protein binding and increased toxicity of some highly protein-bound drugs such as phenytoin and prednisolone.

REDUCED CLOTTING. Reduced hepatic synthesis of blood-clotting factors, indicated by a prolonged prothrombin time, increases the sensitivity to oral anticoagulants such as warfarin and phenindione.

HEPATIC ENCEPHALOPATHY. In severe liver disease many drugs can further impair cerebral function and may precipitate hepatic encephalopathy. These include all sedative drugs, opioid analgesics, those diuretics that produce hypokalaemia, and drugs that cause constipation.

FLUID OVERLOAD. Oedema and ascites in chronic liver disease may be exacerbated by drugs that give rise to fluid retention, e.g. NSAIDs, corticosteroids, and carbenoxolone.

HEPATOTOXIC DRUGS. Hepatotoxicity is either dose-related or unpredictable (idiosyncratic). Drugs causing dose-related toxicity may do so at lower doses than in patients with normal liver function, and some drugs producing reactions of the idiosyncratic kind do so more frequently in patients with liver disease. These drugs should be avoided.

Table of drugs to be avoided or used with caution in liver disease

The list of drugs given below is not comprehensive and is based on current information concerning the use of these drugs in therapeutic dosage. Products introduced or amended since publication of BNF No. 31 (March 1996) are underlined.

Drug	Comment	Drug	Comment
Acamprosate	Avoid in severe liver disease	Anastrozole	Avoid in moderate to severe liver disease
Acarbose	Avoid	Androgens	Preferably avoid— dose-related toxicity with some, and produce fluid retention
ACE Inhibitors	Use of prodrugs such as cilazapril, enalapril, fosinopril, moexipril, perindopril, quinapril, ramipril, and trandolapril requires close monitoring in patients with impaired liver function		
		Antacids	In patients with fluid retention, avoid those containing large amounts of sodium, e.g. magnesium trisilicate mixture, Gaviscon®
Aceclofenac	Halve dose initially; see also NSAIDs		Avoid those causing constipation—can precipitate coma
Acemetacin see NSAIDs			
Acitretin	Avoid—further impairment of liver function may occur	Anticoagulants, Oral	Avoid, especially if prothrombin time is already prolonged
Acrivastine see Antihistamines			
Acrosoxacin see 4-Quinolones		Antidepressants, MAOI see MAOIs	
Alfentanil see Opioid Analgesics		Antidepressants, SSRI	Reduce dose or avoid in severe liver disease
Alfuzosin	Reduce dose in mild to moderate liver disease; avoid if severe	Antidepressants, Tricyclic (and related)	Tricyclics preferable to MAOIs but sedative effects increased (avoid in severe liver disease)
Alprazolam see Anxiolytics and Hypnotics			
Aminophylline see Theophylline			
Amitriptyline see Antidepressants, Tricyclic			
Amlodipine	Reduce dose	Antihistamines	Avoid—may precipitate coma; astemizole and terfenadine, see also p. 138
Amoxapine see Antidepressants, Tricyclic			
Anabolic Steroids	Preferably avoid—dose-related toxicity		
Analgesics see Aspirin, NSAIDs, Opioid Analgesics and Paracetamol			

Table of drugs to be avoided or used with caution in liver disease (*continued*)

Drug	Comment	Drug	Comment
Antipsychotics	All can precipitate coma; phenothiazines are hepatotoxic; with clozapine monitor liver function in liver disease	Cholestyramine	Interferes with absorption of fat-soluble vitamins and may aggravate malabsorption in primary biliary cirrhosis; likely to be ineffective in complete biliary obstruction
Anxiolytics and Hypnotics	All can precipitate coma; small dose of oxazepam or temazepam probably safest; reduce oral dose of chlormethiazole; reduce dose of zopiclone (avoid if severe)	Choline Theophyllinate *see* Theophylline	
		Cilazapril *see* ACE Inhibitors	
		Cimetidine	Increased risk of confusion; reduce dose
Aspirin	Avoid—increased risk of gastro-intestinal bleeding	Cinnarizine *see* Antihistamines	
		Cinoxacin *see* 4-Quinolones	
Astemizole *see* Antihistamines		Ciprofibrate	Avoid in severe liver disease
Auranofin *see* Gold		Ciprofloxacin *see* 4-Quinolones	
Aurothiomalate *see* Gold		Cisapride	Halve dose initially
Azapropazone *see* NSAIDs		Citalopram	Use doses at lower end of range
Azatadine *see* Antihistamines		Clarithromycin	Hepatic dysfunction including jaundice reported
Azathioprine	May need dose reduction		
Azithromycin	Avoid; jaundice reported	Clavulanic Acid [ingredient] *see* Co-amoxiclav and *Timentin*®	
Bambuterol	Avoid in severe liver disease		
Bendrofluazide *see* Thiazides		Clemastine *see* Antihistamines	
Benorylate [aspirin-paracetamol ester] *see* Aspirin		Clindamycin	Reduce dose
Benperidol *see* Antipsychotics		Clobazam *see* Anxiolytics and Hypnotics	
Benzodiazepines *see* Anxiolytics and Hypnotics		Clofibrate	Avoid in severe liver disease
Beta-blockers *see* individual drugs		Clomiphene	Avoid in severe liver disease
Bezafibrate	Avoid in severe liver disease	Clomipramine *see* Antidepressants, Tricyclic	
Bicalutamide	Increased accumulation possible in moderate to severe impairment	Clopamide *see* Thiazides	
		Clorazepate *see* Anxiolytics and Hypnotics	
		Clozapine *see* Antipsychotics	
Bromazepam *see* Anxiolytics and Hypnotics		Co-amoxiclav	Monitor liver function in liver disease. Cholestatic jaundice, see p. 234
Brompheniramine *see* Antihistamines			
Buclizine *see* Antihistamines		Codeine *see* Opioid Analgesics	
Bumetanide *see* Loop Diuretics		Contraceptives, Oral	Avoid in active liver disease and in patients with a history of pruritus or cholestasis during pregnancy
Bupivacaine *see* Lignocaine			
Buprenorphine *see* Opioid Analgesics			
Cabergoline	Avoid in liver disease	Cyclizine *see* Antihistamines	
Carbamazepine	Metabolism impaired in advanced liver disease. For advice on counselling for all patients, see p. 205	Cyclofenil	Avoid in severe liver disease
		Cyclopenthiazide *see* Thiazides	
		Cyclosporin	May need dose adjustment
		Cyproheptadine *see* Antihistamines	
Carbenoxolone	Produces sodium and water retention and hypokalaemia	Cyproterone Acetate	Dose-related toxicity; *see also* CSM advice on p. 371
		Dalteparin *see* Heparin	
Carvedilol	Avoid	Danaparoid *see* Heparin	
Ceftriaxone	Reduce dose and monitor plasma concentration if both hepatic and severe renal impairment	Dantrolene	Avoid—may cause severe liver damage
		Demeclocycline *see* Tetracyclines	
		Desflurane	Reduce dose
Certoparin *see* Heparin		Desipramine *see* Antidepressants, Tricyclic	
Cetirizine *see* Antihistamines		Desogestrel *see* Progestogens	
Chenodeoxycholic Acid	Avoid in chronic liver disease; patients with non-functioning gall-bladder do not respond	Dexfenfluramine	Manufacturer advises avoid
		Dextromethorphan *see* Opioid Analgesics	
		Dextromoramide *see* Opioid Analgesics	
Chloral Hydrate *see* Anxiolytics and Hypnotics		Dextropropoxyphene *see* Opioid Analgesics	
Chloramphenicol	Avoid—increased risk of bone-marrow depression	Diamorphine *see* Opioid Analgesics	
		Diazepam *see* Anxiolytics and Hypnotics	
Chlordiazepoxide *see* Anxiolytics and Hypnotics		Diclofenac *see* NSAIDs	
Chlormethiazole	Reduce oral dose; *see* Anxiolytics and Hypnotics	Didanosine	Reduce initial dose
		Diflunisal *see* NSAIDs	
Chlorothiazide *see* Thiazides		Dihydrocodeine *see* Opioid Analgesics	
Chlorpheniramine *see* Antihistamines		Diltiazem	Reduce dose
Chlorpromazine *see* Antipsychotics		Dimenhydrinate *see* Antihistamines	
Chlorpropamide *see* Sulphonylureas		Diphenoxylate *see* Opioid Analgesics	
Chlortetracycline *see* Tetracyclines			
Chlorthalidone *see* Thiazides			

Table of drugs to be avoided or used with caution in liver disease (*continued*)

Drug	Comment	Drug	Comment
Diphenylpyraline *see* Antihistamines		Gold (auranofin, aurothiomalate)	Avoid in severe liver disease—hepatotoxicity may occur
Dipipanone *see* Opioid Analgesics		Haloperidol *see* Antipsychotics	
Docetaxel	Monitor liver function – reduce dose according to liver enzymes	Halothane *see* p. 522	
		Heparin	Reduce dose in severe disease
Dothiepin *see* Antidepressants, Tricyclic		Hydrochlorothiazide *see* Thiazides	
Doxepin *see* Antidepressants, Tricyclic		Hydroflumethiazide *see* Thiazides	
Doxorubicin	Reduce dose according to bilirubin concentration	Hydroxyprogesterone Hexanoate *see* Progestogens	
		Hydroxyzine *see* Antihistamines	
Doxycycline *see* Tetracyclines		Hypnotics *see* Anxiolytics and Hypnotics	
Doxylamine *see* Antihistamines		Ibuprofen *see* NSAIDs	
Droperidol *see* Antipsychotics		Idarubicin	Reduce dose according to bilirubin concentration
Dydrogesterone *see* Progestogens		Imipramine *see* Antidepressants, Tricyclic	
Enalapril *see* ACE Inhibitors		Indapamide *see* Thiazides	
Enoxaparin *see* Heparin		Indomethacin *see* NSAIDs	
Epirubicin	Reduce dose according to bilirubin concentration	Interferon alfa	Close monitoring in mild to moderate impairment; avoid if severe
Ergometrine	Avoid in severe liver disease	Interferon beta	Avoid in decompensated liver disease
Ergotamine	Avoid in severe liver disease—risk of toxicity increased	Isocarboxazid *see* MAOIs	
Erythromycin	May cause idiosyncratic hepatotoxicity	Isoniazid	Avoid if possible—idiosyncratic hepatotoxicity more common; *see also* p. 255
Ethacrynic Acid *see* Loop Diuretics			
Ethinyloestradiol *see* Oestrogens		Isotretinoin	Avoid—further impairment of liver function may occur
Ethynodiol Diacetate *see* Progestogens		Isradipine	Reduce dose
Etodolac *see* NSAIDs		Itraconazole	Avoid—toxicity with related drugs
Famciclovir	Usual dose in well compensated liver disease (information not available on decompensated)	Ketoconazole	Induces hepatitis-like reaction; may accumulate in severe liver disease; contra-indicated unless no alternative; *see also* p. 262
Felodipine	Reduce dose		
Fenbufen *see* NSAIDs			
Fenofibrate *see* Clofibrate			
Fenoprofen *see* NSAIDs		Ketoprofen *see* NSAIDs	
Fentanyl *see* Opioid Analgesics		Ketorolac *see* NSAIDs	
Flecainide	Avoid (or reduce dose) in severe liver disease	Ketotifen *see* Antihistamines	
		Labetalol	Avoid—severe hepatocellular injury reported
Flucloxacillin	Cholestatic jaundice, see p. 231	Lacidipine	Reduce dose
Fluconazole	Toxicity with related drugs	Lamotrigine	Manufacturer advises avoid
Flunitrazepam *see* Anxiolytics and Hypnotics		Lansoprazole	In severe liver disease dose should not exceed 30 mg daily
Fluoxetine *see* Antidepressants, SSRI			
Flupenthixol *see* Antipsychotics		Levonorgestrel *see* Progestogens	
Fluphenazine *see* Antipsychotics		Lignocaine	Avoid (or reduce dose) in severe liver disease
Flurazepam *see* Anxiolytics and Hypnotics			
Flurbiprofen *see* NSAIDs		Lofepramine *see* Antidepressants, Tricyclic	
Fluvastatin	Avoid in active liver disease or unexplained persistent elevations in serum transaminases	Loop Diuretics	Hypokalaemia may precipitate coma; potassium-sparing diuretic should be used to prevent this; increased risk of hypomagnesaemia in alcoholic cirrhosis
Fluvoxamine *see* Antidepressants, SSRI			
Fosfestrol *see* Oestrogens			
Fosinopril *see* ACE Inhibitors		Loprazolam *see* Anxiolytics and Hypnotics	
Frusemide *see* Loop Diuretics		Lorazepam *see* Anxiolytics and Hypnotics	
Fusidic Acid	Impaired biliary excretion; may be increased risk of hepatotoxicity; avoid or reduce dose	Lormetazepam *see* Anxiolytics and Hypnotics	
		Losartan	Consider lower dose
		Loxapine *see* Antipsychotics	
Gemcitabine	Monitor liver function	Lymecycline *see* Tetracyclines	
Gemfibrozil	Avoid in liver disease	Magnesium Salts	Avoid in hepatic coma if risk of renal failure
Gestodene *see* Progestogens			
Gestronol *see* Progestogens		MAOIs	May cause idiosyncratic hepatotoxicity
Glibenclamide *see* Sulphonylureas			
Gliclazide *see* Sulphonylureas			
Glipizide *see* Sulphonylureas			
Gliquidone *see* Sulphonylureas			

Table of drugs to be avoided or used with caution in liver disease (*continued*)

Drug	Comment	Drug	Comment
Maprotiline *see* Antidepressants, Tricyclic (and related)		NSAIDs	Increased risk of gastro-intestinal bleeding and can cause fluid retention; avoid in severe liver disease
Medroxyprogesterone Acetate *see* Progestogens			
Mefenamic Acid *see* NSAIDs			
Mefloquine	Avoid for prophylaxis in severe liver disease	Oestradiol *see* Oestrogens	
		Oestriol *see* Oestrogens	
Mefruside *see* Thiazides		Oestrogens	Avoid; *see also* Contraceptives, Oral
Megestrol Acetate *see* Progestogens			
Meprobamate *see* Anxiolytics and Hypnotics		Ofloxacin *see* 4-Quinolones	
Meptazinol *see* Opioid Analgesics		Omeprazole	In liver disease not more than 20 mg daily should be needed
Mequitazine *see* Antihistamines			
Meropenem	Monitor transaminase and bilirubin concentrations	Ondansetron	Reduce dose; not more than 8 mg daily in severe liver disease
Mesterolone *see* Androgens			
Mestranol *see* Oestrogens		Opioid Analgesics	Avoid or reduce dose—may precipitate coma
Metformin	Avoid—increased risk of lactic acidosis		
		Oral Contraceptives *see* Contraceptives, Oral	
Methadone *see* Opioid Analgesics		Oxazepam *see* Anxiolytics and Hypnotics	
Methohexitone	Avoid or reduce dose	Oxprenolol	Reduce dose
Methotrexate	Dose-related toxicity—avoid in non-malignant conditions (e.g. psoriasis)	Oxypertine *see* Antipsychotics	
		Oxytetracycline *see* Tetracyclines	
		Paclitaxel	Avoid in severe liver disease
Methotrimeprazine *see* Antipsychotics		Papaveretum *see* Opioid Analgesics	
Methoxsalen	Avoid or reduce dose	Paracetamol	Dose-related toxicity—avoid large doses
Methyldopa	Avoid—increased risk of hepatotoxicity		
		Paroxetine *see* Antidepressants, SSRI	
Metoclopramide	Reduce dose	Pentazocine *see* Opioid Analgesics	
Metolazone *see* Thiazides		Pericyazine *see* Antipsychotics	
Metoprolol	Reduce oral dose	Perindopril *see* ACE Inhibitors	
Metronidazole	Reduce dose in severe liver disease	Perphenazine *see* Antipsychotics	
		Pethidine *see* Opioid Analgesics	
Mexiletine	Avoid (or reduce dose) in severe liver disease	Phenazocine *see* Opioid Analgesics	
		Phenelzine *see* MAOIs	
Mianserin *see* Antidepressants, Tricyclic (and related)		Phenindamine *see* Antihistamines	
		Pheniramine *see* Antihistamines	
Minocycline *see* Tetracyclines		Phenobarbitone	May precipitate coma
Mivacurium	Reduce dose	Phenoperidine *see* Opioid Analgesics	
Moclobemide	Reduce dose in severe liver disease	Phenothiazines *see* Antipsychotics	
		Phenylbutazone *see* NSAIDs	
Moexipril *see* ACE Inhibitors		Phenytoin	Reduce dose to avoid toxicity
Monoamine-oxidase Inhibitors *see* MAOIs		Pholcodine *see* Opioid Analgesics	
Morphine *see* Opioid Analgesics		Pilocarpine	Reduce oral dose
Moxonidine	Avoid in severe liver disease	Pimozide *see* Antipsychotics	
Nabumetone *see* NSAIDs		Piperazine	Manufacturer advises avoid
Nalbuphine *see* Opioid Analgesics		Piperazine Oestrone Sulphate *see* Oestrogens	
Nalidixic Acid *see* 4-Quinolones		Pipothiazine *see* Antipsychotics	
Nandrolone *see* Anabolic Steroids		Piracetam	Avoid
Naproxen *see* NSAIDs		Piretanide *see* Loop Diuretics	
Narcotic Analgesics *see* Opioid Analgesics		Piroxicam *see* NSAIDs	
Nefazodone	Reduce dose	Polyoestradiol *see* Oestrogens	
Nicardipine	Reduce dose	Polythiazide *see* Thiazides	
Nifedipine	Reduce dose	Pravastatin	Avoid in active liver disease or unexplained persistent elevations in serum transaminases
Niridazole	Increased CNS toxicity in patients with cirrhosis or portal-systemic shunts		
Nitrazepam *see* Anxiolytics and Hypnotics		Prednisolone	Side-effects more common
Nitrofurantoin	Cholestatic jaundice and chronic active hepatitis reported	Prednisone	Prednisolone is preferable (prednisone needs conversion to prednisolone by liver before active)
Nitroprusside	Avoid in severe liver disease		
Norethisterone *see* Progestogens		Primidone	Reduce dose; may precipitate coma
Norfloxacin *see* 4-Quinolones			
Norgestimate *see* Progestogens		Procainamide	Avoid or reduce dose
Norgestrel *see* Progestogens		Prochlorperazine *see* Antipsychotics	
Nortriptyline *see* Antidepressants, Tricyclic			

Table of drugs to be avoided or used with caution in liver disease (*continued*)

Drug	Comment	Drug	Comment
Progesterone *see* Progestogens		Tenoxicam *see* NSAIDs	
Progestogens	Avoid; *see also* Contraceptives, Oral	Terbinafine	Reduce dose
Promazine *see* Antipsychotics		Terfenadine *see* Antihistamines	
Promethazine *see* Antihistamines		Testosterone *see* Androgens	
Propafenone	Reduce dose	Tetracyclines	Avoid (or use with caution)—dose-related toxicity by i/v route; SLE syndrome and hepatic damage reported with minocycline
Propranolol	Reduce oral dose		
Protriptyline *see* Antidepressants, Tricyclic			
Pyrazinamide	Avoid—idiosyncratic hepatotoxicity more common; *see also* p. 255		
		Theophylline	Reduce dose
Quinapril *see* ACE Inhibitors		Thiazides	Avoid in severe liver disease; hypokalaemia may precipitate coma (potassium-sparing diuretic can prevent); increased risk of hypomagnesaemia in alcoholic cirrhosis
4-Quinolones	See section 5.1.12; hepatitis with necrosis reported with *ciprofloxacin*; hepatitis also reported for *norfloxacin; nalidixic acid* partially conjugated in liver; reduce dose of *ofloxacin* in severe liver disease		
		Thiopentone	Reduce dose for induction in severe liver disease
Ramipril *see* ACE Inhibitors		Thioridazine *see* Antipsychotics	
Ranitidine	Increased risk of confusion; reduce dose	Tiaprofenic acid *see* NSAIDs	
		Tibolone	Avoid in severe liver disease
Rifabutin	Reduce dose in severe hepatic impairment	*Timentin*®	Cholestatic jaundice, see p. 236
Rifampicin	Impaired elimination; may be increased risk of hepatotoxicity; avoid or do not exceed 8mg/kg daily; *see also* p. 256	Tinzaparin *see* Heparin	
		Tocainide	Avoid (or reduce dose) in severe liver disease
Risperidone *see* Antipsychotics		Tolazamide *see* Sulphonylureas	
Rocuronium	Reduce dose	Tolbutamide *see* Sulphonylureas	
Salsalate *see* Aspirin		Tolmetin *see* NSAIDs	
Sertraline *see* Antidepressants, SSRI		Torasemide *see* Loop Diuretics	
Simvastatin	Avoid in active liver disease or unexplained persistent elevations in serum transaminases	Tramadol *see* Opioid Analgesics	
		Trandolapril *see* ACE Inhibitors	
		Tranylcypromine *see* MAOIs	
Sodium Aurothiomalate *see* Gold		Trazodone *see* Antidepressants, Tricyclic (and related)	
Sodium Bicarbonate *see* Antacids			
Sodium Fusidate *see* Fusidic Acid		Triclofos *see* Anxiolytics and Hypnotics	
Sodium Nitroprusside *see* Nitroprusside		Trifluoperazine *see* Antipsychotics	
Sodium Valproate *see* Valproate		Trimeprazine *see* Antihistamines	
Stanozolol *see* Anabolic Steroids		Trimipramine *see* Antidepressants, Tricyclic	
Stilboestrol *see* Oestrogens		Triprolidine *see* Antihistamines	
Sulindac *see* NSAIDs		Tulobuterol	Avoid
Sulphonylureas	Increased risk of hypoglycaemia in severe liver disease; avoid or use small dose; can produce jaundice	Valproate	Avoid if possible—hepatotoxicity and liver failure may occasionally occur (usually in first 6 months); *see also* p. 208
Sulpiride *see* Antipsychotics			
Sumatriptan	Use half oral dose	Venlafaxine	Halve dose in moderate hepatic impairment; avoid if severe
Suxamethonium	Prolonged apnoea may occur in severe liver disease due to reduced hepatic synthesis of pseudocholinesterase		
		Verapamil	Reduce oral dose
		Xipamide *see* Thiazides	
Tacrolimus	Reduce dose	Zalcitabine	Further impairment of liver function may occur
Temazepam *see* Anxiolytics and Hypnotics		Zidovudine	Accumulation may occur
		Zolpidem *see* Anxiolytics and Hypnotics	
		Zopiclone *see* Anxiolytics and Hypnotics	
		Zuclopenthixol *see* Antipsychotics	

Appendix 3: Renal Impairment

The use of drugs in patients with reduced renal function can give rise to problems for several reasons:

  failure to excrete a drug or its metabolites may produce toxicity;

  sensitivity to some drugs is increased even if elimination is unimpaired;

  many side-effects are tolerated poorly by patients in renal failure;

  some drugs cease to be effective when renal function is reduced.

Many of these problems can be avoided by reducing the dose or by using alternative drugs.

Principles of dose adjustment in renal impairment

The level of renal function below which the dose of a drug must be reduced depends on whether the drug is eliminated entirely by renal excretion or is partly metabolised, and on how toxic it is.

For many drugs with only minor or no dose-related side-effects very precise modification of the dose regimen is unnecessary and a simple scheme for dose reduction is sufficient.

For more toxic drugs with a small safety margin dose regimens based on glomerular filtration rate should be used. For those where both efficacy and toxicity are closely related to plasma concentrations recommended regimens should be seen only as a guide to initial treatment; subsequent treatment must be adjusted according to clinical response and plasma concentration.

The total daily maintenance dose of a drug can be reduced either by reducing the size of the individual doses or by increasing the interval between doses. For some drugs, if the size of the maintenance dose is reduced it will be important to give a loading dose if an immediate effect is required. This is because when a patient is given a regular dose of any drug it takes more than five times the half-life to achieve steady-state plasma concentrations. As the plasma half-life of drugs excreted by the kidney is prolonged in renal failure it may take many days for the reduced dosage to achieve a therapeutic plasma concentration. The loading dose should usually be the same size as the initial dose for a patient with normal renal function.

Nephrotoxic drugs should, if possible, be avoided in patients with renal disease because the consequences of nephrotoxicity are likely to be more serious when the renal reserve is already reduced.

Use of dosage table

Dose recommendations are based on the severity of renal impairment. This is expressed in terms of glomerular filtration rate (GFR), usually measured by the **creatinine clearance**. The serum-creatinine concentration can usually be used instead as a measure of renal function but is only a rough guide unless corrected for age, weight, and sex. Nomograms are available for making the correction and should be used where accuracy is important.

For prescribing purposes renal impairment is arbitrarily divided into 3 grades:

Grade	GFR	Serum creatinine (approx.)
Mild	20–50 mL/min	150–300 µmol/litre
Moderate	10–20 mL/min	300–700 µmol/litre
Severe	<10 mL/min	> 700 µmol/litre

Note. Conversion factors are:
  Litres/24 hours = mL/minute × 1.44
  mL/minute = Litres/24 hours × 0.69

Renal function declines with age; many elderly patients have a glomerular filtration rate below 50 mL/minute which, because of reduced muscle mass, may not be indicated by a raised serum creatinine. It is wise to assume at least mild impairment of renal function when prescribing for the elderly.

The following table may be used as a guide to drugs which are known to require a reduction in dose in renal impairment, and to those which are potentially harmful or are ineffective. Drug prescribing should be kept to the minimum in all patients with severe renal disease.

If even mild renal impairment is considered likely on clinical grounds, renal function should be checked before prescribing **any** drug which requires dose modification.

Table of drugs to be avoided or used with caution in renal impairment

Products introduced or amended since publication of BNF No. 31 (March 1996) are underlined.

Drug and Degree of impairment	Comment	Drug and Degree of impairment	Comment
Acamprosate		Acebutolol *see* Beta-blockers	
Mild	Avoid; excreted in urine	Aceclofenac *see* NSAIDs	
Acarbose		Acemetacin *see* NSAIDs	
Moderate to severe	Manufacturer advises avoid —no information available	Acetazolamide	
		Mild	Avoid; metabolic acidosis

Table of drugs to be avoided or used with caution in renal impairment (*continued*)

Drug and Degree of impairment	Comment
Aciclovir	
Moderate to severe	Reduce dose; possible transient increase in plasma urea
Acipimox	
Mild	Reduce dose
Acitretin	
Mild	Avoid; increased risk of toxicity
Acrivastine	
Moderate	Avoid; excreted by kidney
Alendronic Acid	
Moderate to severe	Avoid
Alfentanil *see* Opioid Analgesics	
Alfuzosin	
Moderate	Reduce dose
Allopurinol	
Moderate	100 mg daily; increased toxicity; rashes
Severe	100 mg on alternate days
Alprazolam *see* Anxiolytics and Hypnotics	
Alteplase	
Moderate	Risk of hyperkalaemia
Aluminium Salts	
Severe	Aluminium is absorbed and may accumulate
Note. Absorption of aluminium from aluminium salts is increased by citrates, which are contained in many effervescent preparations (such as effervescent analgesics)	
Amantadine	
Mild to moderate	Reduce dose; excreted by kidney
Severe	Avoid
Amikacin *see* Aminoglycosides	
Amiloride *see* Potassium-sparing Diuretics	
Aminoglycosides	
Mild	Reduce dose; monitor plasma concentrations; ototoxic; nephrotoxic; *see also* p. 244
Amoxycillin	
Severe	Reduce dose; rashes more common
Amphotericin	
Mild	Use only if no alternative; nephrotoxicity may be reduced with use of complexes (*see also* p. 262)
Ampicillin	
Severe	Reduce dose; rashes more common
Amylobarbitone	
Severe	Reduce dose; active metabolite accumulates
Analgesics *see* Opioid Analgesics and NSAIDs	
Anastrozole	
Moderate to severe	Avoid—no information available
Antipsychotics	
Severe	Start with small doses; increased cerebral sensitivity; *see also* Sulpiride
Anxiolytics and Hypnotics	
Severe	Start with small doses; increased cerebral sensitivity
Aspirin	
Severe	Avoid; sodium and water retention; deterioration in renal function; increased risk of gastro-intestinal bleeding
Atenolol *see* Beta-blockers	
Auranofin *see* Gold	
Aurothiomalate *see* Gold	
Azapropazone *see* NSAIDs (excreted by kidney)	

Drug and Degree of impairment	Comment
Azathioprine	
Severe	Reduce dose
Azithromycin	
Moderate to severe	No information available
Azlocillin	
Moderate	Reduce dose
Aztreonam	
Moderate	Reduce dose
Bacampicillin	
Severe	Reduce dose; rashes more common
Baclofen	
Mild	Use smaller doses (e.g. 5 mg daily); excreted by kidney
Bambuterol	
Mild	Reduce dose
Bendrofluazide *see* Thiazides	
Benorylate [aspirin-paracetamol ester] *see* Aspirin	
Benperidol *see* Antipsychotics	
Benzodiazepines *see* Anxiolytics and Hypnotics	
Benzylpenicillin	
Severe	Max. 6 g daily; neurotoxicity—high doses may cause convulsions
Beta-blockers	
Moderate	Start with small dose of acebutolol (active metabolite accumulates); reduce dose of atenolol, nadolol, pindolol, sotalol (all excreted unchanged)
Severe	Start with small dose; higher plasma concentrations after oral administration; may reduce renal blood flow and adversely affect renal function in severe impairment; manufacturer advises avoid celiprolol and sotalol
Betaxolol *see* Beta-blockers	
Bethanidine	
Moderate	Avoid; increased postural hypotension; decrease in renal blood flow
Bezafibrate	
Mild to moderate	Reduce dose; further deterioration in renal function
Severe	Avoid
Bicarbonate *see* Sodium Bicarbonate	
Bismuth Chelate	
Severe	Avoid
Bisoprolol *see* Beta-blockers	
Bleomycin	
Moderate	Reduce dose
Bromazepam *see* Anxiolytics and Hypnotics	
Bumetanide	
Moderate	May need high doses
Buprenorphine *see* Opioid Analgesics	
Calcitonin	
Moderate	Reduce dose
Capreomycin	
Mild	Reduce dose; nephrotoxic; ototoxic
Captopril	
Mild	Reduce dose and monitor response; avoid if possible; excreted by kidney; hyperkalaemia and other side-effects more common (but specialised role in some forms of renal disease, see section 6.1.5); *see also* p. 87
Carbamazepine	Manufacturer advises caution

Table of drugs to be avoided or used with caution in renal impairment (*continued*)

Drug and Degree of impairment	Comment
Carbenicillin	
Moderate	Reduce dose; neurotoxic; may produce bleeding diathesis; 1 g contains 5.4 mmol sodium
Carbenoxolone	
Moderate	Avoid; fluid retention
Carboplatin *see* Cisplatin	
Cefadroxil	
Moderate	Reduce dose
Cefixime	
Moderate	Reduce dose
Cefodizime	
Moderate	Reduce dose
Cefotaxime	
Severe	Use half dose
Cefoxitin	
Mild	Reduce dose
Cefpirome	
Mild	Usual initial dose, then use half dose
Moderate to severe	Usual initial dose, then one-quarter dose
Cefpodoxime	
Moderate	Reduce dose
Cefsulodin	
Moderate	Reduce dose
Ceftazidime	
Mild	Reduce dose
Ceftibuten	
Mild	Reduce dose
Ceftizoxime	
Mild	Reduce dose
Ceftriaxone	
Severe	Reduce dose; also monitor plasma concentration if both severe renal and hepatic impairment
Cefuroxime	
Moderate to severe	Reduce parenteral dose
Celiprolol *see* Beta-blockers	
Cephalexin	
Severe	Max. 500 mg daily
Cephamandole	
Mild	Reduce dose
Cephazolin	
Mild	Reduce dose
Cephradine	
Mild	Reduce dose
Certoparin *see* Heparin	
Cetirizine	
Moderate	Use half dose
Chloral Hydrate *see* Anxiolytics and Hypnotics	
Chloramphenicol	
Severe	Avoid unless no alternative; dose-related depression of haematopoiesis
Chlordiazepoxide *see* Anxiolytics and Hypnotics	
Chlormethiazole *see* Anxiolytics and Hypnotics	
Chloroquine	
Mild to moderate	Reduce dose; only on prolonged use
Severe	Avoid
Chlorothiazide *see* Thiazides	
Chlorpromazine *see* Antipsychotics	
Chlorpropamide	
Mild	Avoid; tolbutamide and gliquidone suitable alternatives
Chlortetracycline *see* Tetracyclines	
Chlorthalidone *see* Thiazides	
Cilastatin [ingredient] *see* *Primaxin*®	

Drug and Degree of impairment	Comment
Cilazapril	
Mild	Reduce dose and monitor response; avoid if possible; *see also* Captopril
Cimetidine	
Mild to moderate	600–800 mg daily; occasional risk of confusion
Severe	400 mg daily
Cinoxacin	
Moderate	Avoid; nausea, rashes
Ciprofibrate	
Moderate	100 mg on alternate days
Severe	Avoid
Ciprofloxacin	
Moderate	Use half dose
Cisapride	
Moderate	Start with half dose
Cisplatin	
Mild	Avoid if possible; nephrotoxic and neurotoxic
Citalopram	
Moderate to severe	No information available
Citrates	Absorption of aluminium from aluminium salts is increased by citrates, which are contained in many effervescent preparations (such as effervescent analgesics)
Clarithromycin	
Moderate to severe	Use half dose
Clavulanic acid [ingredient] *see* Co-amoxiclav, *Timentin*®	
Clobazam *see* Anxiolytics and Hypnotics	
Clodronate sodium	
Mild to moderate	Use half dose and monitor serum creatinine
Severe	Avoid
Clofibrate	
Mild to moderate	Reduce dose; further deterioration in renal function; myopathy
Severe	Avoid
Clopamide *see* Thiazides	
Clorazepate *see* Anxiolytics and Hypnotics	
Clozapine *see* Antipsychotics	
Co-amoxiclav	
Moderate	Reduce dose
Codeine *see* Opioid Analgesics	
Colchicine	
Severe	Avoid or reduce dose if no alternative
Colistin	
Mild	Reduce dose; nephrotoxic; neurotoxic
Co-trimoxazole	
Moderate	Reduce dose; rashes and blood disorders; may cause further deterioration in renal function
Cyclopenthiazide *see* Thiazides	
Cyclophosphamide	
Moderate	Reduce dose
Cycloserine	
Mild to moderate	Reduce dose
Severe	Avoid
Cyclosporin *see* p. 363 (*see also* p. 471 if used in atopic dermatitis or psoriasis and p. 421 if used in rheumatoid arthritis)	
Dalteparin *see* Heparin	
Danaparoid *see* Heparin	
Debrisoquine	
Moderate	Avoid; increased postural hypotension; decrease in renal blood flow
Demeclocycline *see* Tetracyclines	

Table of drugs to be avoided or used with caution in renal impairment (*continued*)

Drug and Degree of impairment	Comment
De-Nol®, De-Noltab®	
Severe	Avoid
Desflurane	
Moderate	Reduce dose
Desmopressin	Antidiuretic effect may be reduced; **important:** *see also* p.319
Dexfenfluramine	Manufacturer advises avoid
Dextromethorphan *see* Opioid Analgesics	
Dextromoramide *see* Opioid Analgesics	
Dextropropoxyphene *see* Opioid Analgesics	
Diamorphine *see* Opioid Analgesics	
Diazepam *see* Anxiolytics and Hypnotics	
Diazoxide	
Severe	75–150 mg i/v; increased sensitivity to hypotensive effect
Diclofenac *see* NSAIDs	
Didanosine	
Mild to moderate	Reduce dose; excreted by kidney
Diflunisal *see* NSAIDs (excreted by kidney)	
Digitoxin	
Severe	Max. 100micrograms daily; *see also* Digoxin
Digoxin	
Mild	Reduce dose; toxicity increased by electrolyte disturbances; *see also* p. 58
Dihydrocodeine *see* Opioid Analgesics	
Diltiazem	Start with smaller dose
Dimenhydrinate	
Severe	Manufacturer advises may accumulate
Diphenoxylate *see* Opioid Analgesics	
Dipipanone *see* Opioid Analgesics	
Disodium Etidronate *see* Etidronate Disodium	
Disodium Pamidronate *see* Pamidronate Disodium	
Disopyramide	
Mild	100mg every 8 hours *or* 150mg every 12 hours
Moderate	100mg every 12 hours
Severe	150mg every 24 hours
Domperidone	
Severe	Reduce dose by 30–50%
Doxycycline *see* Tetracyclines	
Droperidol *see* Antipsychotics	
Effervescent preparations *see* Citrates	
Enalapril	
Mild	Reduce dose and monitor response; avoid if possible; *see also* Captopril
Enflurane	
Severe	Avoid
Enoxaparin *see* Heparin	
Ephedrine	
Severe	Avoid; increased CNS toxicity
Ergometrine	
Severe	Manufacturer advises avoid
Ergotamine	
Moderate	Avoid; nausea and vomiting; risk of renal vasoconstriction
Erythromycin	
Severe	Max. 1.5g daily (ototoxicity)
Esmolol *see* Beta-blockers	
Ethacrynic Acid	
Severe	Avoid; ototoxic
Ethambutol	
Mild	Reduce dose; optic nerve damage
Etidronate Disodium	
Mild	Max. 5mg/kg daily; excreted by kidney
Moderate	Avoid

Drug and Degree of impairment	Comment
Etodolac *see* NSAIDs	
Etoposide	
Mild	Reduce dose
Famciclovir	
Mild to moderate	Reduce dose
Famotidine	
Severe	Reduce dose
Fenbufen *see* NSAIDs	
Fenofibrate	
Mild	200mg daily
Moderate	100mg daily
Severe	Avoid
Fenoprofen *see* NSAIDs	
Fentanyl *see* Opioid Analgesics	
Flecainide	
Mild	Max. initial dose 100mg daily
Fluconazole	
Mild	Reduce dose for multiple dose therapy
Flucytosine	
Mild	Reduce dose
Fludarabine	
Mild	Reduce dose and monitor response
Moderate	Avoid
Flunitrazepam *see* Anxiolytics and Hypnotics	
Fluoxetine	
Mild to moderate	Reduce dose(give on alternate days)
Severe	Avoid
Flupenthixol *see* Antipsychotics	
Fluphenazine *see* Antipsychotics	
Flurazepam *see* Anxiolytics and Hypnotics	
Flurbiprofen *see* NSAIDs	
Fluvastatin	
Severe	Avoid
Fluvoxamine	
Moderate	Start with smaller dose
Foscarnet	
Mild	Reduce dose; consult data sheet
Fosfomycin	
Severe	Avoid—therapeutic urinary concentrations not achieved
Fosinopril	
Mild	Start with 10mg daily; *see also* Captopril
Frusemide	
Moderate	May need high doses; deafness may follow rapid i/v injection
Fybogel Mebeverine®	
Severe	Avoid; contains 7mmol potassium per sachet
Gabapentin	
Mild	Reduce dose; consult data sheet
Gallamine	
Moderate	Avoid; prolonged paralysis
Ganciclovir	
Mild	Reduce dose; consult data sheet
Gaviscon®	
Severe	Avoid; high sodium content
Gemcitabine	
Mild	Monitor renal function
Gemfibrozil	
Severe	Start with 900mg daily
Gentamicin *see* Aminoglycosides	
Glibenclamide	
Severe	Avoid; increased risk of prolonged hypoglycaemia

Table of drugs to be avoided or used with caution in renal impairment (*continued*)

Drug and Degree of impairment	Comment
liclazide	
Severe	Start with small dose; increased risk of hypoglycaemia
lipizide	
Severe	Start with small dose; increased risk of hypoglycaemia
liquidone	
Severe	May need dose reduction; increased risk of hypoglycaemia
old (auranofin, aurothiomalate)	
Mild	Avoid; nephrotoxic
uanethidine	
Moderate	Avoid; increased postural hypotension and decrease in renal blood flow
laloperidol *see* Antipsychotics	
eparin	
Severe	Risk of bleeding increased
letastarch	
Severe	Avoid; excreted by kidney
examine	
Mild	Avoid; ineffective
ydralazine	
Moderate	Start with small dose; increased hypotensive effect
ydrochlorothiazide *see* Thiazides	
ydroflumethiazide *see* Thiazides	
ydroxychloroquine	
Mild to moderate	Reduce dose; only on prolonged use
Severe	Avoid
ypnotics *see* Anxiolytics and Hypnotics	
uprofen *see* NSAIDs	
larubicin	
Mild	Reduce dose
osfamide	
Moderate	Reduce dose
nipenem *see* Primaxin®	
ndapamide *see* Thiazides	
ndomethacin *see* NSAIDs	
nosine Pranobex	
Mild	Avoid; metabolised to uric acid
nsulin	
Severe	May need dose reduction; insulin requirements fall; compensatory response to hypoglycaemia is impaired
nterferon alfa	
Mild to moderate	Close monitoring required
Severe	Avoid
nterferon beta	No information available— monitoring advised
soniazid	
Severe	Max. 200mg daily; peripheral neuropathy
sotretinoin	
Mild	Avoid; increased risk of toxicity
anamycin *see* Aminoglycosides	
etoprofen *see* NSAIDs	
etorolac *see* NSAIDs and p. 527	
amotrigine	
Moderate to severe	Metabolite may accumulate
evocabastine	
Severe	Manufacturer advises avoid
isinopril	
Mild	Reduce dose and monitor response; *see also* Captopril

Drug and Degree of impairment	Comment
Lithium	
Mild	Avoid if possible or reduce dose and monitor plasma concentration carefully
Moderate	Avoid
Loprazolam *see* Anxiolytics and Hypnotics	
Lorazepam *see* Anxiolytics and Hypnotics	
Lormetazepam *see* Anxiolytics and Hypnotics	
Losartan	
Moderate to severe	Start with 25 mg once daily
Loxapine *see* Antipsychotics	
Lymecycline *see* Tetracyclines	
Magnesium Salts	
Moderate	Avoid or reduce dose; increased risk of toxicity; magnesium carbonate mixture and magnesium trisilicate mixture also have high sodium content
Mefenamic Acid *see* NSAIDs	
Mefloquine *see* p. 273 [text]	
Mefruside *see* Thiazides	
Melphalan	
Moderate	Reduce dose
Severe	Avoid high intravenous doses
Meprobamate *see* Anxiolytics and Hypnotics	
Meptazinol *see* Opioid Analgesics	
Mercaptopurine	
Moderate	Reduce dose
Meropenem	
Mild	Increase dose interval to every 12 hours
Moderate	Half dose every 12 hours
Severe	Half dose every 24 hours
Mesalazine	
Mild	Avoid; nephrotoxic
Metformin	
Mild	Avoid; increased risk of lactic acidosis
Methadone *see* Opioid Analgesics	
Methocarbamol	
Mild	Avoid; increased plasma urea and acidosis due to solvent in injection
Methotrexate	
Mild	Reduce dose; accumulates; nephrotoxic
Moderate	Avoid
Methotrimeprazine *see* Antipsychotics	
Methyldopa	
Moderate	Start with small dose; increased sensitivity to hypotensive and sedative effect
Metoclopramide	
Severe	Avoid or use small dose; increased risk of extrapyramidal reactions
Metolazone *see* Thiazides	
Metoprolol *see* Beta-blockers	
Midazolam *see* Anxiolytics and Hypnotics	
Milrinone	
Mild	Reduce dose and monitor response
Minocycline *see* Tetracyclines	
Mivacurium	
Severe	Reduce dose; prolonged paralysis
Morphine *see* Opioid Analgesics	
Moxonidine	
Mild	Max. single dose 200 micrograms and max. daily dose 400 micrograms
Moderate to severe	Avoid
Nabumetone *see* NSAIDs	

Table of drugs to be avoided or used with caution in renal impairment (*continued*)

Drug and Degree of impairment	Comment
Nadolol *see* Beta-blockers	
Nalbuphine *see* Opioid Analgesics	
Nalidixic Acid	
Moderate	Avoid; increased risk of nausea, vomiting, rashes, photosensitivity; ineffective because of inadequate urine concentration
Naproxen *see* NSAIDs	
Narcotic Analgesics *see* Opioid Analgesics	
Nefazodone	
Severe	Reduce dose
Neomycin	
Mild	Avoid; ototoxic; nephrotoxic
Neostigmine	
Moderate	May need dose reduction
Netilmicin *see* Aminoglycosides	
Nicardipine	
Moderate	Start with small dose
Nifedipine	
Moderate	Start with small dose; reversible deterioration in renal function has been reported
Nitrazepam *see* Anxiolytics and Hypnotics	
Nitrofurantoin	
Mild	Avoid; peripheral neuropathy; ineffective because of inadequate urine concentrations
Nitroprusside	
Moderate	Avoid prolonged use
Nizatidine	
Mild	Use half dose
Moderate	Use one-quarter dose
Norfloxacin	
Severe	Use half dose
NSAIDs	
Mild	Avoid if possible; deterioration in renal function (**important**: see p. 408; also p. 527 (ketorolac)); sodium and water retention; deterioration also reported after topical use
Ofloxacin	
Mild	Usual initial dose, then use half dose
Moderate	Usual initial dose, then 100 mg every 24 hours
Olsalazine	
Mild	Manufacturer advises avoid if significant renal impairment
Opioid Analgesics	
Moderate to severe	Reduce doses or avoid; increased and prolonged effect; increased cerebral sensitivity
Oxazepam *see* Anxiolytics and Hypnotics	
Oxprenolol *see* Beta-blockers	
Oxypertine *see* Antipsychotics	
Oxytetracycline *see* Tetracyclines	
Pamidronate Disodium	
Moderate to severe	Max. infusion rate 20 mg/hour
Pancuronium *see* Tubocurarine	
Papaveretum *see* Opioid Analgesics	
Paroxetine	
Moderate	Usual initial dose; small increments if necessary
Penicillamine	
Mild	Avoid if possible or reduce dose; nephrotoxic
Pentamidine	
Mild	Reduce dose; consult data sheet

Drug and Degree of impairment	Comment
Pentazocine *see* Opioid Analgesics	
Pericyazine *see* Antipsychotics	
Perindopril	
Mild	Reduce dose and frequency and monitor response; *see a* Captopril
Perphenazine *see* Antipsychotics	
Pethidine *see* Opioid Analgesics	
Phenazocine *see* Opioid Analgesics	
Phenobarbitone	
Severe	Avoid large doses
Phenoperidine *see* Opioid Analgesics	
Phenothiazines *see* Antipsychotics	
Phenylbutazone *see* NSAIDs	
Pholcodine *see* Opioid Analgesics	
Pimozide *see* Antipsychotics	
Pindolol *see* Beta-blockers	
Piperacillin	
Moderate	Reduce dose
Piperazine	
Severe	Reduce dose; neurotoxic
Pipothiazine *see* Antipsychotics	
Piracetam	
Mild	Use half dose
Moderate	Use one-quarter dose
Severe	Avoid
Pirenzepine	
Moderate	Reduce dose
Piroxicam *see* NSAIDs	
Pivampicillin	
Severe	Reduce dose; rashes more common
Polythiazide *see* Thiazides	
Potassium Salts	
Moderate	Avoid routine use; high risk hyperkalaemia
Potassium-sparing Diuretics	
Mild	Monitor plasma K⁺; high r of hyperkalaemia in renal impairment; amiloride excreted by kidney unchan
Moderate	Avoid
Povidone-iodine	
Severe	Avoid regular application t inflamed or broken mucosa
Pravastatin	
Moderate to severe	Start at lower end of dosag range
Prazosin	
Severe	Start with small dose; increased sensitivity to hyp tensive effect and possible CNS toxicity
Primaxin®	
Mild	Reduce dose
Primidone	
Severe	Avoid large doses
Probenecid	
Moderate	Avoid; ineffective and toxicity increased
Procainamide	
Mild	Avoid or reduce dose
Procarbazine	
Moderate	Reduce dose
Prochlorperazine *see* Antipsychotics	
Proguanil	
Mild	100 mg once daily
Moderate	50 mg on alternate days
Severe	50 mg once weekly; increa risk of haematological toxi
Promazine *see* Antipsychotics	
Propranolol *see* Beta-blockers	
Propylthiouracil	
Mild	Reduce dose

Table of drugs to be avoided or used with caution in renal impairment (*continued*)

Drug and Degree of impairment	Comment
Pseudoephedrine	
Severe	Avoid; increased CNS toxicity
Pyridostigmine	
Moderate	Reduce dose; excreted by kidney
Quinapril	
Mild	Start with 2.5 mg daily; *see also* Captopril
Raltitrexed	
Mild	Reduce dose
Moderate to severe	Avoid
Ramipril	
Mild	Start with 1.25 mg daily; *see also* Captopril
Ranitidine	
Severe	Use half normal dose; occasional risk of confusion
Ranitidine Bismuth Citrate	
Severe	Avoid
Regulan®	
Severe	Avoid; contains 6.4 mmol potassium per sachet
Rifabutin	
Moderate	Use half dose
Risperidone *see* Antipsychotics	
Rocuronium	
Moderate	Reduce dose; prolonged paralysis
Salcatonin *see* Calcitonin	
Salicylates *see* Aspirin	
Salsalate *see* Aspirin	
Salt Substitutes	
Moderate	Avoid routine use; high risk of hyperkalaemia (*see* section 9.2.1.1)
Sertraline	Manufacturer advises caution
Simvastatin	
Moderate to severe	Doses above 10 mg daily should be used with caution
Sodium Aurothiomalate *see* Gold	
Sodium Bicarbonate	
Severe	Avoid; specialised role in some forms of renal disease
Sodium Cellulose Phosphate	
Mild to moderate	Reduce dose
Severe	Avoid
Sodium Clodronate *see* Clodronate Sodium	
Sodium Nitroprusside *see* Nitroprusside	
Sodium Salts	
Severe	Avoid
Solpadeine®	
Severe	Avoid; contains 18.5 mmol sodium per tablet
Solpadol®	
Severe	Avoid; contains 18.6 mmol sodium per tablet
Sotalol *see* Beta-blockers	
Spironolactone *see* Potassium-sparing Diuretics	
Streptomycin *see* Aminoglycosides	
Sucralfate	
Severe	Avoid; aluminium is absorbed and may accumulate
Sulfametopyrazine *see* Sulphonamides	
Sulindac *see* NSAIDs (excreted by kidney)	
Sulphadiazine	
Severe	Avoid; high risk of crystalluria
Sulphadimidine *see* Sulphonamides	
Sulphasalazine	
Severe	Ensure high fluid intake; rashes and blood disorders; crystalluria a risk
Sulphinpyrazone	
Moderate	Avoid; ineffective as uricosuric

Drug and Degree of impairment	Comment
Sulphonamides	
Moderate	Ensure high fluid intake; rashes and blood disorders; crystalluria a risk
Sulphonylureas *see under* individual drugs	
Sulpiride	
Moderate	Avoid if possible, or reduce dose
Teicoplanin	
Mild	Reduce dose after 4 days; consult data sheet
Temazepam *see* Anxiolytics and Hypnotics	
Temocillin	
Moderate	Reduce dose
Tenoxicam *see* NSAIDs	
Terbinafine	
Mild	Use half normal dose
Tetracyclines (except doxycycline and minocycline)	
Mild	Avoid—use doxycycline or minocycline if necessary; anti-anabolic effect, increased plasma urea, further deterioration in renal function
Thiazides and Related Diuretics	
Moderate	Avoid; ineffective (metolazone remains effective but risk of excessive diuresis)
Thioguanine	
Moderate	Reduce dose
Thioridazine *see* Antipsychotics	
Tiaprofenic Acid *see* NSAIDs	
Ticarcillin	
Moderate	Reduce dose; 1 g contains 5.3 mmol sodium
Tiludronic Acid	
Moderate to severe	Avoid
Timentin®	
Moderate	Reduce dose
Timolol *see* Beta-blockers	
Tinzaparin *see* Heparin	
Tobramycin *see* Aminoglycosides	
Tocainide	
Mild	Reduce dose
Tolazamide	
Severe	May need dose reduction; increased risk of hypoglycaemia
Tolbutamide	
Severe	May need dose reduction; increased risk of hypoglycaemia
Tolmetin *see* NSAIDs (excreted by kidney)	
Topiramate	
Moderate to severe	Longer time to steady-state plasma concentrations
Torasemide	
Moderate	May need high doses
Tramadol *see* Opioid Analgesics	
Trandolapril	
Mild	Start with 500 micrograms daily and monitor response; *see also* Captopril
Triamterene *see* Potassium-sparing Diuretics	
Triclofos *see* Anxiolytics and Hypnotics	
Trifluoperazine *see* Antipsychotics	
Trimeprazine	
Severe	Avoid
Trimethoprim	
Moderate	Reduce dose
Tripotassium Dicitratobismuthate *see* Bismuth Chelate	

Table of drugs to be avoided or used with caution in renal impairment (*continued*)

Drug and Degree of impairment	Comment	Drug and Degree of impairment	Comment
Tulobuterol		**Vigabatrin**	
Mild	May need dose reduction; excreted by kidney	Mild	Excreted by kidney—lower maintenance dose may be required
Moderate to severe	Avoid		
Tylex®		**Xamoterol**	
Moderate to severe	Avoid effervescent tablets; contain 13.6 mmol sodium per tablet	Moderate	Reduce dose; excreted by kidney
Valaciclovir as for Aciclovir		**Xipamide** *see* Thiazides	
Vancomycin		**Zidovudine**	
Mild	Avoid parenteral use if possible; ototoxic; nephrotoxic	Mild	Excreted by kidney; increase risk of toxicity
Vecuronium		**Zopiclone** *see* Anxiolytics and Hypnotics	
Severe	Reduce dose; duration of block possibly prolonged	**Zuclopenthixol** *see* Antipsychotics	
Venlafaxine			
Moderate	Use half dose		
Severe	Avoid		

Appendix 4: Pregnancy

Drugs can have harmful effects on the fetus at any time during pregnancy. It is important to bear this in mind when prescribing for a woman of *childbearing age*.

During the *first trimester* drugs may produce congenital malformations (teratogenesis), and the period of greatest risk is from the third to the eleventh week of pregnancy.

During the *second* and *third trimesters* drugs may affect the growth and functional development of the fetus or have toxic effects on fetal tissues; and drugs given shortly before term or during labour may have adverse effects on labour or on the neonate after delivery.

The following list includes drugs which may have harmful effects in pregnancy and indicates the trimester of risk. It is based on human data but information on *animal* studies has been included for some newer drugs when its omission might be misleading.

> Drugs should be prescribed in pregnancy only if the expected benefit to the mother is thought to be greater than the risk to the fetus, and all drugs should be avoided if possible during the first trimester. Drugs which have been extensively used in pregnancy and appear to be usually safe should be prescribed in preference to new or untried drugs; and the smallest effective dose should be used.
>
> Few drugs have been shown conclusively to be teratogenic in man but no drug is safe beyond all doubt in early pregnancy. Screening procedures are available where there is a known risk of certain defects.
>
> Absence of a drug from the list does not imply safety. It should be noted that the BNF provides independent advice and may not always agree with the data sheets.
>
> Information on drugs and pregnancy is also available from the National Teratology Information Service (telephone: 0191-232 1525).

Table of drugs to be avoided or used with caution in pregnancy

Products introduced or amended since publication of BNF No. 31 (March 1996) are underlined.

Drug (Trimester of risk)	Comment	Drug (Trimester of risk)	Comment
Acamprosate	Manufacturer advises avoid	Alendronic Acid *see* Bisphosphonates	
Acarbose	Manufacturer advises avoid	Alfentanil *see* Opioid Analgesics	
ACE Inhibitors (1, 2, 3)	Avoid; may adversely affect fetal and neonatal blood pressure control and renal function; also possible skull defects and oligohydramnios; toxicity in *animal* studies	Alprazolam *see* Anxiolytics and Hypnotics	
		Alteplase *see* Streptokinase	
		Amantadine	Avoid; toxicity in *animal* studies
Acebutolol *see* Beta-blockers		Amikacin *see* Aminoglycosides	
Aceclofenac *see* NSAIDs		Amiloride *see* Diuretics	
Acemetacin *see* NSAIDs		Aminoglutethimide	Avoid; toxicity in *animal* studies and may affect fetal sexual development
Acetazolamide *see* Diuretics			
Acetohexamide *see* Sulphonylureas		Aminoglycosides (2, 3)	Auditory or vestibular nerve damage; risk greatest with streptomycin; probably very small with gentamicin and tobramycin, but avoid unless essential (if given, monitor plasma concentration)
Aciclovir	Experience limited—manufacturer advises use only when potential benefits outweigh possibility of unknown risks		
Acitretin (1, 2, 3)	Teratogenic; effective contraception must be used for at least 1 month before treatment, during treatment, and for at least 2 years after stopping	Aminophylline *see* Theophylline	
		Amiodarone (2, 3)	Possible risk of neonatal goitre; use only if no alternative
		Amitriptyline *see* Antidepressants, Tricyclic	
Acrivastine *see* Antihistamines		Amlodipine *see* Calcium-channel Blockers	
Albendazole	Manufacturer advises teratogenic in *animal* studies	Amoxapine *see* Antidepressants, Tricyclic	
		Amphotericin	Not known to be harmful but manufacturer advises avoid unless expected benefit outweighs potential risk
Alclometasone *see* Corticosteroids			
Alcohol (1, 2)	Regular daily drinking is teratogenic (fetal alcohol syndrome) and may cause growth retardation; occasional single drinks are probably safe	Amylobarbitone *see* Barbiturates	
		Anabolic Steroids (1, 2, 3)	Masculinisation of female fetus
		Anaesthetics General (3)	Depress neonatal respiration
(3)	Withdrawal syndrome may occur in babies of alcoholic mothers		

Table of drugs to be avoided or used with caution in pregnancy (*continued*)

Drug (Trimester of risk)	Comment
Anaesthetics, Local (3)	With large doses, neonatal respiratory depression, hypotonia, and bradycardia after paracervical or epidural block; neonatal methaemoglobinaemia with prilocaine and procaine
Analgesics *see* Opioid Analgesics and NSAIDs	
Androgens (1, 2, 3)	Masculinisation of female fetus
Anistreplase *see* Streptokinase	
Anticoagulants	
Heparin (1, 2, 3)	Osteoporosis has been reported after prolonged use
Oral Anticoagulants (1, 2, 3)	Congenital malformations; fetal and neonatal haemorrhage *See also* section 2.8
Antidepressants *see* individual drugs (and groups)	
Antidepressants, SSRI (1, 2, 3)	Manufacturers advise use only if potential benefit outweighs possible risk (no evidence of teratogenicity); adverse effects with sertraline in *animals* (manufacturer recommends avoid)
Antidepressants, Tricyclic (and related) (3)	Tachycardia, irritability, and muscle spasms in neonate reported with imipramine
Antiepileptics	Benefit of treatment outweighs risk to fetus; risk of teratogenicity greater if more than one drug used; **important**: *see also* carbamazepine, ethosuximide, phenobarbitone, phenytoin, valproate, vigabatrin, and p. 204
Antihistamines	No evidence of teratogenicity; some packs of antihistamines sold to the public carry warning to avoid in pregnancy; manufacturer of astemizole advises avoid (see p. 137)
Antimalarials (1, 3)	Benefit of prophylaxis and treatment in malaria outweighs risk; **important**: *see also* individual drugs and p. 273
Antipsychotics	Manufacturer advises avoid clozapine
(3)	Extrapyramidal effects in neonate occasionally reported
Anxiolytics and Hypnotics (1)	Avoid if possible; manu-facturer of buspirone advises toxicity in *animal* studies
(3)	Depress neonatal respiration. Benzodiazepines cause neonatal drowsiness, hypotonia, and withdrawal symptoms; avoid large doses and regular use; short-acting benzodiazepines preferable to long-acting

Drug (Trimester of risk)	Comment
Apomorphine	Avoid
Aspirin (3)	Impaired platelet function and risk of haemorrhage; delayed onset and increased duration of labour with increased blood loss; avoid analgesic doses if possible in last few weeks (low doses probably not harmful); with high doses, closure of fetal ductus arteriosus *in utero* and possibly persistent pulmonary hypertension of newborn; kernicterus in jaundiced neonates
Astemizole *see* Antihistamines	
Atenolol *see* Beta-blockers	
Atovaquone	Information not available
Auranofin *see* Gold	
Aurothiomalate *see* Gold	
Azapropazone *see* NSAIDs	
Azatadine *see* Antihistamines	
Azathioprine *see* p. 352	
Azelastine *see* Antihistamines	
Azithromycin	Not known to be harmful but manufacturer advises use only if adequate alternatives not available
Aztreonam	Manufacturer advises avoid (but no evidence of teratogenicity)
Baclofen	Manufacturer advises toxicity in *animal* studies
Bambuterol *see* section 3.1.1 [text]	
Barbiturates (3)	Withdrawal effects in neonate; *see also* Phenobarbitone
Beclomethasone *see* Corticosteroids	
Bendrofluazide *see* Diuretics	
Benorylate [aspirin-paracetamol ester] *see* Aspirin	
Benperidol *see* Antipsychotics	
Benserazide [ingredient] *see* Madopar®	
Benzodiazepines *see* Anxiolytics and Hypnotics	
Beta-blockers	May cause intra-uterine growth retardation, neonatal hypoglycaemia, and bradycardia; risk greater in severe hypertension *See also* section 2.5
Betamethasone *see* Corticosteroids	
Betaxolol *see* Beta-blockers	
Bethanidine *see* Guanethidine	
Bezafibrate *see* Clofibrate	
Bismuth Chelate	Manufacturer advises avoid on theoretical grounds
Bisoprolol *see* Beta-blockers	
Bisphosphonates	Manufacturers advise avoid
Botulinum Toxin	Manufacturers advise avoid
Bromazepam *see* Anxiolytics and Hypnotics	
Brompheniramine *see* Antihistamines	
Buclizine *see* Antihistamines	
Budesonide *see* Corticosteroids	

Table of drugs to be avoided or used with caution in pregnancy (*continued*)

Drug (Trimester of risk)	Comment
Bumetanide *see* Diuretics	
Bupivacaine *see* Anaesthetics, Local	
Buprenorphine *see* Opioid Analgesics	
Buserelin	Avoid
Buspirone *see* Anxiolytics and Hypnotics	
Cabergoline	Once regular ovulatory cycles have been achieved manufacturer advises discontinuation for one month before intended conception (although no evidence of teratogenicity)
Calcipotriol	Manufacturer advises avoid if possible
Calcitonin	Information not available
Calcium-channel Blockers	May inhibit labour and manufacturers advise that diltiazem and some dihydropyridines are teratogenic in *animals*
Capreomycin	Manufacturer advises teratogenic in *animal* studies
Captopril *see* ACE Inhibitors	
Carbamazepine (1)	Risk of teratogenesis including increased risk of neural tube defects (counselling and screening and adequate folate supplements advised, e.g. 5 mg daily); *see also* Antiepileptics and p. 204
(3)	Because of neonatal bleeding tendency associated with some antiepileptics, manufacturer advises prophylactic vitamin K₁ for mother before delivery (as well as for neonate)
Carbenoxolone (3)	Avoid; causes sodium retention with oedema
Carbimazole (2, 3)	Neonatal goitre and hypo-thyroidism; has been associated with aplasia cutis of the neonate
Carvedilol *see* Beta-blockers	
Celiprolol *see* Beta-blockers	
Cephalosporins	Not known to be harmful
Certoparin *see* Anticoagulants (Heparin)	
Cetirizine *see* Antihistamines	
Chenodeoxycholic Acid (1, 2, 3)	Theoretical risk of effects on fetal metabolism
Chloral *see* Anxiolytics and Hypnotics	
Chloramphenicol (3)	Neonatal 'grey syndrome'
Chlordiazepoxide *see* Anxiolytics and Hypnotics	
Chlormethiazole *see* Anxiolytics and Hypnotics	
Chloroquine *see* Antimalarials	
Chlorothiazide *see* Diuretics	
Chlorpheniramine *see* Antihistamines	
Chlorpromazine *see* Antipsychotics	
Chlorpropamide *see* Sulphonylureas	
Chlortetracycline *see* Tetracyclines	
Chlorthalidone *see* Diuretics	
Choline Theophyllinate *see* Theophylline	

Drug (Trimester of risk)	Comment
Cilastatin [ingredient] *see* Primaxin®	
Cilazapril *see* ACE Inhibitors	
Cinnarizine *see* Antihistamines	
Ciprofibrate *see* Clofibrate	
Ciprofloxacin *see* 4-Quinolones	
Cisapride	Manufacturer advises avoid
Cisatracurium	Information not available
Citalopram	Information not available; *see also* Antidepressants, SSRI
Cladribine *see* Cytotoxic Drugs	
Clarithromycin	Not known to be harmful but manufacturer advises avoid unless expected benefit outweighs potential risk
Clemastine *see* Antihistamines	
Clindamycin	Not known to be harmful
Clobazam *see* Anxiolytics and Hypnotics	
Clobetasol *see* Corticosteroids	
Clobetasone *see* Corticosteroids	
Clodronate Sodium *see* Bisphosphonates	
Clofibrate (1, 2, 3)	Avoid—theoretical possibility of interference with embryonic growth and development due to anticholesterol effect
Clomiphene	Possible effects on fetal development
Clomipramine *see* Antidepressants, Tricyclic	
Clomocycline *see* Tetracyclines	
Clonazepam *see* Antiepileptics	
Clorazepate *see* Anxiolytics and Hypnotics	
Clozapine *see* Antipsychotics	
Co-amoxiclav	No evidence of teratogenicity but manufacturer advises avoid unless essential
Codeine *see* Opioid Analgesics	
Colistin (2, 3)	Avoid—possible risk of fetal toxicity
Contraceptives, Oral	Epidemiological evidence suggests no harmful effects on fetus
Corticosteroids (2, 3)	Benefit of treatment, e.g. in asthma, outweighs risk; high doses (>10 mg prednisolone daily) may produce fetal and neonatal adrenal suppression; corticosteroid cover required by mother during labour; monitor closely if fluid retention
Co-trimoxazole	
(1)	Theoretical teratogenic risk (trimethoprim a folate antagonist)
(3)	Neonatal haemolysis and methaemoglobinaemia; fear of increased risk of kernicterus in neonates appears to be unfounded
Cromoglycate	Not known to be harmful; *see also* section 3.1.1 [text]
Cyclizine *see* Antihistamines	

Table of drugs to be avoided or used with caution in pregnancy *(continued)*

Drug (Trimester of risk)	Comment
Cyclopenthiazide *see* Diuretics	
Cyclosporin *see* p. 352	
Cyproheptadine *see* Antihistamines	
Cyproterone [ingredient] *see Dianette*®	
Cytotoxic Drugs (1)	Most are teratogenic; *see* section 8.1
Dalteparin *see* Anticoagulants (Heparin)	
Danaparoid	Insufficient information available
Danazol (1, 2, 3)	Has weak androgenic effects and virilisation of female fetus reported
Dapsone (3)	Neonatal haemolysis and methaemoglobinaemia; adequate folate supplements should be given to mother
Debrisoquine *see* Guanethidine	
Demeclocycline *see* Tetracyclines	
Desferrioxamine	Manufacturer advises toxicity in *animal* studies
Desflurane *see* Anaesthetics, General	
Desipramine *see* Antidepressants, Tricyclic	
Desmopressin	Has low oxytocic effect
Desogestrel *see* Contraceptives, Oral	
Desonide *see* Corticosteroids	
Desoxymethasone *see* Corticosteroids	
Dexamethasone *see* Corticosteroids	
Dexamphetamine	Manufacturer advises avoid (retrospective evidence of uncertain significance suggesting possible embryotoxicity)
Dexfenfluramine (1,2,3)	No evidence of teratogenicity but not recommended
Dextromethorphan *see* Opioid Analgesics	
Dextromoramide *see* Opioid Analgesics	
Dextropropoxyphene *see* Opioid Analgesics	
Diamorphine *see* Opioid Analgesics	
Dianette® (1, 2, 3)	Feminisation of male fetus (due to cyproterone)
Diazepam *see* Anxiolytics and Hypnotics	
Diazoxide (2, 3)	Prolonged use may produce alopecia and impaired glucose tolerance in neonate; inhibits uterine activity during labour
Diclofenac *see* NSAIDs	
Didanosine	Information not available; manufacturer advises use only when potential benefit outweighs possible risk
Diflucortolone *see* Corticosteroids	
Diflunisal *see* NSAIDs	
Digoxin	May need dosage adjustment
Dihydrocodeine *see* Opioid Analgesics	
Dihydroergotamine *see* Ergotamine	
Diltiazem *see* Calcium-channel Blockers	
Dimenhydrinate *see* Antihistamines	
Diphenhydramine *see* Antihistamines	
Diphenoxylate *see* Opioid Analgesics	
Diphenylpyraline *see* Antihistamines	

Drug (Trimester of risk)	Comment
Dipipanone *see* Opioid Analgesics	
Disodium Etidronate *see* Bisphosphonates	
Disodium Pamidronate *see* Bisphosphonates	
Disopyramide (3)	May induce labour
Distigmine	Manufacturer advises avoid (may stimulate uterine contractions)
Disulfiram (1)	High concentrations of acetaldehyde which occur in presence of alcohol may be teratogenic
Diuretics	Not used to treat hypertension in pregnancy
(1)	Manufacturers advise avoid acetazolamide and torasemide (toxicity in *animal* studies)
(3)	Thiazides may cause neonatal thrombocytopenia
Docetaxel *see* Cytotoxic Drugs	
Domperidone	Manufacturer advises avoid
Dothiepin *see* Antidepressants, Tricyclic	
Doxazosin	No evidence of teratogenicity; manufacturer advises use only when potential benefit outweighs potential risk
Doxepin *see* Antidepressants, Tricyclic	
Doxycycline *see* Tetracyclines	
Doxylamine *see* Antihistamines	
Droperidol *see* Antipsychotics	
Dydrogesterone *see* Progestogens	
Econazole	Not known to be harmful
Eformoterol *see* section 3.1.1 [text]	
Enalapril *see* ACE Inhibitors	
Enflurane *see* Anaesthetics, General	
Enoxaparin *see* Anticoagulants (Heparin)	
Ephedrine	Not known to be harmful
Ergotamine (1, 2, 3)	Oxytocic effects on the pregnant uterus
Erythromycin	Not known to be harmful
Esmolol *see* Beta-blockers	
Ethacrynic acid *see* Diuretics	
Ether *see* Anaesthetics, General	
Ethinyloestradiol *see* Contraceptives, Oral	
Ethionamide (1)	May be teratogenic
Ethosuximide (1)	May possibly be teratogenic; *see* Antiepileptics
Ethynodiol *see* Contraceptives, Oral	
Etidronate Disodium *see* Bisphosphonates	
Etodolac *see* NSAIDs	
Etomidate *see* Anaesthetics, General	
Etoposide *see* Cytotoxic Drugs	
Etretinate (1, 2, 3)	Teratogenic; effective contraception must be used for at least 1 month before treatment, during treatment, and for at least two years after stopping
Famciclovir *see* Aciclovir	

Table of drugs to be avoided or used with caution in pregnancy (*continued*)

Drug (Trimester of risk)	Comment	Drug (Trimester of risk)	Comment

Fansidar®

(1) — Possible teratogenic risk (pyrimethamine a folate antagonist)

(3) — Neonatal haemolysis and methaemoglobinaemia; fear of increased risk of kernicterus in neonates appears to be unfounded
see also Antimalarials

Felodipine *see* Calcium-channel Blockers

Fenbufen *see* NSAIDs

Fenofibrate (1, 2, 3) — Manufacturer advises toxicity in *animal* studies; *see also* Clofibrate

Fenoprofen *see* NSAIDs

Fenoterol *see* section 3.1.1 [text]

Fentanyl *see* Opioid Analgesics

Fenticonazole — Manufacturer advises avoid unless essential

Filgrastim — Toxicity in *animal* studies; manufacturer advises use only if expected therapeutic benefit outweighs possible risk

Finasteride (1, 2, 3) — Avoid unprotected intercourse (see section 6.4.2). May cause feminisation of male fetus

Flavoxate — Manufacturer advises avoid unless no safer alternative

Flecainide — Manufacturer advises toxicity in *animal* studies

Fluclorolone *see* Corticosteroids

Fluconazole — Manufacturer advises avoid (toxicity at high doses in *animal* studies)

Flucytosine (1) — Possible teratogenic risk

Fludarabine *see* Cytotoxic Drugs

Flunisolide *see* Corticosteroids

Flunitrazepam *see* Anxiolytics and Hypnotics

Fluocinolone *see* Corticosteroids

Fluocinonide *see* Corticosteroids

Fluocortolone *see* Corticosteroids

Fluoxetine *see* Antidepressants, SSRI

Flupenthixol *see* Antipsychotics

Fluphenazine *see* Antipsychotics

Flurandrenolone *see* Corticosteroids

Flurazepam *see* Anxiolytics and Hypnotics

Flurbiprofen *see* NSAIDs

Fluticasone *see* Corticosteroids

Fluvastatin *see* Statins

Fluvoxamine *see* Antidepressants, SSRI

Foscarnet — Manufacturer advises avoid

Fosfomycin — Not known to be harmful, but manufacturer advises avoid unless expected benefit outweighs potential risk

Fosinopril *see* ACE Inhibitors

Framycetin *see* Aminoglycosides

Frusemide *see* Diuretics

Gabapentin *see* Antiepileptics

Gamolenic Acid — Manufacturer advises caution (but no teratogenic effects in *animals*)

Ganciclovir — Avoid—teratogenic risk; *see also* p. 270

Gemcitabine *see* Cytotoxic Drugs

Gemfibrozil *see* Clofibrate

Gentamicin *see* Aminoglycosides

Gestodene *see* Contraceptives, Oral

Gestrinone (1, 2, 3) — Avoid

Glibenclamide *see* Sulphonylureas

Gliclazide *see* Sulphonylureas

Glipizide *see* Sulphonylureas

Gliquidone *see* Sulphonylureas

Gold

Auranofin — Manufacturer advises teratogenicity in *animal* studies; effective contraception should be used during and for at least 6 months after treatment

Aurothiomalate (1, 2, 3) — Manufacturer advises avoid

Goserelin — Avoid—manufacturer advises theoretical risk of toxicity

Granisetron — Information not available; manufacturer advises use only when compelling reasons

Griseofulvin — Avoid (fetotoxicity and teratogenicity in *animals*); manufacturer now also states that a man should not father a child within 6 months of treatment

Growth Hormone *see* Somatropin

Guanethidine (3) — Postural hypotension and reduced uteroplacental perfusion; should not be used to treat hypertension in pregnancy

Halcinonide *see* Corticosteroids

Halofantrine (1) — Manufacturer advises toxicity in *animal* studies

Haloperidol *see* Antipsychotics

Halothane *see* Anaesthetics, General

Heparin *see* Anticoagulants

Hydralazine (1) — Manufacturer advises toxicity in *animal* studies

Hydrochlorothiazide *see* Diuretics

Hydrocortisone *see* Corticosteroids

Hydroflumethiazide *see* Diuretics

Hydroxychloroquine — Avoid for rheumatic disease (but for malaria *see* Antimalarials)

Hydroxyprogesterone *see* Progestogens

Hydroxyzine *see* Antihistamines

Hypnotics *see* Anxiolytics and Hypnotics

Ibuprofen *see* NSAIDs

Table of drugs to be avoided or used with caution in pregnancy (*continued*)

Drug (Trimester of risk)	Comment
Idarubicin *see* Cytotoxic Drugs	
Idoxuridine	Manufacturers advise toxicity in *animal* studies
Imipenem [ingredient] *see* *Primaxin*®	
Imipramine *see* Antidepressants, Tricyclic	
Immunosuppressants *see* section 8.1	
Indapamide *see* Diuretics	
Indomethacin *see* NSAIDs	
Insulin (1, 2, 3)	Insulin requirements should be assessed frequently by an experienced diabetic physician
Interferons	Manufacturers recommend avoid unless compelling reasons
Iodine and Iodides (2, 3)	Neonatal goitre and hypothyroidism
Radioactive iodine (1, 2, 3)	Permanent hypothyroidism—avoid
Iodoform *see* Povidone-iodine	
Isocarboxazid *see* MAOIs	
Isoflurane *see* Anaesthetics, General	
Isotretinoin (1, 2, 3)	Teratogenic; effective contraception must be used for at least 1 month before oral treatment, during treatment and for at least 1 month after stopping; also avoid topical treatment
Isradipine *see* Calcium-channel Blockers	
Itraconazole	Manufacturer advises toxicity at high doses in *animal* studies
Kanamycin *see* Aminoglycosides	
Ketamine *see* Anaesthetics, General	
Ketoconazole	Manufacturer advises teratogenicity in *animal* studies; packs carry a warning to avoid in pregnancy
Ketoprofen *see* NSAIDs	
Ketorolac *see* NSAIDs and p. 527	
Ketotifen *see* Antihistamines	
Labetalol *see* Beta-blockers	
Lacidipine *see* Calcium-channel Blockers	
Lamotrigine *see* Antiepileptics	
Lansoprazole	Manufacturer advises avoid
Lenograstim	Toxicity in *animal* studies; manufacturer advises use only if expected therapeutic benefit outweighs possible risk
Levocabastine *see* Antihistamines	
Levodopa	Manufacturers advise toxicity in *animal* studies
Levonorgestrel *see* Contraceptives, Oral	
Lignocaine *see* Anaesthetics, Local	
Lisinopril *see* ACE Inhibitors	

Drug (Trimester of risk)	Comment
Lithium (1, 2, 3)	Dose requirements increased; neonatal goitre reported; lithium toxicity (hypotonia and cyanosis) in neonate if maternal therapy poorly controlled
Lofepramine *see* Antidepressants, Tricyclic	
Loprazolam *see* Anxiolytics and Hypnotics	
Loratadine *see* Antihistamines	
Lorazepam *see* Anxiolytics and Hypnotics	
Lormetazepam *see* Anxiolytics and Hypnotics	
Losartan	As for ACE Inhibitors
Lymecycline *see* Tetracyclines	
Madopar® *see* Levodopa	
Maloprim®	
(1)	Possible teratogenic risk (pyrimethamine a folate antagonist)
(3)	Neonatal haemolysis and methaemoglobinaemia (due to dapsone); adequate folate supplements should be given to mother; *see also* Antimalarials
MAOIs (including moclobemide) (1, 2, 3)	No evidence of harm but manufacturers advise avoid unless compelling reasons
Maprotiline *see* Antidepressants, Tricyclic (and related)	
Mebendazole	Manufacturer advises toxicity in *animal* studies
Mefenamic Acid *see* NSAIDs	
Mefloquine (1)	Manufacturer advises teratogenicity in *animal* studies; avoid for prophylaxis, *see* p. 277
Mefruside *see* Diuretics	
Melphalan *see* Cytotoxic Drugs	
Menadiol (3)	Neonatal haemolytic anaemia, hyperbilirubinaemia and increased risk of kernicterus in jaundiced infants
Meprobamate *see* Anxiolytics and Hypnotics	
Meptazinol *see* Opioid Analgesics	
Meropenem	Information not available; manufacturer advises use only if potential benefit justifies potential risk
Mesalazine	Negligible quantities cross placenta
Mesna	Not known to be harmful; *see also* section 8.1
Mesterolone *see* Androgens	
Mestranol *see* Contraceptives, Oral	
Metaraminol (1, 2, 3)	Avoid—may reduce placental perfusion
Metformin (1, 2, 3)	Avoid
Methadone *see* Opioid Analgesics	
Methohexitone *see* Anaesthetics, General	

Table of drugs to be avoided or used with caution in pregnancy (*continued*)

Drug (Trimester of risk)	Comment
Methotrexate *see* Cytotoxic Drugs; for additional advice relating to women and men, *see also* p. 472	
Methotrimeprazine *see* Antipsychotics	
Methylphenidate	Limited experience; manufacturer advises avoid unless potential benefit outweighs risk
Methylphenobarbitone *see* Antiepileptics	
Methylprednisolone *see* Corticosteroids	
Metoclopramide	Not known to be harmful but manufacturer advises use only when compelling reasons
Metolazone *see* Diuretics	
Metoprolol *see* Beta-blockers	
Metronidazole	Manufacturer advises avoidance of high-dose regimens
Metyrapone	Avoid (may impair biosynthesis of fetal-placental steroids)
Mianserin *see* Antidepressants, Tricyclic (and related)	
Mifepristone	Manufacturer advises that if treatment fails, essential that pregnancy be terminated by another method
Minocycline *see* Tetracyclines	
Minoxidil (3)	Neonatal hirsutism reported
Misoprostol (1, 2, 3)	Avoid; increases uterine tone
Mitomycin *see* Cytotoxic Drugs	
Moclobemide *see* MAOIs	
Moexipril *see* ACE Inhibitors	
Molgramostim	Manufacturer advises toxicity in *animal* studies
Moracizine	Information not available
Morphine *see* Opioid Analgesics	
Moxonidine	Information not available
Mycophenolate Mofetil	Avoid; effective contraception required during and for 6 weeks after discontinuation of treatment
Nabumetone *see* NSAIDs	
Nadolol *see* Beta-blockers	
Nafarelin	Avoid
Nalbuphine *see* Opioid Analgesics	
Nalidixic acid *see* 4-Quinolones	
Naloxone	Manufacturer advises use only if expected benefit outweighs potential risk
Nandrolone *see* Anabolic Steroids	
Naproxen *see* NSAIDs	
Narcotic Analgesics *see* Opioid Analgesics	
Nedocromil *see* section 3.1.1 [text]	
Nefazodone	Information not available; manufacturer advises use only if clearly needed

Drug (Trimester of risk)	Comment
Nefopam	Information not available; manufacturer advises avoid unless no safer treatment
Neomycin *see* Aminoglycosides	
Neostigmine (3)	Neonatal myasthenia with large doses
Netilmicin *see* Aminoglycosides	
Nicardipine *see* Calcium-channel Blockers	
Nicorandil	Information not available
Nicotine (1,2,3)	Avoid
Nicoumalone *see* Anticoagulants, Oral	
Nifedipine *see* Calcium-channel Blockers	
Nimodipine *see* Calcium-channel Blockers	
Nitrazepam *see* Anxiolytics and Hypnotics	
Nitrofurantoin (3)	May produce neonatal haemolysis if used at term
Nitrous oxide *see* Anaesthetics, General	
Nizatidine	Manufacturer advises toxicity at high doses in *animal* studies
Noradrenaline (1, 2, 3)	Avoid—may reduce placental perfusion
Norethisterone *see* Contraceptives, Oral	
Norfloxacin *see* 4-Quinolones	
Norgestimate *see* Contraceptives, Oral	
Nortriptyline *see* Antidepressants, Tricyclic	
NSAIDs	Most manufacturers advise avoid (or avoid unless expected benefit outweighs potential risk)
(3)	With regular use closure of fetal ductus arteriosus *in utero* and possibly persistent pulmonary hypertension of the newborn. Delayed onset and increased duration of labour *See also* ketorolac, p. 527
Nystatin	Information not available, but absorption from gastro-intestinal tract negligible
Octreotide (1, 2, 3)	Avoid; possible effect on fetal growth
Oestrogens *see* Contraceptives, Oral	
Ofloxacin *see* 4-Quinolones	
Omeprazole	Manufacturer advises toxicity in *animal* studies
Opioid Analgesics (3)	Depress neonatal respiration; withdrawal effects in neonates of dependent mothers; gastric stasis and risk of inhalation pneumonia in mother during labour
Orphenadrine	Information not available
Oxazepam *see* Anxiolytics and Hypnotics	
Oxprenolol *see* Beta-blockers	
Oxybutynin	Manufacturer advises toxicity at high doses in *animal* studies
Oxypertine *see* Antipsychotics	
Oxytetracycline *see* Tetracyclines	
Paclitaxel *see* Cytotoxic Drugs	

Table of drugs to be avoided or used with caution in pregnancy (*continued*)

Drug (Trimester of risk)	Comment
Pamidronate Disodium *see* Bisphosphonates	
Pancreatin	Not known to be harmful
Papaveretum *see* Opioid Analgesics	
Paroxetine *see* Antidepressants, SSRI	
Penicillamine (1, 2, 3)	Fetal abnormalities reported rarely; avoid if possible
Penicillins	Not known to be harmful
Pentazocine *see* Opioid Analgesics	
Pericyazine *see* Antipsychotics	
Perindopril *see* ACE Inhibitors	
Perphenazine *see* Antipsychotics	
Pethidine *see* Opioid Analgesics	
Phenelzine *see* MAOIs	
Phenindamine *see* Antihistamines	
Phenindione *see* Anticoagulants, Oral	
Pheniramine *see* Antihistamines	
Phenobarbitone (1, 3)	Congenital malformations. Neonatal bleeding tendency—prophylactic vitamin K_1 for mother before delivery (as well as for neonate); *see also* Antiepileptics
Phenoperidine *see* Opioid Analgesics	
Phenothiazines *see* Antipsychotics	
Phentolamine	Information not available
Phenytoin (1, 3)	Congenital malformations (screening advised); adequate folate supplements should be given to mother (e.g. folic acid 5 mg daily). Neonatal bleeding tendency—prophylactic vitamin K_1 for mother before delivery (as well as for neonate). Caution in interpreting plasma concentrations—bound may be reduced but free (i.e. effective) unchanged; *see also* Antiepileptics
Pholcodine *see* Opioid Analgesics	
Pilocarpine	Avoid—smooth muscle stimulant
Pimozide *see* Antipsychotics	
Pindolol *see* Beta-blockers	
Piperazine	No clinical evidence of harm but packs sold to the general public carry a warning to avoid in pregnancy except on medical advice
Pipothiazine *see* Antipsychotics	
Piracetam	Manufacturer advises avoid
Pirbuterol *see* section 3.1.1 [text]	
Piroxicam *see* NSAIDs	
Podophyllotoxin	Avoid
Podophyllum resin (1, 2, 3)	Avoid—neonatal death and teratogenesis have been reported
Polythiazide *see* Diuretics	

Drug (Trimester of risk)	Comment
Povidone-iodine (2, 3)	Sufficient iodine may be absorbed to affect the fetal thyroid
Pravastatin *see* Statins	
Prazosin	No evidence of teratogenicity; manufacturer advises use only when potential benefit outweighs potential risk
Prednisolone *see* Corticosteroids	
Prednisone *see* Corticosteroids	
Prilocaine (3)	Neonatal methaemoglobinaemia; *see also* Anaesthetics, Local
Primaquine (3)	Neonatal haemolysis and methaemoglobinaemia; *see also* Antimalarials
Primaxin®	Manufacturer advises toxicity in *animal* studies
Primidone *see* Phenobarbitone	
Probucol *see* Clofibrate	
Procaine (3)	Neonatal methaemoglobinaemia; *see also* Anaesthetics, Local
Prochlorperazine *see* Antipsychotics	
Progestogens (1)	High doses may possibly be teratogenic
Proguanil	Adequate folate supplements should be given to mother; *see also* Antimalarials
Promazine *see* Antipsychotics	
Promethazine *see* Antihistamines	
Propafenone	Information not available; manufacturer advises avoid
Propofol *see* Anaesthetics, General	
Propranolol *see* Beta-blockers	
Propylthiouracil (2, 3)	Neonatal goitre and hypothyroidism
Prothionamide (1)	May be teratogenic
Protriptyline *see* Antidepressants, Tricyclic	
Pseudoephedrine	Not known to be harmful
Pyridostigmine (3)	Neonatal myasthenia with large doses
Pyrimethamine (1)	Theoretical teratogenic risk (folate antagonist); adequate folate supplements should be given to mother; *see also* Antimalarials
Quinagolide	Manufacturer advises discontinue when pregnancy confirmed unless medical reason for continuing
Quinapril *see* ACE Inhibitors	
Quinine (1)	High doses are teratogenic; but in malaria benefit of treatment outweighs risk
4-Quinolones (1, 2, 3)	Arthropathy in *animal* studies
Raltitrexed *see* Cytotoxic Drugs	
Ramipril *see* ACE Inhibitors	
Reproterol *see* section 3.1.1 [text]	
Rifabutin	Information not available

Table of drugs to be avoided or used with caution in pregnancy (*continued*)

Drug (Trimester of risk)	Comment	Drug (Trimester of risk)	Comment
Rifampicin		Sulphonamides (3)	Neonatal haemolysis and methaemoglobinaemia; fear of increased risk of kernicterus in neonates appears to be unfounded
(1)	Manufacturers advise very high doses teratogenic in *animal* studies; *see also* p. 254		
(3)	Risk of neonatal bleeding may be increased	Sulphonylureas (3)	Neonatal hypoglycaemia; insulin is normally substituted in all diabetics; if oral drugs are used therapy should be stopped at least 2 days before delivery
Rimiterol *see section 3.1.1 [text]*			
Risperidone *see Antipsychotics*			
Ritodrine	For use in premature labour see section 7.1.3		
Salbutamol	For use in asthma *see* section 3.1.1 [text]	Sulpiride *see Antipsychotics*	
(3)	For use in premature labour *see* section 7.1.3	Sumatriptan	Limited experience—manufacturer advises avoid unless expected benefit to mother outweighs any possible risk to fetus
Salcatonin *see Calcitonin*			
Salicylates *see Aspirin*			
Salmeterol *see section 3.1.1 [text]*			
Salsalate *see Aspirin*		Tacrolimus	Avoid; manufacturer advises toxicity in *animal studies*
Sertraline *see Antidepressants, SSRI*			
Sevoflurane *see Anaesthetics, General*		Tamoxifen	Avoid—possible effects on fetal development; effective contraception must be used during treatment and for 2 months after stopping
Simvastatin *see Statins*			
Sodium Aurothiomalate *see Gold*			
Sodium Clodronate *see Bisphosphonates*			
Sodium Cromoglycate *see Cromoglycate*		Temazepam *see Anxiolytics and Hypnotics*	
Sodium Valproate *see Valproate*		Tenoxicam *see NSAIDS*	
Somatropin	Discontinue if pregnancy occurs—no information available but theoretical risk	Terbinafine	Information not available
		Terbutaline	For use in asthma *see* section 3.1.1 [text]
Sotalol *see Beta-blockers*		(3)	For use in premature labour *see* section 7.1.3
Spironolactone	Manufacturers advise toxicity in *animal* studies		
		Terfenadine *see Antihistamines*	
Stanozolol *see Anabolic Steroids*		Testosterone *see Androgens*	
Statins	Avoid—congenital anomalies reported; decreased synthesis of cholesterol possibly affects fetal development	Tetracyclines	
		(1)	Effects on skeletal development in *animal* studies
Stilboestrol (1)	High doses associated with vaginal carcinoma, urogenital abnormalities, and reduced fertility in female offspring	(2, 3)	Dental discoloration; maternal hepatotoxicity with large parenteral doses
		Theophylline (3)	Neonatal irritability and apnoea have been reported
Streptokinase (1, 2, 3)	Possibility of premature separation of placenta in first 18 weeks; theoretical possibility of fetal haemorrhage throughout pregnancy; avoid postpartum use—maternal haemorrhage	Thiabendazole (1)	Teratogenic in *animal* studies
		Thiazides (3)	May cause neonatal thrombocytopenia; *see also* Diuretics
		Thiopentone *see Anaesthetics, General*	
Streptomycin *see Aminoglycosides*		Thioridazine *see Antipsychotics*	
Sulfadoxine *see Sulphonamides*		Thymoxamine	Manufacturer advises avoid
Sulfametopyrazine *see Sulphonamides*		Thyroxine *see section 6.2.1*	
Sulindac *see NSAIDs*		Tiaprofenic Acid *see NSAIDs*	
Sulphadiazine *see Sulphonamides*		Tiludronic Acid *see Bisphosphonates*	
Sulphadimidine *see Sulphonamides*		Timolol *see Beta-blockers*	
Sulphasalazine (3)	Theoretical risk of neonatal haemolysis; adequate folate supplements should be given to mother	Tinidazole	Manufacturer advises avoid in first trimester
		Tinzaparin *see Anticoagulants (Heparin)*	
		Tobramycin *see Aminoglycosides*	
		Tocainide	Manufacturer advises toxicity in *animal* studies
		Tocopheryl Acetate (1, 2, 3)	No evidence of safety of high doses

Table of drugs to be avoided or used with caution in pregnancy (*continued*)

Drug (Trimester of risk)	Comment
Tolbutamide *see* Sulphonylureas	
Tolmetin *see* NSAIDs	
Topiramate	Manufacturer advises avoid unless potential benefit outweighs potential risk; *see also* Antiepileptics
Torasemide *see* Diuretics	
Tramadol	Information not available; *see also* Opioid Analgesics
Trandolapril *see* ACE Inhibitors	
Tranylcypromine *see* MAOIs	
Trazodone *see* Antidepressants, Tricyclic (and related)	
Tretinoin	Avoid; other retinoids teratogenic
Triamcinolone *see* Corticosteroids	
Triamterene *see* Diuretics	
Tribavirin	Manufacturer advises avoid
Triclofos *see* Anxiolytics and Hypnotics	
Trifluoperazine *see* Antipsychotics	
Trilostane (1, 2, 3)	Interferes with placental sex hormone production
Trimeprazine *see* Antihistamines	
Trimetaphan (3)	Avoid; risk of paralytic ileus in newborn
Trimethoprim (1)	Theoretical teratogenic risk (folate antagonist)
Trimipramine *see* Antidepressants, Tricyclic	
Tripotassium Dicitratobismuthate *see* Bismuth Chelate	
Triprolidine *see* Antihistamines	
Tropisetron	Manufacturer advises toxicity in *animal* studies
Tulobuterol *see* section 3.1.1 [text]	
Urokinase (1, 2, 3)	Avoid; possibility of premature separation of placenta in first 18 weeks; theoretical possibility of fetal haemorrhage throughout pregnancy; also avoid postpartum use—maternal haemorrhage

Drug (Trimester of risk)	Comment
Vaccines (live) (1)	Theoretical risk of congenital malformations, but need for vaccination may outweigh possible risk to fetus (*see also* p. 501)
Valaciclovir	Information not available; *see also* Aciclovir
Valproate (1, 3)	Increased risk of neural tube defects (counselling and screening advised—**important**: see also p. 204); neonatal bleeding and neonatal hepatotoxicity also reported; *see also* Antiepileptics
Vancomycin	Little information available; manufacturer advises avoid unless expected benefit outweighs potential risk
Venlafaxine	Information not available
Verapamil *see* Calcium-channel Blockers	
Vigabatrin	Congenital anomalies reported—manufacturer advises avoid; *see also* Antiepileptics
Viloxazine *see* Antidepressants, Tricyclic (and related)	
Vitamin A (1)	Excessive doses may be teratogenic; *see also* p. 399
Warfarin *see* Anticoagulants, Oral	
Xamoterol	Manufacturer advises toxicity in *animal* studies
Xipamide *see* Diuretics	
Zalcitabine	Limited information available; use only if potential benefit to mother justifies potential risk to fetus
Zidovudine	Limited information available; manufacturer advises use only if clearly indicated; *see also* p. 268
Zolpidem *see* Anxiolytics and Hypnotics	
Zopiclone *see* Anxiolytics and Hypnotics	
Zuclopenthixol *see* Antipsychotics	

Appendix 5: Breast-feeding

Administration of some drugs to nursing mothers may cause toxicity in the infant (e.g. ergotamine), whereas administration of others (e.g. digoxin), has little effect on the neonate. Some drugs inhibit lactation (e.g. bromocriptine).

Toxicity to the infant can occur if the drug enters the milk in pharmacologically significant quantities. Milk concentrations of some drugs (e.g. iodides), may exceed those in the maternal plasma so that therapeutic doses in the mother may cause toxicity to the infant. Some drugs inhibit the infant's sucking reflex (e.g. phenobarbitone). Drugs in breast milk may, at least theoretically, cause hypersensitivity in the infant even when concentrations are too low for a pharmacological effect.

The following table lists drugs:

which should be used with caution or which are contra-indicated in breast-feeding for the reasons given above;

which, on present evidence, may be given to the mother during breast-feeding, because they are excreted in milk in amounts which are too small to be harmful to the infant;

which are not known to be harmful to the infant although they are present in milk in significant amounts.

For many drugs there is insufficient evidence available to provide guidance and it is advisable only to administer essential drugs to a mother during breast-feeding. Because of the inadequacy of currently available information on drugs in breast milk the following table should be used only as a guide; absence from the table does not imply safety.

Table of drugs excreted in breast milk

Products introduced or amended since publication of BNF No. 31 (March 1996) are underlined.

Drug	Comment	Drug	Comment
Acamprosate	Manufacturer advises avoid	Androgens	Avoid; may cause masculinisation in the female infant or precocious development in the male infant; high doses suppress lactation
Acarbose	Manufacturer advises avoid		
Acebutolol see Beta-blockers			
Aceclofenac	No information available—manufacturer advises avoid		
Acemetacin	Manufacturer advises avoid	Anthraquinones	Avoid; large doses may cause increased gastric motility and diarrhoea (particularly cascara and danthron)
Acetazolamide	Amount too small to be harmful		
Acetohexamide see Sulphonylureas			
Aciclovir	Significant amount in milk	Anticoagulants, Oral	Risk of haemorrhage; increased by vitamin-K deficiency; warfarin appears safe but phenindione should be avoided
Acitretin	Avoid		
Acrivastine see Antihistamines			
Alcohol	Large amounts may affect infant and reduce milk consumption	Antidepressants, SSRI see individual entries	
Alendronic Acid	No information available	Antidepressants, Tricyclic (and related)	Amount of tricyclic antidepressants (including related drugs such as mianserin and trazodone) too small to be harmful but most manufacturers advise avoid; accumulation of doxepin metabolite may cause sedation and respiratory depression
Alfacalcidol see Vitamin D			
Alprazolam see Benzodiazepines			
Amantadine	Avoid; excreted in milk; toxicity in infant reported		
Amethocaine	No information available		
Amiloride	No information available—manufacturer advises avoid		
Aminoglutethimide	Avoid	Antihistamines	Significant amount of some antihistamines; although not known to be harmful some manufacturers advise avoid; drowsiness in infant reported with clemastine
Aminophylline see Theophylline			
Amiodarone	Avoid; present in milk in significant amounts; theoretical risk from release of iodine; see also Iodine		
Amitriptyline see Antidepressants, Tricyclic		Antipsychotics	Although amount excreted in milk probably too small to be harmful, animal studies indicate possible adverse effects of these drugs on developing nervous system therefore avoid unless absolutely necessary; drowsiness in infant reported with chlorpromazine; significant amount of sulpiride excreted in milk (best avoided); also avoid clozapine
Amoxapine see Antidepressants, Tricyclic			
Amphetamines	Significant amount in milk. Avoid		
Amphotericin	No information available		
Amylobarbitone see Barbiturates			
		Apomorphine	No information available

Table of drugs excreted in breast milk (*continued*)

Drug	Comment
Aspirin	Avoid—possible risk of Reye's syndrome; regular use of high doses could impair platelet function and produce hypoprothrombinaemia in infant if neonatal vitamin K stores low
Astemizole *see* Antihistamines	
Atenolol *see* Beta-blockers	
Atropine	May possibly have antimuscarinic effects in infants
Atovaquone	No information available
Auranofin *see* Gold	
Aurothiomalate *see* Gold	
Azapropazone	Avoid—small amounts in milk
Azatadine *see* Antihistamines	
Azithromycin	No information available
Baclofen	Amount too small to be harmful
Barbiturates	Avoid if possible (*see also* phenobarbitone); large doses may produce drowsiness
Beclomethasone *see* Corticosteroids	
Bendrofluazide *see* Thiazides	
Benperidol *see* Antipsychotics	
Benzodiazepines	Avoid repeated doses; lethargy and weight loss may occur in infant
Beta-blockers and Labetalol	Monitor infant; possible toxicity due to beta-blockade but amount of most beta-blockers excreted in milk too small to affect infant; acebutolol, atenolol, nadolol, and sotalol are present in greater amounts than other beta-blockers; manufacturer advises avoid celiprolol
Betamethasone *see* Corticosteroids	
Betaxolol *see* Beta-blockers	
Bezafibrate	Manufacturer advises avoid
Bisoprolol *see* Beta-blockers	
Botulinum Toxin	Manufacturers advise avoid
Bromazepam *see* Benzodiazepines	
Bromocriptine	Suppresses lactation
Brompheniramine *see* Antihistamines	
Buclizine *see* Antihistamines	
Bumetanide	No information available—manufacturer advises avoid if possible
Bupivacaine	Amount too small to be harmful
Buprenorphine	Amount too small to be harmful
Butobarbitone *see* Barbiturates	
Cabergoline	Suppresses lactation
Caffeine	Regular intake of large amounts can affect infant
Calciferol *see* Vitamin D	
Calcipotriol	No information available
Calcitonin	Avoid; inhibits lactation in *animals*
Calcitriol *see* Vitamin D	
Captopril	Amount probably too small to be harmful, but manufacturer advises avoid

Drug	Comment
Carbamazepine	Amount probably too small to be harmful but severe skin reaction reported in 1 infant
Carbimazole	Amounts in milk may be sufficient to affect neonatal thyroid function therefore lowest effective dose should be used (*see also* section 6.2.2)
Carisoprodol	Concentrated in milk; no adverse effects reported but best avoided
Carvedilol *see* Beta-blockers	
Cascara *see* Anthraquinones	
Celiprolol *see* Beta-blockers	
Cephalosporins	Excreted in low concentrations
Cetirizine *see* Antihistamines	
Chloral Hydrate	Sedation in infant
Chloramphenicol	Use another antibiotic; may cause bone-marrow toxicity in infant; concentration in milk usually insufficient to cause 'grey syndrome'
Chlordiazepoxide *see* Benzodiazepines	
Chlormethiazole	Amount too small to be harmful
Chloroquine	Amount probably too small to be harmful; inadequate for reliable protection against malaria, see section 5.4.1
Chlorothiazide *see* Thiazides	
Chlorpheniramine *see* Antihistamines	
Chlorpromazine	Drowsiness in infant reported; *see* Antipsychotics
Chlorpropamide *see* Sulphonylureas	
Chlortetracycline *see* Tetracyclines	
Chlorthalidone *see* Thiazides	
Cholecalciferol *see* Vitamin D	
Choline Theophyllinate *see* Theophylline	
Cilastatin [ingredient] *see* Primaxin®	
Cilazapril	No information available
Cimetidine	Significant amount—not known to be harmful but manufacturer advises avoid
Ciprofibrate	No information available
Ciprofloxacin	Avoid—high concentrations in breast milk
Cisapride	Although amount in milk small manufacturer advises avoid
Cisatracurium	No information available
Citalopram	No information available
Cladribine *see* Cytotoxic Drugs	
Clarithromycin	Excreted in milk
Clavulanic acid (in co-amoxiclav, Timentin®)	Trace amounts in milk
Clemastine *see* Antihistamines	
Clindamycin	Amount probably too small to be harmful but bloody diarrhoea reported in 1 infant
Clobazam *see* Benzodiazepines	
Clodronate Sodium	No information available
Clofibrate	Excreted in milk—manufacturer advises avoid
Clomipramine *see* Antidepressants, Tricyclic	

Table of drugs excreted in breast milk (*continued*)

Drug	Comment
Clomocycline *see* Tetracyclines	
Clorazepate *see* Benzodiazepines	
Clozapine	Avoid
Co-amoxiclav	Trace amounts in milk
Codeine	Amount too small to be harmful
Colchicine	Caution because of its cytotoxicity
Contraceptives, Oral	Avoid combined oral contraceptives until weaning or for 6 months after birth (adverse effects on lactation); progestogen-only contraceptives do not affect lactation (start 3 weeks after birth or later)
Corticosteroids	Continuous therapy with high doses (>10 mg prednisolone daily) could possibly affect infant's adrenal function—monitor carefully
Cortisone Acetate *see* Corticosteroids	
Co-trimoxazole	Small risk of kernicterus in jaundiced infants and of haemolysis in G6PD-deficient infants (due to sulphamethoxazole)
Cough mixtures containing iodides	Use alternative cough mixtures; *see* Iodine
Cromoglycate	Unlikely to be excreted in milk
Cyclopenthiazide *see* Thiazides	
Cycloserine	Amount too small to be harmful
Cyclosporin	Excreted in milk—manufacturer advises avoid
Cyproheptadine *see* Antihistamines	
Cyproterone Acetate	Caution; possibility of anti-androgen effects in neonate
Cytotoxic Drugs	Discontinue breast-feeding
Danaparoid	No information available
Danazol	No data available but avoid because of possible androgenic effects in infant
Danthron *see* Anthraquinones	
Dapsone	Haemolytic anaemia; although significant amount in milk risk to infant very small
Demeclocycline *see* Tetracyclines	
Desipramine *see* Antidepressants, Tricyclic	
Desogestrel *see* Contraceptives, Oral	
Dexamethasone *see* Corticosteroids	
Dexamphetamine *see* Amphetamines	
Dexfenfluramine	Avoid
Dextropropoxyphene	Amount too small to be harmful
Diamorphine	Therapeutic doses unlikely to affect infant; withdrawal symptoms in infants of dependent mothers; breast-feeding no longer considered best method of treating dependence in offspring of dependent mothers and should be stopped
Diazepam *see* Benzodiazepines	
Diclofenac	Amount too small to be harmful
Didanosine	Manufacturer advises avoid

Drug	Comment
Diflunisal	Manufacturer advises avoid
Digoxin	Amount too small to be harmful
Dihydrotachysterol *see* Vitamin D	
Diltiazem	Significant amount—manufacturers advise avoid
Diphenhydramine *see* Antihistamines	
Diphenylpyraline *see* Antihistamines	
Disodium Etidronate	No information available
Disodium Pamidronate	Manufacturer advises avoid
Disopyramide	Amount probably too small to be harmful—monitor infant for antimuscarinic effects
Docetaxel *see* Cytotoxic Drugs	
Domperidone	Amount probably too small to be harmful
Dothiepin *see* Antidepressants, Tricyclic	
Doxazosin	Accumulates in milk—manufacturer advises avoid
Doxepin *see* Antidepressants, Tricyclic	
Doxycycline *see* Tetracyclines	
Doxylamine *see* Antihistamines	
Droperidol *see* Antipsychotics	
Eformoterol	No information available—manufacturer advises avoid
Enalapril	Amount probably too small to be harmful
Ephedrine	Irritability and disturbed sleep reported
Ergocalciferol *see* Vitamin D	
Ergotamine	Avoid; ergotism may occur in infant; repeated doses may inhibit lactation
Erythromycin	Only small amounts in milk
Esmolol *see* Beta-blockers	
Ethambutol	Amount too small to be harmful
Ethamsylate	Significant amount but not known to be harmful
Ethinyloestradiol *see* Contraceptives, Oral	
Ethosuximide	Avoid—significant amount in milk; hyperexcitability and poor suckling reported
Ethynodiol *see* Contraceptives, Oral	
Etidronate Disodium	No information available
Etodolac	Manufacturer advises avoid
Etoposide *see* Cytotoxic Drugs	
Etretinate	Avoid
Famciclovir	No information available
Famotidine	Amount too small to be harmful
Fansidar®	Small risk of kernicterus in jaundiced infants and of haemolysis in G6PD-deficient infants (due to sulfadoxine)
Fenbufen	Amount too small to be harmful
Fenoprofen	Amount too small to be harmful
Fentanyl	Manufacturer advises avoid
Fenticonazole	No information available
Filgrastim	No information available
Flavoxate	No information available

Table of drugs excreted in breast milk (*continued*)

Drug	Comment
Flecainide	Significant amount but not known to be harmful
Fluconazole	Significant amount—manufacturer advises avoid
Fludarabine *see* Cytotoxic Drugs	
Flunitrazepam *see* Benzodiazepines	
Fluoxetine	Significant amounts in milk reported—manufacturer advises avoid
Flupenthixol *see* Antipsychotics	
Fluphenazine *see* Antipsychotics	
Flurazepam *see* Benzodiazepines	
Flurbiprofen	Amount too small to be harmful
Fluticasone *see* Corticosteroids	
Fluvastatin	Manufacturer advises avoid
Fluvoxamine	Manufacturer advises avoid
Fosfomycin	Excreted in milk—manufacturer advises avoid unless real need
Fosinopril	Excreted in milk—manufacturer advises avoid
Frusemide	Amount too small to be harmful
Gabapentin	No information available
Ganciclovir	Avoid; *see also* p. 270
Gemcitabine *see* Cytotoxic Drugs	
Gemfibrozil	No information available
Gestodene *see* Contraceptives, Oral	
Glibenclamide *see* Sulphonylureas	
Gliclazide *see* Sulphonylureas	
Glipizide *see* Sulphonylureas	
Gliquidone *see* Sulphonylureas	
Glymidine *see* Sulphonylureas	
Gold (auranofin, aurothiomalate)	Caution—excreted in milk; theoretical possibility of rashes and idiosyncratic reactions
Goserelin	Manufacturer advises avoid
Granisetron	No information available
Growth Hormone *see* Somatropin	
Halofantrine	Avoid
Haloperidol *see* Antipsychotics	
Halothane	Excreted in milk
Hepatitis A Vaccine	No information available
Hydrochlorothiazide *see* Thiazides	
Hydrocortisone *see* Corticosteroids	
Hydroflumethiazide *see* Thiazides	
Hydroxychloroquine	Avoid—risk of toxicity in infant
Hydroxyzine *see* Antihistamines	
Hyoscine	Amount too small to be harmful
Ibuprofen	Amount too small to be harmful but some manufacturers advise avoid (including topical use)
Idarubicin *see* Cytotoxic Drugs	
Idoxuridine	May possibly make milk taste unpleasant
Imipenem [ingredient] *see* *Primaxin*®	
Imipramine *see* Antidepressants, Tricyclic	
Indapamide	No information available—manufacturer advises avoid

Drug	Comment
Indomethacin	Amount probably too small to be harmful but convulsions reported in one infant
Insulin	Amount too small to be harmful
Interferons	No information available
Iodine	Stop breast-feeding; danger of neonatal hypothyroidism or goitre; appears to be concentrated in milk
Radioactive iodine	Breast-feeding contra-indicated after therapeutic doses. With diagnostic doses withhold breast-feeding for at least 24 hours
Isoniazid	Monitor infant for possible toxicity; theoretical risk of convulsions and neuropathy; prophylactic pyridoxine advisable in mother and infant
Isotretinoin	Avoid
Itraconazole	Small amounts excreted in milk
Ketoprofen	Amount probably too small to be harmful but manufacturer advises avoid unless essential
Ketorolac	Avoid
Ketotifen *see* Antihistamines	
Labetalol *see* Beta-blockers	
Lamotrigine	No information available
Lansoprazole	No information available
Lenograstim	No information available
Levocabastine	Amount too small to be harmful
Levodopa	No information available
Levonorgestrel *see* Contraceptives, Oral	
Lignocaine	Amount too small to be harmful
Liothyronine	May interfere with neonatal screening for hypothyroidism
Lisinopril	No information available
Lithium salts	Monitor infant for possible intoxication; low incidence of adverse effects but increased by continuous ingestion; good control of maternal plasma concentrations minimises the risk
Lofepramine *see* Antidepressants, Tricyclic	
Loprazolam *see* Benzodiazepines	
Loratadine	Excreted in milk—manufacturer advises avoid
Lorazepam *see* Benzodiazepines	
Lormetazepam *see* Benzodiazepines	
Losartan	No information available
Lymecycline *see* Tetracyclines	
Lysuride	May suppress lactation
Maloprim®	Haemolytic anaemia (due to dapsone); risk to infant very small
Maprotiline *see* Antidepressants, Tricyclic (and related)	
Mebendazole	No information available
Mebeverine	Amount too small to be harmful
Medroxyprogesterone Acetate *see* Progestogens	
Mefenamic Acid	Amount too small to be harmful

Table of drugs excreted in breast milk (*continued*)

Drug	Comment
Mefloquine	Avoid—excreted in milk
Mefruside *see* Thiazides	
Meprobamate	Avoid; concentration in milk may exceed maternal plasma concentrations fourfold and may cause drowsiness in infant
Mequitazine *see* Antihistamines	
Meropenem	Manufacturer advises avoid unless potential benefit justifies potential risk
Mesalazine	Diarrhoea reported but manufacturers advise negligible amounts detected in breast milk
Mestranol *see* Contraceptives, Oral	
Methadone	Withdrawal symptoms in infant; breast-feeding permissible during maintenance but dose should be as low as possible and infant monitored to avoid sedation
Methotrimeprazine *see* Antipsychotics	
Methyldopa	Amount too small to be harmful
Methylphenidate	No information available—manufacturer advises avoid
Methylprednisolone *see* Corticosteroids	
Metoclopramide	Although amount in milk small, avoid unless essential
Metolazone *see* Thiazides	
Metoprolol *see* Beta-blockers	
Metronidazole	Significant amount in milk; manufacturer advises avoid large single doses
Mexiletine	Amount too small to be harmful
Mianserin *see* Antidepressants, Tricyclic (and related)	
Minocycline *see* Tetracyclines	
Minoxidil	Significant amount but not known to be harmful
Misoprostol	No information available—manufacturer advises avoid
Moclobemide	Amount too small to be harmful, but patient leaflet advises avoid
Moexipril	No information available—manufacturer advises avoid
Molgramostim	No information available—manufacturer advises avoid (potential for adverse effects in infant)
Moracizine	Excreted in milk—manufacturer advises avoid
Morphine	Therapeutic doses unlikely to affect infant; withdrawal symptoms in infants of dependent mothers; breast-feeding not best method of treating dependence in offspring and should be stopped
Moxonidine	Excreted in milk—manufacturer advises avoid
Mycophenolate Mofetil	No information available
Nadolol *see* Beta-blockers	
Nafarelin	No information available
Nalidixic Acid	Risk to infant very small but one case of haemolytic anaemia reported
Naloxone	No information available
Naproxen	Amount too small to be harmful
Nefazodone	No information available
Neostigmine	Amount probably too small to be harmful; monitor infant
Nicorandil	No information available—manufacturer advises avoid
Nicoumalone *see* Anticoagulants, Oral	
Nifedipine	Amount too small to be harmful but manufacturer advises avoid
Nitrazepam *see* Benzodiazepines	
Nitrofurantoin	Only small amounts in milk but could be enough to produce haemolysis in G6PD-deficient infants
Nizatidine	Amount too small to be harmful
Norethisterone *see* Contraceptives, Oral	
Norfloxacin	No information available—manufacturer advises avoid
Norgestimate *see* Contraceptives, Oral	
Nortriptyline *see* Antidepressants, Tricyclic	
NSAIDs *see* individual entries	
Nystatin	No information available, but absorption from gastro-intestinal tract negligible
Octreotide	Avoid
Oestrogens	Avoid; adverse effects on lactation; *see also* Contraceptives, Oral
Ofloxacin	Manufacturer advises avoid
Omeprazole	No information available
Opioid Analgesics *see* individual entries	
Orphenadrine	Excreted in milk—manufacturer advises avoid
Oxazepam *see* Benzodiazepines	
Oxitropium	No information available
Oxprenolol *see* Beta-blockers	
Oxypertine *see* Antipsychotics	
Oxytetracycline *see* Tetracyclines	
Pamidronate Disodium	Manufacturer advises avoid
Papaveretum *see* Morphine	
Paracetamol	Amount too small to be harmful
Paroxetine	Manufacturer advises avoid unless potential benefit outweighs possible risk
Penicillins	Trace amounts in milk
Pergolide	May suppress lactation
Pericyazine *see* Antipsychotics	
Perindopril	No information available
Perphenazine *see* Antipsychotics	
Phenindamine *see* Antihistamines	
Phenindione *see* Anticoagulants, Oral	
Pheniramine *see* Antihistamines	
Phenobarbitone	Avoid when possible; drowsiness may occur but risk probably small; one report of methaemoglobinaemia with phenobarbitone and phenytoin
Phenolphthalein	Avoid; increased gastric motility, diarrhoea, and possibly rash

Table of drugs excreted in breast milk (*continued*)

Drug	Comment
Phentolamine	No information available
Phenylbutazone	Avoid—small amounts in milk
Phenytoin	Small amount excreted in milk; manufacturer advises avoid—*but see* section 4.8.1
Pilocarpine	No information available—manufacturer advises avoid
Pimozide *see* Antipsychotics	
Pindolol *see* Beta-blockers	
Piracetam	Manufacturer advises avoid
Pirenzepine	Amount too small to be harmful
Piroxicam	Amount too small to be harmful
Pizotifen	Amount probably too small to be harmful, but patient information leaflet advises avoid
Polythiazide *see* Thiazides	
Povidone-iodine	Avoid; iodine absorbed from vaginal preparations is concentrated in milk
Pravastatin	Small amount excreted in milk—manufacturer advises avoid
Prazosin	Amount probably too small to be harmful
Prednisolone *see* Corticosteroids	
Prednisone *see* Corticosteroids	
Primaxin®	No information available—manufacturer advises avoid
Primidone *see* Phenobarbitone	
Prochlorperazine *see* Antipsychotics	
Procainamide	Excreted in milk—manufacturer advises avoid
Progestogens	High doses suppress lactation but *see also* Contraceptives, Oral
Proguanil *see* Chloroquine	
Promazine *see* Antipsychotics	
Promethazine *see* Antihistamines	
Propafenone	No information available—manufacturer advises avoid
Propranolol *see* Beta-blockers	
Propylthiouracil	Monitor infant's thyroid status but amounts in milk probably too small to affect infant; high doses might affect neonatal thyroid function
Protriptyline *see* Antidepressants, Tricyclic	
Pseudoephedrine	Amount too small to be harmful
Pyrazinamide	Amount too small to be harmful
Pyridostigmine	Amount probably too small to be harmful
Pyrimethamine	Significant amount—avoid administration of other folate antagonists to infant
Quinagolide	Suppresses lactation
Quinalbarbitone *see* Barbiturates	
Quinapril	No information available
Quinidine	Significant amount but not known to be harmful
Raltitrexed *see* Cytotoxic Drugs	
Ramipril	Manufacturer advises avoid
Ranitidine	Significant amount but not known to be harmful

Drug	Comment
Ranitidine Bismuth Citrate	No information available—manufacturer advises avoid
Rifabutin	No information available
Rifampicin	Amount too small to be harmful
Risperidone *see* Antipsychotics	
Senna *see* Anthraquinones	
Sertraline	No information available
Simvastatin	No information available—manufacturer advises avoid
Sodium Clodronate	No information available
Sodium Cromoglycate *see* Cromoglycate	
Sodium Valproate *see* Valproate	
Somatropin	No information available
Sotalol *see* Beta-blockers	
Sulfametopyrazine *see* Sulphonamides	
Sulindac	Manufacturer advises avoid
Sulphadiazine *see* Sulphonamides	
Sulphadimidine *see* Sulphonamides	
Sulphasalazine	Small amounts in milk (1 report of bloody diarrhoea and rashes); theoretical risk of neonatal haemolysis especially in G6PD-deficient infants
Sulphinpyrazone	No information available
Sulphonamides	Small risk of kernicterus in jaundiced infants particularly with long-acting sulphonamides, and of haemolysis in G6PD-deficient infants
Sulphonylureas	Caution; theoretical possibility of hypoglycaemia in infant
Sulpiride	Best avoided; significant amounts in milk; *see also* Antipsychotics
Sumatriptan	No information available
Tacrolimus	Avoid—excreted in milk
Tamoxifen	No information available—manufacturer advises avoid
Teicoplanin	No information available
Temazepam *see* Benzodiazepines	
Tenoxicam	No information available
Terbinafine	Excreted in milk— manufacturer advises avoid
Terbutaline	Amount too small to be harmful
Terfenadine *see* Antihistamines	
Tetracyclines	Avoid (although absorption and therefore discoloration of teeth in infant probably prevented by chelation with calcium in milk)
Theophylline	Irritability in infant reported; modified-release preparations probably safe
Thiamine	Severely thiamine-deficient mothers should avoid breast-feeding as toxic methylglyoxal excreted in milk
Thiazides	Amount too small to be harmful; large doses may suppress lactation
Thioridazine *see* Antipsychotics	
Thyroxine	May interfere with neonatal screening for hypothyroidism

Table of drugs excreted in breast milk (*continued*)

Drug	Comment
Tiaprofenic Acid	Amount too small to be harmful
<u>Tiludronic Acid</u>	No information available
Timolol *see* Beta-blockers	
Tolazamide *see* Sulphonylureas	
Tolbutamide *see* Sulphonylureas	
Tolmetin	Amount too small to be harmful
Topiramate	Manufacturer advises avoid
Torasemide	No information available
Tramadol	Amount probably too small to be harmful, but manufacturer advises avoid
Trandolapril	Manufacturer advises avoid
Trazodone as for Antidepressants, Tricyclic	
Tretinoin	No information available
Triamcinolone *see* Corticosteroids	
Trifluoperazine *see* Antipsychotics	
Trimeprazine *see* Antihistamines	
Trimethoprim	Excreted in milk—short-term use not known to be harmful
Trimipramine *see* Antidepressants, Tricyclic	
Triprolidine *see* Antihistamines	
Tropisetron	No information available
Tulobuterol	No information available
Valaciclovir	No information available; *see also* Aciclovir

Drug	Comment
Valproate	Amount too small to be harmful
Vancomycin	Excreted in milk—manufacturer advises avoid
Venlafaxine	No information available
Verapamil	Amount too small to be harmful
Vigabatrin	No information available—manufacturer advises avoid
Viloxazine *see* Antidepressants, Tricyclic (and related)	
Vitamin A	Theoretical risk of toxicity in infants of mothers taking large doses
Vitamin D (and related compounds)	Caution with high doses; may cause hypercalcaemia in infant
Warfarin *see* Anticoagulants, Oral	
Xipamide	No information available
Zalcitabine	No information available
Zidovudine	No information available
Zolpidem	Small amounts excreted in milk—manufacturer advises avoid
Zopiclone	Excreted in milk—manufacturer advises avoid
Zuclopenthixol *see* Antipsychotics	

Appendix 6: Intravenous Additives

INTRAVENOUS ADDITIVES POLICIES. A local policy on the addition of drugs to intravenous fluids should be drawn up by a multi-disciplinary team in each Health Authority and issued as a document to the members of staff concerned.

Centralised additive services are provided in a number of hospital pharmacy departments and should be used in preference to making additions on wards.

The information that follows should be read in conjunction with local policy documents.

Guidelines

1. Drugs should only be added to infusion containers when constant plasma concentrations are needed or when the administration of a more concentrated solution would be harmful.

2. In general, only one drug should be added to any infusion container and the components should be compatible. Ready-prepared solutions should be used whenever possible. Drugs should not normally be added to blood products, mannitol, or sodium bicarbonate. Only specially formulated additives should be used with fat emulsions or amino-acid solutions (see section 9.3).

3. Solutions should be thoroughly mixed by shaking and checked for absence of particulate matter before use.

4. Strict asepsis should be maintained throughout and in general the giving set should not be used for more than 24 hours.

5. The infusion container should be labelled with the patient's name, the name and quantity of additives, and the date and time of addition (and the new expiry date or time). Such additional labelling should not interfere with information on the manufacturer's label that is still valid. When possible, containers should be retained for a period after use in case they are needed for investigation.

6. It is good practice to examine intravenous infusions from time to time while they are running. If cloudiness, crystallisation, change of colour, or any other sign of interaction or contamination is observed the infusion should be discontinued.

Problems

MICROBIAL CONTAMINATION. The accidental entry and subsequent growth of micro-organisms converts the infusion fluid pathway into a potential vehicle for infection with micro-organisms, particularly species of Candida, Enterobacter, and Klebsiella. Ready-prepared infusions containing the additional drugs, or infusions prepared by an additive service (when available) should therefore be used in preference to making extemporaneous additions to infusion containers on wards etc. However, when this is necessary strict aseptic procedure should be followed.

INCOMPATIBILITY. Physical and chemical incompatibilities may occur with loss of potency, increase in toxicity, or other adverse effect. The solutions may become opalescent or precipitation may occur, but in many instances there is no visual indication of incompatibility. Interaction may take place at any point in the infusion fluid pathway, and the potential for incompatibility is increased when more than one substance is added to the infusion fluid.

Common incompatibilities. Precipitation reactions are numerous and varied and may occur as a result of pH, concentration changes, 'salting-out' effects, complexation or other chemical changes. Precipitation or other particle formation must be avoided since, apart from lack of control of dosage on administration, it may initiate or exacerbate adverse effects. This is particularly important in the case of drugs which have been implicated in either thrombophlebitis (e.g. diazepam) or in skin sloughing or necrosis caused by extravasation (e.g. sodium bicarbonate and certain cytotoxic drugs). It is also especially important to effect solution of colloidal drugs and to prevent their subsequent precipitation in order to avoid a pyrogenic reaction (e.g. amphotericin).

It is considered undesirable to mix beta-lactam antibiotics, such as semi-synthetic penicillins and cephalosporins, with proteinaceous materials on the grounds that immunogenic and allergenic conjugates could be formed.

A number of preparations undergo significant loss of potency when added singly or in combination to large volume infusions. Examples include ampicillin in infusions that contain glucose or lactates, mustine hydrochloride in isotonic saline and gentamicin/carbenicillin combinations. The breakdown products of dacarbazine have been implicated in adverse effects.

Blood. Because of the large number of incompatibilities, drugs should not normally be added to blood and blood products for infusion purposes. Examples of incompatibility with blood include hypertonic mannitol solutions (irreversible crenation of red cells), dextrans (rouleaux formation and interference with cross-matching), glucose (clumping of red cells), and oxytocin (inactivated).

If the giving set is not changed after the administration of blood, but used for other infusion fluids, a fibrin clot may form which, apart from blocking the set, increases the likelihood of microbial growth.

Intravenous fat emulsions may break down with coalescence of fat globules and separation of phases when additions such as antibiotics or electrolytes are made, thus increasing the possibility of embolism. Only specially formulated products such as Vitlipid N® (see section 9.3) may be added to appropriate intravenous fat emulsions.

Other infusions that frequently give rise to incompatibility include amino acids, mannitol, and sodium bicarbonate.

Bactericides such as chlorocresol 0.1% or phenylmercuric nitrate 0.001% are present in some injection solutions. The total volume of such soluions added to a container for infusion on one occasion should not exceed 15 mL.

Method

Ready-prepared infusions should be used whenever available. **Potassium chloride** is usually available in concentrations of 20, 27, and 40 mmol/litre in sodium chloride intravenous infusion (0.9%), glucose intravenous infusion (5%) or sodium chloride and glucose intravenous infusion. **Lignocaine hydrochloride** is usually available in concentrations of 0.1 or 0.2% in glucose intravenous infusion (5%).

When addition is required to be made extemporaneously, any product reconstitution instructions such as those relating to concentration, vehicle, mixing, and handling precautions should be strictly followed using an aseptic technique throughout. Once the product has been reconstituted, addition to the infusion fluid should be made immediately in order to minimise microbial contamination and, with certain products, to prevent degradation or other formulation change which may occur; e.g. reconstituted ampicillin injection degrades rapidly on standing, and also may form polymers which could cause sensitivity reactions.

It is also important in certain instances that an infusion fluid of specific pH be used (e.g. **frusemide** injection requires dilution in infusions of pH greater than 5.5).

When drug additions are made it is important to mix thoroughly; additions should not be made to an infusion container that has been connected to a giving set, as mixing is hampered. If the solutions are not thoroughly mixed a concentrated layer of the additive may form owing to differences in density. **Potassium chloride** is particularly prone to this 'layering' effect when added without adequate mixing to infusions packed in non-rigid infusion containers; if such a mixture is administered it may have a serious effect on the heart.

A time limit between addition and completion of administration must be imposed for certain admixtures to guarantee satisfactory drug potency and compatibility. For admixtures in which degradation occurs without the formation of toxic substances, an acceptable limit is the time taken for 10% decomposition of the drug. When toxic substances are produced stricter limits may be imposed. Because of the risk of microbial contamination a maximum time limit of 12 hours should be imposed for additions made elsewhere than in hospital pharmacies offering central additive service.

Certain injections must be protected from light during continuous infusion to minimise oxidation, e.g. amphotericin, dacarbazine, and sodium nitroprusside.

Dilution with a small volume of an appropriate vehicle and administration using a motorised infusion pump is advocated for preparations such as heparin where strict control over administration is required. In this case the appropriate dose may be dissolved in a convenient volume (e.g. 24 to 48 mL) of sodium chloride intravenous infusion (0.9%).

Use of table

The table lists preparations given by three methods:
continuous infusion,
intermittent infusion, and
addition via the drip tubing.

Drugs for **continuous infusion** must be diluted in a large volume infusion. Penicillins and cephalosporins are not usually given by continuous infusion because of stability problems and because adequate plasma and tissue concentrations are best obtained by intermittent infusion. Where it is necessary to administer them by continuous infusion, detailed literature should be consulted.

Drugs that are both compatible and clinically suitable may be given by **intermittent infusion** in a relatively small volume of infusion over a short period of time, e.g. 100 mL in 30 minutes. The method is used if the product is incompatible or unstable over the period necessary for continuous infusion; the limited stability of ampicillin or amoxycillin in large volume glucose or lactate infusions may be overcome in this way.

Intermittent infusion is also used if adequate plasma and tissue concentrations are not produced by continuous infusion as in the case of drugs such as carbenicillin, dacarbazine, gentamicin, and ticarcillin.

An in-line burette may be used for intermittent infusion techniques in order to achieve strict control over the time and rate of administration, especially for infants and children and in intensive care units. Intermittent infusion may also make use of the 'piggy-back' technique provided that no additions are made to the primary infusion. In this method the drug is added to a small secondary container connected to a Y-type injection site on the primary infusion giving set; the secondary solution is usually infused within 30 minutes.

Addition *via* the drip tubing is indicated for a number of cytotoxic drugs in order to minimise extravasation. The preparation is added aseptically *via* the rubber septum of the injection site of a fast-running infusion. In general, drug preparations intended for a bolus effect should be given directly into a separate vein where possible. Failing this, administration may be made *via* the drip tubing provided that the preparation is compatible with the infusion fluid when given in this manner.

Table of drugs given by intravenous infusion

Covers addition to Glucose 5 and 10%, Sodium chloride 0.9%, Compound sodium chloride (Ringer's solution), and Compound sodium lactate (Hartmann's solution). Compatibility with glucose 5% and with sodium chloride 0.9% indicates compatibility with any strength of sodium chloride and glucose infusion. Infusion of a large volume of hypotonic solution should be avoided therefore care should be taken if water for injections is used. The information in the Table relates to the proprietary preparations indicated; for other preparations suitability should be checked with the manufacturer

Abciximab (ReoPro®)
Continuous in Glucose 5% or Sodium chloride 0.9%
Withdraw from vial (through a non-pyrogenic low protein-binding 0.2 or 0.22 micron filter), dilute in infusion fluid and give via infusion pump through a non-pyrogenic low protein-binding 0.2 or 0.22 micron filter

Acetylcysteine (Parvolex®)
Continuous in Glucose 5%
See Emergency Treatment of Poisoning

Aclarubicin hydrochloride (Aclacin®)
Intermittent in Glucose 5% or Sodium chloride 0.9%
Dissolve initially in 10 mL water for injections or sodium chloride 0.9% then dilute with 200–500 mL infusion fluid to a concentration of 200–500 micrograms/mL; give over 30–60 minutes and protect from light during administration; pH of glucose infusion should be between 5 and 6

Aciclovir sodium (Zovirax IV®)
Intermittent in Sodium chloride 0.9% or Sodium chloride and glucose or Compound sodium lactate
Initially reconstitute to 25 mg/mL in water for injections or sodium chloride 0.9% then dilute to not more than 5 mg/mL with the infusion fluid; minimum volume 50 mL; to be given over 1 hour; alternatively, may be administered in a concentration of 25 mg/mL using a suitable infusion pump and given over 1 hour

Aldesleukin (Proleukin®)
Continuous in Glucose 5%
Reconstitute each vial with 1.2 mL water for injections (do not shake or allow to foam); dilute in up to 500 mL glucose 5% containing albumin 0.1% (albumin added and thoroughly mixed in glucose 5% solution before adding aldesleukin); polypropylene, PVC, polyolefin, or glass containers with polyethylene or PVC giving sets may be used; do not use in-line filter

Alfentanil hydrochloride (Rapifen® preparations)
Continuous or intermittent in Glucose 5% or Sodium chloride 0.9% or Compound sodium lactate

Alprostadil (Prostin VR®)
Continuous in Glucose 5% or Sodium chloride 0.9%
Add directly to the infusion solution avoiding contact with the walls of plastic containers

Alteplase (Actilyse®)
Continuous or intermittent in Sodium chloride 0.9%
Dissolve in water for injections to a concentration of 1 mg/mL and infuse intravenously; alternatively dilute the solution further in the infusion fluid to a concentration of not less than 200 micrograms/mL; not to be infused in glucose solution

Amikacin sulphate (Amikin®)
Intermittent in Glucose 5% or Sodium chloride 0.9% or Compound sodium lactate
To be given over 30 minutes

Aminophylline
Continuous in Glucose 5% or Sodium chloride 0.9% or Compound sodium lactate

Amiodarone hydrochloride (Cordarone X®)
Continuous or intermittent in Glucose 5%
Suggested initial infusion volume 250 mL given over 20–120 minutes; for repeat infusions up to 1.2 g in max. 500 mL; infusion in extreme emergency see section 2.3.2; should not be diluted to less than 600 micrograms/mL; incompatible with sodium chloride infusion

Amoxycillin sodium (Amoxil®)
Intermittent in Glucose 5% or Sodium chloride 0.9%
Reconstituted solutions diluted and given without delay; suggested volume 100 mL given over 30–60 minutes
via drip tubing in Glucose 5% or Sodium chloride 0.9% or Ringer's solution or Compound sodium lactate
Continuous infusion not usually recommended

Amphotericin (colloidal) (Amphocil®)
Intermittent in Glucose 5%
Initially reconstitute with water for injections (50 mg in 10 mL, 100 mg in 20 mL), shaking gently to dissolve (fluid may be opalescent) then dilute to a concentration of 625 micrograms/mL (1 volume of reconstituted solution with 7 volumes of infusion fluid); give at a rate of 1–2 mg/kg/hour (or slower if not tolerated); incompatible with sodium chloride or other electrolyte solutions, flush existing intravenous line with glucose 5% or use separate line

Amphotericin (liposomal) (Abelcet®)
Intermittent in Glucose 5%
Allow suspension to reach room temperature, shake gently to ensure no yellow settlement, withdraw requisite dose (using 17–19 gauge needle) into one or more 20-mL syringes; replace needle on syringe with a 5-micron filter needle provided (fresh needle for each syringe) and dilute to a concentration of 1 mg/mL; preferably give via an infusion pump at a rate of 2.5 mg/kg/hour (initial test dose of 1 mg given over 15 minutes); an in-line filter (pore size no less than 5 micron) may be used; do not use sodium chloride or other electrolyte solutions, flush existing intravenous line with glucose 5% or use separate line

Amphotericin (liposomal) (AmBisome®)
Intermittent in Glucose 5%
Reconstitute each vial with 12 mL water for injections and shake vigorously to produce a preparation containing 4 mg/mL; withdraw requisite dose from vial and introduce into infusion fluid through the 5 micron filter provided to produce a final concentration of 0.2–2 mg/mL; infuse over 30–60 minutes; incompatible with sodium chloride solutions, flush existing intravenous line with glucose 5% or use separate line

Amphotericin sodium deoxycholate complex (Fungizone®)
Continuous in Glucose 5%
Dissolve thoroughly at reconstitution stage; preparation must be diluted in a large volume infusion; pH of the glucose must not be below 4.2 (check each container); protect from light; suggested infusion time 6 hours

Ampicillin sodium (*Penbritin®*)
Intermittent *in* Glucose 5% *or* Sodium chloride 0.9%
Reconstituted solutions diluted and given without delay;
suggested volume 100 mL given over 30–60 minutes
via drip tubing *in* Glucose 5% *or* Sodium chloride
0.9% *or* Ringer's solution *or* Compound sodium lactate
Continuous infusion not usually recommended

Ampicillin/cloxacillin (sodium salts)
(*Ampiclox®*)
Intermittent *in* Glucose 5% *or* Sodium chloride 0.9%
Reconstituted solutions diluted and given without delay;
suggested volume 100 mL given over 30–60 minutes
via drip tubing *in* Glucose 5% *or* Sodium chloride
0.9% *or* Ringer's solution *or* Compound sodium lactate

Amsacrine (*Amsidine®*)
Intermittent *in* Glucose 5%
Reconstitute with diluent provided and dilute to suggested volume 500 mL; give over 60–90 minutes; use glass syringes; incompatible with sodium chloride infusion

Atenolol (*Tenormin®*)
Intermittent *in* Glucose 5% *or* Sodium chloride 0.9%
Suggested infusion time 20 minutes

Atracurium besylate (*Tracrium®*)
Continuous *in* Glucose 5% *or* Sodium chloride 0.9% *or* Compound sodium lactate
Stability varies with diluent

Azathioprine (sodium salt) (*Imuran®*)
via drip tubing *in* Glucose 5% *or* Sodium chloride 0.9%

Azlocillin sodium (*Securopen® 5 g*)
Intermittent *in* Glucose 5 and 10% *or* Sodium chloride 0.9% *or* Ringer's solution
Intermittent infusion suggested for doses over 2 g; to be given over 20–30 minutes

Aztreonam (*Azactam®*)
Intermittent *in* Glucose 5% *or* Sodium chloride 0.9% *or* Ringer's solution *or* Compound sodium lactate
Dissolve initially in water for injections (1 g per 3 mL) then dilute to a concentration of less than 20 mg/mL; to be given over 20–60 minutes

Benzylpenicillin sodium (*Crystapen®*)
Intermittent *in* Glucose 5% *or* Sodium chloride 0.9%
Suggested volume 100 mL given over 30–60 minutes
Continuous infusion not usually recommended

Betamethasone sodium phosphate (*Betnesol®*)
Continuous *or* intermittent *or via* drip tubing *in* Glucose 5% *or* Sodium chloride 0.9%

Bleomycin sulphate Intermittent *in* Sodium chloride 0.9%
To be given slowly; suggested volume 200 mL

Bumetanide (*Burinex®*)
Intermittent *in* Glucose 5% *or* Sodium chloride 0.9%
Suggested volume 500 mL given over 30–60 minutes

Calcium folinate (*Calcium Leucovorin®*, *Refolinon®*)
Continuous *in* Sodium chloride 0.9%
Calcium Leucovorin® can also be infused in Glucose 5 and 10% or Compound sodium lactate

Calcium gluconate
Continuous *in* Glucose 5% *or* Sodium chloride 0.9%
Avoid bicarbonates, phosphates, or sulphates

Carbenicillin sodium (*Pyopen®*)
Intermittent *in* Glucose 5% *or* Water for injections
Suggested volume 100 mL given over 30–40 minutes

Carboplatin (*Paraplatin®*)
Continuous *in* Glucose 5% *or* Sodium chloride 0.9%
Final concentration as low as 500 micrograms/mL; give over 15–60 minutes

Carmustine (*BiCNU®*)
Intermittent *in* Glucose 5% *or* Sodium chloride 0.9%
Reconstitute with diluent provided; give over 1–2 hours

Cefodizime sodium (*Timecef®*)
Intermittent *in* Glucose 5% *or* Sodium chloride 0.9% *or* Ringer's solution *or* Compound sodium lactate *or* Water for injections
Dissolve in 40 mL infusion fluid and give over up to 30 minutes

Cefotaxime sodium (*Claforan®*)
Intermittent *in* Glucose 5% *or* Sodium chloride 0.9% *or* Compound sodium lactate *or* Water for injections
Suggested volume 40–100 mL given over 20–60 minutes

Cefoxitin sodium (*Mefoxin®*)
Intermittent *or via* drip tubing *in* Glucose 5 and 10% *or* Sodium chloride 0.9%
Continuous infusion not usually recommended

Ceftazidime pentahydrate (*Fortum®*, *Kefadim®*)
Intermittent *or via* drip tubing *in* Glucose 5 and 10% *or* Sodium chloride 0.9% *or* Compound sodium lactate
Dissolve 2 g initially in 10 mL (3 g in 15 mL) infusion fluid; for *Fortum®* dilute further to a concentration of 40 mg/mL; for *Kefadim®* dilute further to a concentration of 20 mg/mL; give over up to 30 minutes

Ceftizoxime sodium (*Cefizox®*)
Continuous *or* intermittent *or via* drip tubing *in* Glucose 5 and 10% *or* Sodium chloride 0.9% *or* Ringer's solution *or* Compound sodium lactate
Suggested volume 50–100 mL

Ceftriaxone (sodium salt) (*Rocephin®*)
Intermittent *or via* drip tubing *in* Glucose 5 and 10% *or* Sodium chloride 0.9%
Give intermittent infusion of 2 g (50 mg/kg or more for children) over at least 30 minutes; not to be given with infusion fluids containing calcium

Cefuroxime sodium (*Zinacef®*)
Intermittent *or via* drip tubing *in* Glucose 5% *or* Sodium chloride 0.9% *or* Compound sodium lactate
Dissolve initially in water for injections (at least 2 mL for each 250 mg, 15 mL for 1.5 g); suggested volume 50–100 mL given over 30 minutes

Cephamandole nafate (*Kefadol®*)
Intermittent *or via* drip tubing *in* Glucose 5 and 10% *or* Sodium chloride 0.9%
Continuous infusion not usually recommended

Cephazolin sodium (*Kefzol®*)
Intermittent *or via* drip tubing *in* Glucose 5 and 10% *or* Sodium chloride 0.9% *or* Compound sodium lactate
Continuous infusion not usually recommended

Cephradine (*Velosef®*)
Continuous *or* intermittent *in* Glucose 5 and 10% *or* Sodium chloride 0.9% *or* Ringer's solution *or* Compound sodium lactate

Chloramphenicol sodium succinate (*Kemicetine®*)
Intermittent *or via* drip tubing *in* Glucose 5% *or* Sodium chloride 0.9%

Chloroquine sulphate (*Nivaquine®*)
Continuous *in* Sodium chloride 0.9%
   See also section 5.4.1

Cimetidine (*Tagamet®*)
Continuous *or* intermittent *in* Glucose 5% *or* Sodium chloride 0.9%
   For intermittent infusion suggested volume 100 mL given over 30–60 minutes

Cisatracurium (*Nimbex®, Nimbex Forte®*)
Continuous *in* Glucose 5% *or* Sodium chloride 0.9%
   Solutions of 2 mg/mL and 5 mg/mL may be infused undiluted; alternatively dilute with infusion fluid to a concentration of 0.1–2 mg/mL

Cisplatin *Cisplatin* (Lederle), *Cisplatin powder for injection* (Lederle)
Continuous *in* Sodium chloride 0.9% *or* Sodium chloride and glucose
   Reconstitute cisplatin powder for injection with water for injections (10 mg in 10 mL, 50 mg in 50 mL); suggested volume 2 litres given over 6–8 hours

Cladribine (*Leustat®*)
Continuous *in* Sodium chloride 0.9%
   Dilute with 100–500 mL and give over 24 hours; glucose solutions are unsuitable

Clarithromycin (*Klaricid® I.V.*)
Intermittent *in* Glucose 5% *or* Sodium chloride 0.9% *or* Ringer's solution *or* Compound sodium lactate
   Dissolve initially in water for injections (500 mg in 10 mL) then dilute to a concentration of 2 mg/mL; give over 60 minutes

Clindamycin phosphate (*Dalacin C®*)
Continuous *or* intermittent *in* Glucose 5% *or* Sodium chloride 0.9%
   Dilute to a concentration of 300 mg in 50 mL; give each 300 mg over at least 10 minutes (1.2 g over at least 45 minutes)

Clomipramine hydrochloride (*Anafranil®*)
Intermittent *in* Glucose 5% *or* Sodium chloride 0.9%
   See data sheet for details of initial dose to test tolerance; suggested volume 125–500 mL given over 45–180 minutes

Clonazepam (*Rivotril®*)
Intermittent *in* Glucose 5 and 10% *or* Sodium chloride 0.9%
   Suggested volume 250 mL

Cloxacillin sodium (*Orbenin®*)
Intermittent *in* Glucose 5% *or* Sodium chloride 0.9%
   Suggested volume 100 mL given over 30–60 minutes
via drip tubing *in* Glucose 5% *or* Sodium chloride 0.9% *or* Ringer's solution *or* Compound sodium lactate
   Continuous infusion not usually recommended

Co-amoxiclav (*Augmentin®*)
Intermittent *in* Sodium chloride 0.9% *or* Water for injections; see also package leaflet
   Suggested volume 50–100 mL given over 30–40 minutes and completed within 4 hours of reconstitution
via drip tubing *in* Glucose 5% *or* Sodium chloride 0.9%

Co-fluampicil (sodium salts) (*Magnapen®*)
Intermittent *in* Glucose 5% *or* Sodium chloride 0.9%
   Reconstituted solutions diluted and given without delay; suggested volume 100 mL given over 30–60 minutes
via drip tubing *in* Glucose 5% *or* Sodium chloride 0.9% *or* Ringer's solution *or* Compound sodium lactate

Colistin sulphomethate sodium (*Colomycin®*)
Continuous *or* intermittent *in* Glucose 5% *or* Sodium chloride 0.9% *or* Ringer's solution
   Max. 6 hours between addition and completion of administration

Co-trimoxazole (*Septrin® for infusion*)
Intermittent *in* Glucose 5 and 10% *or* Sodium chloride 0.9% *or* Ringer's solution
   Dilute contents of 1 ampoule (5 mL) to 125 mL, 2 ampoules (10 mL) to 250 mL or 3 ampoules (15 mL) to 500 mL; suggested duration of infusion 90 minutes (but may be adjusted according to fluid requirements); if fluid restriction necessary, 1 ampoule may be diluted with 75 mL glucose 5%

Cyclophosphamide (*Endoxana®*)
Intermittent *or via* drip tubing *in* Glucose 5% *or* Sodium chloride 0.9% *or* Water for injections
   For intermittent infusion suggested volume 50–100 mL given over 5–15 minutes
via drip tubing in Glucose 5%

Cyclosporin (*Sandimmun®*)
Continuous *in* Glucose 5% *or* Sodium chloride 0.9%
   Dilute to a concentration of 50 mg in 20–100 mL; give over 2–6 hours; not to be used with PVC equipment

Cytarabine (*Alexan®, Cytosar®*)
Continuous *or* intermittent *or via* drip tubing *in* Glucose 5% *or* Sodium chloride 0.9%
   Reconstitute *Cytosar®* with the diluent provided; check container for haze or precipitate during administration

Dacarbazine (*DTIC-Dome®*)
Intermittent *in* Glucose 5% *or* Sodium chloride 0.9%
   Suggested volume 125–250 mL given over 15–30 minutes; protect infusion from light

Dactinomycin (*Cosmegen Lyovac®*)
Intermittent *or via* drip tubing *in* Glucose 5% *or* Sodium chloride 0.9%
   Reconstitute with water for injections

Daunorubicin (liposomal) (*DaunoXome®*)
Intermittent *in* Glucose 5%
   Dilute to a concentration of 0.2–1 mg/mL; give over 30–60 minutes; incompatible with sodium chloride solutions; in-line filter not recommended (if used, pore size should be no less than 5 micron)

Desferrioxamine mesylate (*Desferal®*)
Continuous *or* intermittent *in* Glucose 5% *or* Sodium chloride 0.9%
   Dissolve initially in water for injections (500 mg in 5 mL) then dilute with infusion fluid

esmopressin (*DDAVP®*)
termittent *in* Sodium chloride 0.9%
Dilute with 50 mL and give over 20 minutes

examethasone sodium phosphate
Decadron®; *Dexamethasone*, Organon)
ontinuous *or* intermittent *or* via drip tubing *in* Glu-
se 5% *or* Sodium chloride 0.9%
Dexamethasone (Organon) can also be infused in
Ringer's solution *or* Compound sodium lactate

iamorphine hydrochloride (*Diamorphine Injec-
n*, CP)
ontinuous *in* Glucose 5% *or* Sodium chloride 0.9%
Glucose is preferred as infusion fluid

iazepam (solution) (*Valium®*)
ontinuous *in* Glucose 5% *or* Sodium chloride 0.9%
Dilute to a concentration of not more than 40 mg in
500 mL; max. 6 hours between addition and completion
of administration; adsorbed to some extent by the plastics of the infusion set

iazepam (emulsion) (*Diazemuls®*)
ontinuous *in* Glucose 5 and 10%
May be diluted to a max. concentration of 200 mg in
500 mL; max. 6 hours between addition and completion
of administration; adsorbed to some extent by the plastics of the infusion set
a drip tubing *in* Glucose 5 and 10% *or* Sodium chlor-
e 0.9%
Adsorbed to some extent by the plastics of the infusion
set

iclofenac sodium (*Voltarol®*)
ontinuous *or* intermittent *in* Glucose 5% *or* Sodium
iloride 0.9%
Dilute 75 mg with 100–500 mL infusion fluid (previously buffered with 0.5 mL sodium bicarbonate 8.4%
solution *or* with 1 mL sodium bicarbonate 4.2% solution); for intermittent infusion give over 30–120 minutes

igoxin (*Lanoxin®*)
ontinuous *in* Glucose 5% *or* Sodium chloride 0.9%
To be given slowly; see also section 2.1.1

igoxin-specific antibody fragments
Digibind®)
termittent *in* Sodium chloride 0.9%
Dissolve initially in water for injections (4 mL/vial) then
dilute with the sodium chloride 0.9% and give through a
0.22 micron sterile, disposable filter over 30 minutes

inoprostone (*Prostin E2®*)
ontinuous *or* intermittent *in* Glucose 5% *or* Sodium
iloride 0.9%

isodium etidronate (*Didronel IV®*)
ontinuous *in* Sodium chloride 0.9%
Dilute in large-volume infusion, suggested minimum
volume 250 mL; minimum period of infusion 2 hours

isodium pamidronate (*Aredia®*)
ontinuous *in* Sodium chloride 0.9%
Reconstitute initially with water for injections (15 mg in
5 mL, 30 mg or 90 mg in 10 mL); dilute with infusion
fluid to a concentration of not more than 60 mg in
250 mL; give at a rate not exceeding 1 mg/minute; not to
be given with infusion fluids containing calcium

Disopyramide phosphate (*Rythmodan®*)
Continuous *or* intermittent *in* Glucose 5% *or* Sodium
chloride 0.9% *or* Ringer's solution *or* Compound sodium lactate
Max. rate by continuous infusion 20–30 mg/hour (or
400 micrograms/kg/hour)

Dobutamine hydrochloride (*Dobutrex®*, *Posiject®*)
Continuous *in* Glucose 5% *or* Sodium chloride 0.9%
Dilute to a concentration of 0.5–1 mg/mL and give via a
controlled infusion device; give higher concentration
(max. 5 mg/mL) with infusion pump; incompatible with
bicarbonate

Docetaxel (*Taxotere®*)
Intermittent *in* Glucose 5% *or* Sodium chloride 0.9%
Stand docetaxel vials and solvent at room temperature
for 5 minutes; add solvent to produce a concentrate containing 10 mg/mL; dilute the requisite dose with 250 mL
infusion fluid to a final concentration of 300–
900 micrograms/mL; infuse over 1 hour

Dopamine hydrochloride (*Intropin®*)
Continuous *in* Glucose 5% *or* Sodium chloride 0.9% *or*
Compound sodium lactate
Dilute to a concentration of 1.6 mg/mL; incompatible
with bicarbonate

Dopexamine hydrochloride (*Dopacard®*)
Continuous *in* Glucose 5% *or* Sodium chloride 0.9%
Dilute to a concentration of 400 or 800 micrograms/mL;
give via infusion pump or other device which provides
accurate control of rate; contact with metal should be
minimised; incompatible with bicarbonate

Doxorubicin hydrochloride (*Doxorubicin Rapid
Dissolution, Doxorubicin Solution*) (both Pharmacia)
via drip tubing *in* Glucose 5% *or* Sodium chloride
0.9%
Reconstitute *Doxorubicin Rapid Dissolution* with water
for injections or sodium chloride 0.9% (10 mg in 5 mL,
50 mg in 25 mL); give over 2–3 minutes

Electrolytes (*Addiphos®*)
Continuous *in* Glucose 5 and 10%
Suggested volume 500 mL

Enoximone (*Perfan®*)
Continuous *or* intermittent *in* Sodium chloride 0.9% *or*
Water for injections
Dilute to a concentration of 2.5 mg/mL; incompatible
with glucose solutions; use only plastic containers or
syringes

Epirubicin hydrochloride (*Pharmorubicin® Rapid
Dissolution, Pharmorubicin® Solution*)
via drip tubing *in* Sodium chloride 0.9%
Reconstitute *Pharmorubicin® Rapid Dissolution* with
sodium chloride 0.9% or with water for injections
(10 mg in 5 mL, 20 mg in 10 mL, 50 mg in 25 mL); give
over 3–5 minutes

Epoetin beta (*Recormon®*)
Intermittent *in* Sodium chloride 0.9%
Reconstitute with water for injections provided and
dilute in at least 100 mL infusion fluid; complete administration within 2 hours of preparation; avoid glass, use
only plastic materials for infusion

Epoprostenol (*Flolan®*)
Continuous *in* Sodium chloride 0.9%
Reconstitute with the diluent provided (pH 10.5) to
make a concentrate; use this concentrate within 12 hours
and store at 2–8°C; dilute with not more than 6 times the
volume of sodium chloride 0.9% before use

Erythromycin lactobionate
Continuous *or* intermittent *in* Glucose 5% (neutralised with sodium bicarbonate) *or* Sodium chloride 0.9%
> Dissolve initially in water for injections (1 g in 20 mL) then dilute to a concentration of 1 mg/mL for continuous infusion and 1–5 mg/mL for intermittent infusion

Esmolol hydrochloride (*Brevibloc*®)
Continuous *or* intermittent *in* Glucose 5% *or* Sodium chloride 0.9%
> Dilute to a concentration of 10 mg/mL; for continuous infusion use a suitable infusion control device; incompatible with bicarbonate

Ethacrynic acid (sodium salt) (*Edecrin*®)
via drip tubing *in* Glucose 5% *or* Sodium chloride 0.9%
> pH of glucose infusion should be adjusted to above 5

Ethanol
Continuous *in* Glucose 5% *or* Sodium chloride 0.9% *or* Ringer's solution *or* Compound sodium lactate
> Dilute to a concentration of 5–10%

Etoposide (*Vepesid*®; *Etoposide*, Du Pont)
Intermittent *in* Sodium chloride 0.9%
> For *Vepesid*® dilute to a concentration of not more than 250 micrograms/mL and give over not less than 30 minutes; for *Etoposide* (Du Pont) dilute with either sodium chloride 0.9% or glucose 5% to a concentration of 200 micrograms/mL and give over 30–60 minutes; check container for haze or precipitate during infusion

Filgrastim (*Neupogen*®)
Continuous *or* intermittent *in* Glucose 5%
> For a filgrastim concentration of less than 1 500 000 units/mL (15 micrograms/mL) albumin solution (human serum albumin) is added to produce a final albumin concentration of 2 mg/mL; should not be diluted to a filgrastim concentration of less than 200 000 units/mL (2 micrograms/mL) and should not be diluted with sodium chloride solution

Flecainide acetate (*Tambocor*®)
Continuous *or* intermittent *in* Glucose 5% *or* Sodium chloride 0.9% *or* Compound sodium lactate
> Minimum volume in infusion fluids containing chlorides 500 mL

Flucloxacillin sodium (*Floxapen*®)
Intermittent *in* Glucose 5% *or* Sodium chloride 0.9%
> Suggested volume 100 mL given over 30–60 minutes
via drip tubing *in* Glucose 5% *or* Sodium chloride 0.9% *or* Ringer's solution *or* Compound sodium lactate
Continuous infusion not usually recommended

Fludarabine phosphate (*Fludara*®)
Intermittent *in* Sodium chloride 0.9%
> Reconstitute each 50 mg with 2 mL water for injections and dilute requisite dose in 100 mL; give over 30 minutes

Flumazenil (*Anexate*®)
Continuous *in* Glucose 5% *or* Sodium chloride 0.9%

Fluorouracil sodium
Continuous *or via* drip tubing *in* Glucose 5%
> For continuous infusion suggested volume 500 mL given over 4 hours

Foscarnet trisodium (*Foscavir*®)
Continuous *in* Glucose 5%
> Dilute to a concentration of 12 mg/mL or less for infusion into peripheral vein (undiluted solution *via* central venous line only)

Frusemide (sodium salt) (*Lasix*®)
Continuous *in* Sodium chloride 0.9% *or* Ringer's solution
> Infusion pH must be above 5.5 and rate should not exceed 4 mg/minute; glucose solutions are unsuitable

Fusidic acid (sodium salt) (*Fucidin*®)
Continuous *in* Glucose 5% (but see below) *or* Sodium chloride 0.9%
> Reconstitute with the buffer solution provided and dilute to 500 mL; give through central venous line over 2 hours (or over 6 hours if superficial vein used); incompatible in solution of pH less than 7.4

Ganciclovir (sodium salt) (*Cymevene*®)
Intermittent *in* Glucose 5% *or* Sodium chloride 0.9% *or* Ringer's solution *or* Compound sodium lactate
> Reconstitute initially in water for injections (500 mg in 10 mL) then dilute to not more than 10 mg/mL with infusion fluid (usually 100 mL); give over 1 hour

Gemcitabine (*Gemzar*®)
Intermittent *in* Sodium chloride 0.9%
> Reconstitute initially with sodium chloride 0.9% (200 mg in at least 5 mL, 1 g in at least 25 mL); may be diluted further with infusion fluid; give over 30 minutes

Gentamicin sulphate (*Cidomycin*®)
Intermittent *or via* drip tubing *in* Glucose 5% *or* Sodium chloride 0.9%
> Suggested volume for intermittent infusion 50–100 mL given over 20 minutes

Glyceryl trinitrate (*Nitrocine*®, *Nitronal*®, *Tridil*®)
Continuous *in* Glucose 5% *or* Sodium chloride 0.9%
> For *Tridil*® dilute to a concentration of not more than 400 micrograms/mL; for *Nitrocine*® suggested infusion concentration 100 micrograms/mL; incompatible with polyvinyl chloride infusion containers such as *Viaflex*® or *Steriflex*®; use glass or polyethylene containers; give *via* a syringe pump

Granisetron hydrochloride (*Kytril*®)
Intermittent *in* Glucose 5% *or* Sodium chloride 0.9% *or* Compound sodium lactate
> Dilute 3 mL in 20–50 mL infusion fluid (up to 3 mL in 10–30 mL for children); give over 5 minutes

Heparin sodium
Continuous *in* Glucose 5% *or* Sodium chloride 0.9%
> Administration with a motorised pump advisable

Hydralazine hydrochloride (*Apresoline*®)
Continuous *in* Sodium chloride 0.9% *or* Ringer's solution
> Suggested infusion volume 500 mL

Hydrocortisone sodium phosphate (*Efcortesol*®)
Continuous *or* intermittent *or via* drip tubing *in* Glucose 5% *or* Sodium chloride 0.9%

Hydrocortisone sodium succinate (*Efcortelan Soluble*®, *SoluCortef*®)
Continuous *or* intermittent *or via* drip tubing *in* Glucose 5% *or* Sodium chloride 0.9%

Idarubicin hydrochloride (*Zavedos®*)
via drip tubing *in* Sodium chloride 0.9%
Reconstitute with water for injections; give over 5–10 minutes

Ifosfamide (*Mitoxana®*)
Continuous *or* intermittent *or via* drip tubing *in* Glucose 5% *or* Sodium chloride 0.9%
For continuous infusion, suggested volume 3 litres given over 24 hours; for intermittent infusion, give over 30–120 minutes

Imipenem/cilastatin (sodium salt) (*Primaxin®*)
Intermittent *in* Glucose 5% *or* Sodium chloride 0.9%
Dilute to a concentration of 5 mg (as imipenem)/mL; infuse 250–500 mg (as imipenem) over 20–30 minutes, 1 g over 40–60 minutes
Continuous infusion not usually recommended

Insulin (soluble) Continuous *in* Sodium chloride 0.9% *or* Compound sodium lactate
Adsorbed to some extent by plastics of infusion set; see also section 6.1.3; ensure insulin is not injected into 'dead space' of injection port of the infusion bag

Isoprenaline hydrochloride (*Saventrine IV®*)
Continuous *in* Glucose 5% *or* Sodium chloride and glucose
Dilute in a large-volume infusion; suggested minimum volume 500 mL; pH of the infusion must be below 5

Isosorbide dinitrate (*Isoket 0.05%®*, *Isoket 0.1%®*)
Continuous *in* Glucose 5% *or* Sodium chloride 0.9%
Adsorbed to some extent by polyvinyl chloride infusion containers; preferably use glass or polyethylene containers or give *via* a syringe pump; *Isoket 0.05%®* can alternatively be administered undiluted using a syringe pump with a glass or rigid plastic syringe

Kanamycin sulphate (*Kannasyn®*)
Intermittent *in* Glucose 5% *or* Sodium chloride 0.9%
Dilute to 2.5 mg/mL and give at a rate of 3–4 mL/minute

Ketamine hydrochloride (*Ketalar®*)
Continuous *in* Glucose 5% *or* Sodium chloride 0.9%
Dilute to 1 mg/mL; microdrip infusion for maintenance of anaesthesia

Labetalol hydrochloride (*Trandate®*)
Intermittent *in* Glucose 5% *or* Sodium chloride and glucose
Dilute to a concentration of 1 mg/mL; suggested volume 200 mL; adjust rate with in-line burette

Lenograstim (*Granocyte®*)
Intermittent *in* Sodium chloride 0.9%
Initially reconstitute with 1 mL water for injection provided (do not shake vigorously) then dilute content of each vial with up to 100 mL infusion fluid; give over 30 minutes

Magnesium sulphate
Continuous *in* Glucose 5% *or* Sodium chloride 0.9%

Melphalan (*Alkeran®*)
Intermittent *or via* drip tubing *in* Sodium chloride 0.9%
Reconstitute with the solvent-diluent provided then dilute with infusion fluid; max. 90 minutes between addition and completion of administration; incompatible with glucose infusion

Meropenem (*Meronem®*)
Intermittent *in* Glucose 5 and 10% *or* Sodium chloride 0.9%
Dilute in 50–200 mL infusion fluid and give over 30 minutes

Mesna (*Uromitexan®*)
Continuous *or via* drip tubing *in* Glucose 5% *or* Sodium chloride 0.9%

Metaraminol tartrate (*Aramine®*)
Continuous *or via* drip tubing *in* Glucose 5% *or* Sodium chloride 0.9% *or* Ringer's solution *or* Compound sodium lactate
Suggested infusion volume 500 mL

Methocarbamol (*Robaxin®*)
Intermittent *in* Glucose 5% *or* Sodium chloride 0.9%
Dilute to a concentration of not less than 1 g in 250 mL

Methotrexate sodium (*Methotrexate*) (Lederle)
Continuous *or via* drip tubing *in* Glucose 5% *or* Sodium chloride 0.9% *or* Compound sodium lactate *or* Ringer's solution
Dilute in a large-volume infusion; max. 24 hours between addition and completion of administration

Methyldopate hydrochloride (*Aldomet®*)
Intermittent *in* Glucose 5%
Suggested volume 100 mL given over 30–60 minutes

Methylprednisolone sodium succinate (*Solu-Medrone®*)
Continuous *or* intermittent *or via* drip tubing *in* Glucose 5% *or* Sodium chloride 0.9%
Reconstitute initially with water for injections; doses up to 250 mg should be given over at least 5 minutes, high doses over at least 30 minutes

Metoclopramide hydrochloride (*Maxolon High Dose®*)
Continuous *or* intermittent *in* Glucose 5% *or* Sodium chloride 0.9% *or* Compound sodium lactate
Continuous infusion recommended; loading dose, dilute with 50–100 mL and give over 15–20 minutes; maintenance dose, dilute with 500 mL and give over 8–12 hours; for intermittent infusion dilute with at least 50 mL and give over at least 15 minutes

Mexiletine hydrochloride (*Mexitil®*)
Continuous *in* Glucose 5% *or* Sodium chloride 0.9%

Milrinone (*Primacor®*)
Continuous *in* Glucose 5% *or* Sodium chloride 0.9%
Dilute to a suggested concentration of 200 micrograms/mL

Mitozantrone hydrochloride (*Novantrone®*)
via drip tubing *in* Glucose 5% *or* Sodium chloride 0.9%
Suggested volume at least 50 mL given over at least 3–5 minutes

Mivacurium chloride (*Mivacron®*)
Continuous *in* Glucose 5% *or* Sodium chloride 0.9%
Dilute to a concentration of 500 micrograms/mL; may also be given undiluted

Molgramostim (*Leucomax®*)
Intermittent *in* Glucose 5% *or* Sodium chloride 0.9%
  Reconstitute each vial with 1 mL water for injections; dilute with 25–100 mL infusion fluid to a concentration of not less than 80 000 units/mL; give over 4–6 hours; infusion through low protein binding 0.2 or 0.22 micron filter recommended; some infusion sets (e.g. *Port-A-Cath®*) adsorb molgramostim and should not be used

Mustine hydrochloride (Knoll)
via drip tubing *in* Glucose 5% *or* Sodium chloride 0.9%

Naloxone (*Min-I-Jet® Naloxone Hydrochloride, Narcan®*)
Continuous *in* Glucose 5% *or* Sodium chloride 0.9%
  Dilute to a concentration of 4 micrograms/mL

Netilmicin sulphate (*Netillin®*)
Intermittent *or via* drip tubing *in* Glucose 5 and 10% *or* Sodium chloride 0.9%
  For intermittent infusion suggested volume 50–200 mL given over 90–120 minutes

Nimodipine (*Nimotop®*)
via drip tubing *in* Glucose 5% *or* Sodium chloride 0.9% *or* Ringer's solution
  Not to be added to infusion container; administer *via* an infusion pump through a Y-piece into a central catheter; incompatible with polyvinyl chloride giving sets or containers; protect infusion from light

Nizatidine (*Axid®*)
Continuous *or* intermittent *in* Glucose 5% *or* Sodium chloride 0.9% *or* Compound sodium lactate
  For continuous infusion, dilute 300 mg in 150 mL and give at a rate of 10 mg/hour; for intermittent infusion, dilute 100 mg in 50 mL and give over 15 minutes

Noradrenaline acid tartrate (*Levophed®*)
Continuous *in* Glucose 5% *or* Sodium chloride and glucose
  Give *via* controlled infusion device; for administration *via* syringe pump, dilute 4 mg noradrenaline acid tartrate (2 mL solution) with 48 mL; for administration *via* drip counter dilute 40 mg (20 mL solution) with 480 mL; give through a central venous catheter; incompatible with alkalis

Ondansetron hydrochloride (*Zofran®*)
Continuous *or* intermittent *in* Glucose 5% *or* Sodium chloride 0.9% *or* Ringer's solution

Oxytocin (*Syntocinon®*)
Continuous *in* Glucose 5%
  Preferably given *via* a variable-speed infusion pump in a concentration appropriate to the pump; if given by drip infusion for *induction or enhancement of labour*, dilute 5 units in 500 mL infusion fluid; for *postpartum uterine haemorrhage* dilute 5–20 units in 500 mL; if high doses given for prolonged period (e.g. for inevitable or missed abortion or for postpartum haemorrhage), use low volume of an electrolyte-containing infusion fluid (not Glucose 5%) given at higher concentration than for induction or enhancement of labour; close attention to patient's fluid and electrolyte status essential

Paclitaxel (*Taxol®*)
Continuous *in* Glucose 5% *or* Sodium chloride 0.9%
  Begin infusion within 3 hours of dilution; dilute to a concentration of 0.3–1.2 mg/mL and give through a 0.22 micron in-line filter over 3 hours; not to be used with PVC equipment (short PVC inlet or outlet on filter may be acceptable)

Pentamidine isethionate (*Pentacarinat®*)
Intermittent *in* Glucose 5% *or* Sodium chloride 0.9%
  Dissolve initially in water for injections (300 mg in 3–5 mL) then dilute in 50–250 mL; give over at least 60 minutes

Pentostatin (*Nipent®*)
Intermittent *in* Glucose 5% *or* Sodium chloride 0.9%
  Dilute with 25–50 mL and give over 20–30 minutes

Phenoxybenzamine hydrochloride (*Dibenyline®*)
Intermittent *in* Sodium chloride 0.9%
  Dilute in 200–500 mL infusion; give over at least 2 hours; max. 4 hours between dilution and completion of administration

Phentolamine mesylate (*Rogitine®*)
Intermittent *in* Glucose 5% *or* Sodium chloride 0.9%

Phenylephrine hydrochloride
Intermittent *in* Glucose 5% *or* Sodium chloride 0.9%

Phenytoin sodium (*Epanutin®*)
Intermittent *in* Sodium chloride 0.9%
  Flush intravenous line with Sodium chloride 0.9% before and after infusion; dilute in 50–100 mL infusion fluid (final concentration not to exceed 10 mg/mL) and give through an in-line filter (0.22–0.50 micron) at a rate not exceeding 50 mg/minute (neonates, give at a rate of 1–3 mg/kg/minute); complete administration within 1 hour of preparation

Phytomenadione (in mixed micelles vehicle) (*Konakion® MM*)
Intermittent *in* Glucose 5%
  Dilute with 55 mL; may be injected into lower part of infusion apparatus

Piperacillin sodium (*Pipril®*)
Intermittent *in* Glucose 5% *or* Sodium chloride 0.9% *or* Compound sodium lactate *or* Water for injections
  Minimum volume 50 mL given over 20–40 minutes

Piperacillin/tazobactam (sodium salts) (*Tazocin®*)
Intermittent *in* Glucose 5% *or* Sodium chloride 0.9% *or* Water for injections
  Reconstitute initially with water for injections or sodium chloride infusion 0.9% (2.25 g in 10 mL, 4.5 g in 20 mL) then dilute with 50 mL infusion fluid; give over 20–30 minutes

Potassium canrenoate (*Spiroctan-M®*)
Intermittent *in* Glucose 5% *or* Sodium chloride 0.9%
  Suggested volume 250 mL

Potassium chloride
Continuous *in* Glucose 5% *or* Sodium chloride 0.9%
  Dilute in a large-volume infusion; mix thoroughly to avoid 'layering', especially in non-rigid infusion containers; use ready-prepared solutions when possible

Procainamide hydrochloride (*Pronestyl®*)
Continuous *or* intermittent *in* Glucose 5%
  For maintenance, dilute to a concentration of *either* 2 mg/mL and give at a rate of 1–3 mL/minute *or* 4 mg/mL and give at a rate of 0.5–1.5 mL/minute

Propofol (emulsion) (*Diprivan®*)
via drip tubing *in* Glucose 5% *or* Sodium chloride 0.9%
> Not to be mixed with other therapeutic agents or infusion fluids; to be administered *via* a Y-piece close to injection site

Continuous *in* Glucose 5%
> Dilute to a concentration not less than 2 mg/mL; administer using suitable device to control infusion rate; use glass or PVC containers (if PVC bag used it should be full—withdraw volume of infusion fluid equal to that of propofol to be added); give within 6 hours of preparation; propofol may alternatively be infused undiluted using a suitable infusion pump

Quinine dihydrochloride
Continuous *in* Sodium chloride 0.9%
> To be given over 4 hours; see also section 5.4.1

Ranitidine hydrochloride (*Zantac®*)
Intermittent *in* Glucose 5% *or* Sodium chloride 0.9% *or* Compound sodium lactate

Rifampicin (*Rifadin®*, *Rimactane®*)
Intermittent *in* Glucose 5 and 10% *or* Sodium chloride 0.9% *or* Ringer's solution
> Reconstitute with solvent provided then dilute with 250 mL (*Rimactane®*) or 500 mL (*Rifadin®*) infusion fluid; give over 2–3 hours

Ritodrine hydrochloride (*Yutopar®*)
Continuous *in* Glucose 5%
> Give *via* controlled infusion device, preferably a syringe pump; if syringe pump available dilute to a concentration of 3 mg/mL; if syringe pump not available dilute to a concentration of 300 micrograms/mL; close attention to patient's fluid and electrolyte status essential

Rocuronium bromide (*Esmeron®*)
Continuous *or via* drip tubing *in* Glucose 5% *or* Sodium chloride 0.9%

Salbutamol sulphate (*Ventolin® For Intravenous. Infusion*)
Continuous *in* Glucose 5%
> For *bronchodilatation* dilute 5 mg with 500 mL glucose 5% or sodium chloride 0.9%; for *premature labour* dilute with glucose 5% to a concentration not exceeding 500 micrograms/mL (preferable to use low volume); give *via* controlled infusion device; close attention to patient's fluid and electrolyte status essential

Salcatonin (*Miacalcic®*)
Continuous *in* Sodium chloride 0.9%
> Diluted solution given without delay; dilute in 500 mL and give over at least 6 hours; glass or hard plastic containers should not be used; approx. 20% loss of potency on dilution (take into account when calculating dose)

Sodium calciumedetate (*Ledclair®*)
Continuous *in* Glucose 5% *or* Sodium chloride 0.9%
> Dilute to a concentration of not more than 3%; suggested volume 250–500 mL given over at least 1 hour

Sodium clodronate (*Bonefos® Concentrate, Loron®*)
Continuous *in* Sodium chloride 0.9%
> Dilute 300 mg in 500 mL and give over at least 2 hours or 1.5 g in 500 mL and give over at least 4 hours; *Bonefos®* Concentrate can also be diluted in Glucose 5%

Sodium nitroprusside (*David Bull*)
Continuous *in* Glucose 5%
> Reconstitute 50 mg with 2–3 mL glucose 5% then dilute immediately with 250–1000 mL infusion fluid; preferably infuse *via* infusion device to allow precise control; protect infusion from light

Sodium valproate (*Epilim®*)
Continuous *or* intermittent *in* Glucose 5% *or* Sodium chloride 0.9%
> Reconstitute with solvent provided then dilute with infusion fluid

Sotalol hydrochloride (*Sotacor®*)
Continuous *or* intermittent *in* Glucose 5% *or* Sodium chloride 0.9%
> Dilute to a concentration of between 0.01–2 mg/mL

Streptokinase (*Kabikinase®*, *Streptase®*)
Continuous *or* intermittent *in* Glucose 5% *or* Sodium chloride 0.9%
> Reconstitute *Kabikinase®* with water for injections and *Streptase®* with sodium chloride 0.9% then dilute further with infusion fluid

Sulphadiazine sodium
Continuous *in* Sodium chloride 0.9%
> Suggested volume 500 mL; ampoule solution has a pH of over 10

Suxamethonium chloride (*Anectine®*, *Scoline®*)
Continuous *in* Glucose 5% *or* Sodium chloride 0.9%

Tacrolimus (*Prograf®*)
Continuous *in* Glucose 5%
> Give over 24 hours; sodium chloride 0.9% may be used as diluent with polyethylene containers; incompatible with PVC

Teicoplanin (*Targocid®*)
Intermittent *in* Glucose 5% *or* Sodium chloride 0.9% *or* Compound sodium lactate
> Reconstitute initially with water for injections provided; infuse over 30 minutes

Continuous infusion not usually recommended

Temocillin sodium (*Temopen®*)
Intermittent *in* Glucose 5% *or* Sodium chloride 0.9% *or* Ringer's solution *or* Compound sodium lactate
> Dissolve initially in water for injections (500 mg in 10 mL; 1–2 g in 20 mL) then dilute with infusion fluid and give over 30–40 minutes

Terbutaline sulphate (*Bricanyl®*)
Continuous *in* Glucose 5%
> For *bronchodilatation* dilute 1.5–2.5 mg with 500 mL glucose 5% or sodium chloride 0.9% and give over 8–10 hours; for *premature labour* dilute in glucose 5% and give *via* controlled infusion device preferably a syringe pump; if syringe pump available dilute to a concentration of 100 micrograms/mL; if syringe pump not available dilute to a concentration of 10 micrograms/mL; close attention to patient's fluid and electrolyte status essential

Tetracycline hydrochloride (*Achromycin® Intravenous*)
Continuous *in* Glucose 5% *or* Sodium chloride 0.9% *or* Compound sodium lactate
> Reconstitute initially with water for injections (250 mg in 5 mL, 500 mg in 10 mL) then dilute to at least 100 mL (max. 1 litre) and give at a rate not exceeding 100 mL in 5 minutes preferably through a 0.22 micron filter

Ticarcillin sodium (*Ticar*®)
Intermittent *in* Glucose 5% *or* Water for injections
  Suggested volume 100–150 mL given over 30–40 minutes

Ticarcillin sodium/clavulanic acid (*Timentin*®)
Intermittent *in* Glucose 5% *or* Water for injections
  Suggested volume glucose 5%, 50–150 mL (depending on dose) or water for injections, 25–100 mL; given over 30–40 minutes

Tobramycin sulphate (*Nebcin*®)
Intermittent *or via* drip tubing *in* Glucose 5% *or* Sodium chloride 0.9%
  For adult intermittent infusion suggested volume 50–100 mL (children proportionately smaller volume) given over 20–60 minutes

Tramadol hydrochloride (*Zydol*®)
Continuous *or* intermittent *in* Glucose 5% *or* Sodium chloride 0.9% *or* Ringer's solution *or* Compound sodium lactate

Treosulfan (*Treosulfan*) (Medac)
Intermittent *in* Water for injections
  Infusion suggested for doses above 5 g; dilute to a concentration of 5 g in 100 mL

Trimetaphan camsylate (*Arfonad*®)
Intermittent *in* Sodium chloride 0.9% *or* Sodium chloride and glucose
  Dilute to a concentration of 0.05–0.1% (0.25% if fluid restriction necessary)

Trimethoprim lactate (*Monotrim*®)
via drip tubing *in* Glucose 5% *or* Sodium chloride 0.9% *or* Compound sodium lactate *or* Ringer's solution

Trisodium edetate (*Limclair*®)
Continuous *in* Glucose 5% *or* Sodium chloride 0.9%
  Dilute to a concentration of 10 mg/mL; give over 2–3 hours

Tropisetron hydrochloride (*Navoban*®)
Intermittent *or via* drip tubing *in* Glucose 5% *or* Sodium chloride 0.9% *or* Ringer's solution
  Suggested volume for infusion 100 mL

Urokinase (*Urokinase*) (Leo), (*Ukidan*®)
Continuous *in* Sodium chloride 0.9%

Vancomycin hydrochloride (*Vancocin*®)
Intermittent *in* Glucose 5% *or* Sodium chloride 0.9%
  Reconstitute 500 mg with 10 mL water for injections and dilute to 100–200 mL with infusion fluid; give over at least 60 minutes (rate not to exceed 10 mg/minute for doses over 500 mg); use continuous infusion only if intermittent not feasible
Continuous infusion not usually recommended

Vasopressin, synthetic (*Pitressin*®)
Intermittent *in* Glucose 5%
  Suggested concentration 20 units/100 mL given over 15 minutes

Vecuronium bromide (*Norcuron*®)
Continuous *in* Glucose 5% *or* Sodium chloride 0.9% *or* Ringer's solution
  Reconstitute with the solvent provided

Vinblastine sulphate (*Velbe*®)
via drip tubing *in* Sodium chloride 0.9%
  Reconstitute with the diluent provided; give within approx. 1 minute

Vincristine sulphate (*Oncovin*®)
via drip tubing *in* Glucose 5% *or* Sodium chloride 0.9%

Vindesine sulphate (*Eldisine*®)
via drip tubing *in* Glucose 5% *or* Sodium chloride 0.9%
  Reconstitute with the diluent provided

Vitamins B & C (*Pabrinex*® *I/V High potency*)
Intermittent *or via* drip tubing *in* Glucose 5% *or* Sodium chloride 0.9%
  Ampoule contents should be mixed, diluted, and administered without delay; give over 10 minutes (see CSM advice, section 9.6.2)

Vitamins, multiple

(*Cernevit*®)
Intermittent *in* Glucose 5% *or* Sodium chloride 0.9%
  Dissolve initially in 5 mL water for injections (or infusion fluid)
(*Multibionta*®)
Intermittent *in* Glucose 5% *or* Sodium chloride 0.9%
  Dilute 10 mL in not less than 250 mL of infusion fluid (adults); see also section 9.3
(*Solivito N*®)
Intermittent *in* Glucose 5 and 10%
  Suggested volume 500–1000 mL given over 2–3 hours; see also section 9.3

Zidovudine (*Retrovir*®)
Intermittent *in* Glucose 5%
  Dilute to a concentration of 2 mg/mL or 4 mg/mL and give over 1 hour

Appendix 7: Borderline Substances

In certain conditions some foods (and toilet preparations) have characteristics of drugs and the Advisory Committee on Borderline Substances advises as to the circumstances in which such substances may be regarded as drugs. Prescriptions issued in accordance with the Committee's advice and endorsed 'ACBS' will normally not be investigated.

General Practitioners are reminded that the ACBS recommends products on the basis that they may be regarded as drugs for the management of specified conditions. Doctors should satisfy themselves that the products can safely be prescribed, that patients are adequately monitored and that, where necessary, expert hospital supervision is available.

FOODS WHICH MAY BE PRESCRIBED ON FP10

Note. This is a list of food products which the ACBS has approved. The clinical condition for which the product has approval follows each entry.

Advera® (Abbott)
Liquid, providing protein 14.2 g, carbohydrate 48.3 g, fat 5.4 g, energy 1262 kJ (299 kcal)/237 mL, with vitamins and minerals. Gluten-free. Orange and chocolate flavours. Net price 237-mL can = £2.43. For use as a necessary nutritional supplement prescribed on medical grounds for: short-bowel syndrome, intractable malabsorption, pre-operative preparation of patients who are undernourished, proven inflammatory bowel disease, following total gastrectomy, bowel fistulas, disease-related malnutrition. Not to be prescribed for any child under 5 years of age

Aglutella® (Ultrapharm)
Rice, low protein. Net price 500 g = £3.95. For inherited metabolic disorders, renal or liver failure requiring a low-protein diet

AL 110® (Nestlé)
Powder, protein 14 g, fat 25 g, carbohydrate 55.3 g, energy 2100 kJ (502 kcal)/100 g with vitamins and minerals. Net price 400 g = £7.27. For proven lactose intolerance in pre-school children, galactosaemia, and galactokinase deficiency

Alcoholic Beverages *see under* Rectified Spirit

Alembicol D® (Alembic Products)
Fractionated coconut oil. Net price 5 kg = £123.00. For steatorrhoea associated with cystic fibrosis of the pancreas, intestinal lymphangiectasia, surgery of the intestine, chronic liver disease, liver cirrhosis, other proven malabsorption syndromes; and in a ketogenic diet in the management of epilepsy

Alfare® (Nestlé)
Powder, protein 16.5 g, fat 24 g, carbohydrate 51.7 g, energy 2010 kJ (480 kcal)/100 g with vitamins and minerals. Net price 400 g = £5.49. For disaccharide and/or whole protein intolerance, or where amino acids or peptides are indicated in conjunction with medium chain triglycerides

Aminex® (Gluten Free Foods)
Rusks, low-protein. Net price 200 g = £3.75. For inherited metabolic disorders, renal or liver failure requiring a low-protein diet

Amino Acid Modules (Scientific Hospital Supplies)
Leucine-Free Amino Acid Mix, powder, essential and non-essential amino acids 93%, except leucine. Net price 200 g = £49.59. For isovaleric acidaemia
Methionine-Free Amino Acid Mix, powder, essential and non-essential amino acids 93%, except methionine. Net price 200 g = £49.59. For homocystinuria or hypermethioninaemia
Methionine, Threonine, Valine-Free and Isoleucine-Low Amino Acid Mix, powder, essential and non-essential amino acids 93%, except methionine, threonine, and valine, with trace amounts of isoleucine. Net price 200 g = £49.59. For methylmalonic acidaemia or propionic acidaemia
Phenylalanine, Tyrosine, and Methionine-Free Amino Acid Mix, powder, essential and non-essential amino acids 93%, except methionine, phenylalanine, and tyrosine. Net price 200 g = £49.59. For tyrosinaemia type I where plasma concentrations are above normal
Tyrosine and Phenylalanine-Free Amino Acid Mix, powder, essential and non-essential amino acids 93%, except phenylalanine and tyrosine. Net price 200 g = £52.07. For tyrosinaemia where plasma concentrations are normal

Aminogran® (UCB Pharma)
Food Supplement, powder, containing all essential amino acids except phenylalanine, for use with mineral mixture (see below). Net price 500 g = £42.77. For phenylketonuria
Mineral Mixture, powder, containing all appropriate minerals for use with the above food supplement and other synthetic diets. Net price 250 g = £7.24. For phenylketonuria and as a mineral supplement in synthetic diets

Analog® (Scientific Hospital Supplies)
Note. Analog products are generally intended for use in children up to 1 year
MSUD Analog, powder, essential and non-essential amino acids 15.5% except isoleucine, leucine and valine, with carbohydrate, fat, vitamins, minerals, and trace elements. Net price 400 g = £24.00. For maple syrup urine disease
RVHB Analog, powder, essential and non-essential amino acids 15.5% except methionine, with carbohydrate, fat, vitamins, minerals, and trace elements. Net price 400 g = £24.00. For hypermethioninaemia; homocystinuria
XLeu Analog, powder, essential and non-essential amino acids 15.5% except leucine, with carbohydrate, fat, vitamins, minerals, and trace elements. Net price 400 g = £24.00. For isovaleric acidaemia
Ingredients: include arachis oil (peanut oil)
XLys Analog, powder, essential and non-essential amino acids 15.5% except lysine, with carbohydrate, fat, vitamins, minerals, and trace elements. Net price 400 g = £24.00. For hyperlysinaemia
XMet, Thre, Val, Isoleu, Analog, powder, essential and non-essential amino acids 15.5% except methionine, threonine, valine and low isoleucine, with carbohydrate, fat, vitamins, minerals, and trace elements. Net price 400 g = £24.00. For methylmalonic acidaemia or propionic acidaemia
XP Analog, powder, essential and non-essential amino acids 15.5% except phenylalanine, with carbohydrate, fat, vitamins, minerals, and trace elements. Net price 400 g = £16.00. For phenylketonuria
XPhen, Tyr, Analog, powder, essential and non-essential amino acids 15.5% except phenylalanine and tyrosine, with carbohydrate, fat, vitamins, minerals and trace elements. Net price 400 g = £24.00. For tyrosinaemia

Aproten® (Ultrapharm)

Gluten-free. Flour. Net price 300 g = £1.84. For gluten-sensitive enteropathies including steatorrhoea due to gluten sensitivity, coeliac disease, and dermatitis herpetiformis

Low protein. Low Na^+ and K^+. Net prices: anellini 500 g = £3.95; biscuits 180 g (36) = £2.80; bread mix 250 g = £2.00; cake mix 300 g = £2.10; crispbread 260 g = £3.95; ditalini 500 g = £3.95; rigatini 500 g = £3.95; spaghetti 500 g = £3.95; tagliatelle 250 g = £2.10. For inherited metabolic disorders, renal or liver failure requiring a low-protein diet

Arnott® (Ultrapharm)

Rice Cookies, gluten-free. Net price 200 g = £1.68. For gluten-sensitive enteropathies including steatorrhoea due to gluten sensitivity, coeliac disease, and dermatitis herpetiformis

Barkat® (Gluten Free Foods)

Bread mix, gluten-free. Net price 500 g = £4.12. For gluten-sensitive enteropathies including steatorrhoea due to gluten sensitivity, coeliac disease, and dermatitis herpetiformis

Bi-Aglut® (Ultrapharm)

Biscuits, gluten-free. Net price 180 g (36) = £2.60

Cracker toast, gluten-, lactose-, and milk-protein-free. Net price 240 g (40) = £3.60

Both for gluten-sensitive enteropathies including steatorrhoea due to gluten sensitivity, coeliac disease, dermatitis herpetiformis

Calogen® (Scientific Hospital Supplies)

Emulsion, arachis oil (peanut oil) 50% in water. Net price 250 mL = £3.67; 1 litre = £13.26. For renal failure and other conditions requiring a high-energy, low-fluid, low-electrolyte diet, disorders of amino acid metabolism or carbohydrate absorption; in a ketogenic diet in the management of epilepsy

Caloreen® (Clintec)

Powder, water-soluble dextrins, with less than 1.8 mmol of Na^+ and 0.3 mmol of K^+/100 g. Net price 250 g = £1.51; 5 kg = £24.79. For renal failure; liver cirrhosis; disaccharide intolerance (without isomaltose intolerance), disorders of amino acid metabolism (and other similar disorders) and/or whole protein intolerance; malabsorption states and other conditions (including proven hypoglycaemia) requiring a high energy, low fluid intake, whether or not sodium and/or potassium restriction is essential

Calsip® (Fresenius)

Liquid, maltodextrin 50%. Flavours: apple, pineapple, neutral. Net price 200-mL Tetrabrik® = 89 p. For renal failure, liver cirrhosis, disaccharide intolerance (without isomaltose intolerance), hypoglycaemia, disorders of amino acid metabolism, whole protein intolerance, malabsorption states, other conditions requiring a high energy, low fluid diet, whether or not sodium and/or potassium restriction is essential

Caprilon® (Cow & Gate)

Powder, protein 11.8%, carbohydrate 55.1%, fat 28.3% (medium chain triglycerides 21.3%). Low in lactose, gluten- and sucrose-free. Used as a 12.7% solution. Net price 420 g = £10.10. For disorders in which a high intake of MCT is beneficial

Note. Caprilon replaces MCT (1) powder

Carobel, Instant® (Cow & Gate)

Powder, carob seed flour. Net price 45 g = £2.63. For thickening feeds in the treatment of vomiting

Casilan 90® (Crookes)

Powder, whole protein, containing all essential amino acids, 90% with less than 0.1% Na^+. Net price 250 g = £4.58. For biochemically proven hypoproteinaemia

Clinifeed® (Clintec)

Clinifeed 400, protein 15 g, carbohydrate 55 g, fat 13.4 g, energy 1674 kJ (400 kcal)/375 mL, with vitamins and minerals, vanilla flavour. Fructose-free. Net price 375-mL can = £1.80

Clinifeed Protein Rich, protein 30 g, carbohydrate 70 g, fat 11 g, energy 2092 kJ (500 kcal)/375 mL, with vitamins and minerals, vanilla flavour. Fructose- and lactose-free. Net price 375-mL can = £2.00

Both for use as necessary nutritional supplements prescribed on medical grounds for: short bowel syndrome, intractable malabsorption, pre-operative preparation of patients who are undernourished, proven inflammatory bowel disease, following total gastrectomy, dysphagia, bowel fistulas, disease-related malnutrition, continuous ambulatory peritoneal dialysis (CAPD), and haemodialysis. Neither to be prescribed for any child under one year; use with caution for young children up to 5 years of age

[1]*Clinifeed 1.0*, protein 14.1 g, carbohydrate 49.9 g, fat 14.6 g, energy 1575 kJ (375 kcal)/375 mL, with vitamins and minerals, neutral flavour. Lactose-, fructose-, and sucrose-free. Net price 375-mL can = £1.80; 500-mL Dripac = £2.60

1, Formerly Clinifeed Favour

Clinifeed Iso, protein 10.5 g, carbohydrate 49.2 g, fat 15.4 g, energy 1575 kJ (375 kcal)/375 mL, with vitamins and minerals, vanilla flavour. Fructose- and sucrose-free, and low sodium. Net price 375-mL can = £1.80

Both for use as the sole source of nutrition or as necessary nutritional supplements prescribed on medical grounds for: short bowel syndrome, intractable malabsorption, pre-operative preparation of patients who are undernourished, proven inflammatory bowel disease, following total gastrectomy, dysphagia, bowel fistulas, disease-related malnutrition. Neither to be prescribed for any child under one year; use with caution for young children up to 5 years of age

Comminuted Chicken Meat (Cow & Gate)

Suspension (aqueous). Net price 150 g = £2.01. For carbohydrate intolerance in association with possible or proven intolerance of milk; glucose and galactose intolerance

Corn flour and corn starch For hypoglycaemia associated with glycogen-storage disease

Corn oil (maize oil). Net price 100 mL = 26p. For familial hypercholesterolaemia

Dextrose *see* Glucose

Dialamine® (Scientific Hospital Supplies)

Powder, essential amino acids 30%, with carbohydrate 62%, energy 1500 kJ (360 kcal)/100 g, with ascorbic acid, minerals, and trace elements. Flavour: orange. Net price 200 g = £20.13. For oral feeding where essential amino acid supplements are required; e.g. chronic renal failure, hypoproteinaemia, wound fistula leakage with excessive protein loss, conditions requiring a controlled nitrogen intake, and haemodialysis

dp® (Nutricia Dietary)

Cookies, low-protein, butterscotch- or chocolate-flavoured chip cookies. Net price 170 g = £5.64. For inherited metabolic disorders, renal or liver failure requiring a low-protein diet

Duobar® (Scientific Hospital Supplies)

Bar, protein-free (phenylalanine nil added), carbohydrate 56 g, fat 42 g, energy 2450 kJ (600 kcal)/100 g. Low sodium and potassium. Strawberry and vanilla flavours. Net price 100-g bar = £2.02. For children and adults on protein-restricted diets and for conditions where there is a need for energy fortification and where fluid intake is restricted, such as renal disease, disorders of amino-acid metabolism, and liver disease

Duocal® (Scientific Hospital Supplies)

Liquid, emulsion providing carbohydrate 23.4 g, fat 7.1 g, energy 628 kJ (150 kcal)/100 mL. Low-electrolyte, gluten-, lactose-, and protein-free. Net price 250 mL = £1.96; 1 litre = £6.99

Super Soluble Powder, carbohydrate 72.7 g, fat 22.3 g, energy 1988 kJ (473 kcal)/100 g. Low electrolyte,

---

gluten-, protein-, and lactose-free. Net price 400 g = £11.26

Both for renal failure; liver cirrhosis; disaccharide intolerance (without isomaltose intolerance), disorders of amino acid metabolism (and other similar disorders), and/or whole protein intolerance; malabsorption states and other conditions requiring a high energy, low fluid intake, whether or not sodium and/or potassium restriction is essential

Elemental 028® (Scientific Hospital Supplies)

028 Powder, amino acids 12%, carbohydrate 70.5–72%, fat 6.64%, energy 1544–1568 kJ (364–370 kcal)/100 g with vitamins and minerals. For preparation with water before use. Net price 100-g box (orange flavoured or plain) = £4.08

028 Extra powder, amino acids 15%, carbohydrate 59%, fat 17.45%, energy 1860 kJ (443 kcal)/100 g, with vitamins, minerals, and trace elements. For preparation with water before use. Net price 100 g (plain) = £4.08; also available orange-flavoured (carbohydrate 55%, energy 1793 kJ (427 kcal)/100 g), 100 g = £4.08

028 Extra liquid, amino acids 7.5 g, carbohydrate 27.5 g, fat 8.7 g, energy 896 kJ (215 kcal)/250 mL, with vitamins, minerals, and trace elements. Flavours: grapefruit, orange and pineapple, summer fruits. Net price 250-mL carton = £2.30

All for use as the sole source of nutrition or as a necessary nutritional supplement prescribed on medical grounds for: short-bowel syndrome, intractable malabsorption, proven inflammatory bowel disease, bowel fistulas. Not to be prescribed for any child under one year; use with caution for young children up to 5 years of age

Emsogen® (Scientific Hospital Supplies)

Powder, amino acids 15%, carbohydrate 60%, fat 16.4%, energy 1839 kJ (436 kcal)/100 g, with vitamins, minerals, and trace elements. For preparation with water before use. Net price 100 g = £4.08; also available orange-flavoured (carbohydrate 55%, energy 1754 kJ (418 kcal)/100 g), 100 g = £4.08. For use as the sole source of nutrition or as a necessary nutritional supplement prescribed on medical grounds for short bowel syndrome, intractable malabsorption, proven inflammatory bowel disease, bowel fistulas. Not to be prescribed for any child under one year; use with caution for young children up to 5 years of age

Ener-G® (General Dietary)

Gluten-free. Rice bread (sliced), brown, net price 200 g = £1.80, 474 g = £3.75; white, 200 g = £1.80, 456 g = £3.75. Rice loaf, 612 g = £3.75. Brown rice and maize bread, 742 g = £3.75. Tapioca bread (sliced), 200 g = £1.80, 480 g = £3.75. Rice pasta (macaroni, shells, small shells, and lasagne), 454 g = £3.45; spaghetti, 447 g = £3.45; tagliatelle, 400 g = £3.45; vermicelli, 300 g = £3.45; cannelloni, 284 g = £3.45. Brown rice pasta: lasagne, 454 g = £3.45; macaroni, 454 g = £3.45; spaghetti, 447 g = £3.45. For gluten-sensitive enteropathies including steatorrhoea due to gluten sensitivity, coeliac disease, and dermatitis herpetiformis

Enlive® (Abbott)

Liquid, protein 9.6 g, carbohydrate 65.4 g, energy 1274 kJ (300 kcal)/240 mL, with vitamins and minerals; fat-free. Flavours: apple, lemon and lime, peach, orange, pineapple, strawberry. Net price 240-mL tetrapak = £1.50. For use as a necessary nutritional supplement prescribed on medical grounds: for short bowel syndrome, intractable malabsorption, pre-operative preparation of patients who are undernourished, proven inflammatory bowel disease, following total gastrectomy, dysphagia, bowel fistulas, disease-related malnutrition. Not to be prescribed for any child under 1 year; use with caution for young children up to 5 years of age

Enrich® (Abbott)

Liquid with dietary fibre, providing protein 9.4 g, carbohydrate 34.9 g, fat 8.8 g, fibre 3.4 g, energy 1079 kJ

(256 kcal)/250 mL with vitamins and minerals. Lactose- and gluten-free. Vanilla and chocolate flavours. Net price 250-mL can = £1.86. For use as the sole source of nutrition or as a necessary nutritional supplement prescribed on medical grounds for: short-bowel syndrome, intractable malabsorption, pre-operative preparation of patients who are undernourished, proven inflammatory bowel disease, following total gastrectomy, dysphagia, disease-related malnutrition. Not to be prescribed for any child under one year; use with caution for young children up to 5 years of age

Ensure® (Abbott)

Liquid, protein 10.0 g, fat 8.4 g, carbohydrate 33.9 g, energy 1057 kJ (251 kcal)/250 mL with minerals and vitamins, lactose- and gluten-free. Vanilla flavour. Net price 237-mL bottle = £1.71; 250-mL can = £1.58. Chocolate, coffee, eggnog, nut, chicken, mushroom, and asparagus flavours. Net price 250-mL can = £1.51

Powder, same composition as Ensure liquid when reconstituted. Net price 400 g = £11.06

Both for use as the sole source of nutrition or as a necessary nutritional supplement prescribed on medical grounds for: short bowel syndrome, intractable malabsorption, pre-operative preparation of patients who are undernourished, proven inflammatory bowel disease, following total gastrectomy, dysphagia, bowel fistulas, disease-related malnutrition. Neither to be prescribed for any child under one year; use with caution for young children up to 5 years of age

Ensure Plus® (Abbott)

Liquid, protein 12.5 g, fat 10.0 g, carbohydrate 40.0 g, with vitamins and minerals, lactose- and gluten-free, energy 1260 kJ (300 kcal)/250 mL. Vanilla flavour. Net price 250-mL can = £1.81; 500-mL bottle = £3.25; 1-litre bottle = £6.50. Caramel, chocolate, strawberry, banana, fruit of the forest, raspberry, orange, coffee, black currant and vanilla flavours. Net price 200-mL Tetrapak = £1.45. As a necessary nutritional supplement prescribed on medical grounds for: short bowel syndrome, intractable malabsorption, pre-operative preparation of patients who are undernourished, proven inflammatory bowel disease, following total gastrectomy, dysphagia, bowel fistulas, disease-related malnutrition, continuous ambulatory peritoneal dialysis (CAPD), and haemodialysis. Not to be prescribed for any child under one year; use with caution for young children up to 5 years of age

Entera® (Fresenius)

Liquid, protein 11.3 g, carbohydrate 37.6 g, fat 11.66 g, energy 1260 kJ (300 kcal)/200 mL, with vitamins and minerals. Net price 200-mL Tetrabrik = £1.40 (flavours: vanilla, strawberry, butterscotch, blackcurrant, banana, orange, pineapple, chocolate-mint, vegetable cream, and neutral): 500-mL bottle = £3.10 (flavour: neutral). For use as sole source of nutrition or as a necessary nutritional supplement prescribed on medical grounds for: short-bowel syndrome, intractable malabsorption, pre-operative preparation of patients who are undernourished, proven inflammatory bowel disease, following total gastrectomy, dysphagia, bowel fistulas, disease-related malnutrition. Not to be prescribed for any child under one year; use with caution for young children up to 5 years of age

Farley's Soya Formula (Farley)

[formerly OsterSoy®]

Powder, providing protein 2%, carbohydrate 7%, fat 3.8% with vitamins and minerals when reconstituted. Gluten-, sucrose-, and lactose-free. Net price 450 g = £3.53. For proven lactose and associated sucrose intolerance in pre-school children, galactokinase deficiency, galactosaemia, and cow's milk protein intolerance

Flexical® (Bristol-Myers)

Powder, protein 9.9%, carbohydrate 67%, fat 15% with vitamins and minerals. Gluten- and lactose-free. Net price 454 g = £10.20. For use as the sole source of nutrition or as a necessary nutritional supplement prescribed on medical grounds for: short-bowel syndrome, intractable malabsorption, proven inflammatory bowel disease, bowel fistulas. Not to be prescribed for any child under one year; use with caution for young children up to 5 years of age

Forceval Protein® (Unigreg)

Powder, calcium caseinate 60%, carbohydrate 30%, with vitamins and minerals, providing not less than 55% protein, not more than 1% of fat, not more than 0.12% of Na+. Lactose- and gluten-free. Neutral flavour. Net price 300 g = £12.00; 8 × 15-g sachets = £5.12. For biochemically proven hypoproteinaemia

Formance® (Abbott)

Semi-solid, protein 6.8 g, carbohydrate 34.0 g, fat 9.7 g, energy 1052 kJ (250 kcal)/142 g with vitamins and minerals. Gluten-free. Vanilla, chocolate, and butterscotch flavours. Net price 142-g can = £1.76. As a necessary nutritional supplement prescribed on medical grounds for: short bowel syndrome, intractable malabsorption, pre-operative preparation of patients who are undernourished, proven inflammatory bowel disease, following total gastrectomy, dysphagia, bowel fistulas, disease-related malnutrition, continuous ambulatory peritoneal dialysis (CAPD), and haemodialysis. Not to be prescribed for any child under one year; use with caution for young children up to 5 years of age

Fortical® *see* Polycal® Liquid

Fortijuce® (Nutricia Clinical)

Liquid, protein 8 g, carbohydrate 56.8 g, energy 1046 kJ (250 kcal)/200 mL, with vitamins, minerals and trace elements. Fat-free. Flavours: lemon and lime, peach and orange, summer fruit. Net price 200-mL carton = £1.50. As a necessary nutritional supplement prescribed on medical grounds for: short-bowel syndrome, intractable malabsorption, pre-operative preparation of patients who are undernourished, proven inflammatory bowel disease, following total gastrectomy, dysphagia, bowel fistulas, disease-related malnutrition. Not to be prescribed for any child under 1 year; use with caution for young children up to 5 years of age

Fortimel® (Nutricia Clinical)

Liquid, protein 19.4 g, carbohydrate 20.8 g, fat 4.2 g, energy 840 kJ (200 kcal)/200 mL with vitamins and minerals. Vanilla, strawberry, chocolate, coffee, apricot, and forest fruits flavours. Net price 200-mL carton = £1.16. As a necessary nutritional supplement prescribed on medical grounds for: short bowel syndrome, intractable malabsorption, pre-operative preparation of patients who are undernourished, proven inflammatory bowel disease, following total gastrectomy, dysphagia, bowel fistulas, disease-related malnutrition. Not to be prescribed for any child under one year; use with caution for young children up to 5 years of age

Fortipudding® (Nutricia Clinical)

Semi-solid, protein 15.3 g, carbohydrate 24 g, fat 4.5 g, energy 840 kJ (198 kcal)/150 g with vitamins and minerals. Vanilla, chocolate, and coffee flavours. Net price 150-g tub = £1.31. As a necessary nutritional supplement prescribed on medical grounds for: short bowel syndrome, intractable malabsorption, pre-operative preparation of patients who are undernourished, proven inflammatory bowel disease, following total gastrectomy, dysphagia, bowel fistulas, disease-related malnutrition, continuous ambulatory peritoneal dialysis (CAPD) and haemodialysis. Not to be prescribed for any child under one year; use with caution for young children up to 5 years of age

Fortisip® (Nutricia Clinical)

Liquid, protein 10 g, carbohydrate 35.8 g, fat 13 g, energy 1260 kJ (300 kcal)/200 mL, with vitamins, minerals and trace elements. Gluten-free and low lactose. Vanilla, banana, orange, strawberry, tropical fruits, toffee, chicken, mushroom, and neutral flavours. Net price 200 mL = £1.46. As a necessary nutritional supplement

prescribed on medical grounds for: short-bowel syndrome, intractable malabsorption, pre-operative preparation of patients who are undernourished, proven inflammatory bowel disease, following total gastrectomy, dysphagia, bowel fistulas, disease-related malnutrition. Not to be prescribed for any child under one year; use with caution for young children up to 5 years of age

Fresenius OPD® (Fresenius)

Liquid, protein 22.5 g, carbohydrate 75 g, fat 13 g, energy 2100 kJ (500 kcal)/500 mL, with vitamins, minerals, and trace elements. Gluten-free, and low lactose. Net price 500-mL bottle = £3.99. As a necessary nutritional supplement prescribed on medical grounds for: short bowel syndrome, intractable malabsorption, pre-operative preparation of patients who are undernourished, proven inflammatory bowel disease, following total gastrectomy, dysphagia, bowel fistulas, disease-related malnutrition. Not to be prescribed for any child under one year; use with caution for young children up to 5 years of age

Fresubin® (Fresenius)

Liquid, protein 7.6 g, carbohydrate 27.6 g, fat 6.8 g, energy 840 kJ (200 kcal)/200 mL with vitamins and minerals. Gluten-free, low lactose and cholesterol. Net price 200-mL Tetrabrik (nut, peach, black currant, chocolate, mocha, vanilla, and neutral flavours) = £1.15; 500-mL bottle (nut, peach, vanilla and neutral flavours) = £2.60. For use as the sole source of nutrition or as a necessary nutritional supplement prescribed on medical grounds for: short-bowel syndrome, intractable malabsorption, pre-operative preparation of patients who are undernourished, proven inflammatory bowel disease, following total gastrectomy, dysphagia, bowel fistulas, disease-related malnutrition, and Refsum's disease. Not to be prescribed for any child under one year; use with caution for young children up to 5 years of age

High Energy Liquid, replaced by Entera® 500 mL bottle

Fresubin Isofibre® (Fresenius)

Liquid with dietary fibre, protein 19 g, carbohydrate 69 g, fat 17 g, energy 2100 kJ (500 kcal)/500 mL, with vitamins and minerals. Net price 500-mL bottle = £3.10. Neutral flavour. For use as sole source of nutrition or as a necessary nutritional supplement prescribed on medical grounds for: short-bowel syndrome, intractable malabsorption, pre-operative preparation of patients who are undernourished, proven inflammatory bowel disease, following total gastrectomy, dysphagia, disease-related malnutrition. Not to be prescribed for any child under 2 years; use with caution for young children up to 5 years of age

Fresubin Plus F® (Fresenius)

Liquid foods with dietary fibre in 2 formulations. For use as the sole source of nutrition or as a necessary nutritional supplement prescribed on medical grounds for: short-bowel syndrome, intractable malabsorption, pre-operative preparation of patients who are undernourished, proven inflammatory bowel disease, following total gastrectomy, dysphagia, disease-related malnutrition. Not to be prescribed for any child under 1 year; use with caution for young children up to 5 years of age

Muesli-flavour, milk protein, cereals, coconut, sunflower oil, vitamins and minerals providing protein 19 g, fat 17 g, carbohydrate 69 g, fibre 5 g, energy 2100 kJ (500 kcal)/500 mL. Low sodium, lactose, and cholesterol. Net price 200-mL carton = £1.15; 500-mL bottle £2.65

Vegetable soup-flavour, milk protein, beef fat and protein, sunflower oil, maize starch, vitamins and minerals providing protein 19 g, fat 17 g, carbohydrate 69 g, fibre 3 g, energy 2100 kJ (500 kcal)/500 mL. Gluten-free, low sodium, lactose, and cholesterol. Net price 200-mL bottle = £1.30

Fresubin 750® (Fresenius)

Liquid, protein 37.5 g, carbohydrate 85 g, fat 30 g, energy 3150 kJ (750 kcal)/500 mL with vitamins, minerals, and trace elements. Gluten-free and low lactose. Vanilla flavour. Net price 500-mL bottle = £2.75. As a necessary nutritional supplement prescribed on medical grounds for: short bowel syndrome, intractable malabsorption, pre-operative preparation of patients who are undernourished, proven inflammatory bowel disease, following total gastrectomy, dysphagia, bowel fistulas, disease-related malnutrition, continuous ambulatory peritoneal dialysis (CAPD), and haemodialysis. Not to be prescribed for any child under one year; use with caution for young children up to 5 years of age

Fructose (laevulose). For proven glucose/galactose intolerance

Galactomin® (Cow & Gate)

Formula 17, powder, protein 14.5 g, fat 25.9 g, carbohydrate 56.9 g, mineral salts 3.4 g/100 g. Used as a 13.1% solution with additional vitamins in place of milk. Net price 400 g = £9.30. For proven lactose intolerance in preschool children, galactosaemia and galactokinase deficiency

Formula 19, powder, protein 14.6 g, fat 30.8 g, carbohydrate 49.7 g (fructose as carbohydrate source), mineral salts 2.1 g/100 g, with vitamins. Used as a 12.9% solution in place of milk. Net price 400 g = £24.50. For glucose plus galactose intolerance

Generaid® (Scientific Hospital Supplies)

Powder, whey protein and additional branched-chain amino acids (protein equivalent 81%). Net price 200 g (unflavoured) = £20.39. For patients with chronic liver disease and/or porto-hepatic encephalopathy

Plus Powder, whey protein and additional branched-chain amino acids (protein equivalent 11%) carbohydrate 62%, fat 19% with vitamins, minerals and trace elements. Net price 400 g = £13.75. For children over one year of age with hepatic disorders

Glucose (dextrose monohydrate). Net price 100 g = 20p. For glycogen storage disease and sucrose/isomaltose intolerance

Glutafin® (Nutricia Dietary)

Gluten-free. Bread (whole or sliced), net price 400-g loaf = £2.30. Fibre bread (whole or sliced), 400-g loaf = £2.30. Bread with soya bran (dispensed in tin), 280 g = £1.56. White loaf (sliced or unsliced), 400 g = £2.59. White rolls, 400 g = £2.59. Mix, 500 g = £4.83. Baking mix, 500 g = £4.83. Fibre mix, 500 g = £4.83. Biscuits, savoury or tea, 125 g = £1.43. Biscuits, digestive or sweet, 150 g = £1.43. Biscuits, 200 g = £3.21. Crackers, 200 g = £2.34. High fibre crackers, 200 g = £1.96. Pasta (macaroni, pasta spirals, spaghetti short cut), 500 g = £4.88; (lasagne, tagliatelle), 250 g = £2.56. For gluten-sensitive enteropathies including steatorrhoea due to gluten sensitivity, coeliac disease, and dermatitis herpetiformis

Glutano® (Gluten Free Foods)

Gluten-free. Biscuits, net price 125 g = £1.09. Crackers, 150 g = £1.43. Flour mix, 750 g = £4.12. Pasta (macaroni, spaghetti, spirals, tagliatelle), 250 g = £1.68. Wholemeal bread (sliced or par-baked), 500 g = £2.24. For gluten-sensitive enteropathies including steatorrhoea due to gluten sensitivity, coeliac disease, and dermatitis herpetiformis

Hycal® (SmithKline Beecham Healthcare)

Liquid, protein-free, low-electrolyte, glucose syrup solids 49.5%. Flavours: blackcurrant, lemon, orange, and raspberry. Net price 171 mL = 73p. For renal failure; liver cirrhosis or other conditions requiring a high-energy, low-fluid, low-electrolyte diet

InfaSoy® (Cow & Gate)

Powder, carbohydrate 7.1%, fat 3.6%, and protein 1.8% with vitamins and minerals when used as a 12.7% solution. Net price 450 g = £3.42; 900 g = £6.60. For proven lactose and associated sucrose intolerance in preschool

children, galactokinase deficiency, galactosaemia, and proven whole cow's milk sensitivity

Instant Carobel® see **Carobel, Instant**®

Isomil® (Abbott)

Powder, protein 1.8%, carbohydrate 6.9%, fat 3.7% with vitamins and minerals when reconstituted. Lactose-free. Net price 400 g = £3.38. For proven lactose intolerance in preschool children, galactokinase deficiency, galactosaemia, and proven whole cow's milk sensitivity

Jevity® (Abbott)

Liquid, protein 4 g, fat 3.5 g, carbohydrate 13.1 g, dietary fibre 1.4 g, energy 421 kJ (100 kcal)/100 mL, with vitamins and minerals. Gluten-, lactose-, and sucrose-free. Net price 500-mL bottle = £3.10, 1-litre bottle = £6.20. For use as the sole source of nutrition or as a necessary nutritional supplement prescribed on medical grounds for: short bowel syndrome, intractable malabsorption, pre-operative preparation of patients who are undernourished, proven inflammatory bowel disease, following total gastrectomy, dysphagia, disease-related malnutrition. Not to be prescribed for any child under 1 year; use with caution for young children up to 5 years of age

Juvela® (Scientific Hospital Supplies)

Gluten-free. Corn mix, fibre mix, and flour mix, net price 500 g = £4.80. Bread (whole or sliced), 400-g loaf = £2.28. Fibre bread (sliced and unsliced), 400-g loaf = £2.28. Bread rolls, 3 × 5 = £7.74, fibre bread rolls, 3 × 5 = £7.74. Crispbread, 360 g = £4.60. Digestive biscuits, 160 g = £1.69. Tea biscuits, 160 g = £1.69. For gluten-sensitive enteropathies including steatorrhoea due to gluten sensitivity, coeliac disease, and dermatitis herpetiformis

Low Protein. Mix, net price 500 g = £4.80. Bread, (whole or sliced) 400-g loaf = £2.28. Bread rolls, 3 × 5 rolls = £7.56. Biscuits, orange and cinnamon flavour, 150 g = £4.48; chocolate chip, 130 g = £4.48. For inherited metabolic disorders, renal or liver failure requiring a low-protein diet

Kindergen PROD® (Scientific Hospital Supplies)

Powder, protein 7.6 g, carbohydrate 60.6 g, fat 26.1 g, energy 2060 kJ (492 kcal)/100 g with vitamins and minerals. Net price 400 g = £14.06. For complete nutritional support or supplementary feeding for infants and children with chronic renal failure who are receiving peritoneal rapid overnight dialysis

Leucine-Free Amino Acid Mix *see* Amino Acid Modules

Lifestyle® (Ultrapharm)

Gluten-free. Brown bread (sliced and unsliced). Net price 400-g loaf = £2.16. White bread (sliced and unsliced), 400-g loaf = £2.16. High fibre bread (unsliced), 400 g = £2.16. Bread rolls, 400 g = £2.16. For gluten-sensitive enteropathies including steatorrhoea due to gluten sensitivity, coeliac disease, and dermatitis herpetiformis

Liga® (Jacobs)

Rusks, gluten-free, low sugar. Net price 6 = 88p. For gluten-sensitive enteropathies including steatorrhoea due to gluten sensitivity, coeliac disease, and dermatitis herpetiformis

Liquigen® (Scientific Hospital Supplies)

Emulsion, medium chain triglycerides 52%. Net price 250 mL = £5.58; 1 litre = £20.60. For steatorrhoea associated with cystic fibrosis of the pancreas; intestinal lymphangiectasia, surgery of the intestine; chronic liver disease and liver cirrhosis; other proven malabsorption syndromes; ketogenic diet in the management of epilepsy; type I hyperlipoproteinaemia

Liquisorbon MCT® (Nutricia Clinical)

Liquid, protein 25 g, carbohydrate 61.5 g, fat 16.5 g, energy 2095 kJ (500 kcal)/500 mL with vitamins and minerals. Gluten- and fructose-free, low-lactose. Vanilla flavour. Net price 500 mL = £2.80. As a necessary nutritional supplement prescribed on medical grounds for: short bowel syndrome, intractable malabsorption, pre-operative preparation of patients who are undernourished, proven inflammatory bowel disease; following total gastrectomy, dysphagia, bowel fistulas, disease-related malnutrition. Not to be prescribed for any child under one year; use with caution for young children up to 5 years of age

Locasol® (Cow & Gate)

Powder, protein 14.6 g, carbohydrate 56.5 g, fat 26.1 g, mineral salts 1.9 g, not more than 55 mg of Ca^{2+}/100 g and vitamins. Used as a 13.1% solution in place of milk. Net price 400 g = £12.93. For calcium intolerance

Lofenalac® (Bristol-Myers)

Powder, protein 15%, carbohydrate 60%, fat 18%, phenylalanine not more than 0.1% with vitamins and minerals. Gluten-, sucrose-, and lactose-free. Net price 450 g = £8.48. For phenylketonuria

Loprofin® (Nutricia Dietary)

Low protein. Sweet biscuits, net price 150 g = £1.43; chocolate cream-filled biscuits, 125 g = £1.43; cookies (chocolate chip or cinnamon), 100 g = £4.70; wafers (orange, vanilla, or chocolate), 100 g = £1.40. Egg replacer, 250 g = £4.01. Bread (sliced or whole), net price 400-g loaf = £2.30. Bread (white, with or without salt), 227 g = £1.56. Mix, 500 g = £4.83. Crackers, 150 g = £1.96. Pasta (macaroni, pasta spirals, spaghetti, vermicelli), 250 g = £2.56. For inherited metabolic disorders, renal or liver failure requiring a low-protein diet

PKU Drink, protein 1 g (phenylalanine 30 mg), lactose 9.4 g, fat 4 g, energy 300 kJ (72 kcal)/200 mL. Net price 200-mL bottle = 47p. For phenylketonuria

Lorenzo's Oil (Scientific Hospital Supplies)

Liquid, glycerol trioleate oil 4 parts, glycerol trierucate oil 1 part. Net price 710 mL = £78.10. For biochemically proven and/or clinically manifest adrenoleukodystrophy

Low protein drink (Milupa)

Powder, protein 0.4%, carbohydrate 5.1%, fat 2% when reconstituted. Net price 400 g = £7.06. For inherited disorders of amino acid metabolism in childhood

Note. Termed Milupa lpd by manufacturer

Maxamaid® (Scientific Hospital Supplies)

Note. Maxamaid products are generally intended for use in children aged 1 to 8 years

MSUD Maxamaid, powder, essential and non-essential amino acids 30% except isoleucine, leucine, and valine, with carbohydrate, fat less than 0.5%, vitamins, minerals, and trace elements. Net price 500 g = £51.22. For maple syrup urine disease

RVHB Maxamaid, powder, essential and non-essential amino acids 30% except methionine, with carbohydrate, fat less than 0.5%, vitamins, minerals, and trace elements. Net price 500 g = £51.22. For hypermethioninaemia, homocystinuria

XLeu Maxamaid, powder, essential and non-essential amino acids 28.6% except leucine, with carbohydrate, fat less than 0.5%, vitamins, minerals, and trace elements. Net price 454 g = £46.51. For isovaleric acidaemia

XLys Maxamaid, powder, essential and non-essential amino acids 30% except lysine, with carbohydrate, fat less than 0.5%, vitamins, minerals, and trace elements. Net price 500 g = £51.22. For hyperlysinaemia

XLys,Try, Maxamaid, powder, essential and non-essential amino acids 30% except lysine and tryptophan, with carbohydrate, fat less than 0.5%, vitamins, minerals, and trace elements. Net price 500 g = £51.22. For glutaric aciduria

XMet, Thre, Val, Isoleu Maxamaid, powder, essential and non-essential amino acids 30% except methionine, threonine, valine and low isoleucine, with carbohydrate, fat less than 0.5%, vitamins, minerals, and trace elements. Net price 500 g = £51.22. For methylmalonic acidaemia or propionic acidaemia

XP Maxamaid, essential and non-essential amino acids 30% except phenylalanine, with carbohydrate, vitamins, minerals, and trace elements. Net price 25-g bar = £1.35; powder (unflavoured), 500 g = £32.29; (orange-fla-

voured), 500 g = £32.29. For phenylketonuria. Not to be prescribed for children under 2 years of age

Ingredients: of 25-g bar include arachis oil (peanut oil)

XP Maxamaid Concentrate, powder, essential and non-essential amino acids 65% except phenylalanine, with carbohydrate, fat less than 0.5%, vitamins, minerals, and trace elements. Unflavoured. Net price 200 g = £38.50. For phenylketonuria. Not to be prescribed for children under 2 years of age

XPhen, Tyr Maxamaid, powder, essential and non-essential amino acids 30% except phenylalanine and tyrosine, with carbohydrate, fat less than 0.5%, vitamins, minerals, and trace elements. Net price 500 g = £51.22. For tyrosinaemia

Maxamum® (Scientific Hospital Supplies)

Note. Maxamum products are generally intended for use in children over 8 years

MSUD Maxamum, powder, essential and non-essential amino acids 47% except isoleucine, leucine, and valine, with carbohydrate, fat less than 0.5%, vitamins, minerals, and trace elements. Orange-flavoured or unflavoured. Net price 500 g = £82.12. For maple syrup urine disease

RVHB Maxamum, powder, essential and non-essential amino acids 47% except methionine, with carbohydrate, fat less than 0.5%, vitamins, minerals, and trace elements. Unflavoured. Net price 500 g = £82.12. For hypermethioninaemia, homocystinuria

XMet, Thre, Val, Isoleu Maxamum, powder, essential and non-essential amino acids 47% except methionine, threonine, valine, and low isoleucine, with carbohydrate, fat less than 0.5%, vitamins, minerals, and trace elements. Unflavoured. Net price 500 g = £82.12. For methylmalonic acidaemia or propionic acidaemia

XP Maxamum, powder, essential and non-essential amino acids 47% except phenylalanine, with carbohydrates, vitamins, minerals, and trace elements. Orange flavoured or unflavoured. Net price 500 g = £49.90. For phenylketonuria. Not to be prescribed for children under 8 years

Maxijul® (Scientific Hospital Supplies)

Liquid, carbohydrate 50%, with potassium 0.004%, sodium 0.023%. Gluten-, lactose-, and fructose-free. Flavours: black currant, lemon and lime, orange, and natural. Net price 200 mL = 78p

Super Soluble Powder, glucose polymer, potassium 0.004%, sodium 0.046%. Gluten-, lactose-, and fructose-free. Net price 4 × 132-g sachet pack = £2.89, 200 g = £1.48, 2.5 kg = £12.31

Both for renal failure; liver cirrhosis; disaccharide intolerance (without isomaltose intolerance); disorders of amino acid metabolism (and other similar disorders) and/or whole protein intolerance; malabsorption states and other conditions, including proven hypoglycaemia, requiring a high-energy, low-fluid intake

Maxijul LE® (Scientific Hospital Supplies)

Powder, modification of Maxijul® with lower concentrations of sodium and potassium. Net price 200 g = £2.84, 2 kg = £18.86. For indications, see under Maxijul where sodium and/or potassium restriction is also essential

Maxipro Super Soluble® (Scientific Hospital Supplies)

Powder, whey protein and additional amino acids (protein equivalent 80%). Net price 200 g = £6.07; 1 kg = £24.28. For biochemically proven hypoproteinaemia. Not to be prescribed for any child under one year; unsuitable as a sole source of nutrition

Maxisorb® (Scientific Hospital Supplies)

Powder, protein 12 g, carbohydrate 9 g, fat 6 g, energy 565 kJ (135 kcal)/30 g with minerals. Vanilla, strawberry and chocolate flavours. Net price 5 x 30-g sachets = £2.61. As a necessary nutritional supplement prescribed on medical grounds for: short bowel syndrome, intractable malabsorption, pre-operative preparation of patients who are undernourished, proven inflammatory bowel disease, following total gastrectomy, dysphagia, bowel fistulas, disease-related malnutrition, continuous ambulatory peritoneal dialysis (CAPD) and haemodialysis. Not to be prescribed for any child under one year; use with caution for young children up to 5 years of age

MCT Oil

Triglycerides from medium chain fatty acids. For steatorrhoea associated with cystic fibrosis of the pancreas; intestinal lymphangiectasia; surgery of the intestine; chronic liver disease and liver cirrhosis; other proven malabsorption syndromes; in a ketogenic diet in the management of epilepsy; in type I hyperlipoproteinaemia

Available from Bristol-Myers (net price 950 mL = £8.50); Cow & Gate (net price 500 mL = £7.27)

MCT (1) replaced by Caprilon Formula®

MCT Pepdite® (Scientific Hospital Supplies)

Powder, essential and non-essential amino acids, peptides, medium chain triglycerides, monoglyceride of sunflower oil, with carbohydrate, fat, vitamins, minerals, and trace elements.

MCT Pepdite 0–2. Net price 400 g = £11.43

MCT Pepdite 2+. Net price 400 g = £11.43

Both for disorders in which a high intake of medium chain triglyceride is beneficial

Metabolic Mineral Mixture® (Scientific Hospital Supplies)

Powder, essential mineral salts. Net price 100 g = £7.10. For mineral supplementation in synthetic diets

Methionine-Free Amino Acid Mix see Amino Acid Modules

Methionine, Threonine, Valine-Free and Isoleucine-Low Amino Acid Mix see Amino Acid Modules

Milupa® Low Protein Drink see under Low Protein Drink

Milupa® PKU2 and PKU3 see under PKU2 and PKU3

MSUD Aid III® (Scientific Hospital Supplies)

Powder, containing full range of amino acids except isoleucine, leucine, and valine, with vitamins, minerals, and trace elements. Net price 200 g = £49.59. For maple syrup urine disease and related conditions where it is necessary to limit the intake of branched chain amino acids

Neocate® (Scientific Hospital Supplies)

Powder, essential and non-essential amino acids, maltodextrin, fat, vitamins, minerals, and trace elements. Net price 400 g = £17.75. For proven whole protein intolerance, short bowel syndrome, intractable malabsorption, proven inflammatory bowel disease, and bowel fistulas

Nepro® (Abbott)

Liquid, protein 16.6 g, carbohydrate 51.1 g, fat 22.7 g, energy 1991 kJ (475 kcal)/237 mL with vitamins and minerals. Net price 237-mL can = £2.28. For patients with chronic renal failure who are on haemodialysis or continuous ambulatory peritoneal dialysis (CAPD), or patients with cirrhosis or other conditions requiring a high energy, low fluid, low electrolyte diet

Nestargel® (Nestlé)

Powder, carob seed flour 96.5%, calcium lactate 3.5%. Net price 125 g = £3.46. For thickening feeds in the treatment of vomiting

Nutramigen® (Bristol-Myers)

Powder, protein 13%, carbohydrate 62%, fat 18% with vitamins and minerals. Gluten-, sucrose-, and lactose-free. Net price 425 g = £7.21. For disaccharide and/or whole protein intolerance where additional medium chain triglyceride is not indicated

Nutrison® (Nutricia Clinical)

Energy Plus, liquid, protein 30 g, carbohydrate 92 g, fat 29 g, energy 3200 kJ (755 kcal)/500 mL. Net price 500 mL = £3.09; 1 litre (Steriflo®) = £6.18. As a necessary nutritional supplement prescribed on medical grounds for: short bowel syndrome, intractable malabsorption, pre-operative preparation of patients who are undernourished, proven inflammatory bowel disease, following total gastrectomy, dysphagia, bowel fis-

tulas, disease-related malnutrition. Not to be prescribed for any child under one year; use with caution for young children up to 5 years of age

Fibre, liquid, protein 20 g, carbohydrate 61.5 g, fat 19.5 g, fibre 7.5 g, energy 2125 kJ (505 kcal)/500 mL. Net price 500-mL bottle = £2.99; 1 litre (Steriflo®) = £5.98. For use as the sole source of nutrition or as a necessary nutritional supplement prescribed on medical grounds for: short bowel syndrome, intractable malabsorption, pre-operative preparation of patients who are undernourished, proven inflammatory bowel disease, following total gastrectomy, dysphagia, disease-related malnutrition. Not to be prescribed for any child under one year; use with caution for young children up to 5 years of age

Soya, liquid, protein 20 g, carbohydrate 61.5 g, fat 19.5 g, energy 2125 kJ (505 kcal)/500 mL, with vitamins and minerals. Gluten-free. Net price 500 mL = £2.87; 1 litre (Steriflo®) = £6.00. For milk intolerance and lactose intolerance. Not to be prescribed for any child under one year; unsuitable as a sole source of nutrition for young children up to 5 years of age

Standard, liquid, protein 20 g, carbohydrate 61.5 g, fat 19.5 g, energy 2125 kJ (505 kcal)/500 mL, with vitamins and minerals. Net price 500 mL = £2.73; 1 litre (Steriflo®) = £5.46. For use as the sole source of nutrition or as a necessary nutritional supplement prescribed on medical grounds for: short bowel syndrome, intractable malabsorption, pre-operative preparation of patients who are undernourished, proven inflammatory bowel disease, following total gastrectomy, dysphagia, bowel fistulas, disease-related malnutrition. Not to be prescribed for any child under one year; use with caution for young children up to 5 years of age

Nutrison Paediatric® (Nutricia Clinical)

Energy Plus, liquid, protein 6.8 g, carbohydrate 37.6 g, fat 13.6 g, energy 1260 kJ (300 kcal)/200 mL. Net price 200-mL bottle = £2.19. For use as the sole source of nutrition or as a necessary nutritional supplement prescribed on medical grounds for: disease-related malnutrition and growth failure

Standard, liquid, protein 5.5 g, carbohydrate 24.4 g, fat 9 g, energy 840 kJ (200 kcal)/200 mL. Net price 200-mL bottle = £1.82. For use as the sole source of nutrition or as a necessary nutritional supplement prescribed on medical grounds for: short bowel syndrome, intractable malabsorption, pre-operative preparation of patients who are undernourished, dysphagia, bowel fistulas, disease-related malnutrition and/or growth failure. Not to be prescribed for any child under one year

Osmolite® (Abbott)

Liquid, protein 10.0 g, carbohydrate 34 g, fat 8.5 g, energy 1060 kJ (253 kcal)/250 mL with vitamins and minerals. Gluten- and lactose-free. Net price 250-mL can = £1.37; 500-mL bottle = £2.73, 1-litre bottle = £5.46. For use as the sole source of nutrition or as a necessary nutritional supplement prescribed on medical grounds for: short-bowel syndrome, intractable malabsorption, pre-operative preparation of patients who are undernourished, proven inflammatory bowel disease, following total gastrectomy, dysphagia, bowel fistulas, disease-related malnutrition. Not to be prescribed for any child under one year; use with caution for young children up to 5 years of age

OsterSoy® see Farley's Soya Formula

Paediasure® (Abbott)

Liquid, protein 7.5 g, fat 15.5 g, carbohydrate 27.4 g, with minerals and vitamins, gluten-free, energy 1054 kJ (252 kcal)/250 mL. Vanilla flavour. Net price 250-mL can = £2.26. For use as the sole source of nutrition or as a necessary nutritional supplement prescribed on medical grounds for: short-bowel syndrome, intractable malabsorption, pre-operative preparation of patients who are undernourished, dysphagia, bowel fistulas, and disease-related malnutrition and/or growth failure. Not to be prescribed for any child under one year

Paediatric Seravit® (Scientific Hospital Supplies)

Powder, vitamins, minerals, low sodium and potassium, and trace elements. Net price 200 g (unflavoured) = £10.00; pineapple flavour, 200 g = £10.66. For vitamin and mineral supplementation in restrictive therapeutic diets in infants and children

Pepdite® (Scientific Hospital Supplies)

Powder, essential and non-essential amino acids, peptides, with carbohydrate, fat, vitamins, minerals, and trace elements.

Pepdite 0–2. Providing 1925 kJ (460 kcal)/100 g. Net price 400 g = £10.39

Ingredients: include arachis oil (peanut oil)

Pepdite 2+. Providing 1787 kJ (425 kcal)/100 g. Net price 400 g = £10.39

Both for disaccharide and/or whole protein intolerance, or where amino acids or peptides are indicated in conjunction with medium chain triglycerides

Peptamen® (Clintec)

Liquid, protein 4%, carbohydrate 12.7%, fat 3.9%, energy 420 kJ (100 kcal)/100 mL, with vitamins and minerals. Lactose- and gluten-free. Vanilla flavour. Net price 250-mL can = £2.95; 1 litre (spike and hang) = £13.50. For use as the sole source of nutrition or as a necessary nutritional supplement prescribed on medical grounds for: short bowel syndrome, intractable malabsorption, proven inflammatory bowel disease, bowel fistulas. Not to be prescribed for any child under one year; use with caution for young children up to 5 years of age

Flavour sachets, citrus, chocolate, vanilla, strawberry, cappucino flavours. Net price 24-sachet pack = £7.50. For use with vanilla Peptamen®

Pepti-2000 LF® (Nutricia Clinical)

Liquid, protein 20 g, fat 5 g, carbohydrate 94 g, energy 2100 kJ (500 kcal)/500 mL with vitamins and minerals. Gluten-free. Net price 500 mL = £3.87; 1 litre (Steriflo®) = £7.74

Powder, same composition as Pepti-2000 LF® liquid when reconstituted. Net price 126-g sachet = £4.60

Both for use as the sole source of nutrition or as a necessary nutritional supplement prescribed on medical grounds for: short bowel syndrome, intractable malabsorption, proven inflammatory bowel disease, bowel fistulas. Not to be prescribed for any child under one year; use with caution for young children up to 5 years of age

Pepti-Junior® (Cow & Gate)

Powder, protein 15.3 g, fat 28.3 g, carbohydrate 55.1 g, energy 2140 kJ (507 kcal)/100 g with vitamins and minerals. Used as a 13.1% solution in place of milk. Net price 450 g = £8.22. For disaccharide and/or whole protein intolerance or where amino acids and peptides are indicated in conjunction with medium chain triglycerides

Perative® (Abbott)

Liquid, providing protein 15.8 g, carbohydrate 42 g, fat 8.8 g, energy 1308 kJ (310 kcal)/237 mL, with vitamins and minerals. Gluten-free, unflavoured. Net price 237-mL can = £2.49, 1-litre bottle = £9.96. For use as a necessary nutritional supplement prescribed on medical grounds for: short-bowel syndrome, intractable malabsorption, pre-operative preparation of patients who are undernourished, proven inflammatory bowel disease, following total gastrectomy, bowel fistulas, disease-related malnutrition. Not to be prescribed for any child under 5 years of age

Phenylalanine, Tyrosine and Methionine-Free Amino Acid Mix *see* Amino Acid Modules

Phlexy-10® Exchange System (Scientific Hospital Supplies)

Bar, essential and non-essential amino acids except phenylalanine 8.33 g, carbohydrate 20.5 g, fat 4.5 g/42-g bar. Citrus fruit flavour. Net price per bar = £3.61

Capsules, essential and non-essential amino acids except phenylalanine 416 mg/capsule. Net price 200-cap pack = £23.69

Drink Mix, powder, containing essential and non-essential amino acids except phenylalanine 10 g, carbohydrate 6.8 g/20-g sachet. Blackcurrant and apple flavour. Net price 20-g sachet = £2.37

All for phenylketonuria

PK Aid 3® (Scientific Hospital Supplies)

Powder, containing essential and non-essential amino acids except phenylalanine. Net price 500 g = £81.84. For phenylketonuria

PKU 2® (Milupa)

Granules, containing essential and non-essential amino acids except phenylalanine; with vitamins, minerals, trace elements, 7.1% sucrose. Flavour: vanilla. Net price 500 g = £49.73. For phenylketonuria

PKU 3® (Milupa)

Granules, containing essential and non-essential amino acids except phenylalanine, vitamins, minerals, and trace elements, with 3.4% sucrose. Flavour vanilla. Net price 500 g = £49.73. For phenylketonuria, not recommended for child under 8 years

Polial® (Ultrapharm)

Biscuits. Gluten- and lactose-free. Net price 200-g pack = £2.85. For gluten-sensitive enteropathies including steatorrhea due to gluten sensitivity, coeliac disease, and dermatitis herpetiformis

Polycal® (Nutricia Clinical)

Powder, glucose, maltose, and polysaccharides, providing 161 kJ (380 kcal)/100 g. Net price 400 g = £2.73. For renal failure; liver cirrhosis; disaccharide intolerance (without isomaltose intolerance); disorders of amino acid metabolism (and other similar disorders) and/or whole protein intolerance; malabsorption states and other conditions, including proven hypoglycaemia, requiring a high-energy, low-fluid intake, whether or not sodium and/or potassium restriction is essential

Liquid [formerly Fortical® liquid], glucose polymers providing carbohydrate 61.5 g/100 mL. Low-electrolyte, protein-free. Flavours: apple, black currant, lemon, orange, and neutral. Net price 200 mL = £1.07. For renal failure; liver cirrhosis, disaccharide intolerance (without isomaltose intolerance), disorders of amino acid metabolism, and/or whole protein intolerance, malabsorption states, or other conditions including proven hypoglycaemia requiring a high-energy, low-fluid, low-electrolyte diet

Polycose® (Abbott)

Powder, glucose polymers, providing carbohydrate 94 g, energy 1598 kJ (376 kcal)/100 g. Net price 350-g can = £3.22. For renal failure; liver cirrhosis; disaccharide intolerance (without isomaltose intolerance); disorders of amino acid metabolism (and other similar disorders) and/or whole protein intolerance; malabsorption states and other conditions, including proven hypoglycaemia, requiring a high-energy, low-fluid intake, whether or not sodium and/or potassium restriction is essential

Portagen® (Bristol-Myers)

Powder, protein 16.5%, carbohydrate 54%, fat 22% with vitamins and minerals. Gluten- and lactose-free. Net price 454 g = £6.23. For disorders in which a high intake of medium chain triglycerides is beneficial

Pregestimil® (Bristol-Myers)

Powder, protein 12.8%, carbohydrate 61.6%, fat 18.3% with vitamins and minerals. Gluten-, sucrose-, and lactose-free. Net price 450 g = £8.25. For disaccharide and/or whole protein intolerance or where amino acids or peptides are indicated in conjunction with medium chain triglycerides

Prejomin® (Milupa)

Granules, protein 13.3 g, carbohydrate 57 g, fat 24.2 g, energy 2090 kJ (499 kcal)/100 g, with vitamins and minerals. Gluten-free. For preparation with water before use. Net price 400 g = £9.22. For disaccharide and/or

---

whole protein intolerance where additional medium chain triglyceride is not indicated

ProMod® (Abbott)

Powder, protein 75 g, carbohydrate 7.5 g, fat 6.9 g/100 g. Gluten-free. Net price 275-g can = £8.60. For biochemically proven hypoproteinaemia

Prosobee® (Bristol-Myers)

Liquid concentrate, protein 4.1%, carbohydrate 13.7%, fat 7.2% with vitamins, minerals. Gluten-, sucrose-, and lactose-free. Net price 385 mL = £1.28

Powder, protein 15.6%, carbohydrate 51.4%, fat 27.9% with vitamins and minerals. Gluten-, sucrose-, and lactose-free. Net price 400 g = £3.22

Both for proven lactose and associated sucrose intolerance in pre-school children, galactokinase deficiency, galactosaemia, and proven whole cow's milk sensitivity

Protein Forte® (Fresenius)

Liquid, protein 20 g, carbohydrate 19 g, fat 5.2 g, energy 840 kJ (200 kcal)/200 mL, with vitamins, minerals, and trace elements. Gluten-free. Vanilla, strawberry, and chocolate flavours. Net price 200-mL Tetrabrik = £1.10. As a necessary nutritional supplement prescribed on medical grounds for: short bowel syndrome, intractable malabsorption, pre-operative preparation of patients who are undernourished, proven inflammatory bowel disease, following total gastrectomy, dysphagia, bowel fistulas, disease-related malnutrition, continuous ambulatory peritoneal dialysis (CAPD) and haemodialysis. Not to be prescribed for any child under one year; use with caution for young children up to 5 years of age

Protifar® (Nutricia Clinical)

Powder, protein 88.5%. Low lactose, gluten- and sucrose-free. Net price 225 g = £5.46. For biochemically proven hypoproteinaemia

Provide® (Fresenius)

Liquid, protein 9 g, carbohydrate 28 g, fat less than 1 g, energy 630 kJ (150 kcal)/250 mL with vitamins and minerals. Gluten- and lactose-free. Apple, black currant, lemon and lime, and tropical fruit flavour. Net price 250-mL Tetrabrik = £1.20. As a necessary nutritional supplement prescribed on medical grounds for: short bowel syndrome, intractable malabsorption, pre-operative preparation of patients who are undernourished, proven inflammatory bowel disease, following total gastrectomy, dysphagia, bowel fistulas, disease-related malnutrition. Not to be prescribed for any child under one year; use with caution for young children up to 5 years of age

Reabilan® (Clintec)

Liquid, protein 11.8 g, carbohydrate 49.3 g, fat 14.6 g, energy 1575 kJ (375 kcal)/375 mL with vitamins and minerals. Gluten- and lactose-free. Net price 375-mL can = £3.07; 500-mL Dripac = £4.57. For use as the sole source of nutrition or as a necessary nutritional supplement prescribed on medical grounds for: short bowel syndrome, intractable malabsorption, proven inflammatory bowel disease, bowel fistulas. Not to be prescribed for any child under 1 year; use with caution for young children up to 5 years of age

Rectified Spirit. Where the therapeutic qualities of alcohol are required rectified spirit (suitably flavoured and diluted) should be prescribed

Renamil® (Kimal)

Powder, protein 4.7 g, carbohydrate 70.2 g, fat 18.7 g, 1984 kJ (468 kcal)/100 g, with vitamins and minerals. Net price 1 kg = £26.60. For chronic renal failure. Not suitable for infants and children under 1 year of age

Renapro® (Kimal)

Powder, whey protein providing protein 92 g, carbohydrate < 300 mg, fat 500 mg, 1562 kJ (367 kcal)/100 g. Net price 100 g = £9.28. For dialysis and hypoproteinaemia. Not suitable for infants and children under 1 year of age

Rite-Diet® (Nutricia Dietary)

Gluten-free. Flour mix, net price 500 g = £4.83. Bread mix (brown and white), 500 g = £4.83. White bread (sliced and unsliced), 400 g = £2.30. Fibre bread (sliced and unsliced), 400 g = £2.30. White rolls, 4 = £2.30. Fibre rolls, 4 = £2.30. For gluten-sensitive enteropathies including steatorrhoea due to gluten sensitivity, coeliac disease, and dermatitis herpetiformis

Low protein. Baking mix. Net price 500 g = £4.83. Flour mix. 400 g = £4.83. White bread (with added fibre). 400 g = £2.30. For inherited metabolic disorders, renal or liver failure requiring a low-protein diet

Schar® (Ultrapharm)

Gluten-free. Bread. Net price 250 g = £1.41. Baguette (french bread), 400 g = £2.39. Bread rolls, 150 g = £1.41. Bread mix, 500 g = £3.95. Cake mix, 500 g = £3.95. Crackers, 200 g = £2.15. Crispbread, 250 g = £2.82. Pasta (fusilli, penne, rigatoni, tagliatelle), 250 g = £1.90; lasagna, 250 g = £2.80; spaghetti, 500 g = £3.41. Pizza bases, 250 g = £4.12. Savoy biscuits, 200 g = £2.15. For gluten-sensitive enteropathies including steatorrhoea due to gluten sensitivity, coeliac disease, and dermatitis herpetiformis

SHS Modjul® Flavour System (Scientific Hospital Supplies)

Powder, black currant, orange, pineapple, and savoury tomato flavours. Net price 100 g = £6.50. For use with any unflavoured products based on peptides or amino acids

Scandishake® (Scientific Hospital Supplies)

Powder, for reconstitution with milk. Flavours: chocolate, strawberry, vanilla. Net price 85 g sachet = £1.71. For malabsorption states and disease-related malnutrition

Sno-Pro® (Scientific Hospital Supplies)

Drink, protein 220 mg (phenylalanine 12.5 mg), carbohydrate 8 g, fat 3.8 g, energy 272 kJ (65 kcal)/100 mL. Net price 200 mL = 57p. For phenylketonuria, chronic renal failure, and other inborn errors of metabolism

Sunflower oil. Net price 100 mL = 39p. For familial hypercholesterolaemia (non-drug for multiple sclerosis)

Sunnyvale® (Everfresh)

Mixed grain bread, gluten-free. Net price 400 g = £1.31. For gluten-sensitive enteropathies including steatorrhoea due to gluten sensitivity, coeliac disease and dermatitis herpetiformis

Suplena® (Abbott)

Liquid, protein 6%, carbohydrate 51%, fat 43%, energy 1994 kJ (476 kcal)/237 mL. Flavour: vanilla. Net price 237-mL can = £2.28. For patients with chronic or acute renal failure who are not undergoing dialysis, chronic or acute liver disease with fluid restriction, other conditions requiring a high-energy, low-electrolyte, low-volume enteral feed

Thick and Easy® (Fresenius)

Powder. Modified maize starch. Net price 225-g can = £3.75. For thickening of foods in dysphagia. Not to be prescribed for children under one year except in cases of failure to thrive

Thixo-D® (Sutherland)

Powder, modified maize starch, gluten-free. Net price 375-g tub= £4.81. For thickening of foods in dysphagia. Not to be prescribed for children under one year except in cases of failure to thrive

Triosorbon® (Nutricia Clinical)

Powder, protein 19%, carbohydrate 56%, fat 19%, with vitamins and minerals. Gluten-free. Net price 85-g sachet = £1.74. For use as the sole source of nutrition or as a necessary nutritional supplement prescribed on medical grounds for: short-bowel syndrome, intractable malabsorption, pre-operative preparation of patients who are undernourished, proven inflammatory bowel disease, following total gastrectomy, dysphagia, bowel fistulas, disease-related malnutrition. Not to be prescribed for any child under one year; use with caution for young children up to 5 years of age

Trufree® (Cantassium)

Gluten-free, wheat-free flours. For gluten-sensitive enteropathies including steatorrhoea due to gluten sensitivity, coeliac disease, and dermatitis herpetiformis

No. 1, net price 1 kg = £5.06. *No. 2 with rice bran*, 1 kg = £5.40. *No. 3 for Cantabread®*, 1 kg = £5.78. *No. 4 white*, 1 kg = £5.06. *No. 5 brown*, 1 kg = £5.06. *No. 6 plain*, 1 kg = £4.88. *No. 7 self-raising*, 500 g = £2.63, 1 kg = £5.21

Tyrosine and Phenylalanine-Free Amino Acid Mix

see Amino Acid Modules

Ultra® (Ultrapharm)

Gluten-free. Bread, net price 400 g = £2.39. High-fibre bread, 500 g = £3.26. Bread rolls, 280 g = £2.39. Crackerbread, 100 g = £1.72. For gluten-sensitive enteropathies including steatorrhoea due to gluten sensitivity, coeliac disease and dermatitis herpetiformis

Low protein. Brown bread (canned). Net price 500 g = £3.80. White bread (canned), 350 g = £2.75. PKU bread, 400 g = £2.10. PKU flour, 500 g = £2.98. PKU biscuits, 200 g = £2.15. PKU cookies, 250 g = £2.25. PKU pizza base, 400 g = £2.15. PKU savoy biscuits, 150 g = £2.00. For inherited metabolic disorders, renal or liver failure requiring a low-protein diet

Valpiform® (General Dietary)

Gluten-free. Bread mix (wheat free). Net price 1 kg = £5.18. Pastry mix, 1 kg = £5.18. For gluten-sensitive enteropathies including steatorrhoea due to gluten sensitivity, coeliac disease, and dermatitis herpetiformis

Low protein. Shortbread biscuits. Net price 120 g = £3.38. For inherited metabolic disorders, renal or liver failure requiring a low-protein diet

Vitajoule® (Vitaflo)

Powder, glucose polymers, providing carbohydrate 96 g, energy 1610 kJ (380 kcal)/100 g. Net price 40 × 125 g = £31.20, 500 g = £2.21. For renal failure, liver cirrhosis, disaccharide intolerance (without isomaltose intolerance), disorders of amino acid metabolism (and other similar disorders), and/or whole protein intolerance, malabsorption states and other conditions, including proven hypoglycaemia, requiring a high energy, low fluid intake, whether or not sodium and/or potassium restriction is essential

Vitapro® (Vitaflo)

Powder, whole milk proteins, containing all essential amino acids, 75%. Net price 250 g = £4.38. For biochemically proven hypoproteinaemia

Vitaquick® (Vitaflo)

Powder. Modified maize starch. Net price 50 × 10-g sachet = £16.20, 100 g = £1.99, 250 g = £3.41; 1 kg = £10.79. For thickening of foods in dysphagia. Not to be prescribed for children under one year old except in cases of failure to thrive

Wysoy® (Wyeth)

Powder, carbohydrate 6.9%, fat 3.6%, and protein 2.1% with vitamins and minerals when reconstituted. Net price 430 g = £3.88; 860 g = £7.42. For proven lactose and associated sucrose intolerance in preschool children, galactokinase deficiency, galactosaemia and proven whole cow's milk sensitivity

CONDITIONS FOR WHICH FOODS MAY BE PRESCRIBED ON FP10

Note. This is a list of clinical conditions for which the ACBS has approved food products. It is essential to check the list of products (above) for availability.

Adrenoleukodystrophy: Lorenzo's Oil.

Amino acid metabolic disorders and similar protein disorders: low protein drink (Milupa); see also phenylketonuria; histidinaemia; homocystinuria; maple syrup urine disease; tyrosinaemia; synthetic diets; low-protein products.

Bowel fistulas:

Complete foods: Clinifeed Favour and Iso; Elemental 028; Elemental 028 Extra; Emsogen; Enrich; Ensure; Ensure Powder; Entera; Flexical; Fresubin Liquid and Sip Feeds, Plus F; Jevity; Nutrison Fibre, Paediatric and Standard; Osmolite; Paediasure; Peptamen; Pepti-2000 LF; Reabilan; Triosorbon.

Nutritional supplements: Advera; Clinifeed 400 and Protein Rich; Enlive; Ensure Plus; Formance; Fortijuce; Fortimel; Fortipudding; Fortisip; Fresenius OPD; Fresubin 750; Liquisorbon MCT; Maxisorb; Nutrison Energy Plus, Perative; Protein Forte; Provide.

Calcium intolerance: Locasol New Formula.

Carbohydrate malabsorption: Calogen. See also synthetic diets; malabsorption states.

Disaccharide intolerance (without isomaltose intolerance): Alfare; Caloreen; Calsip; Duocal Super Soluble and Duocal Liquid; Maxijul LE, Liquid, Super Soluble; Nutramigen; Pepdite; Pepti-Junior; Polycal; Polycal Liquid; Polycose powder; Pregestimil; Prejomin; Vitajoule. See also lactose intolerance; lactose with sucrose intolerance.

Glucose and galactose intolerance: Comminuted chicken meat (Cow & Gate); Fructose; Galactomin Formula 19 (fructose formula).

Isomaltose intolerance: Glucose (dextrose).

Lactose intolerance: AL 110; Comminuted chicken meat (Cow & Gate); Farley's Soya Formula; Galactomin Formula 17 (new formula); InfaSoy; Isomil powder; Nutramigen; Nutrison Soya; Pepdite; Portagen; Pregestimil; Prejomin; Prosobee; Wysoy.

Note. Defined as a condition of intolerance to an intake of the relevant disaccharide confirmed by demonstrated clinical benefit of the effectiveness of the disaccharide-free diet, and presence of reducing substances and/or excessive acid in the stools, a low concentration of the corresponding disaccharidase enzyme on intestinal biopsy, or by breath tests or lactose tolerance tests

Lactose with sucrose intolerance: Comminuted Chicken Meat (Cow & Gate); Farley's Soya Formula; Galactomin Formula 17 (new formula); InfaSoy; Nutramigen; Pepti-Junior; Pregestimil; Prejomin; Prosobee; Wysoy.

Note. Defined as a condition of intolerance to an intake of the relevant disaccharide confirmed by demonstrated clinical benefit of the effectiveness of the disaccharide-free diet, and presence of reducing substances and/or excessive acid in the stools, a low concentration of the corresponding disaccharidase enzyme on intestinal biopsy, or by breath tests or lactose tolerance tests

Sucrose intolerance: Glucose (dextrose) and see also synthetic diets; malabsorption states; lactose with sucrose intolerance.

Note. Defined as a condition of intolerance to an intake of the relevant disaccharide confirmed by demonstrated clinical benefit of the effectiveness of the disaccharide-free diet, and presence of reducing substances and/or excessive acid in the stools, a low concentration of the corresponding disaccharidase enzyme on intestinal biopsy, or by breath tests or lactose tolerance tests

Coeliac disease: see gluten-sensitive enteropathies.

Continuous Ambulatory Peritoneal Dialysis (CAPD): see dialysis.

Cystic fibrosis: see malabsorption states.

Dermatitis Herpetiformis: see gluten-sensitive enteropathies.

Dialysis: nutritional supplements for haemodialysis or continuous ambulatory peritoneal dialysis (CAPD) patients: Clinifeed 400 and Protein Rich; Ensure Plus; Formance; Fortipudding; Fresubin 750; Kindergen PROD; Maxisorb; Nepro; Protein Forte; Renapro; Suplena.

Disaccharide intolerance: see carbohydrate malabsorption.

Dysphagia:

Complete foods: Clinifeed Favour and Iso ; Enrich; Ensure; Ensure Powder; Entera; Fresubin Liquid and Sip Feeds, Isofibre, and Plus F; Jevity; Nutrison Fibre, Paediatric and Standard; Osmolite; Paediasure; Triosorbon.

Nutritional supplements: Advera; Clinifeed 400 and Protein Rich; Enlive; Ensure Plus; Formance; Fortijuce; Fortimel; Fortipudding; Fortisip; Fresenius OPD; Fresubin 750; Liquisorbon MCT; Maxisorb; Nutrison Energy Plus; Protein Forte; Provide.

Thickeners: Thick & Easy; Thixo-D; Vitaquick.

Note. Defined as that associated with intrinsic disease of the oesophagus, e.g. oesophagitis; neuromuscular disorders, e.g. multiple sclerosis and motor neurone disease; major surgery and/or radiotherapy for cancer of the upper digestive tract; protracted severe inflammatory disease of the upper digestive tract, e.g. Stevens-Johnson syndrome and epidermolysis bullosa

Epilepsy (ketogenic diet in): Alembicol D; Calogen; Liquigen; Medium-Chain Triglyceride Oil (MCT).

Flavouring for use with any unflavoured product based on peptides or amino acids: SHS Flavour Modjul

Galactokinase deficiency and galactosaemia:

AL 110; Farley's Soya Formula; Galactomin Formula 17 (new formula); InfaSoy; Isomil powder; Prosobee; Wysoy.

Gastrectomy (total):

Complete foods: Clinifeed Favour and Iso; Enrich; Ensure; Ensure Powder; Entera; Fresubin Liquid and Sip Feeds, Isofibre, and Plus F; Jevity; Nutrison Fibre and Standard; Osmolite; Triosorbon.

Nutritional supplements: Advera; Clinifeed 400 and Protein Rich; Enlive; Ensure Plus; Formance; Fortijuce; Fortimel; Fortipudding; Fortisip; Fresenius OPD; Fresubin 750; Liquisorbon MCT; Maxisorb; Nutrison Energy Plus; Perative; Protein Forte; Provide.

Glucose/galactose intolerance: Comminuted Chicken Meat (Cow & Gate); Galactomin Formula 19 (fructose formula); also see carbohydrate malabsorption.

Glutaric aciduria: XLys, Try Maxamaid

Gluten-sensitive enteropathies: Aproten flour; Arnott gluten-free rice cookies; Barkat gluten-free bread mix; Bi-Aglut biscuits, and gluten-free cracker toast; Bi Nua; Ener-G brown and white bread, gluten-free tapioca bread, gluten-free rice pasta (cannelloni, lasagna, macaroni, shells, small shells, spaghetti, tagliatelli, vermicelli); brown rice pasta (lasagna, macaroni, spaghetti); Glutafin bread, bread with soya bran (dispensed in tin), wheat-free white loaf (sliced or unsliced), wheat-free white rolls, fibre bread, baking mix, fibre mix, biscuits (digestive, savoury, sweet (without chocolate or sultanas), tea), crackers, high fibre crackers and pasta (spirals, macaroni, spaghetti , vermicelli); Glutano gluten-free biscuits, crackers, flour mix, pastas (macaroni, spaghetti, spirals, tagliatelle), wholemeal bread (sliced or par-baked); Juvela gluten-free corn mix, loaf and high-fibre loaf (sliced and unsliced), bread rolls, fibre bread rolls, crispbread, and fibre mix; digestive biscuits and tea biscuits; Lifestyle gluten-free bread rolls; Lifestyle brown and white bread; Liga gluten-free rusks (Jacobs); Polial gluten-free biscuits; Rite-Diet gluten-free fibre rolls, high-fibre bread (sliced and unsliced), white bread (sliced and unsliced), mixes (brown bread, flour, white bread), white rolls; Schar gluten-free bread, bread mix, bread rolls, cake mix, crackers, crispbread, pasta (fusilli, lasagna, penne, rigatoni, spaghetti, tagliatelli), pizza base, savoy biscuits; Sunnyvale gluten-free bread; Trufree special dietary flours No. 1, No. 2 with rice bran, No. 3 for Cantabread, No. 4 white, No. 5 brown, No. 6 plain, No. 7 self-raising; Ultra gluten-free high-fibre bread; Ultra gluten-free crackerbread; Valpiform bread mix, pastry mix.

Glycogen storage disease: Caloreen; Corn Flour or Corn Starch; Glucose (dextrose); Maxijul LE, Liquid (orange flavour), and Super Soluble; Polycal; Polycal Liquid; Polycose; Vitajoule.

Growth Failure (disease related): Nutrison Paediatric Standard and Energy Plus; Paediasure.

Haemodialysis: see dialysis.

Histidinaemia: see low-protein products; synthetic diets.

Homocystinuria: Analog RVHB; Methionine-Free Amino Acid Mix; RVHB Maxamaid; RVHB Maxamum, and see also low-protein products; synthetic diets.

Hypercholesterolaemia (familial): Corn oil; Sunflower oil.

Hyperlipoproteinaemia type 1: Liquigen; Medium Chain Triglyceride Oil.

Hyperlysinaemia: Analog XLys; XLys Maxamaid

Hypermethioninaemia: Analog RVHB; Methionine-Free Amino Acid Mix; RVHB Maxamaid; RVHB Maxamum.

Hypoglycaemia: Caloreen; Calsip; Corn Flour or Corn Starch; Maxijul LE, Liquid (orange flavour), and Super Soluble; Polycal; Polycal Liquid; Polycose; Vitajoule; and see also glycogen storage disease.

Hypoproteinaemia: Casilan; Dialamine; Forceval Protein; Maxipro Super Soluble; ProMod; Protifar; Renapro; Vitapro.

Inflammatory Bowel Disease:

Complete foods: Clinifeed Favour and Iso ; Elemental 028; Elemental 028 Extra; Emsogen; Enrich; Ensure; Ensure Powder; Entera; Flexical; Fresubin Liquid and Sip Feeds, Isofibre, and Plus F; Jevity; Nutrison Fibre and Standard; Osmolite; Peptamen; Pepti-2000 LF; Reabilan; Triosorbon.

Nutritional supplements: Advera; Clinifeed 400 and Protein Rich; Enlive; Ensure Plus; Formance; Fortijuce; Fortimel; Fortipudding; Fortisip; Fresenius OPD; Fresubin 750; Liquisorbon MCT; Maxisorb; Nutrison Energy Plus; Perative; Protein Forte; Provide.

Intestinal lymphangiectasia: see malabsorption states.

Intestinal surgery: see malabsorption states

Isomaltose intolerance: see carbohydrate malabsorption.

Isovaleric acidaemia: Leucine-Free Amino Acid Mix; X Leu Analog; XLeu Maxamaid.

Lactose intolerance: see carbohydrate malabsorption.

Liver failure: Aglutella low-protein rice; Alembicol D; Aminex low-protein rusks; Aproten products (anellini, biscuits, bread mix, cake mix, crispbread, ditalini, rigatini, spaghetti, tagliatelle); Caloreen; Calsip; dp Low-Protein butterscotch-flavoured or chocolate-flavoured chip cookies; Duobar; Duocal Super Soluble, and Duocal Liquid; Generaid; Generaid Plus; Hycal; Juvela low-protein (chocolate chip, orange, and cinnamon flavour) cookies, loaf (sliced and unsliced), bread rolls, mix; Liquigen; Loprofin egg replacer; Loprofin low-protein bread (sliced and unsliced), bread (with or without salt), mix, pasta (macaroni, spaghetti short-cut, pasta spirals, tagliatelle nests, vermicelli), sweet biscuits, chocolate cream-filled biscuits, crackers, cookies (chocolate chip, cinnamon), wafers (orange, chocolate, vanilla); Maxijul LE, Liquid, and Super Soluble; Medium Chain Triglyceride Oil; Nepro; Polycal; Polycal Liquid; Polycose; Portagen; Rite-Diet low-protein white bread (with added fibre), baking mix, flour mix; Suplena; Ultra low-protein, canned bread (brown and white); Ultra PKU biscuits, PKU bread, PKU cookies, PKU flour, PKU pizza base, PKU savoy biscuits; Valpiform shortbread biscuits; Vitajoule.

Low-protein products: Aglutella low-protein rice; Aminex low-protein rusks; Aproten products (anellini, biscuits, bread mix, cake mix, crispbread, ditalini, rigatini, spaghetti, tagliatelle); dp Low-Protein butter-scotch-flavoured or chocolate-flavoured chip cookies; Juvela low-protein (chocolate chip, orange, and cinnamon flavour) cookies, loaf (sliced and unsliced), mix, bread rolls; Loprofin egg replacer; Loprofin low-protein bread (sliced and unsliced), bread (with or without salt), mix, pasta (macaroni, spaghetti short-cut, pasta spirals, tagliatelle nests, vermicelli); sweet biscuits, chocolate cream-filled biscuits, crackers, cookies (chocolate chip, cinnamon), wafers (orange, chocolate, vanilla); Rite-Diet low-protein white bread (with added fibre), flour mix, baking mix; Ultra low-protein, canned bread (brown and white); Ultra PKU biscuits, PKU bread, PKU cookies, PKU flour, PKU pizza base, PKU savoy biscuits, Valpiform shortbread biscuits.

Malabsorption states: (see also gluten-sensitive enter-opathies; liver failure; carbohydrate malabsorption; intestinal lymphangiectasia; milk intolerance and synthetic diets).

(a) Protein sources: Caprilon Formula; Comminuted Chicken Meat (Cow & Gate); Duocal Super Soluble and Liquid; Forceval Protein; Maxipro Super Soluble; MCT Pepdite; Neocate; Pepdite.

(b) Fat sources: Alembicol D; Calogen; Caprilon Formula; Liquigen; MCT Pepdite; Medium Chain Triglyceride Oil.

(c) Carbohydrate: Caloreen; Calsip; Hycal; Maxijul LE, Liquid (orange flavour), and Super Soluble; Polycal; Polycal Liquid; Polycose; Vitajoule.

(d) Complete Feeds. For use as the sole source of nutrition or as a necessary nutritional supplement prescribed on medical grounds: Caprilon Formula; Clinifeed Favour and Iso; Elemental 028; Elemental 028 Extra; Emsogen; Enrich; Ensure; Ensure Powder; Entera; Flexical; Fresubin Liquid and Sip Feeds, Isofibre, and Plus F; Jevity; MCT Pepdite; Nutrison Fibre, Paediatric and Standard; Osmolite; Paediasure; Pepdite; Peptamen; Pepti-2000 LF; Pepti-Junior; Portagen; Pregestimil; Reabilan; Triosorbon.

(e) Nutritional supplements. Necessary nutritional supplements prescribed on medical grounds: Advera; Clinifeed 400 and Protein Rich; Enlive; Ensure Plus; Formance; Fortijuce; Fortimel; Fortipudding; Fortisip; Fresenius OPD; Fresubin 750; Liquisorbon MCT; Maxisorb; Nutrison Energy Plus; Perative; Protein Forte; Provide; Scandishake.

(f) Minerals: Aminogran Mineral Mixture; Metabolic Mineral Mixture.

(g) Vitamins: As appropriate, and see synthetic diets.

(h) Vitamins and Minerals: Paediatric Seravit

Malnutrition (disease-related):

Complete foods: Clinifeed Favour and Iso; Enrich; Ensure; Ensure Powder; Entera; Fresubin Liquid and Sip Feeds, Isofibre, and Plus F; Jevity; Nutrison Fibre, Paediatric and Standard; Osmolite; Paediasure; Triosorbon.

Nutritional supplements: Advera; Clinifeed 400 and Protein Rich; Ensure Plus; Formance; Fortijuce; Fortimel; Fortipudding; Fortisip; Fresenius OPD; Fresubin 750; Liquisorbon MCT; Maxisorb; Nutrison Energy Plus; Perative; Protein Forte; Provide; Scandishake.

Maple syrup urine disease: Analog MSUD; MSUD Maxamaid; MSUD Maxamum; MSUD Aid III, and see also low-protein products; synthetic diets.

Methylmalonic acidaemia: Analog XMet, Thre, Val, Isoleu; XMet, Thre, Val, Isoleu Maxamaid; XMet, Thre, Val, Isoleu Maxamum; Methionine, Threonine, Valine-Free and Isoleucine-Low Amino Acid Mix.

Milk protein sensitivity: Comminuted Chicken Meat (Cow & Gate); Farley's Soya Formula; InfaSoy; Isomil powder; Nutramigen; Nutrison Soya; Prosobee; Wysoy, and see also synthetic diets.

Nutritional support for adults (for precise conditions for which these products have ACBS approval, see products above):

A. **Nutritionally complete feeds.** For use as the sole source of nutrition or as a necessary nutritional supplement prescribed on medical grounds:

(i) Gluten-Free: Clinifeed Iso; Entera; Fresubin Liquid, Sip Feeds, and Plus F (vegetable soup flavour only); Nutrison Fibre and Standard; Triosorbon.

(ii) Lactose-free: Clinifeed Favour.

(iii) Lactose- and Gluten-Free: Enrich; Ensure, Ensure Powder; Fresubin Isofibre; Osmolite.

(iv) Containing fibre: Enrich; Fresubin Isofibre; Fresubin Plus F; Jevity; Nutrison Fibre.

(v) Elemental Feeds: Elemental 028; Elemental 028 Extra; Emsogen; Flexical; Peptamen; Pepti-2000 LF.

B. **Nutritional source supplements**: see synthetic diets; malabsorption states.

(a) General supplements. Necessary nutritional supplements prescribed on medical grounds: Advera; Clinifeed 400 and Protein Rich; Ensure Plus; Formance; Fortijuce; Fortimel; Fortipudding; Fortisip; Fresenius OPD; Fresubin 750; Liquisorbon MCT; Maxisorb; Nutrison Energy Plus; Perative; Protein Forte; Provide.

(b) Carbohydrates: lactose-free and gluten-free; Caloreen*; Duocal Super Soluble and Liquid*; Hycal*; Maxijul LE*, Liquid, and Super Soluble; Polycal; Polycal Liquid; Polycose; Vitajoule.
*Have low electrolyte content.

(c) Fat: Alembicol D; Calogen; Liquigen; MCT Oil.

(d) Nitrogen sources: Casilan (whole protein based, low-sodium); Forceval Protein (whole protein based, low-sodium); Maxipro Super Soluble (whey protein based, low-sodium); Pro-Mod (whey protein based, low-sodium).

(e) Minerals: Aminogran Mineral Mixture; Metabolic Mineral Mixture.

Phenylketonuria: Aglutella low-protein rice; Aminex low-protein rusks; Aminogran Food Supplement and Mineral Mixture; Analog XP; Aproten products (annellini, biscuits, bread mix, cake mix, crispbread, ditalini, rigatini, spaghetti, tagliatelle); Calogen; Caloreen; dp Low-Protein butterscotch-flavoured or chocolate-flavoured chip cookies; Juvela low-protein loaf (sliced and unsliced), bread rolls, cookies (chocolate chip, orange, and cinnamon flavour), mix; Lofenalac; Loprofin egg replacer; Loprofin low-protein bread (sliced and unsliced), bread (with or without salt), mix and pasta (macaroni, spaghetti short-cut, pasta spirals, tagliatelle nests, vermicelli), sweet biscuits, chocolate cream-filled biscuits, crackers, cookies (chocolate chip, cinnamon), wafers (orange, chocolate, vanilla); Loprofin PKU drink; XP Maxamaid ; XP Bar Maxamaid; XP Concentrate Maxamaid; XP Maxamum; Metabolic Mineral Mixture; Milupa PKU2 and PKU3; Phlexy-10 drink; PK Aid IV; Polycal; Polycose powder; Rite-Diet low-protein white bread (with added fibre), baking mix, flour mix; Sno-Pro; Ultra low-protein, canned white bread; Ultra PKU biscuits, PKU bread; PKU cookies, PKU flour, PKU pizza base; PKU savoy biscuits; Vitajoule, and see low-protein products and synthetic diets

Propionic acidaemia: Analog XMet, Thre, Val, Isoleu; XMet, Thre, Val, Isoleu Maxamaid; XMet Thre, Val, Isoleu Maxamum; Methionine, Threonine, Valine-Free and Isoleucine-Low Amino Acid Mix.

Protein intolerance: see milk protein sensitivity, whole protein sensitivity, low-protein products, synthetic diets, and amino acid metabolic disorders.

Refsum's Disease: Fresubin Liquid and Sip Feeds.

Renal dialysis: see Dialysis.

Renal failure: Aglutella low-protein rice; Aminex low-protein rusks; Aproten products (annellini, biscuits, bread mix, cake mix, crispbread, ditalini, rigatini, spaghetti, tagliatelle); Calogen; Caloreen; Calsip; Dialamine; dp Low-Protein butterscotch-flavoured or chocolate-flavoured chip cookies; Duobar; Super-Soluble Duocal and Duocal Liquid; Hycal; Juvela low-protein (chocolate chip, orange, and cinnamon flavour) cookies, loaf (sliced and unsliced) and flour mix; Kindergen PROD; Loprofin egg replacer; Loprofin low-protein bread (sliced and unsliced), bread (with or without salt), mix and pasta (macaroni, macaroni elbows, spaghetti short-cut, pasta spirals, tagliatelle, vermicelli; sweet biscuits, chocolate cream-filled biscuits, crackers, cookies (chocolate chip, cinnamon), wafers (orange, chocolate, vanilla); Nepro; Polycal; Polycose powder; Renamil; Rite-Diet low-protein white bread (with added fibre), flour mix, baking mix, Sno-Pro Drink; Suplena; Ultra low-protein, canned bread (brown and white); Ultra PKU biscuits, PKU cookies, PKU flour, PKU pizza base, PKU savoy biscuits; Valpiform shortbread biscuits; Vitajoule.

Short bowel syndrome: *see* Malabsorption states.

Sicca Syndrome: Glandosane; Luborant; Saliva Orthana; Salivace; Saliveze; Salivix.

Sucrose intolerance: *see* Carbohydrate malabsorption.

Synthetic diets:

(a) Fat: Alembicol D; Calogen; Liquigen; Medium Chain Triglyceride Oil.

(b) Carbohydrate: Caloreen; Hycal; Maxijul LE, Liquid, Super Soluble; Polycal; Polycal Liquid; Polycose powder; Vitajoule.

(c) Minerals: Aminogran Mineral Mixture; Metabolic Mineral Mixture.

(d) Protein sources: see malabsorption states, complete feeds.

(e) Vitamins: as appropriate and see malabsorption states, nutritional support for adults.

(f) Vitamins and Minerals: Paediatric Seravit.

Tyrosinaemia: Analog XPhen, Tyr; Analog XPhen, Tyr, Met; XPhen, Tyr Maxamaid; Phenylalanine, Tyrosine and Methionine-Free Amino Acid Mix; Tyrosine and Phenylalanine-Free Amino Acid Mix.

Vomiting in infancy: Instant Carobel, Nestargel.

Whole protein sensitivity: Alfare; Caprilon Formula; MCT Pepdite; Neocate; Nutramigen; Pepdite; Pepti-Junior; Pregestimil; Prejomin.
   Note. Defined as intolerance to whole protein, proven by at least two withdrawal and challenge tests, as suggested by an accurate dietary history

Xerostomia: Glandosane; Luborant; Saliva Orthana; Salivace; Saliveze; Salivix.

CONDITIONS FOR WHICH TOILET PREPARATIONS MAY BE PRESCRIBED ON FP10

Note. This is a list of clinical conditions for which the ACBS has approved toilet preparations. For details of the preparations see Chapter 13.

Birthmarks: see disfiguring skin lesions.

Dermatitis (includes contact, atopic and infective dermatoses, eczema and pruritic dermatoses): Aveeno Bath Oil; Aveeno Cream; Aveeno sachets (regular and oilated); Bath E45; Vaseline Dermacare Cream and Lotion; Wash E45.

Dermatitis herpetiformis: see gluten-sensitive enteropathies.

Disfiguring skin lesions (birthmarks, mutilating lesions and scars): Boots Covering Cream; Covermark classic foundation and finishing powder; Dermablend Cover Creme, Leg Cover, and Setting Powder; Dermacolor Camouflage cream and fixing powder; Keromask masking cream and finishing powder; Veil Cover cream and Finishing Powder. (Cleansing Creams, Cleansing Milks, and Cleansing Lotions are excluded.)

Disinfectants (antiseptics): drugs only when ordered in such quantities and with such directions as are appropriate for the treatment of patients. Not to be regarded as drugs if ordered for general hygienic purposes.

Eczema: see dermatitis.

Photodermatoses (skin protection in): Coppertone Ultrashade 23; Piz Buin Sunblock Lotion 20; RoC Total Sunblock Cream SPF 25 (Colourless and tinted); Spectraban 25; Spectraban Ultra 28; Sun E45 Cream SPF 25 and Lotion SPF 15; Uvistat Babysun Cream 22; Uvistat Lipscreen 15; Uvistat Sun Block Cream 20; Uvistat Tinted Lotion 25; Uvistat Ultrablock Sun Cream 30.

Pruritus: see dermatitis.

Appendix 8: Urinary and Stoma Appliances

This Appendix includes incontinence appliances, urethral catheters, and stoma products. Other products such as dressings, elastic hosiery, and glucose monitoring reagents are included in the relevant BNF chapters.

Incontinence appliances and urethral catheters

Incontinence appliances are listed in Part IXB of *Drug Tariff* or Part 5 of *Scottish Drug Tariff*; urethral catheters are included in Part IXA of *Drug Tariff* or Part 3 of *Scottish Drug Tariff*

DRAINABLE DRIBBLING APPLIANCES

Re-usable for at least 1 month (with exception of Alexa®)

Body's Surgical range
Bag (Body's Surgical)
Dribbling bag with loops and tapes. Net price 1 = £15.94
Urinal (Body's Surgical)
Drip male urinal with tap. Net price 1 = £42.80; 1 replacement belt = £10.56

Bullen range
Bags (Bullen)
Net price 10 Dribblet® bags = £21.09; 10 Dribblet® sheath bags = £47.34

DePuy range
Aquadry® (DePuy)
Drip type urinal. Net price 1 = £47.64

Henleys range
Alexa® dribbler bag (Henleys)
Plain bag, with draw strings. Net price 100 bags = £4.22; 100 bags with non-reflux valve = £16.25

Rüsch range
Peoplecare® (Rüsch)
Male drip urinal. Net price 1 = £48.49

Ward range
Bags (Ward)
Male dribbling bag with diaphragm and belt. Net price 1 = £26.48

INCONTINENCE BELTS

Average life 6 months

Body's Surgical range
Waist belt for kipper bags (Body's Surgical)
Net price 1 = £5.27; 1 (with webbing band) = £5.27

Rüsch range
Peoplecare® (Rüsch)
Waist and support strap for kipper bag. Net price 1 = £6.28

Simcare range
Belts (Simcare)
Rubber belt. Net price 1 = £5.22
Web belt (small, medium, or large) = £10.82

Ward range
Belts (Ward)
Waist belt for black kipper bag. Net price 1 = £4.85
Rubber belt for PP (pubic pressure) urinal. Net price 1 £4.20

INCONTINENCE SHEATHS

Unless otherwise indicated the incontinence sheaths (also known as penile sheaths or external catheters) listed below are of the soft, flexible, latex type. Each sheath may be left in place for 1 to 3 days between changes

Bard range
Integrity® (Bard)
Incontinence sheath, self-adhesive. Net price 30 sheaths (25, 30, or 35 mm) = £38.72
Reliasheath® (Bard)
Incontinence sheath with adhesive strip. Net price 3 sheaths (20, 25, 30, 35, or 40 mm) = £35.50
Uriplan® (Bard)
Incontinence sheath. Net price 30 sheaths (20, 25, 30, 35 or 40 mm) = £23.77
Uro sheath® (washable; may be used many times). Net price 1 (25, 35, or 40 mm) = £4.96

Camp range
Posey® (Camp)
Incontinence sheath. 'Fastflow' incontinence sheath. Net price 10 sheaths (25, 30, or 35 mm) = £6.38

Cliniflex range
Medimates® (CliniFlex)
Incontinence sheath with single-sided adhesive strip. Net price 30 sheaths (straight, 20, 25, 30, 35, or 40 mm; bulb, 25, 30, or 35 mm) = £29.35
Incontinence sheath with double-sided adhesive strip. Net price 30 sheaths (straight, 20, 25, 30, or 40 mm; bulb, 25, 30, or 35 mm) = £31.31

Coloplast range
Conveen® (Coloplast)
Incontinence sheath, with anti-kink design and Uriliner® adhesive strip. Net price 30 sheaths (20, 25, 30, 35, o 40 mm) = £42.12
Conveen self-sealing Urisheath® (Coloplast)
Incontinence sheath. Net price 30 sheaths (25, 30, o 35 mm) = £41.49

DePuy range
Aquadry® (DePuy)
Incontinence sheath. Net price 10 sheaths (small medium, large, or extra-large) = £9.56; 30 sheaths with bulbous end (small, medium, standard, large, or extra large) = £28.40
Aquadry Freedom® (DePuy)
Freedom® incontinence sheath, self-adhesive. Net price 30 sheaths (small, medium, standard, large, or extra large) = £39.94
Freedom Plus® incontinence sheath, self-adhesive. Net price 30 sheaths (small, medium, standard, large, o extra-large) = £39.94

Clear Advantage® (DePuy)

Incontinence sheath, silicone, self-adhesive . Net price 30 sheaths (small, medium, standard, large, extra-large) = £39.94

EMS Medical range
Sheaths (EMS)

Incontinence sheath. Net price 100 sheaths (25, 30, or 35 mm) = £43.00; 30 sheaths (with liner; 25, 30, or 35 mm) = £30.98

Fry range
Uridom® (Fry)

Incontinence sheath, including adhesive strip. Net price 30 sheaths = £27.07

Hollister range
InCare® (Hollister)

Incontinence sheath, self-adhesive. Net price 30 sheaths (22–25 mm; 26–30 mm; 31–35 mm; 36–39 mm) = £39.30

Hospital Management and Supplies range
Macrodom® (Hospital Management & Supplies)

Incontinence sheath, including adhesive strip. Net price 30 sheaths (with 2-inch tube) = £22.30; 25 sheaths (with 5-inch tube) = £23.33

Macrodom Plus® (Hospital Management & Supplies)

Incontinence sheath, including adhesive strip. Net price 30 sheaths (small, medium, or large) = £23.00

North West Medical range
Uridrop® (North West)

Incontinence sheath. Net price 30 sheaths (paediatric = 42 or 55 mm; sizes 1, 2, 3, or 4 = 70, 80, 100, or 107 mm) = £12.35

Incontinence sheath, with Uristrip® adhesive strip. Net price 30 sheaths (paediatric = 42 or 55 mm; sizes 1, 2, 3, or 4 = 70, 80, 100, or 107 mm) = £24.70

Payne range
Incontiaid® (Payne)

Incontinence sheath. Net price 10 sheaths, with adhesive strip (sizes 20, 25, 30, 35 or 40 mm) = £12.73; 1 sheath, without adhesive strip (sizes 20, 25, 30, 35 or 40 mm) = 79p; 10 adhesive strips = £4.14

Rüsch range
Dryaid® (Rüsch)

Incontinence sheath. Net price 20 sheaths (with adhesive strip; small, medium, large, or extra-large) = £26.13; 20 sheaths (without adhesive strip; small, medium, large, or extra-large) = £15.14

Portasheath® (Rüsch)

Incontinence sheath. Net price 25 sheaths (25, 30, or 35 mm) = £21.25

Secure external catheter kit, with adhesive strip. Net price 10 sheaths (25, 30, or 35 mm) = £8.70

Salts range
Heritage Cohesive /Sheath Pack® (Salts)

Incontinence sheath, with adhesive. Net price 30 sheaths (17, 22, 25, 32, or 34 mm) = £32.60

Male continence sheath (Salts)

Incontinence sheath. Net price 10 sheaths (17, 22, 25, 32, or 34 mm) = £7.35

Seton range
Incontinence sheath (Seton)

Incontinence sheath. Net price 30 sheaths (small, medium, large, or extra-large) = £31.39; 30 sheaths with self-adhesive liner (small, medium, large, or extra-large) = £37.40

Sherwood range
Texas Catheter® (Sherwood)

Incontinence sheath, with adhesive strip. Net price 12 sheaths = £8.64

Uri Drain® (Sherwood)

Incontinence sheath, with double-sided adhesive strap (25, 30, or 35 mm). Net price 10 = £8.00

Simcare range
Continence sheath (Simcare)

Incontinence sheath. Net price 1 sheath (small, medium, large, or extra-large) = £1.35

Uro Flo® (Simcare)

Incontinence sheath, straight, including adhesive liner. Net price 30 sheaths (small, medium, or large) = £39.30

Uro Flo Mk2® (Simcare)

Incontinence sheath, bulbous, with adhesive liner. Net price 30 sheaths (small, medium or large) = £39.30

Male incontinence sheath (Simcare)

Incontinence sheath. Net price 100 sheaths = £65.11

Simpla range
U-Sheath Plus® (Simpla)

Incontinence sheath, with external liner. Net price 30 sheaths (small, medium, large, or extra-large) = £27.64

Incontinence sheath, with Uriseal® liner. Net price 30 sheaths (small, medium, large, or extra-large) = £39.37

U-Sheath® (Simpla)

Incontinence sheath, with Uriseal® liner. Net price 30 sheaths (small, medium, large, or extra-large) = £35.83

FIXING STRIPS AND ADHESIVES

Bio Diagnostics®
Urifix® tape. Net price 5 m = £4.90

Camp®
Posey® sheath holder. Net price 12 (adult) = £13.25; 12 (paediatric) = £10.20

CliniFlex®
MediMates® adhesive strips. Net price 30 = £10.00

ConvaTec®
Urihesive® strips. Net price 15 = £6.21

DePuy
Aquadry® penile liners. Net price 20 = £7.78

EMS Medical
Urifix® tape. Net price 5 m = £5.88

North West Medical
Uristrip® adhesive strip. Net price 30 = £12.35

Payne
Incontiaid® sheath holder. Net price 1 = 94p

Rüsch
Dryaid® strip. Net price 20 strips = £10.99

Salts
Heritage® sheath collar pack. Net price 30 = £3.75
NHS Cohesive® strips for use with sheaths. Net price 10 = £4.97

LEG BAGS

Most plastic bags suitable for use for 5–7 days; rubber bags re-usable for 4–6 months

Bard range
Uriplan® (Bard)

Leg bag, plastic, shaped, with tap outlet and elastic Velcro straps. Net price 10 bags (350 mL, direct inlet) = £24.24; 10 bags (350 mL, 12 inch inlet tube) = £24.02; 10 bags (500 mL, direct inlet) = £24.48; 10 bags (500 mL, 4 or 12 inch inlet tube) = £24.57; 10 bags (750 mL, direct inlet, or 4, 12, or 15 inch inlet tube) = £24.72

Seton Urisac® (Bard)

Leg bag, plastic. Net price 10 bags (350 mL, short tube) = £12.18; 10 bags (350 mL, long tube) = £12.54; 10 bags (500 mL, short tube) = £13.26; 10 bags (500 mL, long tube) = £13.63; 10 bags (750 mL, short tube) = £13.98; 10 bags (750 mL, long tube) = £14.58

Body's Surgical range

Leg bags (Body's Surgical)

Kipper bag, black, white, or clear. Net price 1 bag = £24.25

Leg drainage bag, plastic, with tap outlet. Net price 10 bags (350 or 500 mL) = £20.80; 10 bags (750 mL) = £21.70

Coloplast range

Conveen® (Coloplast)

Security leg bag, plastic. Net price 10 bags (500 mL, 25 or 50 cm tube) = £19.79

Contour leg bag, plastic, shaped, sterile with sample port. Net price, with 1 set Velcro bands, 10 bags (600 mL, 5 or 30 cm tube; 800 mL, 45 cm tube) = £24.51; 10 non-sterile bags (600 mL, 45 cm adjustable tube) = £24.51

ConvaTec range

Accuseal® (ConvaTec)

Leg bag, plastic. Net price 10 bags (500 mL) = £17.82

DePuy range

Aquadry® (DePuy)

Catheter drainage bag, plastic. Net price 10 bags (small) = £21.32; 10 bags (large) = £21.88

Leg bag, plastic. Net price 10 bags (350, 500, or 750 mL, short or long tube) = £21.36

EMS Medical range

Leg drainage bags (EMS)

Leg bag, plastic. Net price 10 bags (500 mL, short or long tube) = £15.09

Incare range

Urinary leg bag (Incare)

Leg bag, plastic. Net price 10 bags (540 mL, 37 cm tube) = £24.06; 10 bags (540 mL, direct in-let) = £23.48

Maersk range

Careline® (Maersk)

Leg bag, plastic, with tap outlet and overnight connection tube. Net price, with 1 pair Velcro straps, 10 bags (350 mL, short or long tube) = £21.44; 10 bags (500 mL, short or long tube) = £22.01; 10 bags (750 mL, short or long tube) = £22.47

Manfred Sauer range

Sauer leg bag (Manfred Sauer)

Leg bag, plastic, with tap outlet and overnight connection tube and fabric/velcro leg straps. Net price 10 bags (700 or 1300 mL, short or long tube) = £19.31; 10 bags, sterile (700 or 1300 mL, short or long tube) = £22.30

Payne range

Incontiaid® (Payne)

Leg bag, plastic. Net price 1 bag (500 or 750 mL) = £2.38

Single-chambered GU Black Kipper Bags (Payne)

Leg bag, single-chambered. Net price 1 bag (rubber, with box outlet tap) = £46.44; 1 rubber bag (for night use) = £50.72; 1 bag (for female use) = £37.68; 1 bag (rubber, kipper-style) = £37.68; 1 bag (rubber, Ross type) = £43.00

Leg bags (formerly Willis range)

Rubber bag, for catheter drainage, short neck leg strap. Net price 1 bag = £25.82; 1 bag with web belt and support strap) = £30.22

Rubber bag, female, drainage bag, with conical mount. Net price 1 bag = £24.51; 1 bag (with web belt and support strap) = £28.90

Rüsch range

Leg bag (Rüsch)

Leg bag, plastic. Net price 10 bags (short tube, 350 or 500 mL) = £13.48; 10 bags (long tube, 350 or 500 mL) = £14.41; 10 bags (750 mL) = £17.50

Kipper bags (Rüsch)

Leg bag. Net price 1 bag (clear/white plastic or all black plastic or rubber, with strap and buckle) = £26.24; 1 bag (clear/white plastic, without strap and buckle) = £21.51

Salts range

Heritage® (Salts)

Leg bag, plastic. Net price 10 bags (500 mL, short tube) = £13.58; 10 bags (500 mL, long tube) = £13.82; 10 bags (750 mL, short tube) = £15.13; 10 bags (750 mL, long tube) = £15.49; 5 leg bag packs = £9.69

Sherwood range

Argyle® (Sherwood)

Leg bag, plastic. Net price (350, 500 or 750 mL, short or long tube) = £21.30

Simcare range

Leg bags (Simcare)

Leg bag, with valve outlet, natural latex straps, and plastic tube. Net price 10 bags (350 mL, short tube) = £23.28; 10 bags (350 mL, long tube) = £23.75; 10 bags (500 mL, short tube) = £23.78; 10 bags (500 mL, long tube) = £24.40; 10 bags (750 mL, short tube) = £24.14; 10 bags (750 mL, long tube) = £24.28

Leg bag, with twist tap, elastic straps, and plastic tube. Net price 10 bags (750 mL, short tube) = £24.18; 10 bags (750 mL, long tube, 30 cm) = £24.32

Tri-form® leg bag, plastic. Net price 10 bags (500 mL, short tube) = £23.53; 10 bags (500 mL, medium tube) = £23.80; 10 bags (500 mL, long tube) = £24.01

NHS Meredith® (Simcare)

Top outlet bag. Net price 25 bags (2 litres) = £47.28

PVC drainage bag (Simcare)

Leg bag, plastic. Net price 1 bag (small or large) = £3.68

Rubber bags (Simcare)

Leg bag, rubber, with leg strap. Net price = £34.10

Uro-Flo® (Simcare)

Standard leg bag, plastic. Net price 10 bags (350, 500 or 750 mL, 5 or 30 cm tube) = £14.37

Simpla range

Trident® (Simpla)

Leg bag, plastic. Net price 10 bags (350 mL, short tube) = £24.31; 10 bags (500 mL, short or long tube) = £24.57; 10 bags (750 mL, short, long, or adjustable long tube) = £24.68

Trident Plus® (Simpla)

Leg bag, plastic. Net price 10 bags (350 mL, short tube) = £24.43; 10 bags (500 mL, short tube or adjustable long tube) = £24.69; 10 bags (750 mL, adjustable long tube) = £24.81

Universal range

Unicorn® (Universal)

Leg bag, plastic. Net price 10 bags (350 mL, short tube) = £17.60; 10 bags (500 mL, short or long tube) = £17.80; 10 bags (750 mL, short or long tube) = £18.00

Ward range

Kipper bag (Ward)

Leg bag, kipper type, rubber. Net price 1 bag (black, clear, or white) = £22.09

Leg drainage bag (Ward)

Leg bag, plastic. Net price 10 bags (350 mL) = £10.67; 10 bags (500 mL) = £11.00; 10 bags (750 mL) = £11.65

St Peters Pattern (Ward)

Leg bag. Net price 5 bags = £29.52

Comfort® (Ward)

Leg bag, plastic. Net price 10 bags (350 mL) = £10.71; 10 bags (500 mL) = £11.02; 10 bags (750 mL) = £11.58

NIGHT DRAINAGE BAGS

Suitable for night-time use for collection of urine from indwelling catheters or from incontinence sheaths; bag hangers normally supplied through community nursing service.

Drainage bags have life of 5–7 nights

Bard

Uriplan® drainage bag. Net price 10 bags = £10.99; Collection bag (non-drainable), 10 bags = £2.15

Body's Surgical

2 litre drainage bag with tap outlet. Net price 1 bag = £1.40

Coloplast

Conveen® 1.5 litre drainage bag with 90 cm tube. Net price 10 bags = £12.32

ConvaTec

Surgicare System® 2 litre drainage bag. Net price 5 bags (Accuseal®) = £7.35; 5 bags (night) = £7.35

Dansac

Dansac® 2 litre night drainage bag. Net price 10 bags = £10.30

DePuy

Aqua® range 2 litre urine drainage bag. Net price 10 bags (Aqua® 2, non-drainable) = £1.96; 10 bags (Aqua® 4) = £9.24

Maersk

Careline® range, 2 litre urine drainage bag with 90 cm inlet tube. Net price 10 bags (Careline® E1, non-drainable) = £1.86; 10 bags (Careline® E2, non-drainable, with non-reflux valve) = £2.00; 5 bags (Careline® E4, with non-reflux valve and tap outlet) = £4.89

Rand Rocket

Urine drainage bag (non-drainable, short or long tube). Net price 25 bags = £3.87

Rüsch

Drainage bags, 2 litre. Net price 10 bags (C) = £10.37; 10 bags with non-reflux valve and plug (CV) = £11.51; 10 bags with non-reflux valve and tap (CVT) = £11.93; 10 bags with non-reflux valve and wide bore tap (DVT) = £11.00

Salts

2 litre H2 urine drainage bag. Net price 10 bags with non-reflux valve and tap = £11.27

Sherwood

Argyle® 2 litre urinary drainage bag. Net price 10 bags = £9.60

Simcare

Inbeds 2 litre drainage bag with twist tap. Net price 10 bags = £12.87

Uro-flo® night drainage bag. Net price 10 bags (female or male) = £14.01

Simpla

S4 Plus® overnight drainage bag. Net price 10 bags = £10.36

Urine drainage bag. Net price 10 bags (S1, non-drainable) = £2.22; 10 bags (S2, non-drainable with non-reflux valve) = £2.36; 10 bags (S4, short tube) = £11.21; 10 bags (S4, long tube) = £11.64

Ward

2 litre drainage bag with push/pull outlet. Net price 10 bags = £11.59

SUSPENSORY SYSTEMS

Drainage bag with support; bags may be used for 5–7 days

Bard

Urisac® Portabag® with belt. Net price 10 bags (plastic) = £11.35; 1 belt = £6.64

EMS Medical

Drainage bag with Shepheard Sporran belt. Net price 10 bags (plastic) = £15.09; 1 belt = £7.69

Rüsch

Portabag® with Portabelt®. Net price 10 bags (plastic) = £15.45; 1 belt = £8.63

Simcare

Holster bag with leg bag holster. Net price 10 bags (400 mL, plastic) = £18.13; 1 holster (24–30, 30–36, or 36–44 inch) = £8.47

TUBING AND ACCESSORIES

Bard

Adaptor for Uro sheath® (penile sheath to leg bag) 8 inch. Net price 1 = £1.01

Uriplan® leg bag straps (washable). Net price 5 pairs = £11.77

Latex leg bag straps. Net price 10 pairs = £2.41

Seton range foam /Velcro leg bag straps. Net price 10 pairs = £4.58

Urisac® tapes. Net price 10 pairs = £5.08

Body's Surgical

Velcro leg straps. Net price 1 pair = £1.71

Leg bag connecting tube. Net price 1 = £1.33; 1 (with mount) = £2.27

Coloplast

Velcro bands (washable). Net price 10 pairs = £34.54

ConvaTec

Accuseal® leg bag extension tube. Net price 10 tubes = £6.58

DePuy

Leg bag connecting tube. Net price 10 = £6.55

Aquadry® leg straps. Net price 5 pairs = £8.75

EMS Medical

Velcro leg straps. Net price 10 = £5.30

Incare

Leg bag straps. Net price 1 pair (14 inch, calf or 23 inch, thigh) = £2.65

Maersk

Careline® leg bag straps. Net price 10 = £11.94

Payne

Rubber extension tube, 6 inch. Net price = £3.19

Rubber leg strap. Net price 1 = £1.11

Velcro leg strap. Net price 1 = 88p

Portex

Paul (Penrose) tubing. Net price 10 (6, 13, 19, or 25 mm) = £12.46; 10 (32, 38, 44, or 51 mm) = £12.46

Tapered adaptor (catheter to leg bag). Net price 1 = £6.00; 1(stepped) = £8.47

Rüsch

Connecting tubes, net price 1 tube for kipper bag = £2.61; 14-inch connecting tube for drip urinal = £2.60; 1 connecting tube for all urinals with female connector = £3.97

Salts

Heritage® leg bag extension tube. Net price 2 tubes = £1.94

Sherwood

Argyle® foam and Velcro strap, washable. Net price 1 (75 cm, leg) = £1.69; 1 (150 cm, abdomen) = £3.17

Argyle Suregrip® general purpose tube, internal diameter 7 mm, length 2.7 m. Net price 50 tubes = £36.00

Argyle Penrose® tubing, internal diameter 6, 8, 10, 13, 16, 19, or 25 mm and length 44 cm. Net price 50 = £30.75

Cautionary label wordings, see inside back cover

Simcare

Stopcock for Chiron plastic urinal bags (in place of screwcap). Net price 1 = £4.35

Rubber extension tube (with mounts). Net price = £4.35

Rubber tubing (length, 1.5 m). Net price 1 = £10.16

Plastic connector with tube. Net price 1 = £2.91

Female connector for Mitcham bag. Net price 1 = £2.01

Night bag connector. Net price 1 = £1.22

Spare 'O' rings for pubic pressure urinal. Net price 5 = £1.15

Uro-Flo® elastic Velcro leg straps. Net price 5 pairs = £4.13

Leg bag extension tube. Net price 10 (30 cm) = £23.46; 10 (60 cm) = £25.80

Silgrip® leg straps. Net price 5 pairs (elasticated or Side-Fix thigh-fitting) = £11.94; 5 pairs (Side-Fix calf-fitting) = £11.35

Simpla

Leg bag straps. Net price 20 pairs (foam) = £12.84; 5 pairs (elasticated, washable) = £12.60

G-Strap. Net price 'adult' or 'short', 5 = £11.49 'abdomen', 5 = £12.66

URINAL SYSTEMS

Patients generally have two urinal systems (one to wash and one to wear). Each appliance should last for 6 months

Bard

Uriplan Maguire® urinal and adaptor. Net price (waist sizes 66–81 cm, 81–96 cm, or 96–112 cm) = £58.05

Male day and night urinal. Net price 1 (14 oz) = £41.79; 1 (20 oz) = £37.01

Mobile paraplegic day and night urinal. Net price 1 = £47.36

Uriplan Maguire® adaptor and tubing. Net price = £7.83

Bell and Croyden

Fridjohn male urinal. Net price 1 = £40.61

Male urinal, day and night use. Net price 1 (with long or short bag) = £37.35

Body's Surgical

Male day and night urinal with tap, covered bag, with band and suspensory, and leg strap with air vent. Net price 1 = £50.24

Male night urinal with tap, covered bag, with band and suspensory. Net price 1 = £61.14

Male day and night urinal with tap, long tube, covered bag, with band and suspensory with air vent. Net price 1 = £59.41

Male day and night urinal with tap, double bag, air vent, inflating rim, with band understraps. Net price 1 = £62.92

Male day and night urinal with tap, covered bag, diaphragm top, and air vent. Net price 1 = £54.37

Male day and night urinal with tap, improved pattern, inflating rim, short air vent, with band and understrap. Net price 1 = £59.67; 1 (with extension tube) = £62.98; 1 (with long bag) = £60.52

Male day and night urinal with tap, air vent, diaphragm top, with band and understrap. Net price 1 (with long bag) = £57.89; 1 (with short bag) = £53.64

Male day and night urinal with tap, air vent, with band and suspensory. Net price 1 (long bag) = £51.55

Male day urinal with tap, to contain penis and scrotum. Net price 1 (short bag, with band and understrap) = £48.60; 1 (with inner sheath and air vent) = £50.49

Male jockey appliance with tap. Net price 1 = £53.76

Spares

Replacement belt. Net price 1 = £10.56

Outer receiver. Net price 1 = £12.30

Inner sheath. Net price 5 = £12.30

Plastic bags. Net price 5 = £13.54

Rubber bag. Net price 1 = £22.58

Ring. Net price 1 = 90p

Stoke Mandeville male urinal with tap (specify sheath size). Net price 1 = £57.07; 1 (with double bag) = £68.52; 1 replacement sheath (specify size) = £5.64

Male pubic pressure urinal with tap (specify sheath size). Net price 1 (with rubber bag) = £61.03; 1 (with 5 plastic bags) = £57.44

Spares

Flange with sheaths. Net price 1 = £28.52

Cone. Net price (curved, small, medium, or large; straight, small, medium, large, or extra-large) = £11.31

Plastic bag. Net price 1 (small or large) = £13.54

Rubber bag. Net price 1 = £22.13

Rubber belt. Net price 1 = £4.06

Progress® long life plastic urinal. Net price 1 (inner sheath or scrotal) = £24.11

Fridjohn urinal. Net price 1 = £72.08

YB wet urinal. Net price 1 = £58.50

Essex appliance. Net price 1 = £48.83

One-piece belt. Net price 1 (rubber or plastic bag coverlet) = £48.98

Bullen

Child urinal. Net price 1 (with transverse bag) = £67.16; 1 (with medium-size long bag) = £64.90

Male urinal. Net price 1 (with large-size long bag) = £72.01

DePuy

Aquadry® urinal. Net price 1 cross cut diaphragm and scrotal support; inner sheath and rubber understrap (1.125, 1.25, 1.375, 1.5, or 1.625 inch); pubic pressure: pressure ring, tapered inner sleeve trimmed to fit and rubber understrap; pressure ring, diaphragm and rubber understrap (1, 1.25, or 1.5 inch); pressure ring, diaphragm and scrotal support (1, 1.25, or 1.5 inch) = £51.16

Spares

Bag (for all standard urinals). Net price 5 (250 or 325 mL) = £11.17; rubber leg bag connecting tube with female attachment, net price 1 = £2.58

Flange (child: 0.5, 0.675, 0.75, 0.875, 1, 1.125, or 1.25 inch; adult: 1, 1.125, 1.25, 1.375, 1.5, 1.625, or 1.75 inch). Net price 1 = £24.47

Cones. Net price 1 (small, medium, or large; curved or straight) = £10.58

Rubber belt. Net price 1 (24, 28, 36, or 44 inch) = £2.94

Ellis

Hallam modular urinal. Net price 1 = £31.63; 1 spare bag = £1.68; 1 spare belt = £3.75

LRC

Dry sheaths. Net price 144 = £14.42

Payne

Male incontinence appliance with rubber belt. Net price 1 (MK1 with combined rubber flange and understraps) = £58.95; 1 (MK2 with rubber flange and fabric facepiece) = £63.39; 1 (MK3 with combined rubber flange, understraps, and coned top) = £52.31; 1 (MK9, with rubber flange and fabric facepiece) = £66.05

Lightweight male incontinence appliance. Net price 1 (MK4 with fabric facepiece and separate long flanged plastic bag with foam pad) = £37.37; 1 (MK5, with fabric facepiece, with belt combined, separate flange, and long flanged plastic bag) = £52.49; 1 (MK6 with combined flange and understraps and long flanged plastic bag with rubber belt) = £46.03; 1 (MK10, with fabric facepiece, with belt combined, separate flange, and long flanged plastic bag) = £55.17

Spares

Rubber flange. Net price 1 (with feathered diaphragm, MK2, MK5, MK9, MK10) = £17.07; 1 (MK1, MK6) = £26.42; 1 (with feathered diaphragm and combined reinforced top, MK3) = £29.97

Material facepiece. Net price 1 facepiece with belt and loop (MK2, MK4, MK5) = £19.79; 1 facepiece with support belt, loop and scrotal = £22.45

Flange support with wide belt and scrotal support (MK9, MK10). Net price 1 = £22.45

Reinforced cone top (MK1, MK2, MK9). Net price 1 = £11.48

Bag (MK1, MK2, MK3, MK9). Net price 1 plastic bag = £2.89; 1 rubber bag = £17.37

Bag, long flange plastic. Net price 1 MK4 bag = £4.43; 1 MK5, MK6, MK10 bag = £3.90

Belt (MK1, MK3, MK6). Net price 1 (elastic) = £7.88; 1 (web) = £5.51; 1 (rubber) = £3.72

Night connector (MK1, MK2, MK3, MK9). Net price 1 = £3.72

Payne's urine director. Net price 1 = £21.09

Stoke Mandeville condom urinal complete. Net price 1 = £48.64

Spares

Kipper bag. Net price 1 = £27.37

Belt. Net price 1 (38, 46, or 60 inch) = £5.80

Rubber tube and connector. Net price 1 = £2.13; rubber tubing = £4.38 per metre; nylon connector (GU or SM) 1 = £1.24

Dry incontinence sheath. Net price 144 = £14.16

Pubic pressure urinal complete with bag. Net price 1 (rubber or plastic bag) = £58.95

Spares

Pubic pressure flange with sheath (1-inch flange with 0.5, 0.625, 0.75, or 0.875 inch sheath; 1.25-inch flange with 0.875 or 1 inch sheath; 1.5-inch flange with 1.125 or 1.25 inch sheath; 1.75-inch flange with 1.375, 1.5, or 1.625 inch sheath). Net price 1 = £26.42

Coned top. Net price 1 (straight or curved: small, medium, or large; straight: extra-large) = £11.48

Replacements

Rubber bag with vent tube (MK1, MK2, MK3, MK9). Net price 1 = £20.85

Reinforced cone top with vent tube (MK1, MK2, MK3, MK9). Net price 1 = £15.10

Latex tubing, 8 or 10 mm bore. Net price per metre = £4.38

GU Condom set. Net price 1 = £50.72; 1 (with 40 oz bag) = £62.93

Urinal replacement parts

Nylon stud (GU or SM). Net price 1 = £1.24; 1 (with latex tube) = £2.13

Waist belt for single-chambered bag. Net price 1 (38, 46, or 60 inch) = £5.80

(formerly Willis range)

Male urinal, day and night, air tube to bag, inner sheath and diaphragm to receiver, web belt and cotton suspensory bag. Net price 1 = £47.72; 1 (long narrow Coutil®-covered bag, web belt and cotton suspensory bag) = £49.67

Male urinal, receiver to contain penis and scrotum, web waist band, and tape understraps. Net price 1 (day, night, or small build) = £45.57

Male urinal, long rubber bag with 2 leg straps, loops and straps, flanged receiver, air tube, diaphragm and short conical inner sheath, web band and cotton suspensory bag. Net price 1 (day and night) = £47.14

Male urinal, short rubber bag, detachable bag and night tube, web belt and cotton suspensory bag. Net price 1 (day and night) = £37.99

Spares for above urinals

Suspension bag. Net price 1 (small, medium, or large) = £4.80

Rüsch

Thames urinal with bag and connecting tube. Net price 1 (standard or long bag) = £76.24

Severn urinal with bag and connecting tube. Net price 1 (standard, long, or 5 plastic bags) = £76.24; 5 Severn spare sheaths = £29.89

Mersey urinal with bag and connecting tube. Net price 1 (standard, long, or 5 plastic bags) = £76.24

Wye, male, MkII, light-weight urinal. Net price 1 (with separate connecting tube and on/off valve) = £24.64; 1 (with long night extension tube) = £28.72; 1 (with short or long bag) = £41.03

Arizona male urinal. Net price 1 = £76.24

'55' male urinal for paraplegic patients. Net price 1 = £75.09; 6 spare sheaths = £34.05

Stoke Mandeville pattern male urinal with double chamber rubber collection bag. Net price 1 (20, 24, 25, 28, 32, 35, 38, 42, 45, 48, 51, 54, 57, 60, or 63 mm sheath) =£76.24; 1 spare sheath = £7.03

Sahara one-piece top pubic pressure urinal with bag. Net price 1 paediatric (with small rubber collection bag or 5 small plastic collection bags) = £72.68; 1 standard or large (with standard or long rubber collection bag or 5 medium plastic collection bags, and connecting tube) = £72.68

Peoplecare® pubic pressure male urinal. Net price 1 paediatric (flange 25 mm and sheath 13, 16, 19, or 22 mm; or flange 29 mm and sheath 22 or 25 mm; or flange 32 mm and sheath 19, 22, or 25 mm) = £23.60; 1 adult (flange 38 mm and sheath 19, 22, 25, 29, or 32 mm; or flange 44 mm and sheath 35, 38, or 41 mm) = £23.60

Spares

Pubic pressure bag, standard. Net price 1 (medium) = £12.18; 1 (large) = £15.10; 1 (curved top, small, medium, or large) = £9.19; 1 (straight top, small, medium, large, or extra-large) = £9.19

Transverse rubber bag with tap. Net price 1 = £24.94

Pubic pressure flange for transverse rubber bag with tap. Net price 1 (double-based) = £23.60; 1 (adult, rubber) = £27.21

Kipper inco set with 1 black rubber kipper bag, 10 penile sheaths, waist and support strap, and connecting tube. Net price 1 = £40.84

Salts

Male pubic pressure urinal with rubber bag or 4 plastic bags. Net price 1 = £48.15

Spares

Pubic pressure flange with sheath (1-inch flange with 0.5, 0.625, 0.75, or 0.875 inch sheath; 1.25-inch flange with 0.75, 0.875, or 1 inch sheath; 1.5-inch flange with 0.75, 0.875, 1, or 1.125 inch sheath; 1.75-inch flange with 1.375, 1.5, or 1.625 inch sheath). Net price 1 = £22.89

Cone. Net price 1 (small, medium, or large: straight or curved; extra-large: straight) = £10.19

Pubic pressure flange belt. Net price 1 = £20.11

Bags. Net price 4 (plastic, child or adult) = £11.20; 1 (rubber, child, adult, or transverse) = £11.20

Belt. Net price = £3.40

Simcare

Male pubic pressure urinal, child, with integral flange. Net price 1 (rubber bag, straight cone, medium) = £57.51; 1 (plastic bag, curved cone, small or medium) = £56.22

Spares

Pubic pressure flange with integral sheath for child. Net price 1 (25-mm flange with 13, 16, 19, or 22 mm sheath; 29-mm flange with 25 mm sheath; 32-mm flange with 25 mm sheath) = £31.65

Cone. Net price 1 (small, medium, or large, straight or curved; extra-large, straight) = £13.39

Pubic pressure flange, double-based. Net price 1 (child, 32 mm; adult, 38 or 44 mm) = £28.30

Chailey male urinal. Net price 1 (child, plastic bag) = £59.18; 1 (adolescent or adult, rubber bag) = £53.06; 1 (adolescent or adult, plastic bag) = £67.21

Spares

Curved top with integral sheath and straps. Net price 1 (child: 22-mm sheath; adult: 22, 25, 29, 32, 35, 38, or 44 mm sheath) = £35.41

Belt, rubber. Net price 1 (61 or 91 cm) = £5.22

Bags, plastic (also suitable for pubic pressure and Chiron® urinals). Net price 1 (wide neck, adult, or child) = £3.48

Bags, rubber (also suitable for pubic pressure and Chiron® urinals). Net price 1 child size = £16.84; 1 adult size = £23.08

Male pubic pressure urinal, adult, with integral flange. Net price 1 (rubber bag, various sizes) = £66.63; 1 (plastic bag, various sizes) = £62.09

Replacement pubic pressure flange. Net price 1 = £31.65

Male pubic pressure urinal, adult, with double-based flange. Net price 1 (rubber bag, various sizes) = £66.63; 1 (plastic bag,various sizes) = £62.09

Replacement sheath. Net price 10 = £1.21

Bag, rubber, for pubic pressure urinals. Net price 1 (adult, with vent tube) = £27.62; 1 (adult, double) = £29.58

Stoke Mandeville urinal. Net price 1 (sheath type) = £60.71; 1 (double rubber bag) = £78.89

Spares

Sheath. Net price 1 = £8.28; 10 (for sheath type) = £3.64

Chiron male rubber urinal with webbing belt. Net price 1 = £54.64

Male one-piece urinal. Net price = £52.02

Surrey model lightweight urinal. Net price (MKI or MKII) = £49.42

Spares

Foam pad. Net price 5 (76 mm /32 mm) = £6.13

Chiron urinal. Net price 1 (male, plastic, rubber sheaths) = £28.27; 1 (geriatric, film-type sheaths) = £41.05; 1 (rubber sheaths) = £41.05

Spares

Sheath. Net price 1 (rubber) = £5.22; 10 (non-allergenic film type) = 96p

Net suspensory. Net price 1 = £12.27

Male urinal for bed use. Net price 1 = £46.12

Pubic flange, large opening. Net price 1 = £21.20

Transverse rubber bag and stopcock. Net price 1 (child) = £31.21

Ward

Jockey male urinal. Net price 1 = £69.28

Varsity male urinal. Net price 1 = £53.48

Male urinal. Net price 1 (day use, covered bag, complete with belt suspensory and thigh strap) = £44.24; 1 (day and night, covered bag, air vent, belt suspensory) = £45.79; 1 (day and night, short bag and belt) = £47.40; 1 (day and night, short covered bag and belt) = £51.38; 1 (day and night, double chamber bag) = £53.40; 1 (day and night, long bag and belt) = £47.40

Paraplegic male urinal. Net price 1 = £64.78

Stoke Mandeville Pattern. Net price 1 = £62.24; 1 (removable rubber sheath, double chamber rubber bag, thigh strap and belt) = £55.90

Spare sheath. Net price 1 = £5.77

Male pubic pressure urinal. Net price 1 (rubber bag) = £58.00; 1 (plastic bag) = £51.39

Spares

Pubic pressure flange. Net price 1 = £26.60

Pubic pressure cone; Net price 1 = £10.51

Bags. Net price 1 (rubber) = £14.41; 1 (plastic) = £2.88

Male urinal. Net price 1 (day, covered bag complete with belt) = £42.12; 1 (day and night or night, covered bag complete with belt, suspensory, and thigh strap) = £55.64; 1 (day and night, long tube, air vent, rubber bag, complete with belt and thigh strap) = £50.51

Male urinal. Net price 1 (night, covered bag complete with belt, suspensory, and thigh strap) = £55.64

Male dribbling bag and tapes. Net price 1 = £20.55

Male urinal. Net price 1 (day and night, short covered bag or short bag and belt) = £47.40

Male urinal. Net price 1 (sheath and disc type with long rubber belt or sheath and suspensory with short or long covered bag) = £51.69

Male urinal. Net price 1 (conical top with short or long rubber bag) = £29.49

Night urinal. Net price 1 (with long tube) = £24.98

Stoke Mandeville sheath-type urinal, with 30 rubber film sheaths, rubber bag, and thigh strap and belt. Net price 1 = £49.49

St Peters pattern suprapubic bag. Net price 1 = £29.52

Webbing belt. Net price 1 = £8.75

Elastic leg strap. Net price 10 = £5.00

Net suspensory. Net price 1 = £11.50

Spare rubber bag with vent. Net price 1 = £25.00

Spare receiver. Net price 1 = £36.00

URETHRAL CATHETERS

Urethral catheter sizes are designated by the Charrière (Ch) gauge system; when the size is not stated by the prescriber the Drug Tariff recommends that size 14 or 16 be supplied. For the Foley catheter, if the balloon size is not stated, the 10 mL size should be supplied for adults, 5 mL for paediatric use (balloon sizes are defined as the amount of fluid required to fully inflate the volume of lumen).

Foley catheters for short-/medium-term use in adults

Bard

Uriplan®, teflon-coated latex, male or female. Net price, male (12-26 Ch: 10-mL balloon; 16-26 Ch: 30-mL balloon), 1 catheter = £2.21; female (Ch 12-22: 10-mL balloon), 1 catheter = £3.30; pre-filled with sterile water (Ch 12-22: 10-mL balloon), 1 catheter = £2.51

Rüsch

Soft Simplastic®, PVC, male or female. Net price, male (12–26 Ch: 10-mL balloon; 16–26 Ch: 30-mL balloon),1 catheter = £4.52; female (12–22 Ch: 10-mL balloon; 16–22 Ch: 30-mL balloon), 1 catheter = £4.52

100 plus®, teflon-coated latex, male or female. Net price male (12–26 Ch: 10-mL balloon; 16–26 Ch: 30-mL balloon), 1 catheter = £1.95; female (12–22 Ch: 10-mL balloon; 16–32 Ch: 30-mL balloon), 1 catheter = £2.48

Simcare

Eschmann Folatex®, latex, male or female. Net price, male (12-28 Ch: 10- or 30-mL balloon), 1 catheter = £2.00; female (12-28 Ch: 10- or 30-mL balloon), 1 catheter = £2.00

Foley catheters for short-/medium-term use in children
All 8-10 Ch: 5-mL balloon

Bard

Uriplan®, teflon-coated latex. Net price 1 catheter = £6.09

Rüsch

100 plus®, teflon-coated latex. Net price 1 catheter = £4.16

Simcare

Eschmann Folatex ®, latex. Net price 1 catheter = £3.69

Foley catheters for long-term use in adults
Bard

Biocath®, hydrogel-coated, male or female. Net price, male (12-26 Ch: 10- or 30-mL balloon), 1 catheter = £6.81; female (12-22 Ch: 10-mL balloon), 1 catheter = £6.90; pre-filled with sterile water, (12-22 Ch: 10-mL balloon), 1 male catheter = £7.06; 1 female catheter = £7.09

Silastic®, silicone-coated. Net price (12-24 Ch: 10-mL balloon; 16-28 Ch: 30-mL balloon), 1 catheter = £7.21

Bard®, silicone elastomer-coated latex, male or female. Net price, male (12-22 Ch: 10-mL balloon; 16-22 Ch: 30-mL balloon), 1 catheter = £7.49; female (16-22 Ch: 30-mL balloon), 1 catheter = £7.49; pre-filled with sterile water, male or female (12-22 Ch: 10-mL balloon), 1 catheter = £8.09

Bard®, all silicone. Net price male (12-22 Ch: 10-mL balloon; 16-22 Ch: 30-mL balloon), 1 catheter = £7.72; female (12-16 Ch: 10-mL balloon), 1 catheter = £7.48

Medasil

All silicone, male or female. Net price, male (12-26 Ch: 10-mL balloon; 16-26 Ch: 30-mL balloon), 1 catheter = £4.62; female (12-26 Ch: 10-mL balloon; 16-26 Ch: 30-mL balloon), 1 catheter = £4.62

Rüsch

Silikon 100®, male or female. Net price, male (12-26 Ch: 10-mL balloon; 18-20 Ch: 20-mL balloon; 22-26 Ch: 30-mL balloon), 1 catheter = £6.50; female (12-22 Ch: 10-mL balloon; 18-20 Ch: 20-mL balloon; 22 Ch: 30-mL balloon), 1 catheter = £6.50

Ultrasil®, silicone elastomer-coated latex, male. Net price (12-26 Ch: 10-mL balloon; 16-26 Ch: 30-mL balloon), 1 catheter = £5.42

Sherwood

Argyle®, all silicone, male or female. Net price, male (12-24 Ch: 10-mL balloon; 16 Ch: 20-mL balloon; 18-26 Ch: 30-mL balloon), 1 catheter = £5.83; female (12-18 Ch: 10-mL balloon), 1 catheter = £5.83

Simpla

All silicone, male or female. Net price, male (12-26 Ch: 10-mL balloon; 16-18 Ch: 20-mL balloon; 20-26 Ch: 30-mL balloon), 1 catheter = £7.63; female (12-18 Ch: 10-mL balloon; 20-26 Ch: 30-mL balloon), 1 catheter = £7.58

Trident®, silicone elastomer-coated latex, male. Net price (12-22 Ch: 10-mL balloon; 16-24 Ch: 30-mL balloon), 1 catheter = £4.82

Foley catheters for long-term use in children
All 8-10 Ch: 5-mL balloon

Bard

Biocath®, hydrogel-coated. Net price 1 catheter = £6.90

Medasil

All silicone. Net price 1 catheter = £4.62

Rüsch

Silikon 100®. Net price 1 catheter = £6.50

Sherwood

Argyle®, all silicone. Net price 1 catheter = £6.29

Simpla

All silicone. Net price 1 catheter = £7.69

Nélaton catheters ('ordinary' cylindrical catheter)

Bard

Reliacath®, teflon-coated latex, 14 Ch. Net price 5-catheter pack = £6.65

Reliacath®, plastic, male, female, or paediatric. Net price, male or female (12-18 Ch), 5-catheter pack = £6.13; paediatric (8-10 Ch), 5-catheter pack = £6.13

EMS

PVC, male, female or paediatric. Net price, male (10-18 Ch), 1 catheter = 98p, 5-catheter pack = £4.67; female (12-18 Ch), 1 catheter = 98p, 5-catheter pack = £5.00; paediatric (6-10 Ch), 1 catheter = 98p, 5-catheter pack = £5.00

Maersk

PVC, male, female or paediatric. Net price, male (12-24 Ch), 5-catheter pack = £5.00; female (12-18 Ch), 5-catheter pack = £5.00; paediatric (6-10 Ch), 5-catheter pack = £5.00

Pennine

Male, female, or paediatric. Net price, male (12-16 Ch), 10-catheter pack = £3.46; female (10-14 Ch), 10-catheter pack = £3.15; paediatric (6-10 Ch), 10-catheter pack = £3.15

Portex

PVC, male or female, 8-14 Ch. Net price, male, 5-catheter pack = £7.02; female, 5-catheter pack = £6.70

Rüsch

Jacques®, soft red rubber, 8-18 Ch. Net price 1 catheter = £1.40, 5-catheter pack = £5.79

Simcare

PVC, male or female, 8-14 Ch. Net price, male, 5-catheter pack = £7.18; female, 5-catheter pack = £6.90

Simpla

Male, female, or paediatric. Net price, male (12-14 Ch), 5-catheter pack = £5.00; female (12-14 Ch), 5-catheter pack = £4.80; paediatric (8-10 Ch), 5-catheter pack = £5.00

Nélaton catheters (single use)

Astra Tech

Lofric®, PVC, single use, male, female, or paediatric. Net price, male (8-24 Ch); female (8-18 Ch); paediatric (6-10 Ch), 25-catheter pack (all) = £30.00

Coloplast

Conveen Easicath®, single use, male, female, paediatric, or Tiemann tip. Net price, male (8-18 Ch); female (8-16 Ch); paediatric (6-10 Ch); Tiemann tip (10-18 Ch), 25-catheter pack (all) = £25.00

Scott catheters (short curved tubular catheter for women and girls)

Simcare

Polyethylene, female, 8-14 Ch. Net price 5-catheter pack = £11.25

STOMA APPLIANCES

Stoma appliances are listed in Part IXC of *Drug Tariff* or Part 6 of *Scottish Drug Tariff*.

It is not necessary to state an **order number** on a prescription for one of these products provided the **full details** as given in the BNF are included on the **prescription**.

CLOSED POUCHES AND COLOSTOMY SETS

Closed pouches are suitable for patients with a **colostomy** and well-formed stools

Body's Surgical range

Rubber bags screwcap (Body's Surgical)

Black butyl, one-piece closed pouch. Net price 1 day pouch = £27.05; 1 night pouch = £31.55

White rubber, one-piece closed pouch. Net price 1 day pouch = £15.03; 1 night pouch = £17.31

Rubber bags spout (Body's Surgical)

Black butyl, one-piece closed pouch. Net price 1 day pouch or night pouch = £28.56

White rubber, one-piece closed pouch. Net price 1 day pouch or night pouch = £13.51

CliniMed range

Biotrol® (CliniMed)

Colo S, one-piece pouch with skin protector adhesive, white. Net price 30 pouches (25, 30, 35, 40, 45, 50, or 60 mm holes) = £61.50

Elite Closed, covered one-piece pouch with skin protector adhesive and filter, white or beige. Net price 30 pouches (starter hole, 25, 30, 35, 40, 45, 50, 60, 70 mm holes) = £65.83; clear (25, 30, 35, 40, 45, 50, 60, 70 mm holes) 30 pouches = £60.56; starter hole, 30 = £61.39

Elite Petite, one-piece pouch with skin protector adhesive and filter, beige. Net price 30 pouches (starter hole, 25, 30, 35, 40 or 45 mm holes) = £56.52

Lockring 2, two-piece pouches with filter and backing, white. Net price 30 pouches (for 35, 50 or 75 mm flanges) = £30.45

Mini S, one-piece pouch with skin protector adhesive and filter, beige. Net price 30 pouches (25, 30, 35, or 40 mm) = £50.99

Integrale, one-piece pouch with skin protector adhesive and filter, white. Net price 30 pouches (starter hole, 25, 30, 35, 40, 45, 50, 60, 70 mm holes) = £65.83

Preference Closed, fabric covered one-piece pouch with skin protector adhesive, porous adhesive collar, and filter, white or beige. Net price 30 pouches (starter hole, 25, 30, 35, 40, 45, 50, 60 mm holes) = £62.00

Coloplast range

Assura® (Coloplast)

Maxi, closed pouches, opaque or clear. Net price 30 one-piece pouches (opaque or clear: 20, 25, 30, 35, 40 mm; clear: also 45 or 50 mm holes; 20 mm can be cut to fit up to 55 mm) = £62.34; 30 two-piece pouches, opaque or clear (to fit 40, 50, or 60 mm base plates) = £34.56

Midi, closed pouches with flatus filter, opaque or clear. Net price 30 one-piece pouches (20, 25, 30, 35, 40, 45, or 50 mm holes) = £62.34; 30 two-piece pouches (to fit 40, 50, or 60 mm base plates) = £34.56; base plate (40, 50, or 60 mm), 5 = £13.77

Minicap, closed pouches, opaque. Net price 30 one-piece pouches (20 mm can be cut to fit up to 55 mm) = £32.43; 30 two-piece pouches (to fit 40 or 50 mm base plates) = £27.54

Conseal® System (Coloplast)

Two-piece pouch. Net price 30 bags (to fit 40 or 50 mm base plates) = £36.60; base plate (40 or 50 mm) 5 = £13.52; colostomy plug (40 × 35 or 45 mm, 50 × 35 or 45 mm) 10 = £12.20; discharge bag (40 or 50 mm) 50 = £2.65

K-Flex® (Coloplast)

One-piece closed pouch with karaya skin protector and filter. Net price 30 pouches (clear: 10, 30, or 40 mm holes; opaque: 30 or 40 mm holes) = £65.73

Extra, one-piece closed pouch. Net price, No. 1 (24 mm hole), 100 pouches = £87.50; No. 2 (30 or 40 mm holes), 100 = £107.10; No. 3 (30 mm hole), 100 = £128.50, 50 mm hole, 100 = £129.50

Regular, one-piece closed pouch. Net price, No. 1 (24 mm hole), 100 pouches = £73.80; No. 2 (30 mm hole), 100 = £87.50; No. 3 (30 mm hole) = £105.00; No. 5 (24 mm hole), 100 = £98.40

mc2000® (Coloplast)

One-piece pouch with double seal and filter, opaque or clear. Net price 30 pouches (25, 30, 35, 40, 45, 50, 55, or 60 mm holes) = £68.04

mc2002® (Coloplast)

Two-piece pouch with filter, opaque or clear. Net price 30 pouches (to fit 40 or 60 mm base plates) = £38.46; base plate (40 mm × 15 or 25 mm, 60 × 35 or 45 mm) 5 = £14.19; belt plate (40 or 60 mm) 10 = £5.70

pc3000® (Coloplast)

One-piece pouch, opaque or clear. Net price 30 pouches (25, 30, 35, 40, 45, 50, or 55 mm holes; 25 mm can be cut to fit up to 60 mm) = £63.93

ConvaTec range

Colodress® (ConvaTec)

Colodress, one-piece closed pouch with textured backing, opaque beige. Net price 30 pouches (19, 32, 38, 45, or 50 mm holes; 19 mm can be cut to fit) = £62.03

Colodress Plus, one-piece closed pouch with single-release paper and filter. Net price 30 pouches (opaque or clear: 19, 25, 32, 38, 45, 50, or 64 mm holes; opaque: 19 mm can be cut to fit) = £62.03; Mini pouches, 30 pouches (19, 25, 32, 38, or 45 mm holes) = £55.95

Colodress Plus Lite, one-piece closed pouch, standard, opaque. Net price 30 pouches (25, 32, 38, 45 or 50 mm holes; 19 mm can be cut to fit) = £57.30

Combihesive Natura® (ConvaTec)

Two-piece pouch with filter, opaque. Net price 30 pouches (to fit 32, 38, 45, 57 or 70 mm flanges) = £32.07; Mini pouches, 20 pouches (to fit 32, 38, 45 or 57 mm flanges) = £17.58

Natures® (ConvaTec)

Naturess, closed pouches. Net price 50 pouches (standard opaque pouch: 19 mm starter hole, 25, 32, 38, 45 or 50 mm hole; standard clear pouch: 19 mm starter hole) = £94.50; 50 pouches (small opaque pouch: 19 mm starter hole, 25, 32, 38, 45 or 50 mm holes) = £84.00

Surgicare System ® 2 (ConvaTec)

System 2, two-piece closed pouch, white. Net price 30 pouches (to fit 38, 45, 57, or 70 mm flanges) = £31.05

System 2 Combihesive, two-piece closed pouch with textured backing, beige. Net price 30 pouches (to fit 38, 45, 57, or 70 mm flanges) = £31.05; with filter, 30 pouches (to fit 32, 38, 45, 57, or 70 mm flanges) = £32.07 ; Mini pouches, 20 pouches (to fit 32, 38, 45, or 57 mm flanges) = £17.58

Dansac range

Dansac® (Dansac)

Combi Colo F, one-piece pouch with filter, opaque or clear. Net price 100 pouches (standard pouch: 25, 30, 38, 44, 50, or 63 mm holes; small pouch: 25, 30, or 38 mm holes) = £156.01

CombiMicro C + S, one-piece pouch with porous adhesive, filter, skin barrier ring, and fabric backing, opaque or clear. Net price 30 pouches (25, 32, 38, 44, 50, 63 mm or cut-to-fit; 10-38 mm; 38-63 mm holes) = £65.37

Standard Colo, one-piece pouch with filter, clear. Net price 100 pouches (22, 30, 32, or 38 mm holes) = £140.12

Unique, one-piece closed pouch, opaque or clear. Net price 30 pouches (25, 30, 35, 40, 45, 50, 60 mm or cut-to-fit holes) = £56.50; oval flange, opaque or clear, starter hole, net price 30 = £56.50

Unique 2, two-piece closed pouch, opaque or clear. Net price 30 pouches (to fit 36, 43, 55 or 80 mm flange) = £31.00; flange, 36, 43, or 55 mm, net price 5 = £12.75; 80 mm, net price, 5 = £13.00

Unique Light, one-piece closed pouch with filter and comfort backing, opaque. Net price 30 pouches (25, 30, 35, 40, 45, 50 or 60 mm holes; 20 mm can be cut to fit up to 60 mm) = £57.60

Unique Mini, one-piece closed pouch, opaque. Net price 30 pouches (25, 30, 35, or 40 mm holes; 20 mm can be cut to fit up to 50 mm) = £53.33

DePuy range

Schacht® (DePuy)

Colostomy bag (= pouch), one-piece closed pouch. Net price 100 pouches = £32.30

Colostomy appliance. Net price 1 appliance = £27.85

Eurocare range

Eurocare® (EuroCare)

One-piece closed pouch, opaque. Net price 30 pouches (13 mm starter hole, 25, 32, 38, 45, or 52 mm holes) = £56.40

Mini, closed pouches. Net price 30 pouches (13 mm starter hole, 25, 32, 38, 45 or 52 mm holes) = £44.44

One-piece closed pouch with transparent front. Net price 30 pouches (13 mm starter hole) = £54.00

Second Nature® (EuroCare)

Second Nature, two-piece closed pouch. Net price 30 pouches (opaque: 32, 38, 45 or 57 mm; clear: 45 or 57 mm) = £32.05

Hollister range

Classic® (Hollister)

All with 25, 32, 38, 44, 51, 64, or 76 mm holes

Adhesive (series 217), one-piece closed pouch with adhesive and filter, clear. Net price 50 pouches = £62.77

Karaya seal (series 716), one-piece pouch with karaya skin protector (without filter), must be worn with belt, clear. Net price 30 pouches = £53.38

Karaya seal with filter (series 211), one-piece closed pouch with karaya skin protector and filter, must be worn with belt, opaque. Net price 30 pouches = £53.38

Karaya 5® Seal (series 331 and 332), one-piece closed pouch with porous adhesive, karaya skin protector seal, and filter, may be worn with belt, opaque or clear. Net price 30 pouches = £64.71

Microporous adhesive (series 314), one-piece compact closed pouch with porous adhesive and filter, may be worn with belt, clear. Net price 50 pouches = £67.92

Compact® (Hollister)

Closed, one-piece pouch with filter and comfort backing. Net price 30 pouches (beige or clear: 13-64 mm cut-to-fit; 25, 32, 38, 44, 51, or 64 mm) = £60.00

Prices are **net**, see p. 1

Guardian® (Hollister)

All with 25, 38, 51, or 64 mm holes

Guardian (series 451 and 450), two-piece closed pouch with filter, opaque (with double side comfort backing) or clear (with single side comfort backing). Net price 15 pouches = £15.33

Guardian mini-pouch (series 452), two-piece compact closed pouch with filter, opaque. Net price 15 pouches = £15.03

Flanges. Net price 'F' floating flange (25, 38, 51, 64 mm) 5 = £12.47, (102 mm) 5 = £13.20; 'S' stationary flange (25, 38, 51, or 64 mm) 5 = £12.26

Stoma cap, with filter, opaque. Net price 30 (38, 51, or 64 mm) = £28.44

Belt adaptor. Net price 10 = £8.70

HolliGard® (Hollister)

All with 25, 32, 38, 44, 51, 64, or 76 mm holes

Microporous adhesive (series 411), one-piece closed pouch with porous adhesive, HolliGard® seal, and filter, may be worn with belt, opaque. Net price 30 pouches = £67.15

Without adhesive (series 416), one-piece closed pouch with HolliGard® seal and filter, must be worn with belt, clear. Net price 30 pouches = £61.64

Impression C® (Hollister)

Closed, one-piece pouch with wafer, filter and bridge, comfort backing, beige. Net price 10 pouches (19, 22, 25, 29, 32, 35, 38, 41, 44 or 51 mm holes) = £21.20

Impression CPL® (Hollister)

Closed, two-piece pouch with filter and comfort backing, clear or beige. Net price 30 pouches (38, 44, 57 or 70 mm holes) = £30.90

Mini, two-piece closed pouch with filter, opaque. Net price 30 pouches (38, 44, 57 or 70 mm holes) = £26.70

Premium® (Hollister)

All with 25, 32, 38, 44, 51, 64, or 76 mm holes

Karaya 5® Seal (series 355 and 353), one-piece closed pouch with porous adhesive, karaya skin protector and filter, may be worn with belt, opaque or clear. Net price 15 pouches = £32.64

Synthetic Seal (series 354 and 356), one-piece closed pouch with porous adhesive, synthetic skin protector seal and filter, opaque or clear. Net price 15 pouches = £33.70

Marlen range

Ultra® (Marlen)

All with 12, 16, 19, 22, 25, 29, 32, 34, 38, 41, 44, 48, 50, 54, 57, 60, 63, 70, 73, 76 mm or cut-to-fit holes; opaque or clear; flat or shallow convex.

Closed, one-piece pouch. Net price 15 pouches = £28.80

Pelican range

Pelican® (Pelican)

Closed, one-piece pouch (formerly Simplaseel®). Net price 30 pouches (26, 32, 40, 45, 50 mm or cut-to-fit holes) = £69.93; 30 casual pouches (32, 40, or 45 mm holes) = £65.71

Pelican Select® (Pelican)

Closed, one-piece pouch with skin protector, filter, fabric front and back. Net price 30 pouches, clear or opaque, 20-65 mm (cut-to-fit) = £59.28; opaque (27, 34, 41, 48, or 55 mm holes), 30 = £59.28

Phoenix® (Pelican)

Closed, one-piece closed pouch. Net price (both 32, 40, or 45 mm holes) 100 pouches = £155.79; 100 casual pouches = £144.91

Sassco® (Pelican)

Closed, one-piece closed pouch. Net price 100 pouches (32, 40, or 45 mm holes) = £148.38

Rüsch range

Ostopore® (Rüsch)

Colo AV-opaque, one-piece pouch with adhesive and vent. Net price 30 pouches (25, 32, 38, or 45 mm holes) with 2 belt flanges = £40.56

Colo KAV-opaque, one-piece closed pouch with karaya seal skin protector, adhesive, and vent. Net price 30 pouches (25, 32, 38, 45, or 51 mm holes) with 5 belt flanges = £55.22

Colo KAV-transparent, one-piece closed pouch with karaya seal skin protector, adhesive, and vent. Net price 30 pouches (32, 38, 45, or 51 mm holes) with 30 belt flanges = £70.51

Rubber bags (Rüsch)

White rubber, one-piece closed pouch with spout outlet. Net price (both 19, 25, or 28 mm holes), 1 day pouch = £11.51; 1 night pouch = £12.42

Translet® (Rüsch)

Premier colostomy set, 1 adhesive ring with 6 bags. Net price 15 (27, 40, or 57 mm hole) = £63.90; spare bags 10 (18 or 28 cm length) = £6.90; spare adhesive rings or microporous spare adhesive rings (27, 40, or 57 mm) 5 = £6.54

Royal colostomy set, 1 adhesive ring and 6 odourproof bags. Net price 15 (27, 40, or 57 mm) = £88.80; spare bags (18 or 28 cm length) 10 = £7.76

Salts range

Cohflex® (Salts)

Closed, one-piece pouch with single-release paper, wafer, and filter, fabric front and back, flesh. Net price 30 pouches (all may be cut to fit; 25, 30, 35, 40, 45, 50, 55, 60 mm or 10–60 mm cut-to-fit holes) = £57.30

Coloset® (Salts)

Closed, one-piece pouch. Net price 30 pouches (medium: 713655) = £14.80; (small: 713656) = £9.74; (large: 713658) = £12.28; (medium: 713659) = £11.20

Eakin® (Salts)

Closed, one-piece pouch, white or clear. 32, 45, or 64 mm holes, net price 20 pouches = £41.33; 90 mm hole, 20 pouches = £49.81

Kombo® (Salts)

Kombo closed, one-piece pouch with karaya skin protector seal and adhesive, clear. Net price (30, 40, 50, or 60 mm holes), 30 pouches = £58.75; with filter, 30 pouches = £70.05

Simplicity® (Salts)

Closed, two-piece closed pouch, clear or pink, medium. Net price, clear (40, 50, 60, or 70 mm) 30 = £15.46; pink (40, 50, or 60 mm holes) 30 = £15.30; flange, standard (30, 40, 50, or 60 mm hole) 5 = £2.80; flange with cohesive washer (30 or 40 mm) 5 = £11.90, (50 mm) 5 = £13.42

Simplicity 1® (Salts)

Anatomical, closed one-piece pouch. Net price, clear (cut-to-fit), 30 = £62.05; opaque (30, 40, 50, 60 mm, or cut-to-fit holes), 30 = £62.05

Closed, one-piece pouch with porous adhesive, skin protector seal, and filter, fabric front and back. Net price 30 pouches (all may be cut to fit; opaque or pink: 30, 40, 50, or 60 mm holes; opaque, clear or pink: cut-to-fit holes) = £64.32

Paediatric, closed one-piece pouch with single-release paper, porous adhesive, clear. Net price 30 pouches (13 mm cut-to-fit hole) = £43.14

Simplicity 2® (Salts)

Closed, two-piece closed pouch (may also be applied directly to skin). Net price 30 pouches (40, 50, 60, or 70 mm holes, also 30 mm only for direct application to skin) = £33.17; flange (30, 40, 50, or 60 mm) 5 = £13.84

Solo® (Salts)

Solo closed, one-piece pouch with single-release paper, and adhesive flange, clear. Net price (30, 40, 50, or 60 mm holes), 30 pouches = £17.72; with filter, 30 pouches = £26.75

Supasac® (Salts)

Closed, one-piece pouch. Net price 30 (medium) = £23.09

Shannon range
Colostomy (Shannon)

Adhesive appliance. Net price, 1 (TJS 948B) = £48.25
Appliance. Net price, 1 appliance (TJS 962) = £16.81
Day bag (= pouch). Net price 1 pouch, TJS 948f =
£22.13; TJS 948j = £25.32
Disposable bag (= pouch). Net price TJS 948g, 100
pouches = £10.96
Night bag (= pouch). Net price 1 pouch, TJS 948e =
£25.32; TJS 948k = £27.61
Outfit. Net price 1 TJS 948A = £74.72, 1 TJS 948NA =
£72.36; 1 TJS 948T = £39.62
Easychange® (Shannon)

Appliance. Net price 1 appliance = £4.43
Spare bag (= pouch). Net price 100 pouches = £44.22
Shannon (Shannon)

Disposable bag (= pouch), closed pouches with plasters.
Net price 12 pouches = £6.05
Elastic necks. Net price 50 pouches = £22.11

Shaw range
Hainsworth® (Shaw)

Hainsworth® bag (= pouch), one-piece closed pouch.
Net price (both 25, 32, 38, or 51 mm holes), 20 pouches
with body mould adhesive = £40.11; 20 pouches with
Healwell® adhesive = £21.05
Shaw (Shaw)

Colostomy outfit, comprising, 4-inch wide elastic belt
with grainstrap (26- to 42-inch), 1 flange and 100 colostomy pouches. Net price one NSI 6 outfit with 11 × 6-
inch pouches = £37.17; one NSI 7 outfit with 12× 8-inch
pouches = £37.92; one NSI 8 outfit with 11× 6-inch
pouches = £40.60
Double seal, one-piece closed pouch. Net price 100 11 ×
6-inch pouches = £9.59; 100 12 × 8-inch pouches =
£10.50
Stick-on bag (= pouch), one-piece closed pouch with
plasters. Net price 10 pouches = £7.98

Simcare range
Adhesive (Simcare)

Stomabag, one-piece closed pouch with adhesive,
opaque. Net price (25, 32, 38, 44, 51, or 64 mm holes),
90 pouches = £123.18; with filter, 90 pouches = £138.44
Beta® (Simcare)

Closed, two-piece pouch with filter. Net price, 1 kit comprising 30 pouches and 8 Seel-a-peel sheets (100 ×
100 mm) = £51.15; 90 spare pouches = £140.83
Chiron® (Simcare)

Adhesive appliance with spout bag. Net price 1 appliance
(Mk I and Mk III) = £67.52
Clearseal bag (= pouch), one-piece closed pouch. Net
price 10 pouches (305 ×127 mm: 22 mm hole) = £14.51
Closed bag (= pouch). Net price 10 pouches (305
× 127 mm or 230 × 127 mm: 38 mm hole) = £14.51
Disposable bag (= pouch), one-piece closed pouch. Net
price 10 pouches (305 × 102 mm or 305 × 127 mm:
19 mm hole) = £9.67
Reinforced, one-piece disposable pouch. Net price 10
pouches = £14.51
Chironseal® (Simcare)

Closed bag (= pouch), one-piece closed pouch. Net price
10 pouches (305 × 102, 305 × 127, 230 × 127, or 305 ×
150 mm: 22 or 38 mm holes) = £10.89; 10 pouches (305
× 205 or 305× 255 mm: 22 or 38 mm hole) = £12.50
Reinforced, one-piece disposable pouch. Net price 10
pouches (305 × 102 mm: 25 or 38 mm holes or 305 ×
127 mm: 38 mm hole) = £14.51
EC1® (Simcare)

Colo Classic, one-piece closed pouch with wafer, comfort backing, and filter, opaque or clear. Net price 30
pouches (25, 32, 38, 44, 51, 64 mm or 15–64 mm cut-to-
fit holes) = £67.14

Omni® (Simcare)

Closed, one-piece pouch with wafer, porous adhesive, filter. Net price 30 pouches (opaque: 25, 32, 38, 44, or
51 mm; opaque or clear: 15–44 mm cut-to-fit holes) =
£68.11
Redifit® (Simcare)

Continuation bag (= pouch), one-piece closed pouch with
karaya skin protector, may be worn with belt, opaque.
Net price 20 pouches (32, 38, 44, 51, 64, or 75 mm
holes) = £70.14
Non-adhesive bag (= pouch), one-piece closed pouch,
opaque, must be worn with belt. Net price 20 pouches
with karaya skin protector (44 mm hole) = £70.14; without karaya, 20 pouches (38 mm hole) = £53.23
Rediseal® (Simcare)

Small bag (= pouch), one-piece PVC compact closed
pouch, opaque. Net price 10 pouches (38, 44, or 51 mm
holes) = £13.70
Serenade® (Simcare)

WC Disposable, two-piece closed pouch. Net price 30
pouches (25, 32, 38, 44, or 51 mm holes) with filter =
£33.10; 30 pouches (25, 32, 38, 44, or 51 mm holes)
with soft-backing and filter = £34.77; Mini pouches, 30
pouches (15–51 mm) with soft backing and filter =
£27.05; base plate (25, 32, 38, 44 or 51 mm), 10 =
£27.58
Symphony® (Simcare)

WC Disposable, one-piece closed pouch with wafer and
filter. Net price 30 pouches (opaque or clear: 25, 32, 38,
44, or 51 mm holes; opaque: 15–44 mm cut-to-fit holes)
= £70.60
Symphony Classic® (Simcare)

WC Disposable, one-piece closed bag with soft backing,
beige. Net price 30 pouches (25, 32, 38, 44, 51 mm or
15–51 mm cut-to-fit holes) = £70.60

Ward range
Ward (Ward)

Disposable bag (= pouch), one-piece closed pouch. Net
price 10 pouches (12 × 4-inch) with 4 × 3-inch plasters =
£8.40; 10 pouches (12 × 5-inch) with 4 × 4-inch plasters
= £8.40
Celluloid colostomy cup, with sponge or solid rim. Net
price 1 (small, medium, or large) cup = £34.88; with belt
fitting, 1 cup = £39.80; 1 pouch with mount outlet =
£14.50

Welland range
Impact® (Welland)

Colostomy bag (= pouch), one-piece closed pouch with
wafer, filter and disposable liner, opaque. Net price 30
pouches (19, 25, 32, 38, 44 or 51 mm holes) = £61.00
Vogue® shorter closed bag (Welland)

Colostomy bag (= pouch), one-piece pouch, opaque or
clear. Net price 30 pouches (25, 32, 38, 44, 51 mm or
10 mm cut-to-fit holes) = £52.27
Welland (Welland)

Colostomy bag (= pouch), one-piece closed pouch with
wafer and filter, opaque or clear. Net price 30 pouches
(25, 32, 38, 44, 51, 60 mm, or 10 mm cut-to-fit holes) =
£57.70
Softback colostomy bag, one-piece closed pouch with
wafer, filter, and soft backing, opaque or clear. Net price
30 pouches (25, 32, 38, 44, 51, 60 mm or 10 mm cut-to-
fit holes) = £59.25
Oval flange closed bag, one-piece pouch with oval
shaped wafer, filter and soft backing, opaque or clear.
Net price 30 pouches (10 mm cut-to-fit holes) = £61.26

Abbreviations and symbols, see inside front cover

Prices are **net**, see p. 1

DRAINABLE POUCHES AND ILEOSTOMY SETS

Drainable pouches are suitable for patients with an **ileostomy** or a **colostomy** with fluid effluent.

Body's Surgical range
Rubber bags screwcap (Body's Surgical)

Black butyl, one-piece pouch. Net price 1 day pouch = £27.05; 1 night pouch = £31.55

White rubber, one-piece pouch. Net price 1 day pouch = £15.03; 1 night pouch = £17.31

Rubber bags spout (Body's Surgical)

Black butyl, one-piece pouch. Net price 1 day or night pouch = £28.56

White rubber, one-piece pouch. Net price 1 day pouch = £13.51; 1 night pouch = £13.51

Bullen range
Denbul® (Bullen)

Bag, with one-piece flange. Net price 1 pouch (25 or 51 mm holes) = £27.83; 1 lightweight pouch (25 or 51 mm holes) = £1.60

Day bag (= pouch), one-piece pouch. Net price 1 pouch with screwcap outlet = £12.13; 1 pouch with screwcap outlet and larger opening = £12.60; 1 pouch with metal strip = £14.56; 1 pouch with tap outlet = £14.09

Night bag (= pouch), one-piece pouch. Net price 1 pouch with screwcap outlet = £13.36; 1 pouch with screwcap outlet and larger opening = £13.87; 1 pouch with metal strip = £14.56; 1 pouch with tap outlet = £16.10

CliniMed range
Biotrol® (CliniMed)

Elite, fabric covered one-piece pouch with skin protector adhesive and clamp closure, white or beige. Net price 30 pouches (starter hole, 20, 25, 30, 35, 40, 45, 50, 60, 70 mm holes) = £67.36; 30 clear pouches (20, 25, 30, 35, 40, 45, 50, 60, 70 mm or cut-to-fit holes) = £61.18; starter hole, 30 = £62.93

Elite Petite, one-piece pouch with skin protector adhesive and fabric backing, beige. Net price 30 pouches (starter hole, 25, 30, 35, 40 or 45 mm holes) = £58.38

Lockring 2, two-piece pouches with backing. Net price 30 pouches (for 35, 50 or 75 mm flanges) = £30.45

Ileo S, one-piece pouch with skin protector adhesive, white. Net price 30 pouches (starter hole, 20, 25, 30, 35, 40, 45, 50, 60, 70 mm holes) = £67.36

Post-op, one-piece pouch with skin protector adhesive, for temporary or permanent colostomies or ileostomies, clear. Net price (cut-to-fit holes) small, 30 pouches = £69.50; large, 30 pouches = £97.63

Preference, fabric covered one-piece pouch with skin protector adhesive, porous adhesive collar, beige. Net price 30 pouches (starter hole, 20, 25, 30, 35, 40, 45, 50, 60 mm or cut-to-fit holes) = £67.36

Coloplast range
Assura® (Coloplast)

Maxi, one-piece pouch, opaque or clear. Net price 30 pouches (10, 25, 30, 35, or 40 mm holes); 10 mm can be cut to fit up to 55 mm) = £63.03; two-piece pouch, opaque or clear. Net price 30 pouches (to fit 40, 50, or 60 mm base plates) = £34.56

Midi, one-piece pouch, opaque or clear. Net price 30 pouches (10, 25, 30, 35, 40, 45 or 50 mm holes; 10 mm can be cut to fit up to 55 mm) = £63.03; two-piece pouch, opaque or clear. Net price 30 pouches (to fit 40, 50 or 60 mm base plates) = £34.56

Mini, one-piece pouch, opaque. Net price 30 pouches (10, 25, 30, 35, or 40 mm holes; 10 mm can be cut to fit up to 55 mm) = £63.03

Ileo B® (Coloplast)

One-piece pouch with zinc oxide adhesive, clear or white. Net price 100 pouches (20 mm hole) = £159.60

Mini, one-piece compact pouch with zinc oxide adhesive, white. Net price 100 pouches (20 mm hole) = £158.60

K-Flex® (Coloplast)

One-piece pouch with karaya skin protector, clear. Net price 30 pouches (10 or 40 mm holes) = £73.02

mc2000® (Coloplast)

One-piece pouch with double seal, opaque or clear. Net price 30 pouches (20, 25, 30, 35, 40, 45, 50, 55, 60 mm holes or clear pouch with cut-to-fit hole) = £72.09

Mini, one-piece compact pouch, opaque. Net price 30 pouches (20, 25, 30, 35, or 40 mm holes) = £68.04

mc2002® (Coloplast)

Two-piece pouch, opaque or clear. Net price 30 open pouches (to fit 40 or 60 mm base plates) = £38.46; 30 closed pouches (to fit 40 or 60 mm base plates) = £42.42

pc3000® (Coloplast)

One-piece pouch, opaque or clear. Net price 30 pouches (20, 25, 30, 35, 40, 45, 50, 55, or 60 mm holes; 20 mm can be cut to fit up to 60 mm) = £64.86

Mini starter hole, one-piece pouch. Net price 30 pouches = £58.74

Sterile post-op bag, one-piece pouch. Net price 20 pouches (2200) = £48.00; (2202) = £31.26

ConvaTec range
Combihesive Natura® (ConvaTec)

Two-piece drainable pouch. Net price 10 standard pouches, clear or opaque; small pouches, opaque (to fit 32, 38, 45, 57 or 70 mm flanges) = £10.62

Ileodress® (ConvaTec)

Ileodress, one-piece pouch with textured backing. Net price 10 standard pouches with clip (opaque or clear: 19, 38, 45, 50, or 64 mm holes; 19 mm can be cut to fit; opaque only: 25 and 32 mm holes) = £21.37; 10 small pouches with clip, opaque (19, 25, 32, 38, 45, 50, or 64 mm holes; 19 mm can be cut to fit) = £20.92

Ileodress Plus, one-piece pouch single-release paper. Net price 10 standard pouches with clip (opaque or clear: 19, 38, 45, 50, or 64 mm holes; 19 mm can be cut to fit; opaque only: 25 and 32 mm holes) = £21.37; 10 small pouches with clip, opaque (19, 25, 32, 38, 45, or 50 mm holes; 19 mm can be cut-to-fit) = £18.70

Little Ones® (ConvaTec)

Paediatric, one-piece pouch. Net price 15 pouches (8 mm cut-to-fit hole) = £29.41

Stomadress® (ConvaTec)

One-piece pouch, clear. Net price 10 pouches (8 mm cut-to-fit hole) = £21.00

Surgicare System® 2 (ConvaTec)

System 2, two-piece pouches, white. Net price 10 pouches with clip (to fit 32, 38, 45, 57, or 70 mm flanges) = £10.53

System 2 Combihesive, two-piece pouches with textured backing. Net price 10 standard or small pouches with clip, beige (to fit 32, 38, 45, 57, or 70 mm flanges) = £10.62; 10 standard pouches with clip, clear, to fit 45, 57, or 70 mm flanges = £10.62, to fit 100 mm flanges = £18.77

Dansac range
Dansac® (Dansac)

CombiMicro D + S, one-piece pouch with porous adhesive, skin barrier ring, and fabric backing. Net price 30 pouches (25, 32, 38, 44, 50, 63 mm), opaque = £66.91; clear, 30 pouches = £65.66; cut-to-fit holes: 10–38 mm, 38–63 mm, opaque, 30 = £65.66; clear, 30 pouches = £65.66

CombiMicro Infant, one-piece pouch, opaque or clear. Net price 30 pouches (cut-to-fit holes: 10–25 mm) = £56.98

Supersquare System, two-piece pouch, opaque or clear. Net price 30 standard or small pouches to fit 50 mm base plate = £38.04; 30 standard pouches to fit 80 mm base plate = £54.96

Unique, one-piece pouch, opaque or clear. Net price 30 pouches (20, 25, 30, 35, 40, 45, 50, 60 mm or cut-to-fit holes) = £57.74; oval flange, opaque or clear, starter hole, 30 = £57.74

Unique 2, two-piece pouch, opaque or clear, regular or large. Net price 10 pouches (to fit 36, 43, 55 or 80 mm flange) = £10.25

Unique Infant, one-piece pouch, clear or opaque. Net price 30 pouches (10 mm can be cut to fit 40 mm) = £56.56

Unique Maxi, one-piece pouch. Net price 10 pouches (10 mm can be cut to fit up to 90 mm) = £21.00

Unique Mini, one-piece pouch. Net price 30 pouches (opaque: 20, 25, 30, or 35 mm holes; opaque or clear: 15 mm can be cut to fit up to 50 mm) = £56.10

DePuy range
Raymed® (DePuy)
Butyl day bag (= pouch), one-piece pouch. Net price 1 pouch with screwcap outlet = £23.28; 1 pouch with tap outlet = £24.46

Schacht® (DePuy)
Ileostomy, one-piece pouches. Net price 50 pouches = £19.80

Ileostomy appliance, odourproof. Net price 1 = £29.25

Drew range
Drew® (Drew)
Ileostomy bag (= pouch), one-piece pouch. Net price 50 D1/1 pouches = £61.85; 50 D1/6 pouches = £44.15

Ileostomy appliance. Net price 1 appliance (D1/1) = £32.52; 1 appliance (D1/6) = £27.86

Eurocare range
Confidence® (EuroCare)
Confidence, one-piece pouch, opaque. Net price 30 pouches (13 mm starter hole, 25, 32, 38, 45, or 52 mm holes) = £56.40

Confidence, one-piece pouch, small. Net price 30 pouches (13 mm starter hole, 25, 32, 38, 45 or 52 mm holes) = £45.00

Confidence, one-piece pouch with transparent front. Net price 30 pouches standard (13 mm starter hole) = £54.00; large (13 mm starter hole) = £56.40

Second Nature® (EuroCare)
Second Nature, two-piece drainable pouch. Net price 30 pouches (opaque: 32, 38, 45 or 57 mm; clear: 45 or 57 mm) = £31.50; secu-ring® to fit 32, 38, 45 or 57 mm flange, 10 = £9.80; wafer (110 × 100 mm to fit 32, 38 or 45 mm flange; 134 × 124 mm to fit 57 mm flange), 5 = £10.99

Hollister range
Classic® (Hollister)
Karaya seal (series 721), one-piece pouch with karaya skin protector seal, must be worn with belt, clear. Net price 30 pouches with 1 clamp (25, 32, 38, 44, 51, 64, or 76 mm hole) = £65.71

Karaya 5® transparent, one-piece pouch with karaya skin protector seal, may be worn with belt. 30- or 40-cm clear pouch with microporous adhesive (series 322 and 327), net price 30 pouches with 1 clamp (25, 32, 38, 44, 51, 64, or 76 mm hole) = £72.54; 30-cm pouches with regular adhesive (series 722) = £72.54

Karaya 5® opaque, one-piece pouch with karaya skin protector seal and porous adhesive, may be worn with belt. Net price 30 pouches with 1 clamp, 23-cm pouches (series 313: 25, 32, 38, 44, or 51 mm holes) = £72.54; 30-cm pouches (series 311: 25, 32, 38, 44, 51, 64, or 76 mm holes) = £69.85

Karaya 5® seal (series 360), one-piece pouch with porous adhesive and karaya skin protector seal, clear. Net price 15 pouches (25, 32, 38, 44, 51, 64, or 76 mm holes) with 1 clamp = £35.59

Loop ostomy bag (= pouch). Net price 20 pouches (3.5 or 4.5 inch) = £65.40

Loop ostomy gasket. Net price 10 (3.5 or 4.5 inch) = £65.40

Compact® (Hollister)
Drainable, one-piece pouch with comfort backing. Net price 10 pouches (beige or clear: 13-64 mm cut-to-fit 19, 25, 32, 38, 44, 51, or 64 mm) = £21.00

Mini Drainable, one-piece pouch with comfort backing, beige. Net price 10 pouches (13-51 mm cut-to-fit; 19, 25, 32, 38, 44, or 51 mm) = £19.20

Guardian® (Hollister)
All with 25, 38, 51, or 64 mm holes

Guardian (series 461 and 460), two-piece pouch, opaque (with beige non-woven double side backing) or clear (with beige non-woven single side backing). Net price 10 pouches with 1 clamp = £10.22; larger pouch to fit 102-mm flange, 10 pouches (clear) with 1 clamp = £21.44

Guardian mini-pouch, two-piece compact pouch, opaque. Net price (series 464), 10 pouches = £10.22; NHS : with inner film and replaceable filter (series 463), 10 pouches with pack of filters and 1 clamp

NHS *With replaceable filter* (series 462), two-piece pouch with inner film and replaceable filter, clear. 10 pouches with pack of filters and 1 clamp

Impression® (Hollister)
One-piece pouch with Convex wafer, synthetic seal and Microporous II adhesive, opaque or clear. Net price 10 pouches (19, 22, 25, 29, 32, 35, 38, 41, 44 or 51 mm holes) = £23.03

Impression CPL® (Hollister)
Two-piece pouch with comfort backing, beige or clear. Net price 10 pouches (38, 44, 57 or 70 mm holes) = £10.40; (102 mm hole) = £20.00

Mini Drainable, two-piece pouch with comfort backing, beige. Net price 10 pouches (38, 44, 57 or 70 mm holes) = £10.00

Premium® (Hollister)
Karaya 5® seal with filter (series 366), one-piece pouch with porous adhesive, karaya skin protector seal, and replaceable filter, may be worn with belt, clear. Net price 15 pouches (25, 32, 38, 44, 51, or 64 mm holes) with 1 clamp and filter elements = £38.82

Synthetic seal (series 364), one-piece pouch with porous adhesive and synthetic skin protector seal, clear. Net price 15 pouches (25, 32, 38, 44, 51, or 64 mm holes) with 1 clamp = £35.59

Marlen range
Ultra® (Marlen)
All with 12, 16, 19, 22, 25, 29, 32, 34, 38, 41, 44, 48, 50, 54, 57, 60, 63, 67, 70, 73, 76 mm or cut-to-fit holes; opaque or clear; small or large

Drainable, one-piece pouch. Net price 15 pouches = £32.25; with convex flange, 15 pouches = £33.00

Oakmed range
LOP-F7® (Oakmed)
Ileostomy appliance. Net price 1 appliance = £38.68
OPR-F® (Oakmed)
Ileostomy appliance. Net price 1 appliance = £80.69
SR-F® (Oakmed)
Ileostomy set. Net price 1 set = £55.60

Pelican range
Sassco® (Pelican)
Ileostomy bag (= pouch), one-piece pouch. Net price 100 pouches (26 or 32 mm holes) = £170.35
Pelican® (Pelican)
Drainable bag (= pouch), formerly Simplaseel®, one-piece pouch, opaque. Net price 30 pouches (26, 32, 40, 45, or 50 mm holes) = £71.02

Post-op drainable bag (= pouch), one-piece pouch. Net price 10 pouches (20-80 mm cut-to-fit) = £38.90

Paediatric drainable bag (= pouch), one-piece pouch. Net price 30 pouches (7-40 mm cut-to-fit) = £63.00

üsch range

irkbeck® (Rüsch)

Rubber, one-piece pouch, black or pink. Net price (both 19, 38, or 54 mm holes), 1 day pouch = £26.66; 1 night pouch = £30.49

Disposable, one-piece plastic pouch. Net price 100 pouches = £15.54

Ileostomy appliance. Net price 1 appliance 'A' (19, 38, or 54 mm) = £93.07; 1 appliance 'B' (19, 38, or 54 mm) = £60.06

ostopore® (Rüsch)

Ileo KAV-opaque, one-piece pouch with karaya seal skin protector, adhesive, and vent, opaque. Net price 30 pouches (25, 32, or 38 mm holes) with 30 belt flanges and 10 clips = £61.78

Rubber bag (Rüsch)

White rubber, one-piece pouch. Net price, 1 day pouch (38, 44, or 51 mm holes) = £11.94; 1 screwcap pouch (38 mm hole) = £12.89; 1 pouch with vent (38 mm hole) = £14.28

White rubber child bag (= pouch), one-piece pouch. Net price (both 19, 25, or 28 mm holes), 1 day pouch = £11.51; 1 night pouch = £14.08

Salts range

Cohflex® (Salts)

Drainable, one-piece pouch with single-release paper, wafer, and fabric front and back. Net price 30 pouches with integral closure clip (flesh: 25, 30, 35, 40, 45, 50, 55, or 60 mm, 10–60 mm starter hole) = £61.50

Paediatric drainable, one-piece small pouch with single-release paper, wafer, and fabric backing, opaque/clear/beige. Net price 30 pouches with integral closure clip (10–50 mm cut-to-fit holes) = £54.50

Eakin® (Salts)

Drainable, one-piece pouch, white or clear. Net price 20 small or large pouches (32, 45, or 64 mm holes) = £47.76

Fistula, one-piece pouch with or without remote drainage. Net price 10 infant pouches = £35.00; 10 small pouches = £49.68, 10 medium pouches = £64.26; 10 large pouches = £118.15; 20 wide pouches (90 mm hole) = £98.20

Light White® (Salts)

Drainable, one-piece pouch, white. Net price 30 large, small, or medium pouches (all 25, 32, or 38 mm holes) = £46.95

Drainable self-adhesive, one-piece pouch with adhesive, white. Net price 30 pouches (large: 25, 32, 38, or 44 mm holes; small and medium: 25, 32, or 38 mm holes) = £53.27

Koenig Rutzen® screwcap (Salts)

All with screwcap outlet

Black butyl all rubber, one-piece pouch. Net price 1 pouch (large: 25, 29, 32, 35, 38, 44, or 51 mm holes; small: 25, 32, 38, 44, or 51 mm) = £29.31; with bridge (soft-face Maggie Bag), 1 pouch (large: 25, 32, 38, 44, or 51 mm holes; small: 25, 32, or 38 mm) = £39.32

Black butyl reinforced, one-piece pouch. Net price 1 large or small pouch (both 25, 32, or 38 mm holes) = £32.32; with bridge (hard-face Maggie Bag), 1 pouch (large: 25, 32, 38, 44, or 51 mm holes; small: 25, 32, or 38 mm) = £45.83

Koenig Rutzen® spout (Salts)

All with spout outlet

Black butyl all rubber, one-piece pouch. Net price 1 large or small pouch (both 25, 32, 38, 44, or 51 mm holes) = £27.52; with bridge, 1 pouch (large: 25, 32, 38, 44, or 51 mm holes; small: 25, 32, or 38 mm) = £28.41

Black butyl reinforced, one-piece pouch. Net price 1 large or small pouch (25, 32, or 38 mm holes) = £35.14; with bridge, 1 pouch (large: 25, 32, 38, 44, or 51 mm holes; small: 25, 32, or 38 mm) = £36.28

Kombo® (Salts)

Kombo drainable, one-piece pouch with karaya skin protector seal and adhesive, clear. Net price 30 pouches (30, 40, 50, 60, or 80 mm holes) = £56.28; with filter, 30 pouches = £67.58

Rubber bags (Salts)

All must be used with flange

Black butyl screw, one-piece bag with screwcap outlet. Net price 1 large or small pouch = £28.99

Black butyl spout, one-piece bag with spout outlet. Net price 1 large or small pouch = £20.91

White screw, one-piece bag with screwcap outlet. Net price 1 large or small pouch = £9.67

White spout, one-piece bag with spout outlet. Net price 1 large or small pouch = £8.06

Salger® (Salts)

Drainable, one-piece pouch. Net price 10 pouches (40 or 57 mm holes) = £10.96

Simplicity® (Salts)

Drainable, two-piece pouch, clear. Net price 30 230 × 137 mm pouches (40, 50, or 60 mm holes) = £17.62

Post-op, two-piece pouch, clear. Net price 30 300 ×125-mm pouches (40, 50, or 60 mm holes) = £15.30

Simplicity 1® (Salts)

Anatomical, one-piece pouch. Net price clear (cut-to-fit), 30 = £66.70; opaque (30, 40, 50, 60 mm or cut-to-fit holes), 30 = £66.70

Drainable, one-piece pouch with porous adhesive and skin protector seal, fabric front and back. Net price 30 pouches with integral closure clip (opaque or pink: 30, 40, 50, or 60 mm, all may be cut to fit; opaque, clear or pink: 10–60 mm cut-to-fit hole) = £69.10

Paediatric drainable, one-piece pouch with porous adhesive and skin protector seal, clear. Net price 30 pouches (cut-to-fit hole) = £43.14

Simplicity 2® (Salts)

Drainable, two-piece pouch (may also be applied directly to skin). Net price 15 pouches (40, 50, 60, or 70 mm holes, also 30 mm only for direct application to skin) = £18.40

Post-op, two-piece pouch (may also be applied directly to skin). Net price 30 pouches (40, 50, 60, or 70 mm holes, also 30 mm only for direct application to skin) = £36.34

Transverse, two-piece pouch (may also be applied directly to skin). Net price 10 pouches (cut-to-fit hole) = £41.32; 5 flanges = £20.19

Solo® (Salts)

Drainable, one-piece pouch with single-release paper and adhesive, clear. Net price 30 pouches (30, 40, 50, 60 or 80 mm holes) = £21.04; with filter, 30 pouches = £26.53

NHS United® (Salts)

Soft & Secure drainable, one-piece pouch, opaque or clear. Net price 10 pouches (38, 45, or 57 mm holes) = £8.47

Shaw range

Rubber bags (Shaw)

Black screwcap, one-piece pouch with screwcap outlet. Net price (both 19, 38 or 54 mm holes), 1 day pouch = £22.55; 1 night pouch = £23.89

Simcare range

Adhesive (Simcare)

Stomabag, one-piece pouch with adhesive, opaque. Net price 60 pouches (19, 25, 32, 38, 51 mm or cut-to-fit holes) = £90.05

Cavendish® (Simcare)

Odourproof, one-piece pouch. Net price (all 25, 32, or 38 mm holes), 10 opaque pouches with non-adhesive flange = £30.64; 10 opaque pouches with adhesive flange = £36.91; 10 clear PVC pouches = £30.83

Chiron® screwcap (Simcare)

All with screwcap outlet

Butyl rubber day bag (= pouch), one-piece pouch, black. Net price 1 pouch (38, 44, or 51 mm hole) = £31.72

Butyl rubber night bag (= pouch), one-piece pouch, black. Net price 1 pouch (38 or 44 mm holes) = £38.07

Latex rubber day bag (= pouch), one-piece pouch. Net price 1 pouch (38 mm hole) = £16.04

Latex rubber night bag (= pouch), one-piece pouch. Net price 1 pouch (38 mm hole) = £21.22

White rubber day bag (= pouch), one-piece pouch. Net price 1 pouch (38, 44, or 51 mm) = £18.26, child-size pouch (38 mm hole) = £15.88; body-size outlet, 1 pouch (38 mm hole) = £18.26, child-size pouch (38 mm hole) = £14.42

White rubber night bag (= pouch), one-piece pouch. Net price 1 pouch (38 or 51 mm hole) = £21.22; body-size outlet, 1 pouch (38 mm hole) = £17.45

Chiron® spout (Simcare)

White rubber bag (= pouch), one-piece pouch. Net price 1 day pouch (38 mm hole) = £15.70; 1 night pouch (38 mm hole) = £17.05

EC1® (Simcare)

Ileo classic, one-piece pouch with wafer and comfort backing, opaque. Net price 30 pouches with 1 clamp (19, 25, 32, 38, 44 mm or 10–44 mm cut-to-fit holes) = £70.34

Mini classic, one-piece compact pouch with wafer and comfort backing, opaque or clear. Net price 30 pouches with 1 clamp (10–44 mm cut-to-fit holes) = £70.34

Post-op classic, one-piece pouch with wafer and comfort backing, clear. Net price 30 pouches with 1 clamp, 10–64 mm cut-to-fit holes = £72.54; 10–90 mm cut-to-fit holes = £102.65

Omni® (Simcare)

Drainable, one-piece pouch with porous adhesive wafer and replaceable filter. Net price 20 pouches (opaque: 25, 32, 38, 44 mm; opaque or clear: 10–44 mm cut-to-fit hole) = £46.85; **NHS** opaque (10–44 mm cut-to-fit hole) = £53.39

Redifit® (Simcare)

Opaque, one-piece pouch with karaya skin protector, may be worn with belt. Net price 20 pouches with 2 closure clips (25, 32, 38, 44, 51, or 64 mm holes) = £68.80; small outline pouches, 20 pouches with 2 closure clips (25, 32, or 38 mm) = £68.80

Clear fronted, one-piece pouch with karaya skin protector, may be worn with belt. Net price 20 pouches with 2 closure clips (25, 32, 44, 51, or 64 mm holes) = £68.80

Ward range

Donald Rose® (Ward)

Bag (= pouch), with celluloid collars, solid, flat or fluid rims. Net price 1 pouch = £18.73

Ileostomy appliance. Net price 1 appliance (first stage) = £45.83; 1 appliance (second stage) = £45.33; 1 appliance (new improved) = £48.11

Rubber bags (Ward)

Bag, rubber. Net price 1 pouch, complete with collar = £20.33; 1 pouch, with tap outlet and skirt = £22.72

Night bag (= pouch), shaped rubber with long vertical spring vulcanite screw outlet. Net price 1 pouch = £18.63

Black rubber bag (= pouch), one-piece pouch with screw-cap outlet. Net price (19, 35, or 54 mm hole), 1 day pouch = £17.52; 1 night pouch = £18.30

White rubber ileostomy bag (= pouch) with flange, pouch with St. Mark's flange. Net price 1 pouch = £25.65

White rubber ileostomy bag (= pouch), one-piece pouch. Net price 1 day pouch (screwcap or spout outlet) = £11.97; 1 night pouch (screwcap or spout outlet) = £13.46; tap outlet, 1 day pouch = £17.53; 1 night pouch = £19.44

White rubber transverse ileostomy bag (= pouch), one-piece pouch. Net price 1 pouch = £27.98

Welland range

Vogue® shorter drainable bag (Welland)

Drainable, one-piece pouch, opaque or clear. Net price 30 pouches (25, 32, 38, 44, 51 mm, or 19 mm cut-to-fit holes) = £52.05

Welland® (Welland)

Softback ileostomy bag (= pouch), one-piece with wafer and soft backing, opaque or clear. Net price 30 pouches (25, 32, 38, 44, 51 mm, or 10 mm cut-to-fit holes) = £60.82

Oval drainable, one-piece pouch with wafer, opaque. Net price (both cut-to-fit holes), 30 pouches = £61.26; with soft backing, 30 pouches = £64.05

Post-op, one-piece pouch with soft backing, clear or opaque. Net price (10 mm cut-to-fit hole), 30 pouches = £63.00

UROSTOMY POUCHES

Body's Surgical range

Rubber bags (Body's Surgical)

Black butyl, one-piece pouch, odourless. Net price 1 day pouch (tap outlet) = £30.07; 1 night pouch (tap outlet) = £31.55

White rubber, one-piece pouch. Net price 1 day pouch (tap outlet) = £15.03; 1 night pouch (tap outlet) = £17.31

Bullen range

Lenbul® (Bullen)

Day bag (= pouch), one-piece pouch. Net price 1 pouch with tap outlet = £14.09; 1 pouch with large opening (for 4-inch flange with tap outlet) = £14.62; 1 pouch with metal strip = £15.77

Night bag (= pouch). Net price 1 pouch with tap outlet = £16.10; 1 pouch with large opening = £16.71

One-piece flange and bag (= pouch) with tap outlet. Net price 1 (1-inch hole) = £29.59; (2-inch hole) = £29.60

Baby's bag (= pouch) and flange with tap outlet. Net price 1 (1.25- or 2-inch hole, with or without night tube) = £40.75

Child's rubber cap and bag (= pouch) with non-reflux valve. Net price 1 small, 1 small with metal strip, or 1 large = £27.62; 1 large with metal strip = £29.70

Coloplast range

Assura® (Coloplast)

Maxi, urostomy pouch with soft backing, clear or opaque. Net price 30 (one-piece) pouches (10–55 mm hole) = £117.00; two-piece pouch, 30 pouches (to fit 40, 50 or 60 mm base plates) = £68.70

Midi, urostomy pouch with soft backing, clear. Net price 30 (one-piece) pouches (10–55 mm hole) = £117.00; two-piece pouch, 30 pouches (to fit 40 or 50 mm base plates) = £68.70

Paediatric, urostomy pouches with soft backing, clear or opaque. Net price 30 (one-piece) pouches (10–35 mm hole) = £117.00; two-piece pouch, 30 pouches (to fit 40 mm base plate) = £68.70; 5 paediatric (40 mm) = £13.50

Stoma Urine (Coloplast)

Maxi, one-piece pouch with zinc oxide adhesive. Net price 30 pouches (13-mm hole) = £76.98

Midi, one-piece pouch with zinc oxide adhesive. Net price 30 pouches (13-mm hole) = £76.98

URO 2002® (Coloplast)

Two-piece pouch. Net price 20 small pouches (100 mL, to fit 40 mm base plate) = £55.78; 20 large pouches (375 mL, to fit 40 or 60 mm base plate) = £55.78

Base plate. Net price 5 plates (40 mm, to fit 10–35 mm stoma) or 5 plates (60 mm, to fit 10–55 mm stoma) = £14.54

Night drainage system. Net price 10 pouches (1.65 litre), 1 tube, and 2 connectors = £14.14; hospital pack, 10 pouches (1.65 litre), 5 tubes, and 10 connectors = £17.60

ConvaTec range

Surgicare System® 2 (ConvaTec)

Two-piece pouch, with non-reflux valve, clear. Net price 10 (small or standard) pouches (32, 38, 45, or 57 mm flange) = £22.92; 10 standard pouches (70 mm flange) = £24.82, (100 mm flange) = £37.38

Surgicare System® 2 Combihesive (ConvaTec)

Two-piece pouch with Accuseal® tap, and textured backing, clear. Net price 10 standard pouches (32, 38, 45, or 57 mm flange) = £23.49

Urodress® (ConvaTec)

One-piece pouch with Stomahesive® and tap. Net price 10 pouches (19, 25, 32, 38, or 45 mm holes) = £43.16

Dansac range

Unique® 2 (Dansac)

Two-piece pouch, with 1 Dansac® drain tube adaptor, opaque or clear. Net price 10 pouches (to fit 30, 36, 43 or 55 mm flange) = £22.90

DePuy range

Raymed® (DePuy)

Butyl night bag (= pouch), one-piece pouch. Net price 1 pouch with screwcap outlet = £24.95; 1 pouch with tap outlet = £25.80

Drew range

Urostomy bags (Drew)

Urostomy bag (= pouch), one-piece pouch. Net price 50 pouches (D1/2, OSTO 06) = £76.34

Rubber bags (Drew)

Rubber bag (= pouch), one-piece pouch. Net price 1 pouch screwcap outlet (OSTO 16) = £13.03; 1 pouch (OSTO 17) tap outlet = £13.67

Ureterostomy appliance (Drew)

Ureterostomy appliance. Net price 1 appliance, 1–1.25 inch (D1/2, OSTO 05) = £38.83

Hollister range

Classic® (Hollister)

Karaya 5® seal and regular adhesive with attachment for optional belt, one-piece pouch, clear. Net price 20 pouches (series 741, 23-cm pouch: 19, 25, 32, 38, 44, or 51 mm holes; series 746, 40-cm pouch and series 748, 30-cm pouch: 25, 32, 38, 44, or 51 mm holes) including 1 standard drain tube = £63.47

Regular adhesive with attachment for optional belt, one-piece pouch, clear. Net price 20 pouches (series 740, 23-cm pouch: 19, 25, 32, 38, 44, or 51 mm holes; series 745, 40-cm pouch and series 747, 30-cm pouch: 25, 32, 38, 44, or 51 mm holes) including 1 standard drain tube = £48.29

Regular adhesive only (beltless), one-piece pouch, clear. Net price 20 pouches (series 744, 23-cm pouch: 19, 25, 32, 38, 44, or 51 mm holes), including 1 standard drain tube = £48.29

Compact® (Hollister)

Urostomy pouch with comfort backing. Net price 10 pouches (13-64 mm cut-to-fit; 13, 16, 19, 25, 32, 38, 44 or 51 mm) = £42.00

First Choice® (Hollister)

Urostomy pouch with synthetic skin barrier and Microporous II adhesive (series 146). Net price 10 pouches (13–64 mm starter hole, 19, 25, 32, 38, 44, or 51 mm holes) = £44.13

Guardian® (Hollister)

Guardian, two-piece pouch with wide-bore tap and non-reflux valve, clear (with beige, non-woven single side backing) (series 470). Net price 10 pouches (25-cm for max. 25, 38, or 51 mm stomas), including 1 drain tube adaptor = £23.50

Impression® (Hollister)

One-piece pouch with Convex wafer, synthetic seal and Microporous II® adhesive, clear. Net price 10 pouches (13, 16, 19, 22, 25, 29, 32, 35, 38 or 44 mm holes) = £44.13

Impression C® (Hollister)

Closed, one-piece pouch with Convex wafer, comfort backing, clear. Net price 10 pouches (13, 16, 19, 22, 25, 29, 32, 35, 38, 44 or 51 mm holes) = £38.00

Impression CPL® (Hollister)

Two-piece pouch with comfort backing. Net price 10 pouches (38, 44, 57 or 70 mm holes) = £22.90

Lo-profile® (Hollister)

Karaya 5® seal and Microporous II® adhesive with gasket for optional belt, one-piece pouch, with non-reflux valve, clear (series 143). Net price 10 pouches (25-cm pouch: 19, 25, 32, 38, 44, or 51 mm gasket), including 1 Lo-profile drain tube = £48.40

Microporous II® adhesive only (beltless) one-piece pouch with non-reflux valve (series 142). Net price 10 pouches (25-cm pouch: 19, 25, 32, 38, 44, or 51 mm holes), including 1 Lo-profile® drain tube = £40.55

Marlen range

Ultra® (Marlen)

Urostomy pouch, clear. Net price 10 (small or large; flat or shallow convex) pouches (12 mm starter hole, 12, 16, 19, 22, 25, 29, 32, 34, 38, 41, 44, 48, 50, 54, 57, 60, 63, 67, 70, 73, or 76 mm holes) = £38.00

Oakmed range

Urostomy sets (Oakmed)

Urostomy sets. Net price 1 LOP-U appliance (wire ring retainer with 1.5-inch elastic belt for small flange, 10 one-piece flanges and lightweight bags with 1-inch hole, 30 3.5 × 3.5-inch double-sided adhesive plasters) = £38.68; 1 OPR-U appliance (waterproof canvas retaining shield waistband, 2 one-piece flanges and bags with 1- or 2-inch hole and tap outlet, 30 3.5 × 3.5-inch double-sided adhesive plasters) = £80.69; 1 SR-U appliance (plastic retainer ring shield with 1-inch elastic belt for medium flange, Lenbul® 1.5-inch diameter flange, 1 Lenbul® day and 1 night bag with tap outlet, 30 3.5 × 3.5-inch double-sided adhesive plasters) = £60.60

Rüsch range

Rubber bags (Rüsch)

Black rubber (Birkbeck®), one-piece pouch with tap outlet. Net price 1 day pouch (19 mm hole) = £30.49; 1 night pouch (19 mm hole) = £33.26

Pink rubber, one-piece pouch with tap outlet. Net price 1 day pouch (19 mm hole) = £30.49; 1 night pouch (19 mm hole) = £33.26

White rubber, one-piece pouch with tap outlet. Net price 1 day pouch (19, 25, or 28 mm hole) = £16.56; 1 night pouch (19, 25, or 28 mm hole) = £17.01

White rubber (Glasgow), one-piece pouch. Net price 1 pouch (small or large tap) = £20.23

White rubber transverse, one-piece pouch. Net price 1 left or right pouch (small, medium, or large) = £20.23

Salts range

Koenig Rutzen® (Salts)

All rubber white rubber tap bag (= pouch), one-piece pouch with tap outlet. Net price 1 small or medium pouch (both 25, 32, or 38 mm holes) or 1 large pouch (25, 32, 38, 44, or 51 mm holes) = £15.67

All rubber black butyl bag (= pouch), one-piece pouch with tap outlet and non-reflux valve. Net price 1 medium or large pouch (both 19, 25, 32, or 38 mm holes) = £37.84; special size holes also available to order

---

All rubber MB black butyl bag (= pouch), one-piece pouch with tap outlet, bridge, and non-reflux valve. Net price 1 small, medium, or large pouch (all 19, 25, 32, or 38 mm holes) = £44.25; special size holes also available to order

Black butyl, reinforced bag (= pouch), one-piece pouch with tap outlet and non-reflux valve. Net price 1 medium or large pouch (both 19, 25, 32, or 38 mm holes) = £46.38; special size holes also available to order

MB black butyl, reinforced bag (= pouch), one-piece pouch with tap outlet and non-reflux valve. Net price 1 medium or large pouch (both 19, 25, 32, or 38 mm holes) = £53.13; special size holes also available to order

Rubber bags (Salts)

Black rubber bag (= pouch) (for use with flange), two-piece pouch with tap outlet. Net price 1 small, medium, or large pouch = £38.42; special size holes also available to order

White rubber bag (= pouch) for use with flange, two-piece pouch with tap outlet. Net price 1 small, medium, or large pouch = £10.13

Light White® (Salts)

Urostomy pouch with Realistic® washer, one-piece pouch, white. Net price 20 large pouches (all 25, 32, or 38 mm holes) = £104.88

Urostomy pouch with Realistic® washer, one-piece pouch, clear. Net price 20 large or small pouches (all 25, 32, or 38 mm holes) = £105.08

Urostomy pouch, one-piece pouch, white. Net price 20 large pouches (25, 32, or 38 mm holes) = £78.83

Urostomy pouch, one-piece pouch, clear. Net price 20 large or small pouches (25, 32, or 38 mm holes) = £78.83

Urostomy pouch, one-piece pouch with adhesive, white. Net price 20 large pouches (25, 32, or 38 mm holes) = £83.23

Urostomy pouch, one-piece pouch with adhesive, clear. Net price 20 large or small pouches (both 25, 32, or 38 mm holes) = £83.23

Simplicity 1® (Salts)

Paediatric Uri-bag, one-piece pouch, 13 mm starter hole. Net price 15 pouches = £39.88

Simcare range

Carshalton® (Simcare)

Bag (= pouch), one-piece pouch. Net price 10 oval or triangular pouches (both 25, 32, or 38 mm) with acrylic plaster = £19.25

Set, one-piece pouch. Net price 20 oval or triangular pouches with plasters, bodyplate, clamp, connector, and medium belt (both 25, 32, or 38 mm holes) = £64.87

Chiron® Non-disposable (Simcare)

Butyl rubber bag (= pouch), one-piece pouch with stopcock outlet, odourless, black. Net price 1 day bag (22 mm) = £34.46

Latex rubber bag (= pouch), one-piece pouch with stopcock outlet. Net price (both 38 mm) 1 day bag = £23.87; 1 night bag = £27.07

Rubber child-size bag (= pouch), one-piece pouch with stopcock outlet, white. Net price 1 = £20.03

Rubber day bag (= pouch), one-piece pouch, white with stopcock outlet. Net price 1 (38 mm) = £23.87

Rubber night bag (= pouch), one-piece, white. Net price 1 (38, 44, or 51 mm) = £27.07

Chiron® (Simcare)

Ileal bladder appliance, set comprises 1 web and elastic belt 25 mm wide, 1 wire pressure frame, 1 St Mark's pattern rubber flange (without diaphragm), 2 rubber day pouches with stopcock outlet, 30 double-sided plasters. Net price = £75.12

Mitcham® (Simcare)

Maxi, one-piece pouch. Net price 10 pouches with adhesive flange (25, 32, or 38 mm) = £39.24, 10 pouches with nonadhesive flange (25, 32, or 38 mm) = £32.04

Mini, one-piece pouch. Net price 10 pouches with adhesive flange (19, 25, or 32 mm) = £39.24, 10 pouches with nonadhesive flange (25 mm or 32 mm) = £32.04

Standard, one-piece pouch. Net price 10 pouches with adhesive flange (19, 25, 32 or 38 mm) = £39.24, 10 pouches with nonadhesive flange (19, 25, 32, or 38 mm) = £32.04, 1 pouch with nonadhesive flange and foam pads (25, 32, or 38 mm) = £5.48

Rediflow® (Simcare)

Adhesive set, may be worn with belt. Net price 20 pouches (19, 25, 32, 38, 44, or 51 mm) = £57.65

Ward range

Ward® (Ward)

Ureterostomy bag (= pouch) with tap outlet. Net price 1 night pouch = £19.13; 1 day pouch (19, 35, or 54 mm hole) = £17.91

ADHESIVE PREPARATIONS, ADHESIVE REMOVERS AND DEODORANTS

Adhesive preparations

Hollister® (Hollister)

Medical adhesive spray (with silicones). Net price 170-g aerosol spray = £13.51

Latex adhesive solution (Salts)

Net price per tube = £1.86. Label: 15

Adhesive removers

Clear Peel® (CliniMed)

Adhesive remover. Net price 50 mL = £2.10

Hollister® (Hollister)

Adhesive remover spray. Net price 170-g spray = £11.32

Salts 'SPR' Plaster Remover (Rezolve)® (Salts)

Adhesive remover spray. Net price 70-g aerosol spray = £2.78. Label: 15

Deodorants

Atmocol® is used as a deodorising spray when emptying the appliance. The other deodorants listed are placed in the appliance.

Atmocol® (DePuy)

Aerosol deodorant. Net price 1 unit (400 sprays) = £1.90

Chironair Odour Control Liquid® (Simcare)

Deodorant solution. Net price 113 g = £5.60

Colostomy Plus® (Shannon)

Deodorant. Net price 1 unit = £2.68

Day-drop® (Loxley)

Deodorant solution. Net price 7.5 mL = £1.04; 15 mL = £1.73; 30 mL = £2.95 (7.5 and 15 mL also available as Lemon Day-drop®)

Dor® (Pelican)

Deodorant solution. Net price 7 mL = £1.79

Forest Breeze® (Shaw)

Deodorant. Net price 1 unit = £3.18

LiMone® (CliniMed)

Deodorant spray. Net price 50 mL = £4.00

NaturCare® (AlphaMed)

Deodorant spray. Net price 50 mL = £3.37

Ostobon® (Coloplast)

Deodorant powder. Net price 22 g = £3.92

Saltair No-Roma® (Salts)

Deodorant solution. Net price 28 mL = £2.21; 227 mL = £7.23

Sween® (Bullen & Smears)

Deodorant. Net price 36 mL = £3.95

Translet Plus One® (Rüsch)

Deodorant solution for men. Net price 7 mL = £2.88

Translet Plus Two® (Rüsch)

Deodorant solution for women. Net price 7 mL = £2.88

ADHESIVE DEVICES AND RINGS

Bullen range
Adhesive plaster, double-sided. Net price 10 zinc oxide plasters 3.5 × 3.5 inch = £3.91, 4 × 4 inch = £4.82, 5 × 5 inch = £8.15; 10 acrylic base plasters 3.5 × 3.5 inch = £3.62, 4 × 4 inch = £4.65, 5 × 5 inch = £7.83

Flange retention strips. Net price 50 strips 4 × 1 inch = £1.75, 4 × 2 inch = £2.37

3M range
Stomaseal® (3M)
Adhesive discs. Net price 12 discs (10 cm diameter) = £4.41

Rüsch range
Ostomy plasters, double-sided. Net price 25 plasters (25 mm hole, or no hole) = £6.49

Salts range
Kidney seals. Net price 10 = £4.17
Reliaseal® (Salts)
Adhesive discs, double-sided, round, hypo-allergic. Net price 10 discs (13, 19, 22, 25, 29, 32, or 38 mm) = £16.19
Transacryl® (Salts)
Adhesive plasters, double-sided. Net price 10 plasters (25, 32, or 38 mm) = £5.30
Zopla® (Salts)
Adhesive plasters, double-sided. Net price (both 25, 32, or 38 mm) 10 square plasters = £3.98; 10 round plasters = £4.62

Shannon range
Adhesive plasters, double-sided. Net price 25 plasters = £14.91
Rings. Net price 5 rubber retaining rings = £5.96; 1 plastic locking ring = £2.22
Easychange® (Shannon)
Adhesive plasters, with rings (spare). Net price 5 plasters = £5.90

Shaw range
Adhesive plasters, double-sided, hole cut-to-size. Net price 10 plasters, 4 × 4 inch = £7.13; 5 × 5 inch = £7.40

Simcare range
Adhesive discs, double-sided (76 mm diameter: 19 or 25 mm opening; 90 mm diameter: 32 or 38 mm opening) = £4.40
Rings, elastic, for use with spout bags. Net price 3 rings = £2.17
Carshalton® (Simcare)
Adhesive plasters, double-sided. Net price both (25, 32, or 38 mm) 10 acrylic plasters = £4.67; 10 zinc oxide plasters = £7.40
Chiron® (Simcare)
Adhesive plasters, double-sided. Net price 10 plasters (90 mm square: 19 or 35 mm hole) = £5.97, (102 mm square: 19 or 35 mm hole) = £6.86, (127 mm square: 19 or 35 mm hole) = £7.56, (150 mm square and 102 × 76 mm: both 19 mm hole) = £8.45, (90 and 102 mm square: both 25 mm hole) = £8.45, (125 mm square: 25 mm hole) = £9.27
Clearseal plasters. Net price 10 plasters (100 mm square: 19 or 35 mm hole) = £6.86
Kidney seals, adhesive flange retaining strips. Net price 10 strips (small or large) = £4.71

Ward range
Adhesive plasters, double-sided with opening. Net price 10 plasters = £4.26

BAG CLOSURES

Clamps
Available from *CliniMed* (Biotrol® for post-op or for drainage pouches, 1 clamp = 98p), *Hollister,* (for drainable pouches, 1 clamp = £1.00, 20 = £16.41; for Premium® pouches, 1 clamp = £1.04, 20 = £17.38), *Simcare* (10 clamps = £8.28; Carshalton®, 5 clamps = £9.63), *Simpla* (for Ileo® pouches, 20 clamps = £5.50)

Clips
Available from *ConvaTec* (10 beige clips = £2.76; for Surgicare System® 2, 10 white clips = £2.76; drainable, 10 curved clips = £5.00); *Drew* (10 clips = 60p), *Eurocare* (for drainable pouches, 10 clips = £6.40), *Pelican* (drainable, 20 = £5.67), *Salts* (5 clips = £1.77), *Simcare* (for odourproof pouches, 10 = £6.33)

Closing Tape
Available from *Shannon* (1 reel = £1.44)

Fastening Ring
Rubber pouch fastening ring. Available from *Shaw* (1 ring = £1.04)

Ties
Available from *CliniMed* (30 soft-end ties, white or beige for drainable pouches = £2.39), *ConvaTec* (50 soft wire ties = £4.87)

BAG COVERS

Body's Surgical
Bag cover, cloth. Net price 1 cover = £4.18
Bullen
Bag cover, cloth, for day or night bags. Net price 1 cover = £7.86
CliniMed
Bag cover, cloth for closed or drainable Biotrol® pouches. Net price 5 covers = £7.78
Coloplast
Bag cover, cloth for closed or drainable mc2000® or mc2002® pouches (white or flesh), for mc2000® Mini pouches (decorated: white or flesh), for Ileo B® standard pouches, or for URO2002® pouches (white). Net price 5 covers = £21.37
Cover Care
Bag cover, formerly Surgicare System® 2 pouch covers. Net price 3 covers (for 32/38 mm Mini pouches or 45/57 mm pouches) = £6.34; 3 covers (for standard drainable pouches, urostomy pouches, large urostomy pouches, small closed 38/45 mm pouches: small drainable pouches, combihesive closed pouches, medium closed pouches: 57 and 70 mm) = £6.71
Drew
Bag cover, cotton. Net price 1 cover = £1.34
Hollister
Bag cover, non-woven. Net price 5 covers (for closed or non-drainable pouch) = £4.15
Impharm
Ostocover® bag cover, cloth, white or coloured. Net price 3 covers = £6.86
Pelican
Bag cover, cotton, for closed pouch. Net price 5 covers, normal = £10.27, casual = £10.21; for drainable pouch, 5 covers = £10.61
Rüsch
Bag cover, cloth for Ostopore® pouches. Net price 5 covers (small or large) = £17.06
Salts
Bag covers, cotton, appliance to be stated. Net price 1 cover = £3.46. Cloth, for Eakin® pouches, 1 cover small or large (both 32, 45 or 64 mm) = £4.15
Shaw
Bag covers, cloth. Net price 1 day pouch cover, cotton = £4.68; lycra = £4.94. 1 night cover, cotton = £4.94; lycra = £5.30

Simcare

Bag cover. Net price 1 day or night cotton pouch cover = £10.41; 5 stomabag covers (white or coloured) = £23.25; for Redifit® pouches, 1 cotton cover (25 and 32 mm, 38, 44, and 51 mm, 64, and 75 mm holes) = £7.43; for Symphony® pouches, 5 polyethylene covers = £4.30

Ward

Bag cover, white linen. Net price 1 cover = £6.17

Welland

Bag shields, spunbonded polypropylene. Net price 10 (small: 25–44 mm; large: 10, 51, or 60 mm) = £2.99

BELTS

Body's Surgical

Belts. Net price 3-inch belt = £14.16: 3-inch one-piece belt, = £18.48; 4-inch one-piece belt = £18.67; 1-inch web and elastic with button and buckle fastening = £7.86; 2-inch belt = £9.30; 3-inch belt = £10.72; 1 girdle and panti-brief with hole for stoma and suspenders or understrap = £45.84; 1 St Mark's (male or female) = £54.11; 1 St Mark's Coutil ostomy = £37.03

Bullen

Belts. Net price 1.5-inch belt with aluminium retaining shield (small, medium, or large) = £9.31; 1.5-inch elastic belt with wire or plastic ring retainer (wire; small, medium, or large) = £9.50; 4-inch (wire; small, medium, or large) = £13.92; 1-inch elastic belt with plastic ring shield = £10.05: 1 waterproof canvas retaining shield (small, medium, or large) = £15.03; 1 St Mark's = £39.01

Bullen & Smears

Girdles. Net price 1 Camila® panty girdle = £18.00; 1 Cloe® roll on girdle = £15.00; 1 Constance® panty girdle = £23.80

J. Chawner

Girdles. Net price 1 ostomy girdle = £31.95; 1 ostomy-panty girdle = £28.90; 1 colostomy belt with understraps = £31.30

CliniMed

Waist belt for Biotrol® pouches. Net price 1 belt = £3.94

Coloplast

Belts. For Ileo B® pouches, net price 1 belt = £7.26 or for K-Flex® pouches, 1 belt = £5.54

ConvaTec

Belt, for Surgicare System® 2. Net price 1 belt = £2.76

Dansac

Belt with plates for Combi® pouches. Net price 1 belt plus 5 plates (50–63 mm) = £33.60

DePuy

Belts. Net price 1 ostomy girdle or panty girdle (white or pink colour) = £28.90; 1 4-inch nightbelt with waterproof backing = £9.55; for Schacht® pouches, 1 36-inch belt = £5.05

Drew

Belts. Net price 1 waistband with metal ends = £2.62, with plastic ends = £8.17; 1 day belt = £19.14; 1 night belt = £13.02; 1 × 4 inch belt (deep stoma hole) = £6.24; stoma/bones = £6.85

Hollister

Belt. Net price 1 adjustable ostomy belt (small, medium, or large) = £6.35; 10 = £52.82

Marlen

Belt. Net price 1 adjustable elastic waist belt = £2.65

Orthotic

Belt. Net price 1 ostomy girdle with hole, zip and suspenders (white) = £31.95

Peacock

Belts. Net price 1 St Mark's belt = £38.15

Rüsch

Belts. Net price 5 elastic waistbands (Birkbeck®) = £33.84; 5 elastic waistbands with shields = £44.52; 5 retaining rings (19, 38, or 54 mm) = £8.44. 1 narrow or

normal width belts (Ostopore®, waist: 17–34 inch or 28–56 inch) = £5.44. White rubber belting 28 mm = £3.70/metre, 72 mm = £7.64/metre. White sausage belt per metre = £7.61. 1 waist and support strap = £6.28

Sallis

Belts. Net price 1 night belt, 14b = £10.27; 14c = £5.37; 1 day belt, 15a = £28.29. 1 zipped pocket (to fit 15a and 16) = £4.80; 1 St Mark's = £25.94, 1 shield = £9.40; 1 ostomy girdle/pantie brief, with hole and suspenders,15c = £36.05

Salts

Belts. Net price 25 mm elastic belt (single), with 2 loops (standard 35 inch or extra-large 42 inch) = £3.20; with suspender ends = £3.75; double elastic with 4 loops = £5.43; with waterproof panel 102 mm = £13.13, 150 mm = £16.03; with 4 loops and retaining ring = £17.26. 1 rubber belt with straps and buckles = £6.28; with 2 fastening studs = £3.68. 25 mm button belt with or without loop = £3.20. 1 baby lycra belt = £12.93; with Velcro fastening (standard 35 inch or extra-large 42 inch) = £3.23. 1 colostomy belt = £67.23. 1 ileostomy girdle (Saltair®) = £42.94; 1 ileostomy elastic night belt (Saltair®) = £12.80. For Eakin® pouches, 1 elastic belt (small or large) = £3.26. For Salger® pouches, 1 elastic adjustable belt with or without Velcro fastening = £3.28

Shannon

Belt. Net price 1 elastic belt with shield and Velcro fastening = £7.32; with button and buckle fastening = £4.45

Shaw

Belts, colostomy, all made to measure. Net price 4 inch elastic web belt = £13.39; with under-strap or suspenders, 6 inch = £17.94, 8 inch = £25.76; with lace fastenings, 6 inch = £24.27; 8 inch = £30.75; 10 inch = £29.24; 12 inch = £32.14; 14 inch (made to measure) = £32.77; with zip panel, 10 inch = £36.90; 12 inch = £39.15; 14 inch = £40.97; elastic with nylon fronts, 10 inch = £34.32; 12 inch = £36.05; 14 inch = £38.35. 1 inch adjustable colostomy/ileostomy belt = £7.77; 4 inch (3 sections) = £19.65; 6 inch (3 sections) = £24.74. 1 colostomy night belt (net or rayon, no hole, for use with dressing pad), 4 inch = £14.29. 4 inch ostomy belt with groin strap = £15.32; with lace fastenings = £16.28; with wire spring = £15.00; double zip panel = £7.77

Simcare

Belts. Net price 25 mm web and elastic belt (WL002 range) = £10.05; 51 mm = £11.72; 75 mm = £13.12; (WL008) 25 mm = £10.98; 1 belt, child (25 mm) = £8.45, 38 mm = £11.77. 1 web end belt with buckle (short) = £6.78. 1 narrow belt (flange diameter: 32, 38, or 51 mm) = £20.89. 1 Redifit adjustable belt (small, medium, or large) = £8.45. 1 non-slip belt = £17.22; 1 elastic non-slip belt = £11.77. 1 rubber belt ('sausage' or tubular) = £21.94; 1 narrow belt = £6.38. 1 two-way stretch night belt (small, medium, large, or extra-large) = £23.55. 1 stoma belt (small: 17–26 inch or medium: 26–43 inch) = £5.58. 1 Carshalton® belt (small, medium, or large) = £8.91

Ward

Belts. Made to measure, all sizes. Net price 1 day belt = £38.99; 1 night belt = £28.70. 1 nylon elastic colostomy belt, with hook and eye fastening and 2 pairs of suspenders or understraps = £40.27. 1 wide rubberised ileostomy belt with 2 straps and buttonholed ends for use with ileostomy boxes or with celluoid hook ends for use with ileostomy bags = £22.87. 1 belt with understraps or suspenders = £25.72. 1 colostomy belt, with 2 pairs of understraps or suspenders (Gabriel®) = £45.51. 1 web and elastic belt with button and buckle fastening. 1 belt (1 inch) = £7.19; 2 inch = £9.26; 3 inch = £10.52. 1 plastic elastic belt with hook end = £10.02. 1 belt with windows for use with ileostomy bags or colostomy cups or 4 stiched holes for studs of colostomy cups or shields. Net price 35 = £4.15

FILTERS AND BRIDGES

Filters

Available from *CliniMed* (Biotrol®, 50 filters = £11.23), *Coloplast* (Filtrodor®, 50 filters = £18.70; Maclet®, 20 filter washers = £25.70), *ConvaTec* (Surgicare System® 2 for closed pouches, 30 filters = £7.93), *Cuxson* (50 patches = £3.02), *Hollister* (replacement filter elements for series 366 drainable bags, 20 = £2.80, 100 = £13.78), *Simcare* (for Beta® and mini bags, 20 = £7.12; Doublesure®, 10 filters = £3.38)

Bridges

Available from *Salts* (20 metal bridges ready fixed to lightweight and LWU disposable bags = £8.48; 30 bridges for use with other disposable bags = £12.72), *Simcare* (20 bridges = £3.02)

FLANGES

Jody's Surgical

Flanges. Net price 1 St Mark's soft rubber = £12.77; with diaphragm = £12.85

Bullen

Flanges. Net price 1 lightweight, plastic flange (small, medium, or large) = £3.59. 1 flange for Lenbul® pouches (1 inch diameter, 2 inch base) = £8.84; 1.5 inch diameter, 3 inch base = £13.04; 2 inch diameter, 4 inch base = £15.22

CliniMed

Flanges. Net price 5 flanges for Biotrol® Lockring 2 pouches (35, 50 or 75mm) = £12.23

ConvaTec

Flanges for Surgicare System® 2. Net price 10 Accordion flanges, 100 × 100 mm (70 mm hole) = £38.27; 127 ×127 mm (100 mm hole), 10 = £67.55. Combihesive flexible flanges, 100 × 100 mm (32, 38, or 45 mm hole), 5 = £13.25; 127 × 127 mm (57 or 70 mm hole), 5 = £14.42. Stomahesive flexible flanges, 100 × 100 mm (32, 38, 45, 57 or 70 mm holes), 5 = £11.68; Stomahesive flanges, 100 × 100 mm (32, 38, 45, 57 or 70 mm holes) 10 = £23.37; 127 ×127 mm (70 mm hole), 10 = £47.34; 152 × 152 mm (100 mm hole), 20 = £56.83. For Combihesive Natura pouches, 5 flexible flanges (32, 38, 45, 57 or 70 mm holes) = £13.25

Pansac

Flanges for Unique® 2 urostomy pouches. Net price 5 (30 mm flange, 15 mm hole or cut-to-fit 10–22 mm hole) = £12.61; 5 (36 mm flange, 20, 25 mm hole or cut-to-fit 15–28 mm hole) = £12.61; 5 (43 mm flange, 30 mm hole or cut-to-fit 15–35 mm hole) = £12.61; 5 (55 mm flange, 35, 40 mm hole or cut-to-fit 15–47 mm hole) = £12.61

DePuy

Flanges. Net price 1 Ileo B® standard rubber flange (0.75, 1.0, 1.25, 1.375, 1.5 inch) = £8.00. For Schacht® pouches, 1 flange (with locking ring) = £5.10; 1 ileo flange (with locking ring) = £5.10. St Mark's flange with inner sheath. Net price 1 flange, all 16 mm deep (76 mm base, 25 or 32 mm diameter; 100 mm base, 35, 38, 45 or 50 mm diameter) = £12.00

Drew

Flange. Net price 1 kapok flange (1–1.5 inch) = £14.01

Hollister

Flanges for Impression® pouch. Net price 5 Convex flanges with synthetic seal and Microporous adhesive (13, 16, 19, 22, 25, 29, 32, 35, 38, 41, 44 or 51 mm holes) = £13.42; Impression® CPL convex flange (13, 16, 19, 22, 25, 29, 32, 35, 38, 41, 44 or 51 mm holes), 5 = £13.42; Tandem floating flanges with either barrier and adhesive (19, 25, 32, 38, 44, 51 or 57 mm hole) or barrier only (25, 32, 44, 57 cut-to-fit hole), net price 5 = £12.54 or barrier only (89 mm cut-to-fit hole) 5 = £13.00

Rüsch

Flange. Net price 2 Birkbeck® white rubber flanges (75 mm base, 16 mm deep, 20 mm diameter); 90 mm base, 16 mm deep, 38 mm diameter; 110 mm base, 16 mm deep, 58 mm diameter = £22.36; St Mark's, in two rubbers with hard centre (76 mm base, 10 or 16 mm deep, 32 or 38 mm diameter), 2 flanges = £33.50; 76 mm base, 13 or 16 mm deep, 25 mm diameter, 2 flanges = £33.50; 102 mm base, 16 mm deep, 44 or 51 mm diameter, 2 flanges = £33.50; in soft honey coloured rubber (51 or 76 mm base, 13 mm deep, 25 mm diameter), 2 flanges = £19.54; (76 mm base, 10 or 16 mm deep, 32 or 38 mm diameter), 2 flanges = £19.54; 102 mm base, 16 mm deep, 44 or 51 mm diameter, 2 flanges = £19.54; with diaphragm, cowl, or dressing retainer at extra cost = £3.24: black, firm rubber (51 mm base, 13 mm deep, 25 mm diameter), 2 flanges = £22.36; 76 mm base, 10 or 16 mm deep, 32 or 38 mm diameter, 2 flanges = £22.36; 102 mm base, 16 mm deep, 44 or 51 mm diameter, 2 flanges = £22.36

Salts

Flange. Net price 1 flange (SF1, soft rubber, 25 mm) = £6.74; SF2, semi-rigid, 25 mm = £10.83; SF3, hard rubber, 25 mm = £7.70; SF4, soft rubber, 38 mm = £6.84; SF5, semi-rigid, 38 mm = £11.73; SF6, semi-rigid, hard rubber = £7.82; SF7, soft rubber, 51 mm = £8.61; SF8R, flexible, recessed, 32 mm = £10.83. 1 flange with diaphragm (19 mm) = £8.97. 1 Latex foam diaphragm flange = £38.24; 1 sheath for use with flange = £6.37. For Salger® pouches, 1 polythene flange (40 or 57 mm) = £1.90

Shannon

Flange ring. Net price 1 = £2.23

Shaw

Flange. Net price 1 rubber, adhesive = £5.62; rubber, non-stick = £6.80; with diaphragm = £8.84; non-stick inner diaphragm £2.63; 1 colostomy rubber foam facepiece (face hole diameter: 1.75, 2, 2.5, or 3 inch) = £10.28

Simcare

Flange. Net price 1 rubber flange (16 mm deep, 38 mm diameter) = £15.77; double base hole (38 mm diameter) = £20.91; blue rubber (51 mm base, 13 mm deep, 25 mm diameter or 76 mm base, 10 or 16 mm deep, 38 mm diameter) = £14.27; blue and brown, (76 mm base, 13 mm deep, 25 mm diameter; 10 or 16 mm deep, 38 mm diameter) = £20.72. 1 belt flange (19, 25, 32, 38, 44, 51, or 64 mm) = 26p. For Chiron® pouches, 1 flange (10 or 16 mm deep, 38 mm diameter) = £15.77; 13 mm deep, 25 mm diameter = £15.77; 16 mm deep, 32 mm diameter = £15.77; plastic without diaphragm (13 mm deep, 32 or 38 mm diameter) = £7.89. For Redifit® pouches, 1 belt flange = 63p; St Mark's pattern, 1 flange (51 mm base: 13 mm deep, 25 mm diameter; 76 mm base, 13 mm deep, 25 mm diameter; 76 mm base, 10 or 16 mm deep, 32 or 38 mm diameter; 102 mm base, 16 mm deep, 44 or 51 mm diameter) = £13.44: with dressing retainer or with 16 mm canopy, 38 mm = £16.97

Ward

Flange. Net price 1 plastic/rubber air-filled flange = £16.89; 1 St Mark's standard = £11.12; 1 St Mark's with diaphragm = £13.59

IRRIGATION AND WASH-OUT APPLIANCES

Available from *Astra Tech* (Medena® 5 ileostomy catheters = £4.38), *CliniMed* (Biotrol®, 50 irrigation sleeves = £36.09 or 1 cone = £2.55), *Coloplast* (30 disposable sleeves (1540 or 1560) = £31.50; 1 colotip = £5.97; 1 irrigator bag = £11.30; 1 supporting plate = £5.68; 1 irrigation belt = £5.54), *Dansac* (1 water container = £16.23; 1 clamp = £7.03; 1 cone = £10.43; 1 brush = £1.77; 1 tube = £1.24; 1 belt = £33.60; Irri-drain® with ring holder for silicone ring, 20 = £20.75 or adhesive, 20 = £20.75; silicone ring, 1 = £4.17), *Hollister* (irrigator drain for use with Guardian® Two-Piece system, 5 (flange: 38, 51, 64, or 102 mm) = £6.13; 1 stoma cone/irrigator kit = £18.50; 20 irrigator drains = £25.90; 10 replacement cones = £65.63; 1 = £8.02; 1 stoma lubricant = £4.54), *Ward* (1 belt = £7.94)

PRESSURE PLATES, SHIELDS

Coloplast (1 supporting plate = £5.68; Assura® convex inserts for use with two-piece base plates 40, 50, 60 mm, 5 = £1.25), *ConvaTec* (5 System 2® convex inserts for Combihesive®, Stomahesive®, and flexible flanges, 38, 45, or 57 mm) = £1.25, *De Puy* (cotton facepiece with non-slip belt for St. Mark's flange, 45 mm diameter) = £18.00, *Drew* pressure plate (oval or round) = £2.68; pressure plate (4 slot) = £4.02; *Salts* (plastic retaining shield, single = £3.00, double = £4.62, large = £3.66; S S Wire retaining ring, large = £3.00, medium = £2.85, small = £2.78; light white anti-sag ring = £1.19, for belt use = £1.35, for velcro belt fastening = £1.54; convex plate for light white bag (32, 38, or 44 mm), 5 = £12.93; pressure plate for Kombo®, Simplicity®, or Solo® pouches (30, 40, 50, or 60 mm) = £1.86; Eakin® support frame (32, 45, 64, or 90 mm) = £1.20, *Shannon* (faceplate = £7.53), *Simcare* (plastic pressure plates, Surrey model: 25 or 32 mm or Standard model with attached flange for use with lightweight bags: 25, 32, or 38 mm = £7.11; stainless wire pressure frame, hook, lug, to fit 25, 32, 38, 44, or 51 mm flange) = £8.66; cotton facepiece = £21.54; pressure plates (25, 32, or 38 mm) = £4.96, *Ward* (celluloid colostomy cup with sponge or solid rim, small, medium, or large = £34.88, with sponge rubber or solid rim, belt fitting = £39.80; St Mark's shield, celluloid with 4 studs = £7.58)

SKIN PROTECTIVES, FILLERS, AND CLEANSERS

Balspray® (Bullen)
Aerosol. Net price 1 unit = £6.74
Bullen Karaya Gum Powder® (Bullen)
Powder. Net price 70 g = £4.34
Chiron® (Simcare)
Barrier cream (with antiseptic). Net price 52 g = £4.73
CliniShield Wipes® (CliniMed)
Barrier wipes. Net price 50 = £11.53
Comfeel® (Coloplast)
Barrier cream. Net price 60 g = £3.82
Protective film. Net price 30 sachets = £8.85; applicator = £4.18
Dansac® (Dansac)
Karaya paste. Net price 50 g = £2.44
Soft paste. Net price 50 g = £2.90
Day-Drop® (Loxley)
Barrier Cream. Net price 50 g = £2.09
Derma-gard® (Simcare)
Protective skin wipes. Net price 50 = £13.85

Hollister® (Hollister)
Karaya paste. Net price 128 g = £6.70
 Do not apply to severely excoriated skin
Karaya powder. Net price 71 g = £7.95
Premium paste. Net price 57 g = £3.00
Skin gel. Net price 28 g = £5.82. Label: 15
 Do not apply to severely excoriated skin
Orabase® (ConvaTec)
Paste, see section 12.3.1
Orahesive® (ConvaTec)
Powder (with adherent properties), see section 12.3.1
Payne® (Payne)
Barrier cream. Net price 50 g = £3.36
Pelican® (Pelican)
Paste (formerly Simpla® gel). Net price 1 pack = £6.31
Saltair® (Salts)
Karaya gum powder. Net price per puffer pack = £4.18
Ostomy cleansing soap (soap spirit). Net price 110-mL = £2.51
Peri-Prep wipes. Net price 50 = £13.58
Seel-a-peel® (Simcare)
Paste. Net price 50 mL = £2.70
Simcare® (Simcare)
Karaya gum powder. Net price 100 g = £6.79
Karaya gum sheet. Net price 1 = £6.80
Stomahesive® (ConvaTec)
Paste. Net price 60 g = £6.51. For filling and sealing skin creases
Stomosol® (DePuy)
Skin shield. Net price 50 = £7.73
Translet® (Rüsch)
Wipes. Net price 30 = £5.64

SKIN PROTECTORS

Bullen
Karaya gum washers, regular or extra hard. Net price 1
washers (2 inch diameter: 2 × 0.875 inch or 2 × 1.12.
inch hole) = £11.80; 2.5 inch diameter: regular 2.5
1.25 inch or extra hard 2.5 × 1.5 inch hole = £13.68;
inch diameter: 3 × 0.875 inch, 3 × 1.125 inch, 3 × 1.
inch, or 3 × 2 inch hole = £15.68
CliniMed®
Biotrol® skin protectors. Net price 20 × 20 cm, 5
£36.76; 10 × 10 cm or 10 cm diameter, 10 = £15.81
Coloplast
Protective sheets. Net price 10 non-sterile sheets (10
10 cm) = £19.96; 5 (15 × 15 cm) = £23.18; 5 (20 ×
20 cm) = £42.17; 30 rings (10, 15, 20, 25, 30, 40, o
50 mm) = £33.99
ConvaTec
Wafers. Net price 5 Stomahesive® wafers (100 ×
100 mm) = £9.80; 3 (200 × 200 mm) = £23.91; 10 Vari
hesive® wafers (100 × 100 mm) = £8.36
DePuy
Schacht® rings. Net price 10 foam, colostomy or ileo
stomy rings = £7.10
Drew
Washers. Net price 20 K-Seal® karaya gum washer
(small) = £8.53; large = £10.09
Hollister
Skin barrier. Net price 5 Hollister® skin barriers (4 ×
4 inch) = £9.86; 5 (8 × 8 inch) = £30.56
Pelican
Protectors (formerly Simplaseel® wafers). Net price 1
(100 × 100 mm) = £18.05

Salts

Protectors. Net price 10 karaya gum washers (small) = £7.18; 10 (large) = £11.70; 5 foam cushions (25, 32, 38, or 51 mm) = £2.38; 5 dri pads (40 mm) = £2.34; 20 Cohesive® washers (small: 50 mm) = £30.55; 10 (large: 95 mm) = £20.40; 10 Realistic® washers (13, 19, 22, 25, 29, 32, or 38 mm) = £14.63; 1 Saltair® twinpack (small) = £8.79; large = £12.30; 10 foam seals (as in twin packs) = £1.79; 5 United® skin barrier wafers (10 × 10 cm) = £9.67; 3 = £22.43; for Salger® pouches, 5 karaya washers with foam (40 or 57 mm) = £12.44

Shannon

Protectors. Net price 1 foam sponge ring = 73p; 10 Kaygee® washers (2.5 inch base: 0.875 or 1.125 inch hole or 2.75 inch base: 0.875 or 1.375 inch hole) = £6.60

Shaw

Protectors. Net price 5 Body Mould® squares (1.0, 1.25, or 1.5 inch hole) = £10.34; 10 washers (1.0 or 1.25 inch hole) = £9.48; 5 rings (1.0, 1.25, or 1.5 inch hole) = £9.48; 5 Healwell® squares (1.0, 1.25 or 1.5 inch hole) = £9.81; 12 rings (1.0, 1.25 or 1.5 inch hole) = £8.47

Simcare

Protectors. Net price 5 foam pads, white (76 mm diameter: 25 mm hole) = £4.61; 76 mm diameter: 29, 32, or 38 mm hole or 90 mm diameter: 32 or 38 mm hole = £6.31; black (25 mm hole) = £5.90: 1 karaya gum sheet (300 × 100 mm) = £6.80: 20 rings (19, 25, 32, 38, or 44 mm) = £22.68; karaya rings (19, 25, 32, 38, or 51 mm) = £24.80: 10 Down's® adhesive karaya gum washers (51 mm base: 22 or 29 mm hole) = £11.04; 70 mm base: 22 or 29 mm hole = £13.62; 10 Redifit® karaya gum washers (25, 32, 38, 44, or 51 mm) = £13.62: 20 Seel-a-peel® squares (100 mm sq) = £38.42; 5 squares (150 mm sq) = £23.66

STOMA CAPS AND DRESSINGS

Available from *Bullen* (1 stoma cap = £4.22), *Coloplast* (100 Colocap® stomacaps = £107.10; Assura Minicap®, 30 opaque stomacaps, 20 mm starter hole, cut to fit up to 55 mm hole = £32.43), *ConvaTec* (Colodress Plus®, 30 stoma caps (19 mm hole cut-to-size) = £31.89, *Dansac* (50 Dansac® Mini caps (30 or 44 mm) = £51.95; 30 Dansac® Unique Mini caps, 20 mm starter hole, cut to fit up to 50 mm hole; also 30, 40 or 50 mm = £31.41), *Eurocare* (50 Confidence® stoma caps with filter, 13 mm starter hole = £49.00), *Hollister* (50 stoma caps (51 or 76 mm) = £54.43), *Salts* (30 stoma caps for Simplicity 1® pouches = £32.13), *Simcare* (20 leisure pouches = £22.54), *Ward* (2 zip fasteners fitted to colostomy belt = £7.53; 1 waterproof front fitted to colostomy belt = £6.21; 1 pair woven understraps with buttonholed ends = £2.88; 1 Donald Rose® ileostomy/colostomy bath belt with internal chamber for dressings and stud fastenings for adjustment = £18.66))

TUBING

Available from *Hollister* (10 urostomy drain tubes = £22.95; 8 tubes for fitting to Lo-Profile® urostomy bags = £21.35; for Premium® urostomy pouches, 10 drain tube adaptors = £18.28), *Salts* (2 night tube adaptors = 90p), *Simcare* (for Carshalton® urostomy pouches, 10 connectors = £3.98), *Ward* (1 metal spring tubing clip = £2.10)

Appendix 9: Cautionary and Advisory Labels for Dispensed Medicines

Numbers following the preparation entries in the BNF correspond to the code numbers of the cautionary labels that pharmacists are recommended to add when dispensing. It is also expected that pharmacists will counsel patients when necessary.

Counselling needs to be related to the age, experience, background, and understanding of the individual patient. The pharmacist should ensure that the patient understands how to take or use the medicine and how to follow the correct dosage schedule. Any effects of the medicine on driving or work, any foods or medicines to be avoided, and what to do if a dose is missed should also be explained. Other matters, such as the possibility of staining of the clothes or skin by a medicine should also be mentioned.

For some preparations there is a special need for counselling, such as an unusual method or time of administration or a potential interaction with a common food or domestic remedy, and this is indicated where necessary.

ORIGINAL PACKS. Many preparations are now dispensed in unbroken original packs that bear complete instructions for the patient or provide a leaflet addressed to the patient. These labels or leaflets should not normally be obscured or removed. Where it is known that such instructions are provided with an original pack intended for the patient no label has been listed under the preparation. Label 10 may be used where appropriate. Leaflets are available from various sources advising on the administration of preparations such as eye-drops, eye ointments, inhalers, and suppositories.

SCOPE OF LABELS. In general no label recommendations have been made for injections on the assumption that they will be administered by a health professional or a well-instructed patient. The labelling is not exhaustive and pharmacists are recommended to use their professional discretion in labelling new preparations and those for which no labels are shown.

Individual labelling advice is not given on the administration of the large variety of antacids. In the absence of instructions from the prescriber, and if on enquiry the patient has had no verbal instructions, the directions given under 'Dose' should be used on the label.

It is recognised that there may be occasions when pharmacists will use their knowledge and professional discretion and decide to omit one or more of the recommended labels for a particular patient. In this case counselling is of the utmost importance. There may also be an occasion when a prescriber does not wish additional cautionary labels to be used, in which case the prescription should be endorsed 'NCL' (no cautionary labels). The exact wording that is required instead should then be specified on the prescription.

Pharmacists have traditionally labelled medicines with various wordings in addition to those directions specified on the prescription. Such labels include 'Shake the bottle', 'For external use only' and 'Store in a cool place', as well as 'Discard . . . days after opening' and 'Do not use after . . . .' which apply particularly to antibiotic mixtures, diluted liquid and topical preparations, and to eye-drops. Although not listed in the BNF these labels should continue to be used when appropriate; indeed, 'For external use only' is a legal requirement on external liquid preparations, while 'Keep out of the reach of children' is a legal requirement on all dispensed medicines.

It is the usual practice for patients to take standard tablets with water or other liquid and for this reason no separate label has been recommended.

The label or labels for each preparation are recommended after careful consideration of the information available. However, it is recognised that in some cases this information may be either incomplete or open to a different interpretation. The Executive Editor will therefore be grateful to receive any constructive comments on the labelling suggested for any preparation.

Recommended label wordings

Wordings which can be given as separate warning are labels 1–19 and labels 29–33. Wordings which can be incorporated in an appropriate position in the directions for dosage or administration are label 21–28. A label has been omitted for number 20.

If separate labels are used it is recommended that the wordings be used without modification. If changes are made to suit computer requirements care should be taken to retain the sense of the original.

(1) Warning. May cause drowsiness

To be used on *preparations for children* containing antihistamines, or other preparations given to children where the warnings of label 2 on driving or alcohol would not be appropriate.

(2) Warning. May cause drowsiness. If affected do not drive or operate machinery. Avoid alcoholic drink

To be used on *preparations for adults that can cause drowsiness*, thereby affecting the ability to drive and operate hazardous machinery; label 1 is more appropriate for children. *It is an offence to drive while under the influence of drink or drugs.*

Some of these preparations only cause drowsiness in the first few days of treatment and some only cause drowsiness in higher doses.

In such cases the patient should be told that the advice applies until the effects have worn off. However many of these preparations can produce a slowing of reaction time and a loss of mental con centration that can have the same effects as drowsiness.

Avoidance of alcoholic drink is recommended because the effects of CNS depressants are enhanced by alcohol. Strict prohibition however could lead to some patients not taking the medicine. Pharmacists should therefore explain the risk and encourage compliance, particularly in patients who may think they already tolerate the effects of alcohol (see also label 3). Queries from patients with epilepsy regarding fitness to drive should be referred back to the patient's doctor.

Side-effects unrelated to drowsiness that may affect a patient's ability to drive or operate machinery safely include *blurred vision, dizziness, or nausea*. In general, no label has been recommended to cover these cases, but the patient should be suitably counselled.

(3)   Warning. May cause drowsiness. If affected do not drive or operate machinery

To be used on *preparations containing monoamine-oxidase inhibitors*; the warning to avoid alcohol and dealcoholised (low alcohol) drink is covered by the MAOI treatment card.

Also to be used as for label 2 but where alcohol is not an issue.

(4)   Warning. Avoid alcoholic drink

To be used on *preparations where a reaction such as flushing may occur if alcohol is taken* (e.g. metronidazole and chlorpropamide). Alcohol may also enhance the hypoglycaemia produced by some oral antidiabetic drugs but routine application of a warning label is not considered necessary.

(5)   Do not take indigestion remedies at the same time of day as this medicine

To be used with label 25 on *preparations coated to resist gastric acid* (e.g. enteric-coated tablets). This is to avoid the possibility of premature dissolution of the coating in the presence of an alkaline pH.

Label 5 also applies to drugs such as ketoconazole *where the absorption is significantly affected by antacids*; the usual period of avoidance recommended is 2 to 4 hours.

(6)   Do not take iron preparations or indigestion remedies at the same time of day as this medicine

To be used on *preparations containing ciprofloxacin, doxycycline, minocycline, and penicillamine*. These drugs chelate iron and calcium ions and are less well absorbed when given with iron or calcium-containing antacids. If necessary these incompatible preparations may be given about two hours apart.

(7)   Do not take milk, iron preparations or indigestion remedies at the same time of day as this medicine

To be used on *preparations containing tetracyclines that chelate iron, calcium, and magnesium* and are thus less available for absorption; if it is necessary to give milk, iron or antacids, the usual period of avoidance is about 2 hours. Doxycycline and minocycline are less liable to form chelates and therefore only require label 6 (see above).

(8)   Do not stop taking this medicine except on your doctor's advice

To be used on *preparations that contain a drug which is required to be taken over long periods without the patient necessarily perceiving any benefit* (e.g. antituberculous drugs).

Also to be used on *preparations that contain a drug whose withdrawal is likely to be a particular hazard* (e.g. clonidine for hypertension). Label 10 (see below) is more appropriate for corticosteroids.

(9)   Take at regular intervals. Complete the prescribed course unless otherwise directed

To be used on *preparations where a course of treatment should be completed* to reduce the incidence of relapse or failure of treatment.

The preparations are antimicrobial drugs given by mouth. Very occasionally, some may have severe side-effects (e.g. diarrhoea in patients receiving clindamycin) and in such cases the patient may need to be advised of reasons for stopping treatment quickly and returning to the doctor.

(10)   Warning. Follow the printed instructions you have been given with this medicine

To be used particularly on *preparations containing anticoagulants, lithium, monoamine-oxidase inhibitors, and oral corticosteroids*. The appropriate treatment card should be given to the patient and any necessary explanations given.

This label may also be used on other preparations to remind the patient of the instructions that have been given.

(11)   Avoid exposure of skin to direct sunlight or sun lamps

To be used *on preparations that may cause phototoxic or photoallergic reactions* if the patient is exposed to ultraviolet radiation. Many drugs other than those listed (e.g. phenothiazines and sulphonamides) may on rare occasions cause reactions in susceptible patients. Exposure to high intensity ultraviolet radiation from sunray lamps and sunbeds is particularly likely to cause reactions.

(12)   Do not take anything containing aspirin while taking this medicine

To be used *on preparations containing probenecid and sulphinpyrazone* whose activity is reduced by aspirin.

Label 12 should not be used for anticoagulants since label 10 is more appropriate.

(13)   Dissolve or mix with water before taking

To be used on *preparations that are intended to be dissolved in water* (e.g. soluble tablets) or *mixed with water* (e.g. powders, granules) before use. In a few cases other liquids such as fruit juice or milk may be used.

(14)   This medicine may colour the urine

To be used on *preparations that may cause the patient's urine to turn an unusual colour*. These include phenolphthalein (alkaline urine pink), triamterene (blue under some lights), levodopa (dark reddish), and rifampicin (red).

(15)   Caution flammable: keep away from fire or flames

To be used on *preparations containing sufficient flammable solvent to render them flammable if exposed to a naked flame.*

(16)   Allow to dissolve under the tongue. Do not transfer from this container. Keep tightly closed. Discard eight weeks after opening

To be used on *glyceryl trinitrate tablets* to remind the patient not to transfer the tablets to plastic or less suitable containers.

(17)   Do not take more than . . . in 24 hours

To be used on *preparations for the treatment of acute migraine* except those containing ergotamine, for which label 18 is used. The dose form should be specified, e.g. tablets or capsules.

It may also be used on preparations for which no dose has been specified by the prescriber.

(18)   Do not take more than . . . in 24 hours or . . . in any one week

To be used on preparations containing ergotamine. The dose form should be specified, e.g. tablets or suppositories.

(19)   Warning. Causes drowsiness which may continue the next day. If affected do not drive or operate machinery. Avoid alcoholic drink

To be used on *preparations containing hypnotics (or some other drugs with sedative effects) prescribed to be taken at night.* On the rare occasions (e.g. nitrazepam in epilepsy) when hypnotics are prescribed for daytime administration this label would clearly not be appropriate. Also to be used as *an alternative to the label 2 wording* (the choice being at the discretion of the pharmacist) *for anxiolytics prescribed to be taken at night.*

It is hoped that this wording will convey adequately the problem of residual morning sedation after taking 'sleeping tablets'.

(21)   . . . with or after food

To be used on *preparations that are liable to cause gastric irritation,* or *those that are better absorbed with food.*

Patients should be advised that a *small amount of food is sufficient.*

(22)   . . . half to one hour before food

To be used on some preparations *whose absorption is thereby improved.* Most oral antibiotics require label 23 instead (see below).

(23)   . . . an hour before food or on an empty stomach

To be used on *oral antibiotics whose absorption may be reduced by the presence of food and acid in the stomach.*

(24)   . . . sucked or chewed

To be used on *preparations that should be sucked or chewed.*

The pharmacist should use discretion as to which of these words is appropriate.

(25)   . . . swallowed whole, not chewed

To be used on *preparations that are enteric-coated or designed for modified-release.*

Also to be used on *preparations that taste very unpleasant or may damage the mouth* if not swallowed whole.

(26)   . . . dissolved under the tongue

To be used on *preparations designed for sublingual use.* Patients should be advised to hold under the tongue and avoid swallowing until dissolved. The buccal mucosa between the gum and cheek is occasionally specified by the prescriber.

(27)   . . . with plenty of water

To be used on *preparations that should be well diluted* (e.g. chloral hydrate), *where a high fluid intake is required* (e.g. sulphonamides), or *where water is required to aid the action* (e.g. methylcellulose). The patient should be advised that 'plenty' means at least 150 mL (about a tumblerful). In most cases fruit juice, tea, or coffee may be used.

(28)   To be spread thinly . . .

To be used on *external corticosteroid preparations.*

(29)   Do not take more than 2 at any one time. Do not take more than 8 in 24 hours

To be used on containers of dispensed *solid dose preparations containing paracetamol for adults when the instruction on the label indicates that the dose can be taken on an 'as required' basis.* The dose form should be specified, e.g. tablets or capsules.

This label has been introduced because of the serious consequences of overdosage with paracetamol.

(30)   Contains paracetamol

To be used on containers of dispensed *preparations containing paracetamol when the name on the label does not include the word 'paracetamol'.*

(31)   Contains aspirin and paracetamol

To be used on containers of dispensed *preparations containing aspirin and paracetamol (e.g. benorylate), when the name on the label does not include the words 'aspirin' and 'paracetamol'.*

(32)   Contains aspirin

To be used on containers of dispensed *preparations containing aspirin when the name on the label does not include the word 'aspirin'.*

(33)   Contains an aspirin-like medicine

To be used on containers of dispensed *preparations containing a salicylate derivative.*

Products and their labels

Products introduced or amended since publication of BNF No. 31 (March 1996) are <u>underlined</u>.
Proprietary names are in *italic*.
C = counselling advised; see BNF = consult product entry in BNF

Ferrous sulphate paed mixt, 27
Fesovit Z, 25
Filair, 8, C, dose
Filair Forte, 8, 10 steroid card, C, dose
Flagyl S, 4, 9, 23
Flagyl supps, 4, 9
Flagyl tabs, 4, 9, 21, 25, 27
<u>*Fleet Phospho-soda*</u>, 10 patient information leaflet, C, administration
Flexin Continus preps, 21, 25, C, driving
Flixotide, 8, 10 steroid card (250-microgram and 500-microgram only), C, dose
<u>*Flomax MR*</u>, 3, 25, C, dose, see BNF
Florinef, 10 steroid card
Floxapen, 9, 23
Fluanxol, C, administration, see BNF
Flucloxacillin, 9, 23
Flucloxacillin sachets, 9, 13, 23
Fluconazole 50 and 200mg, 9
Fluconazole susp, 9
Fludrocortisone, 10 steroid card
Flunitrazepam, 19
Fluocinolone external preps, 28
Fluocinonide external preps, 28
Fluocinonide scalp lotion, 15, 28
Fluocortolone external preps, 28
Fluorigard mouthwash, C, food and drink, see BNF
Fluoxetine, C, driving, see BNF
Flupenthixol, see preps
Fluphenazine, 2
Flurandrenolone external preps, 28
Flurazepam, 19
Flurbiprofen, 21
Flurbiprofen m/r, 21, 25
Fluticasone inhalations, 8, 10 steroid card (250-microgram and 500-microgram only), C, dose
<u>*Fluvastatin*</u>, C, muscle effects, see BNF
Fluvoxamine, C, driving, see BNF
Foradil, C, dose, see BNF
Fortagesic, 2, 21, 29, 30
Fortespan, 25
Fortral caps and tabs, 2, 21
Fortral supps, 2
<u>*Fosamax*</u>, C, administration, see BNF
Fosfomycin gran, 13, 23
Franol, 21
Franol Plus, 21
Frisium, 2 *or* 19, C, driving (see BNF, p. 204)
Froben, 21
Froben SR, 21, 25
Frusene, 14 (urine blue in some lights), 21
Fucibet, 28
Fucidin susp, 9, 21
Fucidin tabs, 9
Fucidin H, 28
Fulcin, 9, 21, C, driving
Full Marks lotion, 15
Fungilin loz, 9, 24, C, after food
Fungilin susp (g.i.), 9, C, use of pipette
Fungilin susp (mouth), 9, C, use of pipette, hold in mouth, after food
Fungilin tabs, 9
Furadantin, 9, 14 (urine yellow or brown), 21
Furamide, 9
Fybogel, 13, C, administration, see BNF
Fybogel Mebeverine, 13, 22, C, administration, see BNF

Gabapentin, 3, 5, C, driving (see BNF, p. 204)
Galake, 21, 29, 30
Gamanil, 2
Gamolenic acid in evening primrose oil, C, administration, see BNF

Ganciclovir, 21
Gastrobid Continus, 25
Gastromax, 22, 25
Gastrozepin, 22
Glucobay, C, administration, see BNF
Glucophage, 21
Glyceryl trinitrate patch, see preps
Glyceryl trinitrate m/r, 25
Glyceryl trinitrate tabs, 16
Glytrin Spray, 10 patient information leaflet
Gregoderm, 28
Griseofulvin, 9, 21, C, driving
Grisovin, 9, 21, C, driving
GTN 300 mcg, 16
Guar gum, 13, C, adminstration, see BNF
Guarem, 13, C, administration, see BNF

Haelan, 28
Halciderm Topical, 28
Halcinonide external preps, 28
Haldol, 2
Halfan, 23
Halofantrine, 23
Half-Inderal LA, 8, 25
Half-Securon SR, 25
Half-Sinemet CR, 14 (urine reddish), 25
Haloperidol, 2
Heminevrin, 19
Hexamine, 9
Hiprex, 9
Hismanal, C, driving, alcohol, see BNF
Hollister skin gel, 15
Hydergine, 22
Hydrocal, 28
Hydrocortisone inj, 10 steroid card
Hydrocortisone external preps, 28
Hydrocortisone tabs, 10 steroid card, 21
Hydrocortisone butyrate external preps, 28
Hydrocortisone butyrate scalp lotion, 15, 28
Hydrocortistab inj, 10 steroid card
Hydrocortisyl, 28
Hydrocortone, 10 steroid card, 21
Hydromet, 3, 8
Hydroxychloroquine, 5
Hydroxyzine, 2
Hyoscine, 2 (patches, 19)
Hypolar Retard, 25
Hypovase, 3, C, dose, see BNF
Hytrin, 3, C, dose, see BNF

Ibuprofen, 21
Ibuprofen gran, 13, 21
Ibuprofen m/r, 25, 27
Ibuspray, 15
Idarubicin caps, 25
Ilosone, 9
Imdur, 25
Imigran, 3, 10 patient information leaflet
Imipramine, 2
Imperacin, 7, 9, 23
Imunovir, 9
Imuran, 21
Inderal, 8
Inderal-LA, 8, 25
Inderetic, 8
Inderex, 8, 25
Indocid caps and susp, 21, C, driving
Indocid-R, 21, 25, C, driving
Indolar SR, 21, 25, C, driving
Indomethacin caps and mixt, 21, C, driving
Indomethacin m/r, see preps
Indomethacin supps, C, driving
Indomod, 25, C, driving
Indoramin, 2
Industrial methylated spirit, 15
Infacol, C, use of dropper
Inosine pranobex, 9

Insulin, C, see BNF
Intal Spincaps and inhalers, 8
Iodine Solution, Aqueous, 27
Ionamin, 25, C, driving
Ipral, 9
Ipratropium inhalations, C, dose, see BNF
<u>*Isib 60X*</u>L, 25
Ismo Retard, 25
Ismo tabs, 25
Isocarboxazid, 3, 10 MAOI card
Isogel, 13, C, administration, see BNF
Isoket Retard, 25
Isoniazid elixir and tabs, 8, 22
Isoprenaline sulphate tabs, 26
Isordil (sublingual), 26
Isordil Tembids, 25
Isosorbide dinitrate m/r, 25
Isosorbide mononitrate, 25
Isosorbide mononitrate m/r, 25
Isotrate, 25
Isotretinoin, 10 patient information card, 21
Isotretinoin gel, 10 patient information leaflet
Isotrex, 10 patient information leaflet
Ispaghula, 13, C, administration, see BNF
Itraconazole, 5, 9, 21, 25

Junifen, 21

Kalspare, 14 (urine blue in some lights), 21
Kalten, 8
Kapake, 2, 29, 30
Kay-Cee-L, 21
Keflex, 9
Kelfizine W tabs, 9,13
Kemadrin, C, driving
Kenalog (systemic), 10 steroid card
Kerlone, 8
Ketoconazole tabs and susp, 5, 9, 21
Ketoprofen caps, 21
Ketoprofen CR, 21, 25
Ketoprofen m/r caps, 21, 25
Ketotifen, 2, 8, 21
Ketorolac tabs, 17, 21
Ketovail, 21, 25
Kinidin Durules, 25
Klaricid, 9
Klean-Prep, C, administration, see BNF
Kloref, 13, 21
Kloref-S, 13, 21
Konakion tabs, 24
Konsyl, 13, C, administration, see BNF

Labetalol, 8, 21
Laboprin DL, 13, 21, 33
Labrocol, 8, 21
Lacidipine, 21
Lactitol, C, administration, see BNF
Lamictal dispersible tabs, 13, C, driving (see BNF, p.204)
Lamital tabs, C, driving (see BNF, p. 204)
Lamisil, 9
Lamotrigine dispersible tabs, 13, C, driving (see BNF, p. 204)
Lamotrigine tabs, C, driving (see BNF, p. 204)
Lamprene, 8, 14 (urine red), 21
Lanoxin-PG elixir, C, use of pipette
Lansoprazole, 5, 23, 25
Largactil, 2, 11
Lariam, 21, 25, 27, C, driving, malaria prophylaxis, see BNF
Larodopa, 14 (urine reddish), 21
Lasikal, 25, 27, C, posture, see BNF
Lasix + K, 25, 27, C, posture, see BNF
Lasma, 25
Ledercort tabs, 10 steroid card, 21
Lederfen, 21

Nerisone, 28
Nerisone Forte, 28
Neulactil, 2
Neurontin, 3, 5, C, driving (see BNF, p. 204)
Nicardipine m/r, 25
Niclosamide, 4, 24, C, administration, see BNF
Nicotinic acid tabs, 21
Nicoumalone, 10 anticoagulant card
Nidazol, 4, 9, 21, 25, 27
Nifedipine caps, 21, C, administration, see BNF
Nifedipine m/r, see preps
Nifelease, 25
Nifensar XL, 21, 25
Niferex elixir, C, infants, use of dropper
Nitoman, 2
Nitrazepam, 19
Nitrocontin Continus, 25
Nitrofurantoin, 9, 14 (urine yellow or brown)
Nitrofurantoin m/r, 9, 14 (urine yellow or brown), 21, 25
Nivaquine, 5, C, malaria prophylaxis, see BNF
Nizoral, 5, 9, 21
Noctec, 19, 27
Nootropil, 3
Nordox, 6, 9, 11, 27, C, posture, see BNF
Norfloxacin, 6, 9
Normacol preps, 25, 27, C, administration, see BNF
Normax, 14 (urine red)
Normison, 19
Norprolac, 21, C, hypotensive reactions, see BNF
Nortriptyline, 2
Nozinan, 2
Nuelin, 21
Nuelin SA preps, 25
Nu-Seals Aspirin, 5, 25, 32
Nutrizym preps, C, administration, see BNF
Nycopren, 5, 25
Nystadermal 28
Nystaform-HC, 28
Nystan pastilles, 9, 24, C, after food
Nystan susp (g.i.), 9, C, use of pipette
Nystan susp (mouth), 9, C, use of pipette, hold in mouth, after food
Nystan tabs, 9
Nystatin mixt (g.i.), 9, C, use of pipette
Nystatin mixt (mouth), 9, C, use of pipette, hold in mouth, after food
Nystatin pastilles, 9, 24, C, after food
Nystatin tabs, 9

Occlusal, 15
Ocusert Pilo, C, method of use
Oestriol, 25
Oestrogel, 10 patient information leaflet, C, administration, see BNF
Ofloxacin, 6, 9, 11, C, driving
Olbetam, 21
Olsalazine, 21, C, blood disorder symptoms, see BNF
Omeprazole, 25
Opilon, 21
Opium tincture, 2
Optimax, 3
Optimine, 2
Oramorph preps, 2
Oramorph SR, 2, 25
Orap, 2
Orbenin, 9, 23
Orciprenaline inhalation, C, dose, see BNF
Orelox, 5, 9, 21
Orovite-7 gran, 13
Orphenadrine, C, driving
Orudis caps, 21
Oruvail, 21, 25

Ostram, 13
Ovestin, 25
Oxatomide, 2
Oxazepam, 2
Oxerutins, 21
Oxitropium, C, dose
Oxivent, C, dose
Oxpentifylline m/r, 21, 25
Oxprenolol, 8
Oxprenolol m/r, 8, 25
Oxybutynin, 3
Oxypertine, 2
Oxytetracycline, 7, 9, 23

Paludrine, 21, C, malaria prophylaxis, see BNF
Pameton, 29, 30
Panadol tabs, 29, 30
Panadol Soluble, 13, 29, 30
Panadol susp, 30
Pancrease preps, C, administration, see BNF
Pancreatin, C, administration, see BNF
Pancrex gran, 25, C, dose, see BNF
Pancrex V Forte tabs, 5, 25, C, dose, see BNF
Pancrex V caps, 125 caps and pdr, C, administration, see BNF
Pancrex V tabs, 5, 25, C, dose, see BNF
Paracetamol liq and supps, 30 (if 'paracetamol' not on label)
Paracetamol tabs, 29, also 30 (if 'paracetamol' not on label)
Paracetamol tabs, soluble, 13, 29, also 30 (if 'paracetamol' not on label)
Paradote, 29, 30
Paramax sachets, 13, 17, 30
Paramax tabs, 17, 30
Parlodel, 21, C, hypotensive reactions, see BNF
Parnate, 3, 10 MAOI card
Paroven, 21
Paroxetine, 21, C, driving, see BNF
Parstelin, 3, 10 MAOI card
Paxofen, 21
Pecram, 25
Penbritin caps and syrup, 9, 23
Penbritin paed syrup, 9, 23, C, use of pipette
Pendramine, 6, 22, C, blood disorder symptoms, see BNF
Penicillamine, 6, 22, C, blood disorder symptoms, see BNF
Pentaerythritol tetranitrate, 22
Pentaerythritol tetranitrate m/r, 22, 25
Pentasa tabs, C, administration, blood disorder symptoms, see BNF
Pentasa enema and supps, C, blood disorder symptoms, see BNF
Pentazocine caps and tabs, 2, 21
Pentazocine supps, 2
Pentobarbitone, 19
Peppermint oil caps, 5, 22, 25
Percutol, C, administration, see BNF
Pergolide, C, hypotensive reactions, see BNF
Periactin, 2
Pericyazine, 2
Perindopril, 22
Permethrin dermal cream, 10 patient information leaflet
Perphenazine, 2
Persantin, 22
Pertofran, 2
Pethidine, 2
Pevaryl TC, 28
Phenazocine, 2
Phenelzine, 3, 10 MAOI card
Phenergan, 2
Phenethicillin, 9, 23
Phenindamine, 2

Phenindione, 10 anticoagulant card, 14 (urine pink)
Pheniramine m/r, 2, 25
Phenobarbitone elixir and tabs, 2, C, driving (see BNF, p. 204)
Phenolphthalein, 14 (alkaline urine pink)
Phenothrin lotion, 15
Phenoxymethylpenicillin, 9, 23
Phentermine m/r, 25, C, driving
Phenylbutazone, e/c, 5, 21, 25, C, blood disorder symptoms, see BNF
Phenytoin caps and tabs, 27, C, administration, blood or skin disorder symptoms (see BNF), driving (see BNF, p. 204)
Phenytoin chewable tabs, 24, C, blood or skin disorder symptoms (see BNF), driving (see BNF, p. 204)
Phenytoin susp, C, administration, blood or skin disorder symptoms (see BNF), driving (see BNF, p. 204)
Phosphate-Sandoz, 13
Phyllocontin Continus, 25
Physeptone, 2
Physiotens, 3
Phytomenadione, 24
Picolax, 10 patient information leaflet, 13, C, solution, see BNF
Pilocarpine tabs, 21, 27, C, driving
Pimozide, 2
Pindolol, 8
Piperazine powder, 13
Piracetam, 3
Pirbuterol inhalation, C, dose, see BNF
Pirenzepine, 22
Piretanide, 21
Piriton, 2
Piroxicam caps, 21
Piroxicam dispersible tabs, 13, 21
Pivampicillin susp and tabs, 5, 9, 21
Pizotifen, 2
Plaquenil, 5
Platet, 13, 32
Plendil, 25
Podophyllin paint cpd, 15, C, application, see BNF
Ponderax Pacaps, 2, 25, C, exercise
Pondocillin susp and tabs, 5, 9, 21
Ponstan, 21
Potaba caps and tabs, 21
Potaba Envules, 13, 21
Potassium chloride m/r, see preps
Potassium citrate mixt, 27
Potassium effervescent tabs, 13, 21
Pranoxen Continus, 25
Pravastatin, C, muscle effects, see BNF
Praxilene, 25, 27
Prazosin, 3, C, dose, see BNF
Precortisyl, 10 steroid card, 21
Precortisyl Forte, 10 steroid card, 21
Prednesol, 10 steroid card, 13, 21
Prednisolone inj, 10 steroid card
Prednisolone tabs, 10 steroid card, 21
Prednisolone e/c, 5, 10 steroid card, 25
Prednisone, 10 steroid card, 21
Preferid, 28
Prefil, 22, 27, C, administration, see BNF
Prepulsid, C, administration, see BNF
Preservex, 21
Prestim, 8
Prestim Forte, 8
Priadel liq, 10 lithium card, C, fluid and salt intake, see BNF
Priadel tabs, 10 lithium card, 25, C, fluid and salt intake, see BNF
Primalan, 2

Synarel, 10 patient information leaflet, C, nasal decongestants, see BNF
Synflex, 21

Tacrolimus, 23, C, driving, see BNF
Tagamet effervescent tabs, 13
Tamsulosin m/r, 3, 25, C, dose
Tarcortin, 28
Tarivid, 6, 9, 11, C, driving
Tavegil, 2
Tegretol Chewtabs, 3, 21, 24, C, blood, hepatic or skin disorder symptoms (see BNF), driving (see BNF, p. 204)
Tegretol liq, supps and tabs, 3, C, blood, hepatic or skin disorder symptoms (see BNF), driving (see BNF, p. 204)
Tegretol Retard, 3, 25, C, blood, hepatic or skin disorder symptoms (see BNF), driving (see BNF, p. 204)
Temazepam, 19
Temgesic, 2, 26
Tenif, 8, 25
Tenoret 50, 8
Tenoretic, 8
Tenormin, 8
Tenoxicam tabs, 21
Terazosin, 3, C, dose, see BNF
Terbinafine, 9
Terbutaline inhalations, C, dose, see BNF
Terbutaline m/r, 25
Terfenadine, C, driving, alcohol, see BNF
Terra-Cortril oint, 28
Terra-Cortril Nystatin, 28
Terramycin, 7, 9, 23
Testosterone undecanoate caps, 21, 25
Tetrabenazine, 2
Tetrachel, 7, 9, 23, C, posture
Tetracycline, 7, 9, 23, C, posture
Tetracycline mouthwash, see BNF
Tetralysal preps, 6, 9
Theo-Dur, 25
Theophylline, 21
Theophylline m/r, see preps
Thephorin, 2
Thiabendazole, 3, 21, 24
Thioridazine, 2
Thymoxamine, 21
Tiaprofenic acid tabs, 21
Tiaprofenic acid m/r, 25
Tilade, 8
Tildiem preps, 25
<u>Tiludronic acid</u>, C, food and calcium
Timodine, 28
Timolol, 8
Tinidazole tabs, 4, 9, 21, 25
Tinset, 2, 21
Tofranil, 2
Tolectin, 21
Tolmetin, 21
Topamax, 3, C, driving (see BNF p.204)
Topiramate, 3, C, driving (see BNF p.204)

Toradol tabs, 17, 21
Tramadol, 2
Tramadol m/r, 2, 25
<u>*Tramake*</u>, 2
Trandate, 8, 21
Tranxene, 2 or 19
Tranylcypromine, 3, 10 MAOI card
Trasicor, 8
Trasidrex, 8, 25
Traxam foam, 15
Trazodone, 2, 21
Trazodone m/r, 2, 21, 25
Trental m/r, 21, 25
Treosulfan, 25
Tri-Adcortyl external preps, 28
Triamcinolone inj, 10 steroid card
Triamcinolone tabs, 10 steroid card, 21
Triamco, 14 (urine blue in some lights), 21
Triamterene, 14 (urine blue in some lights), 21
Triclofos sodium, 19
Trientine, 6, 22
Trifluoperazine, 2
Trifyba, C, administration, see BNF
Trilostane, 21
Triludan, C, driving, alcohol, see BNF
Trimeprazine, 2
Trimethoprim mixt and tabs, 9
Trimipramine, 2
Trimopan, 9
Trimovate, 28
Tripotassium dicitratobismuthate, C, administration, see BNF
Triprolidine m/r, 2, 25
Triptafen preps, 2
Tropisetron, 23
Tropium, 2
Tryptizol mixt and tabs, 2
Tryptophan, 5
Tuinal, 19
Tylex caps, 2, 29, 30
Tylex effervescent tabs, 2, 13, 29, 30
Typhoid vaccine, oral, 23, 25, C, administration, see BNF

Ubretid, 22
Ucerax, 2
Ultralanum Plain, 28
Uniphyllin Continus, 25
Unipine XL, 23, 25
Univer, 25
Uriben, 9, 11
Ursodeoxycholic acid, 21
Ursofalk, 21
<u>*Utinor*</u>, 6, 9, C, driving

Valaciclovir, 9
Valium, 2 or 19
Vallergan, 2
Valoid, 2
Valtrex, 9
Velosef, 9
Venlafaxine, 21, C, driving, skin reactions
Ventide, 8, C, dose
Ventodisks, C, dose, see BNF

Ventolin inhalations, C, dose, see BNF
Verapamil m/r, 25
Vibramycin caps, 6, 9, 11, 27, C, posture, see BNF
Vibramycin-D, 6, 9, 11, 13
Videx, 23, C, administration, see BNF
Vigabatrin sachets, 3, 13, C, driving (see BNF, p. 204)
Vigabatrin tabs, 3, C, driving (see BNF, p. 204)
Viloxazine, 2
Vioform-Hydrocortisone, 28
Visclair, 5, 22, 25
Viskaldix, 8
Visken, 8
Vivalan, 2
Vivotif, 23, 25, C, administration, see BNF
Volmax, 25
Voltarol dispersible tabs, 13, 21
Voltarol tabs, 5, 25
Voltarol 75mg SR and Retard, 21, 25

Warfarin, 10 anticoagulant card
Warfarin WBP, 10 anticoagulant card
Warticon, 15
Welldorm, 19, 27
Wellvone, 21

Xanax, 2
Xatral, 3, C, dose, see BNF
Xatral SR, 3, 25, C, dose, see BNF

Yomesan, 4, 24, C, administration, see BNF

Z Span, 25
Zaditen, 2, 8, 21
Zadstat supps, 4, 9
Zantac effervescent tabs, 13
Zarontin, C, blood disorder symptoms (see BNF), driving (see BNF, p. 204)
Zavedos caps, 25
Zidovudine syrup, C, use of oral syringe
Zimovane, 19
Zinamide, 8
Zinc sulphate, see preps
Zinnat sachets, 9, 13, 21
Zinnat susp, 9, 21
Zinnat tabs, 9, 21, 25
Zirtek, C, driving, alcohol, see BNF
Zithromax, 5, 9, 23
<u>*Zocor*</u>, C, muscle effects, see BNF
Zopiclone, 19
Zoton, 5, 23, 25
Zovirax susp and tabs, 9
Zuclopenthixol, 2
Zydol, 2
Zydol SR, 2, 25
Zyloric, 8, 21, 27

Dental Practitioners' Formulary

List of Dental Preparations

The following list has been approved by the appropriate Secretaries of State, and the preparations therein may be prescribed by dental practitioners on form P14 (GP14 in Scotland).

Sugar-free versions, where available, are preferred.

Aciclovir Cream, BP
Aciclovir Oral Suspension, BP, 200 mg/5 mL
Aciclovir Tablets, BP, 200 mg
Amoxycillin Capsules, BP
Amoxycillin Oral Powder, DPF
Amoxycillin Oral Suspension, BP
Amoxycillin Tablets, Dispersible, DPF
Amphotericin Lozenges, BP
Amphotericin Oral Suspension, DPF
Ampicillin Capsules, BP
Ampicillin Oral Suspension, BP
Artificial Saliva, DPF
Ascorbic Acid Tablets, BP
Aspirin Tablets, Dispersible, BP[1]
Benzydamine Mouthwash, DPF
Benzydamine Oral Spray, DPF
Carbamazepine Tablets, BP
Carmellose Gelatin Paste, DPF
Cephalexin Capsules, BP
Cephalexin Oral Suspension, BP
Cephalexin Tablets, BP
Cephradine Capsules, BP
Cephradine Oral Solution, DPF
Chlorhexidine Gluconate 1% Gel, DPF
Chlorhexidine Mouthwash, DPF
Chlorhexidine Oral Spray, DPF
Chlorpheniramine Tablets, BP
Choline Salicylate Dental Gel, BP
Clindamycin Capsules, BP
Clindamycin Oral Suspension, Paediatric, DPF
Diazepam Oral Solution, BP, 2 mg/5 mL
Diazepam Tablets, BP
Diflunisal Tablets, BP
Dihydrocodeine Tablets, BP, 30 mg
Doxycycline Capsules, BP, 100 mg
Ephedrine Nasal Drops, BP
Erythromycin Ethyl Succinate Oral Suspension, BP
Erythromycin Ethyl Succinate Tablets, BP
Erythromycin Stearate Tablets, BP
Erythromycin Tablets, BP
Fluconazole Capsules, 50 mg, DPF
Fluconazole Oral Suspension, 50 mg/5 mL, DPF

> Preparations in this list which are not included in the BP or BPC are described on next page

Hydrocortisone Cream, BP, 1%
Hydrocortisone Lozenges, BPC
Hydrocortisone and Miconazole Cream, DPF
Hydrocortisone and Miconazole Ointment, DPF
Hydrogen Peroxide Mouthwash, DPF
Ibuprofen Oral Suspension, BP, sugar-free
Ibuprofen Tablets, BP
Lignocaine 5% Ointment, DPF
Menthol and Eucalyptus Inhalation, BP 1980[2]
Metronidazole Oral Suspension, DPF
Metronidazole Tablets, BP
Miconazole Oral Gel, DPF
Mouthwash Solution-tablets, DPF
Nitrazepam Tablets, BP
Nystatin Ointment, BP
Nystatin Oral Suspension, BP
Nystatin Pastilles, DPF
Oxytetracycline Capsules, BP
Oxytetracycline Tablets, BP
Paracetamol Oral Suspension, BP[3]
Paracetamol Tablets, BP
Paracetamol Tablets, Soluble, BP
Pethidine Tablets, BP
Phenoxymethylpenicillin Oral Solution, BP
Phenoxymethylpenicillin Tablets, BP
Povidone-iodine Mouthwash, DPF
Probenecid Tablets, BP
Promethazine Hydrochloride Tablets, BP
Promethazine Oral Solution, BP
Sodium Chloride Mouthwash, Compound, BP
Sodium Fluoride Oral Drops, DPF
Sodium Fluoride Tablets, DPF
Sodium Fusidate Ointment, BP
Sodium Perborate Mouthwash, DPF
Temazepam Oral Solution, DPF
Temazepam Tablets, DPF
Tetracycline Capsules, BP
Tetracycline Tablets, BP
Thymol Glycerin, Compound, BP 1988[2]
Triamcinolone Dental Paste, BP
Vitamin B Tablets, Compound, Strong, BPC
Zinc Sulphate Mouthwash, DPF

---

1. BP 1993 has directed that when soluble aspirin tablets are prescribed, dispersible aspirin tablets should be dispensed
2. This preparation does not appear in subsequent editions of the BP
3. BP 1993 directs that when Paediatric Paracetamol Oral Suspension or Paediatric Paracetamol Mixture is prescribed and no strength stated Paracetamol Oral Suspension 120 mg/5 mL should be dispensed

Details of DPF preparations

Preparations on the List of Dental Preparations which are specified as DPF are described as follows in the DPF.

Although brand names have sometimes been included for identification purposes preparations on the list should be prescribed by non-proprietary name.

PoM **Amoxycillin Oral Powder** (proprietary product: *Amoxil Sachets SF*), amoxycillin 750 mg and 3 g (as trihydrate) sachet

PoM **Amoxycillin Tablets Dispersible** (proprietary product: *Amoxil Dispersible Tablets*), amoxycillin 500 mg (as trihydrate)

PoM **Amphotericin Oral Suspension** (proprietary product: *Fungilin Suspension*), amphotericin 100 mg/mL

Artificial Saliva, (proprietary product: *Luborant*) consists of sorbitol 1.8 g, carmellose sodium (sodium carboxymethylcellulose) 390 mg, dibasic potassium phosphate 48.23 mg, potassium chloride 37.5 mg, monobasic potassium phosphate 21.97 mg, calcium chloride 9.972 mg, magnesium chloride 3.528 mg, sodium fluoride 258 micrograms/60 mL, with preservatives and colouring agents

Benzydamine Mouthwash (proprietary product: *Difflam Oral Rinse*), benzydamine hydrochloride 0.15%

Benzydamine Oral Spray (proprietary product: *Difflam Spray*), benzydamine hydrochloride 0.15%

Carmellose Gelatin Paste (proprietary product: *Orabase Oral Paste*), gelatin, pectin, carmellose sodium, 16.58% of each in a suitable basis

PoM **Cephradine Oral Solution** (proprietary product: *Velosef Syrup*), cephradine 250 mg/5mL when reconstituted with water

Chlorhexidine Gluconate 1% Gel (proprietary product: *Corsodyl Dental Gel*), chlorhexidine gluconate 1%

Chlorhexidine Mouthwash (proprietary products: *Chlorohex 2000 Mouthwash, Corsodyl Mouthwash*), chlorhexidine gluconate 0.2%

Chlorhexidine Oral Spray (proprietary product: *Corsodyl Spray*), chlorhexidine gluconate 0.2%

PoM **Clindamycin Oral Suspension, Paediatric** (proprietary product: *Dalacin C Paediatric Suspension*), clindamycin 75 mg (as palmitate hydrochloride)/5mL when reconstituted with purified water (freshly boiled and cooled)

PoM **Fluconazole Capsules 50 mg** (proprietary product: *Diflucan*), fluconazole 50 mg

PoM **Fluconazole Oral Suspension 50 mg/5 ml** (proprietary product: *Diflucan*), fluconazole 50 mg 5 mL when reconstituted with water

PoM **Hydrocortisone and Miconazole Cream** (proprietary product: *Daktacort Cream*), hydrocortisone 1%, miconazole nitrate 2%

PoM **Hydrocortisone and Miconazole Ointment** (proprietary product: *Daktacort Ointment*), hydrocortisone 1%, miconazole nitrate 2%

Hydrogen Peroxide Mouthwash consists of hydrogen peroxide solution 6% (≡ approx. 20 volume), BP

Lignocaine 5% Ointment, (proprietary product *Xylocaine Ointment*), lignocaine 5% in a suitable basis

PoM **Metronidazole Oral Suspension** (proprietary product: *Flagyl S*), metronidazole 200 mg (as benzoate)/5mL

PoM[1] **Miconazole Oral Gel** (proprietary product *Daktarin Oral Gel*), miconazole 25 mg/mL
1. For exemption, see p. 266.

Mouthwash Solution-tablets, consist of tablets which may contain antimicrobial, colouring and flavouring agents in a suitable soluble effervescent basis to make a mouthwash suitable for dental purposes

PoM **Nystatin Pastilles** (proprietary product *Nystan Pastilles*), nystatin 100 000 units

Povidone-iodine Mouthwash (proprietary product: *Betadine Mouthwash*), povidone-iodine 1%

Sodium Fluoride Oral Drops, see section 9.5.3

Sodium Fluoride Tablets, see section 9.5.3

Sodium Perborate Mouthwash (proprietary product: *Bocasan Mouthwash*), sodium perborate 68.6%

PoM **Temazepam Tablets,** temazepam 10 and 20 mg

Zinc Sulphate Mouthwash, consists of zinc sulphate lotion, BP. Directions for use: dilute 1 part with 4 parts of warm water

Note. May be difficult to obtain

Nurse Prescribers' Formulary

Nurse Prescribers' Formulary Appendix (Appendix NPF). List of preparations approved by the Secretary of State which may be prescribed on forms FP10(CN) and FP10(PN) by Nurses for National Health Service patients

Preparations on this list which are not included in the BP or BPC are described on p. 659

Medicinal preparations

Almond Oil Ear Drops, NPF
Aqueous Cream, BP
Arachis Oil Enema, NPF
Aspirin Tablets, Dispersible, 300 mg, BP
Bisacodyl Suppositories, BP (includes 5-mg and 10-mg strengths)
Bisacodyl Tablets, BP
Cadexomer–Iodine Ointment, NPF
Cadexomer–Iodine Paste, NPF
Cadexomer–Iodine Powder, NPF
Calamine Cream, Aqueous, BP
Calamine Lotion, BP
Calamine Lotion, Oily, BP 1980
Carbaryl Lotion, BP, alcoholic containing at least 0.5%
Carbaryl Lotion, BP, aqueous containing at least 0.5%
Carbaryl shampoos containing at least 0.5%
Catheter Maintenance Solution, Chlorhexidine, NPF
Catheter Maintenance Solution, Mandelic Acid, NPF
Catheter Maintenance Solution, Sodium Chloride, NPF
Catheter Maintenance Solution, 'Solution G', NPF
Catheter Maintenance Solution, 'Solution R', NPF
Clotrimazole Cream 1%, BP
Co-danthramer Capsules, NPF
Co-danthramer Capsules, Strong, NPF
Co-danthramer Oral Suspension, NPF
Co-danthramer Oral Suspension, Strong, NPF
Co-danthrusate Capsules, BP
Co-danthrusate Oral Suspension, NPF
Dextranomer Beads, NPF
Dextranomer Paste, NPF
Dimethicone barrier creams containing at least 10%
Docusate Capsules, NPF
Docusate Enema, NPF
Docusate Enema, Compound, NPF
Docusate Oral Solution, NPF
Docusate Oral Solution, Paediatric, NPF
Emulsifying Ointment, BP
Glycerol Suppositories, BP
Hydrous Ointment, BP
Ispaghula Husk Granules, NPF

Ispaghula Husk Granules, Effervescent, NPF
Ispaghula Husk Powder, NPF
Ispaghula Husk Powder, Effervescent, NPF
Lactitol Powder, NPF
Lactulose Powder, NPF
Lactulose Solution, BP
Lignocaine Gel, NPF
Lignocaine Ointment, NPF
Lignocaine and Chlorhexidine Gel, BP
Magnesium Hydroxide Mixture, BP
Magnesium Sulphate Paste, BP
Malathion alcoholic lotions containing at least 0.5%
Malathion aqueous lotions containing at least 0.5%
Malathion shampoos containing at least 1%
Mebendazole Tablets, NPF
Mebendazole Oral Suspension, NPF
Miconazole Oral Gel, NPF
Nystatin Oral Suspension, BP
Nystatin Pastilles, NPF
Olive Oil Ear Drops, NPF
Paracetamol Oral Suspension, BP (includes 120 mg/5 mL and 250 mg/5 mL strengths—both of which are available as sugar-free formulations)
Paracetamol Tablets, BP
Paracetamol Tablets, Soluble, BP
Permethrin Cream, NPF
Permethrin Cream Rinse, NPF
Phenothrin Alcoholic Lotion, NPF
Phosphates Enema, BP
Piperazine Citrate Elixir, BP
Piperazine and Senna Powder, NPF
Povidone–Iodine Aqueous Solution, NPF
Senna Granules, Standardised, BP
Senna Oral Solution, NPF
Senna Tablets, BP
Senna and Ispaghula Granules, NPF
Sodium Chloride Solution, Sterile, BP
Sodium Citrate Compound Enema, NPF
Sterculia Granules, NPF
Sterculia and Frangula Granules, NPF
Streptokinase and Streptodornase Topical Powder, NPF
Thymol Glycerin, Compound, BP 1988
Titanium Ointment, NPF
Zinc and Castor Oil Ointment, BP
Zinc Oxide and Dimethicone Spray, NPF

1. Dextranomer Paste Pad Dressings, included as appliance in Part IXA of the Drug Tariff, are also prescribable

This list is currently **only** for the purposes of the **Nurse Prescribing demonstration scheme** which is operating in eight General Practitioner (GP) Fundholding practices and which involves nurses with a District Nurse (DN) or Health Visitor (HV) qualification.

Appliances and Reagents (including Wound Management Products)

Chemical Reagents
The following as listed in Part IXR of the Drug Tariff:
  Detection Tablets for Glycosuria
  Detection Tablets for Ketonuria
  Detection Strips for Glycosuria
  Detection Strips for Ketonuria
  Detection Strips for Proteinuria
  Detection Strips for Blood Glucose
Fertility (Ovulation) Thermometer as listed in Part IXA of the Drug Tariff
Film Gloves, Disposable, EMA as listed in Part IXA of the Drug Tariff
Elastic Hosiery including accessories as listed in Part IXA of the Drug Tariff
Hypodermic Equipment
The following as listed in Part IXA of the Drug Tariff:
  Hypodermic Syringes—U100 Insulin
  Hypodermic Syringe Carrying Case
  Screw cap to convert Hypodermic Syringe Carrying Case for use with Pre-set U100 Insulin Syringe
  Hypodermic Syringe—Single Use or Single-patient Use, U100 Insulin with Needle
  Hypodermic Needles—Sterile, Single-use
  Lancets—Sterile, Single-use
  Needle Clipping Device
Incontinence Appliances as listed in Part IXB of the Drug Tariff
Pessaries, Ring as listed in Part IXA of the Drug Tariff
Stoma Appliances and Associated Products as listed in Part IXC of the Drug Tariff
Urethral Catheters as listed in Part IXA of the Drug Tariff
Urine Sugar Analysis Equipment as listed in Part IXA of the Drug Tariff

Wound Management and Related Products (including bandages, dressings, gauzes, lint, stockinette, etc)
The following as listed in Part IXA of the Drug Tariff:
  Absorbent Cottons
  Absorbent Cotton Gauzes
  Absorbent Cotton and Viscose Ribbon Gauze, BP 1988
  Absorbent Lint, BPC
  Arm Slings
  Cellulose Wadding, BP 1988
  Cotton Conforming Bandage, BP 1988
  Cotton Crêpe Bandage, BP 1988
  Crêpe Bandage, BP 1988
  Elastic Adhesive Bandage, BP
  Elastic Web Bandages
  Gauze and Cellulose Wadding Tissue, BP 1988
  Gauze and Cotton Tissues
  Heavy Cotton and Rubber Elastic Bandage, BP
  High Compression Bandages (Extensible)
  Knitted Polyamide and Cellulose Contour Bandage, BP 1988
  Knitted Viscose Primary Dressing, BP, Type 1
  Multiple Pack Dressing No. 1
  Multiple Pack Dressing No. 2
  Open-wove Bandage, BP 1988, Type 1
  Paraffin Gauze Dressing, BP
  Perforated Film Absorbent Dressing
  Polyamide and Cellulose Contour Bandage, BP 1988
  Povidone–Iodine Fabric Dressing, Sterile
  Skin Closure Strips, Sterile
  Sterile Dressing Packs
  Stockinettes
  Surgical Adhesive Tapes
  Suspensory Bandages, Cotton
  Swabs
  Titanium Dioxide Elastic Adhesive Bandage, BP [Not currently available]
  Triangular Calico Bandage, BP 1980
  Vapour-permeable Adhesive Film Dressing, BP
  Vapour-permeable Waterproof Plastic Wound Dressing, BP, Sterile
  Wound Management Dressings (including gel, colloid and foam)
  Zinc Paste Bandages (including both plain and with additional ingredients)

In the Drug Tariff Appliances and Reagents which may **not** be prescribed by Nurses are annotated ⊗

> This list is currently **only** for the purposes of the **Nurse Prescribing demonstration scheme** which is operating in eight General Practitioner (GP) Fundholding practices and which involves nurses with a District Nurse (DN) or Health Visitor (HV) qualification.

Details of NPF preparations

Preparations on the Nurse Prescribers' Formulary which are not included in the BP or BPC are described as follows in the pilot edition of the Nurse Prescribers' Formulary which has been produced for the Nurse Prescribing demonstration scheme.

Although brand names have sometimes been included for identification purposes preparations on the list should be prescribed by non-proprietary name.

Almond Oil Ear Drops, almond oil 10 mL supplied in a multidose container fitted with an appropriate applicator

Arachis Oil Enema, (proprietary product: *Fletchers' Arachis Oil Retention Enema*), arachis oil

Cadexomer–Iodine Ointment, (proprietary product: *Iodosorb Ointment*), cadexomer–iodine containing iodine 0.9% in an ointment basis

PoM **Cadexomer–Iodine Paste,** (proprietary product: *Iodoflex*), cadexomer–iodine containing iodine 0.9% in a paste basis

PoM **Cadexomer–Iodine Powder,** (proprietary product: *Iodosorb Powder*), cadexomer–iodine containing iodine 0.9%

Carbaryl shampoos, (proprietary products: *Carylderm Shampoo*, carbaryl 1%; *Derbac C Shampoo*, carbaryl 0.5%; *Suleo-C Shampoo*, carbaryl 0.5%), carbaryl 0.5-1% in a shampoo basis

Catheter Maintenance Solution, Chlorhexidine, (proprietary products: *Uro-Tainer Chlorhexidine*; *Uriflex C*), chlorhexidine 0.02%

Catheter Maintenance Solution, Mandelic Acid, (proprietary product: *Uro-Tainer Mandelic Acid*), mandelic acid 1%

Catheter Maintenance Solution, Sodium Chloride, (proprietary products: *Uro-Tainer Sodium Chloride*; *Uriflex-S*), sodium chloride 0.9%

Catheter Maintenance Solution, 'Solution G', (proprietary products: *Uro-Tainer Suby G*, *Uriflex G*), citric acid 3.23%, magnesium oxide 0.38%, sodium bicarbonate 0.7%, disodium edetate 0.01%

Catheter Maintenance Solution, 'Solution R', (proprietary products: *Uro-Tainer Solution R*, *Uriflex R*), citric acid 6%, gluconolactone 0.6%, magnesium carbonate 2.8%, disodium edetate 0.01%

PoM **Co-danthramer Capsules,** co-danthramer 25/200 (danthron 25 mg, poloxamer '188' 200 mg)

PoM **Co-danthramer Capsules, Strong,** co-danthramer 37.5/500 (danthron 37.5 mg, poloxamer '188' 500 mg)

PoM **Co-danthramer Oral Suspension,** (proprietary product: *Codalax*), co-danthramer 25/200 in 5 mL (danthron 25 mg, poloxamer '188' 200 mg/5 mL)

PoM **Co-danthramer Oral Suspension, Strong,** (proprietary product: *Codalax Forte*), co-danthramer 75/1000 in 5 mL (danthron 75 mg, poloxamer '188' 1 g/5 mL)

PoM **Co-danthrusate Oral Suspension,** (proprietary product: *Normax*), co-danthrusate 50/60 (danthron 50 mg, docusate sodium 60 mg/5 mL)

Dextranomer Beads, (proprietary product: *Debrisan Beads*), dextranomer

Dextranomer Paste, (proprietary product: *Debrisan Paste*), dextranomer in a soft paste basis

Dimethicone barrier creams, (proprietary products: *Conotrane Cream*, dimethicone '350' 22%; *Savlon Nappy Rash Cream*, dimethicone '1000' 10%; *Siopel Barrier Cream*, dimethicone '1000' 10%; *Vasogen Barrier Cream*, dimethicone 20%), dimethicone 10–22%

Docusate Capsules, (proprietary product: *Dioctyl Capsules*), docusate sodium 100 mg

Docusate Enema, (proprietary product: *Norgalax Micro-enema*) docusate sodium 120 mg in 10 g

Docusate Enema, Compound, (proprietary product: *Fletchers' Enemette*), docusate sodium 90 mg, glycerol 3.78 g/5 mL with macragol and sorbic acid

Docusate Oral Solution, (proprietary product: *Dioctyl Oral Solution*), docusate sodium 50 mg/5 mL

Docusate Oral Solution, Paediatric, (proprietary product: *Dioctyl Paediatric Oral Solution*), docusate sodium 12.5 mg/5 mL

Ispaghula Husk Granules, (proprietary product: *Isogel*), ispaghula husk 90%

Ispaghula Husk Granules, Effervescent, (proprietary product: *Fybogel Granules*), ispaghula husk 3.5g/sachet

Ispaghula Husk Powder, (proprietary product: *Konsyl*), ispaghula husk 3.4 g or 6 g per sachet

Ispaghula Husk Powder, Effervescent, (proprietary product: *Regulan Powder*), ispaghula husk 3.6 g/6.4-g sachet

Lactitol Powder, lactitol 10 g/sachet

Lactulose Powder, (proprietary products: *Lactulose Dry, Duphalac Dry*), lactulose 10 g/sachet

Lignocaine Ointment, (proprietary product: *Xylocaine Ointment*), lignocaine 5%

Malathion alcoholic lotions, (proprietary products: *Prioderm Lotion*; *Suleo-M Lotion*), malathion 0.5% in an alcoholic basis

Malathion aqueous lotions, (proprietary product: *Derbac-M Lotion*), malathion 0.5% in an aqueous basis

Malathion shampoos, (proprietary product: *Prioderm Cream Shampoo*), malathion 1% in a shampoo basis

PoM[1] **Mebendazole Tablets,** (proprietary products: *Ovex, Vermox*), mebendazole 100 mg

1. For exemption, see p. 282

PoM **Mebendazole Oral Suspension,** (proprietary product: *Vermox*), mebendazole 100 mg/5 mL

PoM[1] **Miconazole Oral Gel,** (proprietary product: *Daktarin Oral Gel*), miconazole 25 mg/mL

1. For exemption, see p. 266

PoM **Nystatin Pastilles,** (proprietary product: *Nystan Pastilles*), nystatin 100 000 units

Olive Oil Ear Drops, olive oil 10 mL supplied in a multidose container fitted with an appropriate applicator

Permethrin Cream, (proprietary product: *Lyclear Dermal Cream*), permethrin 5%

Permethrin Cream Rinse, (proprietary product: *Lyclear Cream Rinse*), permethrin 1%

Phenothrin Alcoholic Lotion, (proprietary product: *Full Marks Lotion*), phenothrin 0.2% in a basis containing isopropyl alcohol

Piperazine and Senna Powder, (proprietary product: *Pripsen Oral Powder*), piperazine phosphate 4 g, sennosides 15.3 mg/sachet

Povidone–Iodine Aqueous Solution, (proprietary product: *Betadine Antiseptic Solution*), povidone–iodine 10%

Senna Oral Solution, (proprietary product: *Senokot Syrup*), sennosides 7.5 mg/5 mL

Senna and Ispaghula Granules, (proprietary product: *Manevac Granules*), senna fruit 12.4%, ispaghula 54.2%

Sodium Citrate Compound Enema, (proprietary products: *Micolette Micro-enema*; *Micralax Micro-enema*; *Relaxit Micro-enema*), sodium citrate 450 mg with glycerol, sorbitol and an anionic surfactant

Sterculia Granules, (proprietary product: *Normacol Granules*), sterculia 62%

Sterculia and Frangula Granules, (proprietary product: *Normacol Plus Granules*), sterculia 62%, frangula (standardised) 8%

PoM **Streptokinase and Streptodornase Topical Powder,** (proprietary product: *Varidase Topical*), streptokinase 100 000 units, streptodornase 25 000 units

Titanium Ointment, (proprietary product: *Metanium Ointment*), titanium dioxide 20%, titanium peroxide 5%, titanium salicylate 3%, titanium tannate 0.1%

Zinc Oxide and Dimethicone Spray, (proprietary product: *Sprilon*), dimethicone 1.04%, zinc oxide 12.5% in a pressurised aerosol unit

Index of Manufacturers

'Special-order' manufacturers—see p. 670

Abbott
Abbott Laboratories Ltd,
Abbott House, Norden Rd,
Maidenhead, Berks SL6 4XE.
(01628) 773355

A&H
Allen & Hanburys Ltd,
see GlaxoWellcome.

Alcon
Alcon Laboratories (UK) Ltd,
Pentagon Park, Boundary Way,
Hemel Hempstead, Herts
HP2 7UD.
(01442) 341234

Alembic Products
Alembic Products Ltd,
River Lane, Saltney,
Chester, Cheshire CH4 8RQ.
(01244) 680147

ALK
ALK (UK),
8 Bennet Rd, Reading,
Berks RG2 0QX.
(01734) 313200

Allerayde
Allerayde,
3 Sanigar Court, Whittle Close,
Newark, Notts NG24 2BW.
(01636) 613444

Allergan
Allergan Ltd,
Coronation Rd, High
Wycombe, Bucks HP12 3SH.
(01494) 444722

Alpha
Alpha Therapeutic UK Ltd,
Howlett Way, Fison Way
Industrial Estate, Thetford,
Norfolk IP24 1HZ.
(01842) 764260

AlphaMed
AlphaMed Ltd,
Bensham House,
340 Bensham Lane,
Thornton Heath,
Surrey CR7 7EQ.
0181-684 0470

Amersham
Amersham International plc,
Amersham Place,
Little Chalfont, Bucks
HP7 9NA.
(01494) 544000

Amgen
Amgen Ltd,
240 Cambridge Science Park,
Milton Rd, Cambridge
CB4 4WD.
(01223) 420305

Anpharm
Anpharm Ltd,
82 Waterloo Rd, Hillside,
Southport PR8 4QW.

Antigen
Antigen Pharmaceuticals (UK),
Trafalgar House,
Union St, Southport,
Merseyside PR9 0QS.
(01704) 545608

APS
Approved Prescription Services
Ltd,
Brampton Rd, Hampden Park,
Eastbourne, East Sussex
BN22 9AG.
(01323) 501111

Armour
Armour Pharmaceutical Co. Ltd,
RPR House,
52 St. Leonards Rd,
Eastbourne, East Sussex
BN21 3YG.
(01323) 410200

Ashbourne
Ashbourne Pharmaceuticals Ltd,
Victors Barns, Hill Farm,
Brixworth, Northampton
NN6 9DQ.
(01604) 882190

ASTA Medica
ASTA Medica Ltd,
168 Cowley Rd, Cambridge
CB4 4DL.
(01223) 423434

Astra
Astra Pharmaceuticals Ltd,
Home Park Estate,
Kings Langley,
Herts WD4 8DH.
(01923) 266191

Astra Tech
Astra Tech Ltd,
Stroudwater Business Park,
Brunel Way, Stonehouse, Glos
GL10 3SW.
(01453) 791763

Aurum
Aurum Pharmaceuticals Ltd,
48–50 High St, Billingshurst,
West Sussex RH14 9NY.
(01403) 786781

Bailey, Robert
Robert Bailey & Son plc,
Dysart St, Great Moor,
Stockport, Cheshire
SK2 7PF.
0161-483 1133

Baker Norton
Division of Norton Healthcare
see Norton.

Bard
Bard Ltd,
Forest House, Brighton Rd,
Crawley, West Sussex
RH11 9BP.
(01293) 527888

Baxter
Baxter Healthcare Ltd,
Caxton Way, Thetford, Norfolk
IP24 3SE.
(01842) 767000

Bayer
Bayer plc,
Pharmaceutical Business
Group, Bayer House,
Strawberry Hill, Newbury,
Berks RG13 1JA.
(01635) 39000

Bayer Diagnostics
Bayer Diagnostics,
Evans House, Hamilton Close,
Houndmills, Basingstoke,
Hants RG21 2YE.
(01256) 29181

Baypharm
see Bayer.

BCM Specials
Boots Contract Manufacturing,
1 Thane Rd West,
Nottingham NG2 3AA.
0500 925935

Becton Dickinson
Becton Dickinson UK Ltd,
Between Towns Rd,
Cowley, Oxford,
Oxon OX4 3LY.
(01865) 748844

Beecham
Beecham Research,
see SmithKline Beecham.

Beecham Products
see SmithKline Beecham
Healthcare.

Beiersdorf
Beiersdorf UK Ltd,
Yeomans Drive, Blakelands,
Milton Keynes,
Bucks MK14 5LS.
(01908) 211444

Bell and Croyden
John Bell and Croyden,
54 Wigmore St, London
W1H 0AU.
0171-935 5555

Bencard
see SmithKline Beecham.

Bengué
Bengué & Co Ltd,
see Syntex.

Berk
Berk Pharmaceuticals,
see APS.

Beta
Beta Medical Products Ltd,
Valley Lodge, Bakewell Rd,
Matlock, Derbyshire
DE4 3BN.
(01629) 582198

BHR

BHR Pharmaceuticals Ltd,
41 Centenary Business Centre,
Hammond Close,
Attleborough Fields, Nuneaton,
Warwickshire CV11 6RY.
(01203) 353742

Bio Diagnostics

Bio Diagnostics Ltd,
Upton Industrial Estate,
Rectory Rd, Upton-upon-
Severn, Worcs WR8 0XL.
(01684) 592262

Biocare

Biocare International Inc.
Belvoir House, Chapel St,
Haconby, Lincs
PE10 0UP.
(01778) 570441

Bioglan

Bioglan Laboratories Ltd,
5 Hunting Gate, Hitchin,
Herts SG4 0TJ.
(01462) 438444

Bio-Medical

Bio-Medical Services,
BMS Laboratories Ltd,
River View Rd, Beverley,
North Humberside HU17 0LD.
(01482) 860228

Biorex

Biorex Laboratories Ltd,
2 Crossfield Chambers,
Gladbeck Way, Enfield,
Middx EN2 7HT.
0181-366 9301

Blake

Thomas Blake & Co,
The Byre House, Fearby,
Nr. Masham, North Yorkshire
HG4 4NF.
(01765) 689042

BM Diagnostics

Boehringer Mannheim
(Diagnostics & Biochemicals)
Ltd,
Bell Lane, Lewes,
East Sussex BN7 1LG.
(01273) 480444

BOC

BOC Gases,
Priestly Rd, Worsley,
Manchester M28 2UT.
0800 111333

Body's Surgical

Body's Surgical Company,
Unit 14, East Hanningfield
Industrial Estate, Old Church
Rd, East Hanningfield,
Chelmsford, Essex CM3 8BG
(01245) 400413

Boehringer Ingelheim

Boehringer Ingelheim Ltd,
Ellesfield Ave, Bracknell, Berks
RG12 4YS.
(01344) 424600

Boehringer Mannheim

Boehringer Mannheim UK
(Pharmaceuticals) Ltd,
Simpson Parkway, Kirkton
Campus, Livingston, West
Lothian EH54 7BH.
(01506) 412512

Boots

The Boots Co plc,
1 Thane Rd West, Nottingham
NG2 3AA.
(0115) 959 5168

BPL

Bio Products Laboratory,
Dagger Lane, Elstree, Herts
WD6 3BX.
0181-905 1818

Braun

B. Braun (Medical) Ltd,
Braun House, 13–14
Farmbrough Close, Aylesbury
Vale Industrial Park, Aylesbury,
Bucks HP20 1DQ.
(01296) 393900

Bristol-Myers

Bristol-Myers Squibb
Pharmaceuticals Ltd,
141–149 Staines Rd, Hounslow,
Middx TW3 3JA.
0181-572 7422

Britannia

Britannia Pharmaceuticals Ltd,
41–51 Brighton Rd, Redhill,
Surrey RH1 6YS.
(01737) 773741

David Bull

David Bull Laboratories,
Spartan Close, Tachbrook Park,
Warwick CV34 6RS.
(01926) 820820

Bullen

C. S. Bullen Ltd,
3–7 Moss St, Liverpool L6 1EY.
0151-207 6995

Bullen & Smears

Bullen & Smears Ltd,
see Bullen.

Burgess

Edwin Burgess Ltd,
see Leo.

Cambridge

Cambridge Laboratories,
Richmond House,
Old Brewery Court,
Sandyford Rd,
Newcastle upon Tyne NE2 1XG.
0191-261 5950

Camp

Camp Ltd,
30–32 Sovereign Rd, Kings
Norton Business Centre,
Birmingham B30 3HN.
0121-451 3016

Cantassium

The Cantassium Company,
Larkhall Laboratories,
225 Putney Bridge Rd,
London SW15 2PY.
0181-874 1130

Centra

Centra Healthcare,
Enterprise House, Station Rd,
Loudwater, High Wycombe
Bucks HP10 9UF.
(01494) 450778

Chancellor

Chancellor Group Ltd,
see Consolidated.

Chauvin

Chauvin Pharmaceuticals Ltd,
Ashton Rd, Harold Hill,
Romford,
Essex RM3 8SL.
(01708) 383838

J. Chawner

J. Chawner Surgical Belts Ltd,
Unit 1B Mayfields
Southcrest, Redditch B98 7DU
(01527) 404353

Chefaro

Chefaro Proprietaries Ltd,
see Organon.
(01223) 420956

Chiron

Chiron UK Ltd,
Salamander Quay West,
Park Lane, Harefield, Middx
UB9 6NY.
(01895) 824087

Chugai

Chugai Pharma UK Ltd,
Mulliner House, Flanders Rd,
Turnham Green, London
W4 1NN
0181-742 0777

Ciba

Ciba Pharmaceuticals,
Wimblehurst Rd, Horsham,
West Sussex RH12 4AB.
(01403) 272827

CIBA Vision

CIBA Vision Ophthalmics,
Flanders Rd, Hedge End,
Southampton SO30 2LG.
(01489) 785399

Cilag

see Janssen-Cilag

Clement Clarke

Clement Clarke International
Ltd,
Airmed House, Edinburgh Way,
Harlow, Essex CM20 2ED.
(01279) 414969

CliniFlex

CliniFlex Ltd,
see CliniMed.

CliniMed

CliniMed Ltd,
Cavell House, Knaves Beech
Way, Loudwater, High
Wycombe, Bucks HP10 9QY.
(01628) 850100

Clintec

Clintec Nutrition Ltd,
Shaftesbury Court,
18 Chalvey Park, Slough,
Berks SL1 2ER.
(01753) 550800

Colgate-Palmolive
Colgate-Palmolive Ltd,
Guildford Business Park,
Middleton Rd, Guildford,
Surrey GU2 5LZ.
(01483) 302222

Coloplast
Coloplast Ltd,
Peterborough Business Park,
Peterborough PE2 0FX.
(01733) 239898

Consolidated
Consolidated Chemicals Ltd,
Abbey Rd,
The Industrial Estate,
Wrexham, Clwyd LL13 9PW.
(01978) 661351

ConvaTec
ConvaTec Ltd,
Harrington House, Milton Rd,
Ickenham, Uxbridge, Middx
UB10 8PU.
(01895) 678888

Co-Pharma
Co-Pharma Ltd,
Talbot House, Church St,
Rickmansworth, Herts
WD3 1DE.
(01923) 710934

Cover Care
Cover Care,
5 Ancaster Gardens, Wollaton
Park, Nottingham NG8 1FR.
(0115) 928 7883

Cow & Gate
Cow & Gate Nutricia Ltd,
Newmarket Ave,
White Horse Business Park,
Trowbridge, Wilts BA14 0XQ.
(01225) 768381

Cox
A. H. Cox & Co Ltd,
Whiddon Valley, Barnstaple,
Devon EX32 8NS.
(01271) 311257

CP
CP Pharmaceuticals Ltd,
Ash Rd North, Wrexham
Industrial Estate, Wrexham,
Clwyd LL13 9UF.
(01978) 661261

Crawford
Crawford Pharmaceuticals,
71a High St, Stony Stratford,
Milton Keynes MK11 1BA.
(01908) 262346

Credenhill
Credenhill Ltd,
10 Cossall Industrial Estate,
Ilkeston, Derbys DE7 5UG.
(0115) 932 0144

Crookes
Crookes Healthcare Ltd,
PO Box 57, Central Park,
Lenton Lane,
Nottingham NG7 2LJ.
(0115) 953 9922

Cupal
Cupal Ltd,
See Seton.

Cupharma
Cupharma Ltd,
Winkton House, Wynnswick Rd,
Seer Green, Beaconsfield,
Bucks HP9 2XW.
(01494) 677055

Cussons
Cussons (UK) Ltd,
Kersal Vale, Manchester
M7 0GL.
0161-792 6111

Cutter
see Bayer.

Cuxson
Cuxson, Gerrard & Co Ltd,
Oldbury, Warley, West Midlands
B69 4BF.
0121-544 7117

Daniels
see Martindale

Dansac
Dansac Ltd,
Victory House, Vision Park,
Histon, Cambridge CB4 2ZR.
(01223) 235100

Davis & Geck
see Lederle.

DDC
DDC (London) Ltd,
6 Clifton Gardens,
London W9 1DT.
0171-266 0056

DDD
DDD Ltd,
94 Rickmansworth Rd,
Watford, Herts WD1 7JJ.
(01923) 229251

DDSA
DDSA Pharmaceuticals Ltd,
310 Old Brompton Rd, London
SW5 9JQ.
0171-373 7884

De Vilbiss
De Vilbiss Health Care UK Ltd,
Airlinks, Spitfire Way, Heston,
Middx TW5 9NR.
0181-756 1133

De Witt
E. C. De Witt & Co Ltd,
Tudor Rd, Manor Park,
Runcorn, Cheshire WA7 1SZ.
(01928) 579029

Delandale
Delandale Laboratories Ltd,
see Lorex.

Dental Health
Dental Health Products Ltd,
Pearl Assurance House,
Mill St, Maidstone,
Kent ME15 6XH.
(01622) 762269

DePuy
DePuy Healthcare,
Millshaw House, Manor Mill
Lane, Leeds LS11 8LQ.
(0113) 270 6000

Dermal
Dermal Laboratories Ltd,
Tatmore Place, Gosmore,
Hitchin, Herts SG4 7QR.
(01462) 458866

Dermalex
see Sanofi Winthrop.

DF
Duncan, Flockhart & Co Ltd,
Division of GlaxoWellcome Ltd
see GlaxoWellcome.

Dista
Dista Products Ltd,
see Lilly.

Dominion
Dominion Pharma Ltd,
Dominion House, Lion Lane,
Haslemere, Surrey GU27 1JL.
(01428) 661078

Downs
see Simcare.

Drew
John Drew (London) Ltd,
433 Uxbridge Rd, Ealing,
London W5 3NT.
0181-992 0381

Du Pont
Du Pont Pharmaceuticals Ltd,
Avenue One, Letchworth
Garden City, Herts SG6 2HU.
(01462) 482648

Dumex
Dumex Ltd,
Tring Business Centre,
Upper Icknield Way,
Tring, Herts HP23 4JX.
(01442) 890090

Durbin
B & S Durbin Ltd,
240 Northolt Rd, South Harrow,
Middx HA2 8DU.
0181-422 1303

Dylade
see Fresenius.

Eastern
Eastern Pharmaceuticals Ltd,
Coomb House, 7 St Johns Rd,
Isleworth, Middx TW7 6NA.
0181-569 8174

Elan
Elan Pharma Ltd,
see P-D.

Elida Gibbs
Elida Gibbs Ltd,
Coal Rd, Seacroft, Leeds
LS14 2AR.
(0113) 273 7473

Ellis
Ellis, Son & Paramore Ltd,
see Camp

EMS
EMS Medical Ltd,
Unit 3, Stroud Industrial Estate,
Stonedale Rd, Oldends Lane,
Stonehouse, Glos GL10 2DG.
(01453) 791791

Ethical Generics Ltd
Ethical Generics Ltd,
West Point, 46–48 West St,
Newbury, Berkshire RG14 1BD.
(01635) 568406

EuroCare
EuroCare (UK) Ltd,
55 Wimpole St, London
W1M 7DF.
0171-935 8560

Euroderma
Euroderma Ltd,
The Old Coach House,
34 Elm Rd, Chessington,
Surrey KT9 1AW.
0181-974 2266

Evans
Evans Medical Ltd,
Evans House, Regent Park,
Kingston Rd, Leatherhead,
Surrey KT22 7PQ.
(01372) 364000

Everfresh
Everfresh Natural Foods,
Gatehouse Close, Aylesbury,
Bucks HP19 3DE.
(01296) 25333

Farillon
Farillon Ltd,
Ashton Rd, Harold Hill,
Romford, Essex RM3 8UE.
(01708) 379000

Farley
Farley Health Products,
Mint Bridge Rd, Kendal,
Cumbria LA9 6NL
(01539) 723815

Ferraris
Ferraris Development &
Engineering Co Ltd,
26 Lea Valley Trading Estate,
Angel Rd, Edmonton, London
N18 3JD.
0181-807 3636

Ferring
Ferring Pharmaceuticals Ltd,
Greville House, Hatton Rd,
Feltham, Middx TW14 9PX.
0181-893 1543

Fisons
Fisons plc,
Pharmaceutical Division,
Coleorton Hall, Ashby Rd,
Coleorton, Coalville, Leics
LE67 8GP.
(01509) 634000

Flynn
Flynn Pharma Ltd,
7 Serlby Court, Addison Rd,
London W14 8EE.
(01438) 820152

Forley
Forley Ltd,
54 Hillbury Ave, Harrow,
Middx HA3 8EW.
0181-665 9169

Fournier
Fournier Pharmaceuticals Ltd,
19–20 Progress Business
Centre, Whittle Parkway,
Slough SL1 6DQ.
(01628) 660552

Fox
C. H. Fox Ltd,
22 Tavistock St, London
WC2E 7PY
0171-240 3111

FP
Family Planning Sales Ltd,
28 Kelburne Rd, Cowley,
Oxford OX4 3SZ.
(01865) 772486

Fresenius
Fresenius Ltd,
6–8 Christleton Court,
Stuart Rd, Manor Park,
Runcorn, Cheshire WA7 1ST.
(01928) 579444

Fry
Fry Surgical International Ltd,
Unit 17, Goldsworth Park
Trading Estate, Woking, Surrey
GU21 3BA.
(01483) 721404

Fujisawa
Fujisawa Ltd,
C P House, 8th Floor,
97–107 Uxbridge Rd,
London W5 5TL.
0181-840 9520

Gainor Medical
Gainor Medical Europe,
Milton Keynes
Distribution Centre,
Bradbourne Drive, Tilbrook,
Milton Keynes MK7 8BN.
(01908) 365361

Galderma
Galderma (UK) Ltd,
Leywood House, Woodside Rd,
Amersham, Bucks HP6 6AA.
(01494) 432606

Galen
Galen Ltd,
Seagoe Industrial Estate,
Craigavon, Northern Ireland
BT63 5UA.
(01762) 334974

Garnier
Laboratoires Garnier,
Golden Ltd,
PO Box 5, Pontyclun, Glam
CF7 8XW.
(01443) 237456

Geigy
Geigy Pharmaceuticals,
see Ciba.

Geistlich
Geistlich Sons Ltd,
Newton Bank, Long Lane,
Chester CH2 2PF.
(01244) 347534

General Dietary
General Dietary Ltd,
PO Box 38,
Kingston upon Thames, Surrey
KT2 7YP.
0181-336 2323

Generics
Generics (UK) Ltd,
12 Station Close, Potters Bar,
Herts EN6 1TL.
(01707) 644556

Gensia
Gensia Europe Ltd,
1 Bracknell Beeches, Bracknell,
Berks RG12 7BW.
(01334) 308803

GF Supplies
see Nutricia.

Glaxo
see GlaxoWellcome

GlaxoWellcome
GlaxoWellcome Ltd,
Stockley Park West, Uxbridge,
Middx UB11 1BT.
0181-990 9444

Glenwood
Glenwood Laboratories Ltd,
Jenkins Dale, Chatham,
Kent ME4 5RD.
(01634) 830535

Gluten Free Foods Ltd
Gluten Free Foods Ltd,
PO Box 178, Stanmore, Middx
HA7 4XN.
0181-954 7348

Goldshield
Goldshield Pharmaceuticals Ltd,
NLA Tower,
12–16 Addiscombe Rd,
Croydon CR9 6BP.
0181-649 8500

Henleys
Henleys Medical Supplies Ltd,
Brownfields, Welwyn Garden
City, Herts AL7 1AN.
(01707) 333164

Hillcross
Hillcross Pharmaceuticals,
Talbot St, Briercliffe, Burnley
BB10 2JY.
(01282) 830042

Hoechst
see Hoechst Roussel

Hoechst Roussel
Hoechst Roussel Ltd,
Broadwater Park, Denham,
Uxbridge, Middx UB9 5HP.
(01895) 834343

Hollister
Hollister Ltd,
Rectory Court, 42 Broad St,
Wokingham, Berks RG11 1AB.
(01734) 775545

**Hospital Management &
  Supplies**
Hospital Management and
Supplies Ltd,
Salthouse Rd, Brackmills,
Northampton, NN4 7UF.
(01604) 704600

Houghs

Houghs Healthcare Ltd,
18–22 Chapel St, Manchester
M19 3PT.
0161-224 3271

Hutchings

Hutchings Healthcare Ltd,
Rede House, New Barn Lane,
Henfield, West Sussex BN5 9SJ.
(01273) 495033

Hypoguard

Hypoguard Ltd,
Dock Lane, Melton,
Woodbridge, Suffolk IP12 1PE.
(01394) 387333

IATRO

IATRO Medical Systems,
35 Quaggy Walk, Blackheath,
London SE3 9EJ.
0181-297 9081

ICN

ICN Pharmaceuticals Inc,
Eagle House, Peregrine
Business Park, Gomm Rd, High
Wycombe, Bucks HP13 7DL.
(01494) 444555

IDIS

IDIS Ltd,
6/7 Canbury Business Park,
Elm Crescent,
Kingston upon Thames, Surrey
KT2 6BR.
0181-549 1355

Immuno

Immuno Ltd,
Arctic House, Rye Lane, Dunton
Green, Nr Sevenoaks, Kent
TN14 5HB.
(01732) 458101

Impharm

Impharm Nationwide Ltd,
PWS Building, Nelson St,
Bolton BL3 2JW.
(01204) 371155

IMS

International Medication
Systems (UK) Ltd,
Foster Ave,
Woodside Park Estate,
Dunstable,
Beds LU5 5TA.
(01582) 475005

Incare

Incare Medical Products,
see Hollister.

Innovex

Innovex Medical,
see Novex.

Intercare

Intercare Products Ltd,
7 The Business Centre,
Molly Millars Lane,
Wokingham, Berks RG41 2QZ.
(01734) 790345

Invicta

see Pfizer.

ISIS

ISIS Products Ltd,
Gough Lane, Bamber Bridge,
Preston, Lancs PR5 6AQ.
(01772) 628311

J&J

Johnson & Johnson Ltd,
Foundation Park, Roxborough
Way, Maidenhead,
Berkshire SL6 3UG.
(01628) 822222

J&J Medical

Johnson & Johnson Medical,
Coronation Rd, Ascot, Berks
SL5 9EY.
(01344) 872626

Jacobs

The Jacobs Bakery Ltd,
Suttons Business Park, Earley,
Reading, Berks RG6 1AZ.
(01734) 492000

Janssen

see Janssen-Cilag

Janssen-Cilag

Janssen-Cilag Ltd,
PO Box 79, Saunderton,
High Wycombe, Bucks
HP14 4HJ.
(01494) 567567

JLB

JLB Textiles Ltd,
Unit 2B, St Columb Industrial
Estate, St Columb Major,
Cornwall TR9 6SF.
(01637) 880065

K & K-Greeff

K & K-Greeff Ltd,
Suffolk House, George St,
Croydon CR9 3QL.
0181-686 0544

K/L

K/L Pharmaceuticals Ltd,
25 Macadam Place, South
Newmoor Industrial Estate,
Irvine KA11 4HP.
(01294) 215951

Kendall

The Kendall Co (UK) Ltd,
2 Elmwood, Chineham Business
Park, Crockford Lane,
Basingstoke, Hants RG24 0WG.
(01256) 708880

Kendall-Lastonet

see Kendall.

Kent

Kent Pharmaceuticals Ltd,
Wotton Rd, Ashford, Kent
TN23 6LL.
(01233) 641802

Kestrel

Kestrel Healthcare Ltd,
21a Hyde St, Winchester,
Hants SO23 7DR.
(01962) 866449

Kimal

Kimal Scientific Products Ltd,
Arundel Rd, Uxbridge, Middx
UB8 2SA.
(01895) 270951

Knoll

Knoll Ltd,
9 Castle Quay,
Castle Boulevard, Nottingham
NG7 1FW
(0115) 912 5000

Kyowa Hakko

Kyowa Hakko UK Ltd,
CP House, 97–107 Uxbridge
Rd, Ealing, London W5 5TL.
0181-840 4600

LAB

Laboratories for Applied
Biology Ltd,
91 Amhurst Park, London
N16 5DR.
0181-800 2252

Laerdal

Laerdal Medical Ltd,
Laerdal House, Goodmead Rd,
Orpington, Kent BR6 0HX.
(01689) 876634

Lagap

Lagap Pharmaceuticals Ltd,
37 Woolmer Way, Bordon,
Hants GU35 9QE.
(01420) 478301

Lamberts

Lamberts (Dalston) Ltd,
Dalston House, Hastings St,
Luton, Beds LU1 5BW.
(01582) 400711

Lederle

Lederle Laboratories,
see Wyeth

Lennon

see Trinity

Leo

Leo Laboratories Ltd,
Longwick Rd, Princes
Risborough, Aylesbury,
Bucks HP27 9RR.
(01844) 347333

LifeScan

LifeScan,
Enterprise House, Station Rd,
Loudwater, High Wycombe,
Bucks HP10 9UF.
(01494) 442211

Lilly

Eli Lilly & Co Ltd,
Dextra Court, Chapel Hill,
Basingstoke, Hants RG21 5SY.
(01256) 315000

Link

Link Pharmaceuticals Ltd,
51 Bishopric, Horsham,
West Sussex RH12 1QJ.
(01403) 272451

Lipha

Lipha Pharmaceuticals Ltd,
see Merck.

Liposome Company

The Liposome Co Ltd,
3 Shortlands, Hammersmith
International Centre,
London W6 8EH.
0181-324 0058

rex
Lorex Synthélabo Ltd,
Lunar House, Globe Park,
Marlow, Bucks SL7 1LW.
(01628) 488011

overidge
J. M. Loveridge plc,
Southbrook Rd, Southampton
SO15 1BH.
(01703) 228411

oxley
Loxley Medical,
Unit 5D, Carnaby Industrial
Estate, Bridlington, North
Humberside YO15 3QY.
(01262) 603979

RC
LRC Products Ltd,
North Circular Rd, Chingford,
London E4 8QA.
0181-527 2377

undbeck
Lundbeck Ltd,
Sunningdale House, Caldecott
Lake Business Park, Caldecott,
Milton Keynes MK7 8LF.
(01908) 649966

M
3M Health Care Ltd,
3M House, Morley St,
Loughborough,
Leics LE11 1EP.
(01509) 611611

aersk
Maersk Medical Ltd,
Thornhill Rd,
North Moons Moat, Redditch,
Worcs B98 9NL.
(01527) 64222

anfred Sauer
Manfred Sauer UK,
Mill Lane, Eastry,
Kent CT13 0QJ.
(01304) 620446

anmed
Mandeville Medicines
Stoke Mandeville Hospital,
Aylesbury, Bucks HP21 8AL.
(01296) 397223

arlen
Marlen (UK) Ltd,
Unit F4C,
Keighley Business Centre,
South St, Keighley,
West Yorkshire BD21 1AG.
(01535) 610300

artindale
Martindale Pharmaceuticals Ltd,
Bampton Rd, Harold Hill,
Romford, Essex RM3 8UG.
(01708) 386660

edac
Medac GmbH,
Fehlandtstraße 3,
D-2000 Hamburg 36, Germany.
(00 49 40) 3509020

edasil
Medasil (Surgical) Ltd,
Medasil House, Hunslet Rd,
Leeds LS10 1AU.
(0113) 243 3491

Medic-Aid
Medic-Aid Ltd,
Hook Lane, Pagham, Sussex
PO21 3PP.
(01243) 267321

Medigas
Medigas Ltd,
Enterprise Drive, Four Ashes,
Wolverhampton WV10 7DF
(01902) 791944

Mediplus
Mediplus Ltd,
Guildmaster Works,
Desborough Rd, High
Wycombe, Bucks HP11 2QA.
(01494) 536222

MediSense
MediSense Britain Ltd,
16–17 The Courtyard,
Gorsey Lane, Coleshill,
Birmingham B46 1JA.
(01675) 467044

Medix
Medix Ltd,
see Clement Clarke.

Medo
Medo Pharmaceuticals Ltd,
see Schwarz.

Mepra-pharm
Mepra-pharm,
PO Box 4, Rickmansworth,
Herts WD3 4AU.

Merck
E. Merck Pharmaceuticals,
Harrier House, High St,
West Drayton, Middlesex,
UB7 7QG.
(01895) 452200

Merrell
Marion Merrell Dow Ltd,
Lakeside House, Stockley Park,
Uxbridge, Middx UB11 1BE.
0181-848 3456

Milupa
Milupa Ltd,
Milupa House, Uxbridge Rd,
Hillingdon, Middx UB10 0NE.
0181-573 9966

MMG
MMG (Europe) Ltd,
157 Redland Rd, Bristol
BS6 6YE.
(0117) 973 6883

Molnlycke
Molnlycke Ltd,
Southfields Rd, Dunstable, Beds
LU6 3EJ.
(01582) 600211

Monmouth
Monmouth Pharmaceuticals,
3/4 Huxley Rd, The Surrey
Research Park, Guildford,
Surrey GU2 5RE.
(01483) 65299

Morson
Thomas Morson
Pharmaceuticals,
see MSD.

MSD
Merck Sharp & Dohme Ltd,
Hertford Rd, Hoddesdon, Herts
EN11 9BU.
(01992) 467272

Napp
Napp Laboratories Ltd,
Cambridge Science Park, Milton
Rd, Cambridge CB4 4GW.
(01223) 424444

Nationwide Ostomy
Nationwide Ostomy Supplies
Ltd,
North West House, 62 Oakhill
Trading Estate, Walkden,
Manchester M28 5PT.
(01204) 709255

Nestlé
Nestlé UK Ltd,
St. George's House, Croydon
CR9 1NR.
0181-686 3333

Network Management
Network Management Ltd,
Christy Estate, North Lane,
Aldershot, Hants GU12 4QP.
(01252) 29911

Neutrogena
Neutrogena Corporation,
see J&J

NeXstar
NeXstar Pharmaceuticals Ltd,
The Quorum, Barnwell Rd,
Cambridge CB5 8RE.
(01223) 571400

Nordic
Nordic Pharmaceuticals Ltd,
see Ferring.
0181-898 8665

Norgine
Norgine Ltd,
Chaplin House, Moorhall Rd,
Harefield, Middx UB9 6NS.
(01895) 826600

Norma
Norma Chemicals Ltd,
see Wallace Mfg.

North West
North West Medical Supplies
Ltd,
Green Arms Rd, Bolton
BL7 0ND.
(01204) 852383

Norton
H. N. Norton & Co. Ltd,
Gemini House, Flex Meadow,
Harlow, Essex CM19 5TJ.
(01279) 426666

Novex
Novex Pharma Ltd,
Innovex House, Marlow Park,
Marlow, Bucks SL7 1TB.
(01628) 491500

Novo Nordisk
Novo Nordisk Pharmaceutical
Ltd,
Novo Nordisk House,
Broadfield Park, Brighton Rd,
Pease Pottage, Crawley, West
Sussex RH11 9RT.
(01293) 613555

Nutricia Clinical
Nutricia Clinical Care,
see Cow & Gate

Nutricia Dietary
Nutricia Dietary Products Ltd,
see Cow & Gate

Nycomed
Nycomed (UK) Ltd,
Nycomed House, 2111 Coventry
Rd, Sheldon, Birmingham
B26 3EA.
0121-742 2444

Oakmed
Oakmed Ltd,
Fleming Rd, Speke,
Liverpool L24 9LS.
0151-486 3551

Omni Triage
Omni Triage Medical Ltd,
131 Tranmere Rd,
London SW18 3QP.
0171-737 7781

Omnicare
The Omnicare Group Ltd,
Enterprise Drive, Four Ashes,
Wolverhampton WV10 7DF.
0500 823773

Opus
Opus Pharmaceuticals
see Trinity.

Oral B Labs
Oral B Laboratories Ltd,
Gatehouse Rd, Aylesbury,
Bucks HP19 3ED.
(01296) 432601

Organon
Organon Laboratories Ltd,
Cambridge Science Park, Milton
Rd, Cambridge, CB4 4FL.
(01223) 423445

Organon-Teknika
Organon-Teknika Ltd,
see Organon
(01223) 423650

Orion
Orion Pharma (UK) Ltd,
1st Floor, Leat House,
Overbridge Square, Hambridge
Lane, Newbury,
Berkshire RG14 5UX.
(01635) 520300

Orphan Europe
Orphan Europe (UK),
Bray Business Centre,
Bray-on-Thames,
Berkshire SL6 2ED.
(01628) 773342

Ortho
Ortho Pharmaceutical Ltd,
see Cilag.

Orthotic
Orthotic Services Ltd
Heartlands House, 19 Catro St,
The Heartlands,
Birmingham B7 4TS.
0121-359 6323

Owen Mumford
Owen Mumford Ltd,
Brook Hill, Woodstock, Oxford
OX20 1TU.
(01993) 812021

Oxford Nutrition
Oxford Nutrition Ltd,
PO Box 110, Witney, Oxon
OX8 7FJ.
(01993) 709752

Oxygen Therapy Co Ltd
The Oxygen Therapy Co Ltd,
Dumballs Rd, Cardiff
CF1 6JE.
0800 373580

Paines & Byrne
Paines & Byrne Ltd,
Brocades House, Pyrford Rd,
West Byfleet,
Surrey KT14 6RA.
(01932) 355405

Panpharma
Panpharma Ltd,
Panpharma House, Repton
Place, White Lion Rd, Little
Chalfont, Amersham,
Bucks HP7 9LP.
(01494) 766866

Parema
Parema Ltd,
Sullington Rd, Shepshed,
Loughborough,
Leics LE12 9JJ.
(01509) 502051

Pari
Pari Medical Ltd,
London House,
243–253 Lower Mortlake Rd,
Richmond,
Surrey TW9 2LL.
0181-332 6513

Pasteur Mérieux
Pasteur Mérieux MSD Ltd,
Clivemont House,
Clivemont Rd, Maidenhead,
Berks SL6 7BU.
(01628) 785291

Payne
S G & P Payne,
Percy House, Brook St, Hyde,
Cheshire SK14 2NS.
0161-367 8561

P-D
Parke-Davis Medical,
Lambert Court, Chestnut Ave,
Eastleigh, Hants SO53 3ZQ.
(01703) 620500

Pelican
Pelican Healthcare Ltd,
see Simpla
(01222) 747787

Penn
Penn Pharmaceuticals Ltd,
Tafarnaubach Industrial Estate
Tredegar, Gwent, NP2 3AA.
(01495) 711222

Pennine
Pennine Healthcare,
Pontefract St, Ascot Drive
Industrial Estate,
Derby DE2 8JD.
(01332) 384489

Perstorp
Perstorp Pharma Ltd,
Wound-Care Division, Intec 2,
Wade Rd, Basingstoke,
Hants RG24 8NE.
(01256) 477868

Pfizer
Pfizer Ltd,
Sandwich, Kent CT13 9NJ.
(01304) 616161

Pfizer Consumer
Pfizer Consumer Healthcare,
Wilsom Rd, Alton,
Hants GU34 2TJ.
(01420) 84801

Pharmacia
see Pharmacia & Upjohn

Pharmacia & Upjohn
Pharmacia & Upjohn Ltd,
Davy Ave, Knowlhill,
Milton Keynes, MK5 8PH.
(01908) 661101

Pharmacia-Leiras
Pharmacia-Leiras Ltd,
see Pharmacia & Upjohn.

Pharmark
Pharmark,
7 Windermere Rd, West
Wickham, Kent BR4 9AN.

Pharmax
Pharmax Ltd,
Bourne Rd, Bexley,
Kent DA5 1NX.
(01322) 550550

Philip Harris
Philip Harris Medical Ltd,
Hazelwell Lane, Birmingham
B30 2PS.
0121-433 3030

Phoenix
Phoenix Pharmaceuticals Ltd,
Glevum Works, Upton St,
Gloucester GL1 4LA.
(01452) 522255

Pickles
J. Pickles & Sons,
Beech House, 62 High St,
Knaresborough, N. Yorks
HG5 0EA.
(01423) 867314

Portex
Portex Ltd,
Hythe, Kent CT21 6JL.
(01303) 260551

Procea
Procea,
Alexandra Road, Dublin 1.
Dublin 741741

octer & Gamble

Procter & Gamble (Health &
Beauty Care) Ltd,
The Heights, Brooklands,
Weybridge, Surrey KT13 0XP.
(01932) 896000

octer & Gamble Pharm.

Procter & Gamble
Pharmaceuticals UK Ltd,
Lovett House, Lovett Rd,
Staines, Middx TW18 3AZ.
(01784) 495000

uinoderm Ltd

Quinoderm Ltd,
Manchester Rd, Hollinwood,
Oldham, Lancs OL8 4PB.
0161-624 9307

nd Rocket

Rand Rocket Ltd,
ABCare House, Hownsgill
Industrial Park, Consett,
County Durham DH8 7NU.
(01207) 591099

&C

Reckitt & Colman Products Ltd,
Dansom Lane, Hull HU8 7DS.
(01482) 326151

gent

Regent Laboratories Ltd,
Cunard Rd, London NW10 6PN.
0181-965 3637

nacare

Renacare Ltd,
Nunn Brook Rd, Huthwaite,
Sutton-in-Ashfield,
Notts NG17 2HU.
(01623) 555809

ône-Poulenc Rorer

Rhône-Poulenc Rorer Ltd,
52 St. Leonards Rd,
Eastbourne, East Sussex
BN21 3YG.
(01323) 534000

chborough

see Pfizer.

ma

Rima Pharmaceuticals Ltd,
214–216 St. James's Rd,
Croydon, Surrey CR0 2BW.
0181-683 1266

binsons

Robinson Healthcare,
Hipper House, Chesterfield,
Derbyshire S40 1YF.
(01246) 220022

C

Laboratoires RoC UK Ltd,
see J & J

che

Roche Products Ltd,
PO Box 8, Welwyn Garden City,
Herts AL7 3AY.
(01707) 366000

che Consumer Health

see Roche.

na

see Lipha.

Rosemont

Rosemont Pharmaceuticals Ltd,
Rosemont House, Yorkdale
Industrial Park, Braithwaite St,
Leeds LS11 9XE.
(0113) 244 1999

Roussel

see Hoechst Roussel

Rüsch

Rüsch UK Ltd,
PO Box 138, Cressex Industrial
Estate, High Wycombe, Bucks
HP12 3NB.
(01494) 532761

Rybar

Rybar Laboratories Ltd,
see Shire

Sallis

E. Sallis Ltd,
Vernon Works, Waterford St,
Basford, Nottingham
NG6 0DH.
(0115) 978 7841

Salts

Salt & Son Ltd,
Saltair House, Lord St,
Heartlands,
Birmingham B7 4DS.
0121-359 5123

Sandoz

Sandoz Pharmaceuticals,
Frimley Business Park, Frimley,
Camberley, Surrey GU16 5SG.
(01276) 692255

Sanofi Winthrop

Sanofi Winthrop Ltd,
One Onslow St, Guildford,
Surrey GU1 4YS.
(01483) 505515

Sara Lee

Sara Lee Household & Personal
Care (UK) Ltd,
225 Bath Rd, Slough SL1 4AU.
(01753) 523971

Schering Health

Schering Health Care Ltd,
The Brow, Burgess Hill,
West Sussex RH15 9NE.
(01444) 232323

Schering-Plough

Schering-Plough Ltd,
Shire Park, Welwyn Garden
City, Herts AL7 1TW.
(01707) 363636

Scholl

Scholl Consumer Products Ltd,
475 Capability Green, Luton,
Beds LU1 3LU.
(01582) 482929

Schwarz

Schwarz Pharma Ltd,
Schwarz House, East St,
Chesham, Bucks HP5 1DG.
(01494) 772071

Scientific Hospital Supplies

Scientific Hospital Supplies
(UK) Ltd,
100 Wavertree Boulevard,
Wavertree Technology Park,
Liverpool L7 9PT.
0151-228 1992

Scotia

Scotia Pharmaceuticals Ltd,
Units 26–29, Surrey Technology
Centre, The Research Park,
40 Occam Rd, Guildford,
Surrey GU2 5YG.
(01483) 462500

Searle

Searle Pharmaceuticals,
PO Box 53, Lane End Rd, High
Wycombe, Bucks HP12 4HL.
(01494) 521124

Serono

Serono Laboratories (UK) Ltd,
99 Bridge Rd East, Welwyn
Garden City, Herts AL7 1BG.
(01707) 331972

Servier

Servier Laboratories Ltd,
Fulmer Hall, Windmill Rd,
Fulmer, Slough SL3 6HH.
(01753) 662744

Seton

Seton Healthcare,
Seton Healthcare Group plc,
Tubiton House, Medlock St,
Oldham, Lancs OL1 3HS.
0161-652 2222

Seton-Prebbles

see Seton.

Seven Seas

Seven Seas Ltd,
Hedon Rd, Marfleet, Hull
HU9 5NJ.
(01482) 375234

Seward

Seward Medical,
131 Great Suffolk St, London
SE1 1PP.
0171-357 6527

Shannon

T. J. Shannon Ltd,
59 Bradford St, Bolton
BL2 1HT.
(01204) 21789

Shaw

A. H. Shaw and Partners Ltd,
Manor Rd, Ossett, West
Yorkshire WF5 0LF.
(01924) 273474

Sherwood

Sherwood Medical Industries
Ltd,
County Oak Way, Crawley, West
Sussex RH11 7YQ.
(01293) 534501

Shire

Shire Pharmaceuticals Ltd,
Fosse House, East Anton Court,
Icknield Way, Andover, Hants
SP10 5RG.
(01264) 333455

Sigma
Sigma Pharmaceuticals plc,
PO Box 233, Watford, Herts
WD2 4EW.
(01923) 250201

Simcare
Simcare,
Peter Rd, Lancing, West Sussex
BN15 8TJ.
(01903) 761122

Simpla
Simpla Plastics Ltd,
Cardiff Business Park,
Cardiff CF4 5WF.
(01222) 747000

Sinclair
Sinclair Pharmaceuticals Ltd,
Borough Rd, Godalming, Surrey
GU7 2AB.
(01483) 426644

S&N Hlth.
Smith & Nephew Healthcare
Ltd,
Healthcare House, Goulton St,
Hull HU3 4DJ.
(01482) 222200

SK&F
Smith Kline & French
Laboratories,
see SmithKline Beecham.

SmithKline Beecham
SmithKline Beecham
Pharmaceuticals,
SmithKline Beecham plc,
Mundells, Welwyn Garden City,
Herts AL7 1EY.
(01707) 325111

**SmithKline Beecham Health-
care**
SmithKline Beecham
Consumer Healthcare,
St. Georges Ave, Weybridge,
Surrey KT13 0DE.
(01932) 822000

SNBTS
Scottish National Blood
Transfusion Service,
Protein Fractionation Centre,
21 Ellen's Glen Rd,
Edinburgh EH17 7QT.
0131-664 2317

Solvay
Solvay Healthcare Ltd,
Hamilton House, Gaters Hill,
West End, Southampton
SO18 3JD.
(01703) 472281

Speywood
Speywood Pharmaceuticals Ltd,
1 Bath Rd, Maidenhead,
Berks SL6 4UH.
(01628) 771417

Squibb
E. R. Squibb & Sons Ltd,
see Bristol-Myers.

Stafford-Miller
Stafford-Miller Ltd,
Broadwater Rd,
Welwyn Garden City, Herts
AL7 3SP.
(01707) 331001

STD Pharmaceutical
STD Pharmaceutical Products,
Fields Yard, Plough Lane,
Hereford HR4 0EL.
(01432) 353684

Steeper
Steeper (Orthopaedic) Ltd,
Unit 4D, Mead Rise,
Temple Gate, Bristol BS3 4RP.
(0117) 971 7436

Sterling Health
see SmithKline Beecham
Healthcare.

Sterwin
see Sanofi Winthrop.

Stiefel
Stiefel Laboratories (UK) Ltd,
Holtspur Lane, Wooburn Green,
High Wycombe, Bucks
HP10 0AU.
(01628) 524966

Storz
Storz Ophthalmics,
154 Fareham Rd, Gosport,
Hants PO13 0AS.
(01329) 224000

Stuart
see Zeneca.

Sussex
Sussex Pharmaceutical Ltd,
Charlwoods Rd,
East Grinstead,
Sussex RH19 2HL.
(01342) 311311

Sutherland
Sutherland Health Ltd,
Unit 5, Rivermead, Pipers Way,
Thatcham, Berks RG13 4EP.
(01635) 874488

Terumo
Terumo Europe N.V.
1st Floor Offices,
62 Mount Pleasant Rd,
Tunbridge Wells,
Kent TN1 1RB.
(01892) 526331

Thackraycare
see DePuy.

Thames
see Consolidated.

Thornton & Ross
Thornton & Ross Ltd,
Linthwaite Laboratories,
Huddersfield HD7 5QH.
(01484) 842217

Tillomed
Tillomed Laboratories Ltd,
Unit 2, Campus 5, Letchworth
Business Park, Letchworth
Garden City, Herts SG6 2JF.
(01462) 480344

Timesco
Timesco of London,
Timesco House
1 Knights Rd, London E16 2AT.
0171-511 1234

Torbet
Torbet Laboratories Ltd,
Pearl Assurance House,
Mill St, Maidstone,.
Kent ME15 6XH.
(01622) 762269

Tosara
Tosara Products Ltd,
Baldoyle Industrial Estate,
Grange Rd, Dublin 13.
Dublin 321199

Trinity
Trinity Pharmaceuticals Ltd,
Tuition House,
27–37 St. George's Rd,
Wimbledon, London
SW19 4DS.
0181-944 9443

Typharm
Typharm Ltd,
14 Parkstone Rd, Poole,
Dorset BH15 2PG.
(01202) 666626

UCB Pharma
UCB Pharma Ltd,
Star House, 69 Clarendon Rd,
Watford, Herts WD1 1DJ.
(01923) 211811

Ultrapharm
Ultrapharm Ltd,
PO Box 18, Henley-on-Thames
Oxon RG9 2AW.
(01491) 578016

Unigreg
Unigreg Ltd,
Enterprise House,
181–189 Garth Rd, Morden,
Surrey SM4 4LL.
0181-330 1421

Unipath
Unipath Ltd,
Norse Rd, Bedford
MK41 0QG.
(01234) 347161

Universal
Universal Hospital Supplies,
313 Chase Rd,
London N14 6JA.
0181-882 6444

Uno Plast
Uno Plast Ltd,
The Wykeham Industrial Estate
Moorside Rd, Winchester, Hant
SO23 7RX.
(01962) 841777

Upjohn
Upjohn Ltd,
see Pharmacia & Upjohn

Vernon-Carus
Vernon-Carus Ltd,
Penwortham Mills, Preston,
Lancs PR1 9SN.
(01772) 744493

Vestric
Vestric Ltd,
West Lane, Runcorn,
Cheshire WA7 2PE.
(01928) 717070

Vitabiotics
Vitabiotics Ltd,
Vitabiotics House, 3 Bashley
Rd, London NW10 6SU.
0181-963 0999

Vitaflo
Vitaflo Ltd,
6 Moss St, Paisley PA1 1BJ.
0800 515174

Vitalograph
Vitalograph Ltd,
Maids Moreton House, Maids
Moreton, Buckingham
MK18 1SW.
(01280) 822811

Vygon
Vygon (UK) Ltd,
Bridge Rd, Cirencester,
Glos GL7 1PT.
(01285) 657051

H G Wallace
H G Wallace Ltd,
Colchester, Essex CO2 8JH.
(01206) 795133

Wallace Mfg
Wallace Manufacturing
Chemists Ltd,
Randles Rd, Knowsley
Industrial Park, Merseyside
L34 9HX.
0151-549 1255

Wanskerne
Wanskerne Ltd,
31 High Cross St, St. Austell,
Cornwall PL25 4AN.
(01726) 69500

Ward
Ward Surgical Appliance Co
Ltd,
57A Brightwell Ave, Westcliffe-
on-Sea, Essex SS0 9EB.
(01702) 354064

Warner Wellcome
Warner Wellcome Consumer
Healthcare
see P-D.

WBP
WB Pharmaceuticals Ltd,
see Boehringer Ingelheim.

Welfare Foods
see Nutricia.

Welland
Welland Medical Ltd,
7 Brunel Centre, Newton Rd,
Crawley, West Sussex
RH10 2TU.
(01293) 615455

Wellcome
see GlaxoWellcome

Whitehall
Whitehall Laboratories Ltd,
Huntercombe Lane South,
Taplow, Maidenhead,
Berks SL6 0PH.
(01628) 669011

Willis
S. R. Willis & Sons Ltd,
176 Albion Rd,
London N16 9JR.
0171-254 7373

Windsor
see Boehringer Ingelheim.

W-L
Warner Lambert UK Ltd,
see P-D.

Wyeth
Wyeth Laboratories,
Huntercombe Lane South,
Taplow, Maidenhead,
Berks SL6 0PH.
(01628) 604377

Wyvern
Wyvern Medical Ltd,
PO Box 17, Ledbury,
Herefordshire HR8 2ES.
(01531) 631105

Yamanouchi
Yamanouchi Pharma Ltd,
Yamanouchi House, Pyrford Rd,
West Byfleet, Surrey
KT14 6RA.
(01932) 345535

Zeal
G. H. Zeal Ltd,
8 Lombard Rd, Merton, London
SW19 3UU.
0181-542 2283

Zeneca
Zeneca Pharma,
King's Court, Water Lane,
Wilmslow, Cheshire SK9 5AZ.
(01625) 712712

Zyma
Zyma Healthcare,
Mill Rd, Holmwood, Dorking,
Surrey RH5 4NU.
(01306) 742800

'Special-order' Manufacturers

The following **companies** manufacture 'special-order' products: BCM Specials, Martindale, Rosemont.
Hospital manufacturing units also manufacture 'special-order' products, details may be obtained from any of the centres listed below.

It should be noted that when a product has a licence *the Department of Health recommends that the licensed product should be ordered* unless a specific formulation is required.

ENGLAND

East Anglian and Oxford

Mr G. Hanson,
Regional Production Pharmacist,
Pharmacy Department,
The Ipswich Hospital,
Heath Rd, Ipswich,
Suffolk IP4 5PD.
(01473) 712233 Extn 5603

Mersey

Dr M. G. Lee,
Regional Quality Control Pharmacist,
Pharmacy Practice Unit,
70 Pembroke Place
Liverpool L69 3BX.
0151-794 8138

North Thames

Mr M. Lillywhite,
Regional Production Pharmacist,
St. Bartholomew's Hospital,
West Smithfield, London
EC1A 7BE.
0171-601 7477

North Western

Mr M.D. Booth,
Production & Aseptic Services Manager,
Stockport Pharmaceuticals,
Stepping Hill Hospital,
Stockport, Cheshire SK2 7JE.
0161-419 5657

Northern

Mr P. W. McKenzie,
Regional Technical Services Pharmacist,
Pharmacy Department,
Newcastle General Hospital,
Westgate Rd,
Newcastle upon Tyne NE4 6BE.
0191-273 8811 Extn 22479

South East Thames

Mr J. Cheetham,
Principal Pharmacist,
Guy's Hospital,
St. Thomas' St,
London SE1 9RT.
0171-955 5000 Extn 5378/3712

South West Thames

Mr S. J. Riley,
Regional Production Pharmacist,
Pharmacy Department,
Lanesborough Wing,
St. George's Hospital,
Blackshaw Rd, Tooting,
London SW17 0QT.
0181-725 1770

South Western

Mr C. W. Lewis,
Director,
Manorpark Pharmaceuticals,
Blackberry Hill Hospital,
Manor Rd, Bristol BS16 2EW.
(0117) 975 4852

Trent

Mr A. C. Moore,
Regional Production Representative, Royal Hallamshire Hospital, Glossop Rd, Sheffield S10 2JF.
(0114) 271 2325

Wessex

Dr E. Brierley,
Regional Manufacturing Unit,
Queen Alexandra Hospital,
Cosham, Portsmouth,
Hants PO6 3LY.
(01705) 286335

West Midlands

Mr P. G. Williams,
Principal Pharmacist,
Pharmacy Manufacturing Unit,
Burton Hospital NHS Trust,
Belvedere Rd,
Burton-on-Trent DE13 0RB
(01283) 566333 Extn 5138

Yorkshire

Mr E. Holt,
Principal Pharmacist,
Production Unit,
The Royal Infirmary,
Acre St, Lindley, Huddersfield,
West Yorks HD3 3EA.
(01484) 422191 Extn 2421

NORTHERN IRELAND

Mrs S. M. Millership,
Principal Pharmacist,
Central Pharmaceutical Production Unit,
CSA Distribution Centre,
77 Boucher Cres, Belfast
BT12 6HU.
(01232) 553407

SCOTLAND

Mr J. A. Cook,
Principal Pharmacist—
Regional Production,
Tayside Pharmaceuticals,
Ninewells Hospital,
Dundee DD1 9SY.
(01382) 632273

WALES

Mr C. Powell
Specialist Principal Pharmacist,
Sterile Products Unit,
Pharmacy Department,
University Hospital of Wales,
The Heath, Cardiff CF4 4XW.
(01222) 747747 Extn 3114

Index

Where an entry is followed by more than one page reference, the principal reference is printed in **bold** type. Proprietary (trade) names are printed in *italic* type.